PRINCIPLES AND PRACTICE OF

PSYCHIATRIC NURSING

PRINCIPLES AND PRACTICE OF
PSYCHIATRIC NURSING

GAIL WISCARZ STUART, R.N., M.S., C.S.

Doctoral Candidate in Behavioral Sciences,
Johns Hopkins University,
School of Hygiene and Public Health;
Psychotherapist and Consultant, Baltimore, Maryland

SANDRA J. SUNDEEN, R.N., M.S.

Program Coordinator, Mental Health Manpower Development Unit,
Maryland Department of Health and Mental Hygiene, Baltimore, Maryland;
Adjunct Assistant Professor, University of Maryland School of Nursing,
Baltimore, Maryland; Adjunct Assistant Professor,
Salisbury State College, Salisbury, Maryland

SECOND EDITION

with **57** illustrations

The C. V. Mosby Company

ST. LOUIS • TORONTO • LONDON   1983

A TRADITION OF PUBLISHING EXCELLENCE

Editor: Alison Miller
Assistant editor: Susan R. Epstein
Manuscript editor: Sandra L. Gilfillan
Designer: Nancy Steinmeyer
Production: Mary Stueck, Carol O'Leary, Gail Morey Hudson

Artwork for the part and chapter openers is by M.C. Escher.
Reprinted with permission of John W. Vermeulen on behalf of the
Escher heirs. Photographs courtesy National Gallery of Art, Washington, D.C.

SECOND EDITION

Copyright © 1983 by The C.V. Mosby Company

Previous edition copyrighted 1979

Printed in the United States of America

The C.V. Mosby Company
11830 Westline Industrial Drive, St. Louis, Missouri 63146

Library of Congress Cataloging in Publication Data

Main entry under title:

Principles and practice of psychiatric nursing.

    Includes index.
    1. Psychiatric nursing. I. Stuart, Gail
Wiscarz, 1949-   . II. Sundeen, Sandra J.,
1940-   . [DNLM: 1. Psychiatric nursing. WY 160
S929p]
RC440.P69   1983   610.73'68   82-12540
ISBN 0-8016-4885-8

GW/VH/VH 9 8 7 6 5 4 3   03/C/312

CONTRIBUTORS

BEVERLY A. BALDWIN, R.N., M.S.

Assistant Professor, Project Director, Gerontology Training Program, University of Maryland School of Nursing, Baltimore, Maryland

E. SUSAN BATZER, R.N., M.S., C.S.

Psychotherapist and Consultant, Fallston and Edgewood, Maryland

RUTH WILDER BELL, R.N., D.N.Sc.

Chairperson, Department of Nursing, Towson State University, Towson, Maryland

SANDRA E. BENTER, R.N., M.S., C.S.

Doctoral Student, Catholic University School of Nursing, Washington, D.C.; Psychotherapist and Consultant, Pikesville, Maryland

THERESA S. FOLEY, R.N., Ph.D., C.S.

Assistant Professor, University of Michigan School of Nursing, Psychiatric–Mental Health Nursing, Ann Arbor, Michigan

KATHRYN G. GARDNER, R.N., M.S.

Psychiatric Nurse Consultant, Rochester General Hospital; Director of Group Psychotherapy Research Team, Department of Psychiatry, University of Rochester, Rochester, New York

PATRICIA E. HELM, R.N., M.S.N.

Assistant Professor, Yale School of Nursing; Clinical Specialist, Connecticut Mental Health Center, New Haven, Connecticut

SUZANNE SAYLE JIMERSON, R.N., M.S., C.S.

Psychotherapist and Consultant, Bethesda, Maryland

I. WADE LANCASTER, Ph.D.

Assistant Professor of Marketing, University of Alabama in Birmingham School of Business Administration, Birmingham, Alabama

JEANETTE LANCASTER, R.N., Ph.D.

Professor, Community Mental Health Nursing, University of Alabama in Birmingham, Birmingham, Alabama

FRANCES G. LEHMANN, R.N., M.S.N., C.S.

Assistant Administrator for Clinical/Patient Services, St. Francis Hospital Center, Beech Grove, Indiana

HELEN R. PEDDICORD, R.N., M.S.

Director of Nursing, Regional Institute for Children and Adolescents, Rockville, Maryland

SUSAN POORMAN, R.N., M.S.N.

Instructor, University of Pittsburgh School of Nursing; Staff Therapist, Persad Mental Health Center, Pittsburgh, Pennsylvania

ELIZABETH ANNE DeSALVO RANKIN, R.N., Ph.D.

Assistant Professor, University of Maryland School of Nursing, Baltimore, Maryland; Psychotherapist and Consultant, Pasadena, Maryland

AUDREY REDSTON, R.N., M.A.

Child Psychiatric Nurse Clinician, Soundview–Throgs Neck Community Mental Health Center; Children's Service of Albert Einstein College of Medicine, Yeshiva University, New York, New York

MARY E. RERES, R.N., Ph.D.

Dean of the School of Nursing, University of California at Los Angeles, Los Angeles, California

RITA RUBIN, R.N., M.S., C.S.

Clinical Nurse Specialist, Springfield Hospital Center, Sykesville, Maryland; Lecturer, University of Maryland School of Nursing, Baltimore, Maryland; Psychotherapist and Consultant, Reisterstown, Maryland

KAY SIENKILEWSKI, R.N., M.S.

Director of Nursing, Springfield Hospital Center, Sykesville, Maryland

PREFACE

In writing the first edition of this text, we felt much like pathfinders, traversing unexplored frontiers. Our first edition reflected both a departure and an evolution. It was a departure from all other texts of psychiatric nursing that organized nursing care, either overtly or covertly, around the medical model and its classifications of psychiatric disorders. Our text was an evolution in that it attempted to identify and refine, for psychiatric nurses, the distinct body of knowledge that is nursing.

This second edition of our text continues to be a departure and an evolution, but also a consolidation. Although other texts may mask the medical model in a nursing vocabulary, its dominance emerges when one considers the variability of their use of nursing diagnoses, the contingency of their nursing interventions on the medical categorizations, and their use of references and research that are primarily outside of nursing. Although departing from a traditional approach, we continue to use nursing's conceptual model, the nursing process, as the basis for defining and describing the practice of psychiatric nursing. This text views humans holistically and behaviorally and derives principles of psychiatric nursing care from a sound theoretical knowledge base, the application of nursing research, and a framework for practice that is the nursing therapeutic process. These principles, the science of psychiatric nursing care, are addressed in Part One. Part Two incorporates and exemplifies these principles as the art and practice of psychiatric nursing in various treatment settings, modalities, and roles.

This second edition also takes one more step down the path of psychiatric nursing science by consolidating the progress made thus far and laying plans for exploring the frontiers ahead. One of our personal goals in undertaking this revision was to clarify the nursing therapeutic process as our framework for practice and examine how it is complementary to the medical model of practice. This second edition therefore contains a separate chapter on our conceptual model of health-illness phenomena, in which theory and practice are integrated and elements of the model are clearly identified, explained, and interrelated. Within this model, nursing and medical diagnoses are presented as being distinct, but complementary, rather than contingent or redundant. Knowledge of both, however, is viewed as being necessary for practice. Thus throughout the text the medical model is presented as a complement, and occasional supplement, to the nursing process model that strives to preserve its unique identity. If this sounds less than absolute, it is because this is a less than absolute endeavor. It is a responsive, emerging, and exciting charting of unexplored territories that we engage in with all of our peers and colleagues who are practicing, teaching, and learning the art and science of psychiatric nursing. Our book is a part of all of you together and a challenge to each of you individually to contribute to the future direction of the principles and practice of psychiatric nursing.

Part One, Principles of Psychiatric Nursing, has a sharpened focus on the professional dimensions of psychiatric nursing practice. It presents a refined analysis of our conceptual model of health-illness phenomena that provides a framework for the nursing therapeutic process. Chapter 1 critically analyzes the roles and functions of psychiatric nurses from the many perspectives of historical evolution, contemporary practice, levels of performance, and issues of professional autonomy. It is intended to describe the present, raise questions about the future, and suggest directions for needed research. Chapter 2 continues to explore models of psychiatric care, while introducing the new diagnostic criteria (DSM-III) of the medical model and a brief perspective of the nursing model used in this text. Chapter 3 has been transformed into a comprehensive analysis of the elements of the therapeutic nurse-patient relationship. New content is included on the personal qualities needed by the nurse to be an effective helper, such as self-awareness, values clarification, and perceptions of altruism and ethics. Theory on facilitative communication has been added relating to levels of communication, the communication process, and therapeutic techniques. With this background, the phases of the relationship, the responsive and action dimensions, and therapeutic impasses are analyzed in depth. Another important addition is a section on the effectiveness of the nurse with a critical focus on supervision and ethics in psychiatric nursing practice. A new Chapter 4 describes the nursing therapeutic process and is a foundational chapter to the text. The chapter elaborates on four components of the nursing therapeutic process, which were derived from the four defining characteristics of nursing as described in "Nursing: A Social Policy Statement." We support this statement and its implications as identified by Peplau. The chapter discusses a model of health-illness phenomena that is inclusive and holistic, yet discrete and relevant to nursing practice. This model views health and illness as a continuum of adaptation and provides an organizing framework for the application of the nursing process. Chapter 4 then describes the phases and needed documentation of the nursing process with application demonstrated in a clinical case analysis. The new 1982 standards of psychiatric and mental health nursing practice are integrated throughout this discussion. Chapters 5 and 6 are also new and unique in psychiatric nursing texts. They respectively address primary prevention and rehabilitative nursing activities—areas of psychiatric nursing practice that have often been neglected. Chapter 5, Preventive Mental Health Nursing, examines conceptual problems in primary prevention, the assessment of vulnerable groups, such as women and families under stress, and prevention strategies related to health education, environmental change, and supporting social systems. Chapter 6, Rehabilitative Psychiatric Nursing, examines rehabilitation as it applies to any person displaying a maladaptive coping response and describes interventions relative to individuals, families, and the community.

Chapters 7 to 14 have all been revised, reorganized, and strengthened from a nursing perspective. Each explores a category of maladaptive coping responses, including the nursing problems of anxiety, alterations in self-concept, disturbances of mood, self-destructive behavior,

disruptions in relatedness, problems with the expression of anger, impaired cognition, and substance abuse. At the beginning of each of these chapters, a continuum of adaptive and maladaptive coping responses is presented relative to the chapter's nursing problem. Each phase of the nursing process is then applied and synthesized with the conceptual model. A consistent approach is used in formulating nursing diagnoses and comparing them with relevant medical diagnoses. Nursing research is used to provide a rationale for nursing interventions. Principles and nursing actions for the interventions are clearly discussed and concisely summarized in each of these chapters. Evaluation is addressed in light of effectiveness, efficiency, and areas in need of further study. The strength of this integrated approach is that it can be applied in any nursing care setting to patients who are responding to any type of stressor, whether physical, psychological, or sociocultural. Thus it is as useful to nurses working on medical units of general hospitals, long-term care facilities, and community health agencies, as it is to nurses working in psychiatric facilities. Chapters 15 and 16 complete Part One with updated analyses of somatic therapies and legal aspects of psychiatric care.

Part Two, Practice of Psychiatric Nursing, has been enhanced by the addition of several chapters that reflect current problems and trends in psychiatric nursing practice. The new chapters include child psychiatric nursing, human sexuality and nursing practice, nursing intervention in family abuse and violence, care of the chronically mentally ill, gerontological psychiatric nursing, and the pragmatics of private practice. All of Part Two reflects the most current thinking on the treatment settings, modalities, and roles of psychiatric nursing.

We have also tried to clarify content and reinforce learning throughout the text. To this end, each chapter contains behaviorally stated learning objectives, expanded illustrations and tables, summaries of important points, suggested cross-references, updated references, and more extensive annotated suggested readings. The second edition of our book is also accompanied by an instructor's manual, which is complete with learning objectives, lecture outlines, chapter glossaries, thought-provoking discussion questions, and multiple choice test questions that include both theoretical aspects and clinical application of the text's content. The instructor's manual further enhances the nursing orientation of the text by identifying nursing research problems that merit additional study by psychiatric nurses.

Visually, this edition is unified with numerous illustrations, all of which are from the collected works of M.C. Escher. The precision, balance, and yet creative perspective that characterize his drawings we feel complement and enhance the content of the text. We hope they stimulate and intrigue you as well.

We end this preface to our second edition with a note of expectancy and a stirring "call to action," complete with images of flying banners, quickened steps, and an assertive stance. Books such as ours make a certain impact on the field by their very presence, but Sir William Osler once observed, "What I read, I forget. What I hear, I remember. What I see, I know." It is therefore imperative that nurses communicate the nature and quality of the art and science of psychiatric nursing through their words, actions, and performance. To such a vision, we dedicate this second edition of our book.

Gail Wiscarz Stuart
Sandra J. Sundeen

CONTENTS

PART ONE

PRINCIPLES OF
PSYCHIATRIC NURSING

The philosophies of one age have become the absurdities of the next, and the foolishness of yesterday has become the wisdom of tomorrow.

Sir William Osler

CHAPTER 1

ROLES AND FUNCTIONS OF PSYCHIATRIC NURSES

Learning objectives

After studying this chapter, the student should be able to:

- describe the early history of psychiatric nursing.

- discuss the evolution of a psychiatric nursing role, including the specific contributions of Peplau.

- relate the influence of the social environment on psychiatric nursing.

- describe the nature, scope, and setting of psychiatric nursing practice.

- identify direct and indirect psychiatric nursing care functions using the concepts of primary, secondary, and tertiary prevention.

- analyze the way in which the psychiatric nurse's level of performance is affected by each of the following factors: laws, qualifications, practice setting, and personal competence and initiative.

- assess the purpose and importance of the American Nurses' Association Standards of Psychiatric–Mental Health Nursing Practice.

- evaluate the position of psychiatric nursing on the six characteristics of the scale of professionalization.

- critique problematic areas for psychiatric nursing and formulate recommendations for future growth.

- identify suggested readings for future study.

Evolutionary perspectives

The function of nursing or caring for the sick has existed since the beginning of civilization. Family members, servants, friends, neighbors, and religious groups have all cared for the ill or infirm throughout the course of history. Before 1860 the emphasis in psychiatric institutions was on custodial care, and this was provided by attendants who were prepared to maintain control of the patients. Frequently these attendants were little more than jailers or cellkeepers with very little training, and psychiatric care was poor.

Nursing, as a profession, began to emerge in the late nineteenth century. In 1873 Linda Richards graduated from the New England Hospital for Women and Children in Boston. She developed better nursing care in psychiatric hospitals and organized nursing services and educational programs in state mental hospitals in Illinois. For these activities she is called the first American psychiatric nurse. The first school to prepare nurses to care for the mentally ill opened at McLean Hospital in Waverly, Massachusetts, in 1882. It was a two-year program, but few psychological skills were addressed. The care was mainly custodial because nurses filled the function of caring for the physical needs of patients. Until the end of the nineteenth century little changed in the role of psychiatric nurses. They had limited special training in psychiatry, and they primarily adapted the principles of medical-surgical nursing to the psychiatric setting. They attended to the physical needs of patients, such as medications, nutrition, hygiene, and ward activities. At that time, psychological care consisted of being kind and tolerant to the patients.

One important contribution of Linda Richards was her ability to assess both the physical and emotional needs of her patients. In this early period of nursing history the emotional and physical needs of patients were separated. Nursing education reflected this division, and nurses were taught either in the general hospital or the psychiatric hospital. Johns Hopkins was the first school of nursing to include a fully developed course for psychiatric nursing in the curriculum. This occurred in 1913, and thereafter other schools began to do likewise. It was not until the late 1930s that nursing education viewed the importance of psychiatric knowledge in general nursing care related to all illnesses.

An important factor influencing the history of psychiatric nursing was the development of various somatic therapies, including insulin shock therapy (1935), psychosurgery (1936), and electroconvulsive therapy (1937). These all required the medical-surgical skills of nurses. Although these therapies did not foster the patient's insight, they did control his behavior and make him more amenable to psychotherapy. Somatic therapies also increased the demand for improved psychological treatment for those patients who did not respond. As nurses became more involved with these therapies, they began their struggle to define their role as psychiatric nurses. An editorial that appeared in the *American Journal of Nursing*[11] in 1940 described the conflict between nurses and physicians as nurses attempted to implement what they saw as appropriate nursing care for the psychiatric patient. This conflict was to continue for many years in the perpetuation of sex-role stereotyping and continues to demand attention in present nursing practice.[27] Another article published in 1933[28] described how psychiatrists were looking for experienced psychiatric nurses to work in psychiatric hospitals. A superintendent of nursing from a state hospital identified the three most pressing needs of psychiatric nurses at that time as (1) more nurses, (2) better prepared nurses, and (3) cooperation and understanding of the nursing organizations.

The period after World War II was one of major growth and change in psychiatric nursing. Because of a large number of service-related psychiatric problems and the increase in treatment programs offered by the Veterans Administration, there was an increased need for psychiatric nurses with advanced preparation. The content of psychiatric nursing had now become an integral part of the generic nursing curriculum, and its principles were applied to other areas of nursing practice, including general medicine, pediatric, and public health nursing. Graduate nursing programs, however, were few in number.

In 1946 the National Mental Health Act was passed by Congress. This act authorized the creation of the National Institute of Mental Health and a program for (1) training professional psychiatric personnel, (2) conducting psychiatric research, and (3) aiding the development of mental health programs at the state level. The purpose of the National Institute of Mental Health, which is located in Bethesda, Maryland, is to research the origins of mental illness and possible methods of treatment. It is also the administrative body that distributes training funds and research grants. Psychiatric nursing was one of the professions specified in the act that paved the way for federal funding of nursing education. Collegiate programs developed at both the baccalaureate and graduate levels. At about the same time the nursing profession endorsed the development of graduate programs that focused on clinical practice in nursing. By 1947 eight graduate programs in psychiatric nursing had been initiated.

Basic nursing programs also continued to grow and change. Many nursing leaders questioned the practice of having specialized hospitals offer training programs to prepare nurses to care for a particular type of patient, such as psychiatric hospitals training psychiatric nurses. The trend was to combine the basic knowledge and various skills needed by nurses into one general education program. In 1948 a report conducted by Brown entitled "Nursing for the Future" recommended the elimination of basic schools of nursing in mental hospitals. The report stated, "We recommend that hospitals for the mentally ill still conducting schools of nursing consider means whereby they can relinquish their schools and, as a substitute, make their clinical facilities more widely available for affiliating students (from general training schools)."[7:136] It also recommended the use of the psychiatric hospital in advanced courses of instruction for graduate nurse specialists. This report was given additional support in 1950 when the National League for Nursing required that a school had to provide an experience in psychiatric nursing to be accredited.

The emergence of a psychiatric nursing role

It was in this developmental period that the role of psychiatric nurses began to emerge. In 1947 Weiss[44] published an article in the *American Journal of Nursing* that reemphasized the shortage of psychiatric nurses and attempted to describe how psychiatric nurses differ from general duty nurses. She described "attitude therapy" as the nurse's directed use of attitudes that contributes to the patient's recovery. In implementing this therapy, the nurse observes the patient for minute and fleeting changes, demonstrates acceptance, respect, and understanding of the patient as a fellow human being, and promotes the patient's interest and participation in reality. She stressed the need to treat each patient as an individual with unique problems. It was also her belief that only physicians should attempt to interpret the patient's behav-

ior and the physician would prescribe the appropriate attitude needed by the nurse based on the patient's problem. More independent functions were described by Santos and Stainbrook[37] in 1949. They believed that nurses should perform "psychotherapeutic tasks" and understand concepts related to therapy, such as transference. They were vague, however, about the exact nature of the nurse's functions.

An article by Bennett and Eaton[6] appeared in the *American Journal of Psychiatry* in 1951 and identified three problems affecting psychiatric nurses: the scarcity of qualified psychiatric nurses, the partial use of their abilities, and the fact that "very little real psychiatric nursing is carried out in otherwise good psychiatric hospitals and units." They described the following functions and responsibilities of the chief psychiatric nurse:

1. To have policy-making authority independent of the psychiatric staff members, hospital administrators, and general nursing staff
2. To decide psychiatric nursing policies
3. To develop all rules and regulations of the department
4. To train an auxiliary staff of assistants to conform to her standards

The role of the nurse in insulin treatment, electroconvulsive therapy, and lobotomy was discussed. Two additional areas were also included —community activities and psychotherapy. They believed it was the responsibility of the psychiatric nurse to join mental health societies, consult with welfare agencies, work in outpatient clinics, practice preventive psychiatry, engage in research, and help educate the public. They took a stand supporting the nurse's participation in individual and group psychotherapy. Bennett and Eaton state, "Despite the fact that most psychiatrists seem to ignore the role of the psychiatric nurse in psychotherapy, all nurses in psychiatric wards do psychotherapy of one kind or another by their contacts with patients."[6:170] They urged that psychotherapy should be used purposefully and believed that nurses, like psychologists and social workers, should be used in "team psychotherapy."

Many of the issues raised in the article would be debated years later. The most controversial one, however, was on nurses conducting psychotherapy. Mellow[23] wrote in the *American Journal of Nursing* of the work she did with schizophrenic patients at Boston State Hospital in 1951. She defined these activities as "nursing therapy" and delineated three phases in the treatment process. The task in phase 1 was to establish contact with the patient and enter his life as a partner in the establishment of a therapeutic symbiotic relationship. In phase 2 the nurse allows the patient to relive his symbiotic attachment to a maternal figure and helps him resolve it. The final task of phase 3 is to help the patient manage his separation anxieties as he assumes more responsibility for his own life. In 1952 Tudor[42] published a study, "Sociopsychiatric Nursing Approach to Intervention in a Problem of Mutual Withdrawal on a Mental Hospital Ward," in which she described the nurse-patient relationships she established, which were characterized by unconditioned care, few demands, and the anticipation of her patients' needs.

As nurses engaged in these kinds of activities, many questions arose. Are these activities therapeutic or are they therapy? What is a therapeutic relationship or a one-to-one nurse-patient relationship? How does it differ from psychotherapy? These questions were addressed by Dr. Hildegard Peplau, a dynamic nursing leader whose ideas and beliefs would shape the future of psychiatric nursing.

In 1952 Peplau[29] published a book, *Interpersonal Relations in Nursing,* in which she described the skills, activities, and role of psychiatric nurses. It was the first systematic, theoretical framework developed for psychiatric nursing. She defined nursing as a "significant, therapeutic process" and believed the nurse-patient relationship was characterized by four overlapping and interlocking phases—orientation, identification, exploitation, and resolution. As she studied the nursing process in nurse-patient situations, she saw various roles emerge. These included the nurse as a resource person, a teacher, a leader in local, national, and international situations, a surrogate parent, and a counselor. She stated, "Counseling in nursing has to do with helping the patient remember and to understand fully what is happening to him in the present situation, so that the experience can be integrated with rather than dissociated from other experiences in life."[29:64]

The use of the nursing process in defining a role for psychiatric nurses was further evident when, in 1953, the National League for Nursing published "A Study of Desirable Functions and Qualifications for Psychiatric Nurses."[30] This report identified the following desirable functions:

1. Collecting significant data relating to the identification of problems (e.g., observing behavior, recording observations)
2. Making inferences and/or judgments based on these data and leading to action (e.g., interpreting the behavior of the patient, seeking to understand patients' needs)
3. Acting or intervening on the basis of inferences (e.g., clarifying with a patient the meaning of a procedure, discussing and acting to solve problems in a work situation)
4. Evaluating the entire process in terms of whether problems identified have been solved (e.g., mutually evaluating experiences and learning)

As nurses continued to describe their qualifications, skills, activities, and responsibilities, the role of the psychiatric nurse began to gain substance and definition.

Two significant developments in psychiatry in the 1950s would affect nursing's role for years to come. The first was Jones[17] publication of *The Therapeutic Community* in 1953. The idea behind this concept was to use the patient's social environment to provide a therapeutic experience for him. The patient was to be an active participant in his own care and become involved in the daily problems of his community. All patients were to help solve problems, plan activities, and develop the necessary rules and regulations. Their independence was increased as they gained control over many of their own personal activities. The environment fostered trust, self-direction, and individual dignity, and patients became aware of how their behavior affected others. Therapeutic communities became the preferred environment for psychiatric patients.

The implications of this development were explored in an article by Gregg[15] published in 1954. She stated that the work of the psychiatric nurse was to "help create an environment in which the patient will have an opportunity to develop new behavior patterns that will enable him to make a more mature adjustment to life." This involved the creation of "nurse-patient relationships that promote emotional growth and are consistent with the therapeutic plan of the doctor-patient relationship." She contrasted this environment to those which are custodial or protective and those which emphasize conformity and acceptable routines. To establish a therapeutic environment, she believed the patient must be allowed to express conflict, the staff must try to understand him, and there should be an opportunity for learning and growth through the development of interpersonal relationships.

The idea of the therapeutic community received support in another significant development in psychiatry—the use of psychotropic drugs in the early 1950s. This allowed more patients to become treatable and required fewer environmental constraints such as locked doors and straightjackets. It also required more personnel to provide therapy and allowed for the expansion of roles of various psychiatric practitioners, including nurses.

An article by Maloney[20] published in 1962 raised the question of whether the psychiatric nurse does have independent functions. She reviewed the spectrum of philosophies of nursing and descriptions of roles and functions. One clear area of independent functioning was identified in the management and supervision of the patient's environment. This function, however, was able to be either therapeutic or mechanical and clerical depending on the nurse's goals in implementation. Hays[16] conducted a review of the literature in 1958 and reported that the following functions of psychiatric nurses were described: dealing with patients' problems of attitude, mood, feeling-tone, and interpretation of reality; exploration of disturbing and conflicting thoughts and feelings; using positive feelings of the patient toward the therapist to bring about psychophysiological homeostasis; counseling patients in emergencies, including panic and fear; and strengthening the well part of patients. She reported that the nurse-patient relationship was referred to by a variety of terms, including the "therapeutic use of self," "therapeutic nurse-patient relationship," "psychiatric nursing therapy," "supportive psychotherapy," "rehabilitation therapies," and "nondirective counseling." The distinction between these terms and the exact nature of the nurse's role remained hazy.

Once again Peplau[31] would clarify psychiatric nursing's position and direct its future growth. In an article entitled "Interpersonal Techniques: The Crux of Psychiatric Nursing" published in 1962, she identified the heart of psychiatric nursing to be in the role of counselor or psychotherapist. The other functions of mother surrogate, technician, manager, socializing agent, and health teacher were seen as subroles. Within this article she differentiated between general practitioners who were staff nurses working on psychiatric units and psychiatric nurses who were specialists and expert clinical practitioners with graduate degrees in psychiatric nursing. Thus, from an undefined role involving primarily physical care, psychiatric nursing was evolving a role of clinical competence based on interpersonal techniques and use of the nursing process. The expanding ideas and clinical experiences of psychiatric nurses would receive an even larger forum in the future with the publication of two new nursing journals in 1963—*Perspectives in Psychiatric Care* and the *Journal of Psychiatric Nursing and Mental Health Services*. Both of these journals continue to explore elements of psychiatric nursing practice at the present time, although the name of the latter journal was changed in 1981 to the *Journal of Psychosocial Nursing and Mental Health Services*. In 1979, a third journal, *Issues in Mental Health Nursing,* was published, which provided nurses with yet another vehicle in which to explore the emerging psychiatric nursing role.

Social-environmental influences

An evolutionary perspective on psychiatric nursing practice would be incomplete without a discussion of its responsiveness to the larger social environment. The more current focus of psychiatric nursing is on primary prevention and implementing care and consultation in the community. This was stimulated by the Community Mental Health Centers Act of 1963, which made federal money available to states to plan, construct, and staff community mental health centers. This legislation was prompted by the growing awareness of the value of treating people in the community and preventing hospitalization whenever possible. It also encouraged the formation of multidisciplinary treatment teams as the skills and expertise of many professions were joined to alleviate illness and promote mental health. This team approach continues to be negotiated at present. The issues of territoriality, professionalism, authority structure, consumer rights, terminology, functioning, labeling, and the use of paraprofessionals are still being debated throughout the country.

The 1978 report of the President's Commission on Mental Health[35] tried to address some of the complex problems and inadequacies of the existing mental health services system. The report emphasized the continued need for community-based services that would provide the following.

1. A range of diagnostic, treatment, rehabilitative, and supportive services that would include long-term and short-term care
2. Easy access and continuity of care
3. Coordination with the network of other human services, such as education, health, income, and social services to provide comprehensive care
4. Adaptation to meet changing circumstances and the needs of special population groups
5. Adequate financing with public and private funds

The report focused on the need to broaden the base of knowledge about the nature and treatment of mental disabilities and called attention to the maldistribution, homogeneity, and tension among mental health professionals that ultimately work to the disadvantage of the patient. Increased mental health funding was proposed in an effort to solve some of these problems.

The Mental Health Systems Act of 1980 was passed to give substance to these recommendations, with particular focus on services for children, youth, the elderly, minority populations, and the chronic mentally ill. It was signed by President Carter who regarded it as landmark legislation because, while it reaffirmed the goal of providing comprehensive mental health services for the United States, it also established a federal role in mental health in the 1980s.

This necessary and commendable role seemed less certain, however, with the change to the Reagan administration in 1981. The Mental Health Systems Act was repealed almost immediately after President Reagan took office. In October of that year, the new Federal Fiscal Budget for 1982 went into effect, in which the funds for psychological and social health services, as well as for the education of health care professionals, had been severely cut. The remaining money was to be dispensed primarily through block grants to the states. Thus the bywords of "fewer services, economic constraints, and less federal regulation" had come to replace those of "comprehensive care, right to health, and government subsidy."

Since 1946 the social environment has greatly changed. At the present time, psychiatric nursing faces drastic cutbacks in federal funding for nursing education, retrenchment in various health care services, and compensation ceilings, amid cries of nursing shortages and unserved patient needs. The challenges to nursing are many; the future is less than clear.

Contemporary practice

The present practice of psychiatric nursing is based on a number of underlying premises or beliefs. Although the following presentation is not exhaustive in scope, it does describe some of the major philosophical beliefs that underlie nursing practice.

■ The individual has intrinsic worth and dignity. Each person is worthy of respect by his nature and presence alone.
■ The goal of the individual is one of growth, health, autonomy, and self-actualization.
■ Every individual has the potential to change and the desire to pursue personal goals.
■ The person functions as a holistic being who acts on, interacts with, and reacts to the environment as a whole person. Each part affects the total response, which is greater than the sum of each separate component.
■ All people have common, basic, and necessary human needs. Maslow[21] has categorized these needs as physical, safety, love and belonging, esteem, and self-actualization. Physical needs include physiological requirements such as food, water, and air. Safety needs pertain to the necessity of a secure physical environment that is free from threat. Love and belonging needs include the desire for intimacy and relatedness. Esteem needs refer to the desire for self-respect and recognition from others that one is a worthwhile and valuable person. Self-actualization needs include the desire for self-fulfillment as one concentrates on realizing one's own potential.
■ All behavior of the individual is meaningful. It arises from personal needs and goals and can only be understood from the person's internal frame of reference and within the context in which it occurs.
■ Behavior consists of perceptions, thoughts, feelings, and actions. These occur in a sequential manner; from one's perceptions thoughts arise, emotions are felt, and actions are conceived. Disruptions may occur in any of these areas and be evident in distorted perceptions, impaired thought processes, alterations in the expression of emotions, and maladaptive or inappropriate actions.
■ Individuals vary in their coping capacities. These are dependent on genetic endowment, environmental influences, nature and degree of stress, and available resources. All individuals have the potential for both health and illness.
■ Illness can be a growth-producing experience for the individual. The goal of nursing care is to maximize the person's positive interactions with his environment, promote his level of wellness, and enhance his degree of self-actualization.

- All people have a right to an equal opportunity for adequate health care regardless of sex, race, religion, ethics, or cultural background. Nursing care is based on the needs of individuals, families, and communities and mutually defined goals and expectations.
- Mental health is a critical and necessary component of comprehensive health care services.
- The individual has the right to participate in decision making regarding his physical and mental health. The person has the right to self-determination. This right allows the individual the choice of changing present behavior or continuing it without modification. It is the decision of the individual to pursue health or illness.
- An interpersonal relationship has the potential for producing change and growth within the individual. It is the vehicle for the application of the nursing process and the attainment of the goal of nursing care.

Present roles and functions

Psychiatric nursing is an interpersonal process that strives to promote and maintain behavior which contributes to integrated functioning. The patient or client system may be an individual, family, group, organization, or community. The American Nurses' Association Division on Psychiatric and Mental Health Nursing defines psychiatric and mental health nursing as follows*:

A specialized area of nursing practice employing theories of human behavior as its science and purposeful use of self as its art. It is directed toward both preventive and corrective impacts upon mental disorders and their sequelae and is concerned with the promotion of optimal mental health for society, the community, and those individuals who live within it.[2,5]

The National Institute of Mental Health officially recognizes psychiatric and mental health nurses as one of the four core mental health disciplines.

The psychiatric nurse uses knowledge from the psychosocial and biophysical sciences and theories of personality and human behavior to derive a theoretical framework on which she bases her practice. The choice of a conceptual model and theoretical framework is an individual one for each nurse. Various theories of psychiatric care are briefly described in Chapter 2.

---

*Quotations in this chapter are from the American Nurses' Association, Division on Psychiatric and Mental Health Nursing Practice: Statement on psychiatric and mental health nursing practice, Kansas City, Mo., 1976. Reprinted by permission.

Some nurses might base their practice on a psychoanalytical framework, others might adopt a family systems orientation, whereas still others may use a behavioral theoretical model. The nurse's choice of a model will depend on her personal philosophy, educational background, setting, and experience in working with patients. Powers[34] believes that one criterion for the selection of a theory base should be its fit as an organized frame of reference for developed nursing models. The selected theoretical framework, she believes, should encompass the following commonalities of nursing models: (1) the holistic view of people, with usually three major interdependent subsystems or components; (2) people as systems in dynamic interaction with the environment; (3) people developing over time; and (4) people adapting continuously to both internal and external forces or variables. The theoretical model selected by the nurse can then be utilized as a framework for nursing practice.

Psychiatric nurses may practice in settings that vary widely in purpose, type, location, and administration. They may be employed by an agency or self-employed in a private practice. Nurses who are employed by an agency are remunerated for their services on either a salaried or fee-for-service basis. The majority of nurses work in such organized settings, and the administrative policies of these organizations can either foster or limit the full utilization of the nurse's potential. Nurses who are self-employed receive remuneration for their services through third-party payment and direct patient fees. Some of these self-employed specialists maintain staff privileges with institutional facilities. The settings in which nurses work can focus on either acute or long-term care. Some examples of settings include psychiatric hospitals, community mental health centers, general hospitals, community health agencies, outpatient clinics, homes, schools, prisons, private organizations, crisis care units, day and night care centers, offices, camps, and industrial centers.

Within these settings, psychiatric nurses may assume various roles. They may be staff nurses, administrators, consultants, in-service educators, clinical practitioners, researchers, or program evaluators. Thus the settings of practice range from institutional to community based to independent practice, and the corresponding roles can include both direct and indirect nursing functions.

The following nine major activities involved in the practice of psychiatric nursing were identified by the American Nurses' Association:

1. Providing a therapeutic milieu
2. Working with the here-and-now problems of clients
3. Using the surrogate parent role
4. Caring for the somatic aspects of the client's health problems
5. Teaching factors related to emotional health
6. Acting as a social agent
7. Providing leadership to other personnel
8. Conducting psychotherapy
9. Engaging in social and community action related to mental health[2]

It is possible to more specifically describe the various functions or activities engaged in by psychiatric nurses. The distinction of direct and indirect nursing care functions is helpful in this regard. "Direct nursing care functions presume that the nurse's actions and reflections are focused on a particular client or family and that the nurse has personal responsibility and is accountable to the client or family for the outcome of such actions."[2:15] Indirect nursing care roles are those in which some other person actually carries out the patient's care. The nursing responsibilities inherent in these roles require the qualifications of a psychiatric and mental health nursing specialist. All of the direct and indirect nursing functions are actions for which the nurse is directly responsible. They are carried out whether or not the patient is under medical care and in any setting agreed on by the nurse and the patient.

The concepts of primary prevention, secondary prevention, and tertiary prevention provide a framework for discussing these activities.[41] Primary prevention is a community concept that involves lowering the incidence of illness in a community by altering the causative factors before they have an opportunity to do harm. It is a concept that precedes disease and is applied to a generally healthy population. It includes health promotion, illness prevention, and protection against disease. Within this area lie many of nursing's independent functions that have as their goal decreasing the vulnerability of the individual to illness and strengthening his capacity to withstand stressors. Direct nursing care functions in this area include the following:

1. Health teaching regarding principles of mental health
2. Affecting changes in improved living conditions, freedom from poverty, and better education
3. Consumer education in such areas as normal growth and development and sex education
4. Initiating appropriate referrals before mental disorder occurs based on assessment of potential stressors and life changes
5. Assisting patients in a general hospital setting to avoid future psychiatric problems
6. Working with families to support family members and group functioning
7. Becoming active in community and political activities related to mental health

Secondary prevention involves the reduction of actual illness by early detection and treatment of the problem. Following are direct nursing care functions in this area:

1. Intake screening and evaluation services
2. Home visits for preadmission or treatment services
3. Emergency treatment and psychiatric services in the general hospital
4. Providing a therapeutic milieu
5. Supervising patients receiving medication
6. Suicide prevention services
7. Counseling on a time-limited basis
8. Crisis intervention
9. Psychotherapy with individuals, families, and groups of various ages ranging from children to older adults
10. Intervening with communities and organizations based on an identified problem

Tertiary prevention involves reducing the residual impairment or disability resulting from the illness. Direct nursing care functions in this area include the following:

1. Promoting vocational training and rehabilitation
2. Organizing aftercare programs for patients discharged from psychiatric facilities to facilitate their transition from the hospital to the community
3. Providing partial hospitalization options for patients

In addition to these direct nursing care functions, psychiatric nurses engage in indirect activities that affect all three levels of prevention. These activities include educating nursing personnel in in-service, continuing, generic, or advanced educational programs; administrating in mental health settings to facilitate the provision of optimal nursing care; supervising nursing personnel to improve the quality of nursing services; consulting with colleagues, other professionals, consumer groups, community care givers, and local and national agencies; and researching clinical nursing problems.

Level of performance

This description of various nursing activities and functions is also indicative of the wide variation in levels of performance. Not all psychiatric nurses are able to perform each of these functions. Individual nurses have primary responsibility and accountability for their own practice and one aspect of accountability is that nurses define and adhere to the legitimate scope of their practice. Four major factors play a role in determining the level at which the nurse functions and the types of activities she engages in. The first is the *law*. Each state has its own nurse practice act, which defines the legal limits of nursing practice and must be adhered to by all licensed nurses.

The second factor is the *qualifications of the nurse, including her education, work experiences, and certification status*. The American Nurses' Association has identified two types of practitioners: nurses who are generalists and are called psychiatric and mental health nurses, and nurses who are specialists and are called psychiatric and mental health specialists.[2] The recommended educational preparation for the generalist role is a baccalaureate degree in nursing. One also needs to demonstrate the profession's standards of knowledge, experience, and quality of care through formal review processes. Generalists provide most of the care for most of the people served by nursing.

In contrast, specialization involves adding to the generic base of nursing practice an organized and systematized body of knowledge and competencies within a discrete area of nursing, applied through specialized practice. The specialist in psychiatric and mental health nursing is characterized by graduate education, supervised clinical experience, and depth of knowledge, competence, and skill in practice. This increased depth of knowledge is reflected in the specialist's more refined ability to apply this knowledge to the solution of mental health problems. The minimum level of preparation for the specialist is a master's degree in psychiatric nursing, which is characterized by academically

supervised clinical practice and study in the theoretical bases for therapeutic intervention. Currently there are over 60 master's degree programs in psychiatric nursing and over 10,000 psychiatric and mental health nurses have master's degrees. In addition, there are 23 doctoral programs in nursing. They focus on either research and theory development in nursing or advanced development of the nurse-therapist role with research focused on specific clinical problems. The first type of program usually leads to a Doctor of Philosophy (Ph.D.) degree, whereas the second results in a Doctor of Nursing Science (D.N.Sc.) degree. Doctorally prepared nurses contribute to the advancement of knowledge in the field of psychiatric and mental health nursing through research and scholarship.

Another qualification is the nurse's relevant work experience. Although work experience does not replace education, it does provide an added and necessary dimension to one's level of competence and ability to function therapeutically. Gardner[13] believes that one's role should be determined by the education, experiential level, and personal assets of the nurse. She suggests defining the role of the psychiatric nurse in an ambulatory setting based on three levels of practice. Table 1-1 summarizes the requirements and responsibilities inherent in each level of practice. Level 2 nurses would correspond to the American Nurses' Association's "psychiatric and mental health nurse," and level 3 would correspond to the "nurse specialist."

The final qualification is the certification process, which is a formal review of the clinical practice of the nurse specialist that has evolved within the professional organization, the American Nurses' Association. This process requires that the specialist evidence a "high degree of proficiency in interpersonal skills, in the use of the nursing process, and in psychiatric, psychological, and milieu therapies."[2:11-12] Following are six requirements for certification in psychiatric and mental health nursing:

1. Current involvement in direct clinical nursing practice at least 4 hours per week
2. A master's or higher degree in nursing, with a specialization in psychiatric and mental health nursing *or* one may apply for individual consideration if one possesses a baccalaureate degree in nursing and a master's degree in a related field,

TABLE 1-1. **Levels of practice for psychiatric nurses in ambulatory settings***

	Level 1	Level 2	Level 3
Education requirements	No formal education is necessary other than current state licensure	Baccalaureate degree in nursing	Master's degree in psychiatric nursing
Experience requirements	Minimum of 1 year experience in acute psychiatric nursing care	Minimum of 2 years of experience in acute psychiatric care settings	Advanced knowledge and expertise in psychiatric care and principles of supervision and consultation
Nature of practice	Supportive treatment	Supportive treatment	Insight treatment
Therapeutic functions	Communicating with other professionals and agencies relative to patient care	Primary responsibility for supportive therapy	Primary responsibility for insight-oriented psychotherapy
	Assisting in assessment and data collection	Assessment of patient functioning	Responsibility for patients cared for by nurses in levels 1 and 2 of practice
	Assisting patient to use environmental resources	Initiation and attendance at all conferences regarding her patients	Assessment of patient pathology
	Assisting in community primary prevention programs	Assignment to interdisciplinary teams responsible for delivery of primary mental health care in ambulatory units	Supervision of other health team members
			Participation in primary community prevention programs
			Responsibility for obtaining supervision consultation
			Responsible for assumption of nursing leadership

*Modified from Gardner, K.: J. Psychiatr. Nurs. **15:**26, Sept. 1977.

such as psychology, sociology, social work, human relations, or counseling and guidance, *or* a master's or higher degree in nursing, plus a baccalaureate in any field and a diploma in nursing.

3. Practice in psychiatric and mental health nursing after receiving a master's degree with direct patient/client contact for either 8 hours a week for 2 years *or* 4 hours a week for 4 years
4. Access to clinical supervision or consultation
5. Experience in at least two different treatment modalities
6. At least 100 hours of supervision/consultation by a certified member of the core mental health disciplines (clinical specialist in psychiatric and mental health nursing, psychiatrist, psychologist, or psychiatric social worker) after receiving a master's degree

On successful completion of the certification examination and written documentation, the nurse can identify herself as a Certified Specialist (C.S.) and be listed in the *Directory of Certified Nurses* published by the American Nurses' Association. Although any specialist nurse may be certified, it is expected that the nurse who is self-employed in the practice of psychotherapy will obtain certification to assure the public of her ability to perform as a competent nurse psychotherapist.

The third factor influencing the psychiatric nurse's level of performance is the *setting in which she practices.* According to Peplau, a basic consideration here is the philosophy of the health care system and the way in which the setting defines mental illness. From this definition will emerge the work of the patient and the role of the nurse as illustrated in Table 1-2. If the setting is that of an organization, additional constraints may be imposed on the nurse

TABLE 1-2. **Different definitions of mental illness and therefore of the work of the patient and the role of the nurse***

Definition	Work of the patient	Role of the nurse
Socially inacceptable behavior of the patient has previously been "rewarded"; he has unfortunately been "conditioned" to behave in these ways	Submit to treatment using behavior modification (reconditioning) techniques	Surveillance of patient following treatment plan; pass out rewards; general nursing routine care
Inacceptable behavior is the result of genetic inheritance	Submit to whatever ameliorative treatment of symptoms is ordered	Surveillance and custody; reporting; general nursing routine care
Inacceptable behavior is due to a biochemical imbalance	Submit to tests and prescribed treatment drugs to rectify the imbalance	Surveillance; reporting; pass medications, such as tranquilizers, stimulants, lithium, hormones, etc.; observe effects; general nursing routine care
Inacceptable behavior is due to some unknown but adverse brain activity	Submit to prescribed treatment (electrostimulation, electroshock, lobotomy, etc.)	Surveillance; reporting; pretreatment and posttreatment "preparation"; general nursing (and surgical nursing) care
Inacceptable behavior reflects problems in living with people and lack in intellectual and interpersonal competencies to understand and solve those problems	Participate in psychotherapy sessions and in ad hoc talking sessions with the available professionals, so as to investigate, understand, and resolve those problems and in the process gain new intellectual and interpersonal competencies on an experiential/educative basis	Use all "activities of daily living" as a basis for observation, discussion, and intervention in ways that enhance the patient's intellectual and interpersonal competencies to change his own behavior; also general nursing care Using "situational counseling" to aid patients involved in disputes, violence, and other grossly inacceptable behavior to investigate the problem inherent in the acting-out situation Referral for other professional services, such as clergy, and coordination and follow-up on discharge
The inacceptable behavior is due to "lack of insight" into intrapsychic causes	Seek psychoanalysis for those who can afford it	

*From Peplau, H.: Int. Nurs. Rev. **25**(2):45, 1978.

due to administrative policies, staff norms, or nursing service expectations. A study done by Sloboda[38] determined that inpatient nurses ranked their functions as primarily those of a "nurse clinician" followed by "change agent" and finally "therapist." Nurses in outpatient settings ranked all three functions fairly equally. Lieb, Underwood, and Glick[19] suggest that inpatient staff nurses are limited in providing primary therapy because of the ready supply of other professionals and a concern for appropriate preparation. The nurse's relationship with other health professionals thus emerges as an important influence on her level of functioning.

An essential part of nursing service is cooperation and collaboration with other health care providers. Nurses may be members of three different types of teams—unidisciplinary, having all team members of the same discipline; multidisciplinary, having members of different disciplines who each provide specific services to the patient; and interdisciplinary, having mem-

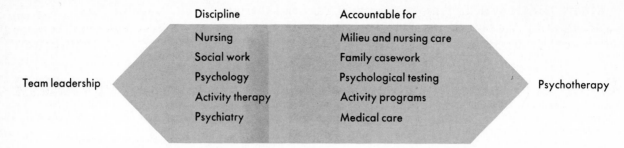

Discipline	Accountable for
Nursing	Milieu and nursing care
Social work	Family casework
Psychology	Psychological testing
Activity therapy	Activity programs
Psychiatry	Medical care

Team leadership   Psychotherapy

FIG. 1-1
Roles assumed by mental health team members. (Modified from Benfer, B.: Perspect.
Psychiatr. Care **18**(4):167, 1980.)

bers of different disciplines involved in a formal arrangement to provide patient services while maximizing educational interchange. Most organized mental health settings employ an interdisciplinary team approach, which requires highly coordinated and frequently interdependent planning. This may or may not proceed smoothly. Given and Simmons[14] describe seven barriers to interdisciplinary team formation: educational preparation, role ambiguity and incongruent expectations, authority, power, status, autonomy, and personal characteristics of members. Benfer[5] has followed up on these by identifying three specific problems related to team functioning. First, is the problem of identifying role and function. Second, there are the difficulties in resolving overlapping problems. Third, there are problems in communication within the team.

If the roles and functions of the various team members are not clarified and agreed on, then confusion, crossing of boundaries, resentment, and underutilization of health professionals is likely to occur. Some overlapping of roles and functions among psychiatric professionals is to be expected, since all mental health disciplines have access to the same body of knowledge on which professional education and improvement of practice is based. Thus, all of the mental health team's members may be competent in providing psychotherapy, although some may prefer group therapy, others individual therapy, and still others family therapy. There are also some discrete role functions among team members as evident in Fig. 1-1 and the subsequent discussion.[5]

The *physician,* whether or not the team leader, carries the medical responsibility for diagnosis, medical orders, medication, admis-

sion, discharge, and accountability for medical treatment. The *activity therapist* carries the responsibility and accountability for activity programming, although aspects of it may be shared with nursing. The *social worker* is accountable and responsible for family casework. The *psychologist* is accountable and responsible for psychological assessment and testing. The *nursing staff* is accountable and responsible for the patient's milieu and for implementing the nursing process with all of its ramifications, ranging from assessing and planning care, providing a safe environment, dealing with the daily activity of patients and evaluating the outcome of care.

In addition to a discrete role description, certain personal characteristics essential to teamwork are seen in the professional members who are able to tolerate frustration and are flexible in their adjustment to new situations. Appropriate members and adequate time are also important to the interdisciplinary team functioning. Table 1-3 summarizes these elements.

Partially in response to vested interests among mental health professionals and lack of cooperation, the Joint Commission on Interprofessional Affairs was founded in 1975. The members are representatives of the American Nurses' Association, the American Psychiatric Association, the American Psychological Association, and the National Association of Social Workers. A major effort of the Commission has been the development of the following guidelines for interprofessional ethics:

1. Seek to achieve interprofessional unity and cooperation.
2. Recognize and respect the autonomy and specialized competency of each profession.
3. Know the facts before speaking or issuing public positions about interprofessional

TABLE 1-3. Analysis of interdisciplinary teams*

Personal qualities vital to interdisciplinary team function	Activities necessary for interdisciplinary team function
Accept differences/perspectives of others	Establish new professional interaction patterns
Function interdependently	Accept changes in authority and status
Negotiate role with other team members	Develop modes of conflict resolution and decision making
Form new values, attitudes, and perceptions	
Tolerate constant review and challenge of ideas	
Take risks	
Possess personal identity and integrity	
Accept team philosophy of care	

*From Given, B., and Simmons, S.: Nurs. Forum **16**(2):165, 1977.

issues and utilize the facts in a responsible and appropriate fashion.

4. Attempt to resolve issues through direct discussion, debate, and negotiation.
5. Pursue joint actions toward mutually acceptable goals.

The Joint Commission on Interprofessional Affairs recommends that a variety of ways be pursued to facilitate communication and resolution of problems at national, state, and local levels, including such undertakings as joint meetings, regular exchange of information, exchange of formal liaison representatives, and organization of local and statewide interprofessional groups. Utilization of these guidelines for interprofessional ethics should enhance the effectiveness of each of the professions in the delivery of mental health services. The Joint Commission on Interprofessional Affairs is presently working on case examples to determine how the professions can better work together regarding autonomy, consultation, collaboration and supervision in relation to legal responsibilities, assessment and diagnosis, treatment planning, and service delivery.

The fourth and final factor affecting the nurse's level of functioning is the *personal competence and initiative* of the individual nurse. These personal qualities will determine how the nurse interprets her role and the success of its implementation. The importance of this final factor should not be ignored, since without a realization of her clinical competence and the assumption of professional initiative, the nurse will be significantly limited in her performance.

The four factors together account for variations in nursing practice. Specifically, these variations will be evident in regard to the following*:

- Assessment and data collection
- Analysis of data
- Application of theory
- Breadth and depth of knowledge base, especially clinical, psychosocial, and pathophysiological theories relating to nursing diagnosis and treatment
- The range of nursing techniques
- Need for, kind, and extent of supervision by other nurses in practice
- Evaluation of effects of practice
- Identification of relationships among phenomena, nursing actions, effects (outcomes for the patients)[3:19-20]

All nurses who are practicing with patients, however, are expected to address the phenomena that form the core of nursing practice. These are identified and described in the Standards of Psychiatric Nursing Practice.

Standards of Psychiatric and Mental Health Nursing Practice

The present Standards of Psychiatric and Mental Health Nursing Practice are a revision of standards enunciated by the Division on Psychiatric and Mental Health Nursing Practice of the American Nurses' Association in 1973. They provide a way of determining the quality of nursing that a patient receives and apply to psychiatric nursing practice in any setting. They are organized around the nursing process. The

*From American Nurses' Association: Nursing: a social policy statement, Kansas City, Mo., 1976. Reprinted by permission.

purpose of the standards is to fulfill nursing's obligation to provide and improve the practice of psychiatric nursing. They are as follows*:

Standard I—Theory The nurse applies appropriate theory that is scientifically sound as a basis for decisions regarding nursing practice.

Standard II—Data collection The nurse continuously collects data that are comprehensive, accurate, and systematic.

Standard III—Diagnosis The nurse utilizes *nursing diagnoses* and standard classification of mental disorders to express conclusions supported by recorded assessment data and current scientific premises.

Standard IV—Planning The nurse develops a nursing care plan with specific goals and interventions delineating nursing actions unique to each client's needs.

Standard V—Intervention The nurse intervenes as guided by the nursing care plan to implement nursing actions that promote, maintain, or restore physical and mental health, prevent illness, and effect rehabilitation.

> **Standard V-A—Psychotherapeutic interventions** The nurse uses *psychotherapeutic interventions* to assist clients to regain or improve their previous coping abilities and to prevent further disability.

> **Standard V-B—Health teaching** The nurse assists clients, families, and groups to achieve satisfying and productive patterns of living through health teaching.

> **Standard V-C—Self-care activities** The nurse uses the activities of daily living in a goal-directed way to foster adequate self-care and physical and mental well-being of clients.

> **Standard V-D—Somatic therapies** The nurse uses knowledge of somatic therapies and applies related clinical skills in working with clients.

> **Standard V-E—Therapeutic environment** The nurse provides, structures, and maintains a therapeutic environment in collaboration with the client and other health care providers.

> **Standard V-F—Psychotherapy** The nurse utilizes advanced clinical expertise in individual, group, and family *psychotherapy*, child psychotherapy, and other treatment modalities to function as a psychotherapist and recognizes professional accountability for nursing practice.

Standard VI—Evaluation The nurse evaluates client responses to nursing actions to revise the data base, nursing diagnoses, and nursing care plan.

---

*From American Nurses' Association, Division on Psychiatric and Mental Health Nursing Practice: Standards of psychiatric and mental health nursing practice, Kansas City, Mo., 1982. Reprinted by permission.

Standard VII—Peer review The nurse participates in peer review and other means of evaluation to assure quality of nursing care provided for clients.

Standard VIII—Continuing education The nurse assumes responsibility for continuing education and professional development and contributes to the professional growth of others.

Standard IX—Interdisciplinary collaboration The nurse collaborates with interdisciplinary teams in assessing, planning, implementing, and evaluating programs and other mental health activities.

Standard X—Utilization of community health systems The nurse participates with other members of the community in assessing, planning, implementing, and evaluating mental health services and community systems that include the promotion of the broad continuum of primary, secondary, and tertiary prevention of mental illness.

Standard XI—Research The nurse contributes to nursing and the mental health field through innovations in theory and practice and participation in research.

The question of professional autonomy

Psychiatric nurses as a group displayed certain personal qualities in a study reported by Mlott.[25] He found that they possessed adequate defenses, a good self-concept, adequate but flexible impulse control, the ability to trust others, and tolerance. They viewed events as products of their own actions and sought information relevant to problems they encountered. He also reported that they were better adjusted and more active, striving, independent, effective, self-confident, persevering, and determined than other nurse subspecialties. His study paints a rather rosy picture of psychiatric nurses as competent, effective, and confident mental health professionals. However, are they truly professionalized?

The professional status of nursing has been a long-debated issue both within nursing and among observers and scholars outside of nursing. Often, in the nursing literature, one sees defensive assertions or soothing assurances that yes, indeed, nursing really is a profession. However, outside the field, nursing is described as a semiprofession, subprofession, or marginal profession. One can only conclude that there is no consensus, and the question is far from resolved. It is helpful, however, to analyze psychiatric nursing's present position on the professionalization continuum because, in so doing, conflicts and roadblocks to future growth can be identified.

Viewed as a continuum, professionalization

"is the evidence of a continuous attempt of a group in any community or society to gain more and more control over certain resources related to an occupational area."[43] The attainment of professional status necessarily involves a struggle. Society alone has the power to grant it, and consensus for it must exist in the body politic. The six characteristics of the scale of professionalization identified by Moore[26] are comprehensive in scope and developmental in nature. They suggest the following sequencing or process of professionalization:

1. *Occupation.* The requirement that the work be a full-time undertaking by a group of individuals.

2. *Calling.* A personal commitment or intention to pursue a stable career in the occupation. It incorporates socialization into the culture of the profession with its values, norms, and symbols.

3. *Organization.* The formation of an association by members because of their recognition of common occupational interests. The organization concerns itself with the occupation's status as a profession, the tasks of its members, the ways to raise the quality of applicants, and political action.

4. *Education.* Preparation by intense study of a systematic "body of theory." This body of theory is a system of abstract propositions that describe in general terms the classes of phenomena which make up the profession's focus of interest and is then practically applied. Theory construction through systematic research is a distinctive professional activity as characterized in the role of researcher-theoretician. In this way, the profession creates, organizes, and transmits its knowledge. The minimal educational requirement is the baccalaureate degree, although many professions have considerably longer educational requirements. A spirit of rationality prevails among the members, as evidenced in its ongoing commitment to learning and the processes of reasoning and the assumption of a critical attitude toward its theory and knowledge base.

5. *Service orientation.* Characterized by rules of competence, conscientious performance, and loyalty or service. Rules of competence require the accreditation of educational programs, establishment of a licensing system, and maintenance and improvement of standards through continuing education. Rules of conscientious performance refer to self-discipline and self-regulation. Rules of service require that the professionals serve the clients' interests first, placing it over personal gain or commercial profit.

6. *Autonomy.* Legitimate control over one's own work. Autonomy is the ultimate value for professionals characterized by professional authority. The outcome of autonomy and authority is power, prestige, and status accorded by society, which in turn expects exemplary behavior from the profession.

Psychiatric nursing has amply met the first two characteristics. The remaining four, however, appear to be problematic.[40]

Organization

The American Nurses' Association was founded in 1896. It is the major professional organization, but approximately only 25% of all licensed nurses belong to it. American Nurses' Association members, furthermore, represent various educational backgrounds and, consequently, various interpretations of the tasks and roles of nursing. They disagree on the uniqueness of their contribution as health care team members, their educational programs and their legal rights and responsibilities.[1] The American Nurses' Association has a Division on Psychiatric and Mental Health Nursing Practice and a specialty subgroup, the Council of Specialists in Psychiatric and Mental Health Nursing. In 1973 it published the *Standards of Psychiatric and Mental Health Nursing Practice* and revised them in 1982. The *Statement on Psychiatric and Mental Health Nursing Practice,*[2] which defines psychiatric nursing, identifies types of practitioners, and describes the scope of practice, was published in 1976. Both of these publications have served to clarify and refine the role, tasks, and functioning of psychiatric nurses.

Since 1948, the American Nurses' Association has had an economic security program, with one of its goals being to upgrade the economic position of registered nurses. To do this, it engages in collective bargaining activities. The majority of nurses appear to accept the validity and necessity of collective action to attain economic goals. What remains in conflict is the mechanism and scope of issues appropriately covered by collective bargaining agreements, specifically, the inclusion of patient care issues in negotiations and the leadership dilemma of a professional organization functioning as a collective bargaining agent.

Underlying the position of the American Nurses' Association toward collective bargaining is the conviction that nurses must speak for nursing. This is a more fundamental issue than the single aspect of salary or scheduling. It is the basis for the difference between a professional organization and a union, and it has particular significance for nursing because of its long history of domination by other groups. No one group represents a majority of nurses; neither is the economic security program the primary purpose of the American Nurses' Association. However, unless nursing accepts its responsibility to control its own practice and to have nurses speak for nursing, the economic security issue may end up being the end, not just the means.

Cleland[8] has described a professional collective bargaining model. She believes that the labor contract can become the legal instrument through which the profession can implement standards of care. To do so, the labor contract should include negotiated clauses relating to wages, hours, and conditions of work. To gain control of nursing practice, she believes the contract should contain provisions on (1) shared governance, (2) individual accountability, and (3) collective professional responsibility. Clearly, the model she advocates is a professional one that would necessitate the active participation and support of nurses. Before it can be widely undertaken, however, nurses need to collectively decide if they wish to be professionals.

In addition to the need for more nurses to support their professional organization, reach some consensus on the tasks of nursing, and exercise more control over their practice, there is also a need for psychiatric nurses to develop a clearer conception of their leadership capabilities. The development of knowledge and strategies for enabling nurses, individually and collectively, to exercise leadership and management in the groups and institutions in which they work is essential to gaining full professional status. It will also serve to strengthen and expand the contribution of psychiatric nursing to the larger mental health care system.

Various theories have been developed regarding the complex social and psychologic phenomena involved in leadership. Most of the studies in this area, however, have focused on men in business organizations and very few on women, let alone nurses. Traditionally women, including nurses, have been considered followers rather than leaders regarding major changes in society. Yet there is much to be gained from greater insight into the factors that promote or inhibit effective leadership among nurses. One might approach this area from two different perspectives: examine the individual who is occupying a position of leadership or explore leadership as a transactional process. The former approach would include the styles and functions of leadership, whereas the latter would include the conditions, processes, and contexts of leadership as a social role or transaction (Table 1-4).[24] Dumas has noted the following:

> Those processes occurring in the groups in which or with which nurses work are of special significance. Pressures to conform to the image of the kind, nurturing, self-sacrificing angel of mercy (the analogue of the good mother) pose a perplexing dilemma for nurse leaders. Those who conform often find themselves deluged by bids from subordinates and colleagues in other disciplines for special attention or assistance to help them deal with the stresses of organizational life. These demands often exceed the responsibilities of their formal positions and drain time and energy that should be used for work tasks. Those who resist run the risk of the opposite stereotype—the cold, rigid, inconsiderate authoritarian leader (the rejecting, depriving, bad mother). There are big prices to pay in either instance.[10:712-713]

There is no question but that psychiatric nurses must utilize their leadership skills and work as change agents to a greater degree than is presently being done. This need derives from the imperative of providing adequate, humane, and socially acceptable care to mental health consumers. To this end, nurses can initiate change; assist in change by supporting, participating, or implementing it; engage in joint ventures for planned change; and evaluate completed change. To do this, however, the following key characteristics are needed by the psychiatric nurse[22]:

1. The ability to take risks. This means to develop the ability to calculate potential risks surrounding the implementation of the change and then to decide whether or not these risks are indeed worth taking.
2. A commitment to the efficacy of the change. The change agent must develop a commitment to investigating the worth, value, effectiveness, and necessity of the change before initiating it.
3. Three areas of competence: knowledge of nursing that combines research findings and basic science information, clinical competence, and interpersonal relationship and communication skills.

This last characteristic requires the use not only

TABLE 1-4. The nature of effective leadership*

Conditions of effective leadership	Social processes underlying effective leadership	Styles of leadership	Functions of effective leadership
Recipient of communication must be able to understand it	Respect expressed *by* leader breeds respect *for* leader	Authoritarian style characterized by firmness, self-assurance, and domination of others	Leaders facilitate adaptive capacity of social systems
Person must have resources and ability to comply with directive	Leader must demonstrate competence in performing own roles	Democratic style characterized by responsiveness, participation, and mutual interaction	Leaders are alert to unanticipated consequences of previous collective action
Person must believe action is consistent with personal beliefs and values	Leader should be in continuing touch with what is going on in work group	Bureaucratic style characterized by strict, adhered to rules	Leaders are both present oriented and future oriented
Person must perceive directive as consistent with purposes and values of organization	Although leader has access to power that coerces, he seldom makes use of it	Laissez-faire style characterized by lack of direction and control	Leaders represent group to its environment
		Paternalistic style characterized by benevolent control	Leaders evaluate resources for system and cope with problems of their allocation
			Leaders express aspirations that evoke resonance among members of group
			Leaders mobilize, guide, coordinate, and control efforts of group members
			Leaders symbolize, extend, and deepen collective unity among members of system
			Leaders enunciate values and ideals of group and give people pride in their group identity
			Leaders arbitrate and mediate inevitable conflicts that emerge in social interaction, so that most members of group believe justice has been done most of time
			Leaders serve as scapegoats for larger group

*Modified from Merton, R.: The social nature of leadership, Am. J. Nurs. **69:**2614, Dec. 1969.

of facilitative communication skills, but also confrontation when appropriate, a skill that nurses have tended to avoid using. Confrontation can only be justified as a precursor to negotiations, which are a foundation for change. It is a process that has two phases. The first requires an assault on the system to be changed. The second requires reconciliation to mend strained relationships or to create new ones. Smoyak believes:

Confrontations are in order when the goals are resolving an issue, improving health care systems, defining changing work roles, revamping licensing and practicing acts, gaining and keeping suitable salary schedules, attaining and maintaining control over professional practice, or any other professional issue, locally defined and carried out, on which there is consensus among nurses who are affected by the issue. They are in order when the group has gathered facts, may have tried other means, and has decided on collective action.[39:1635]

One result of such nursing initiative is that nursing licensure statutes have undergone considerable change and scrutiny in the last decade. Although not all states have revised their nurse practice acts, those which have show nurses assuming responsibility for more complex patient care that involves major independent decision making. Another positive sign is the 1980 publication of the American Nurses' Association entitled, *Nursing: A Social Policy Statement*,[3] which defines and establishes the scope of nursing practice and nursing's social responsibility.

Yet such statements and definitions cannot actually determine the scope of practice, relationships between nurses and other health professionals, needs of the consumer, or interaction between nursing and the government in formulating and implementing health-related policy. Only nurses working together through political processes can make these determinations. Although the impact of nurses on the quality and quantity of health care may be phenomenal, it is largely untapped. Nurses have the potential to be significant forces in the process of shaping the health care future of our society, if they can learn to use their power and resources in the political arena—one of the truly most important targets for nursing actions.

Education

A major challenge to psychiatric nursing in the area of education is in the need for a well-defined body of nursing knowledge. The question "Is psychiatric nursing unique?" has preoccupied the profession for some time now. In so doing, it has siphoned off energy that could better have been applied to clinical or theoretical questions. Nursing's contribution is an outcome of a unique manner of problem conceptualization, the utilization of theoretical models to explain behavior, and a nursing process approach to individuals, families, and communities. Lego[18] asserts that knowledge determines uniqueness, and nursing is distinguished by a holistic approach, crisis orientation, and knowledge of general health matters. The existence of this psychiatric nursing textbook, which incorporates existing nursing research and views the nursing process as the basis for practice, is evidence of the distinct body of knowledge that is

TABLE 1-5. **Doctoral programs in nursing (May-June 1981)**

Institution	Degree	Institution	Degree
University of Alabama in Birmingham Birmingham, AL 35294	D.N.Sc.	University of Pennsylvania Philadelphia, PA 19104	D.N.Sc.
University of Arizona Tucson, AZ 85721	Ph.D.	University of Pittsburgh Pittsburgh, PA 15261	Ph.D.
Boston University Boston, MA 02215	D.N.Sc.	University of Rochester Rochester, NY 14642	Ph.D.
University of California, San Francisco San Francisco, CA 94143	D.N.Sc.	Rush University Chicago, IL 60612	D.N.Sc.
Case Western Reserve University Cleveland, OH 44106	Ph.D.	Teachers College, Columbia University New York, NY 10027	Ed.D.
Catholic University of America Washington, D.C. 20064	D.N.Sc.	University of Texas at Austin Austin, TX 78712	Ph.D.
University of Colorado Denver, CO 80262	Ph.D.	Texas Woman's University Denton, TX 76204	Ph.D.
University of Illinois at the Medical Center Chicago, IL 60612	Ph.D.	University of Utah Salt Lake City, UT 84112	Ph.D.
Indiana University Indianapolis, IN 46202	D.N.Sc.	University of Washington Seattle, WA 98195	Ph.D.
University of Maryland Baltimore, MD 21201	Ph.D.	Wayne State University Detroit, MI 48202	Ph.D.
University of Michigan Ann Arbor, MI 48104	Ph.D.	University of Wisconsin, Madison Madison, WI 53792	Ph.D.
New York University New York, NY 10003	Ph.D.		

TABLE 1-6. Nursing research organizations

State	Organization and address	State	Organization and address
AL	Nursing Research Center, University of Alabama School of Nursing, University of Alabama in Birmingham, University Station, Birmingham, AL 35294	MO	Office for Nursing Research, St. Louis University Medical Center, School of Nursing, 3525 Caroline Street, St. Louis, MO 63104
AZ	Nursing Research Center, University of Arizona, College of Nursing, Tucson, AZ 85721	NE	Nursing Care Research Center, College of Nursing, University of Nebraska, Medical Center, 42nd and Dewey Avenue, Omaha, NE 68105
CA	City of Hope Medical Center, Division of Nursing, 1500 East Duarte Road, Duarte, CA 91010	NY	Department of Nursing Research, Memorial Sloan-Kettering Cancer Center, New York, NY
CA	The Pain Study Group, Department of Nursing in Biological Dysfunction-N611Y, School of Nursing, University of California San Francisco, CA 94143	NY	Nursing Research Center Teachers College, Columbia University, New York, NY 10027
CA	University of California, Irvine—Medical Center, 101 City Drive South, Orange, CA 92668	OH	Center for Nursing Research, Ohio State University, School of Nursing, 1585 Neil Avenue, Columbus, OH 43210
CA	San Diego State University, School of Nursing, College of Human Services, San Diego, CA 92182	PA	Center for Nusing Research, University of Pennsylvania, School of Nursing, 420 Service Drive/S2, Philadelphia, PA 19104
MD	Center for Research, School of Nursing, University of Maryland, 655 West Lombard Street, Baltimore, MD 21201	TX	Center for Nursing Research, University of Texas, School of Nursing, 1700 Red River, Austin, TX 78701
MA	Studies and Research Committee, New England Deaconess Hospital, 185 Pilgrim Road, Boston, MA 02215	UT	Center for Nursing Research, University of Utah, School of Nursing, 25 S. Medical Drive, Salt Lake City, UT 84112
MI	Research Facilitation Office, 4120 School of Nursing, University of Michigan, 1335 East Catherine Street, Ann Arbor, MI 48109	VA	Office of Nursing Research, Medical College of Virginia, School of Nursing, Virginia Commonwealth University, Box 567, Richmond, VA 23298
MI	Center for Health Research, Wayne State University, School of Nursing, 315 Cohn Building, Detroit, MI 48202	WI	Center for Health Sciences, University of Wisconsin-Madison, School of Nursing, 600 Highland Avenue, Madison, WI 53792
MN	Center for Nursing Research, University of Minnesota, School of Nursing, 500 Essex Street SE, Minneapolis, MN 55455		

*From Reflections, Indianapolis, Ind., May-June, 1981, Sigma Theta Tau, p. 3.

nursing. It is the combination of this knowledge base, clinical skills, holistic viewpoint, and behavioral focus that makes the psychiatric nurse's contribution a valuable and unique one.

The development of conceptual models by nursing leaders further attests to the validity of viewing nursing as a unique profession. These theoretical models contribute to the knowledge base of nursing education, the framework for nursing practice, and the direction for nursing research. Over 50% of federally supported nursing research projects deal with investigations into nursing practice, and the development of doctoral programs in nursing suggests that "the science of nursing is coming of age."[4] The momentum in nursing research is steadily increasing, as is evident in the development of programs for the preparation of nurse scientists (Table 1-5); increasing support of federal and interstate agencies; increased acceptance of long-term, research-oriented goals toward enlarging nursing's body of knowledge; development of centers for research (Table 1-6); a rise in the number of consortia and collaborative efforts; change in the nature and number of avenues for reporting research (Table 1-7); and changes in the direction of research from a limited number of studies on curricula, administration, and personal attributes of nurses to more extensive clinical studies that apply the new nursing science to practice.

TABLE 1-7. Overview of contemporary nursing journals published in the United States (1900-1980)*

Journal title	Year of first issue					
	1900-1915	1916-1931	1932-1947	1948-1963	1964-1979	1980-1995
Am. J. Nurs.	●					
Nurs. Outlook	●					
R. N.			●			
Briefs			●			
A.A.N.A.J.			●			
Nurses' Lamp				●		
Perspect. Psych. Care				●		
J. Psychosoc. Nurs.				●		
J. Nurs. Educ.				●		
Nurs. Forum				●		
Regan Rep. Nurs. Law				●		
A.O.R.N.J.				●		
J. Pract. Nurs.				●		
J. Nurse Midwife				●		
Imprint				●		
Occup. Health Nurs.				●		
Nurs. Res.				●		
Cardiovasc. Nurs.					●	
Nurs. Clin. North Am.					●	
Am. Nurse					●	
Image					●	
J. Nurs. Care					●	
J. Neurosurg. Nurs.					●	
J. Contin. Educ. Nurs.					●	
Superv. Nurse					●	
J. Nurs. Admin.					●	
Nursing '82					●	
Heart Lung					●	
J.O.G.N. Nurs.					●	
Matern. Child Nurs. J.					●	
Crit. Care Update					●	
J. Am. Assoc. Nephrol. Nurses Tech.					●	

*From Binger, J.: Image **13**(3):67, 1981. State nurses' association journals are not included here.

Along with these advances, however, have emerged a number of problems identified by Feldman[12]: the need for financial support often outweighs available money; as the quantity of doctoral programs have increased, the quality may have suffered; there are still too few research journals in existence and too few research papers accepted; a rush to produce research has led to inferior quality in some cases; many nurses do not appreciate research, are unable to interpret research findings, and do not use them in practice; and some nurses do not participate in research because they view it as costly, time consuming, and demanding in preparation or because they have poor self-images and are reluctant to ask for help and expose themselves to possible criticism. Rather than simply identifying problems, Feldman[12] offers possible solutions to enhance nursing's growth in this area. All of the following are applicable to psychiatric nursing:

1. *Funding.* If the nursing profession truly supports nursing science, it must contribute to nursing's evolution. Hospital nursing services, professional nursing organizations, and educational facilities should encourage research by contributing a percentage of their income to this endeavor. Also, positions should exist for nurse researchers to be hired in clinical and educational settings.

2. *Collaboration.* Collaboration takes many

TABLE 1-7. Overview of contemporary nursing journals published in the United States (1900-1980)—cont'd

Journal title	\multicolumn{6}{Year of first issue}
	1900-1915	1916-1931	1932-1947	1948-1963	1964-1979	1980-1995
A.P.N.J.					•	
J.E.N.					•	
J. Gerontol. Nurs.					•	
Nurse Pract.					•	
Pediatr. Nurs.					•	
Iss. Com. Ped. Nurs.					•	
M.C.N.					•	
Nurse Educ.					•	
Nurses Drug Alert					•	
Nurs. Adm. Q.					•	
Ad. Nurs. Sci.					•	
Cancer Nurs.					•	
Today's O.R. Nurse					•	
Crit. Care Q.					•	
Iss. Mental Health Nurs.					•	
Nurs. Lead					•	
Res. Nurs. Health					•	
Topics Clin. Nurs.					•	
West J. Nurs. Res.					•	
J. Enterostomal Ther.					•	
Oncology Nurs. Forum					•	
Nephrology Nurse					•	
School Nurse					•	
Life Support Nurse					•	
Emerg. Nurse Legal Bull.					•	
Nurs. Law Ethics						•
Geriatric Nurse						•
Nurs. Health Care						•
Nurs. Insights						•
The Dean's List						•
Modern Nurse Magazine						•
Professional Nurse						•

forms and may occur in developing research questions, designing and implementing studies, providing forums for developing theory and reporting investigative work, and establishing networks for sharing all kinds of information. Symposia must continue to increase, involving nurses at all levels, in all types of practice. A nationwide research network could be established using computers; the technology is available to set up an international network by satellite.

3. *Education*. The process of educating nurses to perform research must be stepped up to meet the demands of a developing science. This involves additional recruitment but not at the expense of quality. Doctoral programs in nursing must have a core of productive nurse scientists who can serve as role models and mentors to students in the in-depth study of specific problems. This would enhance theory development by encouraging greater concentration on concerns of highest priority. It would also involve students in the research process in such a way that their enthusiasm and creativity would be nurtured. However, doctoral preparation for research is just the beginning; postdoctoral work will enable the scientist to pursue particular areas of need and interest and to more fully develop the researcher role.

4. *Marketing*. Enhancing the usefulness of nursing research requires changing the present climate to one of increased receptivity, valuing, learning, and involvement in the process and outcomes of research studies. To accomplish this, Feldman proposes an intensive effort in "marketing" research. She describes the strategies useful in marketing products as segmenting the market, identifying common characteristics within each of the target segments, identifying the needs of those markets, and developing a marketing plan to appeal to the target markets. She then describes how this approach can be adapted to the problem of increasing receptivity to research among nursing professionals.

5. *Reporting*. Increased reporting of research in journals designed for that purpose is advocated. However, new ideas are needed about ways to communicate findings in a fashion acceptable to clinical practitioners. Additionally, prestige must be given to the replication of selected studies, and replication studies must be reported as readily as originals.

The importance of this final suggestion, reporting, should not be minimized. To attain full professional status, the body of nursing knowledge must be accepted as legitimate by other professionals, as well as by society. Many people outside of nursing and some within nursing, still have no concept of this body of knowledge nor of the unique expertise of nursing. To overcome this, psychiatric nurses need to write and publish more and in a greater variety of journals and texts, including multidisciplinary journals and consumer publications. They should also increase their visibility by attending and presenting papers at the meetings of their colleagues, including psychiatrists, psychologists, and social workers. A more assertive and self-confident public stance is both necessary and appropriate for the psychiatric nurse, since knowledge of the role of psychiatric nurses has been found to be correlated with an accepting attitude and greater utilization among other mental health professionals.[9] The gradual implementation of each of these proposed solutions by psychiatric nurses will promote the creation, organization, and transmission of the distinct body of science that is nursing.

Service orientation

There is consensus that nursing is characterized by explicit rules of competence and strong rules of loyalty or service. The rules of performance, however, pertain to self-regulation and accountability for practice that must be demonstrated individually and collectively. The mechanisms within psychiatric nursing to accomplish this include state licensure, certification, primary nursing as a mode of staffing, nursing audit, implementation of standards of practice, and peer review. Sometimes these mechanisms appear more structural than functional.

The dichotomy between nursing theory and nursing practice is not well described in the literature, but it is implied in the sometimes adversarial roles of nursing educators and administrators. Often what is learned in theory is not implemented in practice. For example, direct and indirect psychiatric nursing care functions, although impressive, are often carried out sporadically and inconsistently. One study examined what functions psychiatric nurses employed in an inpatient setting considered to be important and how well nurses were able to perform them.[33] The results indicated the following 5 as the "most important" functions of the 46 listed:

1. To assess patients' emotional needs
2. To respond to patients' crises

3. To intervene to reduce panic of disturbed patients
4. To make sure patients' rights are safeguarded
5. To assess the effect of somatic therapies on patients

Although these functions implied the use of the nursing process, the items to "develop a nursing care plan" and "implement a nursing care plan" were ranked as numbers 18 and 15, respectively. Items related to leadership functions ranked low—providing leadership was ninth, initiating improvements was eleventh, participating in policy making was twenty-fourth, and political involvement was twenty-ninth. Psychotherapy activities were numbered 34, 36, and 38, and research activities were 32, 41, and 46. The ability ratings corresponded closely with the importance ratings. The same questionnaire was given to a group of psychiatrists and psychologists. Significantly, they gave a low ranking compared to that of the nurses to ability to assess emotional needs and develop and implement a nursing care plan, despite the importance they placed on those items. This study raises many questions about the role of the nurse and the contrast between theory and practice.

Traditionally, one response to this perceived dichotomy was an attempt to place blame on either the "ivory-towered" educators, the "non-supportive" nurse administrators, or the "impersonal" hospital organization. However, this type of response is characterized by a passivity and a noticeable lack of accountability. What is needed at present is for psychiatric nurses to assume an active posture of accountability to oneself, one's patients, one's colleagues, one's profession, the public, and nurse administrators.

Accountability means to be answerable to someone for something. It focuses responsibility on the individual nurse for her actions, or perhaps, lack of actions:

Organized nursing services and the professional association carry the leadership responsibility for development, implementation, and evaluation of nursing care systems which assure relevant, high quality nursing to consumers. Individual nurses have primary responsibility and accountability for their own practice, and thus activities to monitor and improve the quality of nursing care form an intrinsic part of the individual's practice.

In the field of psychiatric and mental health nursing, nurses have a particular obligation to define, supervise, and evaluate nursing care. Nursing standards provide authoritative measures for determining the quality of nursing care a client receives, whether services are provided solely by a professional nurse or by a professional nurse and nursing assistants.[2:2]

Accountability includes formal review processes and requirements, but also an attitude of integrity and vigilence—"a quality of the heart and mind of those professionals who are competent and determined that every psychiatric patient will have the best problem-resolving assistance possible."[32]

Autonomy

Autonomy implies self-determination, independence, shared power, and authority and professionals are not likely to achieve it without having met the previous characteristics of professionalization. It is the socially sanctioned condition that allows for the definition and control over a work domain, achieved through a negotiated process. For psychiatric nursing, attaining autonomy means being able to define the domain of nursing and being able to exercise control over psychiatric nursing practice. This idea of shaping destiny, rather than letting outside forces be in control, is the crux of power viewed as a positive force and strength or the capacity to attain goals. Power can be viewed as both a means to an end and a product, the instrument used to attain full professional status and the outcome of achieving professionalization. It involves a conscious decision to identify goals, plan strategy, assume responsibility, exercise authority, and be held accountable.

Autonomy, at an individual level of analysis, has two major and interrelated components. The first is control over nursing tasks, which means the following:

1. Having the opportunity for independent thought and action
2. Having appropriate utilization of one's time, skills, and ability by being able to eliminate, refuse, and delegate nonnursing tasks
3. Having the authority and responsibility necessary for implementing goals related to quality nursing care
4. Being able to initiate changes and innovations in one's practice

The second component of autonomy is that of decision making. It requires the nurse's participation in the following:

1. Determining and implementing standards of quality nursing care

2. Decisions affecting one's nursing job context, including salary, staffing, and professional growth
3. Institutional policies, procedures, and goals

This characteristic of autonomy is particularly problematic for nursing. Most nurses are employed in hospitals in which authority rests primarily with administrators, physicians, and trustees.[36] Furthermore, nurses are frequently expected to do tasks they are overqualified to do, such as housekeeping, dietary, and clerical duties. This results in the underutilization of their many important skills. Nurses are thus caught in the crosswind. They staff the units around the clock, make important clinical decisions, and shoulder major responsibility for coordinating and managing the patient care units; but they lack legitimate decision-making authority as to the allocation of hospital resources. Because nurses are not compensated on a fee-for-service basis, they are not viewed as a source of revenue by hospital administrators and therefore lack a most critical base for power. It is not surprising that if nurses do not have a role in hospital decision making, then they will have only a limited ability to exercise control of their practice. Preliminary recommendations from one national study of nursing, the National Commission on Nursing sponsored by the American Hospital Association, reflects this problem and calls for increased decision-making authority for nurses and collaborative relationships with physicians in providing care.

Nurses should not expect, however, that autonomy and power will be given to them. It is obtained in a negotiated process with other health professionals, consumers, and society at large. It requires increased access to concrete resources, demonstration of expertise, and acknowledgment by other professionals, which is evidenced in interdependent collaboration. Nurses are not yet fully accepted as professionals by other disciplines and often do not function at their full potential. Yet psychiatric nursing is practiced largely in collaboration, coordination, and cooperation with a variety of other professions working with and on behalf of the patient. Nurses will progress in this area as they are able to dialogue with other professionals and as their clinical skills demand recognition and respect. As nurses view themselves in a positive way, they will increase their ability to assert themselves and function effectively.

Benfer[5] has some specific suggestions in this regard. She believes that psychiatric nurses must first assess patients based on their own conceptualization of the patient's emotional difficulties, rather than first checking with the psychiatrist or other team members for their conceptualization. When the nurse has completed her assessment, she must then be able to articulate that information both orally and in writing. This requires an assertiveness in putting forth ideas, observations, and beliefs about treatment, because unless psychiatric nurses define their own role, others will define it for them. Benfer does not believe nurses have done very well in explaining their framework for practice and communicating to other mental health team members what the nursing process is and how it is utilized. Nurses also have a team teaching function to share their knowledge, experience, and perceptions with other team members so that the result is more skilled practitioners. Although nurses have often taught interns and residents, this teaching has seldom been given adequate recognition and importance. Furthermore, some nurses may feel threatened at the thought of teaching other professionals. However, teaching and learning are continuous experiences in life, and nurses have a contribution to make in this area. Finally, for interdisciplinary teams to function well, the members must view themselves as equals. Benfer believes that this is one of the most elusive and difficult issues affecting nurses who must be helped to strengthen their self-concepts by identifying their expertise and the ways in which they can contribute to the common purpose of the team.

Thus, the movement toward professionalization contains complex issues for all psychiatric nurses. Many of these issues are interwoven and all of them are familiar, since they have been repeatedly addressed by nurses over many decades. The prize is professional autonomy, but its attainment, at present, remains a question.

Suggested cross-references

Therapeutic relationship skills, including ethical dimensions of nursing practice, are discussed in Chapter 3. A model of health-illness phenomena and the phases of the nursing process are discussed in Chapter 4. Legal aspects of nursing practice are discussed in Chapter 10. Roles and functions of psychiatric nurses in specific practice settings are discussed in Part two. Issues and future trends in psychiatric nursing practice are discussed in Chapter 34.

SUMMARY

1. Nursing began to emerge as a profession in the nineteenth century. Linda Richards was the first American psychiatric nurse, and the first school for psychiatric nurses opened in 1882. It was not until the late 1930s that nursing education viewed the importance of psychiatric knowledge in general nursing care related to all illnesses. The National Mental Health Act of 1946 provided funds for nursing education. The Brown Report of 1948 recommended the elimination of basic schools of nursing in mental hospitals, and in 1950 the National League for Nursing required that a school had to provide an experience in psychiatric nursing to be accredited.

2. The late 1940s and early 1950s saw nurses struggling to define their roles as psychiatric nurses. The issue of nurses conducting psychotherapy was controversial. A critical development within the profession occurred with the publication of Peplau's book in 1952 in which she presented a theoretical framework for psychiatric nursing. Nursing was influenced by the development of somatic therapies in the mid 1930s, the concept of the therapeutic community in 1953, and effective psychotropic drugs in the early 1950s. By 1962 psychiatric nursing had evolved a role of clinical competence based on interpersonal techniques and use of the nursing process. Counseling was a primary nursing function.

3. The Community Mental Health Centers Act of 1963 influenced the movement of the practice of psychiatric nursing into the community and the formation of multidisciplinary treatment teams. Other influences included the 1978 President's Commission on Mental Health, the Mental Health Systems Act of 1980, and the present environment of fiscal restraint, retrenchment, and budgetary cuts.

4. Psychiatric nursing was defined as an interpersonal process that strives to promote and maintain behavior which contributes to integrated functioning. The patient or client system may be an individual, family, group, organization, or community. It may be practiced in a variety of settings. Various direct and indirect nursing functions were described based on the model of primary, secondary, and tertiary prevention.

5. Four major factors that help to determine the level of functions and types of activities a nurse engages in are the law; qualifications, including education, work experiences, and certification status; practice setting, including team relationships; and personal competence and initiative.

6. The Standards of Psychiatric–Mental Health Nursing Practice as identified by the American Nurses' Association were presented.

7. The question of whether psychiatric nurses are truly professionalized was addressed. The following problematic areas were explored:

  a. Organization, including lack of support for the American Nurses' Association, disagreement over tasks and roles, questions related to collective bargaining issues, need for a clearer conception of leadership capabilities, and greater involvement in political processes.

  b. Education, specifically the need for a well-defined body of nursing knowledge, problems and advances in nursing research, and the need for greater visibility of psychiatric nurses through publishing and presentations.

  c. Service orientation, focusing on the issues of self-regulation, accountability, and the theory-practice dichotomy.

  d. Autonomy, with its elements of self-determination, power, authority, and status as evidenced in control over nursing tasks and involvement in decision making in nursing care, job context, and institutional policies and goals.

References

1. American Nurses' Association: Educational preparation for nurse practitioners and assistants to nurses: a position paper, New York, 1965, The Association.
2. American Nurses' Association, Division on Psychiatric and Mental Health Nursing Practice: Statement on psychiatric and mental health nursing practice, Kansas City, Mo., 1976, The Association.
3. American Nurses' Association: Nursing: a social policy statement, Kansas City, Mo., 1980, The Association.
4. Andreoli, K., and Thompson, C.: The nature of science in nursing, Image 9(2):37, 1977.
5. Benfer, B.: Defining the role and function of the psychiatric nurse as a member of the team, Perspect. Psychiatr. Care 18(4):166, 1980.
6. Bennett, A., and Eaton, J.: The role of the psychiatric nurse in the newer therapies, Am. J. Psychiatry 108:167, Sept. 1951.
7. Brown, E.: Nursing for the future, New York, 1948, Russell Sage Foundation.
8. Cleland, V.: The supervisor in collective bargaining, J. Nurs. Adm. 4(4):33, 1974.
9. Davidson, K., et al.: A descriptive study of the attitudes of psychiatrists toward the new role of the nurse therapist, J. Psychiatr. Nurs. 16(11):24, 1978.
10. Dumas, R.: Expanding the theoretical framework for effective nursing, Nurs. Clin. North Am. 13(4):707, 1978.
11. Editorial, Am. J. Nurs. 40:23, 1940.

12. Feldman, H.: Nursing research in the 1980's: issues and implications, Adv. Nurs. Sci. 3(1):85, 1980.

13. Gardner, K.: Levels of psychiatric nursing practice in an ambulatory setting, J. Psychiatr. Nurs. 15:26, Sept. 1977.

14. Given, B., and Simmons, S.: The interdisciplinary health-care team: fact or fiction? Nurs. Forum 16(2): 165, 1977.

15. Gregg, D.: The psychiatric nurse's role, Am. J. Nurs. 54:848, 1954.

16. Hays, D.: Suggested clinical practice of psychiatric nurses recorded in the literature between 1946 and 1958. In Psychiatric nursing 1946 to 1974: a report on the state of the art, New York, 1975, American Journal of Nursing Co.

17. Jones, M.: The therapeutic community: a new treatment method in psychiatry, New York, 1953, Basic Books, Inc.

18. Lego, S.: Nurse psychotherapists: how are we different? Perspect. Psychiatr. Care 11(4):144, 1973.

19. Leib, A., Underwood, P., and Glick, I.: The staff nurse as primary therapist: a pilot study, J. Psychiatr. Nurs. 14:11, Oct. 1976.

20. Maloney, E.: Does the psychiatric nurse have independent functions? Am. J. Nurs. 62:61, June 1962.

21. Maslow, A.: Motivation and personality, New York, 1954, Harper & Row, Publishers, Inc.

22. Mauksch, I.G., and Miller, M.H.: Implementing change in nursing, St. Louis, 1981, The C.V. Mosby Co.

23. Mellow, J.: Nursing therapy, Am. J. Nurs. 68:2365, 1968.

24. Merton, R.: The social nature of leadership, Am. J. Nurs. 69:2614, Dec. 1969.

25. Mlott, S.: Personality correlates of a psychiatric nurse, J. Psychiatr. Nurs. 14(2):19, 1976.

26. Moore, W.: The professions: roles and rules, New York, 1974, Russell Sage Foundation.

27. Moscato, B.: The traditional nurse-physician relationship. In Kneisl, C.R., and Wilson, H.S., editors: Current perspectives in psychiatric nursing, vol. 1, St. Louis, 1976, The C.V. Mosby Co.

28. Noyes, A.: Nursing needs in the state mental hospitals, Am. J. Nurs. 33:787, 1933.

29. Peplau, H.: Interpersonal relations in nursing, New York, 1952, G.P. Putnam's Sons.

30. Peplau, H.: Historical development of psychiatric nursing. A preliminary statement of some facts and trends, 1956. (Mimeographed.)

31. Peplau, H.: Interpersonal techniques: the crux of psychiatric nursing, Am. J. Nurs. 62:53, June 1962.

32. Peplau, H.: The psychiatric nurse—accountable? To whom? For what? Perspect. Psychiatr. Care 18(3):128, 1980.

33. Plutchik, R., Conte, H., Wells, W., and Karasu, T.: Role of the psychiatric nurse, J. Psychiatr. Nurs. 14(9):38, 1976.

34. Powers, M.: Universal utility of psychoanalytic theory for nursing practice models, J. Psychiatr. Nurs. 18(4): 28, 1980.

35. Report to the president from the President's Commission on Mental Health, vol. 1, Washington, D.C., 1978, U.S. Government Printing Office.

36. Roemer, M., and Friedman, J.: Doctors in hospitals: medical staff organization and hospital performance, Baltimore, 1971, The Johns Hopkins University Press.

37. Santos, E., and Stainbrook, E.: Nursing and modern psychiatry, Am. J. Nurs. 49:107, 1949.

38. Sloboda, S.: What are mental health nurses doing? J. Psychiatr. Nurs. 14:24, 1976.

39. Smoyak, S.: The confrontation process, Am. J. Nurs. 74(9):1632, 1974.

40. Stuart, G.: How professionalized is nursing? Image 13(1):18, 1981.

41. Sundeen, S.J., et al.: Nurse-client interaction: implementing the nursing process, ed. 2, St. Louis, 1981, The C.V. Mosby Co.

42. Tudor, G.: Sociopsychiatric nursing approach to intervention in a problem of mutual withdrawal on a mental hospital ward, Psychiatry 15(2):193, 1952.

43. Unschuld, P.: Medico-cultural conflicts in Asian settings: an exploratory theory, Soc. Sci. Med. 9:304, 1975.

44. Weiss, M.O.: The skills of psychiatric nursing, Am. J. Nurs. 47:174, 1947.

Annotated suggested readings

Aiken, L., editor: Health policy and nursing practice, New York, 1980, McGraw-Hill, Inc.

This multiauthored text traces the evolution of nursing practice from traditional to new, innovative roles. It suggests directions for nursing practice within a complex health care delivery system.

American Nurses' Association, Division on Psychiatric and Mental Health Nursing Practice: Standards of psychiatric and mental health nursing practice, Kansas City, Mo., 1982, The Association.

In this publication the ANA presents the standards of psychiatric nursing, each of which is accompanied by a rationale and structure, process, and outcome criteria. The criteria provide a means by which attainment of the standards may be specifically measured.

American Nurses' Association, Division on Psychiatric and Mental Health Nursing Practice: Statement on psychiatric and mental health nursing practice, Kansas City, Mo., 1976, The Association.

This is the official statement of the American Nurses' Association, which includes a definition and description of setting, types of practitioners, and list of functions. This pamphlet is a resource for all psychiatric nurses.

American Nurses' Association: Power: nursing's challenge for change, Kansas City, Mo., 1979, The Association.

This is a compilation of 20 papers exploring the many areas in which nursing is attempting to acquire and use power to initiate necessary changes in the health care delivery system.

Berger, M.S. et al.: Management for nurses, ed. 2, St. Louis, 1980, The C.V. Mosby Co.

The concepts of leadership and management are the focus of this excellent text. It is a compilation of thought-provoking articles on structural, personnel, and economic factors and their influence on organization functioning. Worthwhile reading for all nurses.

Ducanis, A., and Golin, A.: The interdisciplinary health care team, Germantown, Md., 1980, Aspen Systems Corp.

Research findings and theoretical concepts are incorporated in this book on interdisciplinary health care team functioning. It should prove helpful reading to both practicing and student nurses.

Ehrenwald, J., editor: History of psychotherapy, New York, 1976, Jason Aronson, Inc.

This text reviews the history of psychiatry and the wide variety of approaches to psychotherapy from the mystical to the scientific and from the early influential thinkers to contemporary schools of thought. It is enjoyable reading and is especially recommended for its thoroughness.

Fagin, C.: Psychiatric nursing at the crossroads; quo vadis? Perspect. Psychiatr. Care **19**(3-4):99, 1981.

The author discusses two phases in the development of psychiatric nursing. The first phase is prior to 1952 when psychiatric nursing acquired recognition as a specialty in nursing and a second phase, beginning now, which establishes future directions for psychiatric nursing.

Fagin, C.: Nursing as an alternative to high-cost care, Am. J. Nurs. **82**:56, Jan. 1982.

This address summarizes available research that supports nursing effectiveness and economic viability. Competition and substitution are the key concepts in Fagin's position. A notable need that emerges from this paper is to document the effectiveness and costs of psychiatric nursing care. One might consider this paper as a mandate for action by all nurses.

Given, B., and Simmons, S.: The interdisciplinary health-care team: fact or fiction? Nurs. Forum **16**(2):165, 1977.

An overview of interdisciplinary teams is presented in this article, including discussion of barriers to formation and elements vital to functioning. This is the type of article that should be shared across disciplines.

Greenleaf, N., editor: The politics of self-esteem, Nurs. Digest **6**:1, Fall, 1978.

This is a compilation of 13 articles and an annotated bibliography that focus on the politics and self-esteem of women, particularly nurses. They explore the issues of biology, work, and the psychology of sex roles and suggest some strategies for change. This is important reading for all nurses.

Hamilton, P.A.: Health care consumerism, St. Louis, 1982, The C.V. Mosby Co.

The author, a nurse, demonstrates the depth and breadth of what consumers are saying and feeling about health care in America. Both providers and consumers of health care can benefit from reading this book, which covers the issues of the consumer's role, cost, quality, rights, and ethics in the health care domain. It is not specific to psychiatric care, but provides valuable basic background.

Hardy, M., and Conway, M.: Role theory: perspectives for health professionals, New York, 1978, Appleton-Century-Crofts.

This collection of articles integrates principles of role theory and research and presents a framework from which one can determine role identity and related stressors. Its scholarly approach and thorough bibliography make it a useful reference for advanced study on roles.

Kolin, P.C., and Kolin, J.L.: Professional writing for nurses in education, practice, and research, St. Louis, 1980, The C.V. Mosby Co.

The ability to communicate well in writing is a prime requisite for nurses. This book addresses the wide range of written communication used by nurses from patient records to writing for publication. A good resource text.

Lancaster, J., and Lancaster, W.: Concepts for advanced nursing practice: the nurse as change agent, St. Louis, 1982, The C.V. Mosby Co.

This book identifies, describes, and provides practical ways for dealing with key issues currently facing nursing. It is a collection of articles divided into three major sections, all of which serve to conceptualize the role of the nurse as an agent of change.

Lego, S.: The one-to-one nurse patient relationship. In Psychiatric nursing 1946 to 1974: a report on the state of the art, New York, 1975, The American Journal of Nursing Co.

The author discusses the history and trends, assesses published research, and summarizes patterns in the literature that have reflected and promoted one-to-one psychiatric nursing. The bibliography is quite extensive, and this is an excellent resource article.

Leininger, M., editor: Contemporary issues in mental health nursing, Boston, 1973, Little, Brown & Co.

This is an outstanding book with articles contributed by various nursing leaders. It explores issues in psychiatric nursing related to sociology, anthropology, physiology, clinical practice, historical developments, education, and humanism. It is highly recommended as a resource text.

Lysaught, J.: Action in affirmation toward an unambiguous profession of nursing, New York, 1980, McGraw-Hill, Inc.

This is a follow-up study of the 1970 recommendations of the National Commission for the Study of Nursing and Nursing Education. It is a status report on the pursuit of the goal of nursing as an "unambiguous" profession.

Mauksch, I.G., and Miller, M.H.: Implementing change in nursing, St. Louis, 1981, The C.V. Mosby Co.

This is a valuable resource to all nurses who view their role as change agents. The text covers the nature of change, the nurse's role in change, strategies for implementing it, and ways to make successful change permanent. Valuable learning here for all nurses.

Milio, N.: Promoting health through public policy, Philadelphia, 1981, F.A. Davis Co.

This useful text describes how public policy evolves and its consequences for the health of Americans. The documentation throughout is excellent, and its depth and substance make this a valuable book for all nurses to read.

Moscato, B.: The traditional nurse-physician relationship. In Kneisl, C.R., and Wilson, H.S., editors: Current perspectives in psychiatric nursing, vol. 1, St. Louis, 1976, The C.V. Mosby Co.

The author examines sex-role stereotyping as one element inherent in the traditional nurse-physician relationship. She uses a transactional analysis framework to identify limitations in this relationship and suggests supervision, support, and self-exploration to expand nursing roles beyond tradition.

Peplau, H.: Interpersonal relations in nursing, New York, 1952, G.P. Putnam's Sons.

This book presents the first theoretical framework for the practice of psychiatric nursing. It describes phases and roles in psychiatric nursing, psychological tasks, influences in nursing situations, and methods for studying nursing as an interpersonal process. It had a major impact on psychiatric nursing and is a "classic" in nursing literature.

President's Commission on Mental Health: Report to the president, vol. 1, Washington, D.C., 1978, U.S. Government Printing Office.

This is a government report of a 1-year study commissioned by President Carter to review the mental health needs of the nation. It was completed in April 1978, and volume 1 contains recommendations to the president on how the nation might best meet those needs.

Robitscher, J.: The powers of psychiatry, New York, 1980, Houghton Mifflin Co.

This is a provocative critique of the shortcomings in the field of psychiatry. It expands one's frame of reference regarding psychiatry and poses problems of accountability that all mental health professions need to evaluate.

Sexton, D.: Developing skills in grant writing, Nurs. Outlook **30**(1):31, 1982.

Grant writing is emerging as an essential skill that should be included in nursing curricula. This concise article outlines an approach that will facilitate the preparation and submission of grant proposals. Highly recommended.

Sills, G.: Research in the field of psychiatric nursing 1952-1977, Nurs. Res. **26**:201, 1977.

This review and assessment of research in the area of psychiatric nursing discusses guiding assumptions that have provided the direction for research in the field, a chronological view of the research with comments on the methods of the times, and a discussion of trends and future directions. It is a recommended resource for both its scope and depth in reviewing the field.

CHAPTER 2

CONCEPTUAL MODELS OF PSYCHIATRIC CARE

Though this be madness, yet there is method in't.

William Shakespeare, Hamlet. Act II

Learning objectives

After studying this chapter, the student should be able to:

- *discuss the concepts of mental health and mental illness.*

- *describe the purpose of using a conceptual model as a framework for professional practice.*

- *compare and contrast eight models of mental health care: psychoanalytical, interpersonal, social, existential, communication, behavioral, medical, and nursing.*

- *identify major theorists associated with each model.*

- *describe the roles of the therapist and the patient within the context of each model.*

- *analyze the therapeutic process as it is experienced within each of the models.*

- *critique the advantages and disadvantages of the various models.*

- *compare and contrast the nursing diagnosis and the medical diagnosis.*

- *identify suggested readings for future study.*

Most people believe that they can recognize normal and abnormal behavior in themselves and their associates. In fact, this is true to an extent. Although a person may be unwilling or unable to admit to a serious disturbance of feelings or behavior, most are aware of feeling "nervous" or "irritable" or "depressed" from time to time. This awareness results from a comparison of present behavior to an internalized norm or behavioral self-expectation. Mild or transient disruptions in behavior or feelings are usually experienced as anxiety and resolved by the utilization of coping mechanisms. Each person learns a repertoire of these adaptive mechanisms as he moves through the developmental process. Some are consciously recognized and selected, as when an angry person goes for a walk to "cool down" before confronting the object of the anger. Others are unconscious and take place without the person's awareness. An example of this is the displacement of anger to a spouse when the person is really angry at a supervisor at work. A more complete discussion of conscious and unconscious means of coping with anxiety will be found in Chapter 7.

Personal coping mechanisms are not always adequate to control anxiety. When the person is unable to cope alone, he faces the difficult decision to seek help from another person. The helping person may be a friend or relative, a nonprofessional counselor, or a mental health professional. The choice may depend on the severity of the problem. A young girl wondering how to act on her first date may discuss her concerns with her mother, her older sister, her best friend, or her favorite teacher as she tries to learn new ways to cope with an unfamiliar situation. On the other hand, a woman who is so frightened of crowds that she refuses to leave her house needs to seek help from a professional therapist. Frequently, significant others are instrumental in assisting the troubled person to identify what type of help to consider. Seriously disturbed people may not recognize their need for help. Others may be frightened of the need to see a psychiatrist or other health professional or may think that they will be labeled as "crazy." These people need encouragement and support to reach out for help.

Normalcy may be defined on the basis of the individual's own feelings of anxiety or discomfort. It may also be defined based on the cultural mores, norms, and value system in the society of which the individual is a member. Observable behavior that deviates from the norm may be labeled as deviant or sick, and social pressure may be applied to convince the individual to seek help. In this case, "help" implies the modification of behavior in the direction of compliance with social norms. Clinical example 2-1 gives a brief definition of normal behavior.

CLINICAL EXAMPLE 2-1

Early in the fall semester a black male exchange student from Africa was brought to the psychiatric emergency room. He had been walking around the campus carrying a spear and had been apprehended by the university security patrol. His speech was heavily accented and they could not understand his explanation of his behavior. Later evaluation revealed that in his culture one never went walking at night without a spear to defend against attack by wild beasts or hostile neighboring tribes. He was sent back to his dormitory after being convinced that his spear was not appropriate to the culture of the American college campus.

Behavior may also be defined as normal or deviant for political reasons. Thomas Szasz[17] is a theorist who believes that certain types of behavior are labeled "crazy" for the convenience of society and the political system, even though the behavior may be acceptable to the person involved. According to this frame of reference, the institutionalization of a woman who had been walking nude through her neighborhood could be interpreted as the political system's response to the discomfort of the neighbors. In the Soviet political system, citizens who criticize the government may be labeled mentally ill and hospitalized. In the view of the leadership, such behavior is definitely deviant.

These examples demonstrate that the definition of normal behavior is in no way simple or obvious. Does normality mean conformity? Does it mean an ability to control anxiety? Does it mean acceptability to significant others? Depending on one's frame of reference, it could mean any, all, or none of these. Perhaps the most generally accepted definition of normal behavior at the present time is that the individual is able to function adequately in activities of daily living and to feel reasonably satisfied with his life-style. This is far from precise, but human behavior covers such a range that an exact description of normal behavior is probably impossible. Behavior must be viewed on a continuum with a wide variation of what is accepted as normal. If this is not the case, individual behavior could be unreasonably restricted with resulting limitations on creativity and personal growth. Mental health nurses can often be most helpful by trying to understand the patient's view of his behavior and assisting him to change behaviors that he has defined as unsatisfactory.

Most mental health professionals practice within the framework of a conceptual model. A model is a means of organizing a complex body of knowledge, such as concepts related to human behavior. Utilization of a model assists the practitioner to function rationally and allows for evaluation of the individual's effectiveness as a therapist. Organization of data also facilitates much needed research into human behavior.

At the present time scientific knowledge of behavior is limited. Therefore it is difficult to view any particular conceptual model as right or wrong. Unfortunately, adherents of one model or another do, at times, become embroiled in conflicts about which framework is most accurate. In reality, the only measure of the value of any approach to mental health care is the satisfaction of the person who receives the care. It has not been proved whether the patient's response to care results from the theoretical model utilized or from the relationship with the therapist, irrespective of the model.

In the remainder of this chapter, an overview will be presented of several conceptual models that are commonly utilized by contemporary mental health professionals. The models to be discussed include psychoanalytical, interpersonal, social, existential, communication, behavioral, medical, and nursing models. Information to be discussed relative to each model is the definition of behavioral deviations, the therapy process, the role of the patient, the role of the therapist, and identification of representative theorists. Since it is impossible to provide a thorough exploration of even one of these complex theories in a single chapter, the reader is referred to the annotated suggested readings, which include several basic references for each theoretical framework.

Psychoanalytical model

Psychoanalytical theory was first conceptualized by Sigmund Freud in the late nineteenth and early twentieth centuries. It not only encompassed the nature of deviant behavior but also proposed an entirely new perspective on human development. Many of Freud's ideas were controversial, particularly in the Victorian society into which they were introduced. Sexuality was a central concept in his developmental theory. The emotional response to the assertion that children are sexual beings for a time overshadowed the broader implications of Freudian theory. The effort to observe human behavior objectively was a great contribution of the early psychoanalysts, as was the identification of a mental structure. Such concepts as id, ego, and superego and the ego defense mechanisms are still widely accepted and utilized by many therapists. Most people readily accept the existence of an unconscious level of mental functioning. Due to limitations of space, the psychoanalytical theory of psychosexual development will not be presented here. The focus will be on the analytical method of intervening in deviant behavior, realizing that this must be based on an understanding of the norm. Readers interested in exploring psychoanalytical theories of psychosocial development are referred to the works of Freud and Erik Erikson, a contemporary psychoanalytical theorist and to the discussion in Chapter 26.

Psychoanalytical view of behavioral deviations

Psychoanalysts trace disrupted behavior in the adult back to earlier developmental stages. At each stage of development, there is a task to be accomplished. For instance, the child at the anal stage must learn to accept limits on his behavior and become more independent. If there is undue emphasis on any stage or unusual difficulty in dealing with the associated conflicts, there is a fixation of psychological energy (libido) at that point in an attempt to deal with anxiety. This leaves less libido available to the ego for other tasks, since energy is utilized to maintain repression of early conflicts. At times of stress, when the anxiety level rises, the individual may regress behaviorally to the level of the fixation, utilizing the defenses which were effective at that time. Unfortunately, these are childhood defenses that may not be appropriate to the adult situation. However, since the childhood conflict was not resolved, the adult is not free to implement mature problem-solving techniques.

For example, a young woman was never able to resolve her competitive feelings toward her mother for her father's attention. She repressed this conflict from the phallic stage of development. In addition, she projected her feelings of jealousy and anger to her mother and was never able to relate to her openly. As she reached maturity, she was never able to develop close relationships with other women. She suspected that they were always competing with her for the attention of males. At the same time, her relationships with men were dependent and childlike with constant demands that they prove their devotion to her. Basically, she was lonely and unhappy.

According to psychoanalysts, neurotic symptoms arise when so much energy must be invested to control anxiety that there is serious interference with functional ability. Incidentally, everyone is neurotic to some extent according to this conceptual model. Everyone carries the burden of childhood conflicts and is influenced in adulthood by childhood experiences. For this reason, psychoanalysts in training must undergo a personal analysis so that their neurotic behavior will not hinder their objectivity as therapists.

Symptoms are representative in a symbolic way of the original conflict. For instance, compulsive hand washing may represent the individual's attempt to cleanse himself of impulses that were labeled as unclean by the mothering person during the anal stage of development. This characteristic of a neurotic symptom occurs through the utilization by the ego of the mechanisms of condensation and displacement. Thus the meaning of the behavior is hidden from the conscious awareness of the individual, who is usually upset about these uncontrollable thoughts, actions, and feelings.

Freud developed most of his theories around neurotic symptoms. His theory is less well formulated in the area of psychosis, and it was found that people with psychotic behavior were not responsive to classical psychoanalytical therapy. This position has in more recent times been modified by psychoanalytical theorists such as Harold Searles and Frieda Fromm-Reichmann who have had success in working with psychotic patients. In essence, the psychotic symptom is seen as occurring when the ego must invest most or all of the libido at hand in an effort to defend against primitive id impulses. This leaves little, if any, energy to deal with external reality. This leads to the use of symbolization and the lack of reality testing ability seen in psychosis.

Psychoanalytical process

Psychoanalysis as developed by Freud utilizes the methods of free association and dream analysis to effect reconstruction of the personality. Free association refers to the verbalization of thoughts as they occur without any conscious screening or censorship. Of course, there is always unconscious censorship of thoughts and impulses that are threatening to the ego. The psychoanalyst searches for patterns in the material that is verbalized and in the areas which are unconsciously avoided. The latter areas are identified by comparison to the therapist's knowledge of basic themes of human conflict. Conflictual areas that are not discussed or recognized by the patient are identified as resistances. Additional insight into the nature of the resistances can be derived from the analysis of the patient's dreams, which symbolically communicate areas of intrapsychic conflict.

The therapist attempts to assist the patient to recognize intrapsychic conflicts through the use of interpretation. Interpretation involves explaining to the patient the meaning of dream symbolism and the significance of the issues that are discussed or avoided. The process is complicated by the inevitable occurrence of transference. This refers to the patient's development of strong positive or negative feelings toward the analyst. These feelings are unrelated to the present behavior or characteristics of the analyst. They represent the patient's past response to a significant other, usually a parent. The therapist's reciprocal response to the patient is called countertransference. The transference provides the motivation for a patient to work in therapy. Strong positive transference causes the patient to want to please the therapist and to accept interpretations of his behavior. Strong negative transference may impede the progress of therapy as the patient actively resists the therapist's interventions. Countertransference can also interfere with therapy if the analyst is unaware of it or unable to deal with it.

Since the therapist can temporarily replace the significant other of the patient's early life experience, previously unresolved conflicts can be brought into the therapeutic situation and worked through to a healthier resolution. This releases previously cathected (invested) libido for mature adult functioning. The person is able to conduct his life according to an accurate assessment of external reality and is also able to relate to others uninhibited by neurotic conflicts. Psychoanalytical therapy is a long-term proposition. The patient is seen frequently, usually five times a week and usually over a period of several years. It is therefore time consuming and expensive.

Roles of the patient and the psychoanalyst

The respective roles of the patient and the psychoanalyst were explicitly defined by Freud. The patient was to be an active participant, freely revealing all thoughts exactly as they occurred and describing all dreams. The analytical patient frequently is in a recumbent position during therapy to induce relaxation, which facilitates free association. This also places the patient in a vulnerable position vis-a-vis the therapist, helping to recreate the childhood situation.

The psychoanalyst is a shadow person. Whereas the patient is expected to reveal all his thoughts and feelings, the analyst reveals nothing personal. This is to allow the transference to develop uncontaminated by the reality of the therapist as a person. The analyst usually conducts the therapeutic session outside of the direct line of vision of the patient, so that nonverbal responses do not influence the patient's verbalizations. Verbal responses are noncommittal for the most part and brief so as not to interfere with the associative flow. For instance, the analyst might respond with "Uh huh," "Go on," or "Tell me more." The therapist departs from this communication style when an interpretation of behavior is made. Interpretations are presented for the patient to accept or reject, but rejections are attributed to the operation of resistance. Likewise, any frustration that the patient expresses toward the analyst is interpreted as part of the transference. All the patient's behavior can be defined within the context of the psychoanalytical therapy model. By termination of therapy, the patient should be able to view the analyst realistically as another adult, having worked through his conflicts and dependency needs.

Other psychoanalytical theorists

Much of Freud's basic theory is still utilized by psychotherapists. The theorists who followed him have modified and built on the original psychoanalytical theories. Even some of Freud's contemporaries who later severed relationships with him reveal the basic influence of psychoanalytical theory in their own work. Most prominent among those who left Freud to form their own schools are C.G. Jung, who developed the idea of the "collective unconscious," and Alfred Adler, who evolved the concept of the "inferiority complex."

Several contemporary theorists who are viewed to be psychoanalytical in orientation are listed below with a brief statement identifying their major contribution or area of study:

■ Erik Erikson—expanded Freud's theory of psychosocial development to encompass the entire life cycle; identified an epigenetic progression of developmental tasks; described behavioral disturbances resulting from failure to accomplish developmental tasks
■ Anna Freud—expanded psychoanalytical theory in the area of child psychology; further developed the concept of the mechanisms of defense
■ Melanie Klein—extended use of psychoanalytical techniques to work with young children through development of play therapy
■ Karen Horney—focused on psychoanalytical theory relative to neurotic behavior; related behavior to cultural and interpersonal factors; rejected Freud's view of feminine sexuality
■ Frieda Fromm-Reichmann—utilized psychoanalytical techniques with psychotic individuals; expanded the psychoanalytical theory of psychotic behavior
■ Karl Menninger—applied the concept of dynamic equilibrium to mental functioning; expanded the concept of coping; developed levels of dysfunction

The unique contributions of these theorists can best be understood by reading their works. This, too, will foster an appreciation for the continuing relevance of many aspects of psychoanalytical theory.

Interpersonal model

The origin of the interpersonal model of psychotherapy can be traced clearly to psychoanalytical thought. Karen Horney, Erich Fromm, and Wilhelm Reich have been identified as the first theorists who attempted to incorporate sociocultural influences on human behavior into the psychoanalytical model.[5] However, the theorist who will be presented here as most representative of the interpersonal model is Harry Stack Sullivan, a twentieth century American therapist. In addition, attention will be given to the interpersonal nursing theory of Hildegard Peplau. Her work represents a milestone in the conceptualization of the psychotherapeutic role of the nurse in the context of the interpersonal relationship.

Interpersonal view of behavioral deviations

Interpersonal theorists believe that behavior evolves within the context of interpersonal relationships. Whereas Freudian theory emphasizes the intrapsychic experience of the individual, interpersonal theory shifts the focus to the social or interpersonal experience. Sullivan, like Freud, traced a progression of psychological development. In fact, the psychoanalytical influence can be seen in some of Sullivan's terminology. For instance, the "self-system" bears marked resemblance to the "ego."

Sullivan also places emphasis on early life experiences as extremely influential to the individual's later mental health. He believes that anxiety is first experienced empathically when the infant perceives the anxiety of the mothering person. Later, anxiety is associated with disapproval from significant others. The self-system develops in the context of approval and disapproval. Disapproval causes anxiety because it includes a threat of rejection by the significant other. Security operations are developed to deal with anxiety-provoking areas of disapproval. The most anxiety-laden experiences are dissociated, meaning that they are excluded from the awareness of the self. Note the similarity to the psychoanalytical concept of repression.

If a child is given only disapproving messages about the self, a negative self-system develops. Interestingly, Sullivan states that ". . . one can find in others only that which is in the self."[8:310] Therefore a person who sees himself as untrustworthy will view others with suspicion. The person is then not only burdened with a lack of self-approval, but is also handicapped in establishing supportive relationships with others, which could, theoretically, help modify his self-concept.

Sullivanian theory states that the individual bases his behavior on two complex drives: the drive for satisfaction and the drive for security. Satisfaction refers to the basic human drives, including hunger, sleep, lust, and loneliness.[8] Security relates to culturally defined needs, such as conformity to the social norms and value system of one's particular ethnic group. Sullivan states that when the nature of a person's self-system interferes with his ability to attend to his needs for either satisfaction or security, he is mentally ill.[8]

When Peplau defined nursing as an interpersonal process, she also discussed the importance of basic human needs. She believes that needs must be met if a healthy state is to be achieved and maintained. Health is defined as "forward movement of personality and other ongoing human processes in the direction of creative, constructive, productive, personal and community living."[13:2] Lack of growth, for whatever reason, implies impaired health. The two interacting components of health are physiological demands and interpersonal conditions.[13] These may be viewed as parallel to the drives of satisfaction and security identified by Sullivan. Clinical example 2-2 may clarify this perspective on behavioral deviation.

CLINICAL EXAMPLE 2-2

Ms. Y, an attractive 26-year-old woman, appeared at a psychiatric outpatient clinic requesting therapy. She described her problem as "I can't get close to people." She said that her childhood was happy; that she had loving parents and liked her sister. Her family were devout members of a fundamentalist Protestant church; so most of her activities were church related. She had many friends during childhood and then one close girl friend in early adolescence. She thought that her fear of closeness began when she slept over at her friend's house. During the night her friend began to fondle her in a way that she interpreted as sexual. She became very frightened and felt guilty about this. She did not tell her parents because of her guilt and, in fact, had told no one before entering therapy. Although she attended college, she never dated and would participate only in superficial social contacts. She realized that this was not healthy young adult behavior and, as the behavior continued into her twenties, Ms. Y decided that she needed to seek help.

From an interpersonal frame of reference, Ms. Y was unable to fulfill her needs for friendship and sexual love. Sullivanians would perceive a lack of satisfaction because of the unfulfilled lust dynamism and a lack of security because of her fear that she had deviated from the norm of her cultural group. Her anxiety stemmed from her conviction that her parents would disown her if they heard what had happened. This belief was based on their earlier responses to childhood sexual play. The therapist decided that Ms. Y first needed to experience intimacy at a nonsexual level and this was approached in the therapeutic situation. When she began to feel comfortable sharing closeness with the therapist, she gradually tried to explore friendships and finally was able to begin dating.

Interpersonal therapeutic process

The interpersonal therapist, like the psychoanalyst, explores the patient's life history. The focus of this exploration is on the person's progress through the developmental stages of learning to relate productively to other people. Components of the self-system are identified, including the security operations that are used to defend the self. The therapist also notes areas the patient avoids or claims to have forgotten, since this material may have been dissociated.

The crux of the therapeutic process is the corrective interpersonal experience. The premise is that by experiencing a healthy relationship with the therapist, the patient can learn to have more satisfying interpersonal relationships in general. The therapist actively encourages the development of trust by relating authentically to the patient. This includes the expectation that the therapist share feelings and reactions with the patient. The process of therapy is essentially a process of reeducation, as the therapist helps the patient identify interpersonal problems and then encourages him to try out more successful styles of relating. For example, fear of intimacy is frequently experienced by patients. The therapist allows the patient to become close while clearly communicating that there is no threat of sexual involvement. It is believed that closeness within the therapeutic relationship builds trust, facilitates empathy, enhances self-esteem, and thus fosters growth toward healthy behavior. Peplau[13] describes this process as "psychological mothering," which includes the following steps:

1. The patient is accepted unconditionally as a participant in a relationship that fully satisfies his needs.
2. There is recognition of and response to the patient's readiness for growth as initiated by the patient.
3. Power in the relationship shifts to the patient as he is able to delay gratification and to invest energy in goal achievement.

Therapy is terminated when the patient has developed the ability to establish satisfying human relationships, thereby meeting his basic needs. Termination is viewed as a significant part of the relationship that must be experienced and shared by both the therapist and the patient.

It is through this process that the patient learns that leaving a significant other involves pain but can also be an opportunity for growth.

Roles of the patient and the interpersonal therapist

The patient-therapist dyad is viewed as a partnership by practitioners of interpersonal therapy. Sullivan describes the therapist as a "participant observer" who should not remain detached from the therapeutic situation.[16] The therapist's role is to actively engage the patient, establish trust, and empathize. There is an active effort to provide the patient with consensual validation, thereby helping him to realize that his perceptions and concerns are in many ways similar to those of others. There is an atmosphere of uncritical acceptance to encourage the patient to speak openly. The therapist then interacts as a real person who also has beliefs, values, thoughts, and feelings. The patient's role is to share his concerns with the therapist and to participate in the relationship to the best of his ability. The relationship itself is meant to serve as a model of interpersonal relationships. As the patient matures in his ability to relate, he can then improve and broaden his other life experiences with people outside the therapeutic situation.

Interpersonal nursing roles have been identified by Peplau.[13] They include the following:
1. Stranger—the role assumed by both nurse and patient when they first meet
2. Resource person—provider of health information to a patient who has assumed the consumer role
3. Teacher—assisting the patient as learner to grow and learn from his experience with the health care system
4. Leader—assisting the patient as follower to participate in a democratically implemented nursing process
5. Surrogate—assuming roles that have been assigned by the patient, based on his significant past relationships, similar to the psychoanalytical concept of transference
6. Counselor—helping the patient integrate the facts and feelings associated with an episode of illness into his total life experience

By functioning within these various roles, which may be assumed by the nurse or assigned to others, the practitioner assists the patient to meet the goals of therapy: need satisfaction and personal growth. In addition, the therapist experiences growth as she learns about herself through her role performance. Self-awareness is essential to success as an interpersonal therapist.

Social model

The two preceding models have centered on the individual and his intrapsychic processes and interpersonal experiences as the most significant factors to be considered in psychiatric care. The social model moves beyond the individual to include consideration of the social environment as it impacts on the person and his life experience. A criticism of psychoanalytical theory, in particular, is that it was heavily influenced by Freud's Victorian, Viennese, upper middle-class, Jewish background. It has been suggested that concepts such as the oedipal complex, castration anxiety, and penis envy might not extend to other cultures and times. Likewise, his view of women very much reflects his culture and times and has been repeatedly challenged, particularly by feminists.

There are recent theorists who believe that the culture itself is instrumental in defining mental illness, prescribing the nature of therapy and determining the future of the person who has been assigned the patient role. To represent this point of view, consideration will be given to the theories of Thomas Szasz and Gerald Caplan. In addition, the community mental health plan of the 1960s will be presented as an example of a governmental effort to respond to the philosophy of the social theorists.

Social view of behavioral deviations

According to theorists in this group, social conditions are largely responsible for the existence of deviant behavior. Deviancy is culturally defined. Behavior that is considered to be normal in one cultural setting may be eccentric in another and psychotic in a third. This was exemplified by the experience of the African exchange student mentioned earlier in this chapter. With this point of view, Szasz[17] writes of the "myth of mental illness." He believes that society must find a way of managing "undesir-

ables"; so it labels them as mentally ill. People who are so labeled are usually those who are unable or refuse to conform to social norms. The response to this behavior is generally to institutionalize the person. If he then conforms to social expectations, he is considered to be recovered and is allowed to return to the community. Institutionalization, then, has the dual function of removing deviant members from the community and of exerting social control over their behavior. Szasz states, "Mental illness is coercion concealed as loss of self-control; institutional psychiatry is countercoercion concealed as therapy."[18:100]

The first part of Szasz' statement recognizes that the individual is also responsible for his behavior. The person has control over whether to conform to social expectations. The person who is called mentally ill may be a scapegoat, but the individual participates in the scapegoating process by inviting it or by allowing it to occur. Szasz objects strongly to the designation of deviant behavior as "illness." He believes that illness can occur in the body and that diseases of the body can influence behavior (e.g., brain tumors), but there is no physiological disruption that can be demonstrated to cause most deviancy.[17] He distinguishes between the biological condition that is central to illness and the social role which is the focus of deviancy.

Caplan has also approached the study of deviant behavior from a social perspective. He has extended the public health model of primary, secondary, and tertiary prevention to the mental health field. Primary prevention is the avoidance of occurrence of disease. Secondary prevention is the reduction of the duration of the illness episode; and tertiary prevention is the limitation of impairment resulting from a disease process.[6] Caplan has focused particularly on primary prevention, since much attention has been given in the past to the secondary and tertiary levels. Lack of understanding of causation of deviant behavior has hindered the development of primary prevention techniques.

Caplan believes that social situations can predispose the person to mental illness. These situations include such conditions as poverty, family instability, and inadequate education. Deprivation throughout the life cycle leaves the individual with limited ability to cope with stress. The person has few available environmental supports. This combination results in a predisposition to utilize pathological means of coping.

Crises are viewed as possible precipitating

causes of deviant behavior. When in crisis, a person is vulnerable. If internal coping mechanisms or external supports are inadequate, the person may exhibit pathological behavior. However, a crisis may also be an opportunity for growth if there are adequate resources to help the person learn from the experience and develop improved coping mechanisms. The supports must be available through the social system.

Social therapeutic process

Theorists who see behavioral deviation as intertwined with the social environment believe that therapy is also influenced by this dimension. Szasz is an advocate of freedom of choice for psychiatric patients. He believes that the individual should be allowed without coercion, to select his own therapeutic modality and therapist. This also implies a well-informed consumer who can base this decision on knowledge of available modes of therapy.[8] Szasz does not believe in involuntary institutionalization of the mentally ill and comments, "Involuntary mental hospitalization is like slavery. Refining the standards for commitment is like prettifying the slave plantations. The problem is not how to improve commitment, but how to abolish it."[18:89] He also questions whether any psychiatric hospitalization is truly voluntary. Szasz is not in favor of the recent community mental health trend that purports to place mental health care within the reach of every American. He questions the extension of the involvement of government in what he views as essentially a private concern.

Caplan, on the other hand, has been a great proponent of community psychiatry. He interpreted the 1963 announcement by President Kennedy of the government's intention to become involved in the improvement of mental health care as a challenge to psychiatry. He foresaw a new focus on the reduction of the frequency of mental health problems, which then prompted his elaboration of theories of primary prevention.[6] To a great extent this theorist concentrates on the role of the mental health professional in combating societal problems, thereby indirectly benefiting those who could be future psychiatric patients. This is accomplished through the process of consultation.

The mental health consultant indirectly helps socially deprived individuals who are at risk for developing a mental illness. Examples of such groups might be the poor or minorities. Other people who are at risk and need primary prevention services are those in crisis, for example, mothers of premature babies or the recently widowed. The consultant may intervene on a variety of levels. In consultee-centered case consultation the focus is on an individual client and that person's problems. This approach has relatively narrow impact. Consultee-centered administrative consultation provides advice on program development or on the interpersonal relationships of agency workers. Care must be taken that the focus remain on the work situation rather than an attempt to deal with workers' personal problems. The third type of consultation is program-centered administrative consultation. Attention is paid to a broader perspective of the overall program of an agency or a group of related agencies.[6]

Roles of the patient and the social therapist

In the opinion of Szasz, an individual can be helped to solve his problems only if he requests such help. The patient, then, initiates the therapeutic encounter and defines the problem to be solved. The patient also has the right to approve or disapprove of the therapeutic intervention that is recommended. Therapy is successfully completed when the patient is satisfied with the changes that he has chosen to make in his lifestyle. The therapist collaborates with the patient to promote change. This includes making recommendations to the patient about possible means of effecting behavioral change. It does not include any element of coercion, particularly the threat of hospitalization if the patient does not conform to the therapist's demands. The therapist's role may also include protecting the patient from social demands that he be treated against his will. Szasz feels strongly that the therapist has moral and ethical obligations which are primarily directed toward the patient.

Caplan also takes a moral approach to therapy. However, he believes that society itself has a moral obligation to provide a wide range of therapeutic services covering all three levels of prevention. The patient has a consumer role and selects the level of help that is appropriate from a wide array of available services. Ideally, the client is reached by primary preventive services and thereby avoids the need for secondary or tertiary care. The client, it is hoped, never becomes a patient. For example, a recently widowed woman may be seen by her clergyman, who has received consultative training in counseling techniques. If he is concerned about the course of her grief process, he may refer her to a crisis intervention clinic where she will receive brief psychotherapy from a mental health professional. The person receiving crisis intervention services is viewed as a client who needs support over a short period of time while coping mechanisms and environmental supports are strengthened. The widow may then be referred to a community group of widows who help each other adjust to the shock of widowhood.

Therapists may be professional or nonprofessional with professional consultation. For instance, indigenous supportive people such as clergy, policemen, bartenders, and beauticians can be trained to be helpful listeners and to refer people who need professional help to appropriate resources. The therapist in the social context is not tied to the office but is expected to be involved in the community. Activities may include home visits, lectures to community groups, or consultation to other agencies. The rationale for this is that the more involved the therapist is in the community, the more impact there will be on the mental health of the people. Community involvement also enhances the therapist's ability to understand patients who live in that environment.

Community mental health

A movement of the 1960s that had great significance for psychiatric care was community mental health. It marked the vigorous entry of the federal government into the field of mental health and proved to be a mixed blessing. On the positive side, public attention was brought to the inadequacies of mental health care for the majority of the population. Public funding stimulated the creation of new facilities and the training of additional mental health professionals. Impetus was given to the examination of care delivery systems and, as a result, some modifications were made. For instance, there was interest in establishing a broader range of services with greater accessibility to the community served. There was also an emphasis on making services available to groups that had previously been neglected, such as the mentally retarded,

children, the poor, alcoholics, and drug abusers.

Critics of community mental health point to the enormous amount of money that was spent with no apparent significant impact on the incidence of mental illness. They view it as a bandwagon that was used by some agencies to acquire new physical facilities with little or no commitment to the community mental health philosophy. The pressure to deinstitutionalize chonically hospitalized patients sometimes resulted in the imposition of people without social skills on unprepared communities with inadequate resources. In some cases the utilization of nonprofessional mental health workers led to the suspicion that the disadvantaged were being subjected to yet another type of second-rate care.

There is no doubt that community mental health has had an impact on psychiatric care delivery. It is still too soon to evaluate the total effect in an objective manner. However, the very stimulation of scrutiny of psychiatric services must be viewed as a healthy development, even if all the results did not meet the original high expectations.

Existential model

The existential model of psychiatric care is derived from a philosophical school. These theorists are heavily influenced by the work of such philosophers as Sartre, Heidegger, and Kierkegaard. They are also in agreement with the theory of the I-thou relationship as described by the religious philosopher Martin Buber. The focus is generally on the importance of the individual's experience in the here and now with much less attention being given to the person's past history than is the case with other theoretical models. Among the earliest existentialistic psychiatric thinkers were Karl Jaspers and Ludwig Binswanger. Many contemporary theorists espouse this point of view, including Frederick S. Perls, founder of gestalt therapy; William Glasser, founder of reality therapy; Albert Ellis, rational-emotive therapy; Carl Rogers, particularly in his later work with encounter groups; and R.D. Laing, who combines his existentialist philosophy with an iconoclastic view similar to that of Szasz. Most recently there has also been a growing interest in parapsychology, which is closely allied with existentialism. This is particularly true in the sense that parapsychological experiences are viewed as truly authentic, demonstrating that the person is closely attuned to himself and to the "vibrations" of others as well.

Existentialist view of behavioral deviations

Existentialist theorists tend to believe that behavioral deviations result when the individual is out of touch with himself or his environment. This alienation is the result of inhibitions or restrictions that the person has placed on himself. As a result, he is not free to choose from among all possible alternative behaviors. A deviant behavior is frequently a way of avoiding more socially acceptable, and therefore more responsible, behavior.

The person who is alienated from himself experiences feelings of helplessness, sadness, and loneliness. Lack of self-awareness and self-approbation prevents participation in authentic and rewarding relationships with others. Even though, theoretically, the person has innumerable choices in terms of behavior. Heidegger[8] noted that people tend to avoid being real and instead yield to tradition and the demands of others. This belief has been accepted by the existentialist practitioners of mental health care.

Black[4] has described the psychiatric patient as a person who has either lost or never found the values that can give meaning to his existence. Hence the world seems absurd to him, and its demands appear invalid. Rather than accept the painful realities of life, he gives up. His lack of commitment may lead to a hazy identity and a sense of unreality, which extends to his perception of other people.

Existential therapeutic process

There are several therapies that are basically existential. These include logotherapy and gestalt, rational-emotive, reality, and encounter group therapy. Basic to all of them is the assumption that the patient needs to be able to choose freely from what life has to offer. Although the approaches are somewhat different, the goal is generally to return the patient to an authentic awareness of his being. Laing[12] describes the process of going mad and then returning to sanity. Going mad is compared to death, movement backward, an altered sense of time, self-absorption, and a return to the womb. Recovery is compared to return to life, forward movement, restoration of temporal meaning, the growth of a new ego, and "an existential rebirth." It is the work of therapy for the patient, with the help of the therapist, to find his way from the alienation of madness to the relatedness of a full life.

The existential therapeutic process focuses on the encounter. The encounter is not merely the meeting of two or more persons but is their appreciation of the total existence of each other. As Binswanger has stated, "encounter is a being-with-others in *genuine presence,* that is to say, in the present which is altogether continuous with the *past* and bears within it the possibilities of a *future.*"[8:377] This temporal orientation that takes note of the patient's life as a process of becoming is also basic to most existential theories. Through the encounter, the patient is helped to accept and understand his past, live fully in the present, and look forward to the future.

The actual process of therapy differs somewhat depending on the specific theory being practiced. Following are several of the better known existentially based theories with a brief statement concerning the therapeutic process of each. For further information, the reader is encouraged to explore the writings of these theorists.

- Rational-emotive therapy (Albert Ellis)—an active-directive, cognitively oriented therapy. Confrontation is used to force the patient to assume responsibility for his behavior. The patient is encouraged to accept himself as he is, not because of what he does. He is taught to take risks and try out new behavior. Action is emphasized for both the patient and the therapist.[9]
- Logotherapy (Viktor E. Frankl)—a future-oriented therapy; "the patient is actually confronted with and oriented toward the meaning of his life."[10:153] This search for meaning (*logos*) is viewed as a primary life force. This includes meaning in the spiritual sense. Without a sense of meaning, life becomes an "existential vacuum." The aim of therapy is to help the patient become aware of his responsibleness. In essence, the patient is guided to take control of his own life and to determine its meaning for himself.
- Reality therapy (William Glasser)—central themes are the need for identity reached by loving, feeling worthwhile, and behaving responsibly. The patient is helped to recognize his life goals and the way he keeps himself from accomplishing his goals. He is made aware of the alternatives available to him. Another focus of therapy is the development of the capacity for caring, through the warm acceptance of the therapist. Temporal orientation is to the present. The patient is directed to talk about any topic but to focus on behavior rather than feelings.[11]
- Gestalt therapy (Frederick S. Perls)—emphasizes the here and now. The patient is encouraged to identify feelings by enhancing self-awareness. There is focus on body sensations as they reflect

feelings. The increased awareness makes the patient more sensitive to other aspects of his existence. Self-awareness is expected to lead to self-acceptance. The patient is assisted to deal with unfinished business by becoming aware of the totality of his responses. More attention is focused on the "how" and "what" of behavior, rather than the "why."[11]

■ Encounter group therapy (William C. Schutz, Carl Rogers)—focuses on the establishment of intimate interactions in a group setting. Therapy is oriented to the here and now. The patient is expected to assume responsibility for his own behavior. Feeling is stressed; intellectualization discouraged. Group exercises in relating are frequently utilized. Group members are encouraged to honestly and openly share their thoughts and feelings, thus becoming more self-aware.[11]

Roles of the patient and the existential therapist

The existential theorists emphasize that the therapist and the patient are equal in their common humanity. The therapist is to act as a guide to the patient who has gone astray in his search for authenticity. The therapist is frequently very directive in pointing out areas where the patient should consider changing. However, there is also a focus on caring and warmth. The therapist as well as the patient is to be open and honest. The therapeutic experience is a model for the patient, during which he can test new behaviors prior to risking them in his daily life.

The patient is expected to assume and accept responsibility for his behavior. Dependence on the therapist is generally not encouraged. In this sense, the patient is treated as an adult. Frequently there is a de-emphasis of illness. The patient is viewed as a person who is alienated from himself and others, but for whom there is hope if he can trust and follow the directions of the therapist. The patient is always active in therapy, working to meet the challenge presented by the therapist.

Parapsychology

Parapsychology is not really a therapeutic modality, but it is a phenomenon that has been studied by many psychotherapists, including Freud. It is generally considered to include such experiences as extrasensory perception (ESP), which is the awareness of events that are out of the range of usual sensory functioning, and precognition, which is the foreknowledge of events. Believers in these phenomena state that they emanate from a different level of experience and require special sensitivity to this level to develop an awareness of them.

The level of experience is also described by those who believe in the use of hallucinogenic drugs. The drug-induced experience is supposed to heighten sensory awareness and reveal new vistas of understanding. The intense concentration on the here-and-now experience is compared to the existential knowledge of oneself as a person in the process of becoming.

These phenomena are not scientifically validated and are considered suspect by many reputable theorists. However, knowledge of mental processes is still so limited that there is the possibility of some validity in the claims of these people.

Communication model

A sophisticated system of communication is one of the characteristics that distinguishes human beings from lower orders of animal life. In the eyes of communication theorists, all behavior communicates something. The understanding of the meaning of behavior is based on the clarity of communication between the actor (sender) and observer (receiver). Disruptions in behavior may, then, be viewed as disturbances in the communication process. This point of view is appealing in an information-oriented culture such as the contemporary United States. The prevalence of the use of media for the dissemination of information demonstrates the increasing utilization of communication techniques. At the same time, breakdown in successful transmission of information causes anxiety and frustration.

Theorists who have particularly emphasized the importance of communication are Eric Berne, the founder of transactional analysis, and Paul Watzlawick and his associates who have studied the pragmatics of human communication.

Communications view of behavioral deviations

All behavior is communication, whether verbal or nonverbal. Therefore deviant behavior may be viewed as an attempt to communicate. The message may be masked or distorted; the route may be indirect, but the end result of behavior is still the transmission of a message to others who are able to perceive it.

According to Berne,[3] people communicate from the frame of reference of one of three ego states: parent, adult, or child. These terms do not refer to actual status in life, but refer to the concept that the person acts like a parent, for instance. A communication unit is referred to as a transaction. *Complementary transactions* occur when the message that is directed from one ego state to another is responded to as implicitly expected so the ego state which is addressed actually responds:

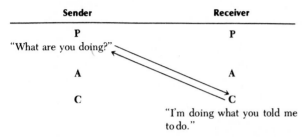

For instance, the sender's parent addresses the receiver's child and then the receiver's child responds to the sender's parent. Problems occur when transactions are crossed. As an example, the sender's adult may address the receiver's adult, but receive a response from the receiver's parent to the sender's child, for instance, "Bring me a glass of milk, please" followed by "Get it yourself, I'm busy." This type of transaction results in a communication block. The four most common crossed communications are the following:

1. Adult to adult—child to parent (the transference reaction)

    Sender   **Receiver**

    P   P
    A ——————→ A
    "I disagree with you. Let's talk about it."
    C   C
    "I hate you."

2. Adult to adult—parent to child (countertransference)

    Sender   **Receiver**

    P   P
        "I know I'm right."
    A ——————→ A
    "I disagree with you. talk about it."
    C   C

3. Child to parent—adult to adult (exasperating)

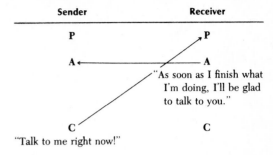

    "Talk to me right now!"

4. Parent to child—adult to adult (impudent)

    Sender   **Receiver**

    P   P
    "I want to speak to you."
    A ←—————— A
        "As soon as I finish what I'm doing, I'll speak with you."
    C   C

In some transactions an ulterior motive is operating. For example, the adult may appear to be addressing the other's adult but may expect a response from the parent or child. In other ulterior transactions there may be superficial social and deeper psychological levels of meaning operating at the same time. According to Berne, the basis of transactional analysis is "rigorous analysis of single transactions into their component specific ego states."[3:20]

Berne further believes that people respond to three drives or hungers: (1) stimulus hunger—the need for sensation, (2) recognition hunger—the need for special interpersonally experienced sensations, and (3) structure hunger—the need to organize. The last drive leads the person to structure his time. He describes six basic types of social behavior that help to provide the needed structure: (1) withdrawal; (2) rituals, which are responses to custom and characterized by strokes or units of recognition; (3) activities, or work; (4) pastimes; (5) games; and (6) intimacy.[3] Two of these in particular, games and intimacy, require further elaboration. He describes games as "sets of ulterior transactions, repetitive in nature, with a well-defined psychological payoff." "Payoff" refers to the feelings that are aroused by the game. Each participant receives a payoff, although the feelings may differ. The other elements of the game are the "con," or bait, which involves the other player; the switch, in which the initiator changes the rules or the character of the game; and the cross-up, in which the other player feels confused and becomes aware of the switch. All these factors are necessary for a game to be played. Intimacy refers to an open relationship in which game playing is avoided. Structure is also accomplished by way of a script, which Berne identifies as a "'life plan' which derives from childhood ideas." Deviant behavior, then, indicates that the person is relating through game playing rather than intimacy and may be living out a script that is irrelevant to his adult life.

Watzlawick[19] and other communications pragmatists believe that deviant behavior is based on disrupted communication patterns. They have identified several such patterns. The first is an effort not to communicate, which is self-defeating because it is impossible. A second is a lack of congruity in levels of communication. In this case the focus is on the content of the message, but the real issue involves the relationship between the communicators. When a person makes a statement about himself, the other may confirm, reject, or disconfirm it. Disconfirmation denies the reality of the other.

Imperviousness is a situation in which each person assumes he understands and is understood when this is not actually the case. Discrepancies in punctuation occur when one party has less information than the other but does not know it, leading to different perceptions of reality. The person who exhibits the self-fulfilling prophecy behaves as he expects others to respond to him, thus reinforcing his (usually negative) self-concept.

Human relationships are either symmetrical or complementary. Symmetry implies equality; whereas complementarity implies difference. One disruption in this area is called symmetrical escalation, which occurs when the participants strive to be "more equal." A disruption of complementarity is folie à deux, in which each partner confirms the pathologic condition of the other. For instance, a rigid, controlling mother and a passive, compliant child may depend on each other for role confirmation.[19] Watzlawick also presents the concept of the pragmatic paradox, which is demonstrated by the double bind. (See Chapter 11.)

Communications therapeutic process

Because communications theorists locate the disruption in behavior within the communication process, interventions are made in patterns of communication. This may take place with individuals, groups, or families. The communication pattern is first assessed and the disruption diagnosed. The patient is then helped to recognize his own disrupted communication. In this sense, there is a definite education component to communication therapy.

Transactional analysts assist patients to recognize ego states in themselves and others and to identify crossed transactions. Analysis of games is an important part of therapy. The patient is helped to see what games he plays repeatedly. He is then assisted to find the elements of these games (i.e., What is the payoff for him? For the other person?). Games that arise during therapy are pointed out, and alternative behavior is presented. As with the existential therapies, the emphasis is on authenticity and responsibility for the self. In addition to the focus on games, the patient also works to discover his script. Once identified, the script can be modified to meet the person's adult needs and to facilitate healthy relationships.

Watzlawick and his colleagues developed the technique of the therapeutic double bind. They contend that there are two ways to induce change in therapy. One is to tell the person to change, which he probably would have done if he were able to do so. The other is to tell him not to change, which enhances his awareness of his behavior, increases tension, and may stimulate him to change. Telling the person to change by not changing creates a paradox in which any behavior is expected to result in a change. The theorists point out that this is a difficult technique to master and should only be attempted by skilled therapists who can deal with the high level of anxiety that might result.

Roles of the patient and the communications therapist

The communications therapist induces change in the patient by intervening in the communication process. Feedback is given about the person's success at communicating. Effective communication is reinforced, and alternatives for ineffective communication are discussed. In group or family settings, patterns are analyzed on a more complex level. The therapist also demonstrates how to relate to others clearly, without playing games or using paradoxes. Nonverbal communication is also emphasized, particularly in terms of congruence with verbal behavior.

The patient must be willing to become involved in an analysis of his style of communicating. If in transactional analysis, he frequently will have to study the communication theory. He is then asked to participate in identifying ego states, games, and scripts. The responsibility for changing rests with the patient. Significant others are often included in communication therapy to deal with their response to change in the identified patient. Change in one participant in a communication system stimulates responses in the other members. These responses are generally directed toward maintaining the status quo. Thus change is more lasting if it takes place at the system level.

Behavioral model

Behavior modification therapy is derived from learning theories. The focus is on the patient's actions, not on thoughts and feelings. It is believed by these theorists that a change in behavior will lead to a change in the cognitive and affective spheres. Behavior therapists emphasize the quantitative aspect of observable behavior. They believe that one of the strengths of this approach is the possibility of conducting research on the effectiveness of therapy. They contend that most other psychotherapies are not compatible with a scientific research process because of the high degree of subjectivity involved in defining the problem and identifying improvement. In addition, there is variation in the therapeutic behavior of psychotherapists who utilize other models. Personality style tends to individualize therapy even among therapists who share the same theoretical framework. Behavior modification therapy, on the other hand, is structured and therefore more reproducible from therapist to therapist.

Prominent theorists of behavioral therapy include H.J. Eysenck, Joseph Wolpe, and B.F. Skinner.

Behavior theorists' view of behavioral deviations

Since the behavioral theorists believe that all behavior is learned, deviations from the norm are viewed as habitual responses that can be modified through application of learning theory. Learning occurs when a stimulus is presented, a response occurs, and the response is reinforced.

The response is strengthened by repetition of the learning sequence. The desirability of the reinforcer to the learner is also important, although even painful (aversive) reinforcers have been found to enhance a behavior more than no response at all.

From the behavioral point of view, then, deviations from behavioral norms occur when undesirable behavior has been reinforced. Clinical example 2-3 illustrates this theory.

CLINICAL EXAMPLE 2-3

Ms. J was a 45-year-old woman who was brought to the mental health center at the insistence of her family. She was actively resisting her 20-year-old son's plan to move to his own apartment by threatening to kill herself. Each time she threatened, he agreed not to move for a few more weeks, thus reinforcing her behavior. The therapeutic plan was that the son would set a date to move and do so. At the same time, Mr. J would give his wife extra attention during the difficult time of their son's leaving.

Behavioral therapeutic process

Behavioral therapy, as described by Wolpe,[7] includes the techniques of reciprocal inhibition. This is based on the premise that the observable behavior, or symptom, is a learned response to anxiety. The symptom is reinforced because it leads to a reduction of anxiety, even though it is not otherwise a productive behavior. Reciprocal inhibition attempts to substitute a more adaptive behavior for the symptom through the learning of an alternative means of reducing the anxiety. One such approach is desensitization or the relaxation technique. The patient establishes a hierarchy of anxiety-provoking experiences from low to high levels of anxiety. He then either actually experiences or fantasizes each experience from lowest to highest. During the fantasy he may practice relaxation exercises with the coaching of the therapist. Sometimes the patient is hypnotized. The whole process takes several therapy sessions, since the patient does not move on to the next level of the hierarchy until the anxiety associated with the lower level has been alleviated. For further discussion of this technique and an example of a hierarchy see Chapter 7.

Another approach that has been advocated by

Wolpe for the alleviation of anxiety is assertiveness training. This is useful when the patient's anxiety arises from interpersonal relationships. Assertiveness implies the ability to stand up for one's own rights while not infringing on the rights of others. It is differentiated from passive behavior, which ignores one's own rights, and aggressive behavior, which violates the other's rights. In therapy the patient identifies his usual mode of behavior. Through role play and practice he works to modify his behavior toward increased assertiveness. This, in turn, increases self-esteem and the sense of self-control, thus reducing interpersonally based anxiety.

Other behavior modification approaches include aversion therapy and the token economy system. Aversion therapy refers to the use of a painful stimulus, usually an electrical shock, to create an aversion to a stimulus. This approach has been tried as an attempt to change homosexual behavior.[7] There has been controversy over the moral-ethical aspects of utilizing a method of therapy that deliberately induces pain to change behavior. Therapists who use this approach believe the end justifies the means. Patients who accept aversion therapy generally do so of their own volition. This gives some indication of the strength of emotional pain so intense that physical pain is accepted to alleviate it.

Token economy systems are positive reinforcement programs that are frequently utilized to encourage socially acceptable behavior in chronically hospitalized patients. The person is rewarded with a token, generally a poker chip, when the desirable behavior occurs and penalized by removal of tokens when undesirable behavior takes place. When enough tokens are accumulated, they may be spent for cigarettes, snacks, grounds passes, or whatever is meaningful to the patient. This pleasurable experience reinforces the future repetition of the desired behavior. For patients with good ability for abstract thinking, points may be substituted for tokens. It is still important, however, to be sure that the reward is highly desirable to the patient. This approach may also be helpful with children and acting-out adolescents.

Roles of the patient and the behavioral therapist

The roles of patient and therapist when a behavioral approach to treatment is used are those of learner and teacher, respectively. The therapist is an expert in behavior who can help the patient unlearn his symptoms and replace them with more satisfying behavior. The therapist utilizes the patient's anxiety as a motivational force toward learning. Behavioral objectives are devised, and careful evaluation takes place.

As a learner, the patient is an active participant in the therapy process. He must produce fantasies or practice uncomfortable behaviors. Behavior modification patients may be well versed in the rationale for the therapy, although this is in no way necessary for this approach to be used. However, the knowledgeable patient is a more cooperative patient. There are frequently homework assignments to further reinforce the teaching done in the therapeutic session. Significant others may also be enlisted to continue the therapy program at home. Therapy is considered to be complete when the symptoms are gone. There is no attempt to unearth an underlying conflict and the patient is not encouraged to explore his past.

Medical model

The medical model refers to psychiatric care that is based on the traditional physician-patient relationship and focuses on the diagnosis of a mental illness. Subsequent treatment is based on this diagnosis. Somatic treatments, including pharmacotherapy, electroconvulsive therapy, and, occasionally, psychosurgery, are important components of the treatment process. The interpersonal aspect of this approach to treatment varies widely, from intensive insight-oriented intervention to brief, superficial medication-supervision sessions.

Much of modern psychiatric care is dominated by the medical model. Other health professionals may be utilized for specific purposes such as interagency referrals, family assessment, and health teaching, but physicians are viewed as the leaders of the team when this model is in effect. In the same way, elements of other models of care may be used in conjunction with the medical model. For instance, a patient may be diagnosed as schizophrenic and treated with phenothiazine medication but may also be on a token economy program to encourage socially acceptable behavior.

Siegler and Osmond[15] believe that the medical model performs two functions. The first is that of treating the ill. The second is to avoid the placing of blame for deviant behavior. This second function is extremely important and may account for the wide acceptance of the medical model. When illness is attributed to disease and a cause is postulated that is external to the patient and his immediate social system, the focus can be on healing rather than blaming. Viewing mental illness in this way helps to remove some of the social stigma that is otherwise attached to it.

Another positive contribution of the medical model has been the continuous exploration for causes of mental illness using the scientific process. Recently there have been great strides in learning about brain and nervous system functioning. This has led to a beginning understanding of the probable physiological components of many behavioral disruptions. This progress will, in turn, lead to increasingly specific and sophisticated approaches to psychiatric care.

Medical view of behavioral deviations

Most adherents of the medical model believe that deviant behavior is a manifestation of a disorder of the central nervous system. At present, the exact nature of the physiological disruption is not well understood. It is suspected that for the psychotic disorders, such as manic-depressive illness, endogenous depression, and schizophrenia, there is an abnormality in the transmission of neural impulses. It is also believed that this difficulty occurs at the synaptic level and involves neurochemicals, such as dopamine, serotonin, and norepinephrine.

Recently a new group of neurochemicals, named endorphins and enkephalins, have attracted a great deal of interest. They have been referred to as natural opiates because they bind to opiate receptors in the brain. Their role in determining behavior is being explored.

Much research is currently taking place to better understand the nature of the brain's involvement in emotional response. Another area of research focuses on stressors and the human response to stress. Researchers are asking the question "Why do some people seem to tolerate great stress and continue to function well and others fall apart when a small problem arises?" They suspect that there may be a physiological stress threshold which may be genetically determined. These research areas are intriguing, but for the present, not well enough defined to provide definitive guidelines for therapy.

Environmental and social factors are also considered in the medical model. They may be either predisposing or precipitating factors in an episode of illness. For example, the person who is unemployed, lonely, and lives near a bar may be predisposed by these factors to develop a drinking problem. In combination with other possible genetic and physiological predispositions this constellation of circumstances could result in alcoholism. In another instance an episode of illness in an alcoholic patient could be precipitated by the social event of separation from his wife.

Medical therapeutic process

The medical process of therapy is well defined and familiar to most patients. The physician examines the patient. The examination includes the history of the present illness, past history, social history, medical history, review of systems, physical examination, and mental status examination. Additional data may be collected from significant others, and past medical records are reviewed, if available. A preliminary diagnosis is then formulated, pending further diagnostic studies and observation of the patient's behavior. This process may take place on an ambulatory or an inpatient basis, depending on the condition of the patient.

The diagnosis is stated and classified according to the *Diagnostic and Statistical Manual of Mental Disorders, third edition (DSM-III)* of the American Psychiatric Association. The names of the various illnesses are augmented by a description of diagnostic criteria, which are tested for reliability on a group of psychiatric practitioners. Changes in the DSM reflect changes in the medical model of psychiatric care. DSM-III is the most recent edition and was published in 1980. One difference between DSM-III and earlier diagnostic manuals is the use in this edition of the concept of multiaxial diagnosis. Five axes are presented as factors to be considered in formulating a psychiatric diagnosis. Axes I and II include the mental disorders and are found on pp. 48 to 51. The diagnostic categories of Personality Disorders and Specific Developmental Disorders are assigned to axis II; all other diagnoses are included in axis I. This was done so that the axis II diagnoses would not be overlooked if they occurred in conjunction with the frequently more dramatic axis I conditions.[2] Axis III is used for documentation of any coexisting physical conditions. These three axes make up the diagnosis that is to be documented for any patient who receives

DSM-III CLASSIFICATION: AXES I AND II CATEGORIES AND CODES*

All official DSM-III codes and terms are included in ICD-9-CM. However, in order to differentiate those DSM-III categories that use the same IC/9-CM codes, unofficial non-ICD-9-CM codes are provided in parentheses for use when greater specificity is necessary.

The long dashes indicate the need for a fifth-digit subtype or other qualifying term.

DISORDERS USUALLY FIRST EVIDENT IN INFANCY, CHILDHOOD, OR ADOLESCENCE
Mental retardation
Code in fifth digit: 1 = with other behavioral symptoms (requiring attention or treatment and not part of another disorder), 0 = without other behavioral symptoms.
317.0(x) Mild mental retardation, _____
318.0(x) Moderate mental retardation, _____
318.1(x) Severe mental retardation, _____
318.2(x) Profound mental retardation, _____
319.0(x) Unspecified mental retardation, _____

Attention deficit disorder
314.01 With hyperactivity
314.00 Without hyperactivity
314.80 Residual type

Conduct disorder
312.00 Undersocialized, aggressive
312.10 Undersocialized, nonaggressive
312.23 Socialized, aggressive
312.21 Socialized, nonaggressive
312.90 Atypical

Anxiety disorders of childhood or adolescence
309.21 Separation anxiety disorder
313.21 Avoidant disorder of childhood or adolescence
313.00 Overanxious disorder

Other disorders of infancy, childhood, or adolescence
313.89 Reactive attachment disorder of infancy
313.22 Schizoid disorder of childhood or adolescence
313.23 Elective mutism
313.81 Oppositional disorder
313.82 Identity disorder

Eating disorders
307.10 Anorexia nervosa
307.51 Bulimia
307.52 Pica
307.53 Rumination disorder of infancy
307.50 Atypical eating disorder

Stereotyped movement disorders
307.21 Transient tic disorder
307.22 Chronic motor tic disorder
307.23 Tourette's disorder
307.20 Atypical tic disorder
307.30 Atypical stereotyped movement disorder

Other disorders with physical manifestations
307.00 Stuttering
307.60 Functional enuresis
307.70 Functional encopresis
307.46 Sleepwalking disorder
307.46 Sleep terror disorder (307.49)

Pervasive developmental disorders
Code in fifth digit: 0 = full syndrome present, 1 = residual state.
299.0(x) Infantile autism, _____
299.9(x) Childhood onset pervasive developmental disorder, _____
299.8(x) Atypical, _____

Specific developmental disorders (coded on axis II)
315.00 Developmental reading disorder
315.10 Developmental arithmetic disorder
315.31 Developmental language disorder
315.39 Developmental articulation disorder
315.50 Mixed specific developmental disorder
315.90 Atypical specific developmental disorder

ORGANIC MENTAL DISORDERS
Section 1. Organic mental disorders whose etiology or pathophysiological process is listed below (taken from the mental disorders section of ICD-9-CM).

Dementias arising in the senium and presenium
Primary degenerative dementia, senile onset,
290.30 with delirium
290.20 with delusions
290.21 with depression
290.00 uncomplicated
Code in fifth digit: 1 = with delirium, 2 = with delusions, 3 = with depression, 0 = uncomplicated.
290.1(x) Primary degenerative dementia, presenile onset, _____
290.4(x) Multiinfarct dementia, _____

*From American Psychiatric Association: Diagnostic and statistical manual of mental disorders, third edition, Washington, D.C., APA, 1980.

Substance-induced mental disorder

Code severity of dementia in fifth digit: 1 = mild, 2 = moderate, 3 = severe, 0 = unspecified.

Alcohol

303.00 intoxication
291.40 idiosyncratic intoxication
291.80 withdrawal
291.00 withdrawal delirium
291.30 hallucinosis
291.10 amnestic disorder
291.2(x) Dementia associated with alcoholism, _____

Barbiturate or similarly acting sedative or hypnotic

305.40 intoxication (327.00)
292.00 withdrawal (327.01)
292.00 withdrawal delirium (327.02)
292.83 amnestic disorder (327.04)

Opioid

305.50 intoxication (327.10)
292.00 withdrawal (327.11)

Cocaine

305.60 intoxication (327.20)

Amphetamine or similarly acting sympathomimetic

305.70 intoxication (327.30)
292.81 delirium (327.32)
292.11 delusional disorder (327.35)
292.00 withdrawal (327.31)

Phencyclidine (PCP) or similarly acting arylcyclohexylamine

305.90 intoxication (327.40)
292.81 delirium (327.42)
292.90 mixed organic mental disorder (327.49)

Hallucinogen

305.30 hallucinosis (327.56)
292.11 delusional disorder (327.55)
292.84 affective disorder (327.57)

Cannabis

305.20 intoxication (327.60)
292.11 delusional disorder (327.65)

Tobacco

292.00 withdrawal (327.71)

Caffeine

305.90 intoxication (327.80)

Other or unspecified substance

305.90 intoxication (327.90)
292.00 withdrawal (327.91)
292.81 delirium (327.92)
292.82 dementia (327.93)
292.83 amnestic disorder (327.94)
292.11 delusional disorder (327.95)
292.12 hallucinosis (327.96)
292.84 affective disorder (327.97)
292.89 personality disorder (327.98)
292.90 atypical or mixed organic mental disorder (327.99)

Section 2. Organic brain syndromes whose etiology or pathophysiological process is either noted as an additional diagnosis from outside the mental disorders section of ICD-9-CM or is unknown.

293.00 Delirium
294.10 Dementia
294.00 Amnestic syndrome
293.81 Organic delusional syndrome
293.82 Organic hallucinosis
293.83 Organic affective syndrome
310.10 Organic personality syndrome
294.80 Atypical or mixed organic brain syndrome

SUBSTANCE USE DISORDERS

Code in fifth digit: 1 = continuous, 2 = episodic, 3 = in remission, 0 = unspecified.

305.0(x) Alcohol abuse, _____
303.9(x) Alcohol dependence (alcoholism), _____
305.4(x) Barbiturate or similarly acting sedative or hypnotic abuse, _____
304.1(x) Barbiturate or similarly acting sedative or hypnotic dependence, _____
305.5(x) Opioid abuse, _____
304.0(x) Opioid dependence, _____
305.6(x) Cocaine abuse, _____
305.7(x) Amphetamine or similarly acting sympathomimetic abuse, _____
304.4(x) Amphetamine or similarly acting sympathomimetic dependence, _____
305.9(x) Phencyclidine (PCP) or similarly acting arylcyclohexylamine abuse, _____ (328.4[x])
305.3(x) Hallucinogen abuse, _____
305.2(x) Cannabis abuse, _____
304.3(x) Cannabis dependence, _____
305.1(x) Tobacco dependence, _____
305.9(x) Other, mixed or unspecified substance abuse, _____
304.6(x) Other specified substance dependence, _____
304.9(x) Unspecified substance dependence, _____
304.7(x) Dependence on combination of opioid and other nonalcoholic substance, _____
304.8(x) Dependence on combination of substances, excluding opioids and alcohol, _____

SCHIZOPHRENIC DISORDERS

Code in fifth digit: 1 = subchronic, 2 = chronic, 3 = subchronic with acute exacerbation, 4 = chronic with acute exacerbation, 5 = in remission, 0 = unspecified.

Schizophrenia,

295.1(x) disorganized, _____
295.2(x) catatonic, _____
295.3(x) paranoid, _____
295.9(x) undifferentiated, _____
295.6(x) residual, _____

DSM-III CLASSIFICATION: AXES I AND II CATEGORIES AND CODES—cont'd

PARANOID DISORDERS
297.10 Paranoia
297.30 Shared paranoid disorder
298.30 Acute paranoid disorder
297.90 Atypical paranoid disorder

PSYCHOTIC DISORDERS NOT ELSEWHERE CLASSIFIED
295.40 Schizophreniform disorder
298.80 Brief reactive psychosis
295.70 Schizoaffective disorder
298.90 Atypical psychosis

NEUROTIC DISORDERS
These are included in affective, anxiety, somatoform, dissociative, and psychosexual disorders. In order to facilitate the identification of the categories that in DSM-II were grouped together in the class of Neuroses, the DSM-II terms are included separately in parentheses after the corresponding categories. These DSM-II terms are included in ICD-9-CM and therefore are acceptable as alternatives to the recommended DSM-III terms that precede them.

AFFECTIVE DISORDERS
Major affective disorders
Code major depressive episode in fifth digit: 6 = in remission, 4 = with psychotic features (the unofficial non-ICD-9-CM fifth digit 7 may be used instead to indicate that the psychotic features are mood incongruent), 3 = with melancholia, 2 = without melancholia, 0 = unspecified.
Code manic or mixed episode in fifth digit: 6 = in remission, 4 = with psychotic features (the unofficial non-ICD-9-CM fifth digit 7 may be used instead to indicate that the psychotic features are mood incongruent), 2 = without psychotic features, 0 = unspecified.
   Bipolar disorder,
296.6(x) mixed, _____
296.4(x) manic, _____
296.5(x) depressed, _____
   Major depression,
296.2(x) single episode, _____
296.3(x) recurrent, _____

Other specific affective disorders
301.13 Cyclothymic disorder
306.40 Dysthymic disorder (or depressive neurosis)

Atypical affective disorders
296.70 Atypical bipolar disorder
296.82 Atypical depression

ANXIETY DISORDERS
Phobic disorders (or phobic neuroses)
300.21 Agoraphobia with panic attacks
300.22 Agoraphobia without panic attacks
300.23 Social phobia
300.29 Simple phobia
   Anxiety states (or anxiety neuroses)
300.01 Panic disorder
300.02 Generalized anxiety disorder
300.30 Obsessive compulsive disorder (or obsessive compulsive neurosis)
   Posttraumatic stress disorder
308.30 acute
309.81 chronic or delayed
300.00 Atypical anxiety disorder

SOMATOFORM DISORDERS
300.81 Somatization disorder
300.11 Conversion disorder (or hysterical neurosis, conversion type)
307.80 Psychogenic pain disorder
300.70 Hypochondriasis (or hypochondriacal neurosis)
300.70 Atypical somatoform disorder (300.71)

DISSOCIATIVE DISORDERS (OR HYSTERICAL NEUROSES, DISSOCIATIVE TYPE)
300.12 Psychogenic amnesia
300.13 Psychogenic fugue
300.14 Multiple personality
300.60 Depersonalization disorder (or depersonalization neurosis)
300.15 Atypical dissociative disorder

PSYCHOSEXUAL DISORDERS
Gender identity disorders
Indicate sexual history in the fifth digit of transsexualism code: 1 = asexual, 2 = homosexual, 3 = heterosexual, 0 = unspecified.
302.5(x) Transsexualism, _____
302.60   Gender identity disorder of childhood
302.85   Atypical gender identity disorder

Paraphilias
302.81 Fetishism
302.30 Transvestism
302.10 Zoophilia
302.20 Pedophilia
302.40 Exhibitionism
302.82 Voyeurism
302.83 Sexual masochism
302.84 Sexual sadism
302.90 Atypical paraphilia

Psychosexual dysfunctions

302.71 Inhibited sexual desire
302.72 Inhibited sexual excitement
302.73 Inhibited female orgasm
302.74 Inhibited male orgasm
302.75 Premature ejaculation
302.76 Functional dyspareunia
306.51 Functional vaginismus
302.70 Atypical psychosexual dysfunction

Other psychosexual disorders

302.00 Ego-dystonic homosexuality
302.89 Psychosexual disorder not elsewhere classified

FACTITIOUS DISORDERS

300.16 Factitious disorder with psychological symptoms
301.51 Chronic factitious disorder with physical symptoms
300.19 Atypical factitious disorder with physical symptoms

DISORDERS OF IMPULSE CONTROL NOT ELSEWHERE CLASSIFIED

312.31 Pathological gambling
312.32 Kleptomania
312.33 Pyromania
312.34 Intermittent explosive disorder
312.35 Isolated explosive disorder
312.39 Atypical impulse control disorder

ADJUSTMENT DISORDER

309.00 with depressed mood
309.24 with anxious mood
309.28 with mixed emotional features
309.30 with disturbance of conduct
309.40 with mixed disturbance of emotions and conduct
309.23 with work (or academic) inhibition
309.83 with withdrawal
309.90 with atypical features

PSYCHOLOGICAL FACTORS AFFECTING PHYSICAL CONDITION

Specify physical condition on axis III.
316.00 Psychological factors affecting physical condition

PERSONALITY DISORDERS (CODED ON AXIS II)

301.00 Paranoid
301.20 Schizoid
301.22 Schizotypal
301.50 Histrionic
301.81 Narcissistic
301.70 Antisocial
301.83 Borderline
301.82 Avoidant
301.60 Dependent
301.40 Compulsive
301.84 Passive-aggressive
301.89 Atypical, mixed or other personality disorder

V CODES FOR CONDITIONS NOT ATTRIBUTABLE TO A MENTAL DISORDER THAT ARE A FOCUS OF ATTENTION OR TREATMENT

V65.20 Malingering
V62.89 Borderline intellectual functioning (V62.88)
V71.01 Adult antisocial behavior
V71.02 Childhood or adolescent antisocial behavior
V62.30 Academic problem
V62.20 Occupational problem
V62.82 Uncomplicated bereavement
V15.81 Noncompliance with medical treatment
V62.89 Phase of life problem or other life circumstance problem
V61.10 Marital problem
V61.20 Parent-child problem
V61.80 Other specified family circumstances
V62.81 Other interpersonal problem

ADDITIONAL CODES

300.90 Unspecified mental disorder (nonpsychotic)
V71.09 No diagnosis or condition on axis I
No diagnosis on axis II
799.90 Diagnosis or condition deferred on axis I
Diagnosis deferred on axis II

TABLE 2-1. Severity of psychosocial stressors (axis IV)

Code	Term	Adult examples	Child or adolescent examples	Code	Term	Adult examples	Child or adolescent examples
1	None	No apparent psychosocial stressor	No apparent psychosocial stressor	6	Extreme	Death of close relative, divorce	Death of parent or sibling, repeated physical or sexual abuse
2	Minimal	Minor violation of law, small bank loan	Vacation with family	7	Catastrophic	Concentration camp experience, devastating natural disaster	Multiple family deaths
3	Mild	Argument with neighbor, change in work hours	Change in schoolteacher, new school year	0	Unspecified	No information or not applicable	No information or not applicable
4	Moderate	New career, death of close friend, pregnancy	Chronic parental fighting, change to new school, illness of close relative, birth of sibling				
5	Severe	Serious illness in self or family, major financial loss, marital separation, birth of child	Death of peer, divorce of parents, arrest, hospitalization, persistent and harsh parental discipline				

*From American Psychiatric Association: Diagnostic and statistical manual of mental disorders, third edition, Washington, D.C., APA, 1980.

psychiatric care. Specialized clinical settings or individuals who are conducting psychiatric research may choose to include axes IV and V as well. Axis IV documents the severity of psychosocial stressors on a scale of one to seven (Table 2-1).[2] Axis V rates the patient's highest level of adaptive functioning in the last year (Table 2-2).[2] The fact that axis IV and V information is not routinely included in the medical diagnosis illustrates one of the important differences between psychiatry and psychiatric nursing. These factors would always be important to include when formulating a nursing diagnosis.

After the diagnosis is formulated, treatment is instituted. The physician-patient relationship is fostered to engender trust in the physician and compliance with the treatment plan. If indicated, the therapist will also assist the patient to look at the stressful situation in his life and his usual style of coping. Other health team members may be enlisted to contribute their expertise to the patient's care. Response to treatment is evaluated on the basis of the patient's subjective assessment of how he is feeling combined with the therapist's objective observations of the occurrence of symptomatic behavior. In some cases therapy may be terminated when the patient returns to a satisfactory functional level. For instance, the person who has experienced a reactive depression may, after a short course of medication and supportive therapy, be able to return to his usual life-style. Other patients will require long-term follow-up therapy, often including pharmacotherapy. For example, the patient with manic-depressive illness will need to take lithium carbonate indefinitely and will also need to see a therapist for observation of behavior and periodic laboratory studies. Still other patients may receive long-term insight-oriented therapy to assist them to learn improved methods of coping with stressors.

Roles of the patient and the medical therapist

The roles of physician and patient have been well defined by tradition and hold true in the psychiatric setting. The physician is the healer. This role entails responsible identification of the patient's illness and instituting a treatment plan

TABLE 2-2. Axis V rating scale

Levels	Adult examples	Child or adolescent examples
1 Superior—Unusually effective functioning in social relations, occupational functioning, and use of leisure time	Single parent living in deteriorating neighborhood takes excellent care of children and home, has warm relations with friends, and finds time for pursuit of hobby	A 12-year-old girl gets superior grades in school, is extremely popular among her peers, and excels in many sports; she does all of this with apparent ease and comfort
2 Very good—Better than average functioning in social relations, occupational functioning, and use of leisure time	A 65-year-old retired widower does some volunteer work, often sees old friends, and pursues hobbies	An adolescent boy gets excellent grades, works part time, has several close friends, and plays banjo in a jazz band; he admits to some distress in "keeping up with everything"
3 Good—No more than slight impairment in either social or occupational functioning	A woman with many friends functions extremely well at a difficult job, but says "the strain is too much"	An 8-year-old boy does well in school, has several friends, but bullies younger children
4 Fair—Moderate impairment in either social relations or occupational functioning or some impairment in both	A lawyer has trouble carrying through assignments, has several acquaintances, but hardly any close friends	A 10-year-old girl does poorly in school, but has adequate peer and family relations
5 Poor—Marked impairment in either social relations or occupational functioning or moderate impairment in both	A man with one or two friends has trouble keeping a job for more than a few weeks	A 14-year-old boy almost fails in school and has trouble getting along with his peers
6 Very poor—Marked impairment in both social relations and occupational functioning	A woman is unable to do any of her housework and has violent outbursts toward family and neighbors	A 6-year-old girl needs special help in all subjects and has virtually no peer relationships
7 Grossly impaired—Gross impairment in virtually all areas of functioning	An elderly man needs supervision to maintain minimal personal hygiene and is usually incoherent	A 4-year-old boy needs constant restraint to avoid hurting himself and is almost totally lacking in skills
0 Unspecified	No information	No information

*From American Psychiatric Association: Diagnostic and statistical manual of mental disorders, third edition, Washington, D.C., APA, 1980.

that will not be harmful to the patient. Although the patient may have input into the plan, the physician prescribes the recommended form of therapy and generally applies the power inherent in his high-status position if the patient refuses to comply with the plan. Patients are frequently not encouraged to question the physician's decision.

The patient is expected to assume the behavior of the sick role. This involves an admission that he is ill, which can be a problem in psychiatry. Patients are sometimes not aware of their disturbed behavior and may actively resist treatment, which is not congruent with the medical model. Another expectation of the patient is that he comply with the treatment program and work hard to get well. Inherent in this expectation is the anticipation that observable improvement will occur. If it does not, there are frequently suspicions expressed by caregivers and significant others that the patient is not trying hard enough. This can be frustrating to a patient who feels he is trying to get well and is disappointed at his own lack of progress. The patient may also have difficulty meeting the expectation that he let people take care of him but also that he try to help himself. These two activities are often not compatible, and it may be difficult to comply with both. The patient who is unable to respond to the therapy offered may be transferred to another physician, another mental health professional, or to a long-term custodial institution where his deviant behavior will be tolerated.

Nursing model

Since nursing is in the process of coming of age as a profession, there is still no one universally accepted theoretical model for the provision of nursing care. However, nursing theorists have proposed several models that are currently being explored and refined. These include models based on general systems theory, developmental theories, and interaction theory.[14] There are some general similarities among these nursing models. They all incorporate a holistic approach to the individual, with attention given to biological, psychological, and social needs. Nursing care delivery is viewed as a collaborative process, with both the nurse and the patient contributing ideas and energy to the therapeutic process. The focus is on the caring functions of nurses, which are distinct from, but complementary to, the curing functions of physicians.

Nurses are experts at observing and interpreting patient's behavior. They also assist the patient to assess his own behavior, identify unfulfilling behaviors, and undertake behavioral change. Caring also implies concern about the patient's emotional response to the problem. The nurse therefore also utilizes comfort measures to ease the patient's pain, emotional as well as physical. To understand the patient as a whole person, time must be spent talking with him and establishing a therapeutic nurse-patient relationship. The nurse also acts as a patient advocate. When appropriate, she represents the patient in the health care system and helps to interpret his needs to significant others and to health team members.

Some prominent nursing theorists who have been developing models for nursing care delivery include Ida Jean Orlando, Hildegard Peplau, Joan Riehl, Sister Callista Roy, and Martha Rogers. The works of all of these nursing leaders are recommended to the reader to gain a broad appreciation of the issues currently being addressed in nursing. The remainder of this chapter reflects our philosophy of nursing. This model is discussed in detail in Chapter 4.

Nursing view of behavioral deviations

The focus of nursing is on the individual's response to potential or actual health problems.[1] The defining characteristics of nursing as related to this focus include the *health-illness phenomena* that are encountered, the *theory base* for nursing care, the *nursing actions* that are carried out, and the *effects* that are identified as a result of nursing intervention.[1]

Behavior is viewed on a continuum from healthy, adaptive responses to maladaptive responses that are indicative of illness. The actual behavior observed is the result of a number of factors. Each individual is predisposed to respond to life events in unique ways. These predispositions are biological, psychological and sociocultural and are the sum of the person's heritage and past experiences. Behavior is the result of the combination of the predisposing factors with precipitating stressors. Stressors are life events that are perceived by the individual as challenging, threatening, or demanding. The nature of the behavioral response depends on the person's primary appraisal of the stressor and secondary appraisal of the coping resources that are available to him. The continuum of coping responses may then include actual health problems that lead to a medical diagnosis or potential health problems. Nursing intervention may take place at any point on the continuum. Nursing diagnoses may focus on behaviors associated with a medical diagnosis or other health behaviors that the patient wishes to change. A nurse may practice primary prevention by intervening in a potential health problem, secondary prevention by intervening in an actual acute health problem, or tertiary prevention by intervening to limit the disability caused by actual chronic health problems.

Human behavior is viewed from a holistic perspective. A stressor that has primary impact on physiological functioning will also affect the person's psychological and sociocultural behavior. For instance, a man who has had a myocardial infarction may also become severely depressed because he fears he will lose his ability to work and to satisfy his wife sexually. On the other hand, the patient who enters the psychiatric inpatient unit with an endogenous depression may be suffering from malnutrition and dehydration because of refusal to eat or drink. The holistic nature of nursing encompasses all these facets of behavior and incorporates them into patient care planning.

The nursing therapeutic process

Psychiatric nurses base their care of patients on the nursing process, including the steps of data collection, formulation of the nursing diagnosis, planning, implementation, and evaluation. Data collection includes the eliciting of a complete health history, learning the patient's perception of his problems and their causes, and assessing strengths and weaknesses of the patient system and the social system. The nurse attempts to identify the predisposing factors and the precipitating stressors to the immediate problem. She also assesses the patient's biopsychosocial behavior in terms of norms for a person of the patient's age, sex, and sociocultural background and consults professional literature. Inferences are validated with the patient to limit the introduction of bias. Other resources for data collection include the patient's health records, significant others, and other health professionals who have provided care to the patient. Data are collected more systematically when the nurse uses a data collection tool that incorporates information about the total health status of the individual.

The nursing diagnosis is formulated on the basis of the collected data. It is a statement of the patient's nursing problem that incorporates the behavioral disruption and the stressor or stressors which are contributing to the actual or potential disruption. The nursing diagnosis provides the focus for nursing care and thus requires the input and concurrence, when possible, of the patient. It is not adequate to take note of the patient's medical diagnosis and use that as a basis for nursing care. Each patient differs from every other, and, although there may be common needs related to the medical diagnosis, there will also be individual needs related to that person's unique life experience.

Nursing care goals are formulated on the basis of the nursing diagnosis. Generally, both long- and short-term goals are developed. Long-term goals describe the health behavior to be accomplished when the identified problem is considered to be resolved. Short-term goals are contributory to the long-term goal.

Nursing actions are planned and implemented on the basis of nursing care goals combined with knowledge and review of nursing theory. Nursing care goals must be mutually developed with understanding of the patient's own goals for his health care. Goals should be stated in behavioral terms. It is important to establish priorities for the nursing care goals that have been mutually agreed on by the nurse and patient. This avoids fragmentation in the provision of nursing care.

Nursing actions may be dependent, based on the physician's order. For example, dispensing medication is a dependent nursing function. Other nursing actions are independent. Deciding to approach a patient who appears upset and allowing him to express his feelings is an independent nursing function. There are also interdependent nursing functions. Requesting the social worker to obtain information for the patient about his medical insurance and reinforcing the social worker's explanation is an interdependent function. All these levels of nursing should be incorporated into the written nursing care plan, since all are important to the total well-being of the patient. Nursing actions should also take advantage of the patient's strengths to build on the healthy aspects of his behavior. All patients have strengths. It is a nursing challenge to discover them and capitalize on them. Well-planned nursing intervention will assist the patient to accomplish the major goals of developing insight and carrying out a plan of positive action.

Nursing actions may also include various psychotherapeutic modalities of care, depending on the nurse's level of professional experience and education. Nurses with advanced psychiatric preparation may be qualified to conduct individual, group, or family psychotherapy, psychodrama, assertiveness training, behavior modification, or other specialized therapies. Many of these therapeutic modalities may be recognized as having been mentioned earlier in this chapter. The nursing model does not preclude the use of any modality of care delivery as long as the nurse is skilled in its application and receives adequate supervision. Nursing care is always implemented with respect for the rights and dignity of the patient and with empathy for the patient as a troubled person who deserves concern and caring. To ensure the highest quality of patient care, the nursing care plan must take into account the potential contributions of the entire health care team and particularly the preferences, wants, and needs of the patient.

Nursing care is continuously evaluated and modified by the patient and the nurse as the nursing process is used. Modifications are made in each phase of the nursing care plan on the basis of the evaluation. The most important factor in the evaluation process is the patient's reaction to the nursing care. Therefore the patient must be an active participant in this process. Validation with the patient is essential to be sure that the nurse's inferences are correct. Ongoing evaluation can add flexibility to nursing care, allowing the nurse and patient to explore alternatives and make choices concerning the most helpful interventions.

Nursing care is terminated mutually by the patient and the nurse. Termination is based on the successful accomplishment of the identified goals. At other times termination results because the patient or the nurse must leave the care delivery system or because the patient chooses not to comply with the identified plan. Whatever the reason for the termination, there should be a final evaluation of the nursing care episode. This serves as a learning and growth experience for the patient and the nurse.

Roles of the patient and the nurse

The nurse-patient relationship is based on mutuality. The needs of the patient are the focus of the relationship. Emphasis is on the strengths of the patient as a person and his growth potential. The patient is an active participant in the nursing care and is asked for feedback about the effectiveness of that care. Modifications in the care plan result from the collaboration of the nurse and patient. Another role assumed by the patient is that of learner, as the nurse strives to make him aware of his health needs and helps him to understand the nature of his health problems.

The nurse coordinates the patient's health care experience. She elicits his needs and, when necessary, interprets these needs to other mental health team members. She applies her knowledge of nursing theory and the biological and social sciences to the patient's health problem and utilizes this knowledge to devise a sophisticated plan of care. She is also responsible for the patient understanding this plan. If he seems puzzled or is noncompliant, the nurse explores his understanding and explains the nursing care plan as needed. Most important, the nurse cares for the patient, in the fullest sense of caring. She listens to his problems nonjudgmentally. She empathizes and helps him to identify and articulate his feelings. She is accessible at the time a need arises and conveys a sense of availability to the patient. She engenders trust by being consistent and reliable and by maintaining confidentiality. She encourages the patient to be as independent as possible but also allows dependency when this is necessary. Through the application of psychomotor and interpersonal skills, the nurse assists the patient to grow and to reach his maximal functional capabilities.

Suggested cross-references

The model of health-illness phenomena, which describes the relationship between nursing and medical diagnosis and the elements of the nursing process, is discussed in Chapter 4 and integrated throughout the other chapters of the book. Medical diagnostic categories are integrated throughout Chapters 7 to 14. Primary intervention strategies based on the medical and behavioral models are discussed in Chapter 5. Community mental health is discussed in Chapter 19. For further discussion of crisis intervention and the consultation process, see Chapters 16 and 23. Behavior modification is discussed in Chapter 21.

SUMMARY

Model	View of behavioral deviation	Therapeutic process	Role of patient and therapist
Psychoanalytical	Based on early development and inadequate resolution of developmental conflicts. Ego defenses inadequate to control anxiety. Symptoms result as effort to deal with anxiety and are related to unresolved conflicts.	Psychoanalysis uses techniques of free association and dream analysis. Interprets behavior. Uses transference to revise earlier traumatic experiences. Identifies problem areas through interpretation of patient's resistances.	Patient verbalizes all thoughts and dreams; considers therapist's interpretations. Long-term commitment to frequent therapy sessions. Therapist remains remote to encourage development of transference. Interprets patient's thoughts and dreams in terms of conflicts, transference, and resistance.
Interpersonal	Anxiety arises and is experienced interpersonally. Symptoms occur when security operations are unable to protect the self from anxiety. Basic fear is fear of rejection. Person needs security and satisfaction that result from positive interpersonal relationships.	Relationship between therapist and patient builds feeling of security. Therapist helps patient experience trusting relationship and gain interpersonal satisfaction. Patient then assisted to develop close relationships outside therapy situation.	Patient shares with therapist anxieties and feelings as he is able. Therapist develops close relationship with patient. Uses empathy to perceive patient's feelings. Uses relationship as a corrective interpersonal experience.
Social	Social and environmental factors create stress, which causes anxiety, resulting in symptom formation. Unacceptable (deviant) behavior is socially defined and meets needs of social and political system.	Patient helped to deal with social system. May use crisis intervention. Environmental manipulation and enlistment of special supports also employed. Peer support encouraged.	Patient actively presents problem to therapist and works with therapist toward resolution. Utilizes community resources. Therapist explores patient's social system and helps patient use resources available. Works to create new resources when needed.
Existential	Life is meaningful when one can fully experience and accept the self. Behavioral deviation is expression of the individual as he is thwarted in his effort to find and accept self. The self can be experienced through authentic relationships with other people.	Person aided to experience authenticity in relationships. Therapy frequently conducted in groups. Patient encouraged to explore and to accept self. Patient helped to assume control of his behavior.	Patient assumes responsibility for behavior. Participates in meaningful experiences to learn about real self. Therapist helps patient to recognize value of self. Clarifies realities of situation. Introduces patient to genuine feelings and expanded awareness.
Communication	Behavioral disruptions occur when messages are not clearly communicated. Language can be used to distort meaning. Messages may be transmitted simultaneously at several levels. Verbal and nonverbal messages may lack congruence. These conditions result in behavioral deviations.	Communication patterns analyzed. Feedback given to clarify problem areas. Family therapy frequently used to help modify lack of congruence or complementarity in communication. Transactional analysis focuses on games and learning to communicate directly without game playing.	Patient looks at communication patterns, including games. Works to clarify own communication and validate messages from others. Therapist interprets communication pattern to patient. Helps him improve communication with significant others. Teaches principles of good communication.

Model	View of behavioral deviation	Therapeutic process	Role of patient and therapist
Behavioral	Behavior is learned. Deviations occur because person has formed undesirable behavioral habits. Since behavior is learned, it can also be unlearned. Deviant behavior may be perpetuated because it reduces anxiety. If so, another anxiety-reducing behavior may be substituted.	Therapy is educational process. Behavioral deviations not rewarded. More productive behaviors reinforced. Reciprocal inhibition involves substituting an acceptable behavior that reduces anxiety for deviance. Relaxation therapy and assertiveness training are behavioral approaches.	Patient practices behavioral technique used. Does homework and reinforcement exercises. Helps develop behavioral hierarchies. Therapist determines behavioral technique. Teaches patient about behavioral approach. Helps develop behavioral hierarchy. Reinforces desired behaviors.
Medical	Behavioral disruptions result from a disease process, probably originating in central nervous system. Symptoms result from a combination of physiological, genetic, environmental, and social factors. Deviant behavior relates to patient's tolerance for stress.	Diagnosis of illness is based on present condition and historical information plus diagnostic studies, and treatment is related to diagnosis. Frequently includes somatic therapies in addition to various interpersonal techniques. Treatment approach adjusted depending on symptomatic response. Other mental health professionals involved when their expertise required.	Patient practices prescribed therapy regimen. Reports effects of therapy to physician. Complies with long-term therapy if necessary. Therapist uses combination of somatic and interpersonal therapies. Diagnoses illness and prescribes therapeutic approach. May teach patient about illness.
Nursing	Person is biopsychosocial entity who responds to stress in an individualized way. Behavioral disruptions affect whole person. Observable behaviors must be related to predisposing factors and precipitating stressors involved. Every person demonstrates strengths as well as weaknesses. Adaptive responses to stress (health) and maladaptive responses (illness) are on a continuum of potential behaviors.	Nursing process includes data collection, formulation of a nursing diagnosis, planning, implementation, and ongoing concurrent evaluation, resulting in modification of care plan. Plan is mutually formulated with patient. Nurse collaborates with other caregivers. Long- and short-term goals specified.	Patient collaborates in development of nursing care plan. Participates in evaluation and modification of treatment. Therapist collaborates with patient and other health team members in developing plan of care. Modifies plan based on patient feedback and own observations. May use many therapeutic modalities within nursing process framework, depending on education, experience, and available supervision.

References

1. American Nurses' Association: Nursing: a social policy statement, Kansas City, Mo., 1980, The Association.
2. American Psychiatric Association: Diagnostic and statistical manual of mental disorders, ed. 3, Washington, D.C., 1980, The Association.
3. Berne, E.: What do you say after you say hello? New York, Grove Press, Inc.
4. Black, Sr. K.M.: An existential model for psychiatric nursing, Perspect. Psychiatr. Care **6:**185, July-Aug. 1968.
5. Brown, J.A.C.: Freud and the post-Freudians, Baltimore, 1961, Penguin Books, Inc.
6. Caplan, G.: Principles of preventive psychiatry, New York, 1964, Basic Books, Inc.
7. Cautela, J.: Behavior therapy. In Hersher, L., editor: Four psychotherapies, New York, 1970, Appleton-Century-Crofts.
8. Ehrenwald, J.: The history of psychotherapy, New York, 1976, Jason Aronson, Inc.
9. Ellis, A.: Rational-emotive therapy. In Hersher, L., editor: Four psychotherapies, New York, 1970, Appleton-Century-Crofts.
10. Frankl, V.: Man's search for meaning, New York, 1959, The Beacon Press.
11. Harper, R.A.: The new psychotherapies, Englewood Cliffs, N.J., 1975, Prentice-Hall, Inc.
12. Laing, R.D.: The politics of experience, New York, 1967, Ballantine Books.

13. Peplau, H.E.: Interpersonal relations in nursing, New York, 1952, G.P. Putnam's Sons.
14. Riehl, J.P., and Roy, C.: Conceptual models for nursing practice, New York, 1974, Appleton-Century-Crofts.
15. Siegler, M., and Osmond, H.: Models of madness, models of medicine, New York, 1976, Harper Colophon Books.
16. Sullivan, H.S.: The psychiatric interview, New York, 1954, W.W. Norton & Co., Inc.
17. Szasz, T.S.: Ideology and insanity, Garden City, N.Y., 1970, Anchor Books, Doubleday Publishing Co.
18. Szasz, T.S.: The second sin, Garden City, N.Y., 1974, Anchor Books, Doubleday Publishing Co.
19. Watzlawick, P., Beavin, J.H., and Jackson, D.D.: Pragmatics of human communication, New York, 1967, W.W. Norton & Co., Inc.

Annotated suggested readings

The following selections are representative works of respected psychiatric theorists. All are recommended as resources of classical approaches to psychiatry.

Adler, A.: The practice and theory of individual psychology, New York, 1929, Harcourt, Brace & Co.
Berne, E.: Transactional analysis in psychotherapy, New York, 1961, Grove Press, Inc.
Berne, E.: Games people play, New York, 1964, Grove Press, Inc.
Caplan, G.: Principles of preventive psychiatry, New York, 1964, Basic Books, Inc.
Ellis, A., and Harper, R.A.: A guide to rational living, Englewood Cliffs, N.J., 1961, Prentice-Hall, Inc.
Erikson, E.: Childhood and society, ed. 2, New York, 1963, W.W. Norton & Co., Inc.
Frankl, V.: Man's search for meaning, New York, 1959, The Beacon Press.
Freud, A.: The ego and the mechanisms of defense, New York, 1966, International Universities Press.
Freud, S.: In Strachey, J., editor: The standard edition of the complete psychological works of Sigmund Freud, London, 1953-1974, Hogarth Press.
Fromm-Reichmann, F.: Principles of intensive psychotherapy, Chicago, 1950, The University of Chicago Press.
Fromm-Reichmann, F.: In Bullard, D.M., editor: Psychoanalysis and psychotherapy, selected papers, Chicago, 1959, The University of Chicago Press.
Glasser, W.: Reality therapy: a new approach to psychiatry, New York, 1965, Harper & Row, Publishers.
Horney, K.: The collected works of Karen Horney, vols. 1 and 2, New York, 1937-1950, W.W. Norton & Co., Inc.
Jung, C.G., Mayman, M., and Pruyser, P.: The psychogenesis of mental disease, New York, 1960, Pantheon Books.
Klein, M.: The psychoanalysis of children, London, 1949, Hogarth Press.
Laing, R.D.: The politics of experience, New York, 1967, Ballantine Books.
Menninger, K.A.: The vital balance, New York, 1963, Viking Press.
Peplau, H.E.: Interpersonal relations in nursing, New York, 1952, G.P. Putnam's Sons.
Perls, F.S.: In and out of the garbage pail, Lafayette, Calif., 1969, Real People Press.
Rogers, C.R.: Client-centered therapy, Boston, 1951, Houghton Mifflin Co.
Rogers, C.R.: Carl Rogers on encounter groups, New York, 1970, Harper & Row, Publishers, Inc.
Schutz, W.C.: Joy, New York, 1967, Grove Press, Inc.
Sullivan, H.S.: In Perry, H.S., and Gawel, M.L., editors: The interpersonal theory of psychiatry, New York, 1953, W.W. Norton & Co., Inc.
Sullivan, H.S.: In Perry, H.S., and Gawel, M.L., editors: The psychiatric interview, New York, 1954, W.W. Norton & Co., Inc.
Szasz, T.: The myth of mental illness, New York, 1961, Hoeber-Harper.
Watzlawick, P., Beavin, J.H., and Jackson, D.D.: Pragmatics of human communication, New York, 1967, W.W. Norton & Co., Inc.
Wolpe, J.: The practice of behavior therapy, ed. 2, New York, 1973, Pergamon Press.

The following selections include anthologies of theoretical approaches to psychiatry. There are also several selections of interest to the nurse who is developing a conceptual approach to psychiatry.

Black, Sr. K.: An existential model for psychiatric nursing, Perspect. Psychiatr. Care **6:**178, July-Aug. 1968.
This article discusses the concept of the existential encounter as it applies to the therapeutic nurse-patient relationship. A basic respect for the dignity of the patient is conveyed and the model is illustrated with a clinical example.
Brown, J.A.C.: Freud and the post-Freudians, Baltimore, 1961, Penguin Books, Inc.
This book presents a review of the works of the major post-Freudian theorists, allowing the reader to compare them with Freud and each other.
Clark, C.C.: Combining therapeutic approaches, J. Psychiatr. Nurs. **15:**18, Oct. 1977.
This author compares and contrasts two apparently incompatible approaches to psychotherapy: psychoanalysis and behavioral therapy. She demonstrates that a combination of these approaches may be used very effectively with some patients. She also identifies several commonalities between these models.
Clark, M.D.: Carl Rogers revisited, Can. J. Psychiatr. Nurs. **22:**14, Jan.-March 1981.
This article is a concise review of the principles of Rogers' approach to counseling. It is a good example of the application of a theoretical frame of reference to the therapy process.
Critchley, D.L.: The adverse influence of psychiatric diagnostic labels on observation of child behavior, Am. J. Orthopsychiatry **49:**157, Jan. 1979.
The author found that informing a student nurse of a psychiatric diagnosis for a child influenced the perception of the child's behavior. Children diagnosed as not normal were not perceived to behave normally, even when the

child was not, in reality, mentally ill. This demonstrates
the value of nursing research in model development and
also points out the dangers inherent in labeling behavior.

He also points out the problems of focusing on pathologic conditions rather than health, thereby reinforcing
sick behavior.

Ehrenwald, J.: The history of psychotherapy, New York,
1976, Jason Aronson, Inc.

This is a fascinating description of the historical development of models of psychotherapy, including both mysti-
cal/religious and scientific approaches. Theories are illustrated with lengthy and informative quotes from the
original theorist.

Frank, J.D.: Persuasion and healing, Baltimore, 1973, The
Johns Hopkins University Press.

This thought-provoking comparison of psychotherapy to
other forms of persuasion, such as religious revivalism,
and thought reform considers several models of psychiatric care in terms of this frame of reference. It is particularly useful for those who are engaged in psychotherapy.

Haley, J.: The art of psychoanalysis. In Haley, J.: The power
tactics of Jesus Christ, New York, 1969, Avon Books.

The author takes a provocative look at psychoanalysis
as a power relationship that is set up to enhance the superior position of the therapist. It is amusing reading, but
very thought-provoking.

Hall, C.S., and Lindzey, G.: Theories of personality, ed. 3,
New York, 1978, John Wiley & Sons, Inc.

This work is a thorough discussion of a wide range of
personality theories, primarily from a psychological approach. It is particularly useful as a reference on the behavioral models of therapy.

Harper, R.A.: The new psychotherapies, Englewood Cliffs,
N.J., 1975, Prentice-Hall, Inc.

This book is a concise and clearly written overview of
a variety of contemporary approaches to psychotherapy.
It would be most useful as an introduction to the basic
assumptions of the theories included.

Hersher, L.: Four psychotherapies, New York, 1970, Appleton-Century-Crofts.

This edited volume includes good descriptions of client-
centered, rational-emotive, behavior, and psychoanalytical therapies and provides an opportunity to compare and
contrast basic concepts of these theoretical approaches to
psychotherapy.

Mansfield, E.: A conceptual framework for psychiatric–
mental health nursing, J. Psychiatr. Nurs. **18:**34, June
1980.

This article describes a conceptual model for a graduate
program in psychiatric nursing. It incorporates theoretical concepts of general systems, human development,
communication, and self-esteem into a nursing process
model. Of particular interest are the author's suggestions
about the utility of the model for generating nursing
research.

Powers, M.E.: Universal utility of psychoanalytic theory for
nursing practice models, J. Psychiatr. Nurs. **18:**28, April
1980.

This author demonstrates that a nursing practice
model can accommodate the adaptation of a particular
theoretical concept. She applies classical psychoanalytical
theory to nursing in a way that challenges the reader
to agree or disagree with her assertion.

Riehl, J.P., and Roy, C.: Conceptual models for nursing practice, New York, 1974, Appleton-Century-Crofts.

This excellent discussion of the status of the development of models for nursing practice presents several nursing models in a format that allows the reader to make
comparisons. It is highly recommended for nurses at all
levels of experience and education.

Rosenhan, D.L.: On being sane in insane places, Science
179:250, 1973.

This report of admission of several pseudopatients to
psychiatric hospitals raises interesting questions about
the implications of labeling people as mentally ill. The
experiential aspect of being a psychiatric patient is also
recounted. The article is worthwhile reading for any
nurse.

Scheff, T.J.: Being mentally ill: a sociological theory, Chicago, 1966, Aldine Publishing Co.

The author discusses the definition of insanity from a
sociological framework and presents interesting material
on the experience of being a psychiatric patient and the
role of society in defining the conditions of insanity.

Siegler, M., and Osmond, H.: Models of madness, models of
medicine, New York, 1976, Harper Colophon Books.

This comparison of the medical model to other models
of psychiatric care presents the case for the continued use
of the medical model as the most helpful framework for
psychiatry.

Sundeen, S.J., et al.: Nurse-client interaction, ed. 2, St.
Louis, 1981, The C.V. Mosby Co.

This book provides discussion of nursing process and
includes a clinical example of the utilization of this
means of organizing nursing care planning.

Wolberg, L.R.: The techniques of psychotherapy, parts I
and II, ed. 2, New York, 1967, Grune & Stratton, Inc.

This is an extremely thorough presentation of basic
theories of psychotherapy, followed by a discussion of the
practice of psychotherapy. It is an excellent resource for
the experienced practitioner of psychiatric nursing. There
is also a discussion of psychosocial development, including
the theories of Freud, Erikson, and Sullivan.

CHAPTER 3

THE
THERAPEUTIC
NURSE-PATIENT
RELATIONSHIP

When we treat man as he is,
we make him worse than he is.
When we treat him as if he already were
what he potentially could be,
we make him what he should be.

Johann Wolfgang von Goethe

Learning objectives

After studying this chapter, the student should be able to:

- *state the nature and goals of the therapeutic nurse-patient relationship.*

- *discuss six personal qualities needed by the nurse to be an effective helper.*

- *describe the tasks of the nurse and particular problems that may arise in each of the four phases of the relationship process.*

- *relate the relevance of communication theory to nursing.*

- *compare and contrast the verbal and nonverbal levels of communication in types of behavior, effectiveness, factors limiting correct interpretation, and implications for nursing care.*

- *identify the three elements of the communication process.*

- *analyze the structural and transactional analysis models of the communication process with respect to the components of each and the communication problems they reveal.*

- *define and give examples of 12 therapeutic communication techniques.*

- *describe how each of the responsive dimensions of genuineness, respect, empathic understanding, and concreteness can be demonstrated by the nurse in a therapeutic relationship.*

61

■ *describe how each of the action dimensions of confrontation, immediacy, nurse self-disclosure, catharsis, and role playing can be demonstrated by the nurse in a therapeutic relationship.*

■ *define the following therapeutic impasses and identify nursing interventions that can effectively deal with them: resistance, transference, and counter-transference.*

■ *discuss the goals of supervision and the ways in which therapy and supervision are parallel processes.*

■ *assess the role of ethics in psychiatric nursing.*

■ *define an ethical dilemma and relate one that arises in psychiatric nursing practice.*

■ *apply the model for ethical decision making to a personally encountered ethical dilemma.*

■ *demonstrate increasing effectiveness in using therapeutic relationship skills with psychiatric patients.*

■ *identify suggested readings for future study.*

The therapeutic nurse-patient relationship is a mutual learning experience and a corrective emotional experience for the patient. It is predicated on Sullivan's observation "We are all more human than otherwise." In this relationship the nurse uses herself and specified clinical techniques in working with the patient to bring about behavioral change. In general, the goals of a therapeutic relationship are directed toward the growth of the patient and include the following:

1. Self-realization, self-acceptance, and an increased genuine self-respect
2. A clear sense of personal identity and an improved level of personal integration
3. An ability to form intimate, interdependent, interpersonal relationships with a capacity to give and receive love
4. Improved functioning and increased ability to satisfy needs and achieve realistic personal goals

To achieve these goals, various aspects of the patient's life experiences will be explored during the course of the relationship. The nurse will allow for the patient's expression of perceptions, thoughts, and feelings and relate these to observed and reported actions. Areas of conflict and anxiety will be clarified. It is also important for the nurse to identify and maximize the ego strengths of the patient and to encourage socialization and family relatedness. Problems of communication will be corrected and maladaptive behavior patterns modified as the patient tests out new patterns of behavior and coping mechanisms.

The nature of the nurse-patient relationship is characterized by the mutual growth of two individuals who "dare" to become related to discover love, growth, and freedom. It is an I-thou relationship,[11] or an authentic relationship between two people who are in the process of becoming. The uniqueness of each is valued, and there is respect for differing values. There is mutual satisfaction derived and the world of each is enlarged and enriched by the other. The communication is a dialogue or discussion, not a monologue, as deeply significant convictions are shared. The reality and worth of the patient are affirmed, which allows him to grasp and more fully define his ego identity. This requires the nurse to be open to experiences and willing to disclose aspects of her own being to the patient. Rogers summarizes the characteristics of helping relationships that facilitate growth in the following series of questions:

1. Can I *be* in some way which will be perceived by the other person as trustworthy, as dependable or consistent in some deep sense?
2. Can I be expressive enough as a person that what I am will be communicated unambiguously?
3. Can I let myself experience positive attitudes toward this other person—attitudes of warmth, caring, liking, interest, and respect?
4. Can I be strong enough as a person to be separate from the other?
5. Am I secure enough within myself to permit him his separateness?
6. Can I let myself enter fully into the world of his feelings and personal meaning and see these as he does?
7. Can I be acceptant of each facet of the other person which he presents to me? Can I receive him as he is? Can I communicate this attitude? Or can I only receive him conditionally, acceptant of some aspects of his feelings and silently or openly disapproving of others?
8. Can I act with sufficient sensitivity in the relationship that my behavior will not be perceived as a threat?
9. Can I free him from the threat of external evaluation?
10. Can I meet this other individual as a person who is in the process of *becoming,* or will I be bound by his past and my past?[51:50-51]

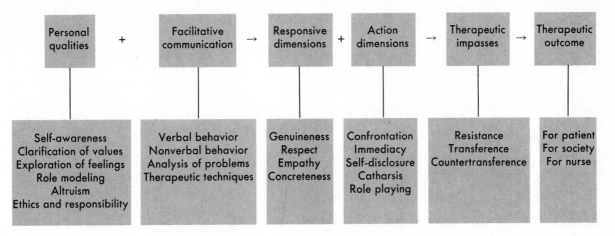

FIG. 3-1
Elements affecting the nurse's ability to be therapeutic.

All nurses working with patients may ask themselves these questions and must accept responsibility for the progress of the relationship. The therapeutic nurse-patient relationship is a complex one that can be analyzed in many different ways. Various elements and therapeutic dynamics of it merit further exploration. These include the nurse as helper, phases of the relationship, facilitative communication, responsive and action dimensions, therapeutic impasses, and effectiveness of the nurse. The interplay among the elements that produce a therapeutic outcome is shown in Fig. 3-1. The rest of this chapter will analyze each of these elements.

The nurse as helper

Helping others is a function of all concerned people, and it is not limited to health professionals. Neither is there a cluster of traits that describes a helping person who is universally effective. Nurses, however, as helpers, must be therapeutic in their care, since the goal of nursing is to facilitate the patient's positive adaptation as a unique individual to the stress he is experiencing.

The principal helping tool the nurse can use in her practice is herself. Thus self-analysis becomes the first building block in being able to provide quality nursing care. It has been suggested that nurses as professionals have become impersonal and detached. Is it possible that nurses are alienated from their true selves and do not allow patients the freedom to express all aspects of themselves? Jourard believes that dur-

ing the socialization process into nursing, the nurse's spontaneity is destroyed and she becomes detached from her real self:

> Now, if a nurse is afraid or even ignorant of her own self, she is highly likely to be threatened by a patient's real-self expressions. . . . A nurse who is more aware of the breadth and depth of her own real self is in a much better position to empathize with her patients and to encourage (or at least not block) their self-disclosures.[31:184]

Research on counselor and teacher effectiveness suggests some essential qualities associated with being able to help others. These can be viewed as necessary characteristics for all nurses who wish to be therapeutic. It is hoped that by describing these qualities in some detail, the nurse will be able to set goals for her future growth.

Awareness of self

There is universal agreement among theorists and practitioners that helpers need to be able to answer the question "Who am I?" The nurse who cares for the biological, psychological, and sociological needs of her patients will be exposed to a broad range of human experiences. She must learn to deal with anxiety, anger, sadness, and joy in helping patients at all intervals of the health-illness continuum. Her goal is the attainment of authentic, open, and personal communication. In her nursing care, she must be able to examine her own feelings and reactions as a person, as well as her actions as a professional pro-

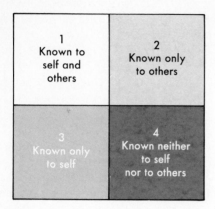

FIG. 3-2
Johari Window. Each quadrant, or windowpane, describes one aspect of the self. (From Sundeen, S.J. et al.: Nurse-client interaction: implementing the nursing process, ed. 2, St. Louis, 1981, The C.V. Mosby Co.)

vider of care. A firm understanding and acceptance of her own self will allow the nurse to acknowledge a patient's differences and uniqueness.

As an individual, no one ever completely knows his inner self. The Johari Window shown in Fig. 3-2 illustrates this idea.[39] Quadrant 1 is the open quadrant, which includes the behaviors, feelings, and thoughts known to the individual and those around him. Quadrant 2 is called the blind quadrant because it includes all those things which others know, but the individual does not know. Quadrant 3 is the hidden quadrant, and it includes those things which only the individual knows about himself. Quadrant 4 is the unknown quadrant, which contains aspects of the self unknown to the individual and others. Altogether, these quadrants represent the total self. The following three principles may help one understand how the self functions in this representation:

1. A change in any one quadrant will affect all other quadrants.
2. The smaller the first quadrant, the poorer the communication.
3. Interpersonal learning means that a change has taken place so that quadrant 1 is larger, and one or more of the other quadrants are smaller.[39:14]

The process of increasing self-awareness is now evident. The goal is to enlarge the area of quadrant 1, while reducing the size of the other three quadrants. The process of increasing

knowledge of self is begun by *listening to oneself.* This means allowing oneself to experience genuine emotions, identify and accept personal needs, and move one's body in free, joyful, and spontaneous ways. It includes exploring one's own thoughts, feelings, memories, and impulses:

> I am most alive when I am open to all the many facets of my inner living—desires, emotions, the flow of ideas, body sensations, relationships, reasoning, forethought, concern for others, my sense of values and all else within me. I am most alive when I can let myself experience and genuinely realize all of these facets even as I am truly feeling and expressing my wholeness.[12:276]

The next step in the process is to reduce the size of quadrant 2 by *listening to and learning from others.* Knowledge of oneself is not possible without association with other people. As a person relates to others, he broadens his perception of self. But such learning requires active listening and openness to the feedback others provide. The final step involves reducing the size of quadrant 3 by *self-disclosing,* or revealing to others important aspects of oneself. As Jourard states, "No man can come to know himself except as an outcome of disclosing himself to another person. Self-disclosure is a symptom of personality health and a means of achieving healthy personality."[31:6]

Compare *A* and *B* of Fig. 3-3. *A* represents a person with little self-awareness. His behaviors and feelings would tend to be limited in variety and scope. *B*, however, shows an individual with great openness to the world. Much of his potential is being developed and realized. He has an increased capacity for experiences of all kinds—joy, hate, work, and love. He has few defenses and can interact more spontaneously and honestly with others. This configuration represents a worthy goal for the nurse to attain for herself and others.

The consequences of being attuned with the inward sense of self are greater integration of the many aspects of one's being, greater feelings of vitality, better mobilization for action, more committed choices, and more authenticity in relationships.

It is frequently assumed that because a nursing student has taken some courses in the behavioral sciences, she is able to use herself in a therapeutic manner in the clinical setting. Most nursing textbooks that describe the nursing process include a paragraph or two, stressing the importance of self-awareness in quality nursing care. The process and components of self-

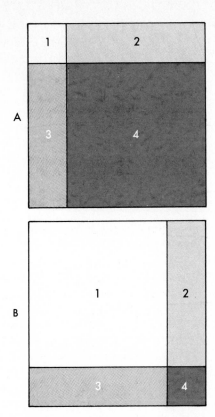

FIG. 3-3
Johari Windows showing varying degrees of self-awareness. **A,** Person with little self-understanding. **B,** Individual with great self-awareness. (From Sundeen, S.J. et al.: Nurse-client interaction: implementing the nursing process, ed. 2, St. Louis, 1981, The C.V. Mosby Co.)

growth for the nurse are never described. If a student took the initiative to seek out this information, she would discover that the nursing literature is seriously lacking in references which develop in depth the concept of self-awareness and its application to nursing. The self-concept of the patient is treated in a similarly cursory and general way. These omissions convey an implicit message to the nursing student: self-analysis is commendable, but a token assessment will suffice. To further reinforce this message, the student's curriculum is burdened with tasks and reports that allow little time for quiet contemplation leading to self-growth.

It is necessary that nurses have the time to explore and define the many facets of their personalities. If nursing does involve perceiving, feeling, and thinking, nursing students should have the time and opportunity to study the basics of their experiences. Authenticity in relationships must be learned. For the nurse to do

this, it is first necessary that she experience openness and authenticity in her relationships with instructors and supervisors. Rogers has stated that one might enhance another's personal growth by accepting this person as an individual and by viewing the world as it appears through his eyes.[51] The student and instructor can mutually participate in a relationship that accepts and respects individual differences. By acting as role models, instructors can facilitate students' self-awareness, increase their level of functioning, stimulate more self-direction, and enable them to cope more effectively with the stressors of life.

Authenticity also involves being truthful and open to exploring one's thoughts, needs, emotions, values, defenses, actions, communications, problems, and goals. In the process of becoming a nurse, the student has many new experiences providing opportunities for self-learning. Feelings about them should be focused on and discussed. The student might enter her clinical settings with high ideals and unrealistic images. Perhaps she views nurses as "miracle workers" who are all knowing and all caring in their mission. During her initial encounters she may feel fearful, anxious, and inadequate, and she may wonder how she will ever acquire the necessary knowledge. The student might devalue her ability and feel that she is imposing on her patients. Both her expectations and abilities should be analyzed to raise her self-esteem and reinforce her capabilities. At another time, she may identify closely with the patient and feel anger at the impersonal system and unresponsive personnel. Her anger should be identified, verbalized, and accepted. Only then can she analyze how she expresses anger and how she can resolve her feelings in a constructive manner.

It is not easy to embark on a career in nursing while still in adolescence. As a nurse, the student will be faced with many adult responsibilities. The student will be forced to face disease, bizarre behavior, complex problems, and even death when most of her friends are focusing on youth, enjoyment, and the future. This might alienate her from some friends and trigger feelings of despair and self-doubt. Her feelings of loneliness and sadness should be shared, so that she can experience the benefit of an interpersonal relationship in working through her own needs.

The development of self-awareness by the nurse must be a self-initiated process. She is an active participant in analyzing her thoughts, communications, and relationships with others. Because it is difficult to be participant and observer at the same time, other ways of collecting data should be used. Tape recordings provide an opportunity for the student to review her communications and study them more closely. Videotapes give feedback regarding nonverbal messages as well as tone and inflection. Maintaining a diary allows for the expression of feelings, the description of perceptions of the student's self-concept, and comments on the student's level of self-esteem.

This introspection should also be accompanied by self-disclosure. Sharing perceptions with others allows the nurse to gain new information and evolve new insights. The interaction with the analysis may be written in the form of a processed recording.[64] This disciplines the nurse to look beyond the obvious and take the time to explore her feelings. Her instructor can review the recording with her and identify areas that the student overlooked or blocked. Throughout her growing process, the student needs the support and guidance of her instructor. Together, they can analyze the student's behavior; the student can then assess her own strengths and limitations. It is often helpful to share these experiences with a peer group. Because students are all in a similar situation, they are able to empathize, criticize, and support each other as they learn, together, more about themselves.

Finally, the process of self-awareness is a painful one. It is not easy or pleasant to objectively examine one's self, particularly when what one finds conflicts with one's self-ideal. But, like many painful experiences, it presents a challenge: accept these limitations of the self or change the behaviors that support them. Choices such as this are the catalysts for growth and stimulate new responses to the question "Who am I?"

Clarification of values

In addition to knowing who they are, nurses should be able to describe "What is important to me?" This awareness aids the nurse in being honest with herself and avoiding the unwarranted and unethical use of patients to meet her own needs. Although the nurse-patient relationship involves mutual growth and satisfaction, the needs of the patient always take precedence. Nurses should have enough sources of satisfaction and security in their nonprofessional life to avoid the temptation of using their patient for the pursuit of personal satisfaction or security. If they do not have sufficient personal fulfillment, they should realize it, and their sources of dissatisfaction should be clarified so that they do not interfere with the success of the nurse-patient relationship.

Values are the concepts that a person holds worthy in his own personal life. They are formed as a result of one's life experiences with family, friends, culture, education, work, and relaxation. The word "value" has positive connotations, since it denotes worth or significance. Yet values also imply negatives. If we value one thing, such as honesty, then it follows that we do not value its opposite, such as dishonesty. Areas in which people are likely to hold strong values include religious beliefs, sexual preferences, family ties, other ethnic groups, and sex-role beliefs.

Value systems, however, are more than statements of what one treasures or highly regards. They provide the framework, either consciously or unconsciously, for many of one's daily decisions and actions. By being aware of one's value system, the nurse can more readily identify situations in which she is involved in a value system conflict. Clarification of values also provides some insurance against the tendency to project values onto another. Many therapeutic relationships test the nurse's values. If a patient is describing a sexual behavior that the nurse finds unacceptable, or if the patient is talking about divorce and the nurse strongly believes that marriage contracts should not be broken, or if the patient is a "born-again" Christian but the nurse has no belief in God or religion, how does the nurse respond? Can she maintain her own values and still accept those of the patient? Can she empathize and help the patient problem solve, while being aware of her own values and natural tendency to project those values?

Understanding one's values may be promoted by *value clarification*. It is a method developed by Raths, Harmin, and Simon[50] and adapted to nursing by Uustal,[67] whereby a person can discover his own values by assessing, exploring, and determining what one's personal values are and what priority they hold in one's personal decision making. It is a growth-producing process that promotes self-understanding and permits one to behave in ways appropriate to one's personal value priorities. Value clarification does not tell an individual what his values should be or what values he should live by. To avoid the imposition of values, value clarification focuses exclusively on the process of valuing or how people come to have the values they have.

Seven criteria have been identified by Raths to be used in determining whether a person is actually holding a value or not. These criteria should be considered in relation to a person's strongest value and tested against his own definition of a value. They are broadly grouped into the following three steps:

Choosing	1.	Freely
	2.	From alternatives
	3.	After thoughtful consideration of the consequences of each alternative
Prizing	4.	Cherishing, being happy with the choice
	5.	Willing to affirm the choice publicly
Acting	6.	Doing something with the choice
	7.	Repeatedly, in some pattern of life[50]

The first three criteria, those of choosing, rely on the person's cognitive abilities; the next two criteria, prizing, emphasize the emotional or affective level; the last two criteria, acting, have a behavioral focus.

It has been found that simple exposure to the value clarification process causes change in people. Rokeach[54] contends that change takes place when the person becomes disturbed emotionally as a result of realizing the existence of certain contradictions in his value system. To eliminate the inevitable self-dissatisfaction that follows such a realization, the person will realign his values to coincide with his new self-conception.

Rogers has described the valuing process in the mature person. He does not view it as an easy or simple thing. Rather, the process is complex, the choices often perplexing and difficult, and there is no guarantee that the choice made will prove to be self-actualizing. The valuing process in the mature person has the following characteristics[34]:

1. It is fluid and flexible, based on the particular moment and the degree to which the moment is experienced as enhancing, enriching, and actualizing. Values are not held rigidly but are continually changing.

2. The valuing experience is highly differentiated, that is, tied to a particular time and experience.

3. The locus of evaluation in the valuing process is firmly established within the person. It is his own experience that provides the value information. Although he is open to all the evidence that he can obtain from other sources, he views it as outside evidence that is not as significant as his own responses. The psychologically mature adult trusts and uses the wisdom of himself.

4. In the valuing process, the person is open to the immediacy of his experiences, trying to sense and clarify all its complex meanings. However, the immediate impact of the moment is colored by experiences from the past and conjecture about the future. Thus past and future are in the present moment and enter into the valuing process.

Exploration of feelings

It is often assumed that helping others requires complete objectivity and detachment from one's feelings. This is definitely not true. Complete objectivity and detachment from one's feelings describes someone who is unresponsive, false, unapproachable, impersonal, and alienated from oneself—qualities that impede or prohibit the establishment of a therapeutic relationship. What is desired is that the nurse be open to her feelings, aware of them, and in control of them so that she may use them in helping patients.

Nurses, as people, are feeling all the time, and these feelings serve an important purpose. They are barometers for feedback about ourselves and our relationships with others. They are useful, serve adaptive purposes, and are part of our learning experience. Gaylin believes:

Feelings are the instruments of rationality. . . . They are fine tunings directing the ways in which we will meet and manipulate our environment. . . . Mental illness is usually a mere disarray of the ingredients of survival. All that is necessary is rearrangement. Feelings are internal directives essential for human life.[23:3-7]

While helping others, nurses will experience many feelings—elation at seeing a patient improve, disappointment when a patient regresses, unappreciation when a patient refuses help, and anger in response to the patient who is demanding or manipulative. Feelings of power can arise when patients express strong dependence on the nurse or indicate that the nurse has influence over them. When patients express profuse gratitude to the nurse, she must wonder if they believe they helped themselves or whether the nurse did it for them.

If the nurse is open to her own feelings, she has access to two important pieces of information, how she is responding to the patient and how she is appearing to him. While talking to a patient, the nurse should be aware of her response to him. Despite his words, she might perceive a strong sense of despair or anger. Her feelings are valuable clues to the patient's problems and should be incorporated in her care for him. So too, the nurse should be aware of the feeling she is conveying to the patient. Is her mood one of hopelessness or contempt? If the nurse views feelings as barometers and feedback instruments, her effectiveness as a helper will be enhanced.

Ability to serve as model

Formal helping is a strong influence process and nurses do function as models to their patients, whether they want to or not. Much research has shown the power of models for acquiring socially adaptive, as well as maladaptive, behaviors. This imposes the obligation on the nurse to model adaptive and growth-producing behavior. If a nurse has a chaotic personal life, such as one characterized by stormy intimate relationships, drug abuse, or conflictual parental ties, it will be evident in her work with patients. Not only will it decrease the effectiveness of her care, but her credibility as a helper and the validity of her care are likely to be questioned. The nurse may object to this with claims that she is able to separate her personal from her professional life, but in psychiatry, this is not possible because psychiatric nursing *is* the therapeutic use of self.

This is not to imply, however, that the nurse must be totally conforming to local community norms or that she must live an idyllic placid life. What is suggested is that the effective nurse has a fulfilling and satisfying personal life that is not dominated by conflict, distress, or denial and that her approach to life conveys a sense of growing and adapting.

Altruism

It is vital for nurses to have an idea of "Why do I want to help others?" This does not necessi-

tate an extensive analysis of motives, but rather an awareness that one is acting for oneself, as well as for the value of the patient. Obviously, an effective helper is interested in people and tends to help out of a deep love for humanity, which is focused on a particular person or group of people. It is also true that everyone seeks a certain amount of personal satisfaction and fulfillment from their work. The goal is to maintain a balance between these two needs. Helping motives have the potential of becoming destructive tools in the hands of naive or zealous users.

Another danger lies in subscribing to an extreme view of altruism. Altruism can be defined as concern for the welfare of others. It does not mean that because one works out of a sense of altruism, one should not expect adequate compensation and recognition. It does not mean that one must practice extreme denial or self-sacrifice. The desire to help humanity is not in conflict with the desire for a satisfying life. In fact, only if the nurse's personal needs have been appropriately met can she expect to be maximally therapeutic.

Finally, a sense of altruism can also apply to more general social support and change motives. Altruism is necessary for society to survive. Activist helpers are needed who are primarily concerned with changing social conditions to meet human welfare needs. One goal of all helping professionals should be to create a people-serving and growth-facilitating society. As such, a legitimate and necessary role for the nurse is to work to change the larger structure and process of society in ways that will promote the individual's health and welfare.

Sense of ethics and responsibility

Personal beliefs about people and society can serve as conscious guidelines for action. When these ethical principles are shared among helpers, they are written down and codified. The Code for Nurses reflects common values regarding nurse-patient relationships and responsibilities and serves as a frame of reference for all nurses in their judgments about patient welfare and social responsibility.

Related to one's sense of ethics is the need for the nurse to assume responsibility for her own behavior. This involves knowing one's own limitations and strengths and being accountable for them. Since the nurse is a member of a health care team, she has the knowledge and expertise of other people readily available to her and she should use them appropriately. Responsibility implies maturity, and as a quality of an effective nurse it is essential.

Phases of the relationship

A vital characteristic of the nurse-patient relationship is the sharing of behaviors, thoughts, and feelings to establish a context of therapeutic intimacy. Coad-Denton[18] describes this as the use of the nursing process to support the patient as he explores his areas of needs, solves problems, and acquires new coping skills. As such, it is distinct from social superficiality and imposes specific expectations on the nurse. Table 3-1 identifies seven components of relationships in general and contrasts social superficiality and therapeutic intimacy on these components.

This is not to assume, however, that these elements emerge simultaneously or at the same time. Rather, they evolve as the nurse moves through the various phases of the therapeutic

TABLE 3-1. Contrast between social superficiality and therapeutic intimacy*

Components of relationship	Social superficiality	Therapeutic intimacy
Mutual self-disclosure	Variable	Patient: self-disclosure; nurse: self-disclosure in terms of response to patient only
Focus of conversation	Unknown to participants	Known to nurse and patient
Pertinence of topic	Social, business, generalized, impersonal	Personal and relevant to nurse and patient
Relationship of experiences to topic	Sense of uninvolvement and use of indirect knowledge	Sense of involvement and use of direct knowledge
Time orientation	Past and future	Present
Use of feelings	Sharing of feelings discouraged	Sharing of feelings encouraged by nurse
Recognition of individual worth	Not acknowledged	Fully acknowledged

*From Coad-Denton, A.: Therapeutic superficiality and intimacy. In Longo, D., and Williams, R., editors: Psychosocial nursing: assessment and intervention, New York, 1978, Appleton-Century-Crofts.

relationship with the patient. Four sequential phases of the relationship process have been identified: preinteraction phase; introductory, or orientation, phase; working phase; and termination phase. Each phase builds on the preceding one and is characterized by specific tasks. These phases will be described only as they apply to the nurse working with a psychiatric patient. Other sources present detailed information on basic elements of the relationship process.[64,65]

Preinteraction phase

The preinteraction phase begins before the nurse's first contact with the patient. Her initial task is one of self-exploration as she analyzes her own feelings, fantasies, and fears. In her first experience working with psychiatric patients the nurse will bring with her the misconceptions and prejudices of the general public. Some of these feelings and fears are common to all novices, and an overriding one is usually anxiety or nervousness, which is provoked by new experiences of any kind. A related feeling is ambivalence or uncertainty, since the nurse may see the need for working with these patients but feel unclear about her own ability or motivations.

This may be compounded by a threat to the nurse's role identification, which is precipitated by the informal nature of psychiatric settings. Usually psychiatric patients do not wear hospital gowns or clothing, the staff do not wear uniforms, and the staff and patients mingle in a casual, relaxed, and apparently unstructured way. A common first reaction among students is a feeling of panic when they realize that they "can't tell the patients from the staff." The student's discomfort may be made more acute if one of the patients mistakes her for a newly admitted patient. Finally, it is unsettling for many students to give up their uniform, stethoscope, and scissors, since it dramatically emphasizes that, in this nursing setting, the most important tools are one's ability to communicate, empathize, and problem solve. Without a tangible physical illness to care for with treatments and activities, new students are likely to feel acutely self-conscious and hesitant about introducing themselves to a patient and initiating a conversation.

Many nurses express feelings of inadequacy and fears of hurting or exploiting the patient.

They may worry about saying the wrong thing, which might drive the patient "over the brink," or wonder if, with their limited knowledge and experience, they will be of any value. They may wonder how they can help or if they can really make a difference. Some nurses perceive the plight of psychiatric patients as hopeful, others perceive it as hopeless.

A common fear of nurses is related to the stereotype of psychiatric patients as abusive and violent. Because this is the picture portrayed by the media, many nurses are afraid of being physically hurt by a patient's outburst of aggressive behavior. Other nurses fear being psychologically hurt by a patient through rejection or silence. A final fear is related to the nurse's questioning of her own mental health. She may fear mental illness and worry that exposure to psychiatric patients might cause her to lose control of her own grasp on reality. Nurses who are working on their own crises of identity and intimacy may fear overidentifying with patients and using patients to meet their own needs.

Many of these feelings and fears were expressed by one nursing student in the preinteraction phase of self-analysis as reported in the following notes from her diary of her psychiatric rotation:

When first told that I would have a clinical psychiatric nursing experience, I received this information with a blank mind. Mental overload, denial, repression, or whatever it was made me hear the words but put off dealing with it. Then, when given a chance to sort through my thoughts and feelings, I thought more about what this experience would entail. Having never been personally involved with any people who were psychiatrically ill before, I was unable to rely on past personal experiences. I did, however, have quite a "pseudo–knowledge base" from my novels, television, and movie encounters. Do places like the hospital in "One Flew Over the Cuckoo's Nest" really exist? Was the portrayal of "Sybil" accurate? How could I possibly help someone who has so many problems, like the boy in "Ordinary People"? I'm afraid these thoughts have raised more questions in me than they have answered.

Three things scare me the most about this experience. First, I feel that the behavior of a psychiatric patient is quite unpredictable. Would they get violent or aggressive without any warning? Would this aggression be directed toward me? If so, would I be hurt? Did I provoke them and was I wrong in my actions that caused this sudden shift? The second, related to the first, is my feeling of inadequacy. I've been exposed to physically ill people and have learned how

to respond to them. But, the psychologically ill are almost totally alien to me. How can I help? What if I do, or say, or infer something they could take offense to. Will I have the patience to persevere? I just don't know, and my not knowing makes me even more nervous. My third fear is how seeing and being in contact with the psychiatrically ill will affect me. Although I know it's not contagious, the more exposure and knowledge I acquire in this area, the more I may begin to doubt my own stability and sanity. I mean adolescence hasn't been easy for me, and I feel like I'm just now beginning to see things more clearly and feel better about myself. Will this experience stir up any past fears and doubts and, if so, how will I handle it? I am beginning to realize that there is a fine line between sanity and insanity and that the psychiatric patients we'll meet have been unable to gather enough resources from within to cope with their problems. Help, reassurance, and understanding are their needs. I'm hoping I can help meet them . . . but I'm just not sure.

Experienced nurses benefit by analyzing additional aspects of their practice. They may ask themselves the following questions:

■ Do I label patients with the stereotype of a group?
■ Is my need to be liked so great that I become angry or hurt when a patient is rude, hostile, or uncooperative?
■ Am I afraid of the responsibility I must assume for the relationship and do I therefore limit my independent functions?
■ Do I cover feelings of inferiority with a front of superiority?
■ Do I require sympathy, warmth, and protection so much that I err by being too sympathetic or too protective toward patients?
■ Do I fear closeness so much that I am indifferent, rejecting, or cold?
■ Do I need to feel important and keep patients dependent on me?

The type of self-analysis that characterizes the preinteraction phase is a necessary task because, to be effective, nurses should have a reasonably stable self-concept and an adequate amount of self-esteem, engage in constructive relationships with others, and face reality to help patients do likewise. If they are aware of and in control of what they convey to their patients verbally and nonverbally, nurses can function as role models to their patients. To do this, however, some nurses abandon their own personal strengths and assume a facade of "professionalism." This facade is an alienation of their authentic self and, instead of increasing their effectiveness, it immobilizes them and acts as a barrier to establishing mutuality with patients.

All nurses possess professional assets and limitations. Therapeutic use of self means using and maximizing one's assets or strengths and minimizing one's limitations. Promoting a patient's self-realization and self-acceptance is facilitated by the nurse's acceptance of herself and behaving in ways congruent with her own personality. Nurses receive feedback from patients, which can help them identify their strengths and assets. Self-analysis, peer review, and supervision provide opportunities to explore feelings and fears and develop useful insights into one's professional role. The nurse who is therapeutic uses this information and relates to patients in a natural, congruent, and relaxed manner.

Additional tasks of this phase include gathering data about the patient if information is available and planning for the first interaction with the patient. The nursing assessment is begun, but most of the work related to it is accomplished with the patient in the second phase of the rela-

tionship. The nurse reviews general goals of a therapeutic relationship and considers what she has to offer to the patient.

Introductory, or orientation, phase

It is during the introductory phase that the nurse and patient first meet. A primary concern of the nurse is to find out why the patient sought help and if he did so voluntarily. Burgess and Burns[13] described six categories of reasons why people seek psychiatric help and an appropriate nursing approach for each. These are summarized in Table 3-2. Determining the patient's reason will directly influence the establishment of mutuality between the nurse and the patient.

TABLE 3-2. Analysis of why patients seek psychiatric help*

Reasons for patients' seeking psychiatric care	Appropriate nursing approach	Sample response
Environmental change from home to hospital: They desire protection, comfort, rest, and freedom from demands of their usual home and work environments.	Emphasis should be placed on ability of environment to provide protection and comfort while healing process of mind occurs.	"Tell me what it was at home/on the job that made you feel so overwhelmed."
Nurturance: They wish for someone to care for them, cure their illnesses, and make them feel better.	Respond by acknowledging their nurturance needs and assuring them that help and caring are available to them.	"We're here to help you feel better."
Control: They are aware of their destructive impulses to themselves or others but lack internal control.	Offer person sources of internal control such as medication, if prescribed, and reinforce external controls available through services of staff.	"We're not going to let you hurt yourself. Tell us when these thoughts come to mind and someone will stay with you."
Psychiatric symptoms: They describe symptoms of depression, nervousness, or crying spells. They know they need psychiatric help and actively want to help themselves.	Ask for clarification of symptom and strive to understand life experiences of patient.	"I can see that you're nervous and upset. Can you tell me about how things are at home/on the job so I can better understand?"
Problem solving: They identify a specific problem or area of conflict and express desire to reason it out and change.	Help patient look at problem objectively, and utilize problem-solving process with him.	"How has drinking affected your life?"
Advised to come to hospital: Family member, friend, or health professional has convinced them to come to hospital. They may feel angry, ambivalent, or indifferent about being there.	Confirm facts surrounding his seeking of help and set limits appropriate to agency, ward, etc.	"I see that you're angry about being here. Perhaps as you become part of the ward community, you'll feel differently."

*Modified from Burgess, A., and Burns, J.: Am. J. Nurs. **73:**314, 1973.

It forms the basis of the nursing assessment and helps the nurse focus on the patient's presenting problem and determine his motivation.

As the nurse relates with the patient in this phase of the relationship, the tasks are to establish a climate of trust, understanding, acceptance, and open communication and formulate a contract with the patient. The contract begins with the introduction of the nurse and patient, exchange of names, and explanation of roles. This is often omitted by the nurse who has determined the patient's name from another source, such as a chart, family member, or other clinician, and fails to introduce herself because of her anxiety, discomfort, or lack of recognition of the patient as an individual worthy of respect. An explanation of roles includes the responsibilities and expectations of the patient and nurse with a description of what the nurse can and cannot do. This is followed by a discussion of the purpose of the relationship in which the nurse emphasizes that the focus of it will be the patient, his life experiences, and areas of conflict. Because the establishment of the contract is a mutual process, it is a good opportunity to clarify misperceptions held by either the nurse or patient.

With the "who" and the "why" determined, the "where, when, and how long" are discussed. Where will the meetings be held? When and how often will they occur? How long will each be and how long will the series of meetings be? The conditions for termination should be reviewed and may include a specified length of time, attainment of mutual goals, or the discharge of the patient if he is hospitalized. The issue of confidentiality is an important one to discuss with the patient at this time. Confidentiality does not imply secrecy or the exclusive possession of information. Rather, it involves the disclosure of certain information to another specifically authorized person. This means that information about the patient will be shared with people who are directly involved in his care in the form of verbal reports and written notes. This is important in providing for the continuity and comprehensiveness of patient care and should be clearly explained to the patient.

Establishing a contract is a mutual process in which the patient participates as fully as possible. In some cases, such as with the psychotic or severely withdrawn patient, the patient may be unable to fully participate, and the nurse must take the initiative in establishing the contract. As the patient's contact with reality increases, the nurse should review the elements of the contract when appropriate and strive to attain mutuality.

Both the nurse and patient may experience some degree of discomfort and nervousness in this phase of the relationship because of its newness and the future expectations each person brings to it. The nurse may be well aware of her own anxieties and fears, but the difficulty inherent in the patient's role is often overlooked. Receiving help can be difficult from the patient's point of view for the following reasons:

1. It may be hard to admit one's difficulties, first to oneself and then to another, and to see them clearly.
2. It is not easy to trust strangers and be open with them.
3. Sometimes problems seem too large, too overwhelming, or too unique to share them easily.
4. Sharing one's problems with another person can pose a threat to one's sense of independence, autonomy, and self-esteem. Some may view it as a sign of weakness or failure.
5. It is very difficult to commit oneself to change. Solving a problem involves thinking about some things that may be unpleasant, viewing life realistically, deciding on a plan of action, and then, most important, carrying out whatever it takes to actually bring about a change. These activities will place great demands on the energy and commitment of the patient.

If this is the first psychiatric experience for the nursing student, she may feel particularly stressed. Stacklum[62] identified a process that all such new students go through in the beginning of their relationships. In the first stage, they experience a moderate to severe level of anxiety characterized by selective inattention to instructions, obsession with detail, dissociation of theory from practice, and avoidance behavior. Stage two is characterized by the students' use of the defense mechanisms of denial of the patients' problems and strong identification with them. Social conversation with the patients predominate, and nursing actions tend to be concrete and simple. In the next stage, the students question their own ability and experience feelings of anger and omnipotence. Hostility is often projected onto the staff. From these early reactions, students hopefully progress to a beginning adjustment stage, which marks the transition into the working phase of the relationship. Students are now truly able to hear what the patient is saying, their anxiety is decreased, their interactions show more depth and insight, and their nursing actions become more realistic. A therapeutic process has begun.

The tasks of the nurse in the orientation phase of the relationship are to explore the patient's perceptions, thoughts, feelings, actions; identify pertinent patient problems; and mutually define specific goals to pursue. It is not uncommon for patients to display manipulative or testing behavior during this phase as they explore the nurse's consistency and intent. They may also evidence temporary regressions during the sessions as reactions to a large amount of self-disclosure in a previous meeting or to the anxiety created by a particular topic.

Working phase

During this phase the major part of the therapeutic work is carried out. The nurse and patient explore relevant stressors and promote the development of insight in the patient by linking together his perceptions, thoughts, feelings, and actions. These insights should be translated into action and integrated into the life experiences of the individual. The nurse helps the patient to master his anxieties, increase his independence and self-responsibility, and develop constructive coping mechanisms. Actual behavioral change is the focus of this phase of the relationship.

Resistance behaviors are usually displayed by patients during this phase of the relationship because it contains the greater part of the problem-solving process. As the relationship develops, the patient panics when he recognizes his beginning feelings of closeness to the nurse and fears impending disintegration. His response is to cling to his defensive structures, and he resists all attempts of the nurse to move forward. An impasse or plateau in the relationship results. Since overcoming resistance behaviors is crucial to the progress of the therapeutic relationship, they will be discussed in greater detail later in this chapter.

Termination phase

Termination is one of the most difficult, but most critically important, phases of the therapeutic nurse-patient relationship. However, little has been researched or written regarding the process and outcome of termination:

Of all the phases of the psychotherapeutic process, the one which can produce the greatest amount of difficulty and create substantial problems for patient and therapist alike is the phase of termination. It is at this time when the impact of the meaning, in affective terms, of the course of therapy and the nature of the therapist-patient relationship is experienced most keenly, not only by the patient but also by the therapist.[57,77]

During this phase, learning is maximized for both the patient and nurse. It is a time to mutually exchange feelings and memories and to evaluate the patient's progress and goal attainment. Levels of trust and intimacy are heightened, which reflects on both the quality of the relationship and the sense of loss that is experienced by both.

The following criteria can be used to decide if the patient is ready to terminate[14]:

1. The patient experiences relief from the presenting problem.
2. The patient's social function has improved, and his isolation is decreased.
3. The patient has strengthened his own ego functions and attained a sense of identity.
4. The patient employs more effective and productive defense mechanisms.
5. The patient has achieved the planned treatment goals.
6. An impasse has been reached in the therapist-patient relationship because of resistance or countertransference that cannot be worked through.

Although mutuality between the patient and therapist is most often desired in deciding when to terminate, this is not always possible. Sometimes the reason is beyond the control of either person, such as when it is due to an institutional rule, the end of a clinical rotation, or the eventual move of the therapist.

Regardless of the reason, the tasks of the nurse during this phase revolve around establishing the reality of the separation. Together the nurse and patient review the progress made in therapy and the attainment of specified goals. Feelings of rejection, loss, sadness, and anger are expressed and explored. The patient's dependency on the nurse should decrease, and there should be an increase in the interdependence of the patient with his environment and with significant others. It may be helpful to prepare the patient for termination by decreasing the number of visits, incorporating others in the meetings, or changing the location of the meetings. If this is done, the reasons behind the change should be clarified with the patient, so he does not interpret it as rejection by the nurse. It may also be appropriate to make referrals at this time for continued care or treatment.

One's understanding of the feelings that accompany termination can be enhanced by examining Fox, Nelson, and Bolman's comparison[22] of the phases in the termination process to the phases of grief work:

The first phase is a period of denial in which the person attempts to ward off either recognition of the loss or important feelings associated with it. The second, a phase that begins when the denial breaks down, is one of considerable emotional expression, usually of grief and sadness but often including anger and expressions of narcissistic hurt. The third phase is a prolonged period in which the reality of loss and the associated feelings of grief and anger are bit by bit worked through in the multitude of current life experiences that bring up memories of the lost person. To the extent that the mourner is able to perform this grief work successfully, he is gradually able to detach or free the emotional ties that are essential for finding new people or interests.*

In light of this comparison, it becomes evident that successful termination requires that the patient work through those feelings related to separation from emotionally significant persons. The nurse can help the patient to accomplish this by allowing him to experience and feel the effects of the anticipated loss, express those feelings generated by the impending separation, and relate his feelings to former symbolic or real losses.

Patients may react to termination in a variety of ways. They may deny the separation or deny the significance of the relationship and impending separation. The inexperienced nurse might not see the reasons behind this denial and might feel rejected by the patient or believe she has failed him. Patients may express anger and hostility either overtly and verbally or covertly through lateness, missed meetings, or superficial talk. These patients may view the termination as personal rejection, which reinforces their negative self-concept. Patients who feel rejected by the nurse may terminate prematurely. By abruptly ending the relationship, they experience a sense of power and control and assert themselves by rejecting the nurse before she rejects them. It is also common to see the onset of symptoms and maladaptive behavior when termination approaches. In this way the patient re-

gresses to his earlier behavior pattern and hopes to convince the nurse not to terminate because he still needs help.

If the nurse is aware of these possible reactions, she can anticipate them and discuss them with the patient should they occur. For some patients, termination is a critical therapeutic experience because many of their past relationships were terminated in a negative way that left them with unresolved feelings of abandonment, rejection, hurt, and anger. All these patient reactions have a similar goal—to cope with the anxiety about the separation and to delay the termination process.

Levinson[38] has identified five factors that can influence the reaction of the patient to termination:

1. The greater the degree of involvement the patient has had in the treatment and with the therapist, the more intense will be the nature of the reaction to termination.
2. Reaction to termination will vary with the degree of success and satisfaction the patient feels with the treatment.
3. The greater the degree of transference involvement and wished for gratification or fulfillment of childlike wishes, the more intense will be the nature of the patient's reaction to termination.
4. Patients who have sustained earlier losses of significant persons in their lives will reexperience, as termination approaches, the arousal of affects and conflicts from those earlier periods.
5. Whether the patient has experienced key losses or not, his reaction to termination will be influenced by the level at which he has achieved mastery of the early separation–individuation crisis.

In addition to these, the patient's response will be significantly affected by the knowledge, skill, experience and willingness of the nurse to remain open, sensitive, empathic, and responsive to the patient's changing needs. Helping the patient to work through and grow through the termination process is an essential goal of each nurse-patient relationship. It is important therefore that the nurse does not deny the reality of it to herself, nor allow herself to be manipulated by the patient into repeated delays or postponements. Particularly in this phase of the relationship, as in the orientation phase, the patient will be testing the nurse's judgment, and the issues of trust and acceptance will again predominate.

During the course of the relationship and with

---

*Copyright 1969, National Association of Social Workers, Inc. Reprinted with permission from Social Work, vol. 14, no. 4 (October 1969), p. 53.

the attainment of nursing goals, the nurse and patient come to realize a growing sense of equality. The nurse perceives a similarity between herself and the patient, and the impending termination can be as difficult for the nurse as it is for the patient. It is necessary for the nurse to deal with her reaction to the various aspects of termination if she expects to make this a positive learning experience for herself and the patient. If the nurse can take the initiative and begin reviewing her thoughts, feelings, and experiences, she will be more aware of her own motivation, as well as more responsive to the needs of her patient. Schultz states the following:

When the student shares her own feelings and explains how she, too, feels the pain and separation, the patient can learn it is not he alone who needs to be dependent on others and to cling to successful relationships, but that life is a series of making and

breaking relationships. The student and the patient learn that to be involved with other human beings is part of living, often a very satisfying part, but there is a time to love and a time to leave. . . . That allowing another to mourn with you, to share the agony of separation unashamedly, could be an answer to bridging some of the gulf between human beings in need of one another.[58:41-42]

Learning to bear the sorrow of the loss while incorporating positive aspects of the relationship into one's life is the goal of termination for both the nurse and the patient in the therapeutic relationship.

The major tasks of the nurse during each phase of the nurse-patient relationship are summarized in Table 3-3.

Facilitative communication

Communication can facilitate the development of a therapeutic relationship or serve as a barrier to block its development. Nurses should understand the elements of the communication process and utilize specific skills or techniques that help the patient in working through the problem-solving process. According to Carkhoff and Truax, "The central ingredient of the psychotherapeutic process appears to be the therapist's ability to *perceive and communicate,* accurately and with sensitivity, the feelings of the patient and the meaning of those feelings."[17:285]

Every individual communicates constantly from birth until death. As Watzlawick et al.[68] have stated, all behavior is communication and all communication affects behavior. This reciprocity is central to the communication process. One of the most widely respected of the communication theorists is Ruesch. He has defined communication as "all those processes by which people influence one another."[55] Spitz is in agreement with the preceding theorists when he defines communication as "any perceivable behavioral change, intentional or not, directed or not, which helps one or more persons influence the perception, feelings, emotions, thoughts or actions of one or more persons, whether that influence is intentional or not."[61] The most prominent similarity among these three definitions is the focus on behavioral change and interpersonal influence.

The relevance of communication theory to nursing practice is quite apparent. First, communication is the vehicle for establishing a ther-

TABLE 3-3. Nurse's tasks in each phase of the relationship process

Phase	Task
Preinteraction	Explore own feelings, fantasies, and fears
	Analyze own professional strengths and limitations
	Gather data about patient when possible
	Plan for first meeting with patient
Introductory	Determine why patient sought help
	Establish trust, acceptance, and open communication
	Mutually formulate a contract
	Explore patient's thoughts, feelings, and actions
	Identify patient's problems
	Define goals with patient
Working	Explore relevant stressors
	Promote patient's development of insight and use of constructive coping mechanisms
	Overcome resistance behaviors
Termination	Establish reality of separation
	Review progress of therapy and attainment of goals
	Mutually explore feelings of rejection, loss, sadness, and anger and related behaviors

apeutic relationship, since it involves conveying information and exchanging thoughts and feelings. Second, communication is the means by which people influence the behavior of another. Thus, it is critical to the successful outcome of nursing intervention, since the nursing process is directed toward promoting behavioral change in the direction of achieving a maximum level of wellness for the individual. Finally, communication is the relationship itself, since without it, a therapeutic nurse-patient relationship is not possible.

Levels of communication

Communication takes place on two levels: verbal and nonverbal. *Verbal communication* occurs through the medium of words, spoken or written. Taken alone, verbal communication can convey factual information accurately and efficiently. It is a less effective means of communicating feelings or nuances of meaning, and it represents only a small segment of total human communication. Another limitation of verbal communication is that words can change meanings with different cultural groups or subgroups in a society. This is because words have both denotative and connotative meanings. The denotative meaning of a word is the concrete representation of it or its specific meaning. For example, the denotative meaning of the word "bread" is "a food made of a flour or grain dough which is kneaded, shaped, allowed to rise and baked." The connotative meaning of a word, in contrast, is its implied or suggested meaning. Thus the word "bread" can conjure up many different connotative or personalized meanings. Depending on a person's past experiences, preferences, and present frame of reference, he may be thinking of French bread, rye bread, a sesame seed roll, or perhaps pita bread. The phrase, "Give me some bread" can even have another meaning. When used as slang by a particular group of people, it may be commonly understood to mean "give me some money." Once again, the characteristics of the speaker and the context in which it is said influence the specific meaning of verbal language.

When communicating verbally, many people assume that they are both "on the same wavelength." But since words are only symbols, they seldom mean precisely the same thing to two people and, if the word represents an abstract idea such as "depressed" or "hurt," the chance of misunderstanding or misinterpretation may be quite great. In addition, many feeling states or personal thoughts cannot be put into words easily. A nurse who wishes to communicate effectively must be aware of the limitations and possible problems inherent with verbal language. She should strive to overcome them by validating her interpretation and incorporating information from the nonverbal level as well.

Nonverbal communication includes everything that does not involve the spoken or written word, and it involves all of the five senses. It has been estimated that about 7% of meaning is transmitted by words; 38% is transmitted by paralinguistic cues, such as voice; and 55% is transmitted by body cues.[41] Nonverbal communication serves many functions in relating to another: supplementing, substituting, reinforcing, contradicting, and emphasizing verbal language; displaying affect; and regulating the flow of information. This level of communication is often unconsciously motivated and may more accurately indicate a person's meaning than the words he is saying. This is because people tend to verbalize what they think the receiver wants to hear, whereas less acceptable or more honest messages may be communicated simultaneously by the nonverbal route.

Various types of nonverbal behaviors have been identified in the literature. Of these, five categories of nonverbal communication will be briefly described. *Vocal cues*, or paralinguistic cues, include all the noises and sounds that are extraspeech sounds. Some examples include pitch, tone of voice, quality of voice, loudness or intensity, rate and rhythm of talking, and unrelated nonverbal sounds, such as laughing, groaning, nervous coughing, and sounds of hesitation ("um," "uh"). These are particularly vital cues of emotion and can be powerful conveyors of information.

Action cues are body movements that are sometimes referred to as kinetics. They include automatic reflexes, posture, facial expression, gestures, mannerisms, and actions of any kind. Facial movements and posture can be particularly significant in interpreting the mood of the speaker.

Object cues are the speaker's intentional and nonintentional use of all objects. Dress, furnishings, and possessions all communicate something to the observer about the speaker's sense of self. They are often consciously selected by the individual, however, and therefore may be chosen to convey a certain "look" or message. Thus, they can be less accurate than other types of nonverbal communication.

Space provides another clue to the nature of the relationship between two people. Hall[26] extensively researched proxemics, the use of space between communicators. He identified the following four zones of space that are demonstrated interpersonally in North America:

1. Intimate space—up to 45.5 cm (18 inches). This allows for maximum interpersonal sensory stimulation.
2. Personal space— 45.5 to 120 cm (18 inches to 4 feet). This is used for close relationships and touching distance. Visual sensation is improved over the intimate range.
3. Social-consultative space—270 to 360 cm (9 to 12 feet). This is less personal and less dependent. Speech must be louder.
4. Public space—360 cm (12 feet) and over. This is used in speech giving and other public occasions.

Observation of seating arrangements and use of space by patients can yield valuable information to the nurse that has implications for both her assessment of the patient and the way in which her nursing intervention should be implemented.

Touch involves both personal space and action. It is possibly the most personal of the nonverbal messages and one's response to it is influenced by the setting, cultural background, type of relationship, sex of communicators, ages, and expectations. Touch can have many meanings.[66] It can express a striving to connect with another person as a way of meeting them or relating to them. It can be a way of expressing or conveying something to another, such as concern, empathy, or caring. Touch can also be used receptively as a way of sensing, perceiving, or allowing someone else to leave their imprint on another. Finally, Krieger[35] has developed the concept of "therapeutic touch," or the nurse's laying hands on or close to the body of an ill person for the purpose of helping or healing. She believes touch to be the imprimatur of nursing and contends that the therapeutic, comforting effects of touch have been often overlooked in nursing.

Touch is a universal and basic aspect of all nurse-patient relationships and has been described as the first and most fundamental means of communication.[6] Nevertheless, relatively little is really known about touch as it relates to health.[69] This is clearly one area in which many questions exist and many aspects remain unexplored. The therapeutic value of touch truly merits further nursing research.

All of these types of nonverbal messages are important, but interpreting them correctly can present numerous problems to the nurse. Body messages are rapid, often imprecise, and extremely complex. It is impossible to examine nonverbal messages out of context, and there are times when one's body reveals a number of different and perhaps conflicting feelings simultaneously. Cultural background is also a major influence on the meaning of nonverbal behavior. In America, with its diverse ethnic communities, such messages between people of different upbringing can easily be misinterpreted. Certain people may have been taught to suppress hands and facial expressions, whereas others may not show emotional response. For instance, Arabs tend to stand closer together when speaking, and Orientals tend to touch more; touching in America is often minimized because of perceived sexual overtones or one's puritan heritage. Because the meaning attached to nonverbal behavior is so subjective, it is essential that the nurse validate its meaning.

Nurses should respond to the variety of nonverbal behaviors displayed by the patient, particularly voice inflections, body movements, gestures, facial expression, posture and physical energy levels. Incongruent behavior or contradictory messages are especially significant. The nurse should refer to the specific behavior observed and attempt to validate its meaning and significance with the patient. If the nurse's words and tone of voice indicate that she is truly clarifying, suggesting, or validating, she will usually not create a defensive reaction in the patient. Three kinds of responses may be used by the nurse:

1. Questions or statements intended to increase the patient's awareness
2. Content reflections
3. Statements reflecting the responsiveness of the nurse

These possible responses are illustrated in the following interaction.

PATIENT: **(Shifting nervously in her chair, eyes scanning the room and avoiding the nurse) What . . . what do you want to talk about today?**

NURSE: **I sense that you are uncomfortable talking to me. Could you describe to me how you are feeling?**

NURSE: **You're not sure what we should be talking
about and you want me to start us off?**

NURSE: **You look very nervous to me and I can feel
those same feelings in me as I sit here with you.**

The nurse's first possible response is a reflection and attempt to validate the feelings of the patient. The purpose is to communicate to the patient the nurse's awareness of his feelings, to show acceptance of those feelings, and to request that he focus on them and elaborate on them. The nurse's second possible response deals with the content of the patient's message. The nurse here is clarifying what the patient is trying to say. The third possible response shares both the nurse's perception of her patient's feelings and the personal disclosure that she too has some of those same feelings. This type of response may help the patient feel accepted and understood by the nurse.

In addition to responding to the patient's nonverbal behavior, the nurse should incorporate aspects of it in implementing her care. This may be most evident in the use of space in the nurse-patient relationship. A patient who is resistant to closeness will most certainly recoil from entry into his intimate space. The close distance area of personal space may also be intolerable to a patient who fears closeness. The nurse can assess the patient's level of spatial tolerance by observing the distance the patient maintains with other people. The nurse can also be alert to the patient's response when she interacts with him. If she sits next to him on the sofa, does he get up and move to a chair? If she pulls her chair closer to him, does he move his chair away to reestablish the original space? Sometimes increasing the space between the nurse and an anxious patient can alleviate the anxiety enough to allow the interaction to continue. A decrease in the distance that the patient chooses to maintain from others may indicate a decrease in interpersonal anxiety.

Argyle[4] enumerates other spatial parameters that are interpersonally significant. Height may communicate dominance and submission. Communication is facilitated when both participants are at similar levels. Orientation of the participants' body positions is also significant. Face-to-face confrontation is more threatening than oblique body positions. The physical setting also has spatial meaning. Ownership of a space affects the communication context. A patient may be more comfortable in his own room than in the therapist's office, unless the patient's room is also defined as bedroom. Control issues are minimized when communication takes place in a neutral area that belongs to neither participant. However, people rather quickly identify their own turf, even in unfamiliar settings, and then begin to exert ownership rights over this area. A common example of this can be observed in most college classes. At the beginning of the semester, people seat themselves somewhat randomly, but the arrangement usually solidifies after a couple of classes. Students then feel vaguely annoyed if they arrive in class to find another person in "their seat." They are experiencing an invasion of personal space. Awareness of a patient's use of space can add a further dimension to the nurse's ability to understand the patient.

Touch also should be used judiciously. It is a powerful communicative tool. Patients who are sensitive to issues of closeness may experience a casual touch as an invasion or as an invitation to intimacy, which may be even more frightening. Physical contact with a person of the same sex may be experienced by the patient as a homosexual advance and may precipitate a panic reaction. If procedures requiring physical contact must be carried out, careful explanations should be given both before and during the procedure. An efficient, impersonal, but caring, approach to physical nursing care may be least threatening to a patient experiencing interpersonal anxiety.

The last point to be made here regarding nonverbal communication is that the nurse must not only be aware of the patient's nonverbal cues, but she must also be aware of her own. Nonverbal cues of the nurse can communicate interest, respect, and genuineness or disinterest, lack of respect, and an impersonal facade. LaCrosse[36] did a study of nonverbal behaviors to determine which ones promoted relating to someone else and which ones prohibited it. He concluded that affiliative nonverbal behavior included smiles, positive head nods, gestures, 80% eye contact, and a 20% forward body lean. Unaffiliative nonverbal behavior included 40% eye contact, a 20% reclining body lean, and none of the other categories. Furthermore, affiliative counselors were perceived to be more attractive and persuasive than unaffiliative ones. The implication of this type of research is that nurses, as therapeutic helpers, need to be aware of a spectrum of nonverbal behaviors in their patients and themselves and then incorporate them judiciously in their care.

The communication process

Human communication is a dynamic process that is influenced by the psychological and physiological conditions of the participants. Ruesch[56] has identified the elements of the process as perception, evaluation, and transmission. Perception occurs by activation of the sensory end organs of the receiver. The impulse is then transmitted to the brain. Human beings are most reliant on visual and auditory stimuli for communications. Vision is the primary means of perceiving nonverbal communication, and hearing primarily responds to verbal stimuli. However, if one of the primary senses is dysfunctional, the other functional senses accommodate to improve the individual's perception. For instance, the deaf person can learn sign language and lipreading, which rely on vision, to compensate for not being able to hear the verbal component of communication.

When the sensory impulse reaches the brain, evaluation takes place. The message is analyzed and categorized by the individual in terms of its meaning. Past personal experience is the matrix within which new experience is evaluated. If the individual encounters an entirely new experience for which there is no frame of reference, a feeling of confusion results. Evaluation results in a cognitive response that relates to the informational aspect of the message and an affective response that relates to the relationship aspect of the message. Most messages stimulate both types of responses.

When the evaluation of the message is complete, transmission takes place. This is perceived by the sender as feedback, thereby influencing the continued course of the communication cycle. Transmission must take place once communication has been initiated. It is impossible not to transmit some kind of feedback. Even lack of any visible response is feedback to the sender that the message did not get through, was considered unimportant, was an undesirable interruption, or any of a number of other possible interpretations, depending on the context. Feedback stimulates perception, evaluation, and transmission on the part of the original sender, and so the cycle continues until the participants mutually agree to terminate it or one participant physically leaves the setting.

Theoretical models of the communication process help one to visualize its dynamic nature. They show visual relationship more clearly and thus can aid in finding and correcting communication breakdowns or problems. Two models, the structural and transactional analysis models, will be presented, since each gives a valuable, but different, perspective on the communication process.

STRUCTURAL MODEL. The structural model has five functional components in communication: the sender, message, receiver, feedback, and context[64] (Fig. 3-4). The *sender* is the originator of the message, which is then trans-

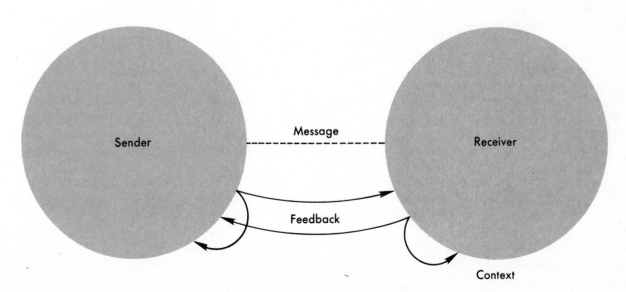

FIG. 3-4
Components of communication.

mitted to the receiver. The *message* is a unit of information that is transmitted from the sender to the receiver. The *receiver,* then, is the perceiver of the message, which influences his behavior in some way. The behavioral response of the receiver is *feedback* to the sender. Feedback, as defined here, functions as described in general systems theory. Positive feedback promotes change within the system, and negative feedback promotes stability. An example of positive feedback might be the receiver unexpectedly telling the sender that the message made him angry, whereas negative feedback might be to respond exactly as the sender anticipated. When viewed structurally, communication is a circular process. The designation of sender and message and receiver and feedback is somewhat arbitrary once the cycle has begun, since feedback is also a new message initiated by the receiver, who then becomes the sender.

The fifth structural element of communication is the *context.* This is the setting in which the communication takes place. Knowledge of context is necessary to understand the meaning of the communication. For example, the phrase "I don't understand what you mean" may have different meanings in the context of a classroom or a courtroom. Context involves more than the physical setting for communication, however. It also includes the psychosocial setting, which encompasses the relationship between the sender and receiver, their past experiences with each other, and past experiences with similar situations, as well as cultural values and norms. Consider again the meaning of "I don't understand what you mean" in the following contexts: two college students discussing a philosophy assignment, a wife responding to her husband's accusation of infidelity, and a Japanese tourist asking directions in San Francisco. Although the content of the message is the same, its meaning is different, depending on the context in which the communication takes place.

If one evaluates the communication process with regard to these five structural elements, specific problems or potential errors become evident. First, the sender must be communicating the same message on both the verbal and nonverbal levels. If so, the sender's communication is termed *congruent.* If, however, the levels are not in agreement, the communication is termed *incongruent,* which can be problematic.

Congruent communication
    Verbal level: I'm pleased to see you.
  Nonverbal level: Voice sounds warm, continuous eye contact, smiling.
Incongruent communication
    Verbal level: I'm pleased to see you.
  Nonverbal level: Voice sounds cold and distant, avoids eye contact, neutral facial expression.

Incongruent, or double-level, messages produce a dilemma for the listener because he does not know to which level he should respond, the verbal or nonverbal. Since he cannot respond to both, he is likely to feel frustrated, angry, or confused. This is a double-bind situation in which one is "damned if you do, and damned if you don't." Obviously, both patients and nurses can display incongruent communication, if they are not aware of their internal feeling states and the nature of their communication.

Another problem initiated by the sender is that of inflexible communication. This is communication that is either too rigid or permissive. A rigid approach is one of exaggerated control by the nurse and may be evident in the overuse of a standardized history or assessment form. It does not allow the patient to spontaneously express himself, nor does it allow him to contribute to the flow or direction of the interaction. Exaggerated permissiveness, on the other hand, refers to a nurse who does not share her thoughts or impressions with the patient and thus the interaction lacks direction and mutuality. The patient may interpret the nurse's behavior as lack of interest or incompetency.

The next element of the communication process, the message, can also pose problems. Basically, these problems are messages that are ineffective, inappropriate, inadequate, or inefficient. Ineffective messages are not goal directed or purposeful. They serve at least to distract, and at most to prevent, the objectives of the nurse-patient relationship from being met. Inappropriate messages are those which are not relevant to the progress of the relationship. They may include failures in timing, stereotyping the receiver, or overlooking important information. Inadequate messages are basically those which lack a sufficient amount of information. The sender assumes the receiver knows more than he actually does. Inefficient messages lack clarity, simplicity, and directness. They use more energy than is necessary to confuse or complicate the message. This can be consciously or unconsciously done by the sender. It may reflect disease in the organ of communication, such as stuttering, or it can be due to lack of knowledge or poor use of language.

The third element, the receiver, is subject to the same problems as the sender but also some additional ones. He may experience errors of perception in which he might miss nonverbal cues, respond only to content and ignore messages of affect, be selectively inattentive to the speaker's message because of his own physical or psychological discomfort, be preoccupied with other thoughts, or have a physiological impairment of hearing organs. All of these errors are fundamentally problems of listening. The receiver may also experience problems in evaluating the message. He may misinterpret the meaning of the message because he is viewing it in terms of his own value system, rather than that of the speakers. In this case, he is not being open to the speaker but is judging him based on his own personal experiences and beliefs. He might also interpret a symbolic message literally or a literal one symbolically.

Errors in the feedback element include all of those which apply to the message. Feedback can also convey incorrect information to the sender about the message. Another serious error exists when the receiver fails to use feedback to validate his understanding of the message. Although feedback is the last step in the cyclical communication process, it has the potential for correcting previous errors and clarifying the nature of the communication.

The fifth element of context can also contribute to communication problems. The setting may be physically noisy, cold, or distracting to one or both parties. So, too, the psychosocial context, or past relationship between the communicators, may be one of mistrust or harbored resentment. From this analysis, the complexity of the communication process is evident, and it may even seem surprising that successful communication can occur, given all of these vulnerable areas. However, it can and does occur among those people who understand the process, have analyzed the elements of it, and use appropriate techniques.

TRANSACTIONAL ANALYSIS MODEL. Transactional analysis (TA) is the study of the communication or transactions that take place between people and of the sometimes unconscious and destructive ways ("games") that people relate to each other. This approach to personality was developed by Berne, a psychiatrist who made

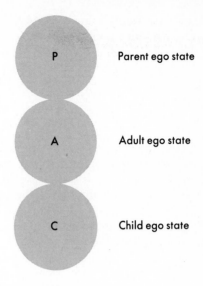

FIG. 3-5
Three ego states as described by Berne's theory of transactional analysis.

transactional analysis a popular theory through his book, *Games People Play: the Psychology of Human Relationships*.[7] It is a method of therapy as well as a model of communication.

The cornerstone of Berne's theory is that each person's personality is made up of three distinct components called *ego states*. An ego state is a consistent pattern of feeling, experiencing, and behaving. The three ego states that make up one's personality are the parent ego state (parent); adult ego state (adult), and child ego state (child) (Fig. 3-5). It is as though there are three "people" inside you: the parent-you, which incorporates all the attitudes and behavior you were taught (directly or indirectly) by your parents; the child-you, which contains all the feelings you had as a child; and the adult-you, which deals with reality in a logical, rational, computer-like manner. These three ego states are distinct, each having a consistent pattern of feeling, experiencing, and behaving.

The parent and child ego states are made up of the feelings, attitudes, and behaviors that are remnants of the past but can be reexperienced under certain conditions. The parent ego state consists of all the nurturing, critical, and prejudicial attitudes, behaviors, and experiences learned from other people, especially parents and teachers. The adult ego state is the reality-oriented part of the personality. It gathers and processes information about the world and is objective, emotionless, and intelligent in its approach to problem solving. The child ego state is the feeling part of the personality. In it resides feelings of happiness, joy, sadness, depression, and anxiety.

Berne's model of communication allows one to diagram transactions using these ego states. Transactional analysis then focuses on the communication between people. A transaction or communication between two people can be complementary, crossed, or ulterior. In a *complementary transaction* (Fig. 3-6), the arrows in the ego state diagram are parallel, and the communication flows smoothly.

COMPLEMENTARY TRANSACTION

PATIENT: **I know that when I get mad at my boss, I take it out on my wife and kids.**

NURSE: **Are you ready to think about some other ways you can handle your anger?**

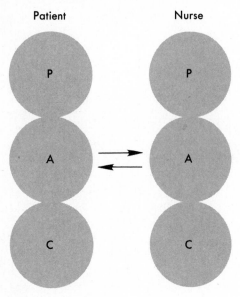

FIG. 3-6
Diagram of complementary transaction.

If the arrows in the ego state diagram *cross,* however, communication breaks down (Fig. 3-7).

CROSSED TRANSACTION

PATIENT: **I know that when I get mad at my boss, I take it out on my wife and kids.**

NURSE: **Men always think that's okay, but the women have to suffer for it.**

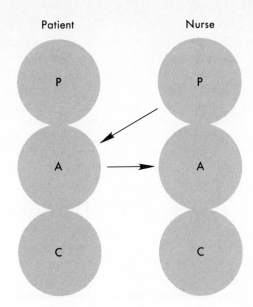

FIG. 3-7
Diagram of a crossed transaction.

The third type of transaction is termed *ulterior* (Fig. 3-8). It takes place on two levels: the social, or overt, level and the psychological, or covert, level. These transactions tend to be destructive because the communicators conceal their true motivations. One of the best known examples of this is the "Why Don't You . . . Yes But" (WDYB) game. This game involves one person asking for a solution to a problem; however, every suggested solution is negated, until the helper is silenced. On the surface, the interaction appears like two adults problem solving, but in reality, one person is using his child to show what a bad parent the other person is.

ULTERIOR TRANSACTION

PATIENT: **I know that when I get mad at my boss, I take it out on my wife and kids but I don't know what else to do.**

NURSE: **Do you think you could let your boss know how you're feeling?**

PATIENT: **He'll fire me for sure.**

NURSE: **Perhaps you could talk it over with someone you work with.**

PATIENT: **I don't have time to chat on the job like that. Besides, no one cares about someone else's beefs.**

NURSE: **Sometimes physical exercise helps people get rid of their anger. Have you ever tried it?**

PATIENT: **Sure. I work out a lot, but it doesn't help.**

NURSE: **Perhaps you can explain all this to your family.**

PATIENT: **My wife's tired of 'all my talk' as she puts it. She says she wants some action.**

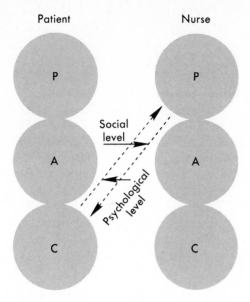

FIG. 3-8
Diagram of an ulterior transaction.

The value of the transactional analysis model
of communication is that it provides a framework
for the nurse to use in exploring the patient's
recurrent behaviors, identifying patterns, postu-
lating causes, and planning alternative ways to
respond. Thus nonproductive communication
patterns can be stopped and new, more healthy,
ones learned.

Therapeutic communication techniques

Ginott[25] believes that the two basic requirements for effective communication are that all
communication be aimed at preserving the self-
respect of both the helper and helpee and that
the communication of understanding precede
any suggestions of information or advice giving.
These lay the groundwork for therapeutic communication, which makes possible the formation
of the nurse-patient relationship and the implementation of the nursing process. The collection
of data and the planning, implementation, and
evaluation activities are carried out with the
patient, not for the patient, when the nurse uses
therapeutic communication skills.

Some nurses reject the notion of therapeutic
communication techniques because they view
them as unnatural, ineffective, or stereotypical.
Like all learned skills, they can be abused, used
too frequently, or incorrectly applied, and knowledge of these skills does not ensure successful
therapeutic communication. These techniques,
although simple on the surface, are, in fact,

difficult and require practice and conscious
thought for mastery. Because they are techniques, they are only as effective as the person
utilizing them. If they are incorporated into the
nurse's existing interpersonal skills, they can
enhance her effectiveness. If they are used as
automatic responses and are inappropriate to the
nurse's manner of personal expression, they will
negate both the nurse's and the patient's individuality and divest them of their dignity.

To ensure that the nurse is using these skills
appropriately and effectively, it will be necessary
for the nurse to record her interactions with the
patient in some way and then analyze them. She
should also seek feedback from others. Many
tools are available to help her in this area. The
nurse can benefit from maintaining a diary of
her thoughts, feelings, and impressions in relation to her clinical work. This can prove to be
valuable in working through difficult aspects of
termination or countertransference reactions.
She may decide to tape record or videotape her
interactions with the patient. These are two of
the most informative recording methods, and
they also allow the nurse the freedom to concentrate on the patient. They do, however, present problems. There is sometimes the need for
another person to operate the equipment, there
is always the possibility of failure, they can be
expensive to obtain and operate, they may be
prohibited by the agency, and they can raise
questions concerning confidentiality. Hand-
written recordings are less expensive and do not
require mechanical devices. They also allow the
nurse to record her thoughts and feelings along
with the verbal and nonverbal behavior. However, they require more physical time and energy. If they are written in the presence of the
patient, they can be very distracting. If they are
written afterward, some aspects of the interaction may be unconsciously forgotten or consciously ignored. Often, these are most significant omissions.

Some of the advantages and disadvantages of
the various methods of recording nurse-patient
interactions are summarized in Table 3-4. These
must be considered, along with the nurse's and
patient's preferences before deciding on a particular method. Some form of recording that is
as objective and comprehensive as possible is
necessary. Only by analyzing the interaction will
the nurse be able to evaluate her degree of suc-

TABLE 3-4. Advantages and disadvantages of various methods of recording nurse-client interactions*

Advantages	Disadvantages
Videotape	
Provides excellent opportunity to see, record, and analyze both nonverbal and verbal levels of communication	Mechanical devices are necessary
Participants are not distracted by writing	Mechanical failure can occur
Can be preserved for comparison with future interactions	At least one other person is necessary to operate equipment
Can provide participants with audiovisual feedback of their responses	Often distracting to participants, at least initially
Possible to see and hear entire interaction for review and supervision	Transcriptions are time consuming
Possible to replay segments for comparison, analysis, and supervision	Unless more than one monitor is available, comparison is time consuming
Tape recording	
Complete verbatim conversation is available	Mechanical devices are necessary
Participants are not distracted by writing	Mechanical failure can occur
Can be preserved for comparison with future interactions	Often distracting to participants, at least initially
Can provide participants with audio feedback of their responses	Transcriptions are time consuming
Possible to hear entire interaction for review and supervision	Unless more than one tape recorder is available, comparison is time consuming
Possible to replay segments for comparison, analysis, and supervision	Nonverbal communication is not available
	With cassette tape recorder, often necessary to disrupt interaction to turn tape over
Verbatim notes	
Possible to record thoughts and feelings during interaction	Difficult to concentrate on interaction until technique of writing without looking is mastered
Messages recorded as said rather than as what was intended	Often distracting to participants, at least initially
Possible to quickly review specific areas for comparison, analysis, and supervision	Requires greater skill in recording
Both verbal and nonverbal levels can be recorded	Segments of the interaction are usually missing or incomplete
No mechanical devices to distract participants	
General outline notes	
Possible to record thoughts and feelings during the interaction	Often distracting to participants, at least initially
Possible to quickly review specific areas for comparison, analysis, and supervision	Necessary to fill in general outline with specific data at a later time
Both verbal and nonverbal levels can be recorded	Often actual messages are distorted by intended messages
No mechanical devices to distract	
Requires less skill than verbatim notes	
Decreases amount of energy needed for writing during interaction, hence increases energy available for communication with client	
Postinteraction notes	
No distractions during interaction	Relies entirely on memory
Possible to focus attention entirely on communication process	Often actual messages are distorted by intended messages
Possible to record information at one's convenience	Often tends to be a more haphazard notation and analysis unless one is well organized

*From Sundeen, S.J. et al.: Nurse-client interaction: implementing the nursing process, ed. 2, St. Louis, 1981, The C.V. Mosby Co.

cess in utilizing therapeutic communication techniques.

Some of the most helpful of these techniques will now be described. Nontherapeutic techniques will not be discussed separately because basically they represent a failure to use an appropriate therapeutic skill. Rather, problems will be discussed relative to some of the therapeutic techniques, and it is hoped that the emphasis of learning will be on a theoretical understanding of therapeutic communication and its appropriate application in a facilitative nurse-patient relationship.

Listening is essential if the nurse is to reach any understanding of the patient. Only the patient can tell the nurse how he feels, what he thinks, and how he sees himself and the world. Only by listening to the patient can the nurse enter his world and see things as he does. Therefore the first rule of a therapeutic relationship is to listen to the patient. It is the foundation on which all other therapeutic skills are built.

Obviously one cannot listen if one is talking, yet inexperienced nurses often find it difficult not to talk. This may be due to their anxiety, need to prove themselves, or habitual manner of social interaction. It is helpful to remember that the patient should be talking more than the nurse during the interaction; the task of the nurse is to listen.

Real listening is difficult. It is an active, not a passive, process. The nurse's complete attention must be given to the patient, and she should not be preoccupied with herself. She should suspend her thinking of her own experiences and problems and her personal judgments of the patient. Listening is a sign of respect for the patient and is a powerful reinforcer. It reinforces verbalization by the patient, without which the relationship could not progress.

Broad openings such as "What are you thinking about?" "Can you tell me more about that?" and "What shall we discuss today?" confirm the presence of the patient and encourage him to select topics to discuss. They can also indicate that the nurse is there, listening to him and following him. Also serving in this way are acceptance responses such as "I understand," "And then what happened?" "Uh huh," or "I follow you."

Restating is the nurse's repeating to the patient the main thought he has expressed. It, too, indicates that the nurse is listening. Sometimes only a part of the patient's statement is repeated. This technique can serve as a reinforcer or bring attention to something important that might otherwise have been passed over.

Clarification occurs when the nurse attempts to put into words vague ideas or thoughts that are implicit or explicit in the patient's talking. It is necessary because statements about emotions and behaviors are rarely straightforward. The patient's verbalizations, especially when he is disturbed or feeling deeply, are not always clear and obvious. They may be confused, jumbled, hesitant, incomplete, disordered, or fragmentary. The nurse should not allow anything to go by that she does not hear or understand. Because of this uncertainty, clarification responses are often tentative or phrased as questions such as "I'm not sure what you mean. Are you saying that . . . ?" or "Could you go over that again?" This technique is important because one of the functions of the nurse-patient relationship is to help clarify feelings, ideas, and perceptions and to provide an explicit correlation between them and the patient's actions.

Reflection goes beyond simple acceptance or restating responses. *Reflection of content* is also called validation, and it lets the patient know that the nurse has heard what he said and understands the content. It consists of repeating in fewer and fresher words the essential ideas of the patient and is like paraphrasing. Sometimes it helps to repeat a patient's statement, emphasizing a key word. Reflecting content is used to clarify the ideas that the patient is expressing and validate that the nurse's understanding is consistent with the patient's meaning.

PATIENT: **When I walked into the room, I felt like I was going to faint. I knew I had tried to do too much, too quickly, and I just wasn't ready for it.**
NURSE: **You thought you were ready to put yourself to the test but when you got there, you realized it was too much, too soon.**

Reflection of feelings consists of responses to the feelings that the patient has about the content. They let the patient know that the nurse is aware of what he is feeling. Broad openings, restatements, clarifications, and reflections of content need not represent empathic understanding. But reflection of feeling signifies understanding, empathy, interest, and respect for the patient. It increases the level of involvement between the nurse and patient.

The purpose of reflecting feelings is to focus on feeling rather than content to bring the patient's vaguely expressed feelings into clear awareness and to help him accept or "own" those feelings as a part of himself. Skillful use of this technique depends on the nurse's ability to identify feelings and cues for feelings from the patient's nonverbal and verbal behaviors. The steps in reflection of feelings are to determine what feelings the patient is expressing, describe these feelings clearly, observe the effect, and judge by the reaction of the patient whether the reflection was correct or not. Sometimes even inaccurate reflections can be facilitative because the patient may correct the nurse and state his feeling more clearly.

Although reflecting techniques are some of the most useful, they can also be used incorrectly by the nurse. One common error is stereotyping one's responses. This means that the nurse begins her reflections in the same monotonous way, such as "You think" or "You feel." A second error is in timing. Some nurses reflect back almost everything the patient says, which provokes feelings of irritation, anger, and frustration in the patient. The nurse appears to be insincere and, in fact, fails to be therapeutic with him. Other nurses may have trouble interrupting patients who continue talking in long monologues. Not only is it difficult to capture a feeling after it has passed, but in this case, the nurse is failing to be a responsible active partner in the relationship. Interruptions may, at times, be productive and necessary. Another error is the inappropriate depth of feeling. The nurse fails by either being too superficial in her assessment of the patient's feelings or too deep. The final error is in the use of language that is inappropriate to the cultural experience and educational level of the patient. Effective language is language that is natural to the nurse and readily understood by the patient.

Focusing helps the patient expand on a topic of importance. It allows him to discuss central issues related to his problem and keeps the communication process goal directed. Intense focusing on an anxiety-producing topic can be detrimental to the relationship if it is not evaluated and balanced with other therapeutic techniques. Effectively used, it can help the patient become more specific, move from vagueness to clarity, and focus on reality.

By avoiding abstractions and generalizations, focusing helps the patient face his problems and analyze them in detail. It helps a patient talk about his situation or problem areas and accept the responsibility for improving them. If a pa-

tient is going to change his thoughts, feelings, or beliefs, he must first identify them as his own. If he fails to "own" them, he has lost control over a part of his life and becomes powerless to change it.

PATIENT: **Women always get put down. It's as if we don't count at all.**
NURSE: **Tell me how *you* feel as a woman.**

Encouraging a description of the patient's perceptions, encouraging comparisons, and placing events in time sequence are focusing techniques that promote specificity and problem analysis.

Sharing perceptions involves asking the patient to verify the nurse's understanding of what he is thinking or feeling. It is a way for the nurse to ask for feedback from the patient, while also possibly providing him with new information. Perception checking can consist of paraphrasing what the patient is saying or doing, asking the patient to confirm your understanding, and allowing him to correct your perception if it was incorrect. "You seem to be very irritated with me. Am I right about that?" It can also note the implied feelings of nonverbal language. When used in this way, it is best to describe the observed behavior first and then reflect on its meaning. "You say you really care about her, but everytime you talk about her, you clench your fists. I wonder if you don't feel betrayed by her?" It is also a way to explore incongruent or double-bind communication. "You're smiling, but I sense that you're really angry with me." Its value as a therapeutic technique lies in the understanding it conveys to the patient and its potential for clearing up confusing communication.

Themes are underlying issues or problems experienced by the patient that emerge repeatedly during the course of the nurse-patient relationship. Once the nurse has identified the patient's basic themes, she can better decide which of the patient's many feelings, thoughts, and beliefs she should respond to and pursue. In this way she can best promote the patient's exploration and understanding. Themes that are important will tend to be repeated throughout the relationship. They can relate to feelings (depression or anxiety), behavior (rebelling against authority or withdrawal), experiences (being loved, hurt, or raped), or combinations of all three.

Silence on the part of the nurse has varying effects, depending on how it is perceived by the patient. To a vocal patient, silence on the part of the nurse may be welcome, as long as he knows the nurse is listening. When the patient pauses in his talk, he often expects and desires a response from the nurse. Not to receive one may be perceived as rejection, hostility, or disinterest by the patient. The nurse's silence with a depressed or withdrawn patient may convey support, understanding, and acceptance. In this case, verbalization by the nurse may be perceived as pressure or frustration. Sharing a patient's silence can be a most difficult task for the nurse but an essential one to furthering the therapeutic relationship.

Silence has several beneficial values.[9] It can make the patient talk. Some introverted people find out that they can be quiet but still be liked. Silence allows the patient time to think and gain insights. And finally, silence can slow the pace of the interaction. In general, the nurse should allow the patient to break a silence, particularly when it has been introduced by the patient. Obviously, sensitivity is called for in this regard, and silence should not develop into a contest. However, if the nurse is unsure how to respond to a patient's comments, a safe approach is to maintain silence. If her nonverbal behavior communicates interest and involvement, the patient will often elaborate on his statement or discuss a related issue.

An ineffective technique would be to begin questioning the patient. As a general technique, direct questioning has limited usefulness in the therapeutic relationship. Repetitive questioning takes on the tone of an interrogation and negates the element of mutuality. "Why" questions are particularly ineffective and are to be avoided, as are questions that can be answered simply by yes or no responses. Excessive questioning tends to be characteristic of inexperienced helpers,[48] and one consequence of it is that patients do not take the initiative and are discouraged or prevented from engaging in the process of exploration.

Humor is a basic part of the personality and has a place within the therapeutic relationship. It resolves paradoxes, tempers aggression, and is a socially acceptable form of sublimation. It is a part of interpersonal relationships and is a constructive coping behavior, and, by learning to express humor, a patient may be able to learn to express other affects. Hutchinson[29] believes that humor can be used in three ways: (1) as an index to the developmental level of the patient, (2) as a planned approach for nursing intervention, and (3) as an indicator of change. As a planned approach to nursing intervention, humor can promote insight by making conscious repressed material, and a change in the expression of humor and the quality of interpersonal relationships may be indicators of significant change in the patient.

Another important feature of humor as described by Heuscher is that it can produce a sudden change or widening in the patient's experiential horizon. He believes that humor is an initial uncomplicated attempt at revealing new and wider visions of one's world and, as such, it can further the growth of the person who is able to integrate some of the new vistas in his world design. "At worst, joking in psychotherapy is a 'playing at change' that allows the therapist and patient to retain their uneasy security in their unchanging individual existences. At best, it is a helpful revelation of new options."[28]

There are no rules, however, for determining how, when, or where humor should be used in the therapeutic relationship. Rather, this depends on the nature and quality of the relationship, the patient's receptivity to such themes, and the relevance of the tale or witticism. Furthermore, the nurse must have insight into why she is using this technique and the dangerous ways it can be used to hide conflicts, ward off anxiety, manipulate the patient, and serve her own need to be liked and admired. Humor must be used cautiously. If it is indiscriminate, it meets only the nurse's needs, may be destructive to the relationship, and frightening to the patient.

Informing, or the skill of information giving, needs little elaboration. It is an essential nursing technique in which the nurse shares simple facts with the patient. It is a skill used by nurses in health teaching or patient education, such as in teaching a patient when to take medication and informing him about necessary precautions and side effects. Giving information, however, must be distinguished from giving suggestions or advice.

Suggesting is the presentation of alternative ideas relative to problem solving. It is an appropriate therapeutic technique if used at the proper time and in a constructive way. As a therapeutic technique, it is a useful intervention in the working phase of the relationship when the patient has analyzed the problem area and is exploring alternative coping mechanisms. At that time, suggestions by the nurse will increase his perceived options and choices.

Suggestion, or giving advice, can also be nontherapeutic. Some patients who seek help do not really expect to work out their own problems, but expect some pronouncement or sound advice on what to do from the health care professional. So too, nursing students often perceive their function as giving "common sense" advice. In these instances, giving advice shifts responsibility to the nurse and reinforces the patient's dependence on her. Another limitation is that the patient may take the nurse's advice and still not have things work out. The patient then returns to blame the nurse for her failure. Most commonly, though, patients do not follow the advice offered by others, as in the transactional analysis model. The request for advice is often a child's expression of dependency, and the patient really knows what to do. If the nurse falls into the trap and responds with advice, she will incur the patient's wrath and contempt. A more productive strategy is for the nurse to deal with the patient's feelings first—feelings of indecision, dependence, and perhaps fear. Then the request for advice can be looked at and responded to in its proper perspective.

Suggestion is also nontherapeutic if it occurs early in the relationship before the patient has analyzed his conflicts or if it is a technique used frequently by the nurse. Then it negates the possibility of mutuality and implies that the patient is not capable of assuming responsibility for his own thoughts and actions. This assumption is also present when suggestion by the nurse is really covert coercion as the nurse tells the patient how he *ought* to live his life.

The nurse's intent in using this technique is to provide feasible alternatives and allow the patient to explore their potential value for himself. The nurse can then focus on facilitating the patient's exploration of the advantages and disadvantages and the meaning and implications of the potential alternatives. In this way suggestions can be offered in a nonauthoritarian manner with such phrases as "Some people have tried. . . . Do you think that would work for you?" When using the technique of suggesting, nurses must be careful about the timing of their intervention as well as their underlying motivation.

SOME ILLNESS-MAINTAINING RESPONSES OF NURSES WITH INPATIENTS*

1. The nurse using a patient (who was similarly exploited at home) to do errands for her (bring coffee, clean office, carry messages).
2. The nurse burdening the patient with tales of her exciting social life—putting the patient in the position of "audience" and at the same time having little interest, if any, in his concerns; to cheer him up by "one-upping" him!
3. The nurse making "pets" of a few patients and thereby reinforcing previous "pet" status for those patients and reinforcing "unfavorable comparison" for other patients. Giving gifts to some but not all patients.
4. Arbitrating siblinglike disputes among two patients, so that one loses and one wins, as in sibling disputes at home.
5. Responding to dependency bids in ways that confirm and reconfirm the patient's self-view: "I am helpless, dependent, etc."
6. Responding to patient bids for derogation or punishment by giving it, thereby confirming and reconfirming these patient self-views.
7. Permitting, inviting, and responding to "tale bearing" in which one patient "tattles" on another, thereby reinforcing the patient's "informer role," which further isolates the patient from constructive interaction with other patients as peers.
8. Allowing or permitting "coalitions across generations"; i.e., participating in nurse/patient discussion to the detriment of some other staff member. This replicates the patient's previous pattern of "pitting one against another," which may have effectively disunited mother and father, who are then reunited in concern for the now "identified patient."
9. Entering into pseudochum relationships with patients.
10. Nonuseful channeling of anxiety into overmedication, seclusion, EST, or work, rather than into investigation of circumstances that evoked the anxiety in a given situation.
11. Using various problematic verbal inputs such as "mixed messages," "double-binds, etc."

*From Peplau, H.: Int. Nurs. Rev. **25**(2):44, 1978.

Responsive dimensions

Certain skills or qualities must be achieved by the nurse to initiate and continue a therapeutic relationship. They incorporate verbal and nonverbal behavior and the attitudes and feelings behind her communication. Truax, Carkhoff, and Berenson[15-17] have identified specific core conditions for facilitative interpersonal relationships. They broadly divided them into responsive dimensions and action dimensions. The responsive dimensions include genuineness, respect, empathic understanding, and concreteness. Many nurses believe that they already demonstrate these qualities with their patients. However, a number of studies have reported that nurses are low in the qualities traditionally associated with therapeutic effectiveness in counseling—genuineness, nonpossessive warmth, and empathy.[49] Furthermore, the helping process can impede the patient's growth rather than enhance it, depending on the level of the nurse's responsive and facilitative skills. Some of the ways in which nurses may consciously or unconsciously do this are given on the facing page.

The responsive dimensions are crucial in the orientation phase of a relationship to establish trust and open communication between the nurse and patient. The nurse's goal at this time is to gain an understanding of the patient and assist him to understand himself or gain insight. These responsive conditions then continue to be useful throughout the working and termination phases. All of the conditions are interrelated and contribute to each other in the therapeutic process, and some degree of all the responsive dimensions is necessary when one is initiating a relationship.

Genuineness

Genuineness implies that the nurse is an open, honest, sincere person who is actively involved in the relationship. She is a "real" person in a "real" encounter who is self-congruent, authentic, or "transparent."[31] Genuineness is the opposite of self-alienation, which occurs when many of one's real, spontaneous reactions to life are repressed or suppressed. Genuineness means that the nurse's response is sincere rather than phony. She is not thinking and feeling one thing and saying something different. She expresses her real feelings rather than presenting a defensive facade. "Being herself" simply means that at the moment the nurse is really

whatever her response denotes. It is an essential quality because the nurse cannot expect openness, self-acceptance, and personal freedom in the patient if she lacks these qualities in the relationship.

Genuineness does not mean that the nurse must disclose her total self, but only that whatever she does show is a real aspect of herself and not merely a "professional" response that has been learned and repeated. It does not imply that the nurse will behave as she does with her family at home, neighborhood friends, or colleagues at a professional meeting. As she focuses on the patient, she puts aside much of her own need system and some of her usual ways of relating to others. Genuineness does not require that the nurse always express all her feelings; it requires only that whatever she does express is congruent. Neither does it imply impulsiveness or "anything goes." Carried to this extreme, genuineness can be destructive and work against the goals of a therapeutic relationship.

Following is an example of genuineness.

PATIENT: **I'd like my parents to give me my freedom and let me do my own thing. If I need them or want their advice, I'll ask them. Why don't they trust what they taught me? Why do parents have to make it so hard—like it's all or nothing?**

NURSE: **I know what you mean. My parents acted the same way. They offered advice, but what they expected was obedience. When they saw I could handle things on my own and used good judgment, they began to accept me as an individual. There are still times when they slip back into their old ways, but we understand each other better now. Do you think you and your parents need to share more openly and honestly your feelings and ideas?**

Respect

The quality of respect has also been called "nonpossessive warmth" or "unconditional positive regard."[16] Positive regard is unconditional in that it does not depend on the patient's behavior. Caring, liking, and valuing are other terms for respect. The patient is regarded as a person of worth; he is respected. The nurse's attitude is nonjudgmental, without criticism, ridicule, depreciation, or reservation. This does not mean that the nurse accepts all aspects of the patient's behavior as desirable or likeable or that she condones it. Yet the patient is accepted for what he is, as he is. She does not demand that he change to be accepted or that he be perfect. Imperfections are accepted along with mistakes and weaknesses as part of the human condition. The inexperienced nurse may have difficulty accepting the patient without transferring her feelings about his thoughts or actions. However, acceptance means viewing his actions as coping behaviors that will change as the patient becomes less threatened and learns more adaptive mechanisms. It involves viewing his behavior as natural, normal, and expected, given his circumstances and perceptions.

Although there should be a basic respect for the patient simply as a person, respect is increased with understanding his uniqueness. Respect can be communicated in many different ways: by sitting silently with a patient who is crying, by genuine laughter with the patient over a particular event, by accepting the patient's request not to share a certain experience, by apologizing for the hurt unintentionally caused by a particular phrase, and by being open enough to communicate one's own anger or hurt caused by the patient. Being genuine with the patient and listening to him are also manifestations of respect for him. The nurse's ability to experience warmth for the patient depends in part on her ability to feel an unconditional positive regard for herself and an acceptance of both her own strengths and liabilities.

When the nurse communicates conditional warmth, she fosters feelings of dependency in the patient because she becomes the evaluator and superior in the relationship, making mutuality impossible. This might occur because of the nurse's need to be in control and dominant, or it might be fostered by the dependent, clinging patient. If dependency feelings should arise in the patient, the nurse can effectively deal with them by acknowledging them and exploring them with the patient.

Empathic understanding

Empathy has been defined by Kalisch as "the ability to enter into the life of another person, to accurately perceive his current feelings and their meanings. It is an essential element of the interpersonal process. When communicated, it forms the basis for a helping relationship between nurse and patient."[32:1548] Without it there is no basis for practice. It is understanding the patient's world from his internal frame of reference rather than from the nurse's own external frame of reference. Rogers described it as "to sense the client's private world as if it were your own, but without losing the 'as if' quality."[51:284] He believes that a high degree of empathy is one of the most potent factors in bringing about change and learning, and it is "one of the most delicate and powerful ways we have of using ourselves."[53:2]

Accurate empathy involves more than knowing what the patient means. It also involves the nurse's sensitivity to the patient's current feelings and her verbal ability to communicate this understanding in a language attuned to the patient. It means frequently checking out with the patient the accuracy of one's perceptions and being guided by the patient's responses. It requires that the nurse lay aside her own views and values to enter another's world without prejudice. This can only be done by a nurse who is secure enough in herself that she knows she will not get lost in what may possibly be the strange or bizarre world of the patient and who can comfortably return to her own world when she wishes.

Empathic understanding consists of a number of stages. If the patient allows the nurse to enter his private world and attempts to communicate his perceptions and feelings to her, the nurse must be receptive to this communication. Next, the nurse must understand the communication of the patient. To do this, she must be able to put herself in the place of the patient and assume his role. She must then be able to step back into her own role and communicate her understanding to the patient. It is not necessary or desirable for the nurse to feel the same emotion as the patient. Empathy does not involve identification with the patient, and it should not be confused with sympathy. It is, instead, an appreciation and awareness of the patient's feelings. At deeper levels, empathy also involves enough understanding of human feelings and experiences to sense feelings that the patient only partially reveals.

A good deal of research has been conducted on empathy.[52] The following discussion of the findings underscores its importance in counseling:

■ Empathy is clearly related to positive outcome.
■ Low empathy is related to a worsening in adjustment or pathologic conditions.
□ The ideal therapist is first of all empathic.
□ Empathy is correlated with self-exploration and process movement.

□ Empathy early in the relationship predicts later success.

□ The patient comes to perceive more empathy in successful cases.

□ Understanding is provided by the therapist, not drawn from her.

□ The more experienced the therapist, the more likely she is to be empathic.

□ Empathy is a special quality in a relationship, and therapists offer definitely more of it than even helpful friends.

■ The better integrated the therapist is within herself, the higher the degree of empathy she exhibits.

□ Experienced therapists often fall far short of being empathic.

□ Brilliance and diagnostic perceptiveness are unrelated to empathy.

■ An empathic way of being can be learned from empathic persons.

The findings highlighted with solid blocks are particularly relevant to improving nursing practice. The last statement indicates that the ability to be accurately empathic is something which can be learned; it is not something one is "born with." This is especially likely to occur if one's nursing educators and supervisors are themselves individuals of sensitive understanding and establish an empathic climate for learning.

The first two findings indicate that, depending on the empathic level of the therapist, therapeutic relationships can be "for better or worse." This is also true among nurses as evident in Williams' study,[70] which found that high and low levels of empathic communication were factors in changing the self-concept of institutionalized aged patients during group therapy. Rogers[53] expands on the profound consequences empathy can have in promoting constructive learning and change. In the first place, it dissolves the patient's sense of alienation by connecting him on some level to a part of the human race. He can perceive that "I make sense to another human being . . . so I must not be so strange or alien. . . . And if I am in touch with somone else, I am not so all alone." On the other hand, if the patient is not responded to empathically, he may believe "If no one understands me, if no one can see what I'm experiencing, then I must be very bad off. . . . I'm sicker than even I thought." Another consequence of empathy for the patient is that he can see that someone values him, cares for him, and accepts him for the person he is. Then perhaps he can come to think "If this other person thinks I'm worthwhile, maybe I could value and care for myself. . . . Maybe I am worthwhile after all."

It is essential that the nurse first provides the contextual base for the relationship by her self-congruence or genuineness and her respect or unconditional positive regard for the patient. Then, the understanding conveyed to the patient through her empathy gives him his personhood or identity. Each of us has the need to have our existence confirmed by another. Empathy gives the needed confirmation that one exists as a separate, valued, and unique person. The patient, as he perceives these new aspects of himself, incorporates them into his changing self-concept. And once his self-concept changes, his behavior changes, thus producing the positive outcome of therapy.

Gazda et al.[24] have described the following guidelines for responding with empathy:

1. Verbal and nonverbal behavior should be focused on by the helper.

2. The helper should formulate responses of empathy in a language and manner that is most easily understood by the helpee.

3. The tone of the helper's response should be similar to that of the helpee.

4. In addition to concentrating on what the helpee is expressing, the helper should also be aware of what is not being expressed.

5. The helper must accurately interpret responses to the helpee and use them as a guide in developing future responses.

A nursing study conducted by Mansfield[40] identified specific verbal and nonverbal behaviors that conveyed high levels of empathy to the patient: having the nurse introduce herself to the patient; head and body positions turned toward the patient and occasionally leaning forward; verbal responses that responded to the patient's previous comments and focused on his strengths and resources; consistent eye contact and response to the patient's nonverbal cues, such as sighs, tone of voice, restlessness, and facial expressions; conveyence of interest, concern, and warmth by the nurse's own facial expressions; a tone of voice consistent with her facial expression and verbal response; and mirror imaging of body position and gestures between the nurse and patient.

Kalisch[32] devised a "Nurse-Patient Empathic Functioning Scale," which describes five levels or categories of empathy (Table 3-5). High levels of empathy (categories 3 and 4) communicate "I am with you," and the nurse's responses fit perfectly with the patient's conspicuous current feelings and content. Her responses also serve

TABLE 3-5. Nurse-patient empathic functioning scale*

Categories of nurse empathic functioning	Level of patient's feelings	
	Conspicuous current feelings	Hidden current feelings
Category 0	Ignores	Ignores
Category 1	Communicates awareness that is accurate at times and inaccurate at other times	Ignores
Category 2	Communicates complete and accurate awareness of essence and strength of feelings	Communicates an awareness of presence of hidden feelings but is not accurate in defining their essence or strength; effort being made to understand
Category 3	Same as category 2	Communicates an accurate awareness of hidden feelings slightly beyond what patient expresses himself
Category 4	Same as category 2	Communicates without uncertainty an accurate awareness of deepest, most hidden feelings

*From Kalisch, B.: Am. J. Nurs. **73**:1548, 1973. Copyright © 1973, American Journal of Nursing Company. Reproduced, with permission, from American Journal of Nursing, September, vol. 73, no. 9.

to expand the patient's awareness of his hidden feelings through the use of clarification and reflection. Such empathy is communicated by the language used, voice qualities, and nonverbal behavior, all of which reflect the nurse's seriousness and depth of feeling.

At low levels of empathy (categories 0 and 1), the nurse ignores the patient's feelings, goes off on a tangent of her own, or misinterprets what the patient is feeling. The nurse, at this low level, may be uninterested in the patient or concentrating on the "facts" of what the patient says rather than his current feelings and experiences. The nurse is doing something other than listening; she may be evaluating the patient, giving advice, sermonizing, or thinking about her own problems or needs.

Empathic responses need to be properly timed within the nurse-patient relationship. Responses from category 4 in the orientation phase may be viewed as too intense and intrusive. Usually a number of category 2 responses are required initially to build an atmosphere of trust and openness. In the later stages of the orientation phase and, most particularly, in the working phase, categories 3 and 4 responses are appropriate and most effective. Responses from categories 0 and 1 are nontherapeutic at all times and block the development of the relationship.

The various levels of empathy are evident in the following example.

PATIENT: **I'm really jittery today, and I hope I can get things out right. It started when I saw Bob on Friday, and its been building up since then.**

NURSE: **You're feeling tense and anxious, and it's related to a talk you had with Bob on Friday. (Category 2.)**

PATIENT: **Yes. He began putting pressure on me to have sex with him again.**

NURSE: **It sounds like you resent it when he pressures you for sex. (Category 3.)**

PATIENT: **I do. Why does he think things always have to be his way? I guess he knows I'm a pushover.**

NURSE: **It makes you angry when he wants his way even though he knows you feel differently. But you usually give in and then you wind up disappointed in yourself and feeling like a failure. (Category 4.)**

PATIENT: **It happens just like that over and over. It's as if I never learn.**

NURSE: **So when the incident's all over, you're left blaming yourself and wallowing in self-pity. (Category 4.)**

PATIENT: **I guess that's right.**

Differences between nurses and patients are barriers to empathy. Differences in sex, age, religion, socioeconomic status, education, and culture can block the development of empathic understanding. Because everyone is unique, no one can completely understand another person. However, the wider a person's background and the more varied one's experiences, the greater will be the potential for understanding people.

Identical or similar experiences are not essential for empathy. No man can really experience what it is like to be a woman; no white can experience what it is like to be black. It is not necessary to be exactly like another, but it is desirable for nurses to prepare themselves in any way they can to understand potential patients. It is also important for nurses to realize that empathy can be learned and enhanced, and staff development programs have been documented as effective in raising a nurse's ability to perceive and respond with empathy.[37]

Concreteness

Concreteness involves the use of specific terminology rather than abstractions in the discussion of the patient's feelings, experiences, and behavior. It avoids vagueness and ambiguity and is the opposite of generalizing, categorizing, classifying, and labeling the patient's experiences. It has three functions: (1) to keep the nurse's responses close to the patient's feelings and experiences, (2) to foster accuracy of understanding by the nurse, and (3) to encourage the patient to attend to specific problem areas.[16] By focusing the patient in specific and concrete terms to his vague ramblings, the nurse helps the patient identify significant aspects of his problems.

The level of concreteness should vary during the various phases of the nurse-patient relationship. In the orientation phase, concreteness should be high and, at this time, it can contribute to empathic understanding. It is essential for the formulation of specific goals and plans. As the patient explores various feelings and perceptions related to his problems in the working phase of the relationship, concreteness should be at a relatively low level to facilitate a thorough self-exploration. At the end of the working phase when the patient is engaging in action and during the termination phase, high levels of concreteness are again desirable.

Concreteness is evident in the following examples.

EXAMPLE 1

PATIENT: I wouldn't have any problems if people would quit bothering me. They like to upset me because they know I'm high strung.
NURSE: What people try to upset you?
PATIENT: My family. People think being from a large family is a blessing. I think it's a curse.
NURSE: Could you give me an example of something someone in your family did that upset you?

EXAMPLE 2

PATIENT: I don't know what the problem is between us. My wife and I just don't get along anymore. We seem to disagree about everything. I think I love her, but she isn't affectionate or caring—hasn't been for a long time.
NURSE: You say you're not sure what the problem is, and you think you love your wife. But the two of you argue often and she hasn't given you any sign of love or affection. Have you felt affectionate toward her, and when was the last time you let her know how you felt?

These four dimensions or conditions facilitate the formation of a therapeutic relationship. Few research instruments have been developed in nursing to objectively evaluate nurse-patient interactions. Aiken and Aiken[1] have adapted the scales developed by Carkhoff and Truax relative to the core dimensions of empathetic understanding, positive regard, genuineness, concreteness, and self-exploration. They divided each dimension into facilitative levels that would allow a practitioner to score herself on them. Methven and Schlotfeldt[43] developed an instrument designed to determine the nature of verbal responses nurses tend to give in emotion-laden situations typically encountered in nursing practice. Stetler[63] analyzed the relationship between empathy as perceived by a helpee and the communication of a helper in a therapeutic interaction. She reported on verbal, nonverbal, and vocal levels of communication. The therapeutic level at which nurses function is unknown at present. Additional research is greatly needed on nurse-patient interactions because there is little empirical evidence on which to base scientific practice in this area.

Action dimensions

Carkhoff identified the action-oriented or initiative conditions of confrontation, immediacy, and therapist self-disclosure. To these will be added the dimensions of catharsis and role playing. The separation of these therapeutic conditions into two groups, the understanding or responsive conditions and the initiating or action conditions, is not a distinct separation. To some extent all the dimensions are present throughout the therapeutic relationship. The action dimensions must have a context of warmth and understanding. This is important for the inexperienced nurse to recall because she may be tempted to move into high levels of action dimensions without having established adequate understanding, empathy, warmth, or respect. The responsive dimensions allow the patient to achieve insight, but this is not enough. With the action dimensions, the nurse moves the therapeutic relationship upward and outward by identifying obstacles to the patient's progress and the need for both internal understanding and external action.

Confrontation

Confrontation is an expression by the nurse of her perceived discrepancies in the patient's behavior. Carkhoff[15] identifies three categories of confrontation:

1. Discrepancy between the patient's expression of what he is (self-concept) and what he wants to be (self-ideal)
2. Discrepancies between the patient's verbal expressions about himself and his behavior
3. Discrepancies between the patient's expressed experience of himself and the nurse's experience of him

Confrontation is an attempt by the nurse to bring to the patient's awareness the incongruence in his feelings, attitudes, beliefs, and behaviors. It may also lead to the discovery of ambivalent feelings in the patient. Confrontation is not limited to negative aspects of the patient. It also includes pointing out discrepancies involving his resources and strengths that are unrecognized and unused. It requires that the nurse collect sufficient data about the patient's history, perceptions, and observations of his verbal and nonverbal communication, so that validation of reality is possible.

Confrontation usually implies venting anger and aggressive behavior. This has the effect of belittling, blaming, and embarrassing the receiver—all of which are harmful and destructive in both social and therapeutic relationships. However, confrontation as a therapeutic action dimension is an assertive, rather than aggressive, action. It requires that the nurse take some risks, avoid venting her own feelings, and help the patient bring his discrepancies into his awareness. The nurse must have developed an understanding of her patient to perceive discrepancies, inconsistencies in word and deed, distor-

tions, defenses, and evasions. The relationship must also contain a bond that will weather the mild or severe crises which confrontation precipitates. The nurse must be willing and capable of working through this crisis after she confronts her patient. Without this commitment, the confrontation lacks therapeutic potential and can be quite damaging to both the nurse and patient. Without question, the effects of confrontation are challenge, exposure, risk, and the possibility for growth. When the nurse uses confrontation, she is modeling an active role to her patient in which she is using insight and understanding to remove ambiguity and inconsistency and thus seek deeper understanding.

Bromley[10] suggests that prior to confrontation, the nurse assess the following factors: the trust level in the relationship, the timing, the patient's stress level, the strength of his defense mechanisms, his perceived need for personal space or closeness, and his level of rage and tolerance for hearing another perception. The patient has the capacity to deny or accept the nurse's observations, and his response to the confrontation can serve as a measure of its success or failure. Acceptance indicates appropriate timing and patient readiness. Denial by the patient serves to allay the threat that the confrontation posed to the patient. It provides additional information to the nurse, since it tells her that the patient is resisting change and is unwilling to enlarge his view of reality at this time.

Confrontation must be appropriately timed to be effective. In the orientation phase of the relationship, the nurse should use confrontation infrequently and pose it as an observation of incongruent behavior. A simple "mirroring" of the discrepancy between a patient's actions and words is the most nonthreatening type of confrontation. The nurse might say, "You seem to be saying two different things." This type of confrontation closely resembles clarification at this time. She might also identify discrepancies between how she and her patient are experiencing their relationship, point out unnoticed strengths or untapped resources of the patient, or provide him with objective, but perhaps different, information about his world.

According to Carkhoff, "Premature direct confrontations may have a demoralizing and demobilizing effect upon an inadequately prepared helpee."[15:93] This is because confrontation requires high levels of empathy and respect to be effective.

In the working phase of the relationship, more

direct confrontations may focus on specific patient discrepancies. The nurse may confront the patient with areas of weaknesses or shortcomings or focus on the discrepancy between her experience of the patient and his own. This expands the awareness of the patient and helps him move to higher levels of functioning. As Carkhoff says, "Confrontation of self and others is prerequisite to the healthy individual's encounter with life."[15:93] Confrontation is especially important to point out when the patient has developed insight but his behavior has not changed. This enables him to see the need to effect actual behavior change. This type of confrontation encourages the patient to act on his world in a reasonable and constructive manner, rather than assuming a dependent and passive stance toward life.

Research indicates that effective counselors use confrontation frequently, confronting patients with their assets more often in earlier interviews and with their limitations in later interviews.[3] Furthermore, Mitchell and Berenson[44] found that therapists who rated significantly higher on empathy, genuineness, respect, and concreteness confronted their patients significantly more often than those therapists who were less facilitative. In the initial interview, these confrontations were based on attempts to clarify the relationship, eliminate misconceptions, provide the patient more objective information about himself and his world, and emphasize the patient's strengths and resources.

Inexperienced nurses frequently avoid confrontation. Certainly it does involve a risk. It can be nontherapeutic when it is not associated with empathy or warmth or when it is used to vent the nurse's negative feelings of anger, frustration, and aggressiveness. However, carefully monitored confrontation can be viewed as an extension of genuineness and concreteness and is a useful therapeutic intervention that can further the patient's growth and progress.

Confrontation is evident in the following examples.

EXAMPLE 1

NURSE: **I see you as someone who has a lot of strength. You've been able to give a tremendous amount of emotional support to your children at a time when they needed it very much.**

EXAMPLE 2

NURSE: **It was my understanding that we were meeting together to talk about the problems that brought you to the hospital. But everytime I come,** you ask me to play cards with you, share a game of table tennis, or toss around a basketball. It seems to me that we're not in agreement on what these meetings are all about.

EXAMPLE 3

NURSE: **The fact that Sue didn't accept your date for Friday night doesn't necessarily mean she never wants to go out with you. She could have had another date or other plans with her family or girl friends. But if you don't ask her, you'll never find out why she refused you or if she'll accept in the future.**

EXAMPLE 4

NURSE: **We've talked three different times now and you've told me how you really don't have a problem or that other people make trouble for you. But I've noticed that on the ward you seldom talk to the other patients and little accidents like the spilled coffee at lunch really seem to upset you.**

EXAMPLE 5

NURSE: **You tell me how your parents don't trust you and never give you any responsibility, but each week you also tell me how you stayed out beyond your curfew or had friends over when your parents weren't home. Do you see a connection between the two?**

EXAMPLE 6

NURSE: **You say you want to feel better and go back to work, but you're not taking your medicine, which will help you to do that.**

EXAMPLE 7

NURSE: **We've been talking for 3 weeks now on how you need to get out and try to meet some people. We even talked of different ways to do that. But so far you haven't made any effort to join aerobics, take a class, or do any of the other ideas we had.**

Immediacy

Immediacy is evident when the current interaction of the nurse and the patient in the relationship is focused on. It is a significant dimension because the patient's behavior and functioning in the relationship are indicative of functioning in other interpersonal relationships. Most patients experience difficulty in interpersonal relationships; so the patient's functioning in the nurse-patient relationship must be evaluated. As Carkhoff states, "The way he relates to the counselor is a snapshot of the way he relates to others. . . . If the counselor does not focus on trying to understand these things, growth possibilities for clients can be missed."[15:192] The nurse has the opportunity to intervene directly with the patient's problem behavior, and the patient has the opportunity to learn and change his behavior. Immediacy may be viewed as empathy, genuineness, or confrontation that involves a particular content—the relationship between the nurse and the patient.

Immediacy connotes sensitivity by the nurse to the feelings of the patient and a willingness to deal with them rather than ignore them. This is particularly difficult when the nurse must recognize and respond to negative feelings expressed by the patient toward her. It is compounded by the fact that patients often express these messages indirectly and conceal them in references to other persons. It is not appropriate or possible for the nurse to focus continually on the immediacy of the relationship. It is most appropriate to do so when the relationship seems to be stalled or is not progressing. Frequently this is due to factors in the immediate nurse-patient relationship, and focusing on them may help. It is also helpful to look at immediacy when the relationship is progressing particularly well. In both instances the patient is actively involved in describing what he feels is helping or hindering the relationship.

As with the other dimensions, high-level immediacy responses should not be suddenly presented to the patient. The nurse must first know and understand him and have developed a good, open relationship. The nurse's initial expressions of immediacy should be tentatively phrased, for example, "Are you trying to tell me how you feel about our relationship?" As the relationship progresses, observations related to immediacy can be made more directly, and, as communication improves, the need for immediacy responses may decrease.

Following are two examples of immediacy:

EXAMPLE 1

PATIENT: **I've been thinking about our meetings, and I'm really pretty busy now to keep coming. Besides, I don't see the point in them, and we don't seem to be getting anywhere.**
NURSE: **Are you trying to say you're feeling discouraged and you feel our meetings aren't helping you?**

EXAMPLE 2

PATIENT: **The staff here could care less about us patients. They treat us like children instead of adults.**
NURSE: **I'm wondering if you feel that I don't care about you or perhaps I don't value your opinion?**

Nurse self-disclosure

Self-disclosures have three characteristics. They are (1) subjectively true, (2) personal statements about the self, and (3) intentionally revealed to another person. In self-disclosure the nurse reveals information about herself, her ideas, values, feelings, and attitudes. She may share that she has had experiences or feelings similar to those of the patient and may emphasize both the similarities and differences. This kind of self-disclosure is an index of the closeness of the relationship and involves a particular kind of respect for the patient. It is an expression of genuineness and honesty by the nurse and is an aspect of empathy.

The rationale for nurse self-disclosure comes from the theoretical and research literature, which provides significant evidence that therapist self-disclosure increases the likelihood of patient self-disclosure. Patient self-disclosure is necessary for a successful therapeutic outcome. It must be emphasized, however, that self-disclosure by the nurse must be used judiciously, and this is determined by the quality, quantity, and appropriateness of her disclosures. The number of self-disclosures appears to be crucial to the success of the therapy. Although too few nurse self-disclosures may fail to produce patient self-disclosures, too many may decrease the time available for patient disclosure or alienate him. There thus appears to be a nonlinear relationship between nurse genuineness and patient disclosure. The problem for the nurse is knowing where the middle ground is. Clinical experience is necessary to determine the optimal therapeutic level.

The appropriateness or relevancy of the nurse's self-disclosure is also important. The nurse should self-disclose in response to statements made by the patient. If her disclosure is far from what the patient is experiencing, it can serve to distract the patient from his problem or make him feel alienated from the nurse. A patient who is experiencing severe or panic levels of anxiety may feel threatened or frightened by the nurse's self-disclosure. She must be careful, in these cases, not to burden a patient with her own self-disclosures. Above all, disclosure by the nurse is always for the patient's benefit. The nurse does not disclose herself to meet her own needs or make herself feel better. She does not impose herself on the patient. When the nurse does self-disclose, she should have a particular therapeutic goal in mind.

Self-disclosure by the nurse is evident in the following example.

PATIENT: **When he told me he didn't want to see me again, I felt like slapping him and hugging him at the same time. But then I knew the problem was really me and no one could ever love me.**
NURSE: **When I broke off with a man I had been seeing, I felt the anger, hurt, and bitterness you just described. I remember thinking I would never date another man.**

In this example the nurse self-disclosed to emphasize that the patient's feelings were natural. She also reinforced the external cause for the separation (boyfriend's decision to leave vs. the patient's inadequacy) and implied that, with time, the patient will be able to resolve the loss.

Even though research has indicated the importance of this dimension for patient growth, it appears to be an area of some discomfort for nurses. Johnson[30] studied the level of reciprocal disclosure occurring between nurses and patients on four clinical units—medical, surgical, psychiatric, and critical care. She found low reciprocal self-disclosure occurring in the psychiatric unit despite the verbal nature of psychiatric therapy and the lack of restrictions placed on talking about oneself. She concluded from her study that nurses and patients need to be assisted in learning to be open and authentic in their interactions with each other.

Emotional catharsis

Emotional catharsis occurs when the patient is encouraged to talk about things that bother him most. Fears, feelings, and experiences are brought out into the open and discussed with the nurse. The expression of feelings can be very therapeutic in itself, even if behavioral change does not ensue. The previously described responsive dimensions create an atmosphere within the nurse-patient relationship in which emotional catharsis is possible. The patient's responsiveness will depend on the confidence and trust he has in the nurse.

The nurse must be able to recognize cues from the patient that he is ready to discuss his problems. It is important that she proceed with the patient at the rate he chooses and support him as he discusses difficult areas. If emotional catharsis is forced on the patient, it could precipitate a panic episode as his defenses are attacked, but sufficient alternative coping mechanisms are not available to him.

Patients are often uncomfortable about expressing feelings because of prohibitive social norms. Nurses may be equally uncomfortable with them, particularly feelings of sadness or anger. Frequently nurses assume they know the patient's feelings and do not attempt to specifically validate them. The dimensions of empathy and immediacy require the attendance to and expression of emotions. Unresolved feelings and feelings that are avoided can cause stalls or barriers in the nurse-patient relationship. Specific examples of this are transference and countertransference phenomena, which will be discussed later in the chapter. If the patient is having difficulty expressing feelings, the nurse may help by suggesting how she might feel in the patient's place or how others might feel in that situation. She might validate with the patient the feeling he seems to be describing in a general way. Some patients respond directly to the question "How did that make you feel?" whereas others intellectualize and avoid the emotional element in their answer. When patients realize they can express their feelings within an accepting relationship, they expand their awareness and potential acceptance of themselves.

The following example illustrates emotional catharsis.

NURSE: **How did you feel when your boss corrected you in front of all those customers?**
PATIENT: **Well, I understood that he needed to set me straight, and he's the type that flies off the handle pretty easily anyhow.**
NURSE: **It sounds like you're defending his behavior. I was wondering how you felt at that moment.**
PATIENT: **Awkward . . . uh . . . upset, I guess (pause).**
NURSE: **That would have made me pretty angry if it happened to me.**
PATIENT: **Well, I was. But you can't let it show, you know. You have to keep it all in because of the customers. But he can let it out. Oh *sure* (emphatically)! He can tell *me* anything he wants. Just *once* I'd like him to know how *I* feel.**

Role playing

Role playing involves the acting out of a particular situation. It functions to increase the patient's insight into human relations and can deepen his ability to see the situation from another person's point of view. Sedgwick[59] identifies the intent of role playing to be a close representation of real life behavior that involves the individual holistically, to focus attention on a problem, and to permit the individual to see himself in action in a neutral situation. It provides a bridge between thought and action in a "safe" environment in which the patient can feel free to experiment with new behavior. It is a method of learning that makes actual behavior the focus of study, is action oriented, and provides immediately available information. Role playing consists of the following steps: defining the problem, creating a readiness for role playing, establishing the situation, casting the characters, briefing and warming up, considering the training design, acting, stopping, involving the audience, analysis and discussion, and evaluation.

When role play is used for attitude change, it relies heavily on role reversal. The patient may be asked to play the role of a certain person in a specific situation or to play the role of someone with opposing beliefs. Research indicates that role reversal can help a person reevaluate the other person's intentions and become more understanding of the other person's position.[8] After role reversal, patients may be more receptive to modifying their own attitudes.

As a method of self-awareness and conflict resolution, role playing may help the patient "experience" a situation, rather than just "talk about it." Role playing can elicit feelings in the patient that are similar in nature and intensity to those experienced in the actual situation. It provides an opportunity for insight and for the expression of affect. For these reasons, it is a useful method for heightening a patient's awareness of his feelings about a situation.

One of the specific ways in which role playing can be used to resolve conflicts and increase self-awareness is through a "dialogue" that requires the patient to take the part of each person or each side of an argument. He is then asked to "play out" the conflict through an imaginary dialogue. If the conflict is internal, the dialogue occurs in the present tense between his conflicting selves until one part of the conflict outweighs the other. If the conflict involves a second person, the patient is instructed to "imagine that the other person is sitting in the chair across from you." The patient is told to begin the dialogue by expressing wants and resentments about the other person. Then the patient changes chairs, assumes the role of the other person, and responds to what was just said. The patient assumes the first role again and responds to the other person. Dialoguing in this way not only serves as practice for the patient in expressing feelings and opinions, but also gives a reality base for the probable response from the other party involved in the conflict. This can often remove the barrier that is keeping the patient from making a decision and implementing the necessary action steps.

Role playing is included as an action dimension because it can facilitate the patient's development of insight. Nurses need a variety of intervention skills. Role playing can be effective when an impasse has been reached in the patient's progress, or when he is having difficulty translating insight into action. In these instances it can reduce tension and allow the patient the opportunity to practice or test out new behaviors for future use.

In concluding this section of therapeutic dimensions, it must be emphasized that the nurse's effectiveness will be based on her openness to learn what works best with particular kinds of patients. Both the use of communication techniques and the therapeutic conditions must be individualized to the nurse's personality and the needs of her patients. Rote application can be destructive. The nurse must be willing to try other approaches and techniques that seem potentially helpful when the present approach seems ineffective at a given time with the patient.

Therapeutic impasses

Therapeutic impasses are blocks in the progress of the nurse-patient relationship. They arise for a variety of reasons and may take many different forms, but they all create stalls in the therapeutic relationship. These impasses provoke intense feelings in both the nurse and patient that may range from anxiety and apprehension to frustration, love, or intense anger. Four specific therapeutic impasses will now be discussed: resistance, transference, countertransference, and gift giving.

Resistance

Resistance is the patient's attempt to remain unaware of anxiety-producing aspects within himself. It is a natural reluctance or learned avoidance of verbalizing or even experiencing the troubled aspects of the self. The term resistance was initially introduced by Freud to mean the patient's unconscious opposition to exploring or recognizing unconscious or even preconscious material. The patient's ambivalent attitudes toward self-exploration, in which he both appreciates and avoids anxiety-producing experiences, are a normal part of the therapeutic process.

Resistance may also be a reaction by the patient to the nurse who has moved too rapidly or too deeply into the patient's feelings or who has intentionally or nonintentionally communicated a lack of respect. It may also simply be the result of a patient who has a nurse working with him who is an inappropriate role model for therapeutic behavior. Secondary gain is another cause of resistance. It can become a powerful force in the perpetuation and propagation of an illness, since it makes the environment more comfortable. Favorable environmental, interpersonal, and situational changes occur and material advantages may be secured as a result of the illness. Types of secondary gain include financial compensation, avoidance of unpleasant situations, the securing of increased sympathy or attention, escape from responsibility, attempted control of people, and lessening of social pressures.

Resistance may take many forms. Wolberg[71] identified some of these:

1. Suppression and repression of pertinent information
2. Intensification of symptoms
3. Self-devaluation and a hopeless outlook on the future
4. Forced flight into health where there is a sudden, but short-lived recovery by the patient
5. Intellectual inhibitions, which may be evident when the patient says he has "nothing on his mind" or that he is "unable to think about his problems" or when he breaks appointments, is late for sessions, or is forgetful, silent, or sleepy
6. Acting out or irrational behavior
7. Superficial talk
8. Intellectual insight in which the patient verbalizes self-understanding with correct use of terminology yet continues destructive behavior or use of the defense of intellectualization where there is no insight
9. Contempt for normality, which is evident when the patient has developed insight but refuses to assume the responsibility for change on the grounds that normality "isn't so great"
10. Transference reactions

Transference

Transference is an unconscious response of the patient in which he experiences feelings and attitudes toward the nurse that were originally associated with significant figures in his early life. Such responses may be triggered by some superficial similarity, such as a facial feature or manner of speech or by the patient's perceived similarity of the relationship. The term transference refers to a group of reactions that attempt to reduce or alleviate anxiety. The outstanding trait defining transference is the inappropriateness of the patient's response in terms of intensity. Transference reduces the patient's self-awareness by helping him maintain a generalized view of the world in which all people are seen in similar terms. Thus the nurse may be viewed as an authority figure from the past, such as a parent figure, or as a lost loved object, such as a former spouse. Transference reactions are harmful to the therapeutic process only if they remain ignored and unexamined.

Two types of transferences present particular resistances in the nurse-patient relationship. The first is the hostile transference. If the patient internalizes his anger and hostility, he may express this resistance as depression and discouragement. He may ask to terminate the relationship on the grounds that he has no chance of getting well. If the patient usually externalizes his hostility, he may become critical, defiant, and irritable. He may express doubts about the nurse's training, experience, or personal adjustment. He may attempt to compete with her by reading books on psychology and challenging her. Hostility may also be expressed by the patient in detachment, forgetfulness, irrelevant chatter, or preoccupation with childhood experiences. An extreme form of uncooperativeness and negativism is evident in prolonged silences. Some of the most frustrating moments for the nurse are those spent in total silence with a patient. This is not the therapeutic silence that communicates mutuality and understanding. Rather, it is the silence that seems to be hostile, eternal, and oppressive. It is particularly disturbing for the nurse in the orientation phase before a relationship has been established. Generally, silences are more uncomfortable for the patient than they are for the nurse, but in this case the reverse may be true. The nurse's task is to understand the meaning of the patient's silence, and decide how to deal with it despite feeling somewhat awkward and useless.

A second difficult type of transference is the dependent reaction. This resistance is characterized by patients who are submissive, subordinate, and ingratiating and who regard the nurse as a "godlike" figure. The patient overvalues the characteristics and qualities of the nurse, and their relationship is in jeopardy because the patient views it as magical. In this reaction the nurse must live up to the overwhelming expectations of the patient, which is impossible because they are completely unrealistic. The patient continues to demand more of the nurse, and when she does not meet his needs, he is filled with hostility and contempt.

Resistances and transferences can pose difficult problems for the nurse. The psychiatric nurse must be prepared to be exposed to powerful negative and positive emotional feelings coming from the patient, often on a highly irrational basis. The relationship can become stalled and nonbeneficial if the nurse is not prepared for the patient's expression of feelings, is not prepared to deal with them, or is so preoccupied by her own needs and problems that she cannot clearly perceive what is happening. Sometimes resistances occur because the nurse and patient have not arrived at mutually acceptable goals or plans of action. Perhaps the patient expected the nurse to give him advice or solve his problems for him. This may occur if the contract was not clearly defined in the orientation stage of the relationship. The appropriate action here is to return to the goals, purpose, and roles of the nurse and patient in the relationship.

Whatever the patient's motivations, the analysis of the resistance or transference is geared toward his gaining awareness of them and the development of his knowledge that he controls his behavior and ultimately he is responsible for all he does and experiences. The first thing the nurse must do in handling resistance or transference is to listen. When she recognizes the resistance, she then uses clarification and reflection of feeling. Clarification helps give the nurse a more focused idea of what is happening. Reflection of content may help the patient to become aware of what has been going on in his own mind. Reflection of feeling acknowledges the resistance and mirrors it back to the patient. The nurse may say, "I sense that you're struggling with yourself. Part of you wants to explore the issue of your marriage and another part says 'No—I'm not ready yet.' "

It is not sufficient, however, to merely identify that resistance is occurring. The behavior must be explored and possible reasons for its occurrence analyzed. The depth of exploration and analysis engaged in by the nurse and patient is related to her experience and knowledge base. The nurse prepared on the master's degree level has the background to review the material of resistance and work through the transference reaction with the patient. The process of supervision will aid her in this endeavor and minimize the effect of any negative reactions she may experience within herself.

Countertransference

Countertransference is a therapeutic impasse created by the nurse. It refers to her specific emotional response generated by the qualities of her patient that is inappropriate to the content and context of the therapeutic relationship or inappropriate in the degree of intensity of emotion. It is transference applied to the nurse. Inappropriateness is the crucial element, as it is with transference, because it is natural that the nurse will have a warmth toward or liking for some patients more than others for realistic reasons. She will also be genuinely angry with the actions of certain patients. But in countertransference her responses are not justified by reality. She will be identifying the patient with individuals from her past, and her own needs will be interfering with her effectiveness. Her unresolved conflicts about authority, sex, assertiveness, and independence will tend to create, rather than solve, problems.

Countertransference reactions are usually one of three types: reactions of intense love or caring, reactions of intense hostility or hatred, and reactions of intense anxiety often in response to reresistance by the patient. Through the use of immediacy the nurse can identify countertransference in one of its various forms. Some of these were described by Menninger[42] and include the following:

1. Inability to empathize with the patient in certain problem areas
2. Depressed feelings during or after the session
3. Carelessness about implementing the contract by being late, running overtime, etc.
4. Drowsiness during the sessions
5. Feelings of anger or impatience because of the patient's unwillingness to change
6. Encouragement of the patient's dependency, praise, or affection
7. Arguing with the patient or a tendency to push the patient before he is ready
8. Trying to help the patient in matters not related to the identified goals
9. Involvement with the patient on a personal or social level
10. Dreaming about or preoccupation with the patient

Forms of countertransference occur because the nurse is involved with the patient as a participant observer and is not a detached bystander. They can be powerful tools in exploration and potent instruments for uncovering inner states. They are destructive only if they are brushed aside, ignored, or not taken seriously. These reactions, if studied objectively, can lead to further information and data about the patient. The analysis of countertransference can bring to light new material of which the nurse was not previously aware. The ability to remain objective does not mean that the nurse may not at times dislike what the patient says or become irritated. The resistance of the patient to acquire insight and transform insight into action and the refusal of the patient to change maladaptive and destructive coping mechanisms can be frustrating. But the capacity of the nurse to understand her feelings will help her to maintain a working relationship with the patient.

One difference between an inexperienced and an experienced psychiatric nurse is that the experienced nurse is constantly on the lookout for countertransference, becomes aware of it when it occurs, and holds it in abeyance or utilizes it to promote the therapeutic goals. In attempting to identify a countertransference the nurse must apply the same standards of honest self-appraisal to herself that she expects of the patient. She should subject herself to self-examination throughout the course of the relationship and particularly when the patient attacks or criticizes her. The following questions may be helpful:

■ How do I feel about the patient?
■ Do I look forward to seeing him?
■ Do I feel sorry for or sympathetic toward him?
■ Am I bored with him and believe that we are not progressing?
■ Am I afraid of him?
■ Do I get extreme pleasure out of seeing him?
■ Do I want to protect, reject, or punish him?
■ Do I dread meeting him and feel nervous during the sessions?
■ Am I impressed by him or do I try to impress him?
■ Does he make me very angry or frustrated?

If any of these questions suggest a problem, the nurse should pursue it. What is the patient doing to provoke these feelings? Who does the patient remind me of? The nurse must discover the source of the problem. Because countertransference can be detrimental to the relationship, it should be dealt with as soon as possible. When recognized, the nurse can exercise control over it. Frequently the nurse needs help in dealing with countertransference. Individual or group supervision can be most beneficial. Weekly clinical seminars, peer consultation, and professional meetings can also offer emotional support.

Countertransference problems are most clearly evident when someone is labeled a "problem patient." Usually such a patient engenders strong negative feelings, such as anger, fear, and helplessness and is often described by nurses as "manipulative, a pain, dependent, inappropriate, and demanding." The label of "problem patient" implies that the patient should change his behavior for the sake of the helper rather than for his own benefit. A common consequence of this labeling is that the patient and nurse become adversaries, and the nurse avoids contact with him. A study of the treatment records of "difficult patients" revealed some interesting findings. As compared to controls, difficult patients were simultaneously involved in or referred to two or more treatment programs, had no one person primarily responsible for coordinating their treatment programs, had incomplete documentation of treatment contacts, and lacked a comprehensive diagnosis and treatment plan.[47]

Rather than viewing him as a "problem patient," it is more productive for a nurse to view him as a patient who poses problems for herself. This turns the responsibility for action away from the patient and back onto the nurse. It forces the nurse to explore her responses to the patient and the behavior she displays that reinforces his unproductive behavior. In this way the nurse also makes the patient responsible for his own behavior. By stepping back and reviewing again the patient's needs and problems, the nurse becomes aware that she is failing to use the responsive dimensions of genuineness, respect, empathic understanding, and concreteness. And, without this therapeutic groundwork, a therapeutic outcome is impossible.

Gift giving

Gift giving is included in this discussion of therapeutic impasses, not because it necessarily precipitates an impasse, but because many nurses perceive it this way. This is partly because there has been a long-accepted taboo in nursing of accepting gifts from patients. Like many traditional taboos, it lacks a sound theoretical rationale, inhibits the independent decision making of the nurse, and creates a feeling of anxiety or guilt.

Gifts can take many forms. They can be tangible or intangible, lasting or temporary. Tangible gifts may include such items as a box of candy, bouquet of flowers, hand-knit scarf, or a hand-painted picture. Intangible gifts can be the expression of thanks to a nurse by a patient who is about to be discharged or a family member's sense of relief and gratitude at being able to share an emotional burden with another caring person. The underlying element among all of these gifts is that something of value is voluntarily offered to another person usually to convey gratitude.

Because gifts can be so varied, it is inappropriate to lump them all together and uniformly arrive at an appropriate nursing action. Rather, the nurse's response to gift giving and the role it plays in the therapeutic relationship depends on the timing of the particular situation, intent of the giver, and contextual meaning of the giving of the gift. Occasionally, it may be most appropriate and therapeutic for the nurse to accept a patient's gift, although on other occasions it may be quite inappropriate and detrimental to the relationship.

The timing of the gift giving is an important consideration. In the introductory, or orientation, phase of the relationship, nurses may be asked, "Do you have a cigarette I can borrow?" or "Will you buy me a cup of coffee?" These seemingly minor requests may make the nurse feel uncomfortable refusing them. She may even rationalize her compliance by thinking that it indicates her interest in the patient and may help him to trust her. But these responses by the nurse indicate her failure to examine the covert, or underlying, need of the patient who is making the request and her own needs in complying with it. Also, in this early phase of the relationship, the nurse may be the one to initiate gift giving by giving the patient a book, plant, or some other item that she believes expresses her interest.

In the orientation phase of the relationship, gift giving can be detrimental because it often meets personal needs rather than therapeutic goals. The patient, for example, may be trying to manipulate the nurse as his way of controlling the relationship and setting interpersonal limits on the level of intimacy he will allow. As such, it can be a form of resistance and act as a therapeutic impasse. The nurse as the gift giver may also be distorting the nature and purpose of the therapeutic relationship by her behavior. By giving gifts to the patient, she is attempting to relate through objects instead of the therapeutic use of self. She is avoiding exploring her own possible feelings of inadequacy of frustration. If the patient accepts the gifts, she may worry that he is relating to her out of a sense of obligation, and this aura of doubt may overshadow the course of the relationship. On the other hand, it may enhance the patient's sense of self to bring to his attention a magazine that has been on the ward and has an article on a topic of interest to him. The distinction lies in the meaning behind the gift and the sense of obligation it implies.

As the relationship progresses, gift giving may take on a different significance. In the working phase, for example, the patient may one day offer to buy the nurse a cup of coffee. This can be an indication of the patient's respect for the nurse and his belief in the mutuality of their work together. As an isolated incident, the nurse's acceptance of it can enhance the patient's confidence, self-esteem, and sense of responsibility.

Gift giving most often arises in the termination phase of the relationship, and it is in this phase that the meaning behind it can be the most complex and difficult to determine. At this time, gift giving can be tangible or intangible and can reflect a patient's need to make the nurse feel guilty, delay the termination process, compensate for feelings of inadequacy, or attempt to transform the therapeutic nurse-patient relationship into a social one that can possibly go on indefinitely. The nurse can initiate gift giving for similar reasons. The feelings evoked during the termination process can be very powerful, and they must be acknowledged and explored if termination is to be a learning experience for both participants. If feelings are identified and clarified, then a small gift that reflects gratitude and rememberance can be exchanged, accepted, and valued. In this case, it becomes not a therapeutic impasse, but a memento of a treasured growth experience.

Effectiveness of the nurse

The nurse's effectiveness in working with psychiatric patients is related to her knowledge base, clinical skills, and capacity for introspection and self-evaluation. The nurse and patient, as participants in an interpersonal relationship, are entwined in a pattern of reciprocal emotions that directly affect the therapeutic outcome. The nurse conveys feelings to the patient. Some of these will be in response to the patient; others will arise from the nurse's personal life and will not necessarily be associated with the patient. For example, a nurse is feeling angry because of an administrative problem involving the nursing service. Her patient may sense these feelings and misconstrue their source as being himself. If he does not have the confidence to discuss this with the nurse, she may be unaware of his misconception.

Many painful feelings arise within the nurse because of the nature of the therapeutic process, which can be stressful. These "normal" stresses are due to a variety of factors. Although the nurse must be a skilled listener, it is inappropriate for her to discuss her own conflicts or personal responses, except when they may help the patient. This bottling up of emotions can be painful. She is expected to empathize with the emotions and feelings of the patient. At the same time, however, she is expected to retain her objectivity and not be caught up in a sympathetic response. This can create a kind of double bind. Termination poses another stress when the nurse must separate from a patient she has come to know well and care for deeply. It is common to experience a grief reaction in response to the loss. Many nurses find it emotionally draining when a patient communicates a prolonged and intense expression of emotion, such as sadness, despair, or anger. Discomfort also arises when the nurse feels unable to help a patient who is in great distress. Suicide dramatizes this situation. Treating suicidal individuals can arouse intense and prolonged anxiety in the nurse.

The painful nature of these emotional responses makes the practice of psychiatric nursing challenging and stressful. The therapeutic use of self involves the nurse's total personality, and total involvement is not an easy task. It is essential that the nurse be aware of her feelings and responses and receive guidance and support in her work.

Supervision

According to Haller, supervision is a "process whereby a therapist, frequently but not always a relative beginner, is helped to become a more effective clinician. The goals of supervision are not only to guide the therapist in the successful handling of the supervised case, but to catalyze the therapist's creative and therapeutic use of self."[27:36] The supervisor serves as a provider of theoretical knowledge and therapeutic techniques, validates the use of the nursing process, and supports the working through of transference and countertransference reactions. Consultation is different from supervision in that it denotes a peer or collegial relationship; it is discussed in detail in Chapter 23.

Supervision also functions as a support system for those providing care and is an essential element in therapeutic relationships. One must care about oneself and experience being cared for before one can give care to others. All practicing psychiatric nurses experience some degree of clinical stress. There are stresses associated with such patient behaviors as hopelessness, self-destruction, and manipulation, as well as the stress inherent in the intimacy, openness, and responsiveness required of the nurse who has established a therapeutic relationship. Supervision provides the nurse with a system of clinical support and contributes greatly, if indirectly, to the quality of nursing care.

In many ways the process of supervision parallels the nurse-patient relationship. Both involve a learning process that takes place in the context of a deep and meaningful relationship which facilitates positive change. Self-exploration is a critical element of both. The supervisor should provide the same responsive and action dimensions present in the nurse-patient relationship to help the supervised nurse become a person who is able to live effectively with herself and others.

The most common forms of supervision are the dyadic or one-to-one relationship, in which the supervisor meets the supervisee in a face-to-face encounter; the triadic relationship, in which a supervisor and two nurses of similar experience and training meet for supervision; and group supervision, in which several supervised nurses meet together for a shared session with the supervisory nurse. All three forms of supervision have a similar purpose of exploring the problem areas and maximizing the strengths of the supervisees.

The process of supervision requires the nurse to record the interactions with her patient. Both written processed recordings and audio recordings have been utilized for this purpose, but neither yields as accurate and complete information as that provided by videotape recordings.[46] Videotaped sessions record both visual and audio elements and minimize distortion of data. The supervised nurse then analyzes her data, extracts themes, and identifies problems relevant to her nursing care. She reviews the literature, draws inferences, evaluates her effectiveness, and formulates plans for her next session. In the supervision conference, she shares this analysis and receives feedback from her supervisor and peers, if it is a group conference.

Supervision can be viewed as either a didactic process in which the theory, concepts, and practice of the individual therapeutic relationship are enunciated, or it can be a quasi-therapeutic process that explores countertransference problems, attitudes, values, and the nurse's emotional needs and personal biases. The more widely accepted view recognizes that the supervisor-therapist relationship is more important than a simple didactic adjunct to the treatment process and that it has a major, if somewhat intangible, bearing on the therapist-patient relationship and the therapeutic process.

Three methods of supervision have been described. The first is *patient centered,* in which the therapist brings her technical problems with the patient to the supervisor and is given advice. The second type is *therapist centered,* in which the focus is on the therapist's blind spots and countertransference reactions, which helps the therapist to see her influence on the therapeutic process. The danger with this method is that when it is used to the extreme, the patient gets

lost from sight, and the supervision evolves into personal therapy for the supervisee. The third approach is *process centered,* in which emphasis is on what is happening between the therapist, patient, and supervisor. The supervisor makes use of the analogy between the therapist-patient relationship and the therapist-supervisor relationship to help the supervisee use her own experience of emotional difficulties in receiving help from her supervisor to facilitate her understanding of the patient's situation.

Ekstein and Wallerstein[21] have developed a process-centered model of supervision that is neither personal therapy nor simply a didactic process of conveying information on theory and technique. In their model, the supervisor is an active participant in an affectively charged learning process, the focus of which is learning and personal growth, rather than psychotherapy for the supervisee. They describe how and in what ways the problems between the therapist and supervisor can shed light on and, in fact, often stand for problems that exist between the therapist and patient. The very problems experienced in the one relationship effect and are reflected in the other relationship, so that a parallel process exists between the supervisor-therapist relationship and therapist-patient relationship.

The goal of supervision, however, is not to eliminate these problems, but to use them to achieve greater understanding of the ongoing dynamic processes at work in therapy. The problems become the vehicles through which therapeutic progress may be made. They propose that the most effective supervision depends on active insight into the interplay of forces in the parallel processes of therapy and supervision.

Little research on the supervisory process is reported in the literature. One of the few studies to explore the nature of the process was conducted by Doehrman.[20] The results of this study highlight an important aspect of supervision—tension in the supervisory relationship is inevitable but when understood and handled skillfully, it is instrumental to the therapist's growth. Learning to be therapeutic inspires fear and resistance in the learner related to change. These are expressed in the supervisee's characteristic way of resisting authority. The therapist's ways of resisting help in supervision are intimately related to her difficulties in giving help to patients. Insight into these resistances will provide the supervisee with insight into her problems as a therapist and particular problems she experiences in the nurse-patient relationship. Deprived of these insights, the supervisee cannot grow as a therapist. There will be no learning, no change, and the status quo will be preserved.

Doehrman's study gives support to the Ekstein and Wallerstein model of supervision, which entails the supervisor's addressing herself to the problems of the supervisee that block her functioning as an effective therapist. Doehrman concludes that the supervisor should deal with the supervisee's feelings toward her and toward the supervisory process when these feelings interfere with the therapist's effectiveness with her patients or her ability to learn from her supervisor. The clarification of these problems requires the supervisor's use of certain therapeutic skills, such as the exploration and expression of feelings and encouraging insight, and this may be intensely therapeutic for the supervisee.

Despite the intensity, however, supervision is not therapy. The essential difference between the two is a difference of purpose. The aim of supervision is the teaching of psychotherapeutic skills, whereas the goal of therapy is to alter the patient's characteristic patterns of coping to function more effectively in all areas of life. In contrast, the supervisee's problems in the supervisory and therapeutic relationships are dealt with only to the extent that they are affecting the nurse's ability to learn from her supervisor and be effective with her patients. Therefore, the problems are limited in scope and depth and do not include all other aspects of the supervisee's life situation. With the resolution of the particular problem, the focus of supervision returns to the teaching of psychotherapeutic skills and their implementation by the nurse with her patients. The therapeutic implications for the supervisee are therefore derivatives of the primary goal of supervision—the teaching of psychotherapeutic skills.

Supervision or consultation is necessary for the practicing psychiatric nurse. Although it is crucial for novices, it is equally as important for experienced practitioners. Personal limitations create a need for assistance in remaining objective throughout the therapeutic process and the "normal" stresses it presents. Obviously supervision is only as helpful as the skill of the supervisor, the openness of the supervised nurse, and the motivation of both to learn and grow.

Ethics and nursing practice

The concept of ethics has different meanings to each individual. It implies what is right and wrong and becomes intermingled with one's ideas on values and morality. An ethic is a standard of valued behavior or beliefs adhered to by an individual or group. It describes what ought to be, rather than what is. It is a goal to which one aspires. These standards of behavior are learned through socialization, growth, and experience. As such, they are not static entities; they evolve and change concurrent with social change. Ethical standards can only be implemented in conjunction with personal value systems. Groups, such as professions, can also hold a code of ethics that reflects the profession's desire to protect its clients. It functions to define behavior that is viewed to be desirable by the profession in its service to consumers, not in service to itself, and it serves as a framework for decision making for members of the profession. Moore[45] has defined two major purposes for a code of ethics as that of "structuring" and "sensitizing." This first has a basically preventive value and aims to hold back impulsive and unethical behavior. The second purpose of sensitizing has an essentially educative value and aims to raise one's ethical consciousness.

The American Nurses' Association published a code of ethics for nurses on p. 106.[2] It places heavy emphasis on the accountability of the nurse for the quality of patient care and the nurse's duty to act as a patient advocate in ensuring the quality of care rendered by others.

These professional standards are intended to be used by nurses in the daily conduct of health care delivery. Knowledge of one's own personal values and implementation of them within the framework of the nursing ethical code can shape the quality of the nursing care one gives patients and increase the satisfaction the nurse receives from her practice.

A discussion of ethics and nursing must take into consideration the crucial element of power. In the psychiatric setting, the nurse can function in many roles, from a custodial keeper of the keys to a skilled therapist. Each of these roles, however, has a certain amount of power inherent in it, since all nurses have the ability to influence the patient's course of treatment. Nurses serve as the major source of information regarding a patient's behavior. This is particularly true in inpatient settings, where longer contacts can occur between a nurse and patient and the nursing staff is the only group to work a 24-hour day. Nurses also participate in team meetings, individual and group psychotherapy,

---

AMERICAN NURSES' ASSOCIATION CODE FOR NURSES*

1. The nurse provides services with respect for human dignity and the uniqueness of the client unrestricted by considerations of social or economic status, personal attributes, or the nature of health problems.
2. The nurse safeguards the client's right to privacy by judiciously protecting information of a confidential nature.
3. The nurse acts to safeguard the client and the public when health care and safety are affected by the incompetent, unethical, or illegal practice of any person.
4. The nurse assumes responsibility and accountability for individual nursing judgments and actions.
5. The nurse maintains competence in nursing.
6. The nurse exercises informed judgment and uses individual competence and qualification as criteria in seeking consultation, accepting responsibilities, and delegating nursing activities to others.
7. The nurse participates in activities that contribute to the ongoing development of the profession's body of knowledge.
8. The nurse participates in the profession's efforts to implement and improve standards of nursing.
9. The nurse participates in the profession's efforts to establish and maintain conditions of employment conducive to high-quality nursing care.
10. The nurse participates in the profession's effort to protect the public from misinformation and misrepresentation and to maintain the integrity of nursing.
11. The nurse collaborates with members of the health professions and other citizens in promoting community and national efforts to meet public health needs.

*From American Nurses' Association: Code for nurses with interpretive statements, Kansas City, Mo., 1976. Reprinted with permission.

---

and behavior modification programs. Finally, nurses can greatly influence decisions about patient medications, such as the type, dosage, and frequency of the prescribed drugs.

The medical literature describes the ethical dilemmas that arise from physicians' "paternalistic" attitude toward their patients. This attitude tends to reduce the adult patient to the status of a child and allows the physician to violate the patient's rights if the physician perceives it to be "for the patient's own good." One might propose that, in a similar way, nurses could assume a "maternalistic" attitude toward their patients that could interfere with a patient's liberty of action. To avoid this potential danger, the nurse should realize that her ethical obligations span a wide range of individuals, including the patient, the patient's family or support system, herself, her own family, other health care professionals, the health care institution or organization in which she works, and the larger social community. Furthermore, her ethical obligations arise within a context of laws and government regulations that may, at times, create ethical dilemmas which involve and affect the nurse. To the extent that she is aware of them, she can examine these problems not only from a clinical perspective, but also from an ethical one.

ETHICAL DILEMMAS. An ethical dilemma exists when moral claims conflict with one another. It can be defined as (1) a difficult problem that seems to have no satisfactory solution or (2) a choice between equally unsatisfactory alternatives. Ethical dilemmas pose such questions as "What should I do?" and "What is the right thing to do?" They can occur both at the nurse-patient-family level of daily nursing care and at the policy-making level of institutions and communities. Although ethical dilemmas arise in all areas of nursing practice, some problems are unique to psychiatric and mental health nursing. Many of these dilemmas come together under the umbrella issue of behavior control.

On first analysis, behavior control may seem like a simple concrete issue—behavior is a personal choice, and any behavior that does not impose on the rights of others is acceptable. Unfortunately, this simple proposition does not help one address complex situations. For example, a severely depressed person may choose suicide as an alternative to an intolerable existence. This is, on one level, an individual choice not directly harming others, yet suicide is strongly prohibited in American society. In many states, suicide is a crime that can be prosecuted. So too, in some states, it is illegal for consenting adults of the same sex to have sexual relations, although it is not illegal for a man to rape his wife. These examples raise some difficult questions: When is it appropriate for society to regulate personal behavior? Who will regulate this behavior? Is the aim of this regulation personal adjustment, personal growth, or adaptation to social norms? And finally, how do we measure the costs and benefits of attempting to control personal freedom in a free society?

One of the most fundamental problems is that psychiatry lacks definitions for mental health, normalcy, mental illness, and insanity. These terms have been debated for hundreds of years, yet society lacks consensus on universally accepted definitions. This is evidence of the blurring boundaries between science and ethics in the field of psychiatry. Theoretically, science and ethics are viewed as two separate entities. Science is descriptive, deals with "what is," and rests on validation; ethics is predictive, deals with "what ought to be," and relies on judgment. However, psychiatry is neither purely scientific nor value free. The fact that psychiatry is not a predictable science is reflected in the existence of over 100 schools of psychotherapy, each with its own theory of causation, treatment goals, and therapeutic practices, which range from screaming cures (Janov's primal therapy), to reasoning cures (Ellis' rational therapy), to realism cures (Glasser's reality therapy), to orgasm cures (Reich's orgone therapy), to profound-rest cures (transcendental meditation), and even to chemical cures (megavitamin therapy).[33] What emerges is the sense that psychiatry represents neither pure science nor pure ethics, but a branch of the healing professions that resides somewhere in between and that often may be affected by culture, chance, and faith.

Despite these ambiguities, each mental health professional must identify the nature of one's professional commitment. Is one committed to the happiness of the individual or the smooth functioning of society? Ideally, these values should not conflict, but in reality they sometimes do. The patient's rights to treatment, to refuse treatment, and to informed consent highlight this conflict-of-interest question and are described in more detail in Chapter 16. As a

nurse, one must consider if one is reinforcing an individual's personal unhappiness to force him to be socially or politically acceptable to society. As such, the nurse may not actually be working for either the patient's best interests or her own; she may be acting as an agent of society and not be really aware of it.

All nurses participate in some therapeutic regimens in psychiatry whose scientific and ethical bases are ambiguous. Any health professional who has witnessed electroconvulsive therapy, for example, has probably questioned the effectiveness, coerciveness, precision, or humaneness of psychiatry. Yet the American health care system continues to apply a medical model of wellness and illness to human behavior. Wellness is socially acceptable behavior, and illness is socially unacceptable behavior. Within this context, it becomes critically important for each nurse to analyze for herself such ethical dilemmas as freedom of choice vs. coercion, defining adequate treatment, deciding on resource allocations, helping vs. imposing values, and focusing on cure vs. prevention.

ETHICAL DECISION MAKING. Ethical decision making involves trying to determine right from wrong in situations where clear guidelines are not evident.

Everything is neither right nor wrong. The right or wrong is the choosing, the keeping, the losing. All paths are light and shadow, and every path is a different thing to each man. The right and the wrong, the good and the evil lie not upon the silent pathway, but in the man that walks it."[52:198]

There are three dimensions to ethical decision making. Each of these dimensions influences one's analysis of the dilemma and decisions related to it:
1. The existence of a code of value judgments or ethics that is known to the individual
2. The awareness of one's personal moral beliefs and values
3. A complex social context with normative and legal implications

It is necessary for the nurse to correlate the code of nursing ethics with her own personal value system and to identify areas of harmony and incongruence. This will allow the nurse to base her ethical decisions on behavior that involves responsibility, accountability, risk, and commitment. Responsibility requires the capac-

ACTION

Societal expectations →

← Legal requirements

Resolution

Application of principles

Options

Ethical agents

Ethical components

Background information

FIG. 3-9
Model for ethical decision making. Societal expectations and legal requirements may sway the resolution of the conflict one way or another. But one must not confuse the notions of what is legal (or expected) with what is good, right, or proper—they may or may not coincide. (From Curtin, L.: Nurs. Forum 17(1):12, 1978.)

ity for rational, moral decision making. Accountability signifies action. Risk involves the undertaking of peril, jeopardy, or chance of loss, and commitment implies loyalty, trust, and a pledge of self. In addition, the nurse's ethical choice must take into consideration the circumstances of the specific situation, social mores, and legal ramifications arising from it.

A decision-making model can be a useful tool in identifying factors that impinge on the decision and principles which need to be clarified. Curtin[19] proposed a model for critical ethical analysis (Fig. 3-9). It describes steps or factors that the nurse needs to consider between encountering an ethical dilemma and resolving it. The first step is *gathering background information* to get as clear a picture as possible of what precisely is the problem. This includes finding out what information is available and what information is needed to clarify one's understanding of the underlying issues. The next

factor is *identifying the ethical components* or the nature of the dilemma, such as freedom vs. coercion or treating vs. accepting the right to refuse treatment. The next step is the *clarification of the rights and responsibilities of all ethical agents,* or those involved in the decision making. This involves the patient, the nurse, and possibly many others, including the patient's family, physician, health care institution, clergyman, social worker, and perhaps even the courts. All involved ethical agents may not agree on how the situation should be handled, but the scope of their rights and duties can be clarified. *All possible options must then be explored* in light of the rights and responsibilities of everyone involved, as well as the purpose and potential result of each option. This step serves to eliminate those alternatives which violate rights or can be certain to produce harm. The nurse then engages in the *application of principles,* which are derived from her philosophy of life and nurs-

TABLE 3-6. Steps and questions in ethical decision making

Steps	Relevant questions
Gathering background information	Does an ethical dilemma exist? What information is known? What information is needed? What is the context of the dilemma?
Identifying ethical components	What is the underlying issue? Who is affected by this dilemma?
Clarification of agents	What are the rights of each involved party? What are the obligations of each involved party? Who should be involved in the decision making? For whom is the decision being made? What degree of consent is needed by the patient?
Exploration of options	What alternatives exist? What is the purpose or intent of each alternative? What are the potential consequences of each alternative?
Application of principles	What criteria should be used? What ethical theories are subscribed to? What scientific facts are relevant? What is one's philosophy of life and nursing?
Resolution into action	What are the social and legal constraints and ramifications? What is the goal of one's decision? How can the resulting ethical choice be implemented? How can the resulting ethical choice be evaluated?

ing, her store of scientific knowledge, and the ethical theory to which she subscribes. Ethical theories suggest ways of structuring or clarifying ethical dilemmas and help one to judge potential solutions. Following are four such positions[5]:

1. *Utilitariansim* focuses on the consequences of actions and on the greatest amount of happiness or the least amount of harm for the greatest number. It is embodied in the idea of "the greatest good for the greatest number."
2. *Egoism* is a position in which one seeks the solution that is best for oneself. The self is of paramount importance, and others are viewed secondarily, if at all.
3. *Formalism* requires the consideration of the nature of the act itself and the principles or rules involved. It involves the universal application of a basic principle, such as "do unto others as you would have them do unto you."
4. *Fairness* is based on the concept of justice, and benefit to the least advantaged in society becomes the norm for decision making.

The final step is the *resolution into action*. Within the context of social expectations and legal requirements, the nurse decides on the goals and methods of implementation. Table 3-6 summarizes the steps the nurse takes in ethical decision making and suggests questions she can ask herself as she deals with the challenge and complexity of ethical choice in psychiatric nursing practice.

Suggested cross-references

This chapter serves as a foundation for formulating principles of psychiatric nursing and implementing psychiatric nursing practice. As such, it is related to all other chapters of this text.

SUMMARY

1. The therapeutic nurse-patient relationship is a mutual learning experience and a corrective emotional experience for the patient. In this relationship the nurse uses herself and specified clinical techniques in working with the patient to bring about behavioral change. General goals of the relationship were identified.

2. Self-awareness was described as the first step in providing quality nursing care through the therapeutic use of self. The following qualities needed by nurses to be effective helpers were analyzed: the awareness of self, the clarification of values, the exploration of feelings, the ability to serve as a role model, altruism, and a sense of ethics and responsibility. All nurses should strive to attain these personal characteristics.

3. The four phases of the relationship process were described. Tasks of the nurse in the preinteraction phase include self-exploration of feelings and fears, gathering data about the patient if information is available, and planning for the first interaction with the patient. Tasks of the nurse in the orientation phase are to establish a climate of trust, understanding, acceptance, and open communication and to formulate a contract with the patient. Problems are identified, and goals are mutually defined. During the working phase the major part of the therapeutic work is carried out. The nurse promotes the development of insight in the patient, the translation of insight into action, and the integration of insight into his life experiences. The tasks of the nurse during the termination phase revolve around establishing the reality of the separation. Learning to bear the sorrow of the loss while incorporating positive aspects of the relationship into one's life is the goal of termination.

4. Communication incorporates the ideas of interpersonal influence and behavioral change and, as such, can play a facilitative role in the therapeutic relationship. Both the verbal and nonverbal levels of it were described, with elaboration on the nonverbal behaviors categorized as vocal cues, action cues, object cues, space, and touch. The elements of the communication process were identified as perception, evaluation, and transmission. The structural and transactional analysis models were used to examine components of the communication process and identify common breakdowns or problems. The following helpful therapeutic communication techniques were also discussed: listening, broad openings, restating, clarification, reflection, focusing, sharing perceptions, themes, silence, humor, informing, and suggesting.

5. The responsive dimensions of genuineness, respect, empathic understanding, and concreteness were presented. They interrelate with each other and contribute to each other in the therapeutic process, and some degree of all of them is necessary when initiating a relationship. Genuineness implies that the nurse is an open person who is self-congruent, authentic, and transparent. Respect implies that the patient is regarded as a person of worth who is valued and accepted without qualification. Empathic understanding is viewing the patient's world from his internal frame of reference. It involves the nurse's sensitivity to the patient's current feelings and the verbal ability to communicate this understanding in a language attuned to the patient. Concreteness involves the use of specific terminology rather than abstractions in the discussion of the patient's feelings, experiences, and behavior. The therapeutic level at which nurses function is unknown at present. Additional research on nurse-patient interactions is greatly needed because there is little empirical evidence on which to base scientific practice in this area.

6. The action dimensions of confrontation, immediacy, nurse self-disclosure, catharsis, and role playing stimulate and contribute to patient insight. Confrontation is an expression by the nurse of her perceived discrepancies in the patient's behavior. Immediacy occurs when the current interaction of the nurse and patient in the relationship is focused on. Nurse self-disclosure is evident when the nurse reveals information about herself, her ideas, values, feelings, and attitudes. Emotional catharsis occurs when the patient is encouraged to talk about things that bother him most. Fears, feelings, and experiences are brought into the open and discussed. Role playing is the acting out of a particular situation.

7. Therapeutic impasses are roadblocks in the progress of the nurse-patient relationship. As such, they should be dealt with by the nurse as soon as possible. One of these, resistance, was defined as the patient's attempt to remain unaware of anxiety-producing aspects within himself. Transference is an unconscious response of the patient in which he experiences feelings and attitudes toward the nurse that were originally associated with significant figures in his early life. Countertransference is the specific emotional response of the nurse, generated by the qualities of her patient, that is inappropriate to the content and context of the therapeutic relationship or inappropriate in the degree of intensity of emotion. It is transference applied to the nurse. Gift giving is often perceived to be a therapeutic impasse but the actual role it plays in the relationship depends on the timing of the situation, the intent of the giver, and the contextual meaning of the giving of the gift.

8. Supervision is a process in which the supervised nurse is helped to become a more effective clinician.

It may occur individually or in groups and is distinct from consultation, which implies a peer relationship. A process-centered model of supervision was described that views therapy and supervision as parallel processes. Although supervision is crucial for novices, it is equally important for experienced practitioners.

9. An ethic is a standard of valued behavior or beliefs adhered to by an individual or group. It describes a goal to which one aspires. An ethical dilemma exists when moral claims conflict with one another. In psy-

chiatric nursing, many of these dilemmas center around the issue of behavior control. Ethical decision making involves trying to determine right from wrong in situations where clear guidelines are not evident. A model for critical ethical analysis was presented and explored.

References

1. Aiken, L., and Aiken, J.: A systematic approach to the evaluation of interpersonal relationships, Am. J. Nurs. **73**:863, 1973.
2. American Nurses' Association: Code for nurses with interpretive statements, Kansas City, Mo., 1976, The Association.
3. Anderson, S.: Effects of confrontation by high- and low-functioning therapists on high- and low-functioning clients, J. Counsel. Psychol. **16**:299, 1969.
4. Argyle, M.: Bodily communication, New York, 1975, International Universities Press, Inc.
5. Aroskar, M.: Anatomy of an ethical dilemma: the theory, Am. J. Nurs. **80**:658, 1980.
6. Barnett, K.: A theoretical construct of the concepts of touch as they relate to nursing, Nurs. Res. **21**:102, March-April 1972.
7. Berne, E.: Games people play: the psychology of human relationships, New York, 1964, Grove Press, Inc.
8. Bohart, A.: Role playing and interpersonal conflict reduction, J. Counsel. Psych. **24**:15, 1977.
9. Brammer, L., and Shostrum, E.: Therapeutic psychology, Englewood Cliffs, N.J., 1977, Prentice-Hall, Inc.
10. Bromley, G.: Confrontation in individual psychotherapy, J. Psychiatr. Nurs. **19**(5):15, 1981.
11. Buber, M.: I and thou, New York, 1958, Charles Scribner's Sons.
12. Bugenthal, J.: The search for existential identity, San Francisco, 1976, Jossey-Bass, Inc., Publishers.
13. Burgess, A., and Burns, J.: Why patients seek care, Am. J. Nurs. **73**:314, 1973.
14. Campaniello, J.: The process of termination, J. Psychiatr. Nurs. **18**(2):29, 1980.
15. Carkhoff, R.: Helping and human relations, vols. 1 and 2, New York, 1969, Holt, Rinehart & Winston, Inc.
16. Carkhoff, R., and Berenson, B.: Beyond counseling and therapy, New York, 1967, Holt, Rinehart & Winston, Inc.
17. Carkhoff, R., and Truax, C.: Toward effective counseling and psychotherapy, Chicago, 1967, Aldine Publishing Co.
18. Coad-Denton, A.: Therapeutic superficiality and intimacy. In Longo, D., and Williams, R., editors: Psychosocial nursing: assessment and intervention, New York, 1978, Appleton-Century-Crofts.
19. Curtin, L.: A proposed model for critical ethical analysis, Nurs. Forum **17**(1):12, 1978.
20. Doehrman, M.: Parallel process in supervision and psychotherapy, Bull. Menninger Clin. **40**:9, 1976.
21. Ekstein, R., and Wallerstein, R.: The teaching and learning of psychotherapy, New York, 1958, Basic Books, Inc., Publishers.
22. Fox, E., Nelson, M., and Bolman, W.: The termination process: a neglected dimension in social work, Social Work **14**:53, Oct. 1969.
23. Gaylin, W.: Feelings, New York, 1979, Harper & Row Publishers, Inc.
24. Gazda, G., et al: Human relations development: a manual for educators, Boston, 1971, Allyn & Bacon, Inc.
25. Ginott, H.: Between parent and child, New York, 1965, Macmillan Co., Publishers.
26. Hall, E.: The silent language, Garden City, N.Y., 1959, Doubleday & Co., Inc.
27. Haller, L.: Clinical psychiatric supervision. In Kneisl, C.R., and Wilson, H.S., editors: Current perspectives in psychiatric nursing, vol. 1, St. Louis, 1976, The C.V. Mosby Co.
28. Heuscher, J.: The role of humor and folklore themes in psychotherapy, Am. J. Psychiatry **137**(12):1546, 1980.
29. Hutchinson, S.: Humor: a link to life. In Kneisl, C.R., and Wilson, H.S., editors: Current perspectives in psychiatric nursing, vol. 1, St. Louis, 1976, The C.V. Mosby Co.
30. Johnson, M.: Self-disclosure: a variable in the nurse-client relationship, J. Psychiatr. Nurs. **18**(1):17, 1980.
31. Jourard, S.: The transparent self, New York, 1971, Litton Educational Publishing, Inc.
32. Kalisch, B.: What is empathy? Am. J. Nurs. **73**:1548, 1973.
33. Karasu, T.: Psychotherapies: an overview, Am. J. Psychiatry **134**:851, 1977.
34. Kirschenbaum, H., and Simon, S., editors: Readings in values clarification, Minneapolis, 1973, Winston Press, Inc.
35. Krieger, D.: The therapeutic touch: how to use your hands to help or to heal, New York, 1979, Prentice-Hall, Inc.
36. La Crosse, M.: Nonverbal behavior and perceived counselor attractiveness and persuasiveness, J. Counsel. Psychol. **22**:563, 1975.
37. La Monica, E., and Karshmer, J.: Empathy: educating nurses in professional practice, J. Nurs. Educ. **17**(2):3, 1978.
38. Levinson, H.: Termination of psychotherapy: some salient issues, paper presented at the Illinois Society for Clinical Social Work, Chicago, Oct. 1975.
39. Luft, J.: Of human interaction, Palo Alto, Calif., 1969, National Press Books.
40. Mansfield, E.: Empathy: concept and identified psychiatric nursing behavior, Nurs. Res. **22**(6):525, 1973.
41. Mehrabian, A.: Nonverbal communication, Chicago, 1972, Aldine Publishing Co.

42. Menninger, K.: Theory of psychoanalytic techniques, New York, 1958, Basic Books, Inc.

43. Methven, D., and Schlotfeldt, R.: The social interaction inventory, Nurs. Res. **11**:83, Spring, 1962.

44. Mitchell, K., and Berenson, B.: Differential use of confrontation by high and low facilitative therapists, J. Nerv. Ment. Dis. **151**(5):303, 1970.

45. Moore, R.: Ethics in the practice of psychiatry: origins, functions, models and enforcement, Am. J. Psychiatry **135**:157, 1978.

46. Muecke, M.: Video-tape recording, Perspect. Psychiatr. Care **8**:200, Sept.-Oct. 1970.

47. Neill, J.: The difficult patient: identification and response, J. Clin. Psychiatry **40**(5):209, 1979.

48. Ornston, P., Cuchetti, D., Levine, J., and Freiman, L.: Some parameters of verbal behavior that reliably differentiate novice from experienced psychotherapists, J. Abnorm. Psychol. **73**:240, 1968.

49. Peitchinis, J.: Therapeutic effectiveness of counseling by nursing personnel, Nurs. Res. **21**(2):138, 1972.

50. Raths, L., Harmin, M., and Simon, S.: Values and teaching, Columbus, Ohio, 1966, Charles E. Merrill Publishing Co.

51. Rogers, C.: On becoming a person, Boston, 1961, Houghton Mifflin Co.

52. Rogers, C.: Nakoa: Blackfoot philosophy, New York, 1972, Warner Books, Inc.

53. Rogers, C.: Empathic: an unappreciated way of being, J. Counsel. Psychol. **5**(2):2, 1975.

54. Rokeach, M.: The nature of human values, New York, 1973, Macmillan, Inc.

55. Ruesch, J.: Communication and human relations: an interdisciplinary approach. In Ruesch, J., and Bateson, G.: Communication: the social matrix of psychiatry, New York, 1968, W.W. Norton & Co., Inc.

56. Ruesch, J.: Disturbed communication, New York, 1972, W.W. Norton & Co., Inc.

57. Schiff, S.: Termination of therapy, Arch. Gen. Psychiatry **6**(1):77, 1962.

58. Schultz, F.: The mourning phase of relationships, J. Psychiatr. Nurs. **2**(1):37, 1964.

59. Sedgwick, R.: Role playing: a bridge between talk and action, J. Psychiatr. Nurs. **14**(11):16, 1976.

60. Sigman, P.: Ethical choice in nursing, Adv. Nurs. Sci. **1**(3):37, 1979.

61. Spitz, R.: No and yes on the genesis of human communication, New York, 1957, International Universities Press, Inc.

62. Stacklum, M.: New student in psychology, Am. J. Nurs. **81**:762, 1981.

63. Stetler, C.: Relationship of perceived empathy to nurses' communication, Nurs. Res. **26**:432, 1977.

64. Sundeen, S. et al.: Nurse-client interaction: implementing the nursing process, ed. 2, St. Louis, 1981, The C.V. Mosby Co.

65. Travelbee, J.: Intervention in psychiatric nursing, Philadelphia, 1969, F.A. Davis Co.

66. Ujhely, G.: Touch: reflections and perceptions, Nurs. Forum **18**(1):18, 1979.

67. Uustal, D.: Values clarification in nursing: application to practice, Am. J. Nurs. **78**:2058, 1978.

68. Watzlawick, P., Beavin, J., and Jackson, D.: Pragmatics of human communication: a study of interactional patterns, pathologies, and paradoxes, New York, 1967, W.W. Norton & Co., Inc.

69. Weiss, S.: The language of touch, Nurs. Res. **28**(2):76, 1979.

70. Williams, C.: Empathic communication and its effect on client outcome, Issues Ment. Health Nurs. **2**(1):16, 1979.

71. Wolberg, L.: The technique of psychotherapy, vol. 2, New York, 1967, Grune & Stratton, Inc.

Annotated suggested readings

Albiez, Sr. A.: Reflecting on the development of a relationship, J. Psychiatr. Nurs. **9**(6):25, Nov.-Dec. 1970.

A nursing student describes her first experience in psychiatric nursing. She shares her feelings, fears, and problems in a way that other beginners can relate to, and this article can reassure the inexperienced nurse.

American Nurses' Association: Ethics in nursing practice and education, Kansas City, Mo., 1980, The Association.

This consists of seven authored papers presented at the 1980 convention that deal with ethical decision making and ethics in nursing educational curricula.

Aroskar, M.: Anatomy of an ethical dilemma: the theory; the practice, Am. J. Nurs. **80**:658, 1980.

In these two articles the author first describes the theory related to ethical dilemmas and decision making and then uses the theory to analyze a specific clinical dilemma. The application to practice makes this reading particularly useful.

Berne, E.: Games people play, New York, 1967, Grove Press, Inc.

The founder of transactional analysis uses it in this text to explore a number of specific "games." This thought-provoking book gives a different slant on relationships and

challenges the reader to find ways to terminate destructive "games."

Carkhoff, R.: Helping and human relations, vols. 1 and 2, New York, 1969, Holt, Rinehart & Winston.

Elements of research and practice in helping relationships are explored in these two volumes. Scales used to rate the "core therapeutic dimensions" are presented.

Claud, E.: The plateau in therapist-patient relationships, Perspect. Psychiatr. Care **10**:112, July-Sept. 1972.

The theoretical basis for resistance is presented, and the author describes her approach in overcoming resistance in a patient she had been working with. Her clinical experiences are clearly related.

Fenner, K.: Ethics and law in nursing, New York, 1980, Van Nostrand Reinhold Co.

The purpose of this book is to help nurses distinguish ethical from unethical practice and be alert to potential problems in exceeding the legal parameters of health care. Theory and case studies are combined to stimulate much needed discussion on ethics and nursing.

Fromer, M.: Paternalism in health care, Nurs. Outlook **29**(5):284, 1981.

The author contends that not only administrators and

physicians, but also nurses exhibit "paternalism"—the tendency to limit the patient's autonomy. One reason for this is because of the socialization process of nurses. This is an excellent, studious, and analytical discussion of a very grave problem of health care practice.

Fromm-Reichmann, F.: Principles of intensive psychotherapy, Chicago, 1950, The University of Chicago Press.

This book presents formulations of principles of intensive psychotherapy with psychoneurotics and psychotics. Written for psychiatrists, it has application to psychiatric nurses as well, and it is a recommended source for nurses with advanced education or experience.

Geach, B., and White, J.: Empathic resonance: a countertransference phenomenon, Am. J. Nurs. **74**:128, 1974.

The authors document a unique countertransference event—presenting characteristics, antecedents, and consequences. They identify a need for nurses to record similar experiences.

Jourard, S.: The transparent self, New York, 1971, Litton Educational Publishing, Inc.

This book proposes that man can attain health only as he gains courage to be himself with others and finds goals that have meaning for him. The author develops the concept of self-disclosure and the implications of it for the therapeutic relationship. Three chapters are specifically addressed to nurses and are highly recommended.

Kalisch, B.: Strategies for developing nurse empathy, Nurs. Outlook **19**:714, 1971.

The author describes her experiment in developing empathic functioning in nursing students. The training includes discussion of the concept, discrimination training, communication practice, role playing, role model of empathy, and an experiential component.

Karasu, T.: The ethics of psychotherapy, Am. J. Psychiatry **137**(12):1502, 1980.

The author addresses the ethics of psychotherapy in terms of the interface between science and ethics, the goals of treatment, the therapeutic relationship, and special issues of confidentiality and therapist-patient sex. It is thought-provoking reading.

Karns, P., and Schwab, T.: Therapeutic communication and clinical instruction, Nurs. Outlook **30**(1):39, 1982.

The premise of this article is that nurse educators rarely apply therapeutic communication in their interactions with students in the clinical area. The need for it is documented, and possible inhibitors are suggested.

Krieger, D.: The therapeutic touch: how to use your hands to help or to heal, New York, 1979, Prentice-Hall, Inc.

This text presents the techniques of therapeutic touch with detailed directions offered for the nurse who wants to expand her healing abilities in this way.

La Monica, E., and Karshmer, J.: Empathy: educating nurses in professional practice, J. Nurs. Educ. **17**(2):3, 1978.

This paper describes in detail a staff development program that was effective in raising nurses' abilities to perceive and respond with empathy. Valuable reading for nurse educators and administrators who wish to design or use programs in behavioral empathy.

Lazare, A. et al.: The walk-in patient as a "customer," Am. J. Orthopsychiatry **42**:872, 1972.

Fourteen categories of patient requests are described, and the article proposes an approach by which the patient is treated as a customer whose requests are usually legitimate and always a key part of the clinical negotiations.

McCann, J.: Termination of the psychotherapeutic relationship, J. Psychiatr. Nurs. **17**(10):37, 1979.

This article discusses the psychodynamics and theories of termination. It also has a good bibliography.

Mihordin, R.: The nunsuch handbook, Perspect. Psychiatr. Care **12**:126, July-Sept., 1974.

This lighthearted article presents "rules" for psychiatric staff. It pokes fun at some common myths and staff prejudices and is fun, enjoyable reading.

Mueller, W., and Kell, B.: Coping with conflict—supervising counselors and psychotherapists, New York, 1972, Appleton-Century-Crofts.

This book explores the goals, relationships, and processes that define supervision. It reviews conflict as the core of supervision and discusses in depth the concepts, principles, and guidelines that characterize supervision. It can be valuable reading to both supervisors and practitioners.

Murphy, K.: Use of territoriality in psychotherapy, J. Psychiatr. Nurs. **19**(3):13, 1981.

This is a brief, but useful, article. The author describes a case report in which she used the concept of territoriality in the therapeutic process.

Raths, L., Harmin, M., and Simon, S.: Values and teaching, Columbus, Ohio, 1966, Charles E. Merrill Publishing Co.

This is the classic text on value clarification. This book includes a theory of values, the value-clarifying method, the use of value theory, and research findings. It is well worth reading and studying.

Sayre, J.: Common errors in communication made by students in psychiatric nursing, Perspect. Psychiatr. Care **16**(4):175, 1978.

This article should be required reading for all students in psychiatric nursing. It identifies many of the communication errors made in each phase of the relationship and gives a clinical example of each. It is a very useful article to enhance student learning.

Sedgwick, R.: Role playing: a bridge between talk and action, J. Psychiatr. Nurs. **14**(11):16, 1976.

The uses and steps of role playing are described in this article. The techniques with a brief description of how they are accomplished are also included.

Sundeen, S. et al.: Nurse-client interaction: implementing the nursing process, ed. 2, St. Louis, 1981, The C.V. Mosby Co.

This text describes the nursing process, including concepts related to self, communication, phases of the nurse-client relationship, and stress and adaptation. It is a useful reference for normative elements of relationship skills.

Termini, M., and Hauser, M.: The process of the supervisory relationship, Perspect. Psychiatr. Care **11**:121, 1973.

This excellent article reviews the basic elements of the supervision relationship with application to the educator and graduate student in psychiatric nursing. Phases of the relationship and transference phenomena are explained.

Uustal, D.: Values clarification in nursing: application to practice, Am. J. Nurs. **78**:2058, 1978.

Value clarification applied to nursing is the focus of this article. Ten strategies in applying the process are described that are helpful in identifying one's own values.

Vidoni, C.: The development of intense positive countertransference feelings in the therapist toward a patient, Am. J. Nurs. **75**:407, 1975.

Transference and countertransference feelings that influence the nurse-patient relationship are described. This is an excellent article that explores this important aspect of therapeutic work.

Walke, M.: When a patient needs to unburden his feelings, Am. J. Nurs. **77**:1164, 1977.

This brief article describes nursing interventions used with a chronically ill patient in a general hospital setting.

It focuses on the nurse's role in creating an atmosphere in which a patient can express his feelings.

Winkler, L., and Fennell, K.: Values and nursing ethics: a bibliography, J. Psychiatr. Nurs. **19**(4):19, 1981.

The authors present a complete bibliography of journal articles on values and nursing ethics. They have done the literature search for us all!

Wolberg, L.: The technique of psychotherapy, vols. 1 and 2, New York, 1967, Grune & Stratton, Inc.

This is a good reference text for the nurse therapist. It describes general principles of psychotherapy and analyzes each phase of treatment in depth. It is clearly written and includes pertinent case examples.

CHAPTER 4

THE NURSING
THERAPEUTIC
PROCESS

To be what we are,
and to become what we are
capable of becoming,
is the only end of life.

Robert L. Stevenson,
Familiar Studies of Men
and Books

Learning objectives

After studying this chapter, the student
should be able to:

- *describe the nursing therapeutic process.*

- *define nursing and its four characteristics as iden-*
  fied by the American Nurses' Association.

- *analyze a model of health-illness phenomena and*
  the five components of it that result in adaptive
  or maladaptive coping responses.

- *critique the significance of stressful life events in*
  precipitating illness based on recent research.

- *discuss the importance of one's primary appraisal*
  of a stressor as it occurs on the cognitive, affec-
  tive, physiological, behavioral, and social levels.

- *describe various types of coping resources.*

- *discuss the importance of one's secondary apprai-*
  sal of coping resources that involve cognitive,
  affective, physiological, behavioral, and social re-
  sponses.

- *distinguish between constructive and destructive*
  coping mechanisms and between neurotic and psy-
  chotic disorders.

- *compare and contrast coping responses, health*
  problems, nursing diagnoses, and medical diag-
  noses.

- *relate the need for a theoretical basis and concep-*
  tual framework for psychiatric nursing practice
  and its implications for the development and re-
  finement of nursing theory.

- *define the nursing process and describe some of the*
  unique challenges it presents when utilized with
  psychiatric patients.

115

■ *evaluate the role of culture in psychiatric care.*

■ *describe the various nursing activities in the
phases of data collection, nursing diagnosis, planning, implementation, and evaluation.*

■ *analyze the ways in which nurses can be involved
in organizational evaluation of patterns of care
through quality assessment measures.*

■ *assess the need for documentation related to each
phase of the nursing process and various tools that
are used by nurses for this purpose.*

■ *describe the three elements of the problem-oriented
medical record and the format used for each.*

■ *incorporate elements of the nursing therapeutic
process in the student's work with psychiatric patients.*

■ *identify suggested readings for future study.*

The nurse-patient relationship is the vehicle
for the application of the nursing process. The
goal of nursing care is to maximize the person's
positive interactions with his environment, promote his level of wellness, and enhance his degree of self-actualization. Through the establishment of a therapeutic nurse-patient relationship and the use of the nursing process, the
nurse strives to promote and maintain patient
behavior that contributes to integrated functioning. This is the essence of the nursing therapeutic process and the framework on which this
text of psychiatric nursing is based.

The simplicity of this concept, however,
should not override its significance. It is, rather,
a complex process with many related components, and it requires a skilled nursing practitioner to utilize it successfully. The American
Nurses' Association defines nursing as "the
diagnosis and treatment of human responses to
actual or potential health problems."[1:9] This
definition suggests four defining characteristics
of nursing*:

1. *Phenomena*. Nursing addresses itself to a
   wide range of health-related responses observed in sick and well people. The actual
   health problem is the focus of the practice

of medicine, whereas a person's response
to the problem is the focus of nursing diagnosis and treatment.
2. *Theory*. Nurses use theory in the form of
   concepts, principles, and processes to
   guide their observations and understand
   the phenomena that are the focus of their
   interventions. This understanding precedes and serves as a basis for determining
   nursing actions to be taken.
3. *Actions*. Nursing actions attempt to prevent illness and promote health. They are
   theoretically related to the observed phenomena and anticipated outcome of care.
4. *Effects*. The aim of nursing actions is to
   produce beneficial effects in relation to
   identified responses. The evaluation of outcomes of nursing actions suggests whether
   or not those actions have been effective in
   improving or resolving the conditions to
   which they were directed.

These characteristics describe nursing as an
applied science in which theory, investigation,
and action are interrelated. They further suggest some essential components of the nursing
therapeutic process that merit further exploration. The characteristic of *phenomena* suggests
that psychiatric nurses need a model of health
and illness so that they may more fully understand the range of actual and potential health
problems which may arise and the possible responses to them. The characteristic of *theory*
maintains that nurses need a theoretical basis
and conceptual framework for psychiatric–mental health nursing practice. The characteristic of
action requires the use of the nursing process
as a problem-solving process, and the characteristic of *effects* relates to the need for standards of nursing practice to evaluate one's practice and the quality of care received by the patient. This chapter will discuss each of these
components of the nursing therapeutic process.
It will also relate them to the 1982 revised Standards of Psychiatric and Mental Health Nursing
Practice* and the process criteria provided with
each standard. The standards are presented in
their entirety, including associated rationale,
structure, process, and outcome criteria, in Appendix A.

Model of health-illness phenomena

Models serve many useful purposes. They
help to clarify relationships, generate hypotheses, and give perspective to an abstract idea or

---

*American Nurses' Association: Nursing: a social policy
statement, Kansas City, Mo., 1980. Reprinted with permission.

*Reprinted with permission from the American Nurses'
Association, Kansas City, Mo., 1982.

concept. Psychiatric nurses can practice more effectively if their actions are based on a model of health-illness phenomena that is inclusive, holistic, and yet discrete and relevant. Such a model must recognize that the presence of health or illness is an outcome of multiple characteristics of a person interacting with a number of interdependent factors in the larger social environment. It assumes that nature is ordered as a social hierarchy or continuum from the simple unit to the most complex (Fig. 4-1). Each level within this hierarchy represents an organized whole with distinctive properties and a level of complex integrated organization. The study of each level therefore requires unique criteria for explanation of structure and function. Additionally, each level is a component of each higher level, so that nothing exists in isolation. Thus the individual is a component of family and community. Material and information flow across levels, and each level is influenced by all the others. For this reason, one level of organization, such as the individual, cannot be characterized as a dynamic system without incorporating the other levels of the social hierarchy.

The most basic level of nursing intervention is the individual level. An exploration of this level must focus on its unique aspects without forgetting its relationship to the whole because "wholeness" is part of the essence of nursing. The model that will serve as the unifying perspective for this text is presented at the level of the individual in Fig. 4-2. It portrays a flow of pertinent events that result in adaptive or maladaptive coping responses, the basis for the health-illness continuum. This model also serves as the focus for the application of the nursing process. Each element of it is important both in itself and in its relation to the larger hierarchy.

Predisposing factors

Predisposing factors are biological, psychological, and sociocultural in nature. They may be viewed as conditioning factors that influence both the type and amount of resources one can elicit to handle stress. Genetic background, nutritional status, biological sensitivities, general health status, and exposure to biological toxins are examples of biological predispositions. Psychological factors include, but are not limited to, intelligence, verbal skills, morale, personality type, past experiences, self-concept, motivation, psychological defenses, and locus of control, or a sense of mastery over one's own fate.

Sociocultural characteristics that act as predisposing factors include age, education, income, occupation, social position, cultural background, religious upbringing and beliefs, political affiliation, socialization experiences, and level of social integration or relatedness. Together these factors provide a link with higher and lower levels of the hierarchy and a back-

FIG. 4-1
Levels of organization that make up the social hierarchy.

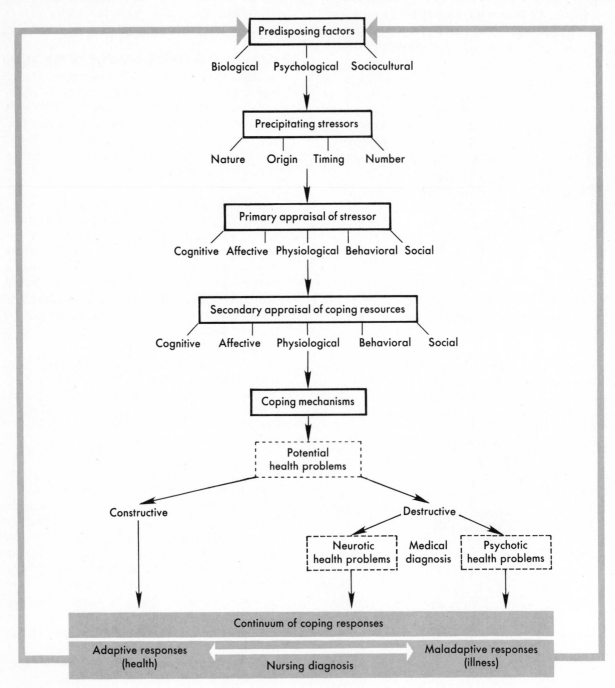

FIG. 4-2
Model of health-illness phenomena.

drop against which all present experiences are given meaning and value.

Precipitating stressors

Stressors are stimuli that the individual perceives as challenging, threatening, or demanding. They require excess energy and produce a state of tension and stress within the individual. They may be biological, psychological, or sociocultural in nature, and they may arise from one's internal or external environment. In addition to describing the nature and origin of a stressor, it is also important to assess the timing of the stressor. This timing has many dimensions, such as when the stressor occurred, the duration or length of time of exposure to the stressor, and the frequency with which it occurs. A final factor to be considered is the number of stressors experienced by the individual within a certain period of time, because events may be more difficult to deal with when they occur close together.

One particular group of stressors that have received a good deal of attention in the health-illness literature are stressful life events. Holmes and Rahe[16] provided the major impetus to the systematic scaling of life events by measuring the correlation of major life events and physical and psychiatric illness. They developed the "Social Readjustment Rating Scale" (Table 4-1). The scale ranks important life events and assigns a specific value to each one on the basis of the amount of coping behavior needed by the individual to deal with the event. As the score of the mean value increases, the likelihood of an illness is similarly hypothesized to increase.

Rahe[37] has also developed a questionnaire called the "Schedule of Recent Experience," which assesses the occurrence of life events for the individual during specific periods of time. The schedule is used to determine the degree of change experienced by the person in a given time period by adding together the mean values of reported life events. Rahe suggests that the schedule is useful in identifying the degree and type of life change experienced.

More recent issues related to life events as stressors focus on the nature of the event and the magnitude of change it represents. There appear to be three ways of categorizing events reported in the literature. The first method is by social activity, which involves family, work, educational, interpersonal, health, financial, legal, or community crises. The second categorization includes the individual's social field. These events are defined as follows: entrances, the

TABLE 4-1. Social readjustment rating scale*

Rank	Life event	Mean value
1	Death of spouse	100
2	Divorce	73
3	Marital separation	65
4	Jail term	63
5	Death of close family member	63
6	Personal injury or illness	53
7	Marriage	50
8	Fired at work	47
9	Marital reconciliation	45
10	Retirement	45
11	Change in health of family member	44
12	Pregnancy	40
13	Sex difficulties	39
14	Gain of new family member	39
15	Business readjustment	39
16	Change in financial state	38
17	Death of close friend	37
18	Change to different line of work	36
19	Change in number of arguments with spouse	35
20	Mortgage over $10,000	31
21	Foreclosure of mortgage or loan	30
22	Change in responsibilities at work	29
23	Son or daughter leaving home	29
24	Trouble with in-laws	29
25	Outstanding personal achievement	28
26	Wife begin or stop work	26
27	Begin or end school	26
28	Change in living conditions	25
29	Revision of personal habits	24
30	Trouble with boss	23
31	Change in work hours or conditions	20
32	Change in residence	20
33	Change in schools	20
34	Change in recreation	19
35	Change in church activities	19
36	Change in social activities	18
37	Mortgage or loan less than $10,000	17
38	Change in sleeping habits	16
39	Change in number of family get-togethers	15
40	Change in eating habits	15
41	Vacation	13
42	Christmas	12
43	Minor violations of the law	11

*Reprinted with permission from Holmes, T., and Rahe, R.: J. Psychosom. Res. **11**:213, 1967, Pergamon Press, Ltd.

introduction of a new person into the individual's social field; and exits, departure of a significant other from the person's social field. A third way of classifying events is by relating them to social desirability. In terms of the currently shared values of American society, one group of events can be considered generally desirable, such as promotion, engagement, and marriage. In contrast, another and proportionately larger group of events can be viewed unfavorably, such as death, financial problems, being fired, and separation.

Unfortunately, conclusions regarding life events are far from definitive. Although they have been correlated with the onset of anxiety and disease symptoms, the methodological and theoretical aspects of research in this area have been the subject of much criticism. Intervening or mediating variables are often not taken into account into the design and execution of empirical studies. The use of unidimensional scales with questionable content validity, internal consistency, and test-retest reliability continues to be a problem. Also, the particular events in the scales may not be the most relevant to certain groups, such as students, working mothers, the elderly, or the poor.

Recent research has shown that social class and ethnic group membership affect the rating of the magnitude of the stress associated with various life events.[3] Also, the life-events approach provides no clues to the specific processes by which the events have an impact on health. In retrospective studies, sources of error in the measurement of life events include selective memory, denial of certain events, and overreporting to justify a current illness. In prospective studies, the subjective evaluation of the significance of the life event to the individual has often been neglected.

Finally, life-events theory is built primarily on the idea of change. However, much stress arises from chronic conditions of living that are unsatisfactory, such as boredom, continuing family tension, job dissatisfaction, and loneliness. This is reflected in the work of Pearlin and Schooler,[34] who wished to explore what people considered potential life strains. In their sample of 2300 people, aged 18 to 65, the following four areas were delineated: (1) marital strains, (2) parental strains associated with teenage and young adult children, (3) strains associated with household economics, and (4) overloads and dissatisfactions associated with the work role. These findings suggest more long-term life dissatisfactions rather than major episodic events.

More recent research by Kanner and Lazarus[25] indicates that small daily hassles or stresses may be more closely linked to and may have a greater effect on one's moods and health than the major misfortunes of life. Hassles are defined by these researchers as irritating, frustrating, or distressing incidents that occur in everyday life. They may include disagreements, disappointments, and unpleasant surprises, such as losing a wallet, getting stuck in a traffic jam, or arguing with one's teenage daughter. In their research, hassles turned out to be better predictors of psychological and physical health than life events. The more frequent and intense the hassles people reported, the poorer their overall mental and physical health. Major events did have some long-term effects, and the authors suggest that these effects may be accounted for by the daily hassles they precipitate.

It has been shown that a certain amount of stress is necessary for survival, and degrees of it can challenge the individual to grow in new ways. However, too much stress that is inappropriately timed can place excessive demands on the individual and interfere with his integrated functioning. So too, it is recognized that stress does not reside within the particular life event itself or within the individual. Rather, it is in the interaction between the individual and situation. The questions that emerge, therefore, are "How much stress is too much?" and "What is a stressful life event?" These questions lead one to explore the significance of the event for the individual's need-value system. The importance of the person's perception or subjective appraisal in determining the stress values of an event has been documented and is crucially important to the implementation of therapeutic activities.

Primary appraisal of a stressor

Primary appraisal of a stressor refers to the processing and comprehension of the stressful situation that takes place on many levels for the individual. Specifically, it involves cognitive, affective, physiological, behavioral, and social responses. Primary appraisal is an evaluation of the significance of an event for one's well-being. It is the step in which the stressor assumes its meaning, intensity, and importance by the unique interpretation and affective significance assigned to it by the person at risk.

Cognitive appraisal is a critical, although inadequately researched, part of this model of health-illness phenomena. Lazarus[24] believes cognitive factors play a central role in adaptation. They affect the impact of stressful events, the choice of coping patterns used, and the emotional, physiological, and behavioral reactions or responses. The process of cognitive appraisal mediates psychologically between the person and the environment in any stressful encounter. That is, the person evaluates whether a situation is damaging, or potentially damaging, on the basis of his understanding of the power of the situation to produce harm and the resources he has available to neutralize or tolerate the harm.

Lazarus[24] describes three types of primary cognitive appraisals to stress: *harm/loss,* referring to damage that has already occurred; *threat,* referring to anticipated or future harm; and *challenge,* in which the focus is placed positively on potential gain, growth, or mastery, rather than on the possible risks. This last perception of challenge may play a crucial role in psychological hardiness or resistance to stress. One longitudinal study showed that people whose attitude on life could be rated high on challenge (viewing change as a challenge rather than a threat), commitment (the opposite of alienation), and control (the opposite of powerlessness) remained healthier than the others.[35] The authors conclude that stress-resistant people have a specific set of attitudes toward life, an openness to change, a feeling of involvement in whatever they are doing, and a sense of control over events. They propose that such differences in cognitive appraisal affect one's response to events. Those who view stress as a challenge are more likely to transform events to their advantage and thus reduce their level of stress. This is in contrast to more passive, avoidance, and self-defeating tactics, in which the source of stress does not go away.

An affective response is the arousal of a feeling state. With regard to the primary appraisal of a stressor, the predominant affective response is a nonspecific or generalized anxiety reaction. Consistent with this is the physiological response associated with the "fight or flight" response. It involves the stimulation of the sympathetic division of the autonomic nervous system and increased activity of the pituitary-adrenal axis. The behavioral response of the individual at the time of primary appraisal is focused on the impact of the stressor. A range of behaviors may be evident, depending on the level of anxiety experienced by the individual and the physiologic changes he is experiencing. They are usually reactive behaviors, rather than goal-directed behaviors, at this time. Chapter 7 explores this area in greater depth.

Finally, Mechanic[29] describes three aspects of a person's social response to stress and illness. The first is the search for meaning, in which individuals seek out information concerning their problem. This is a prerequisite for devising a coping strategy, because only through some formulation of what is occurring can a reasonable response be devised. The second is social attribution, in which the person tries to identify the unique factors that contributed to the present problematic situation. Patients who view their problem as a result of their own negligence may be blocked from assuming an active, adaptive coping response. They may view their problems as a sign of their personal failure and engage in self-blame and passive and withdrawn behavior. Thus the way in which cause is conceptualized by both patients and health professionals can greatly affect successful coping. The third social response is social comparison, in which the individual compares his own skills and capacities with those of other persons with similar problems. How a person comes to assess himself depends very much on those around him with whom comparisons are made. In many situations, feelings and self-esteem may depend as much on this comparison process as on the objective coping capacities of the individual. The outcome of this social response is an evaluation of the need for support from one's social network or social support system. Both one's predisposing factors, such as age, developmental level, and cultural background, and the particular characteristics of the precipitating stressor jointly determine one's perceived need for social support.

In summary, the way a person interprets or appraises an event is the psychological key to understanding his coping efforts in that situation and to understanding the nature and intensity of his stress response. Unfortunately, many nurses and other health professionals ignore this fact when they presume to know how certain stressors will affect an individual and render "routine" care. Not only does this depersonalize the individual, but it also undermines the basis of nursing care. The patient's appraisal of life stressors with its cognitive, affective, physiological, behavioral, and social components must be an essential part of the nurse's assessment.

Secondary appraisal of coping resources

Secondary appraisal is an evaluation of one's coping resources, options, or strategies. Like primary appraisal, it involves cognitive, affective, physiological, behavioral, and social responses. One's cognitive appraisal at this time concentrates on the availability and effectiveness of possible coping strategies. Mechanic[29] identifies five major coping resources that are helpful in assisting individuals in adapting to the stress of illness. These are economic assets, individual abilities and skills, defensive techniques, social supports, and motivational impetus. They incorporate all levels of the social hierarchy represented in Fig. 4-1, and the interrelationships between the individual, family group, and society levels of the hierarchy assume critical importance at this point of the model.

Presently, much research is being conducted regarding these coping resources.[35] Antonovsky is examining what he calls "generalized resistance resources"—characteristics of the person, group, or environment that can encourage more adaptive responses. He believes knowledge and intelligence offer such a resource, since they allow people to see different ways of dealing with their stress. Two other resources he identifies are a strong ego identity and commitment to a stable and continuing social network. Thus, empirical research is lending support to the interrelationship between predisposing factors and coping resources within a strong social community.

Affectively, the previously elicited general anxiety response becomes refined into specific dominant emotions. These may include joy, sadness, fear, anger, acceptance, distrust, anticipation, or surprise.[36] Physiologic responses reflect the interaction of multiple neuroendocrine axes involving growth hormone, prolactin, adrenocorticotropic hormone (ACTH), luteinizing and follicle-stimulating hormones, thyroid-stimulating hormone, vasopressin, oxytocin, epinephrine, norepinephrine, and insulin.[27]

Behavioral responses will reflect both the emotions and physiologic changes experienced by the individual, as well as his cognitive analysis of the stressful situation. Caplan[5] described four interdigitating phases or facets of an individual's

---

DIMENSIONS OF SOCIAL NETWORKS

1. Structural characteristics
   a. Size: The number of individuals with whom the person has direct contact. Criteria used may include frequency of contact or perceptions of importance or closeness.
   b. Density: The extent to which members of a person's social network know and contact each other independent of the focal person.
2. Characteristics of component linkages
   a. Intensity: The strength of the tie as measured by feelings about the other person or exchange of reciprocal services.
   b. Durability: The degree of stability of the person's ties with another.
   c. Multidimensionality: The number of functions (advice, support, and feedback) served by a relationship.
   d. Reciprocity: The degree to which emotional and task-oriented support is both given and received by the focal person.
   e. Relationship density: The degree to which the focal person's relationships serve a variety of functions.
   f. Dispersion: Geographical proximity to members of one's network.
   g. Frequency: The amount of contact through phone, letter, and face-to-face meetings.
   h. Homogeneity: The extent to which members of a network share common social attributes, such as political or religious affiliation, and socioeconomic status.
3. Normative context of the relationship
   a. Nuclear family
   b. Extended family
   c. Friend
   d. Neighbor
   e. Work acquaintance
   f. Community acquaintance

responses to a stressful event. Phase 1 is behavior that changes the stressful environment or enables the individual to escape from it. Phase 2 is behavior to acquire new capabilities for action to change the external circumstances and their aftermath. Phase 3 is intrapsychic behavior to defend against unpleasant emotional arousal. Finally, phase 4 is intrapsychic behavior to come to terms with the event and its sequelae by internal readjustment. Conceptualizing the individual's behavior response in terms of these phases may be helpful to the nurse.

One's social response is that of evaluating the actual social support available to the individual. Numerous studies have documented increased rates of psychiatric disorder and of general medical morbidity and mortality among persons who are socially isolated. So, too, research in the fields of medical sociology, epidemiology, organizational and social psychology, and experimental stress reveal that those members of the social environment who are perceived by the stressed individual as "significant others" do serve health protective and health restorative functions.

Social support for the individual begins in utero and is communicated in a variety of ways to the newborn baby, including the way he is held, fed, and comforted. As life progresses, support is increasingly derived from other members of the family, then from peers at school, work, and in the community. At times of great need, support may be provided by nurses or other health professionals. Although social support systems or social networks are commonly understood terms, they reflect a complexity of dimensions. Some of the major dimensions used to describe social networks are presented at left.

Structural characteristics refer to properties of the overall network, characteristics of component linkages refer to properties of the individual relationships, and normative context refers to the type of relationship.[30]

Given the complexity of the concept, it is not surprising that it is defined differently by various researchers and practitioners. These definitions indicate that different types of support may be provided by social support systems. Some of the functions of social networks that have been identified are shown in Table 4-2. Although phrased differently by each theorist, five common functions of social networks may be described as follows:

1. Emotional support
2. Task-oriented help
3. Feedback and evaluation
4. Social relatedness and integration
5. Access to new information

The value of social networks in providing emotional support has long been recognized. Some believe it is the primary function and equate support with love, affection, and nurturance. Although not minimizing this contribution of social support, Caplan[5] believes that the most important contribution is in the cognitive and educational areas and in helping the person with concrete tasks. Caplan states that a supportive group of family, friends, or community members helps the individual deal with his environment:

This group or network adds to his information; helps him improve his own data collection; aids him in evaluating the situation and working out a sensible plan; and assists him in implementing his plan, assessing its consequences, and replanning in line with the feedback information. It reminds him of his continuing identity and bolsters his positive feelings

TABLE 4-2. Functions of social support systems

Caplan[4]	House[17]	Walker et al.[47]	Weiss[49]
Emotional support	Emotional support	Emotional support	Attachment
Task-oriented assistance	Instrumental support	Material aid and services	Exchange of services
Communication of evaluation and expectation	Appraisal support	Maintenance of social identity	Guidance; social integration
Sense of belonging		Access to new social contacts	Sense of alliance; reassurance of worth
	Informational support	Diverse information	Opportunity to provide nurturance

about himself; assures him that his discomforts are expectable and, although burdensome, can usually be tolerated; and maintains his hope in some form of successful outcome of his efforts, which is a prerequisite to his continuing them.

In effect, a supportive social network complements and supplements those specific aspects of the individual's functioning which are weakened by the effect of the stressful experience.[4:415]

Although relative importance of the functions of social support may be subject to some variation, there is strong agreement with Caplan on its effect. Two areas of its effect are particularly relevant, the relationship of social support to help seeking and to psychological adaptation. In a review article, Gourash[12] outlined the four general ways that social networks influence help seeking:

1. Buffering the experience of stress that obviates the need for help
2. Precluding the necessity for professional assistance through the provision of instrumental and affective support
3. Acting as screening and referral agents to professional services
4. Transmitting atittudes, values, and norms about help seeking

These findings have implications for primary, secondary, and tertiary prevention.

The large number of studies that address the outcome of psychological adaptation prevents discussing each one in detail. Four important review articles, however, outline the historical context and scope of research in this area. In 1974 Cassel[6] explored the topic from an epidemiological perspective and concluded that social support was an important environmental factor affecting human resistance to disease. Cobb[7] in 1976 reviewed social support around the crises of the life cycle, including pregnancy and childhood, hospitalization, recovery from illness, extensive life changes, employment termination, bereavement, aging and retirement, and the threat of death. He suggests that social support functions as a moderating variable that facilitates coping with crises in an adaptive way. Kaplan, Cassel, and Gore's[20] review in 1977 emphasized the importance of social support as protective of health but only in the presence of certain circumstances that they believe need to be better conceptualized and researched. Finally, Mueller[31] in 1980 presented a comprehensive review of the literature on social support and psychiatric disorders.

What one can conclude from all of these studies is that links do exist between social support and outcome coping responses. However, a precise definition of social support, its determinants or conditions, its measurement, the nature of the support process, and the existence of a causal relationship between social support and maladaptation have yet to be established in theoretical or empirical work.

The importance of social support is well documented, but maximizing the benefit it can provide in a specific situation requires a clearer understanding of the dimensions of the social network listed on p. 122; the predisposing factors of the individual, including his needs and attitudes toward using his support network; the nature of the environment; the characteristics of the stressor; and the way in which all of these interact. Future research in this area will be of great value.

Coping mechanisms

It is at this point in the model that coping mechanisms and potential health problems emerge. As such, it is a fertile time for nursing activities directed to primary prevention. Coping mechanisms can be defined as any effort directed at stress management. They can be task oriented and involve direct problem-solving efforts to cope with the threat itself or intrapsychic or ego defense oriented with the goal of regulating one's emotional distress. A more detailed discussion of coping mechanisms used by people experiencing stress can be found in Chapter 7.

Coping mechanisms may be either constructive or destructive in nature. They can be considered constructive when one's anxiety is treated as a warning signal that something is wrong and the individual accepts it as a challenge to clarify and resolve the underlying problem. In this respect, anxiety can be compared to a fever—both serve as warnings that the system is under attack. Once employed successfully, constructive coping mechanisms will modify the way past experiences will be utilized to meet future threats. Destructive coping mechanisms, in contrast, are used to protect oneself from anxiety without resolving the conflict causing it. The mechanism is one of evasion instead of resolution.

Destructive coping mechanisms are often subject to medical evaluation and diagnosis. The *medical diagnosis* of a psychiatric health problem can be broadly differentiated as neurotic or psychotic. In the DSM-III, *neurotic disorders* are distinguished by the following characteristics[2]:

1. A symptom or group of symptoms that is distressing and is recognized as unacceptable and alien to the individual.
2. Reality testing is grossly intact.
3. Behavior does not actively violate gross social norms (although functioning may be significantly impaired).
4. The disturbance is relatively enduring or recurrent without treatment and is not limited to a transitory reaction to stressors.
5. There is no demonstrable organic cause or factor.

In situations of severest conflict, however, the person may be powerless to cope with the threat by such patterns and may be forced to deal with the conflict by distorting reality as in *psychosis*. Psychosis consists of the following characteristics[2]:

1. A severe mood disorder
2. Regressive behavior
3. Personality disintegration
4. A significant reduction in level of awareness
5. Great difficulty in functioning adequately
6. Gross impairment in reality testing

This last characteristic is critical. When there is gross impairment in reality testing, the individual incorrectly evaluates the accuracy of his or her perceptions and thoughts and makes incorrect inferences about external reality, even in the face of contrary evidence. According to the DSM-III, direct evidence of psychosis is the presence of either delusions or hallucinations without insight into their pathological nature. It is obvious, therefore, that psychotic health problems reflect the most severe level of illness and maladaptive coping responses.

Continuum of health-illness coping responses

When a particular event occurs, the person mentally processes the information. Based on specific conditioning factors, the quality of the stressor, his perception of the situation, and his analysis of his resources and needs, he will respond to the stressor. His responses theoretically can be placed on a coping continuum of health and illness. Those responses which support integrated functioning can be viewed as adaptive, or healthy, responses. They lead to growth, learning, and goal achievement. Those responses which block integrated functioning can be viewed as maladaptive, or illness, responses. They can be evident as impaired thought pro-

cesses, alterations in the expression of emotions, physiologic illness, inappropriate behavior, or problems in socialization. These responses to stress, whether actual or potential, are the subject of *nursing diagnoses*. Like the diagnoses, the treatment of these maladaptive responses are a nursing function. Coping responses to stress emerge whether or not a medical diagnosis of an existing health problem has been made. If the individual has been medically diagnosed, the treatment of the medical health problem would be primarily a medical function. It is here that the practice of medicine and nursing mesh and become complementary, while each retains its distinct focus. The practice of nursing does not require a medical diagnosis. A nurse may implement the nursing process for maladaptive responses *whether or not* the diagnosis of a medical health problem has been made. However, all health professionals have an obligation to refer a patient to another practitioner when it is in the patient's best interests.

The final outcome of the model is the emergence of health and illness behaviors. They are seen as a continuum of responses rather than discrete entities. Volumes have been written in the literature with regard to each component of this model. This brief description of it was presented to reveal the organizing framework for this text. Chapters 7 to 14 explore various maladaptive responses. In the beginning of each of these chapters, a continuum of coping or health-illness will be described. This will be followed by a discussion of relevant predisposing or conditioning factors, precipitating stressors, and coping mechanisms. Building on this theoretical knowledge, each phase of the nursing process will be applied to the specific maladaptive response. Medical diagnoses of health problems will be presented when appropriate and related to the nursing diagnoses. Through the consistent use of this framework, the art and science of psychiatric nursing practice will emerge.

Theoretical basis for practice

STANDARD I—THEORY. The nurse applies appropriate theory that is scientifically sound as a basis for decisions regarding nursing practice.
Process criteria
The nurse:
1. Examines basic assumptions on the nature of persons
2. Corrects erroneous beliefs
3. Utilizes theory and critical thinking to:

a. Formulate generalizations, e.g., opinion, speculation, and assumption
b. Generate and test hypotheses
4. Utilizes inferences, principles, and operational concepts
5. Applies relevant theories

All actions of the psychiatric nurse should arise from a theoretical base that includes an understanding of health-illness phenomena and a means for the evaluation of nursing care given. This theoretical basis is partially self-generated and partly drawn from other sciences but is integrated into a conception of nursing practice. The range of theories used by nurses includes intrapersonal, interpersonal, and systems theories. Intrapersonal theories explain within-person phenomena and are focused at the individual level of care. Interpersonal theories elaborate on interactions between two or more people. Systems theories aid the nurse in understanding complex networks or organizations, the dynamics of their parts, and processes in interaction. They are focused at the family, group, or community levels of care. Use of a range of theories is appropriate in nursing because of the great variance in the recipients of nursing care, types of health-illness responses, philosophical backgrounds of individual psychiatric nurses, and settings in which they work. No one theory is universally applicable; the appropriate theory should be selected for its relevance to the tasks at hand.

A conceptual framework is then formulated from relevant theoretical bases. It should reflect an integration of theory and nursing process and stimulate the evolution of a distinct body of nursing science by generating hypotheses, propositions, and relationships that can be empirically tested. In this way, conceptual frameworks provide a basis for the direction of nursing practice, research, and education and contribute to the development of nursing theory. A number of nursing theories have been developed at this time.[11] Flaskerud and Halloran[8] have identified some areas of agreement in nursing theory development. They believe that nurses generally agree on the following central concepts in nursing: man (person), society (environment), health-illness, and nursing. It remains for nurses to concentrate on content analysis and testing of these theories to further the growth of the profession.

STANDARD XI—RESEARCH. The nurse contributes to nursing and the mental health field through innovations in theory and practice and participation in research.
Process criteria
The nurse:
1. Approaches nursing practice with an inquiring and open mind
2. Utilizes research findings in practice
3. Develops, implements, and evaluates research studies as appropriate to level of education
4. Uses responsible standards of research in investigative endeavors
5. Ensures that a mechanism for the protection of human subjects exists
6. Obtains expert consultation and/or supervision as required

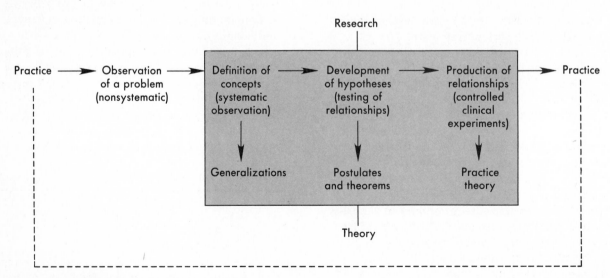

FIG. 4-3
Relationship between theory, practice, and research. (From O'Toole, A.: J. Psychosoc. Nurs. **19**(2):11, 1981.)

Nurses should realize that the relationship between theory, practice, and research is an interactive and reciprocal one.[46] For theory to be useful, it must have implications for practice, and for practice to be tested and validated, it must be theoretical. Theory that arises out of practice is validated by research, which returns to direct practice and has implications for clinical care. This cyclical relationship, as diagrammed by O'Toole,[33] is represented in Fig. 4-3. It shows how the casual, nonsystematic observation of a problem in practice leads to a more systematic observation and a definition of terms, including the nature of the problem and influencing factors. Descriptive, observational, and exploratory research designs are useful at this time in more precisely defining a problem or observation. Following this, hypotheses may be developed concerning relationships between identified variables. They may be tested in correlational or survey research designs. One might then propose causal relationships between the variables and test these predictions in experimental or quasiexperimental designs, in natural or controlled settings, with a specification of the predicted relationship. Only if a causal relationship has been established can one proceed to a prescriptive theoretical level and the testing of specific interventions aimed at changing the clinical problem. In this way, prescriptive studies feed knowledge back into practice to improve the quality of patient care.

This progressive process of observing from practice, theorizing, testing in research, and subsequently modifying practice must become an essential part of psychiatric nursing if it is to survive as a practice discipline.[33] Research about the practice of psychiatric nursing has increased in the past decade, and it is obvious that nurses have the ability to construct sophisticated designs with both theoretical and practical importance. The clinical problems are numerous, and as nurses gain the skills and experience to empirically validate their work, they have the potential of making a significant contribution to psychiatric theory and a substantial impact on practice.

The nursing process

The nursing process is an interactive, problem-solving process used by the nurse as a systematic and individualized way to fulfill the goal of nursing care. It is a deliberate and organized approach requiring thought, knowledge, and experience. The nursing process acknowledges the autonomy of the individual and his freedom to make decisions regarding his own goals and be involved in his own care. Together the nurse and patient emerge as partners in a relationship built on trust and directed toward maximizing the patient's strengths, maintaining his integrity, and promoting his adaptive response to stress.

The problem-solving process is a scientific way of thinking and dealing with problems, and its principles are included in the nursing process. The steps in problem solving include the following:
1. Observation and recognition of the problem
2. Definition of the problem
3. Formulation of hypotheses or possible solutions to the problem
4. Implementation of the hypotheses or possible solutions
5. Formulation of conclusions

The phases of the nursing process are as follows:
1. Data collection
2. Formulation of the nursing diagnosis
3. Planning of nursing care
4. Implementation of nursing actions
5. Evaluation of the nursing assessment, care plan, and actions

When utilized with psychiatric patients, the nursing process presents some unique challenges.[10] Emotional problems are often vague and elusive and are not as tangible or visible as many physiological disruptions. Emotional problems vary in symptomatology or behavior and arise from multiple causes. Conversely, similar past events may be evident in widely differing present behaviors. Many psychiatric patients are initially not able to describe or identify their problems. They may be severely withdrawn, highly anxious, or out of touch with reality. Their ability to participate in the problem-solving process may be limited because of their perception of themselves as powerless victims who deny responsibility for their own behavior.

These factors make the use of the nursing process with psychiatric patients more difficult, but they do not negate it. Geach has identified the following three hallmarks of clinically valid problem solving for psychiatric patients:
1. That the nurse involve the patient in the process
2. That the problem to which the nurse and patient address themselves has immediate relevance to what is happening between them, at least initially

3. That there is some relatedness between the nurse and patient so that the solutions of the problems are experienced from within a relationship, not in isolation[10:12]

It is essential that the nurse and patient become partners in the problem-solving process. There is a great temptation for the nurse to exclude the participation of the patient, particularly if he resists becoming involved. This should be avoided for two reasons. First, learning is most effective when the patient directly participates in the learning experience. Second, the patient's isolation from others and self-alienation is part of his maladaptive life-style that needs to be modified. By including the patient as an active participant in the nursing process, the nurse will be helping to restore his sense of control over life and responsibility for action. It reinforces the message that the patient has been making decisions and continues to make them at present. His choice is between adaptive or maladaptive coping responses. Jourard states:

If a person believes himself to be weak, helpless or doomed to some fate or other, he will tend to behave or suffer in the way expected. If, on the other hand, he has a concept of himself as a being with much untapped potential to cope with problems and contradictions in his life, then when these arise, he will persist in efforts to cope with them long after someone who sees himself as ineffective and impotent has given up.[19:34]

The phases of the nursing process include data collection, formulation of the nursing diagnosis, planning, implementation, and evaluation (Fig. 4-4). Validation is part of each phase, and all phases may overlap or occur simultaneously.

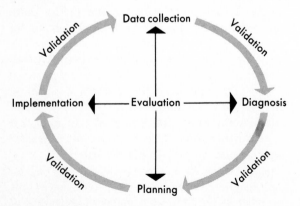

FIG. 4-4
Interrelated phases of the nursing process.

STANDARD X—UTILIZATION OF COMMUNITY HEALTH SYSTEMS. The nurse (specialist) participates with other members of the community in assessing, planning, implementing, and evaluating mental health services and community systems that include the promotion of the broad continuum of primary, secondary, and tertiary prevention of mental illness.
Process criteria
The nurse:
1. Uses knowledge of community and group dymics and systems theory to understand the structure and function of the community system
2. Recognizes current social and political issues that influence the nature of mental health problems in the community
3. Encourages active consumer participation in assessing and planning programs to meet the community's mental health needs
4. Brings the community's needs to the attention of appropriate individuals and groups, including legislative bodies and regional and state planning groups
5. Plans and participates in didactic and experiential educational programs related to the community's mental health
6. Uses consultative skills to facilitate the development and implementation of mental health services
7. Interprets mental health services to others in the community
8. Participates with other health care professionals and members of the community in the planning, implementation, and evaluation of mental health services
9. Participates in the delineation of high-risk population groups in the community and identifies gaps in community services
10. Assesses strengths and coping capacities of individuals, families, and the community in order to promote and increase their mental health
11. Uses knowledge of community resources to assist consumers' referral to and appropriate use of health care resources
12. Collaborates with staff at other agencies to facilitate continuity of service for individuals and families

The focus of this discussion will be primarily at the level of the individual patient. This does not mean, however, that other levels of the hierarchy, such as the family or community, are to be ignored or forgotten when working with the individual. Each level influences all others, and, even though the focus of the psychiatric nurse may be on the individual patient, she must incorporate all other appropriate levels in each phase of the nursing process. Her purpose in working with these other levels, such as the family and community, will be to enhance the resources of her patient and maximize his adaptive healthy responses.

Nurses with advanced experience or education may shift the focus of their care to that of the family system or group. The nursing process will continue to be used at these levels, but the model of health-illness phenomena, theoretical base, and focus of nursing actions will need to be modified to the unique structure and function of these different levels. Nursing intervention in these higher levels of family, group, and community as unique systems is presented in Chapters 5, 19, 24, and 25.

 Data collection

STANDARD II—DATA COLLECTION. The nurse continuously collects data that are comprehensive, accurate, and systematic.

Process criteria

The nurse:

1. Informs the client of their mutual roles and responsibilities in the data-gathering process
2. Uses clinical judgments to determine what information is needed. Health data undergirding the nursing process for psychiatric and mental health clients are obtained through assessing the following:
   a. Biophysical, developmental, mental, and emotional status
   b. Spiritual or philosophical beliefs
   c. Family, social, cultural, and community systems
   d. Daily activities, interactions, and coping patterns
   e. Economic, environmental, and political factors affecting the client's health
   f. Personally significant support systems, as well as unutilized but available support systems
   g. Knowledge, satisfaction, and change motivation regarding current health status
   h. Strengths that can be used in reaching health goals
   i. Knowledge of pertinent legal rights
   j. Contributory data from the family, significant others, the health care team, and pertinent individuals in the community

Data collection may take place as a formal admission procedure outside of an established nurse-patient relationship. In this case, the information will be solicited from the patient in a direct and structured manner. Observing, interviewing, and examining are the basic methods of gathering information. An assessment tool or nursing history form can provide a systematic format that becomes part of the written record of a patient. It provides the facts on which the nurse can assess the patient's level of functioning and serves as a basis for the nursing diagnosis, planning, implementing, and evaluating of nursing care. The use of a specified data collection format helps to ensure that the necessary information will be obtained. It also reduces the patient's repetition of his history and provides a source of information available to all health team members. The mental status examination, as described in Chapter 17, may be included as part of the psychiatric nurse's evaluation.

The assessment tool used by the nurse in collecting data about the patient should, ideally, be derived from her conceptual framework of psychiatric nursing. More frequently, however, it is determined by the setting or program in which she works. Regardless of the format of the tool used, the nurse has the obligation to obtain as complete as picture as possible of the patient's life situation. The process criteria of Standard II identify areas in which data need to be collected. This list includes data relative to all of the components of the model of health and illness utilized in this text. They also identify from whom the data are to be collected and represent various levels of the model of social hierarchy—individual, family, group, and community.

The baseline data should reflect both content and process, and the patient is the ideal source of validation. In collecting the data, the nurse should select a private place, free from noise and distraction, in which to interview the patient. Interviewing is a goal-directed method of communication that is required in a formal admission procedure. It should be focused, but as open ended as possible, progressing from general to specific, and allowing the patient the opportunity to express himself spontaneously. The tasks of the nurse are to maintain the flow of the interview, to listen to the verbal and nonverbal messages being conveyed by the patient, and to be aware of her own responses to the patient.

In an ongoing nurse-patient relationship, data collection may begin in the preinteraction or orientation phases of the relationship. Although the goal is to gather information, it is only one of many goals the nurse will be pursuing at this time. Other tasks of the nurse include establishing trust, acceptance, and open communication; formulating a contract; and exploring the patient's feelings and actions. Her approach, therefore, should be unstructured, flexible, and responsive to the cues of the patient. Rather than working from a formalized data collection tool, the nurse may attempt to focus the patient on observing and describing his present thoughts, feelings, and experiences. To supplement her knowledge of the patient, the nurse can use a variety of secondary sources of information, including the patient's medical record, nursing rounds, change-of-shift reports, nursing care plan, and the evaluation of other health professionals, such as psychologists, social workers, or psychiatrists. In using secondary sources of information, nurses should be cautioned against merely accepting the assessment of another health team member. Rather, the nurse should apply the information she obtains to her nursing framework for data collection and formulate her own impressions and nursing diagnoses. This brings another perspective to the work of the health care team and an unbiased receptivity to the patient and his problems.

A couple of aspects of the data collection phase merit additional discussion. One is the assessment of the patient's cultural, religious, and socioeconomic background. All too frequently these factors are assessed in a cursory way. Yet they exert a powerful influence on the success of the nursing process for two important reasons. The first is because sociocultural factors contribute to a patient's belief system of health and illness. One's religion, sex, race, culture, family ties, and economic status, for example, all have a formative influence on each component of the model of health-illness phenomena. Any one of a variety of sociocultural factors may play a dominant role in an individual's life. Therefore any attempt to promote the well-being of a patient must be based on an understanding of him as a unique individual who lives in a larger social, cultural, and religious community.

The second reason why sociocultural factors are important is that the response of the health care team is framed by the culture of which they are a part. The dominant psychotherapeutic approach of an era reflects the cultural attitudes of its time and place. This helps to explain why there are differences in observed symptoms, frequency, distribution, and outcome of psychiatric illness among countries and cultures throughout the world. For instance, in developing nations like Nigeria and India, the odds favor a fast and complete recovery from major psychoses. In the more technologically advanced countries, such as the United States, the prognosis is worse. This is due, in part, to the cultural stigma against mental illness that is prevalent in the West.

Cultural bias can also affect the process of psychotherapy. One study reported that minority group patients received the least intensive psychotherapy. They were discharged more often or seen for minimal supportive psychotherapy.[51] A study among public health nurses found that different judgments were made about patients as a function of their social class.[21] Still another aspect of this problem has been described as "institutional racism," which involves the notion that those who are not white are inferior.[14] Consequently, rather than viewing some patients as culturally different, they are viewed as disadvantaged, deprived, or underprivileged. Such prejudices do not form on the basis of race alone. They can also be based on a person's sex, religion, age, or ethnic background. However, the result is the same—prejudices influence the nurse's evaluation of the patient and limit the potential effectiveness of her care.

Psychiatry needs to embrace the idea of intercultural psychotherapy. Schlesinger[39] believes this occurs with the acknowledgment of the different cultural backgrounds between the patient and therapist and the resulting interaction of cultural variables. This has ramifications for self-awareness, communications, diagnosis, therapist-patient relations, therapeutic models, and treatment goals. It requires that the nurse have an awareness of her own sociocultural identity and values, an understanding of the roles social systems play in influencing behavior, and a willingness to learn from a patient with another cultural set.

A final important aspect of data collection pertains to the significance of the patient as a family member. If the nurse views the patient as an interacting member of a family unit, it will be necessary for her data base to include the patient's view of the functional state of his family, as well as family resources and strengths. Sedgwick[40] describes the family as both a social organization and an emotional environment. As a social organization, the purpose of the family is to develop within its members sets of skills necessary for productive membership in a larger social system. It is a focal point of interaction for the individual as he relates to other family members, other families, the community, and one's larger social network. So too, the broader social system makes demands, places expectations on the family, and requires it to process

TABLE 4-3. Dimensions of the Family APGAR*

Component	What is measured	Relevant open-ended questions
Adaptation	How resources are shared, or the degree to which a member is satisfied with the assistance received when family resources are needed	How have family members aided each other in time of need? In what way have family members received help or assistance from friends and community agencies?
Partnership	How decisions are shared, or the member's satisfaction with mutuality in family communication and problem solving	How do family members communicate with each other about such matters as vacations, finances, medical care, large purchases, and personal problems?
Growth	How nurturing is shared, or the member's satisfaction with the freedom available within the family to change roles and attain physical and emotional growth or maturation	How have family members changed during the past years? How has this change been accepted by family members? In what ways have family members aided each other in growing or developing independent life-styles? How have family members reacted to your desires for change?
Affection	How emotional experiences are shared, or the member's satisfaction with the intimacy and emotional interaction that exists in a family	How have members of your family responded to emotional expressions, such as affection, love, sorrow, or anger?
Resolve	How time (and space and money) is shared, or the member's satisfaction with the time commitment that has been made to the family by its members	How do members of your family share time, space, and money?

*Modified from Smilkstein, G.: The family APGAR: a proposal for a family function test and its use by physicians, J. Fam. Pract. **6:**1231, 1978.

information, make decisions, attain financial and social productivity, and provide for the personal growth and development of its members.

The larger social context also influences the family's emotional environment. The family must create an atmosphere that is not only conducive to group living and cooperation, but individual development and disagreement as well. Although the emotional environment of the family is constantly changing, it is their mission to create an emotional climate that is trusting, warm, concerned, accepting of differences in opinions and abilities, and adaptable in light of the changes of individual members.

A healthy family unit is considered by Smilkstein[43] to be a nurturing unit that demonstrates integrity in five components: *a*daptability, *p*artnership, *g*rowth, *a*ffection, and *r*esolve. The acronym APGAR was designed by him to refer to these components. To test these area of family functioning, Smilkstein developed a brief screening questionnaire called the Family APGAR. Table 4-3 presents the functional components of the Family APGAR and relevant open-ended questions for family function information. This tool is useful in suggesting areas to be assessed relative to family functioning and potential areas of family strengths and resources.

Various types of family strengths may be noted. These include the ability to acquire resources, such as money or social support, and the productive use of them; the ability to communicate in depth with each other with openness and consensual decision making; the presence of encouragement, ego support, praise, recognition, respect for individuality, and flexibility of family functions and roles; and family unity, loyalty, and cooperation. All of these strengths serve as potential family resources. Other resources may be present in the family's cultural pride, religious affiliation, community ties, economic status, and educational background. The inclusion of these areas in the data collection phase of the nursing process not only gives depth to the nurse's assessment but also suggests actions and resources that will enhance the patient's adaptation.

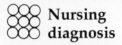 **Nursing diagnosis**

STANDARD III—DIAGNOSIS. The nurse utilizes *nursing diagnoses* and standard classification of mental disorders to express conclusions supported by recorded assessment data and current scientific premises.
Process criteria
The nurse:
1. Identifies actual or potential health problems in regard to:
   a. Self-care limitations or impaired functioning whose general etiology is mental and emotional distress, deficits in the ways significant systems are functioning, and internal psychic and/or developmental issues
   b. Emotional stress or crisis components of illness, pain, self-concept changes, and life process changes
   c. Emotional problems related to daily experiences such as anxiety, aggression, loss, loneliness, and grief
   d. Physical symptoms that occur simultaneously with altered psychic functioning, such as altered intestinal functioning or anorexia
   e. Alterations in thinking, perceiving, symbolizing, communicating, and decision-making abilities
   f. Impaired abilities to relate to others
   g. Behaviors and mental states that indicate the client is a danger to self or others or is gravely disabled
2. Analyzes available information according to accepted theoretical frameworks
3. Makes inferences regarding data from phenomena
4. Formulates a nursing diagnosis subject to revision with subsequent data

On completion of the data collection, the nurse compares the information to documented norms of health and wellness. The psychosocial aspects of a patient's life present some special concerns for the nurse. It is important for her to remember that what is acceptable and appropriate behavior in one social group may be considered deviant or bizarre in another. Since normative standards of behavior are culturally determined, the nurse should make proper allowances for the patient's individual characteristics and the larger social group of which he is a member.

The nurse then uses logical decision making to analyze the collected data and derive a nursing diagnosis. A nursing diagnosis is the independent judgment of a nurse through which the nursing problems of the patient are identified. These nursing problems concern aspects of the patient's health that may need to be promoted or with which the patient needs help in his biopsychosocial adaptation to stress. The subject of nursing diagnoses, therefore, is the patient's behavioral response to stress. This response may lie anywhere on the coping continuum from adaptive, healthy, to maladaptive, ill. Nursing diagnoses identify nursing problems that may be overt, covert, existing, or potential. The responsibility for therapeutic decisions regarding these patients' health responses is assumed by the professional nurse.

The nursing diagnosis is a statement of the patient's nursing problem that includes both the behavioral disruption, or threatened disruption, and contributing stressors. For example, a patient may have paralysis of both legs, resulting from a severe level of anxiety related to her impending wedding, obsessive thoughts of inflicting self-harm related to intense guilt, or disorientation related to alcohol withdrawal.

At the present time, the classification of nursing diagnoses is in its infancy. However, nurses must define and clarify what they do in the psychiatric setting, and this requires the formulation, dissemination, and use of nursing diagnoses. McClosky believes the following:

> In today's world, unless nurses can name the health problems they treat, they are speechless before legislators, third party payers, administrators, other health professionals, and perhaps even nurses themselves. Nursing diagnosis pinpoints what nursing is and what nursing does.[28]

If nurses use nursing diagnoses, record their observations and conclusions, and describe the health responses they treat, the body of nursing knowledge will increase, as will the credibility and value placed on nursing care.

Nursing does not exist in a vacuum, however. Although nurses are the largest group of health care professionals, they must work with other groups, such as physicians, to maximize the health of patients. Each group of health care providers serves as a resource to the others as they collaborate for the improved health status of the patient. Nurses, therefore, while formulating nursing diagnoses and using the nursing process, should also be familiar with medical diagnoses and treatment plans. Medical diagnoses refer to the health problem or disease states of the patient. In the medical model of psychiatry, the health problems are mental disorders, which are classified in the DSM-III.[2] The DSM-III comprehensively describes the manifestations of various mental disorders, but does not attempt to discuss cause or how the disturbances come about. Specific diagnostic criteria, however, are provided for each mental disorder. Chapter 2 discusses the medical model and DSM-III in greater detail.

Nursing and medical diagnoses may complement each other, but one is not a component of another. A patient with one specific medical diagnosis may have a number of complementary nursing diagnoses related to his range of health responses. On the other hand, a patient may have a specific nursing diagnosis without any identified medical diagnosis. The focus of this text is on psychiatric nursing and the identification and treatment of nursing problems. Chapters 7 to 14 are organized on this basis and are developed using a nursing process framework. Because quality nursing care requires an understanding of the patient's medical problems as well, each of these chapters will also incorporate a discussion of the medical diagnoses that may be relevant to the patient's health responses. In these chapters, a repeated format will be used to relate the nursing and medical diagnoses. Table 4-4 shows the format of this presentation and lists the 16 diagnostic classes identified by DSM-III, along with the 9 nursing

TABLE 4-4. Presentation of medical diagnostic classes and nursing problems

Medical diagnostic classes described in DSM-III	Nursing problems
Disorders usually first evident in infancy, childhood, or adolescence	Anxiety
	Alterations in self-concept
	Disturbances of mood
Organic mental disorders	Self-destructive behavior
Substance use disorders	Disruptions in relatedness
Schizophrenic disorders	Problems with expression of anger
Paranoid disorders	
Psychotic disorders not elsewhere classified	Impaired cognition
	Substance abuse
Affective disorders	
Anxiety disorders	
Somatoform disorders	
Dissociative disorders	
Psychosexual disorders	
Factitious disorders	
Disorders of impulse control not elsewhere classified	
Adjustment disorders	
Psychological factors affecting physical condition	
Personality disorders	

problems that are explored in this text. The purpose of including this content is to expand the nurse's understanding of the patient and provide a broader base for her own nursing actions.

Nursing diagnoses are usually formulated in the orientation phase of the relationship. Inexperienced nurses often feel pressured to identify nursing problems quickly and feel confused and frustrated by the withdrawn or noncommunicative patient who does not participate in the relationship and does not share his thoughts or feelings. In this case, the primary nursing problem may be the patient's social isolation related to feelings of inadequacy, or it may be lack of verbalization stemming from fear of interpersonal closeness. Nursing diagnoses describe current health responses of the patient. It is important for the nurse to begin with the behavior and coping responses displayed by the patient at the present time and to work from there. This requires both an acceptance of the patient and a setting of nursing priorities.

Planning

STANDARD IV—PLANNING. The nurse develops a nursing care plan with specific goals and interventions delineating nursing actions unique to each client's needs.

Process criteria
1. The nurse collaborates with clients, their significant others, and team members in establishing nursing care plans
2. In the care plan the nurse:
   a. Identifies priorities of care
   b. States realistic goals in measurable terms with an expected date of accomplishment
   c. Uses identifiable psychotherapeutic principles
   d. Indicates which client needs will be a primary responsibility of the psychiatric and mental health nurse and which will be referred to others with the appropriate expertise
   e. Stresses mutual goal setting and shared responsibility for goal attainment at the level of the client's abilities
   f. Provides guidance for the client care activities performed by others under the nurse's supervision
3. The nurse revises the care plan as goals are achieved, changed, or updated

Careful planning builds on the data collection and nursing diagnosis phases of the nursing process and increases the probability of successful implementation and evaluation. The first step in planning is the development of clearly stated objectives, or goals, for nursing care. In developing methods for writing accurate goals, nursing has built on educational theory. The work of Mager[26] is highly recommended as a resource on this topic.

There are four important aspects of goal setting: mutuality, congruency, realism, and timing. However, before goals can be adequately defined, the nurse must recognize that the patient frequently comes to therapy with goals of his own. Generally, they are expressions of the discomfort he feels and are related to symptom alleviation. Often the patient's goals are not directly stated and may be difficult to clarify. Taking nonspecific concerns and translating them into specific goal statements is no easy task for the nurse. She must understand the nature of the patient's coping responses and the predisposing and precipitating factors that influence them. Some of the difficulties in defining goals have been described as follows by Krumboltz and Thorensen[23]:

1. The patient may view his problem as someone else's behavior. This may be seen in the case of a parent who brings his adolescent son in for counseling. The parent may view the son as the problem, whereas the adolescent may feel his only problem is his father. An approach to handling this type of situation is to help the person who brings the problem into treatment, since he "owns" the problem at that moment. The nurse might suggest, "Let's talk about how I might help you deal with your son. A change in your response might lead to a change in his behavior also."

2. The patient may express his problem as a feeling, such as, "I'm lonely," or "I'm so unhappy." In addition to trying to help the patient clarify what exactly he is feeling, the nurse might ask him "What kinds of things could you do to make yourself feel less alone and more loved by others?" This helps the patient to see the connection between actions and feelings and increases his sense of responsibility for himself.

3. The patient's problem may be that he lacks a goal or an idea of what exactly he desires out of life. It might be helpful for the nurse, in this case, to point out that values and goals are not magically discovered but must be created by people for themselves. The patient can then be engaged in an active exploratory process to construct goals in his life or adopt the goals of a social, service, religious, or political group with whom he identifies.

4. The patient's goals may be inappropriate, undesirable, or unclear. The solution here is not for the nurse to impose her goals on the patient. Rather, even if the patient's goals seem to be against his best interests, the most the nurse can do is to reflect the patient's behavior and the consequences of it back to the patient. If he should then ask for help in setting new goals, the nurse can help him to do so.

5. The patient's problem may be a choice conflict. This is especially common if all of the choices are unpleasant, unacceptable, or unattainable. An example of this is a couple who wishes to divorce, but do not want to see their child hurt or suffer the financial hardship that would result. Although the nurse cannot make undesirable choices desirable, she can help patients use the problem-solving process and identify the full range of alternatives available to them.

6. The patient may have no real problem but just want to talk. Nurses must then decide what role they can play with this person and carefully distinguish between a social and a therapeutic relationship.

It becomes obvious that the process of goal clarification is an essential step in the therapeutic process. Out of this clarification and the nursing diagnoses will emerge the mutually agreed on goals around which the therapeutic relationship will be based. There is often a tendency for the well-intentioned nurse to overlook the patient's goals and devise a care plan leading to an outcome that will be gratifying to herself. However, this imposition of supposedly beneficial goals by others may be one of the conflict-producing situations that the patient has experienced in the past. Therefore the experience of working cooperatively with the nurse to evolve mutually acceptable goals is an extremely beneficial experience. If a goal desired by the nurse cannot be shared by the patient, it may be best to defer it until he is able to share it.

Once the goals are agreed on, the nurse must state them explicitly for herself and the patient. The more specifically one can state the goals of therapy, the more likely one is to achieve them. They also serve to guide later nursing actions and enhance the evaluation of care. It is therefore necessary that the objectives be written in behavioral terms. This means that the verb used in the statement of the objective should represent a behavior that may be observed. They should realistically describe what the nurse wishes to accomplish and within what time span. Often the requirement for explicit goals is avoided through the use of general statements that are applicable to all patients, such as the goals of forming a relationship or relieving depression. They may be valid in general terms, but they are not adequate in and of themselves.

Long- and short-term goals should be developed, with short-term goals contributing to the attainment of the long-term goals. Following are sample goals:

Long-term

The patient will travel about the community independently within 2 months.

Short-term

1. At the end of 1 week the patient will sit on his front steps.
2. At the end of 2 weeks the patient will walk to the corner and back to his house.
3. At the end of 3 weeks the patient, accompanied by the nurse, will walk around the block.
4. At the end of 4 weeks the patient will walk around the block alone.

The hierarchy would continue until the desired goal is accomplished. It should be noted that the goal is stated in terms of observable behavior, includes a period of time in which it is to be accomplished, and incorporates any other conditions applicable to the goal, such as whether the patient is to be alone or accompanied by the nurse.

Most patients exhibit a number of nursing problems, each of which must be incorporated in the plan of care. Several goals may need to be written relative to each nursing diagnosis. As the nurse and patient work together to meet patient needs, new ones often arise. For this reason, it is necessary to make decisions concerning the relative importance or priority of meeting the various nurse-patient goals. Otherwise, care would become haphazard and fragmented, with the focus first on one goal and then on the next, based only on what happened to come up at the time. Important and immediate needs could get lost in the general chaos.

One of the most important tasks of the nurse and patient is to assign priorities to goals. Frequently, a number of goals can be pursued simultaneously. Goals related to the protection of the patient from self-destructive impulses always receive high priority. With the identification of both long- and short-term goals, it is particularly important that the nurse keep the proposed time sequence firmly in mind.

Since the nursing care plan is dynamic and

should ensure responsiveness to the patient's coping responses throughout his contact with the health care system, priorities are constantly changing. If the focus is always kept on the patient's behavioral responses, priorities can be set and modified as the patient changes. Nursing care is then personalized and the patient participates in its planning and implementation.

STANDARD VIII—CONTINUING EDUCATION. The nurse assumes responsibility for continuing education and professional development and contributes to the professional growth of others.

Process criteria

The nurse:

1. Initiates independent learning activities to increase understanding and update skills
2. Participates in inservice meetings and educational programs either as an attendee or as a teacher
3. Attends conventions, institutions, workshops, symposia, and other professional meetings
4. Systematically increases understanding of theories related to psychiatric and mental health nursing
5. Assists others to identify areas of educational needs
6. Communicates formally and informally new knowledge regarding clinical observations and interpretations with professional colleagues and others

Once the goals are formulated, the next task is to outline the plan or method for achieving these goals. The nursing care plan is based on application of theory from nursing and related physical and behavioral sciences to the unique responses of the individual patient. This presupposes that as the nurse identifies areas of patient need, appropriate theoretical resources will again be consulted. Failure to approach nursing care in this scientific manner is likely to result in illogical decision making and a plan based on tradition, intuition, or trial and error. Although use of any of these decision-making methods may result in a valid plan, consistency of depth and accuracy over time will suffer, as will the overall care of the patient. Skill in using the nursing process requires a commitment by the nurse to the ongoing pursuit of knowledge that will enhance professional growth.

Successful care planning is facilitated by the active involvement of the patient. If the nurse collects data, returns to the nurse's station, consults textbooks, and then writes up a plan of care, an important step has been missed. Once the nurse has formulated a tentative care plan, she must validate this plan with her patient. This saves time and effort for them both as they continue to work together and also communicates to the patient his responsibility in getting well. The patient can tell the nurse that a proposed plan is unrealistic regarding financial status, life-style, value system or, perhaps, personal preference. There are usually several possible approaches to a patient problem. Utilizing the one that is most acceptable to the patient enhances the likelihood of goal accomplishment.

If the goal answers the question of "what," the plan of care answers the questions of "how" and "why." The plan chosen obviously will depend on the nursing diagnosis, the nurse's theoretical orientation, and the nature of the goals pursued. In general, the goals will influence the selection of therapeutic techniques. Failure to attain a goal by employing a particular plan can lead to the decision to adopt a new approach or to reevaluate the goal. Mutual planning and implementation activities commonly occur in the working phase of the relationship.

 Implementation

STANDARD V—INTERVENTION. The nurse intervenes as guided by the nursing care plan to implement nursing actions that promote, maintain, or restore physical and mental health, prevent illness, and effect rehabilitation.
Process criteria
The nurse:
1. Acts to ensure that health care needs are met either by using nursing skills or by obtaining assistance from other health care providers when indicated
2. Acts as the client's advocate when necessary to facilitate the achievement of health
3. Reviews and modifies interventions based on patient progress

STANDARD V-A—PSYCHOTHERAPEUTIC INTERVENTIONS. The nurse (generalist) uses psychotherapeutic interventions to assist clients to regain or improve their previous coping abilities and prevent further disability.
Process criteria
The nurse:
1. Identifies the client's responses to health problems
2. Reinforces those responses to health problems that are functional and helps the client modify or eliminate those that are dysfunctional

3. Employs principles of communication, interviewing techniques, problem-solving, and crisis intervention when performing psychotherapeutic interventions
4. Uses knowledge of behavioral concepts such as anxiety, loss, conflict, grief, and anger to assist the client to cope, adapt, and constructively deal with feelings
5. Demonstrates knowledge about and skill in the use of psychotherapeutic interventions specifically useful in the modification of thought, perception, affect, behavior, and motivation
6. Utilizes health team members to help evaluate the outcome of interventions and to formulate modification of psychotherapeutic techniques
7. Reinforces useful patterns and themes in the client's interactions with others
8. Uses crisis intervention to promote growth and to aid the personal and social integration of clients in developmental, situational, or suicidal crisis

STANDARD V-B—HEALTH TEACHING. The nurse assists clients, families, and groups to achieve satisfying and productive patterns of living through health teaching.
Process criteria
The nurse:
1. Identifies health education needs of clients
2. Employs principles of learning and appropriate teaching methods
3. Teaches the basic principles of physical and mental health
4. Teaches communication, interpersonal, and social skills
5. Provides opportunities for clients to learn experientially

STANDARD V-C—SELF-CARE ACTIVITIES. The nurse uses the activities of daily living in a goal-directed way to foster adequate self-care and physical and mental well-being of clients.
Process criteria
The nurse:
1. Respects and protects the client's rights
2. Encourages the client to collaborate in the development of a self-care plan
3. Sets limits in a manner that is humane and the least restrictive necessary to assure safety of the client and others

STANDARD V-D—SOMATIC THERAPIES. The nurse uses knowledge of somatic therapies and applies related clinical skills in working with clients.
Process criteria
The nurse:
1. Utilizes knowledge of current psychopharmacology to guide nursing actions
2. Observes and interprets pertinent responses to somatic therapies in terms of the underlying principles of each therapy
3. Evaluates effectiveness of somatic therapies and recommends changes in the treatment plan as appropriate

4. Collaborates with other team members to provide for safe administration of therapies
5. Supervises the client's chemotherapeutic regimen in collaboration with the physician
6. Provides opportunities for clients and families to discuss, question, and explore their feelings and concerns about past, current, or projected use of somatic therapies
7. Reviews expected actions and side effects of somatic therapies with clients and their families
8. Uses prescribing authority for medications as congruent with the state nursing practice act

STANDARD V-E—THERAPEUTIC ENVIRONMENT. The nurse provides, structures, and maintains a therapeutic environment in collaboration with the client and other health care providers.

Process criteria

The nurse:

1. Assures that clients are adequately oriented to the milieu and are familiar with scheduled activities and rules that govern behavior and daily living
2. Observes, analyzes, interprets and records the effects of environmental forces upon the client
3. Assesses and develops the therapeutic potential of the practice setting on behalf of clients through consideration of the physical environment, the social structure, and the culture of the setting
4. Fosters communications in the environment that are congruent with therapeutic goals
5. Collaborates with others in the development and institution of milieu activities specific to the client's physical and mental health needs
6. Articulates to the client and staff the justification for use of limit setting, restraint, or seclusion and the conditions necessary for release from restriction to the client and staff
7. Participates in ongoing evaluation of the effectiveness of the therapeutic milieu
8. Assists clients living at home to achieve and maintain an environment that supports and maintains health

STANDARD V-F—PSYCHOTHERAPY. The nurse (specialist) utilizes advanced clinical expertise in individual, group, and family *psychotherapy*, child psychotherapy, and other treatment modalities to function as a psychotherapist and recognizes professional accountability for nursing practice.

Process criteria

The nurse:

1. Structures the therapeutic contract with the client in the beginning phase of the relationship, including such elements as purpose, time, place, fees, participants, confidentiality, available means of contact, and responsibilities of both client and therapist
2. Engages in interdisciplinary and intradisciplinary collaboration to achieve treatment goals
3. Engages clients in the process of determining the appropriate form of psychotherapy
4. Identifies the goals of psychotherapy

5. Uses knowledge of growth and development, psychopathology, psychosocial systems, small group and family dynamics, and knowledge of selected treatment modalities as indicated
6. Articulates a rationale for the goals chosen and interventions utilized
7. Fosters increasing personal and therapeutic responsibility on the part of the client
8. Provides for continuity of care for the client in the therapist's absence
9. Determines with the client, when possible, that goals have been achieved and facilitates the termination process
10. Refers clients to other professionals when indicated
11. Respects and protects the client's legal rights
12. Avails self of appropriate opportunities to increase knowledge and skill in the therapies utilized in nursing practice
13. Obtains recognized educational preparation and ongoing supervision for types of psychotherapy utilized, e.g., individual psychotherapy, group and family psychotherapy, child psychotherapy, psychoanalysis, or other forms of therapy
14. Uses clinical judgment in determining whether providing physical care (especially procedures prone to misinterpretation, e.g., injections, enemas) will enhance or impair the therapist-client relationship and delegates such care as needed

Implementation refers to the actual delivery of nursing care to the patient and his response to the care that is given. Good planning maximizes the probability of successful implementation. Such factors as available people, equipment, resources, time, and money must be considered as nursing actions are planned. Well-planned nursing care also takes into account the personalities and experiences of the nurse and the patient, and their interaction.

The most valid basis for nursing action is that which has been investigated by nursing researchers who have applied the scientific method to nursing practice. It is also acceptable to judiciously use theory from the physical and behavioral sciences to provide a rationale for nursing intervention. In most nurse-patient situations, there is more than one possible approach to accomplishing the stated objectives. It is helpful, when planning care, to identify alternative nursing actions that are appropriate to the goal. If this is done, the nurse is not left floundering should the only identified action fail. Consideration of several alternative nursing actions lends a great deal of flexibility to the implementation phase of the nursing process.

The standards of practice and related process criteria presented on pp. 136 and 137 are quite detailed and explicit. They present a thorough analysis of this phase of the nursing process. Nursing interventions should help the psychiatric patient do two things: *develop insight* and resolve problems through *carrying out a plan of positive action*. These two areas for nursing intervention correspond with the responsive and action dimensions of the nurse-patient relationship described in Chapter 3. Insight refers to the development of new emotional and cognitive organizations by the patient. It frequently leads to an increase in anxiety as defense mechanisms are broken down. This is the time when resistances commonly occur. But knowing something on an intellectual level does *not* inevitably lead to a change in behavior. Nurses who terminate their interventions at this point are not fully carrying out the therapeutic process to the patient's benefit. An additional step is needed. The patient must decide if he will revert back to maladaptive coping mechanisms, remain in a resisting, immobilized state, or adopt new, adaptive, and constructive coping mechanisms.

The first step in helping a patient translate insight into action is to build adequate incentives to abandoning old patterns of behavior. The nurse should help the patient see that his old patterns do him more harm than good and inflict much suffering and pain on him. No new patterns can be learned unless the motivation to acquire them is greater than the motivation to retain old ones. Nursing activities therefore must include encouraging any desires the patient expresses for mental health, emotional growth, and freedom from suffering. With sufficient motivation the patient must then be supported as he tests out new behaviors and coping mechanisms. Important in this regard will be the mobilization of the individual's social support system. This is relevant to all levels of nursing intervention—primary, secondary, and tertiary—and all patient populations. Specific strategies for supporting social systems are described in Chapter 5.

Within the context of the nurse-patient relationship, adaptive goals can be actively pursued by the patient in a productive way. It is important for the nurse and patient to allow sufficient time for change. Many of the patient's maladaptive patterns have been building up over months and years and cannot be expected to change in a matter of days or weeks. Finally, the nurse must help the patient evaluate these new patterns, integrate them into his life experiences, and utilize the learning of problem solving as foresight for future experiences. In this way secondary prevention nursing interventions also fulfill primary prevention goals.

STANDARD IX—INTERDISCIPLINARY COLLABORATION. The nurse collaborates with interdisciplinary teams in assessing, planning, implementing, and evaluating programs and other mental health activities. *Process criteria*

The nurse:

1. Participates in the formulation of overall goals, plans, and decisions
2. Includes the client in the collaboration of the mental health team whenever possible and appropriate
3. Recognizes, respects, accepts, and demonstrates trust in colleagues and their contributions
4. Consults with colleagues as needed and is available to be consulted by them
5. Articulates knowledge and skills so that these may be coordinated with the contributions of others working with a client or program
6. Collaborates with other disciplines in teaching, supervision, and research

Planning and implementation of nursing care must not take place in isolation from the patient's other experiences with the health care team and the health care system. The nurse has a responsibility to be sure that the nursing care plan is congruent with the plans of other health care professionals who are involved with the patient. Some degree of conflict can be avoided by personal contact with other professionals to discover how they define their roles and responsibilities. Knowledge of the distribution of responsibility within the health team enables the nurse to consult colleagues appropriately as indicated by the needs of the patient. Although the nurse may have information about these areas, it is a much more efficient and appropriate use of time and energy to refer the patient to team members who specialize in dealing with the patient's needs. Referral should be accompanied by adequate background information so that the assessment process is not duplicated.

 Evaluation

STANDARD VI—EVALUATION. The nurse evaluates client responses to nursing actions in order to revise the data base, nursing diagnoses, and nursing care plan.

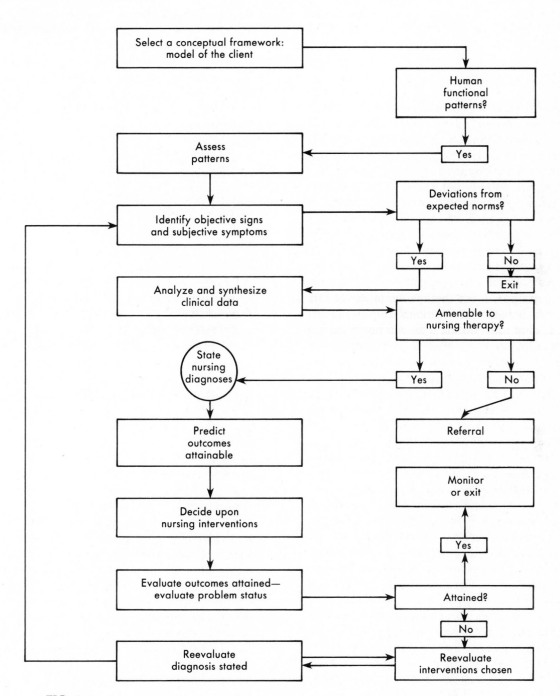

FIG. 4-5

Flowchart of the nursing process. (From Gordon, M.: Nurs. Clin. North Am. **14**:492, 1979.)

Process criteria
The nurse:
1. Pursues validation, suggestions, and new information
2. Discusses observations, insights, and data with colleagues
3. Documents the results of evaluation of nursing care
4. Conducts a nursing audit

When evaluating nursing care, one should review all previous phases of the nursing process and determine the degree of goal achievement by the patient. The overall flow of the nursing process is evident in Fig. 4-5. From this representation, it is evident that many decisions are made by the nurse throughout the process. Evaluation of care requires that the nurse first consider if her conceptual framework was valid and appropriate to the particular patient situation. Next, was the data collection adequate and all relevant patterns of behavior, objective signs, and subjective symptoms identified? The accuracy of the nursing diagnosis may be assessed with relation to the nature of normal parameters used, the analysis and synthesis of data, the application of theory, and its appropriateness for nursing therapy. The nursing goals and plan of care should be examined for their relevancy, priority, mutuality, and consideration of all realistic alternatives. In the area of implementation, the nurse needs to evaluate whether the nursing interventions were appropriate, efficient in use of time and energy and, most important, effective. The timing, relevance, communication, and outcome of the nursing interventions must all be critically analyzed. The achievement of goals is worth noting explicitly. Often progress with psychiatric patients is slow and occurs in imperceptible degrees rather than with dramatic suddenness. Realizing progress has been made can be growth producing in itself and can evoke enthusiasm for further progress on the part of both the patient and the nurse.

Flexibility is needed by the nurse to modify her interventions on the basis of the patient's changing needs and her continuing evaluation. The need to modify a care plan does not connote failure of nursing care. Failure takes place if the plan of care is not relevant to the client's needs and is not revised as the needs change or are clarified. Thus, reassessment, reordering of priorities, new goal setting, and revision of the nursing care plan are all essential evaluation activities.

Evaluation is a mutual process based on the previously identified goals and level of satisfaction expressed by the patient. It is not a cumbersome task left for the termination phase of the relationship. Rather, it is a continuous, active process that begins with the initial phase of the relationship and is present throughout its development and completion. The key words for the evaluation phase of the nursing process can be summarized as mutual, continuous, adequate, effective, appropriate, efficient, and flexible.

STANDARD VII—PEER REVIEW. The nurse participates in peer review and other means of evaluation to assure quality of nursing care provided for clients.
Process criteria
The nurse:
1. Assumes responsibility for review of clinical practice with peers, supervisors, and/or consultants
2. Considers recommendations for change that may arise from review

Evaluation of the nursing process is an ongoing activity that is the professional responsibility of every nurse. It is often difficult, however, for the nurse to evaluate nursing care alone. Supervision by a peer, a group of peers, or a more experienced person is therefore an important part of professional practice. Whether it is conducted formally or informally, evaluation helps the nurse to examine her thinking in planning care and serves as a learning experience for her.

Thus far, this discussion of the evaluation of nursing activities has focused on evaluating the care given by an individual nurse. There is another level of evaluation, however, that nurses need to be knowledgeable about and actively participate in. This is the level of formal, systematic, organizational evaluation of overall patterns of care through *quality assessment measures*. In these activities, the focus is not on the nurse practitioner but on the patient and overall program of care. The present growth and commitment to critically reviewing and analyzing the quality of health care can be attributed to several sources: the demands of the consumer for quality, but reasonable, health care, third party payees for controlled health care costs, the movement toward increased professional accountability, and regulatory and federal groups to monitor the quality of care given to providers. At this higher level of analysis, a comprehensive evaluation should theoretically include the following[42]:

■ Clinical evaluation of treatment outcome and process

■ Consumer evaluation of patient needs and satisfaction

■ Systems evaluation of administration and management of treatment and allocation of resources

Of these three types of evaluation, clinical evaluation is the longest established and most common. Consumer evaluation is gaining attention and acceptance as the public is becoming more educated and assertive. Systems evaluation has primarily been limited to improving operations in private industry, and only recently has it been applied to health care.

Systems evaluation is the evaluation of the organization of the delivery system, which includes patient flow, paperwork, procedures for scheduling patients, staff-patient ratio, disciplinary mix, and the analysis of utilization of resources. It is intended to supplement clinical evaluation. Three components of systems evaluation have been identified: (1) systems analysis, (2) economic analysis, and (3) operations research. Systems analysis attempts to simplify and improve the organization. Economic analysis emphasizes monies spent and what, in turn, they produce. Operations research attempts to develop methods that will help hospital management plan for optimal allocation of the resources available. Together, these analyses bring a new dimension to the institution by evaluating the actual organization of treatment and have the potential for improving the performance of the clinical operation.[42]

Clinical evaluation of ongoing programs is demonstrated in the form of various *quality assurance* activities that include both evaluation and corrective action. Zimmer[52] defines quality assurance as the estimation in degree of excellence in three areas: (1) patient health outcomes, (2) process or activity, and (3) resource cost outcomes. A common method reflecting two of these areas is the patient care audit, which, when restricted to nursing care, is also called the *nursing audit*. The topic of an audit may be a disease, nursing diagnosis, patient behavior, therapeutic measure, or nursing procedure. An audit that focuses on nursing actions is called a *process audit*. In a process audit, data are collected relative to a specific nursing activity, and they are then compared to a preset standard of nursing care, such as the American Nurses' Association Standards of Nursing Practice. If the audit focuses on the behavior of the patient in response to the care that has been provided, it is termed an *outcome audit*. This type of audit

parallels the evaluation phase of the nursing process. Specific examples of nursing audits conducted in the psychiatric setting are described in some of the articles listed in the annotated suggested readings at the end of this chapter.

Both process and outcome audits have advantages, depending on the information desired. Zimmer[52] believes that in quality assurance efforts, nurses should first start with the determination of desired patient health outcomes and the degree to which they are attained. Next, nurses must proceed to the identification of the most powerful and cost-effective activities that cause these outcomes. Finally, when activities are identified and their relationship with specific outcomes is clear, nurses should proceed to the third step, determining the cost of the nursing activities and the related resources used to achieve specific outcomes.

Two important components of quality assurance should be emphasized. The first is the necessity for peer review, which should consist of expert nurse peers who are involved together in the delivery of care. They are the only persons who have the needed nursing knowledge to be able to make judgments about desired patient health outcomes, how patients should progress toward those outcomes, and nursing activities that cause the changes. They are also those people who will be most involved with the other component of quality assurance—the correction of deficiencies or problems of nursing care that the audit reveals. This idea of taking corrective action and actually making improvements is what differentiates quality assurance from simple program evaluation or evaluation research. The reports of quality assurance should reach the highest level of the organization, and it is expected that actions will be taken which will result in improvement. These may take the form of administrative changes in policies or procedures, continuing education programs, reallocation of manpower, changes in activities or procedures, or a need for further research.

Involvement in this level of clinical program evaluation is necessary for all nurses. Through such activities, nurses demonstrate professional accountability. As Zimmer has stated:

Members of the nursing profession will be able to take their place among the disciplines that function in patient health review when and only when they can identify the specific alterations in patient health status secured through nursing activities. The development and the use of nurses' capability to function in quality assurance thus deserves the highest priority in the nursing profession.[52:93]

Clinical case analysis

Clinical example 4-1 is a case study of a long-term relationship that demonstrates the use of the nursing process with a patient. It illustrates the interrelationship of the phases of the nurse-patient relationship, therapeutic dimensions, and various activities of the nurse as she works with the patient to bring about adaptive coping behavior and the more integrated functioning of the patient.

CLINICAL EXAMPLE 4-1

Ms. G came to the psychiatric outpatient department of the local hospital requesting treatment with a female therapist. After consultation with a psychiatrist, the psychiatric nurse specialist agreed to perform the initial screening and evaluation and consider serving as her primary therapist. To collect the initial data, the nurse followed the admission format required by the department. A description of the presenting problem revealed that Ms. G was a 29-year-old single woman who was neat in appearance and markedly overweight. She reported feelings of "confusion and depression" and said that superficially she appeared "outgoing and friendly and played the role of a clown." In reality, however, she said she had few close friends, felt insecure about herself, felt unsuccessful in her job, and believed she "overanalyzed her problems."

Additional information was obtained in other significant areas of her life. Her psychosocial history revealed a disrupted family situation. Her mother died of tuberculosis when she was 11 years of age. Her father, age 73, was alive but had been an alcoholic "for as long as Ms. G could remember." She had one sister, age 20, who married at age 16 and was now divorced. She also had one stepsister, age 45, who was married, had two adopted sons, and lived out of state. In exploring this family information, Ms. G revealed that her stepsister was her natural mother, but she had continued to call her father's wife "mother." After her "mother" died, her stepsister took over the house. Two years later, however, this stepsister married and moved out of state. Ms. G reported feeling closest to this stepsister and felt abandoned when she left. Ms. G then took charge of the house until age 14, when her father placed her and her sister in a group home where she had difficulty making friends.

She completed high school and college. In college she had four good friends who were all married now. Her only close heterosexual relationship was in high school, and this boyfriend eventually married her best friend. Since that time she had never dated and stated she had no desire to marry.

After college she obtained a job as a "girl Friday" for a law firm and expressed much pleasure with it. She then saw the opportunity to make more money as a waitress and switched jobs. She worked at a restaurant at present and her schedule involved day and night rotations as well as weekend shifts. She expressed dissatisfaction with many aspects of her job but an inability to identify alternatives. Her goal in life was to have a fulfilling career.

She lived alone. Her best friend was her immediate supervisor at work. She currently had no male friends and only two other female acquaintances.

Pertinent medical history revealed a major weight problem. She was 36 kg (80 pounds) overweight and extremely conscious of it. She viewed her body negatively and believed others were also "repulsed" by her weight. She was also recently recovered from infectious hepatitis. She drank an occasional beer when out with friends (once or twice a month), denied any drug use, and smoked three fourths of a pack of cigarettes a day.

After consultation the psychiatric nurse agreed to work with Ms. G as primary therapist. In the following session they established a contract for working together, and a moderate fee was set by the agency's financial secretary. At this time they explored her expressed guilt over seeking help, the reason for her request for a female therapist, their mutual roles, and the confidential nature of the relationship. The nurse also shared with Ms. G the behavior patterns she had noted and the inferences she had made. They discussed these areas, and the nursing diagnosis identified the following nursing problems:

1. Negative self-concept related to childhood rejection and unrealistic self-ideals
2. Poor interpersonal relationships with particular ambivalence regarding male-female relations related to lack of socialization skills
3. Job dissatisfaction related to working hours and the nature of the work
4. Negative body image related to weight control problem
5. Ambivalence and anxiety related to the possibility of change and the therapy process

In discussing these areas they agreed that problem 1 was a central one and problems 3 and 4 directly contributed to it. Her coping mechanisms included intellectualization and denial, and she compensated for her self-doubts by an outward appearance that was social, joking, and friendly, yet superficial. Problem 5 presented an immediate demand on the therapeutic relationship. The strengths Ms. G brought to the therapy process included her introspective nature and ability to analyze events, her openness to new ideas, the resource people available to her in her immediate environment, and a genuine sense of humor. They mutually agreed to work on her problem areas in weekly therapy sessions. After 5 months they would evaluate the achievement of the following long-term goals:

1. Aspects of Ms. G's self-ideal will be identified.
2. Factors influencing her self-concept and negative, stereotyped self-perceptions will be evaluated.
3. Interpersonal relationships will be analyzed to include her patterns of relating, her expectations of others, and specific areas of difficulty.
4. Ms. G will describe her expectations of the therapeutic process and her commitment to it.
5. Alternative employment opportunities will be identified.
6. The advantages and disadvantages of a job change will be compared.

Since they were in the introductory phase of the relationship, many of the goals involved areas needing further assessment. During this phase of treatment Ms. G displayed much anxiety, testing behavior, and ambivalence, and the nursing actions were focused on promoting respect, openness, and acceptance and minimizing her anxiety. Through the nurse's use of empathic understanding, Ms. G became less jovial and superficial and began to attain some intellectual insight into her behavior. With guidance she began to appraise her own abilities and became more open in expressing feelings.

She feared intimate personal involvement and could not tolerate physical closeness. The nurse incorporated this into nursing actions by initially minimizing confrontation, setting limits on anxiety-producing topics, and arranging the office seating to allow the patient to select her proximity to the nurse. As they discussed the patient's relationships, the nurse confronted her with the dependent role Ms. G played in them and the unrealistic expectations she placed on others in the exclusiveness and amount of time she demanded from them. Her pattern of relating was also manipulative in that she elicited a sympathetic response and then used it to meet her own needs. She had great difficulty with mutuality and autonomy in relating to others. She was inexperienced in heterosexual relationships and missed many of the normal adolescent growth experiences in this area. Finally, she had much emotion and fear vested in her family of origin. The only trusting relationship Ms. G could recall was with her stepsister-mother. When this stepsister abruptly left home to marry, Ms. G perceived this as a personal rejection. She had since isolated herself from her family and continued to blame herself for her rejection by others, thus lowering her self-esteem and ability to trust others.

At the end of 4 months Ms. G was being considered for a promotion at work to hostess but on the basis of an evaluation by her best friend and supervisor was rejected for it. This precipitated a suicide attempt, which Ms. G revealed at her next regular session. At this point the issue of trust within the relation-

ship became critical, as well as her inability to express anger because of fear of rejection. The nurse now began more actively confronting Ms. G in her areas of ambivalence and inconsistency, setting limits on her self-destructive behavior, and suggesting alternatives. Ms. G then revealed that her relationship with her friend-supervisor was also a sexual one, and she expressed fears of homosexuality and loss of identity.

In later sessions Ms. G's relationship with this friend would become a critical therapeutic issue because many of her conflicts were acted out in it. The therapy process presented a threat to the pathological nature of this relationship, and during the course of therapy Ms. G would need to choose between maladaptive behaviors and more growth-producing ones.

The relationship had now moved into the working phase where focus was placed on specifics, and problem-solving activities were begun. After 5 months the nursing diagnosis was reevaluated to include the following problems:

1. Self-destructive and suicidal tendencies related to perceived rejection by her friend
2. Identity diffusion, including sexual confusion, low self-esteem, and negative body image related to childhood rejection and unrealistic self-ideals
3. Disturbed interpersonal relationships characterized by an inability to trust and by patterns of dependency on others and manipulation of them related to lack of socialization skills and feelings of inadequacy
4. Inability to identify and express feelings, particularly anger, related to fear of rejection by others.
5. Job dissatisfaction related to working hours and the nature of the work

At this time the nurse sought consultation as she further evolved her plan of care. Neither medication nor hospitalization was indicated. These formulations were shared with Ms. G, and together they collaborated about her future progress. They agreed to focus on changing Ms. G's maladaptive behavior by exploring past events and conflicts, and helping her learn more productive patterns of living. Ms. G was now ready to commit herself to the work of therapy and interpersonal change, and she began to assume increased responsibility for this therapeutic work.

Because her self-ideal was unrealistically high, specific short-term goals became essential. The nurse's theoretical orientation incorporated the dynamics of Sullivan's interpersonal theory. Berne's transactional framework, and Glasser's reality therapy. The relationship was focused on frequently through the use of immediacy. It served as a model for examining many of her conflicts. This proved to be an excellent learning opportunity as Ms. G and the nurse dealt with resistance, transference, and countertransference reactions. During the next year Ms. G made much progress, including the following changes:

1. She moved into an apartment with another girl friend.

2. She left her previous job and resumed working in an office where she received more personal satisfaction and a work schedule that would allow her to increase her social activities.

3. She began a diet regimen.

4. She participated in additional activities, such as a dancing class and a health spa.

5. She learned to verbalize her anger more freely with the nurse, friends, and others at work. This included discussing the many relationships in her past that were terminated without her agreement and in which she had internalized the anger.

6. She contacted her stepsister-mother and visited her. This was an important therapeutic goal because it allowed her to review her early experiences and provided her with actual feedback from those involved. Consequently, many of her misperceptions became evident and open to exploration in therapy.

7. She was able to admit her ambivalent feeling about her friend-supervisor and discuss the negative aspects of the relationship. She stopped further sexual contact with her because she felt exploited in this area. Over time, the nature of this relationship changed, and it eventually became a casual acquaintance.

8. She learned about the variety of sexual feelings and responses and saw her needs in this area as appropriate developmental tasks.

9. Her perception of personal space changed, and her tolerance for physical closeness increased.

10. She developed new male and female friends and socialized frequently with them.

The terminating phase of the relationship began after about 18 months. At this time Ms. G was independently solving problems and, in therapy, the nurse primarily validated and supported her thinking. She was now receiving and accepting much positive feedback from others, had lost 15 kg (40 pounds), was continuing to diet, was planning future career goals, and had begun dating men. The mutual goals for therapy had been met.

Terminating was difficult because of the close, trusting bond that developed between them. The nurse had feelings of pleasure in Ms. G's growth, as well as personal satisfaction in her effectiveness as therapist. Ms. G openly described her feelings about terminating and raised the question of a possible social relationship between them. Over the course of 6 months she came to realize that the premise of the relationship was therapy and changing individual perceptions or patterns of relating would not be feasible or desirable. Most important, she had control for terminating this relationship and the opportunity to work it through in a positive way. The sessions were spaced to monthly intervals and considerable time was spent reviewing initial problem areas and the progress she had made in them. After 6 months, or 2 years of therapy, the nurse and patient mutually agreed to terminate regular sessions.

Documentation

The activities of each phase of the nursing process should be documented in writing. Written communication is essential to the successful planning and implementation of nursing care. Documentation by the nurse should begin with her data collection activities. If information obtained from the nurse's data collection is not recorded, there is a tendency for other mental health clinicians to attempt to obtain the same information. This repetition for the patient is unnecessary and inappropriate. By entering all collected data on the patient record, omissions and areas of confusion can be easily identified and clarified with the patient.

An organized and systematic format should be used by the nurse in her data collection activities. The tool used by the nurse for this purpose may be called a *data collection tool, nursing assessment form,* or *nursing history.* It may include elements of the psychiatric evaluation as described in Chapter 17 but goes beyond this evaluation to include subjective and objective data relative to a nursing diagnosis. A variety of such nursing assessment tools for the individual have appeared in the psychiatric nursing literature.* In addition, agencies, nursing departments, psychiatric units, educational programs, and individual nurse clinicians often use a tool that they have developed themselves. These tools may be adapted to the needs of a particular type of patient or institution.

At the present time, there is a need in psychiatric nursing for empirical testing of these tools for validity, reliability, and usefulness in nursing practice. One of the most complete data collection tools is the one developed by Francis and Munjas.[9] It consists of 315 questions divided among the following areas of assessment:

Demographic and vital data
    Name
    Address
    Birth
    Marital status
    Sex
    Race

---

*References 9, 13, 18, 44, 45.

Presenting data
    Nature of the problem
    Time of occurrence
    Reason for seeking care at this time
Family information
    Family system
    Communication patterns
    Interaction patterns
    Crisis response
Socioeconomic status
    Occupation
    Education
    Leisure time
    Residence
    Income
Life values
    Ethnicity
    Religious behavior
    Beliefs about illness
    Attitudes toward life
    Living standards
Social habits
    Eating
    Drinking
    Drug use
    Hygiene
Sexual behavior
    Preference
    Sex role
    Sex activity
Cognition
    Consciousness
    Orientation
    Attention
    Perception
    Apperception
    Thought content
    Thought form
    Thought progress
    Memory
    Self-concept
    Body image
Affect
    Depersonalization
    Continuum of despair to ecstacy
    Affective ambivalence
    Inadequate affect
    Inappropriate affect
    Anxiety
Conation (observed)
    Appearance
    Motor activity
    Communication

The thoroughness of this tool, which is presented in its entirety in Appendix B, makes it a valuable basis for decisions regarding data collection.

Two areas that are not specifically addressed by this tool, however, are the patient's social support network and the patient's past and present physiological status. Although a valid and reliable assessment tool for measuring social support has not yet been developed, Murawski, Penman, and Schmitt[32] suggested some elements that should be included in a current clinical assessment of social support. These elements and the dimensions of social networks described on p. 122 make up the following areas of assessment for social support:

    Size of social network
    Intensity, durability, multidimensionality, dispersion, and frequency of social linkages
    Normative context of the relationships
    Social roles
    Support available to meet role obligations during illness
    Patterns of social affiliation
    Need for social affiliation

An assessment of the patient's past and present physiological status should also be an essential part of the nurse's data collection, since maladaptive coping responses have physiological, as well as psychosocial, manifestations. Furthermore, some physiological imbalances can cause or intensify symptoms indicative of emotional dysfunction. Other tools can be used to assess physiological functioning (Appendix C), and they should include the following areas:

    Medical history
        Development
        Past illnesses and injuries
        Hospitalizations
        Family history
    Physiological status
        Body systems
        Present illnesses
        Medications and ongoing treatments
    Health maintenance
        Health goals

Finally, although the data collection tool of Francis and Munjas does assess family information, there may be occasions when the nurse wishes to focus less on the individual and more on the quality of the family functioning, that is, the degree to which they are able to deal with problems successfully. To do this, she may need to use an assessment tool for family analysis that examines the family as a unit, including its structure, relationships, and coping potential.[40,50] Helm, at Yale University School of Nurs-

ing, developed a useful guide to family analysis
(Appendix D). It assesses the following aspects
of the family unit:

Family's generational structure
Home environment
Physical and mental health
Financial status

Developmental stage in family life cycle
Family structure
Intrafamily relationships
Sociocultural family context
Strengths and weaknesses
Identified problem

If the nurse were to undertake a complete
biopsychosocial assessment of the patient based
on these tools, it would require a number of

SAMPLE NURSING CARE FORMAT

Patient information
  Name _____
  Age _____
  Sex _____
  Marital status _____
  Race or ethnic group _____
  Religion _____
  Occupation _____
  Current living environment _____
  Immediate support system _____

Date of admission _____
Medical diagnosis _____
_____
_____
_____
Nursing diagnosis _____
_____
_____
_____

| Biopsychosocial behaviors | | Nursing problem | Priority | Goals | | Nursing actions | Rationale | Evaluation |
Objective data	Subjective data			Long-term	Short-term			
								Modification:

hours to complete. At times, this might be necessary and appropriate. At other times, however, based on the patient's situation and the use of a team approach to care, the nurse may need to collect data relevant to only a few of these areas. A skilled practitioner, although possessing thorough knowledge of all areas of assessment, would then use her judgment in determining the exact nature and extent of the data needed.

The next type of documentation used by nurses is the *nursing care plan,* which should reflect all of the remaining stages of the nursing process—nursing diagnosis, planning, implementation, and evaluation. Although the precise format of the care plan may differ somewhat among agencies, because it is based on the nursing process, the differences tend to be minor ones. A complete nursing care plan would include pertinent demographic data on the patient, nursing diagnoses, objective and subjective behaviors of the patient, nursing problems identified, priority of the problems, nurse-patient goals, nursing actions, rationale, and evaluation with modifications of the plan. An example of a detailed and comprehensive care plan format is given on the facing page.

There are a number of advantages to formulating a written record of the nursing care plan as it evolves. The nurse who initiates and writes the plan must think through the whole nursing process in a logical and structured manner. The likelihood of basing nursing care on sound rationale is greater, since nursing care plans are generally scrutinized by others, and the reasons for specific components of the plan may be questioned. Self-evaluation by the nurse is also facilitated. A working care plan that is kept up to date requires that application of the nursing process be consistently reviewed and revised. Many agencies are aware that well-written nursing care plans reflect the course of the patient's contact with nursing personnel. It is frequently a practice to include the nursing care plan in the patient's permanent agency record. This can greatly enhance the quality of nursing care if the patient contacts the agency again in the future. Much data from the original assessment need not be collected again, thereby freeing the energy of both the patient and nurse to work on current concerns.

Detailed nursing care plans are useful learning tools. However, the daily use of a care plan by the nursing staff and other personnel working with the patient may require an abbreviated form of the care plan. Recording care plan in-formation in a concise manner can save both time and energy, but the dangers of vague generalities and routine analysis are great. The use of shortened care plans, such as *Kardex forms,* is prevalent in many institutions. A sample format for a psychiatric nursing Kardex form developed by Holden and Bedgio[15] is presented in Fig. 4-6. Nurses using such formats must ensure that patients are given clearly defined and individualized nursing care.

The documentation required in effective use of the nursing process sometimes poses problems for nurses. Transposing ideas into prose is often difficult, and usually the source of the difficulty is the fact that it is hard to crystallize one's thinking and be specific. Krall* suggests the following five guideline questions she found helpful in formulating written mental health treatment plans:

1. What is the exact behavior keeping the patient in the hospital?
2. Is the treatment plan written in behavioral terminology?
3. Is the stated behavior written in such a way that the patient can understand it?
4. Are the stated behaviors written in such a way that all nursing personnel can readily understand them?
5. How is the written treatment plan to be used?[22:236]

Santora and Willer[38] report on a study they conducted that examined the frequency, length, and content of staff's discussions and written reports about ninety hospitalized psychiatric patients. They found that nursing staff, as compared with psychiatrists, were more likely to record patient progress, but they were usually limited to behavioral descriptions; psychiatrists were more likely to focus on treatment goals or plans; and the overall quality of the records and reporting habits of the staff was low.

Partly as a response to such problems and the desire to avoid the duplication and dissatisfaction with traditional record keeping, Weed[48] developed the *problem-oriented medical record.* Traditional medical records have often been repetitive, confusing, and disorganized. Separation of nursing notes from the rest of the chart tended to block communication among various health team members. Nurses were

---

*From Krall, M.L.: Am. J. Nurs. **76:**236, 1976. Copyright by the American Journal of Nursing Co.

TREATMENT PLAN

Treatment goals   [ ] Decrease intensity of symptoms   [ ] Effective functioning
      [ ] Reduction of conflicts   [ ] Improve personal relationships
      [ ] Modify behavior   [ ] Improve grasp on reality

Precautions   [ ] Agitation   [ ] Emotional withdrawal   [ ] Drug use and withdrawal
      [ ] Suicide   [ ] Aggression   [ ] Acting out
      [ ] Self-mutilation   [ ] Assault   [ ] Confusion
      [ ] Elopement   [ ] Manipulation   [ ] Falling

Self-attitudes

Encourage socialization   Yes [ ] No [ ]   Encourage dependence   Yes [ ] No [ ]
Encourage verbalization   Yes [ ] No [ ]   Allow withdrawal   Yes [ ] No [ ]
Encourage responsibility   Yes [ ] No [ ]   Matter of fact attitude   Yes [ ] No [ ]

Socialization and visiting

[ ] Staff   [ ] Immediate family   [ ] Phone
[ ] Staff and patients   [ ] Family   [ ] Limited
      [ ] No restrictions   [ ] Unlimited

Recreation

[ ] Unit only   [ ] Off unit   [ ] Physical activities   [ ] Withhold activities
[ ] Recreational therapy   [ ] Accompanied   [ ] Moderate
      [ ] Unaccompanied   [ ] None

PSYCHIATRIC NURSING CARE PLAN

Background information: _____

Date	Problems and needs	Approach and evaluation

Room number	Patient's name	Age	Doctor	Admit date	Discharge date

FIG. 4-6
Psychiatric nursing Kardex form. (From Holden, M., and Bedgio, R.: J. Psychiatr. Nurs. **19**(5):29, 1981.)

Date	Medications	Date	P.R.N. medications	Diagnostic & psychiatric tests	Req.	Done
		Date	Treatments	Special orders and concerns		

Allergies: Diagnosis: Diet:

FIG. 4-6, cont'd.
For legend see opposite page.

often less motivated to write good notes, especially in settings where it was the practice to destroy nursing notes a given period of time after the patient's discharge. Frequently, incidents that nurses thought were significant enough to record in detail were also recorded by other health team members. In the problem-oriented medical record, this duplication is avoided, because all notes are written chronologically. Therefore each person can concentrate on adding new observations to the chart. It is also convenient to read notes that are arranged sequentially, thus facilitating improved communication.

The problem-oriented medical record is used by many mental health facilities. It consists of three basic elements: (1) the data base, (2) the problem list and treatment plan, and (3) progress notes.[48] The data base is the sum total of information from which the patient's problems can be identified. Many mental health professionals, including nurses, psychiatrists, psychologists, and social workers, may contribute to its collection. The problem list and treatment plan are drawn up as soon after the patient is admitted as possible. Every significant problem of the patient and related treatment plan should be included. Problems may be active or inactive. They should be dated and appropriately labeled, and notation should be made when the problem is resolved.

Progress notes are usually written in SOAP format, and they are preceded by a date, problem number, and problem name. The components of a SOAP note include the following:

S   **Subjective data,** which include verbal comments, complaints, or information obtained from the patient or information obtained from a source other than the patient, such as the family

O   **Objective data,** which may be a factual observation of a patient's behavior, such as his appearance or nonverbal behavior; a physiological measurement, such as height, weight, or blood pressure; or a result of a test, such as an x-ray examination or laboratory data

A   **Assessment,** which is the interpretation of the subjective and objective data

P   **Plan,** which is the specific plan of action for the problem, including diagnostic studies, treatment approaches, and patient education plans.

The following is a sample SOAP note.

TABLE 4-5. Sample problem-oriented medical record

Problem list and treatment plan

Date	Problem list	Treatment plan	Resolved
3-24-81	1. Agitated depression—loss of appetite, loss of interest in housework, difficulty sleeping	1. Amitriptyline (Elavil), 50 mg t.i.d. 2. Group therapy, Tuesdays 3. Explore patient's self-concept and perception of role performance 4. Encourage expression of emotion, particularly feelings of guilt, sadness, and hostility	
3-24-81	2. Marital conflict—states she and her husband are not compatible sexually and feels that he is not interested in her	1. Conjoint marital therapy, Fridays 2. Explore nature of sexual incompatibility 3. Confront patient with her inability to communicate her feelings and thoughts to her husband	

Treatment team progress notes

Date and time	Problem list		Progress notes
3-29-81 4 PM	2. Marital difficulty	S	Patient attended group therapy session today. Talked about difficulties with her husband, feels he doesn't love her.
		O	Appears nervous in group, feigns eye contact, but does participate somewhat.
		A	Still not comfortable with group members. Blames herself for problems at home, feels guilty.
		P	Support her in group, encourage her to express her emotions freely.
			F. Hawkins, R.N.
4-20-81 2 PM	1. Depression	S	Patient stated she was feeling better and liked participating in ward activities.
		O	Appears more enthusiastic and motivated. Increase in appetite and better sleeping habits.
		A	Adjusting to ward well. Appears antidepressants have taken effect.
		P	Continue medication and encourage patient to become even more involved on the unit.
			L. Wilson, M.D.

S "I'm scared to go for a job interview . . . scared of all the strange people looking at me."

O Patient's hand rubbed forehead, biting on fingernails, frequent changes in sitting positions, no eye contact. Patient smoked rapidly and continuously while discussing his employment status.

A Patient experiencing moderate anxiety over the thought of going for a job interview. Strangers continue to make him feel self-conscious and inferior.

P Encourage patient to verbalize his fears and anxiety. He must be approached by staff in a firm but caring manner, since he will not initiate social contacts. He requires persistent encouragement to verbalize feelings.

A sample of the two basic elements of the problem-oriented medical record, the problem list and treatment plan, and related progress notes are shown in Table 4-5.

Various methods of documentation have been presented. The specific format used by the nurse may vary but the important issue is that information about the plan of care be disseminated, so that there can be consistency and continuity in the staff's approach to the psychiatric patient. Written records are subject to review by professional colleagues. Another dimension to the purpose and nature of documentation emerges when one realizes that in some states the identified patient also has access to documentation concerning his case. In one study,[41] patients on a psychiatric unit of a general hospital were given their complete medical records to read daily, and the practice was evaluated to determine its effect on patients and staff. Both medical and nursing staff along with patients found this practice to be an effective way to educate patients, help patients become more actively involved in their treatment, correct inaccuracies in the medical record, and promote thoughtful charting by the professional staff. Committing oneself in writing is a necessary part of implementing the nursing process. The implications of it should be seriously considered by all psychiatric nurses.

Suggested cross-references

This chapter serves as a foundation for formulating principles of psychiatric nursing and implementing psychiatric nursing practice. As such, it is related to all other chapters of this text.

SUMMARY

1. Through the establishment of a therapeutic nurse-patient relationship and the use of the nursing process, the nurse strives to promote and maintain the integrated functioning of the patient. This is the essence of the nursing therapeutic process and the framework for this psychiatric nursing text. The American Nurses' Association defines nursing as "the diagnosis and treatment of human responses to actual or potential health problems." It has four characteristics: phenomena, theory, actions, and effects.

2. A model of health-illness phenomena was presented at the individual level of the social hierarchy. This model serves as the focus for the application of the nursing process. It portrays five components that result in adaptive or maladaptive coping responses.

    a. Predisposing factors that are biological, psychological, and sociocultural in nature.

    b. Precipitating stressors that vary in nature, origin, timing, and number. Research related to stressful life events was critiqued.

    c. Primary appraisal of a stressor involves the processing and comprehension of the stressful situation that takes place on the cognitive, affective, physiological, behavioral, and social levels.

    d. Secondary appraisal of coping resources is an evaluation of one's coping resources or strategies that involve cognitive, affective, physiological, behavioral, and social responses.

    e. Coping mechanisms that may be either constructive or destructive in nature.

The relationship between coping responses, health problems, nursing diagnoses, and medical diagnoses was explored.

3. The need for a theoretical basis and conceptual framework for psychiatric nursing practice was presented, along with its implication for the development and refinement of nursing theory.

4. The nursing process was defined as an interactive problem-solving process used by the nurse as a systematic and individualized way to fulfill the goal of nursing care. It is essential that the nurse and patient become partners in this process. The five phases of the nursing process—data collection, nursing diagnosis, planning, implementation, and evaluation—were described, with the American Nurses' Association's Standards of Nursing Practice used as the organizing framework.

    a. Data collection. Observing and interviewing are the basic method of data collection. It may be facilitated by the use of a systematic assessment tool. Data should reflect both content and process, and information relative to the patient's biopsychosocial world. The patient is the ideal source of validation. The importance of cultural, religious, and socioeconomic data was emphasized, and the idea of intercultural psychiatry was introduced. The data base should also include the patient's view of the functional state of his family, as well as family strengths and resources.

    b. A nursing diagnosis is the independent judgment of a nurse through which the nursing problems of the patient are identified. These may be overt, covert, existing, or potential. The subject of nursing diagnoses is the patient's behavioral response to stress. The statement of a nursing diagnosis should include both the behavioral disruption and contributing stressors.

    c. Planning involves setting goals that are mutual, congruent, realistic, and appropriately timed. Difficulties in defining and writing goals were described. The plan of nursing care also includes priorities and prescribed nursing approaches to achieve the goals derived from the nursing diagnoses.

    d. Implementation refers to the actual delivery of nursing care to the patient. It requires the consideration of alternative courses of action, mobilization of social support systems, collaboration with other health team members, and efficient use of time and energy. With psychiatric patients, nursing interventions should be directed to helping them develop insight and resolve problems through carrying out a plan of positive action.

e. Evaluation requires the review of all previous phases and the determination of the degree of goal achievement by the patient. It is a mutual continuous process that incorporates reassessment and modification of the care plan. Organizational evaluation of overall patterns of care through quality assessment measures was also discussed.

5. A case analysis of a long-term relationship with a patient was used to illustrate the use of the nursing process, phases of the relationship, and various therapeutic dimensions.

6. Activities of each phase of the nursing process should be documented in writing. Examples of various tools that can be utilized by the nurse were presented. The problem-oriented medical record was described.

References

1. American Nurses' Association: Nursing: a social policy statement, Kansas City, Mo., 1980, The Association.
2. American Psychological Association: Diagnostic and statistical manual of mental disorders, ed. 3, Washington, D.C., 1980, The Association.
3. Askenasy, A.R., Dohrenwend, B.P., and Dohrenwend, B.S.: Some effects of social class and ethnic group membership on judgments of the magnitude of stressful life events: a research note, J. Health Soc. Behav. **18**(4):432, 1977.
4. Caplan, G.: Support systems and community mental health, New York, 1974, Behavioral Publications.
5. Caplan, G.: Mastery of stress: psychosocial aspects, Am. J. Psychiatry **138**(4):41, 1981.
6. Cassel, J.: Psychosocial processes and "stress": theoretical formulation, Int. J. Health Serv. **4**:471, 1974.
7. Cobb, S.: Social support as a moderator of life stress, Psychosom. Med. **38**:300, 1976.
8. Flaskerud, J., and Halloran, E.: Areas of agreement in nursing theory development, Adv. Nurs. Sci. **4**:1, 1980.
9. Francis, G., and Munjas, B.: Manual of social psychologic assessment, New York, 1976, Appleton-Century-Crofts.
10. Geach, B.: The problem-solving technique: as taught to psychiatric students, Perspect. Psychiatr. Care **12**:9, Jan.-March 1974.
11. George, J., editor: Nursing theories: the base for professional nursing practice, Englewood Cliffs, N.J., 1980, Prentice-Hall, Inc.
12. Gourash, N.: Help-seeking: a review of the literature, Am. J. Community Psychol. **6**:499, 1978.
13. Green, N.C.: A psychiatric assessment tool for staff and students, J. Psychiatr. Nurs. **17**(4):28, 1979.
14. Hankins-McNary, L.: The effect of institutional racism on the therapeutic relationship, Perspect. Psychiatr. Care **17**(1):25, 1979.
15. Holden, M., and Bedgio, R.: Kardex forms for psychiatric nursing, J. Psychiatr. Nurs. **19**(5):29, 1981.
16. Holmes, T., and Rahe, R.: The social readjustment rating scale, J. Psychosom. Res. **11**:213, 1967.
17. House, J.: Work stress and social support, Reading, Mass., 1981, Addison-Wesley Publishing Co., Inc.
18. Joel, L., and Davis, S.: A proposal for baseline data collection for psychiatric care, Perspect. Psychiatr. Care **11**:48, April-June 1973.
19. Jourard, S.: Toward a psychology of transcendent behavior in explorations. In Otto, H., editor: Human potentialities, Springfield, Ill., 1966, Charles C Thomas, Publisher.
20. Kaplan, B., Cassel, J., and Gore, S.: Social support and health, Medical Care **15**(5):(suppl.):47, 1977.
21. Kini, J.: The effects of patient social class on the judgments of public health nurses, Nurs. Res. **17**(3):261, 1968.
22. Krall, M.L.: Guidelines for writing mental health treatment plans, Am. J. Nurs. **76**:236, 1976.
23. Krumboltz, J., and Thorensen, C.: Behavioral counseling, cases and techniques, New York, 1969, Holt, Rinehart & Winston.
24. Lazarus, R.: Psychological stress and the coping process, New York, 1966, McGraw-Hill, Inc.
25. Lazarus, R.: Little hazards can be hazardous to health, Psychology Today **15**:58, July 1981.
26. Mager, R.: Preparing instructional objectives, Palo Alto, Calif., 1962, Fearon Publishers.
27. Mason, J.: A re-evaluation of the concept of nonspecificity in stress theory, J. Psychol. Res. **8**:323, 1971.
28. McClosky, J.: Nurses' orders: the next professional breakthrough, RN **431**(2):99, 1980.
29. Mechanic, D.: Illness behavior, social adaptation, and the management of illness, J. Nerv. Ment. Dis. **165**(2):79, 1977.
30. Mitchell, R., and Trickett, E.: Task force report: social networks as mediators of social support, Community Ment. Health J **16**(1):27, 1980.
31. Mueller, D.: Social networks: a promising direction for research on the relationship of the social environment to psychiatric disorder, Soc. Sci. Med. **14A**:147, 1980.
32. Murawski, B., Penman, D., and Schmitt, M.: Social support in health and illness: the concept and its measurement, Cancer Nurs. **1**:356, 1978.
33. O'Toole, A.: When the practical becomes theoretical, J. Psychosoc. Nurs. **19**(2):11, 1981.
34. Pearlin, L.I., and Schooler, C.: The structure of coping, J Health Soc. Behav. **19**(3):2, 1978.
35. Pines, M.: Psychological hardiness: the role of challenge in health, Psychology Today **14**:34, Dec. 1980.
36. Plutchik, R., Kellerman, H., and Conte, H.: A structural theory of ego defense and emotions. In Izard, C., editor: Emotions in personality and psychopathology, New York, 1979, Plenum Press.
37. Rahe, R.: Life-change measurement as a predictor of illness, Proc. R. Soc. Med. **61**:1124, 1968.
38. Santora, E., and Willer, B.: The reporting habits of staff in a psychiatric hospital, Hosp. Community Psychiatry **26**:362, June 1975.
39. Schlesinger, R.: Cross-cultural psychiatry: the applicability of Western Anglo psychiatry to Asian-Americans

of Chinese and Japanese ethnicity, J. Psychosoc. Nurs. **19**(9):26, 1981.

40. Sedgwick, R.: Family mental health: theory and practice, St. Louis, 1981, The C.V. Mosby Co.
41. Simonton, M. et al.: The open medical record: an educational tool, J. Psychiatr. Nurs. **15**:25, 1977.
42. Singh, A., May, P., and Messick, J.: The role of operations research and systems analysis in holding down the cost of hospitals and clinics, J. Psychiatr. Nurs. **16**(9):24, 1978.
43. Smilkstein, G.: The family APGAR: a proposal for a family function test and its use by physicians, J. Fam. Pract. **6**:1231, 1978.
44. Smith, L.: A nursing history and data sheet, Nurs. Times **77**:749, 1980.
45. Snyder, J., and Wilson, M.: Elements of a psychological assessment, Am. J. Nurs. **77**:235, 1977.
46. Stevens, B.: Nursing theory, Boston, 1979, Little, Brown & Co.
47. Walker, K., MacBride, A., and Vachon, M.: Social support networks and the crisis of bereavement, Soc. Sci. Med. **11**:35, 1977.
48. Weed, L.: Medical records, medical education and patient care, Cleveland, 1969, The Press of Case Western Reserve University.
49. Weiss, R.: The provisions of social relationships. In Rubin, A., editor: Doing unto others, Englewood Cliffs, N.J., 1974, Prentice-Hall, Inc.
50. Whall, A.: Nursing theory and the assessment of families, J. Psychiatr. Nurs. **19**(1):30, 1981.
51. Yamamoto, J., James, Q., and Palley, N.: Cultural problems in psychiatric therapy, Arch. Gen. Psychiatry **19**:45, July 1968.
52. Zimmer, M.: Quality assurance in the provision of hospital care. A model for evaluating nursing care, Hospitals **48**:91, 1974.

Annotated suggested readings

Adams, G.: The sexual history as an integral part of the patient history, Matern. Child Nurs. J. **1**(3):170, 1976.

A sexual history is often a forgotten or omitted part of the nurse's data collection. This article emphasizes its importance and presents guidelines for effectively integrating it into one's nursing assessment.

American Nurses' Association: Affirmative action: toward quality nursing care for a multiracial society, Kansas City, Mo., 1976, The Association.

Unique needs of ethnic minority patients and suggestions for removing barriers to quality care in a multiracial society are explained in this collection of papers.

American Nurses' Association: Issues in evaluation research, Kansas City, Mo., 1976, The Association.

This is a collection of papers by nursing leaders and researchers that presents a comprehensive view on the subject of evaluation research as it relates to quality assurance.

Apostoles, F., Little, M., and Murphy, H.: Developing a psychiatric nursing audit, J. Psychiatr. Nurs. **15**:9, May 1977.

This article describes the experience of developing the first nursing audit, primarily a process one, in one clinical division of a large psychiatric hospital. Eight specific steps are described in a way that makes it useful reading for nurses involved in a similar process.

Bevilacqua, J.: Voodoo—myth or mental illness? J. Psychiatr. Nurs. **18**(2):17, 1980.

This is a fascinating clinical study of a 14-year-old Haitian girl's experience with what has been diagnosed as mental illness. The author raises many questions on etiology, interventions, and influence of voodoo and causes the reader to consider how the system that we work in perpetuates mental illness rather than relieves it.

Boettcher, E.: Nurse-client collaboration: dynamic equilibrium in the nursing care system, J. Psychiatr. Nurs. **16**:7, Dec. 1978.

This article explores the process of nurse-client collaboration, which parallels the nursing process. It is highly recommended for the clinical example it includes that describes a nursing care plan, including behaviors, nursing diagnosis, mutual goals, specific interventions, rationale, and evaluation.

Bush, M., and Babich, K.: Cultural variation. In Longo, D., and Williams, R., editors: Clinical practice in psychosocial nursing: assessment and intervention, New York, 1978, Appleton-Century-Crofts.

This contributed chapter provides the nurse with an understanding of the importance of cultural diversity, a framework for assessment of needs, and some general principles for intervention that can be used to provide safe and sensitive psychosocial care for ethnic people of color.

Carson, V., and Huss, K.: Prayer: an effective therapeutic and teaching tool, J. Psychiatr. Nurs. **17**(3):34, 1979.

The authors contend that the spiritual components of nursing care are often neglected. The article provides a brief review of the literature on the importance of spirituality in psychiatry. It describes a project conducted at a state mental institution in which actions to meet spiritual needs of patients were implemented and evaluated.

Foreman, M.: Building a better nursing care plan, Am. J. Nurs. **79**(6):1086, 1979.

This article presents a general semantics approach to formulation of a nursing care plan. The author believes that by asking oneself a series of questions, a more specific and more useful plan of care can be developed. This well-written article presents a concise and unique approach to care plan writing.

Francis, G., and Munjas, B.: Manual of social psychologic assessment, New York, 1976, Appleton-Century-Crofts.

This text presents a systematic method for nurses to assess the sociological and psychological aspects of clients. A comprehensive analysis of variables is presented along with suggested questions. It is a valuable resource for nurse practitioners.

George, J.: Nursing theories: the base for professional practice, Englewood Cliffs, N.J., 1980, Prentice-Hall, Inc.

The ideas of 12 nursing theorists and how the work of each relates to the nursing process are described in this text. A useful and logical overview with examples of application and utilization of theory.

Gordon, M.: Symposium on the implementation of nursing diagnosis, Nurs. Clin. North Am. **14**(3):483, 1979.

*This group of articles evolved from presentations at the
Second Northeastern Regional Conference on Nursing Diagnosis held in Newport, Rhode Island. The major themes
contained in all of these valuable papers are that nursing
diagnosis can only be used in the context of nursing practice, that it allows the practitioner to be articulate in
describing nursing practice, and that it is the best vehicle
for providing continuity of care between nurses and care
settings.*

Halleck, S.: The treatment of emotional disorders, New
York, 1978, Jason Aronson, Inc.

*This text is an excellent, yet easy to read conceptual-
ization and integration of various treatment issues and
modalities, including diagnosis and environmental, biological, behavioral, individual, group, and family therapies.*

Hankins-McNary, L.: The effect of institutional racism on
the therapeutic relationship, Perspect. Psychiatr. Care
17(1):25, 1979.

*The author explores the idea of racism and the many
ways it influences the patient-therapist relationship.
This is a topic that is not frequently discussed in the
literature, and this article is thoughtful reading for
blacks and whites alike.*

Hauser, M., and Feinberg, D.: Problem solving revisited,
J. Psychiatr. Nurs. **15**:13, Oct. 1977.

*The authors present a framework consisting of a com-
bination of the problem-solving process and the creative
thinking process. The processes directed in a complementary manner are suggested as a means of solving problems creatively in situations that call for unique and
novel solutions.*

Joel, L., and Davis, S.: A proposal for baseline data collection
for psychiatric care, Perspect. Psychiatr. Care **11**:48, April-
June 1973.

*The authors describe a data collection tool they devel-
oped for the psychiatric unit of a Veterans Administration
general hospital. The article thoroughly discusses the pertinent data, sample questions, and data utilization in
determining goals, problems, and approaches.*

LaMonica, E.L.: The nursing process: a humanistic approach, Menlo Park, Calif., 1979, Addison-Wesley Publishing Co., Inc.

*This is a good resource book on the nursing process.
The author presents general theory relative to each phase,
followed by several articles that present other points of
view or enhance the points that were made. It focuses
on the humanistic approach to client care and includes
a separate section on quality assurance.*

Lucas, M., and Folstein, M.: Nursing assessment of mental
disorders on a general medical unit, J. Psychiatr. Nurs.
18(5):31, 1980.

*The authors of this study found that current nursing
assessments on general medical units failed to identify
cognitive disorders and symptoms of emotional distress.
To correct this omission, the authors suggest the use of
two brief tools to quantitatively measure psychiatric disorder.*

Mager, R.F.: Preparing instructional objectives, Palo Alto,
Calif., 1962, Fearon Publishers.

*This is a classic text on the art of writing behavioral
objectives. It is written in a programmed learning format
and is easy to read, but at the same time, it is very in-*

*formative. This is highly recommended for inexperienced
objective writers.*

Miller, T.: Life events scaling: clinical methodological issues,
Nurs. Res. **30**(5):316, 1981.

*This article examines (1) research evidence addressing
the assessment of life events, (2) prominent scales for
the measurement of stress in life events, and (3) various
issues, problems, and implications for clinical and research application. A good review of a timely issue.*

Miller, T., and Lee, L.: Quality assurance: focus on environmental perceptions of psychiatric patients and nursing
staff, J. Psychiatr. Nurs. **18**(2):9, 1980.

*A unique application of quality assurance is described
in this study, which assessed the ward atmosphere of an
inpatient psychiatric service and utilized this information for the benefit of staff education and enrichment.*

Ness, R., and Wintrob, R.: Folk healing: a description and
synthesis, Am. J. Psychiatry **138**(11):1477, 1981.

*This is an excellent review of four systems of folk
healing that have evolved in different cultural groups in
the United States: faith healing, rootwork, curanderism,
and espiritismo.*

O'Toole, A.: When the practical becomes theoretical, J.
Psychosoc. Nurs. **19**(12):11, 1981.

*The relationship among practice, theory, and research
is explored in this article, and studies in psychiatric
nursing are reviewed with an assessment of the progress
of the field in developing practice theory. Implications
and suggestions for future direction highlight important
areas that psychiatric nursing needs to address to survive.*

Rowan, F.: The chronically distressed client, St. Louis, 1980,
The C.V. Mosby Co.

*Eight in-depth psychiatric case studies are used by the
author to illustrate the application of the nursing process
methodology. It is highly recommended for its consistent
and thorough analysis in a case-specific presentation.*

Schlesinger, R.R.: Cross-cultural psychiatry: the applicability of Western Anglo psychiatry to Asian-Americans of
Chinese and Japanese ethnicity, J. Psychosoc. Nurs.
19(9):26, 1981.

*This excellent study focuses on Asian-Americans of
the East Asian group and investigates the applicability
of Western psychiatry to this particular cultural group.
Stimulating and enlightening reading.*

Schmidt, C.: Withdrawal behavior of schizophrenics: application of Roy's model, J. Psychosoc. Nurs. **19**(11):26, 1981.

*This article describes a study that tested the applica-
bility of Roy's adaptation model to one problem identified
by the nurse—withdrawn behavior of schizophrenic patients. It is an excellent example of the interrelatedness
of theory, research, and clinical practice.*

Sedgwick, R., and Hildebrand, S.: Focus on health: family
health assessment, Nurse Pract. **6**(2):37, 1981.

*This concise but valuable article presents an overview
of the family, an analysis of family mental health, and
a discussion of the clinical assessment of families. Highly
recommended for all nurses.*

Singh, A., May, P., and Messick, J.: The role of operations
research and systems analysis in holding down the costs
of hospitals and clinics, J. Psychiatr. Nurs. **16**(9):24, 1978.

*In this article the applications of operations research
and systems analysis techniques are explored to find ways
to improve clinical operations and contain costs within
medical care facilities.*

Sue, D.: Counseling the culturally different: theory and practice, New York, 1981, John Wiley & Sons, Inc.

Attention all psychiatric nurses who are working with patients from different cultures—this book is necessary reading. It is one of the few texts devoted to this topic that approaches it from an integrated conceptual framework. Specific chapters concern Asian Americans, blacks, Hispanics, and American Indians.

Zimmer, M.J., editor: Symposium on quality assurance, Nurs. Clin. North Am. **9**(2):305, 1974.

Quality assurance is the topic addressed in this group of articles. It is highly recommended reading for those nurses interested in further information on the subject.

CHAPTER 5

PREVENTIVE
MENTAL HEALTH
NURSING

*What is this thing called health?
Simply a state in which the individual
happens transiently to be perfectly
adapted to his environment. Obviously,
such states cannot be common, for the
environment is in constant flux.*

H.L. Mencken, in the American Mercury, March 1930

Learning objectives

*After studying this chapter, the student
should be able to:*

- *define primary, secondary, and tertiary prevention.*

- *discuss why it is difficult to define mental health and conditions that may help in establishing criteria.*

- *describe criteria of mental health and relate these to the concepts of cultural relativism and psychobiological resilience.*

- *compare and contrast a medical model and behavioral model of mental illness and the implications of each for a paradigm of primary prevention.*

- *apply the nursing process model to a behavioral paradigm of primary prevention.*

- *identify developmental stages and tasks of the individual and family life cycles.*

- *assess the vulnerability of the following groups to developing maladaptive coping responses: adolescents, new parents, families, women, and mature adults.*

- *describe the following primary prevention nursing interventions: health education, environmental change, and supporting social systems.*

- *compare and contrast group psychotherapy, therapeutic groups, and self-help groups in relation to group goals, desired outcomes, and role of the nurse.*

- *assess the importance of evaluation of the nursing process when applied to primary prevention.*

- *identify suggested readings for future study.*

Prevention of mental disorders is regarded by
many people, at least in principle, as a desirable
goal that should be actively pursued. Although
this may appear to be straightforward, in fact,
the issues raised in a discussion of prevention
are quite complex and even controversial. The
basic concepts underlying preventive mental
health endeavors were articulated by Caplan in
his classic work, *Principles of Preventive Psychiatry.*[6] In it, he applies the three levels of preventive intervention from the public health
model to mental illness and emotional disturbance. He defined primary prevention as lowering the *incidence* of mental disorders or reducing
the rate at which new cases of a disorder develop. Secondary prevention involves reducing
the *prevalence* of a disorder by reducing its duration. Techniques for the control of a disorder
that focus on early case finding, screening, and
prompt effective treatment can all be considered
secondary prevention activities. Tertiary prevention activities attempt to reduce the *severity* of a
disorder and the disability associated with it.

At the present time the major thrust in the
United States is in secondary prevention activities or the treatment of mental disorders. This
is evident in the allocation of economic resources, the nature of caregiving organizations
and institutions, and the characteristic activities
of psychiatric professionals. Similarly, much of
this textbook is focused on the treatment of
existing mental disorders. Tertiary prevention is
evident in rehabilitative activities that often reflect a chronically ill patient group. This group
is underserved and undervalued and, although
it represents a substantial number of the mentally ill, their needs appear to have a low priority
within present American society. Chapter 6
examines the area of tertiary prevention in more
depth.

Although primary prevention is often es-
poused with such slogans as "An ounce of prevention is worth a pound of cure" or "Curing is
costly—prevention, priceless," it has yet to
evolve as a substantial force in the mental health
movement. This is partly because of the fuzzi-
ness of the concepts and definitions underlying
the issues. For example, primary prevention programs may be aimed at an entire population
or only at persons believed to be at high risk for
developing a disorder. This depends on how one
views primary prevention in general—is it disease prevention or health promotion? This simple but important question raises still another
one, What is mental illness and mental health?

Obviously, there needs to be agreement on what
one is promoting or preventing to best determine
what action should be taken.

Defining mental health and illness

Since the early 1940s, the terms mental health
and mental hygiene have appeared in the literature and in statements of public policy. They
are now common in everyday speech and
thought. However, there have been relatively
few attempts to define "mental health," and
little consensus exists at present. Mental health
is often spoken of as a state of well-being, such
as happiness, contentment, satisfaction, or
achievement. These are difficult terms to apply
and fluctuate according to different situations
and conditions. This is not to deny that happiness is a desirable consequence of mental
health, but it poses problems if used as a criterion. There are similar problems with viewing
mental health statistically as the central tendency or mean of a group. What one derives in
this way is "average," which may not necessarily
mean "healthy."

In seeking the positive signs of mental health,
Jahoda[36] suggested the following conditions:

1. The idea of any single criterion of mental health
   should be abandoned. Good mental health cannot be refined down to a simple concept and a
   simple item of behavior is not adequate.
2. The terms we use to define mental health may
   seem to be abstract but they should be reduced
   to definite operational procedures and there is a
   need to have scales and measures for each criterion.
3. Each of the criteria should be thought of as a
   continuum or as containing continua since there
   are unhealthy trends for an otherwise healthy
   person.
4. These criteria of mental health should operate
   any any point in time to define the state of the
   individual or can be thought of as indicative of
   trends in the individual towards health or disease. Implicit in the criteria is the concept of
   gradients of mental health.
5. The criteria are regarded as relatively enduring
   attributes of the person. They are not merely
   functions of a particular situation the individual
   may find himself in.
6. These criteria are set up as the optimum of
   mental health. They are not to be regarded as
   absolute, and the minimum standard for any

individual to achieve has yet to be determined and may change with age. Each individual has his own limits and no one reaches the ideal in all the criteria. However, the assumption made is that most people can approach the optimum, and below a yet to be determined minimum, most if not all people will break down.

The following six criteria were offered by Jahoda[36] as a recipe for mental health:

1. Positive attitudes toward self
2. Growth, development, and self-actualization
3. Integration
4. Autonomy
5. Reality perception
6. Environmental mastery

Positive attitudes toward self include an acceptance of self and self-awareness. There has to be some objectivity about the self and the acquisition of a realistic level of aspiration that will necessarily change with age. A healthy person must also have a sense of identity, a feeling of wholeness, a sense of belongingness, security, and meaningfulness.

Second, there is the criterion of *growth, development, and self-actualization.* Maslow and Rogers developed extensive theories on the development and realization of the human potential. Maslow describes the concept of "self-actualization," and Rogers emphasizes the "fully functioning person." Both theories focus on the entire range of human adjustment. They describe a self that is engaged in a constant quest, always seeking new growth, new development, and new challenges. Their theories focus on the total person and such considerations as whether a person is adequately in touch with his own self to free the resources that are there, whether he has free access to his feelings and emotions and can integrate them with his intellectual and cognitive functioning, whether he is immobilized by inner conflicts and stresses or can interact freely and openly with his environment, and whether he can share himself with other people and grow from such experiences. Maslow[52] identified fifteen basic personality characteristics that distinguish "self-actualized" individuals—people moving in the direction of achieving and reaching their highest potential. Rogers[63] described seven essential personality traits of the "fully functioning person" who is similarly moving toward self-growth and fulfillment. These are presented in Table 5-1.

TABLE 5-1. Theories on development and realization of human potential

Maslow's "self-actualized" individual	Rogers' "fully functioning" person
Has accurate perception of reality	Moves away from facades that are not true to self
Has a high degree of acceptance of self, others, and human nature	Moves away from others' expectations of what he "ought to be"
Exhibits spontaneity	Moves away from pleasing others who impose artificial goals on him
Is problem-centered as opposed to self-centered	Moves toward becoming autonomous, self-directing, and self-responsible
Has need for privacy	Is open to change and exploring his potential
Demonstrates high degree of autonomy and independence	Is open to his own self and the lives of others
Has freshness of appreciation	Trusts and values himself and dares to express himself in new ways
Has frequent "mystic or peak" experiences	
Shows identification with mankind	
Shares intimate relationships with a few significant others	
Has democratic character structures	
Possesses strong ethical sense	
Demonstrates unhostile sense of humor	
Possesses creativeness	
Exhibits resistance to conformity	

The third criterion involves the concept of *integration,* or the relatedness of all life processes. This involves a balance between what is expressed and what is repressed, between outer and inner conflicts and drives, and a regulation of one's moods and emotions. It includes the concepts of emotional responsiveness and control and a unified philosophy of life. This consistent set of values provides a framework for a certain continuity in all responses. This criterion can at least in part be measured by the person's ability to withstand stress and cope with anxiety. The ability to withstand stress involves a strong but not rigid ego, so that a person is able to handle change and grow from it.

Autonomy is the fourth criterion of mental health. This involves self-determination, a balance between dependence and independence, and the acceptance of the consequences of one's actions. It implies that one is responsible for himself, including decisions, actions, thoughts, and feelings. Consequently, the person is able to respect the autonomy and freedom of choice in others.

The fifth criterion involves *reality perception,* the ability of the individual to test by empirical action his assumptions about the outside world. The mentally healthy person is able to change his perceptions in the light of new information. This criterion also includes the ability of empathy or social sensitivity, a respect for the feelings and attitudes of others.

Finally, there is the criterion of *environmental mastery.* A mentally healthy person feels success in an approved role in his society or group. He can deal effectively with the world, work out his problems of living, and obtain satisfaction from life. It incorporates the idea of social competence as well. The person should have the essential quality of being able to cope with loneliness, aggression, and frustration without being overwhelmed. The mentally healthy person has the ability to respond to other individuals, to love and be loved, and to cope with others in reciprocal relationships. He should maintain the ability to make new friendships and to have satisfactory social group involvement.

Although criteria such as these are helpful in describing qualities of mental health, they are not definitions in themselves. Health and normality emerge within a social context in which *cultural relativism* is a particularly important problem, since the content and form of mental health and mental illness will vary greatly from one culture to another. Different cultures place different kinds of stressors on people. So too, they vary in symbolic interpretation, acceptance of expression and repression, cohesion of social groups, and tolerance of deviation. The danger in ignoring cultural diversity and group norms is that one may equate deviance with illness. When social alternatives are equated with illness, an unusual life-style is regarded as sick, and aberrant behavior is taken as a sign of personal abnormality.

This can potentially be avoided if one recognizes that health-illness and conformity-deviance are two distinctly independent variables. Combining them generates four separate patterns: the healthy conformist, the healthy deviant, the unhealthy conformist, and the unhealthy deviant. This obliges any mental health professional to attend carefully to the meaning of any apparent deviant behavior, to its significance in its social context. It may reflect an adaptation to realistic forces in a person's life or conformity to group norms.

Cautions against cultural relativism also have a corollary in the individual. A person should not be assessed against some vague or ideal notion of health. Rather, he should be seen in a group context, an age context, and an individual context. It is not a matter of how well someone fits an arbitrary age standard, but rather what is reasonable for a particular person with a specific background and life experience. Is there continuity or discontinuity with the past? Is there evidence of evolving adaption to changing needs throughout the person's life cycle? Such a view incorporates the concept of *psychobiological resilience,* which proposes that there is a recurrent human need to weather periods of stress and change throughout life. The ability to successfully weather each period of disruption and reintegration leaves the person better able to deal with the next change. This dimension equates mental health with adaptation and mental illness with maladaptation.

A final point in describing mental health is the fact that the health-illness continuum is asymmetrical. The two poles of health and illness are not equally unclear. Rather, standards of mental health are less clear and less agreed on than those of mental illness. Whereas conceptions of mental health can be extended indefinitely in unbounded potential, conceptions of mental illness are bounded somewhat by greater consensus of symptoms of mental disorders that can be specified and studied. Rosow[65] observes that clinical entities are more problematic and more amenable to useful theory, research, and treatment. He therefore proposes that focus be placed on mental illness and the problems of determining mental health be given the benefit of benign neglect.

Conceptualizing primary prevention

The idea of promoting mental health in general is a very attractive one. Promotion sounds optimistic and positive. It is consistent with the idea of self-help and taking responsibility for one's own health. It implies changing human behavior and draws on a holistic approach to health. A continuing problem, however, with the strategy of promoting mental health is the vastness and vagueness of its goals. As Kessler and Albee note, "Nearly everything, it appears, has implications for primary prevention, for reducing emotional disturbance, for strengthening and fostering mental health."[41:355] Thus goals are frequently ill defined, and evaluation of promotion activities is difficult at best. Even if goals of a project can be identified and measured, their relation to long-term goals and behavior remains questionable. For example, successfully teaching coping skills to schoolchildren may attain one's short-term goals, but what this precisely means for their mental health as adults is unclear and unsupported by empirical evidence.

Lamb and Zusman, in a critique of primary prevention, note the following*:

In the area of mental health, most—if not all—successful primary preventive activities have been aimed at specific diseases. In contast to the situation in large areas of physical illness, there is no evidence that it is possible to strengthen "mental health" and thereby increase resistance to mental illness by general preventive activities. Despite massive efforts to combat poverty (at least partly in the name of mental health), to increase social welfare and Social Security benefits, and to change the educational systems and methods of child rearing, there is no indication of a decrease in frequency of any of the functional mental illnesses. Nor is there obvious evidence that other countries with stronger social welfare systems and different child-rearing practices have different rates of mental illness. Thus, as far as we can see, the major functional mental illnesses (as well as the very frequent diagnosable minor illnesses) remain untouched by primary prevention in the sense of trying to strengthen mental health.[44:13]

This suggests that primary prevention activities are perhaps best focused on illness prevention. If so, attention must be given to specifying what one means by mental illness. Does it mean prevention of unhappiness, lack of social adjustment, problems in living, or discreet clinical and diagnostic disorders? Viewing mental illness as a disease in the medical model perspective allows one to use the classic, epidemiological paradigm in primary prevention. This paradigm consists of the following steps:

1. Identify a disease of sufficient importance to justify the development of a preventive intervention program. Develop reliable methods for its diagnosis so that people can be divided with confidence into groups according to whether they do or do not have the disease.
2. By a series of epidemiological and laboratory studies identify the most likely theory of that disease's path of development.
3. Mount and evaluate an experimental preventive intervention program based on the results of those research studies.[2:182]

Unquestionably this paradigm has been effective for a broad array of communicable diseases, such as smallpox, typhus, malaria, diphtheria, tuberculosis, rubella, and polio, and nutritional diseases, such as scurvy, pellagra, rickets, kwashiorkor, and endemic goiter. It has also proved useful in a variety of mental disorders caused by poisons, chemicals, licit or illicit drugs, electrolyte imbalances, and nutritional deficiencies.

All of these diseases have one thing in common. For each, there is a known necessary, although not always sufficient, causative agent. Many diseases and many disorders, however, do not appear to have a single identified precondition. Mental illnesses in particular may have causative factors that are multiple, interactive, situational, and sociocultural in nature. They thus require that prevention of mental illness be conceptualized in a more behavioral way as the prevention of problems or maladaptive responses. Hollister supports this view. He calls for prevention of the following:

1. *Specific behaviors* that are self-defeating or harmful to others, such as poor or unhealthy habits, overeating, procrastinating, evasiveness, blaming others, and "setting the stage" to fail
2. *Role failures,* as a student, a parent, or an employee
3. *Relationship breakdowns* between husband wife, parent and child, boss and employee, including detection and control of interpersonal "games" that are destructive
4. *Feeling overreactions,* such as panics, new situation anxiety, flights, and temper tantrums
5. *Psychological disabilities,* such as the social deterioration of a confined ill person, decompensation, "going to pieces," or falling into melancholia instead of experiencing normal grieving.

With such a conceptualization, many of the commonsense services already given in the community by mental health and other helping agencies can be identified and publicly acknowledged as prevention efforts.[34:41-48]

By defining problems in this way they can include both single-episode events, such as a divorce, or a long-standing condition, such as marital conflict. They can also reflect either an acute health problem or a chronic health problem. For example, Room[64] has identified the following categories of problems that can arise from the abuse of alcohol:

---

*From Lamb, H., and Zusman, J.: Primary prevention in perspective, The American Journal of Psychiatry, vol. 136, p. 12, 1979. Copyright, 1979, the American Psychiatric Association.

1. Acute health problems, such as overdose or delirium tremens
2. Chronic health problems, such as cirrhosis or head or neck cancer
3. Casualties, such as accidents on the road, in the home or elsewhere, and suicide
4. Violent crime and family abuse
5. Problems of demeanor, such as public drunkenness and use of alcohol by teenagers
6. Default of major social roles—work or school and family roles
7. Problems of feeling state—demoralization and depression and experienced loss of control

This conceptualization requires the use of a new paradigm for primary prevention, which has been developed by Bloom.[2] It assumes that problems are multicausal, that everyone is vulnerable to stressful life events, and that any disability or problem may arise as a consequence of them. For example, four vulnerable persons can face a stressful life event—perhaps the collapse of their marriage, or the loss of their job. One person may become severely depressed, the second may be involved in an automobile accident, the third may head down the road to alcoholism, and the fourth may develop a psychotic thought disorder or coronary artery disease. This paradigm does not search for a cause for each problem. Rather, it attempts to reduce the incidence of stressful life events as outlined in the following steps:

1. Identify a stressful life event that appears to have undesirable consequences in a significant proportion of the population. Develop procedures for reliably identifying persons who have undergone or who are undergoing that stressful experience.
2. By traditional epidemiological and laboratory methods, study the consequences of that event and develop hypotheses related to how one might go about reducing or eliminating the negative consequences of the event.
3. Mount and evaluate experimental preventive intervention programs based on these hypotheses.[2:183]

This paradigm shifts attention from nonspecific predisposing factors of mental illness to more discrete and identifiable precipitating stressors. These factors may be single-episode life events, such as loss of a job, or more long-term life event stressors, such as job dissatisfaction. By narrowing the focus of one's study in this way, one is able to limit the population at risk and allow for a more judicious use of one's financial and program resources.

If primary prevention in mental health is conceptualized in this manner, one can identify specific dimensions needed in a primary prevention project. The nurse can then engage in a systematic application of the nursing process with a focus on primary prevention of problems associated with an identified stressor. This would incorporate the following aspects:

1. *Assessment.* Identification of a stressor that precipitates maladaptive responses and a target or vulnerable population group that is at high risk in relationship to it.
2. *Planning.* Elaboration of specific strategies of prevention and relevant social institutions and situations through which the strategies may be applied.
3. *Implementation.* Application of selected nursing interventions aimed at decreasing maladaptive responses to the identified stressor and enhancing adaptation.
4. *Evaluation.* Determining the effectiveness of the nursing interventions with regard to short- and long-term outcomes, use of resources, and comparison with other prevention strategies.

The nursing process is thereby used in a goal-directed way to decrease the incidence of mental illness and promote mental health.

Assessment of vulnerable groups

Knowledge of normal growth and development is essential for nursing activities in primary prevention, secondary prevention, and tertiary prevention. Other sources[73] describe these stages in some detail, and the nurse should be familiar with normative stages, tasks, and parameters to know what issues the person has faced in the past and what challenges lie ahead. In addition to individual development, knowledge of the family cycle is also important. Many nursing interventions are directed at the family level, ranging from mobilizing their support of an individual patient to interrupting and modifying dysfunctional family patterns. Table 5-2 summarizes the developmental stages of the individual using Erikson's theory[18] of psychosocial development and Duvall's stages[16] of the family life cycle. Streff[72] integrated Erikson's theory with that of Duvall's to define developmental tasks of the family that parallel those of the individual. Such an integrated approach allows

TABLE 5-2. Developmental stages and tasks of the individual and family unit

Erikson's stage of individual psychosocial development [18]	Developmental task of the individual [73]	Duvall's stage of the family life cycle [16]	Developmental task of the family identified by Streff [72]
Trust vs. mistrust (0-2 years)	Oral needs are of primary importance Adequate mothering is necessary to meet infant's needs Acquisition of hope	Premarital-married couple	Establishing relationship Defining mutual goals Developing intimacy Developing appropriate dependence, independence, interdependence pattern Establishing mutually satisfying relationship Negotiating boundaries of couple relationship and with individuals' families of origin Discussing issue of childbearing Making decision to conceive
Autonomy vs. shame (1½-3 years)	Anal needs are of primary importance Father emerges as important figure Acquisition of will	Childbearing	Working out authority and responsibility issues Working out caretaker roles Having children Forming new unit Facilitating child's establishment of trust Acknowledging need for personal time and space while sharing with each other and child
Initiative vs. guilt (3-6 years)	Genital needs are of primary importance Family relationships contribute to early sense of responsibility and conscience Acquisition of purpose	Preschool	Continuing individual development as couple, parent, and family Experiencing changes in energy and time for individual and couple needs Promoting continued growth in each other and the relationship while encouraging child to develop autonomy and retain self-esteem Establishing own family tradition with each other and children without guilt related to breaks with traditions of families or origin
Industry vs. inferiority (6-12 years)	Active period of socialization for child as he moves from family and into society Acquisition of competence	School age	One or both spouses establishing new roles in work settings or community or changes in child-rearing practices and gaining recognition for selves and children Children in school and after-school activities, relating with peers, self-esteem being enhanced or inhibited, and interfacing with activities in family

TABLE 5-2. Developmental stages and tasks of the individual and family unit—cont'd

Erikson's stage of individual psychosocial development[18]	Developmental task of the individual[73]	Duvall's stage of the family life cycle[16]	Developmental task of the family identified by Streff[72]
Identity vs. identity diffusion (13+ years)	Search for self, in which peers play important role Psychosocial moratorium is provided by society to aid adolescent Acquisition of fidelity	Teenage	Parents continue to develop roles in community and interests other than with children Children examine ways to experience freedom while expressing responsibility for actions Struggles evolve with parents as emancipation process proceeds Family's value system may be challenged Couple relationship may be strong or weak, depending on how members respond to each other's needs
Intimacy vs. isolation (adulthood)	Characterized by increasing importance of human closeness and sexual fulfillment Acquisition of love	Launching career	Parents launching young adults with rituals marking rites of passage Change in relationship with children who are becoming adults and/or in new living situations; change in couple's relationship because of children's absence and increased time with one another
Generativity vs. self-absorption (middle-age)	Characterized by productivity creativity, parental responsibility, and concern for new generation Acquisition of care	Middle-age parents	Energy channeled into guiding next generation via family on in community activities, or couple may now be dealing with issues of aging of their own parents Children of middle-age parents may be adolescent
Integrity vs. despair (old age)	Characterized by unifying philosophy of life and more profound love for mankind Acquisition of wisdom	Aging family members	Persons have achieved satisfying relationships and feel sense of accomplishment and desiring to continue to live fully until death instead of existing in state of despair Aging members are coping with bereavement and may now be living alone

one to view life as successive stages marked by critical developmental tasks. This aids the nurse in identifying future changes that may be potential stressors for an individual or family. By acknowledging, understanding, and anticipating them, the nurse can design and implement effective preventive nursing care.

All people and all families face these same developmental tasks. Not everyone adapts to them, however, or copes with them in a positive way. This may be because certain individuals or groups in our society have additional stressors placed on them, inadequate coping resources, and fewer positive experiences to balance out their perceived stress. These people and groups are thus particularly vulnerable or at high risk for developing maladaptive responses. It is extremely helpful if the nurse has an awareness of these vulnerable people. Her increased sensitivity that results from this awareness will affect her assessment of both existing and potential problems and her actual work with people from these high-risk groups. Nurses, as the largest group of health care providers, can make a significant impact in promoting mental health if they would anticipate problems and commit their time and skill to preventing their occurrence. Assessment in primary prevention therefore involves identifying groups of people who are vulnerable to developing mental disorders or maladaptive coping responses to specific stressors or risk factors. To complete such an assessment, the nurse needs to draw on information generated from theory, research, and clinical practice.

Some of these vulnerable groups will now be briefly described. Each group could merit, in itself, a separate chapter or perhaps a textbook. The intent of this discussion, however, is to highlight the unique ways in which some people are particularly vulnerable to maladaptive responses. It should also be noted that these are not the only high-risk groups for developing mental disorders. The actual identification of vulnerable groups is greatly dependent on one's geography and life experiences. And not all individuals within these groups are at equal risk. What these groups do share, however, is the experience of a life event, stressor, or risk factor that represents a loss of some kind or places an excessive demand on one's ability to cope. These broad categories are intended to help one conceptualize common stressful experiences. Utilizing them in clinical research or practice would necessitate a further specification of a particular subgroup within these broad categories based on a particular stressor or risk factor. The more clearly the subgroup can be defined, the more specific the prevention strategies can be researched, identified, and implemented.

Adolescents

Adolescence is an accepted time of tremendous change biologically, psychologically, and socially. The demands placed on the young person are great, and not all adolescents have sufficient resources to cope with them. One usual resource of the adolescent, the peer group, can actually become a stressor by pressuring the young person to participate in experiences, such as drugs or sex, that may not be in his or her best interests. Concerns about sex typing

and homosexuality may develop at this time, as do questions about contraception, pregnancy, abortion, and venereal disease.

Late adolescence may be a time of moving away from home, making an initial career choice, or becoming involved in advanced schooling. All of these occurrences may lead to questions about independence, motivation, competence, control, and capacity for intimacy. The need to develop intimate psychosocial relationships with others may be a major source of stress even though it is considered to be a normal developmental task. Many questions and insecurities may surround the issues of marriage, selecting a mate, conjoint living, and shared decision making. Each of these demands placed on adolescents may come together and compound their level of stress. If this occurs and their coping resources are not adequate, this group will be highly vulnerable to the development of maladaptive responses.

There is a tremendous amount of documentation related to the adolescent's potential for developing maladaptive responses. Reporting the many studies and statistics pertaining to this high-risk group is beyond the scope of this chapter but the problems are self-evident in the large numbers of adolescent suicides, runaways, drug abusers, and school failures, and the tremendous problems posed by juvenile prostitution, unwanted pregnancies, delinquency, and crime. These problems are discussed in Chapter 27. Certainly not all adolescents develop problems, but in the face of additional stressors from peers or family, this is one population group that is particularly vulnerable to a range of social, psychological, and behavioral problems.[66]

New parents

The stress involved in decisions regarding children, conception, birth, and assuming the parental role has been well documented in both the professional literature and popular press. The decision whether or not to have children has become increasingly complex with recent changes in American society. Women now may have more extensive career options, less geographical proximity to their own families of origin, more earning potential, greater medical technology available, changing sex-role perceptions, and a more frequently used option to have children later in their adult years. However, these changes may be at odds with the cultural norms or personal beliefs of the couple, and, rather than serving to increase one's options, they may instead create conflict and dissonance.

How the couple copes with this stress has far-reaching implications for their own health and that of their children. The transition to motherhood is accepted as a stressful period for women of all ages. Pregnancy and the postpartum period are generally regarded as maturational crises for women equal in importance to those of adolescence and midlife. Stressors undergone during this period include the following:

1. Endocrine changes
2. Changes in body image
3. Activation of psychological conflicts pertaining to pregnancy
4. Intrapsychic reorganization of becoming a mother

The result of these stressors is often the experience of a postpartum depression of varying intensity, or with some women, a postpartum psychosis. Studies indicate that from 20% to 40% of women report emotional disturbance or cognitive dysfunction or both in the early postpartum period.[37] Another study found 65% of mothers describing depression postpartum, with 25% of the women reporting symptoms continuing longer than a week.[59] Disturbances of psychotic proportions occur much less frequently but obviously with greater impairment.

The response of men to pregnancy and fatherhood has most often been described in the literature in terms of the benefits of parental involvement to father, mother, and infant. Little attention has been given to their more problematic responses, despite the fact that minor emotional reactions are common, and severe reactions are not rare.[20] Lacoursiere[43] reported that about 2% of hospitalized patients with a diagnosis of paranoid psychosis developed symptoms in relation to fatherhood. An interesting study found that one of the most important factors in female maladjustment to pregnancy was rejection of the pregnancy by the husband or father of the child.[30]

Yet, if one views childbirth as a maturational crisis, it must serve as a stressor for the man as well as the woman. For both, it is a time to recapitulate some of the developmental problems of earlier phases. The following variables have been suggested as significant instigators of psychopathological reactions in men: increased financial responsibility, triggering of latent homosexual conflicts by restriction of heterosexual opportunities during the prenatal period, rearousal of unacceptable childhood anger toward parents or siblings, reactivation of unresolved oedipal conflict, and frustration of dependency demands as the wife's attention is diverted to the baby's needs.[40] Fishbein[20] suggests that the essential determinant of what happens to the man psychodynamically appears to be how satisfactorily the man has resolved his own developmental attachment-individuation-separation processes.

Clearly new parents are at high risk for developing maladaptive responses. Bieber and Bieber[1] describe a psychiatric syndrome that appears not uncommonly in the first year after the birth of a child in both men and women. The signs and symptoms include combinations of acute anxiety, depression, psychosomatic disorders, changes in affectional responses toward the spouse, changes in sexual behavior, the onset of various types of frigidity in the woman, potency difficulties in the man, an apparent loss of interest in the marriage, and the first involvement in extramarital relations, often leading to divorce. Pregnancy thus sets in motion a series of changes and stressors that challenge the coping resources of the man and the woman and can result in either adaptive or maladaptive responses. Furthermore, the mental health of the parents directly affects the health of the infant.

This is demonstrated in a study by Nuckolls, Cassel, and Kaplan,[58] which found that the proportion of women having pregnancy and birth complications was significantly higher among those women who had experienced a high frequency of life changes accompanied by a low degree of social–emotional support during their pregnancies and that when social support was high, there was no increase in complications. Conflict over the acceptance of pregnancy has been associated with increased length of the labor process, as well as increased levels of maternal anxiety,[45] and the degree of wantedness of the pregnancy has been associated with increased risk of low birth weight. Cobb[9] cites several studies which show that wanted children tend to adapt to or cope with the stresses of growing up better than do those who began life under circumstances where the parental preference had been for abortion. Wanted children fared better in terms of the decreased incidence of juvenile delinquency and need for psychiatric treatment and were better able to adapt to the school socialization and educational achievement processes.[21]

Another dimension of stress in this high-risk

group is related to the bonding and attachment process and the development of parent-child relationships. Stressors related to childbirth can place the family at risk for child maltreatment. A number of circumstances, including a medically abnormal pregnancy, difficult labor or delivery, neonatal separation, other separations in the first 6 months, illnesses in the infant during the first year of life, and maternal illness during the first year of life all place a family at risk for child maltreatment. Threats to the parent-infant bond are particularly dangerous. In one study,[50] 66% of the abused children were found to have experienced 48-hour separations from their parents in the first week of life, whereas only 3% of those same children's siblings had been separated. Medically high-risk infants are particularly in danger. In a study[39] of 146 infants who had been in an intensive care nursery, it was found that a lack of parental visits was associated with the likelihood of later maltreatment.

Although these results are not in and of themselves definitive, when combined with other research findings they are persuasive. Disruption in parent-infant bonding predicts greater risk for maltreatment.[25] Where the mother has an active role and high status in the childbirth process, there are fewer medical complications, less resort to medications that suppress infant functioning, fewer cesarean section deliveries, and fewer induced labors.[17] These, in turn, have a positive influence on the child and may serve to reduce the risk of child maltreatment.

The abuse and neglect of children is evidence of parental difficulty in assuming the maternal or paternal role. Both roles are assumed through a complex social and cognitive learning process. They are not intuitive, nor are they universally present in couples who have given birth. Many variables have been identified as having an impact on the maternal role. Mercer[53] identifies these as age, perceptions of the birth experience, early maternal-infant separation, support system, self-concept and personality traits, maternal illness, child-rearing attitudes, infant temperament, infant illness, and socioeconomic status. Although all of these variables have been described in the literature, there is no evidence that one variable is most predictive or how they interact to account for variance in the maternal role. The framework proposed by Mercer for studying these variables is necessary to guide research projects that can identify stressors and suggest prevention strategies.

A similar research paradigm has been developed by Cronenwett and Kunst-Wilson[12] for the transition to fatherhood. They believe that a separate paradigm for fathers is necessary because the experience of becoming a parent differs for men and women, and the stress associated with becoming a parent is least understood for men. The framework they propose for understanding the processes involved in a man's transition to fatherhood incorporates many pertinent variables and can help stimulate the formulation of theoretical questions for further research. More precise knowledge of the nature of the stress and the intervening variables that promote adaptation will be necessary for the nurse to actively work to prevent potential problems.

Three other subgroups of new parents may also be particularly vulnerable. These include teenage parents, unwed parents, and the parents of adopted children. Pregnancy in adolescence brings together two maturational crises, each of which compounds the problems of the other. At this time, the adolescent has not yet achieved his or her own sense of identity and independence and yet must assume the role of parent for an infant who is totally dependent. The unwed mother of any age experiences to some degree a lack of coping resources that may include social support, financial assistance, and shared care-taking responsibilities. The stressor of parenthood thus makes excessive demands on one's coping ability.

Stress is also experienced by parents throughout the process of adoption. The parents who are not able to conceive their own child have undergone an extensive period of testing, waiting, hoping, and accepting one's physiological limitations. Once the decision to adopt has been made, a long waiting period usually follows. The actual arrival of an adopted child of any age requires a readjustment of roles and family dynamics. In addition, the relatively recent phenomena of surrogate mothers may initiate changes and problems that are new to the couple and society at large.

Families

In our society the family unit is of critical importance. It continues to be a primary personal and cultural institution that has undergone some major and minor changes in structure in response to the larger social environment. The majority of Americans continue to seek and contract marriages, desire and have children, and live in households independent of the nuclear family. Important changes have also occurred. Because of increased longevity and fertility control, the "shape" of the family life cycle has changed, so that parenting no longer dominates most of the family's life cycle. Raising a family may only occupy half or a third of a couple's married life. In addition, today over 50% of American mothers work outside the home. This statistic is expected to increase to 75% by 1990. Of all married women with children under the age of 6, 45% are employed.[75] The employment of married women thus appears to be an accepted and perhaps even expected social pattern because of economic and personal fulfillment needs. Of those women who work, two thirds are single, widowed, divorced, or separated, or have husbands who earn less than $10,000.[75] A final important change is the increasing divorce rate, which has given rise to single-parent families. It is estimated that one out of five children lives in a single-parent home. Remarriage is also increasing, with the result that families may have stepparents, stepchildren, and multiple sets of grandparents.

Although it can be argued that none of these changes are necessarily destructive in themselves, they all do place demands on the family's functioning and create a more complex set of needs. For example, all parents need some relief from their child and home care responsibilities. Often these needs can be met through an evening out or an informal arrangement with families and friends. However, in families in which both parents work, child care that is consistent, dependable, and of high quality becomes a necessity. In a similar way, families experiencing separation, divorce, or remarriage have significant stress placed on them and are in need of a broader range and more intense level of coping resources. Another type of family at high risk for developing problems is the one in which there is lack of knowledge of effective parenting. Since parenting is not an established course in educational curriculum and families are more geographically mobile, it is not surprising that this need has emerged. Yet one's child-rearing practices do have a significant effect on one's children and even future generations.

Pratt[60] has observed that the use of the developmental style of child rearing (reasons, information, rewards, and autonomy) tends to be more effective than disciplinary methods in assisting children to develop resources and capacities for coping, learning, and taking care of themselves. Maladaptive behaviors associated with the strongly disciplinary style of child rearing have been identified as social aggressiveness, hostility, and dependency in boys and regressiveness, fearfulness, and social withdrawal in girls. Studies have shown that, when parents have tended to be lax or inconsistent in the use of appropriate rules or controls, their children's failure to develop adequate coping mechanisms in early life can cause subsequent maladjustment in their neurophysical development and lead to lifelong patterns of psychosomatic as well as social complications.[38]

It becomes apparent that there are numerous subgroups of families under stress. Many of these high-risk family groups have been researched, analyzed, and reported on in both the popular literature and that of the psychiatric community. Although the potential problems are significant, there is a major deficit in programs to either prevent them or alleviate them once they develop. The lack of quality day care programs, the government's cancellation of the 1981 White House Conference on Children, and federal reductions in programs aiding children and families all reveal the low priority given to families under stress.

Another major source of stress for all families is illness in any form. The illness of one family member affects all other members and can result in maladaptive responses and a variety of pathological states. The premature birth of a child, the child born with a genetic defect, and the handicapped child all place great and unanticipated demands on the family. Parents of such children, and the children themselves, have special individualized needs. Studies show that parental attitudes about having produced handicapped children vary quite widely (regret, denial, anger, and rejection), since these children may represent parental incompetence both to the parents themselves and to others.[42] Voysey[76] reported that parental coping patterns include the projection of false reports of progress, statements of grief, and the development of cynical acceptance of the disabilities.

Nurses are particularly aware that major and minor illnesses of family members take a significant toll. Illnesses requiring hospitalization and surgery precipitate multiple threats to the family unit. Adapting to a hyperactive child, an alcoholic parent, a psychotic sibling, or an arthritic spouse may be impossible without the extended use of outside resources.

A final well-documented stressor for the individual and family is the death of a member. Bereavement and its sequelae have been studied in various forms—widows, widowers, stillborn death, death of a parent, death of a child, sudden death, sudden infant death, and death after a protracted illness. Research in this area has led to the elaboration of the normal mourning or grieving process and the identification of strategies for anticipatory guidance, support systems, and preventive intervention. These are described in Chapter 9. Perhaps of all of the vulnerable groups discussed in this chapter, the bereaved have been the focus of the most research and the most clearly articulated prevention strategies. The task of adequately implementing these strategies remains to be done.

Women

The mental health of men and women is intimately connected to the idea of equality: "The equal right to participate in all areas of the life of society and to pursue one's unique psychological potential in all of its aspects."[7:1320] Unfortunately American society is one of structured social inequality based on gender, race, and class differences to name a few. Women have a disadvantaged status in this society, which increases their vulnerability to stress and their potential for developing maladaptive responses. The status of women is summarized in the 1978 President's Commission on Mental Health:

1. *Salary*. More than half of all women are now employed outside of the home, but they are clustered in the lowest paying occupations and at the bottom of the achievement ladder. One woman in four compared to one man in 18 lives on an annual income of less than $4000.
2. *Dual roles*. Whether or not a woman is employed outside the home, housework remains largely "women's work." Thus many American women have two full workdays in every 24 hours.
3. *Politics*. Only about 3.5% of the House and 2% of the Senate of the United States and about 9% of the state legislators are women. This greatly reduces the political capacity of women to improve their status.
4. *Business*. It is still unusual to see women in the bastions of financial power and in high corporate echelons.
5. *Law*. In many states when a woman marries, she trades the rights of a person for the duties of a wife. A husband who deserts his wife and takes a temporary job in another state can seriously affect his wife's credit rating, right to vote, serve on juries, run for office, and so on.[61:1027]

The Subpanel on the Mental Health of Women of this commission reported that circumstances and conditions which society accepts as normal and ordinary often lead to despair, anguish, and mental illness in women.[61] The subpanel documented the ways in which inequality creates dilemmas and conflicts for women in the contexts of marriage, family relationships, reproduction, child rearing, divorce, aging, education, and work. These same conditions encourage the frequency of incest, rape, and marital violence, which also heighten women's vulnerability to mental illness. Finally, the epidemiological data that establish conditions associated with mental illness are particularly relevant to women. These include poverty, alienation, and powerlessness. The convergence, therefore, of multiple stressful events with the chronic stressful conditions in which women frequently live, produces a high susceptibility to mental disorders among women.

This susceptibility is substantiated by a high incidence and prevalence of mental illness among women. One of the most consistent findings is that depression is closely associated with being female. The ratio of depressed women to men is about two to one. The data also show that young poor women who head single-parent families and young married women who work at dead-end jobs have shown the greatest rise in the rate of both treated and untreated depression.[27] The most recent research data suggest, however, that the excess of psychological symptoms in women is not intrinsic to femaleness but to the conditions of subordination, stress, and powerlessness that characterize traditional female roles.

Families are usually viewed as providing support networks for people, yet Carmen, Russo, and Miller[7] believe that it is in the traditional construct of marriage that the subjugation of women is the most apparent and destructive. For example, it is in rigidly traditional families that female adults and children are at highest risk for violence and sexual abuse.[61] Violence is said to occur in 50% of American families,[32] and it has been estimated that 1% of all girls have been sexually abused by their fathers.[31] Yet these destructive patterns of family roles and relationships are reinforced by society's pervasive pattern of sex discrimination. Women who leave unhappy or violent homes are denied equal educational, vocational, and economic opportunities; quality and supportive child care facilities, and a legitimate self-supporting role in society. Women are clustered in "female" jobs that are characterized by low pay. In the same occupation, they earn less than men. They are not equally compensated with men for work involving similar education or experience. In 1979, the median annual income of women who worked full time was 60% that of men. The earnings gap is greatest for minority women.[75] Of divorced women, only 14% are awarded alimony, and only 44% are awarded child support. Less than half of these, or only 21% of divorced mothers, collect child support regularly, and even then the payments are generally insufficient.[74] It would appear then, that the alternative to depression in an unhappy marriage can be a life of poverty with a dead-end job and great difficulty in attempting to provide adequate care for one's children.

The idea of powerlessness in the development of psychological distress and mental disorders among women is evident in one study, which reported that women who became depressed had previously made many attempts to cope. Those with the highest rates of depression were continuously faced with multiple and chronic stresses affecting themselves and their children. Efforts to deal with these stresses led to repeated frustration in employment possibilities, housing conditions, protection against violence and crime, child care assistance, and the unhelpful responses of social service and mental health agencies.[26]

If one's goal is illness prevention and health promotion, one cannot overlook this last concern—the responsiveness of the health community. New knowledge about women, men, and sex roles has not generally been incorporated in mental health education or clinical practice. This is evident in the following criticisms:

1. There is a double standard for mental health based on sex-role stereotyping and adjustment to one's environment. Broverman's now classic study[4] of mental health clinicians' attitudes indicates that healthy women are viewed differently from men and adults of unspecified gender in being more submissive, less independent, less adventurous, more suggestible, less competitive, more excitable in minor crises, more likely to have their feelings hurt, more emotional, more conceited about appearance, less objective, and more illogical. Although this study was conducted in 1970, Sherman[70] in 1980 concluded that there is still sex-role stereotyping in mental health standards and that sex role–discrepant behaviors are viewed as more of

a maladjustment. Although nurses were not included in Broverman's study, Davis[14] believes that as a group, they are not very different from others practicing in the mental health field. She notes that despite nurses' perceptions to the contrary, research seems to indicate that as an occupational group, nurses have a traditional view of sex roles.

2. Sexual abuse and exploitation in the male therapist–female patient relationship is more common than has previously been realized. This includes such erotic activities as kissing, hugging, touching, and therapist-patient sex. Some studies have indicated that as many as 10% of men psychiatrists and psychologists in practice report having sexual contact with women patients.[13]

3. A related danger in the male-female therapeutic relationship is that the dyad may replicate rather than remedy the "one-down" position in which women frequently find themselves in life. This may encourage the fantasy that an idealized relationship with a more powerful other is a better solution to life problems than is taking autonomous action. This possibility is strengthened by the predominance of male therapists.[8]

4. Therapeutic theories have often supported stereotypes about sex roles, including the assumption that dependency, masochism, and passivity are normal for women and that assertiveness and aggression should be treated differently for women than for men.[4] Women are also subjected to the theories based on a "blame-the-mother" tradition, particularly in reference to schizophrenic children and a general "antifeminine Freudian" position.

5. A pervasive sex bias has been documented in the therapeutic relationship. There is evidence that therapists' knowledge about issues affecting the lives of women is inadequate.[70] Adjustment to traditional roles is stressed, yet there has been a lack of realistic appraisals of the occupational hazards of the housewife role. Anger in women is often labeled pathological and inappropriate.[46] Thus many women experience conflict about anger and have difficulty expressing it adaptively.

The consequences of these practices affect both the quality and quantity of mental health care available to women. Carmen notes*:

---

*From Carmen, E., Russo, N., and Miller, J.: Inequality and women's mental health: an overview, The American Journal of Psychiatry, vol. 138, pp. 1319-1330, 1981. Copyright 1981, the American Psychiatric Association.

Women can be considered *both* overserved and underserved by mental health delivery systems. For disorders congruent with sex-role stereotypes, such as depression, conversion hysteria, and phobias, women show higher rates of service utilization than do men. In contrast, problems of women that are congruent with societal views of male authority and female devaluation, such as rape, incest, and wife beating, have been ignored. Thus, services for female victims of male aggression have been provided largely through the coordinated efforts of women themselves at a time when mental health professionals were often either blaming the victims or not noticing them. Similarly, for disorders that are incongruent with society's idealized view of women, such as alcoholism and illicit drug abuse, women's service needs have usually been hidden and ignored.[7,1327]

Yet the incidence of alcoholism among women is high, and in the United States more than two thirds of all tranquilizers, stimulants, and antidepressants are used by women.[19] Nonworking housewives over age 35 have been identified as the largest single group of tranquilizer users.[11]

What one can conclude from this discussion is that women at high risk for psychiatric illness are often separated or divorced, nonwhite, poorly educated, of low socioeconomic status, and coping with the stress of raising small children and being a breadwinner on a low income.[28] Furthermore, although the new freedom of emergent feminism has expanded some opportunities, it has also brought problems in work, sexual, and family settings. Four new syndromes have been identified as a result of these changes: (1) reentry anxiety when a long homebound woman returns to work in the outer world, (2) performance anxiety and fear that career success may be viewed as social failure, (3) conflict between social expectations of accommodation and compliance and the need to assert herself and fight for her rights when they have been imposed on, and (4) conflict between a woman's sense of personal identity and her professional identity, in which marriage or family may be viewed as a threat to autonomy.[54] The mental health problems of women are complex and pervasive. Nursing, as a predominantly female profession, has the potential of making a significant impact in health promotion and illness prevention with this high-risk population.

Mature adults

The issues of midlife and advancing age are problematic for some, but not all, adults. As people approach midlife they reflect on the choices they have made and their progress in attaining the goals they had set for themselves. Marriage, life-style, children, career, and quality of life all are subject to scrutiny. Certain types of stressors, including career changes (promotion, change of job, demotion, or being fired), changes in the family unit (death, divorce, or departure of the last child), and the aging process, may precipitate anxiety, depression, or psychosomatic illnesses. In essence, midlife is the time when previous choices in important life areas and one's related success, failure, satisfaction, and disappointment are reviewed and reworked in light of one's previous goals, currently perceived limitations, finiteness of opportunities, and time itself. It combines the sense of "another chance" with that of a "final chance."

Midlife has traditionally been given very little attention in theory, research, or practice. Recent works by Neugarten,[55] Sheehy,[69] Levenson,[47] and Gould[24] have explored it as a time of development and change, rather than a period merely focused on impending aging and death. The middle years range in the 30s to 40s, although precisely defining it by chronological age has been more recently criticized. Neither can it any longer be defined as the time of menopause for the woman. Rather, it relates to a combination of biological, psychological, and sociological events. Notman compares it to the period of adolescence*:

This importance of separation, the change in relationship to family, and the potential for further development of one's own interests, are common to both periods. However, the differences are highly significant. At adolescence the separation is from parents, who are incestuous object choices. At midlife the separation is from children, and the experience often revives some sense of loss. The adolescent perspective of infinite time and choices to be made differs from the midlife sense of the finite and the reassessment of choices that have been made. The reality is that time is limited and that although choices do exist or even increase, there is also a limited range and variety of careers, new physical pursuits, and new relationships.[57,1273]

Important in a discussion of midlife is the fact that it is viewed differently by men and women. According to Levenson's work,[47] men give central importance to the role of work in establishing oneself in the world. Work, not family, ap-

*From Notman, M.: Midlife concerns of women: implications of the menopause, The American Journal of Psychiatry, vol. 136, p. 1270, 1979. Copyright, 1979, the American Psychiatric Association.

pear to be the organizing theme of men's lives. Thus, at midlife, men focus heavily on evaluating their work and their career goals. Women, on the other hand, focus on the world in relation to their family or potential to have one, as well as their work or career goals. Women who have not had children feel a last chance to consider motherhood. Women with children experience a decrease in their absorption in the burdens of child care. One's children may either be launched into the world or functioning quite independently at home. Consequently, these women may feel relieved, renewed, and ready to return to the work world.

Although this can be an exciting time, it can also be viewed negatively if one feels displaced, unprepared, or unaccepted. Extramarital affairs, divorces, and major life changes can result from a midlife crisis and pose problems for the individual, as well as the family.

Another time of increased stress for the individual has, in the past, been largely ignored by researchers and clinicians in the mental health field who focus heavily on the early developmental stages. This is the period of later adulthood and old age. One of the most obvious reasons for this may be evident in the changing distribution of the population. In 1900, only 28% of the American population exceeded the age of 35 and only 3% had reached the age of 65. In contrast, in 1981, 45% exceeded age 35, and 11% of the population were 65 or older. During the same period of time, life expectancy in America has increased from an average of 51 years to 76 years for men.[68] Furthermore, the United States census in 1970 identified more than 106,000 Americans 100 years of age or older.

Although the majority of the present elderly population is not poor (only 14% of those over 65 are under the poverty line) and 95% of those over 65 remain community, rather than institutional, residents,[68] there are noticeable changes that begin to impose constraints on the aging adult. In reviewing the literature, Hefferin[29] identified three life stages of people living beyond age 65. The first stage is between ages 65 and 75, in which most people continue with normal activities unless there is a specific illness. In the second stage, from age 75 to 85, normal activities can also be carried out, although the effects of aging are evident. The final stage occurs after 85, in which most people need some help to maintain normal activities, and some may even require institutionalization.

As these stages reflect, the period of the life course extending from middle age into early old age is often characterized at the outset by the height of social and economic success as well as physical well-being. But slowly changes occur that for most people are simply a somewhat lower level of physical and psychological energy, accompanied by society's subtle and open pressures to make room for the next generation. It has been shown that the documentable quantitative changes in learning ability, intellectual competence, and other contextual behavior are relatively small and often within the realm of individual and environmental compensatory interventions. The evidence is strong, also, that individual differences in the maintenance of behavioral competence are related primarily to the person's state of health and the opportunities and tendencies to be fully involved in a stimulating environment.

Yet the extension of the normative life span into a long period of postparental and postvocational behavior is creating new life stressors and resulting maladaptive responses. For example, certain life events, such as enforced retirement, and loss of friends and family become more likely with increasing age, and loss of a spouse is often perceived as the single greatest loss that an individual can experience throughout the life cycle. The combined physical, social, financial, and psychological changes that result from the loss of a spouse severely tax the coping ability of the bereaved.

Although death of a spouse may be perceived as the greatest stressor, multiple other stressors that are social, psychological, and biological in origin overlap, interact, and enhance the vulnerability of aging adults. These are described in detail by Goodstein.[22] He notes that the social sphere presents a major source of stress, including family-cultural, employment, commercial, logistical, financial, and discriminatory stresses as described in Table 5-3. He observes that the elderly's social status and physical function have decreased at the same time this population has increased.

The elderly also have a bombardment of emotional pressures as they struggle with the issues of integrity and independence. Stressors involving mastery, coping style, generation gap, fears, love cues, self-image, loss, death of family and friends, relocation, money, retirement, deteriorating body functions, attractiveness, visual and auditory acuity, prestige, sex, and cognition (Table 5-3) all pose emotional hardship to the

TABLE 5-3. **Summary of stresses facing the elderly***

Category of stress	Influencing factors	Outcomes
SOCIAL STRESSES		
Family-cultural	Smaller family size	Weakened traditional nuclear family unit
	Increased mobility	Less opportunity for role modeling by elderly
	One fourth of elderly have no children	Shift from family to public responsibility for care of the aged
	One half of elderly have only distant relatives	
Employment	Security not based on ability to work but on government and union pensions	Retirement represents a major change that may be responded to adaptively or maladaptively
	Elderly capable of work function beyond age 65	Some models of part-time work have been developed
	In 1900, 66% of those over 65 still worked	
	Now less than 33% work	
	Retirement age is now 70 by new federal law	
Commercial	Society values youth and views older people and objects as obsolescent	Aging is devalued
	Commercial advertising is aimed at youth and deplores aging in principle	
Logistical	Physical disabilities, costs, fears, access, distances, and weather are all problems affecting the mobility of the elderly	Transportation is difficult for many of the elderly
		Access to activities and health care is often limited
		The elderly are easy targets for robbery and assault
Financial	Pensions are outstripped by the cost of living	Inflation has a severe impact on the elderly
	Health insurance is often inadequate with rising premiums and poor psychiatric coverage	
	Statistics for physical and psychiatric illness demonstrate the elderly's great need for services	
Discriminatory	Negative stereotypes of the elderly are commonly accepted	Ageism, or prejudice toward the elderly, exists in American society
	Providing health care to the elderly lacks prestige and is often avoided by caregivers	Health problems of the elderly often receive inadequate treatment
	Courses in aging and care of the aged are seldom part of the educational curricula of health care professionals	
PSYCHOLOGICAL STRESSES		
Mastery	The elderly experience decreasing influence over their outer life and preoccupation with their inner life	Through denial and projection the elderly evolve a "magical mastery" of their external environment
Coping style	The elderly tend to use coping styles that were effective earlier in life	If previously used and trusted coping styles fail, the elderly may display maladaptive responses
	Denial, somatization, projection, and constructed affect may occur	

*Modified from Goodstein, R.: Am. J. Orthopsychiatry **51**(2):219, 1981.

TABLE 5-3. **Summary of stresses facing the elderly—cont'd**

Category of stress	Influencing factors	Outcomes
Generation gap	At the time of the elderly's need, younger relatives may be at crucial points in their own lives and lack the time and insight to help	Younger relatives have difficulty understanding the aging process
Fears	Common fears include the following: 1. Maintaining control over their lives and environment 2. Maintaining physical functioning 3. Retaining a sense of purpose and productivity 4. Maintaining independence while acknowledging the possible need of a dependent status for survival 5. Failing cognition and senility 6. Death 7. Losing the interest of others	Predictable fears are common among the elderly and may cause significant psychological stress
Love cues	The elderly have acquired skills in interpreting nonverbal communication They easily detect and respond to cues of lack of interest or respect	If the elderly perceive lack of interest or honesty, they believe they are unliked and respond by withdrawing
Self-image	The elderly may dislike their dependent status or interpret it as a sign of their own failures	The elderly may have an aversion to youth or an acceptance of the stereotypes of the aged
Loss	Losses are predictable, steady, numerous, and often arrive in bunches	Losses for the elderly represent the most basic psychological stress
Death of family and friends	Loss of family and friends suggests impending loss of self	Results in loss of security and companionship and depletion of the pool of caregivers
Relocation	Relocation can involve loss of privacy, accustomed diet, favorite belongings, and familiar faces It may be accompanied by a feeling of aloneness or abandonment	Stress is a function of losing the familiar and facing the unsure new environment
Money	Loss of money affects the availability of goods, care, identity, and status	This compounds any other stressor experienced by the elderly
Retirement	Some external sources of gratification may be lost, and the couple may have to deal with changes in privacy and daily routine	Results in changes in income, identity, and lifestyle
Deteriorating body function	This decreases a person's skills	Loss of body functioning may affect one's identity and sense of productivity and usefulness
Attractiveness	Aging produces physical changes The effect of aging on one's physical appearance is subject to personal evaluation	One potential outcome is negative self-image and withdrawal from others
Visual and auditory acuity	Acuity in sensory cues is important for orientation, processing information, and maintaining daily activities	Diminution in sight or hearing can create inaccurate interpretation of the environment and may lead to paranoid or avoiding behavior

Continued.

TABLE 5-3. Summary of stresses facing the elderly—cont'd

Category of stress	Influencing factors	Outcomes
Prestige	The elderly often are retired from membership in decision-making bodies or are given an "honorary" membership without voting privileges	They perceive that their opinions are not valued and that their experience does not count
Sex	Sexual ability is determined by availability of a partner, past sexual activity, physical health, and support from family and health professionals	Natural physiological changes, if explained to the elderly and understood by them, can result in increased closeness, satisfaction, and communication
	The elderly may be embarrassed to discuss their sexual needs or experience side effects from medications	
	One's ability to enjoy sex can be maintained throughout the life cycle	
Cognition	Subtle changes in cognitive ability are detected first by the elderly	Resulting changes and perceptions can affect practical coping abilities and be psychologically disturbing
	Cognitive changes can be compounded by other life stresses	

BIOLOGICAL STRESSES

Illness and accidents	Result in decreased function and pain	Can erode activity, appearance, finances, employability, and self-esteem
Physiological aging	Aging inevitably occurs in body organs, biochemical and metabolic pathways, musculoskeletal systems, and central nervous system	Requires specific and sensitive guidelines for treatments, medications, education, and compliance
	It occurs at different rates in different people and among different organs in the same person	
Medications	The elderly tend to collect large numbers of medications from multiple sources, using an average of 13 prescriptions a year	Prescribing medications must be accompanied by proper discussion, written instructions, and careful monitoring
	They often take higher than prescribed doses and for longer periods of time	
	Of psychogeriatric admissions, 20% are precipitated by adverse effects of psychotropic drugs	
Other ingested substances	Changes in appetite, decreased activity, and poor physical function interfere with proper food intake among the elderly	Nutrition is often a problem for the elderly
	Assessment of caffeine, nicotine, and alcohol is often overlooked in the elderly	Drugs and alcohol may be used as tranquilizers or to allay loneliness
Iatrogenic biological stresses	The negative stereotypes of aging may block the reality of medication side effects and infection sequelae	Major iatrogenic problems arise from failing to diagnose and treat the causes of illness because of stereotyped thinking and an inappropriate prescription of medications to "keep the patient happy"

elderly. Goodstein believes that no matter what the specific psychological stress, the common denominators of sequelae to loss are reduced self-esteem and dignity, plus the implication that life and personal usefulness are slipping away.

Finally, without question, biological stress takes a toll on the elderly. Consider these statistics:

The elderly represent one third of the nation's health bill, one third of the family physician's practice time, two times the number of outpatient visits of other age populations, twice the number of days in the hospital of other age populations, three and a half times the cost of health care in other age populations, and 45% of the elderly have some physical limitations.[22:226]

Major sources of biological stress for the elderly include illness and accidents, physiological aging, medications, other ingested substances, and iatrogenic biological stresses (Table 5-3).

Despite these multiple stresses, most elderly are able to live in the community reasonably secure financially and in social contact with family and friends. However, those older persons experiencing multiple stresses and inadequate coping resources are at greater risk to require some form of institutional support. Access to and use of social support systems has been identified to be an important determinant of an older person's response to stress along with previous life experiences, premorbid coping styles, physical and emotional status, and the approach health professionals provide to the elderly from both a practical and an attitudinal standpoint. Schaie believes that "the quality of life in developed societies can be readily sensed from the manner in which transition from midlife to old age is accomplished with a minimum of stress and the preservation of maximum personal freedom and opportunities."[68:216] If this is true, primary prevention activities directed toward mature adults must command the attention of psychiatric nurses and other health professionals.

 ## Planning and implementing prevention strategies

The model of health-illness continuum as presented in Chapter 4 and represented in Fig. 5-1 is useful for the nurse in planning strategies for primary prevention. It suggests both target areas and types of activities that might be useful. If one's overall nursing goal is to promote constructive coping mechanisms and maximize adaptive coping responses, then the model sug- gests that prevention strategies should be directed toward influencing predisposing factors, precipitating stressors, appraisal of stressors, and coping resources and mechanisms through the following interventions: (1) health education, (2) environmental change, and (3) supporting social systems. Because the process depicted in the model is a dynamic one, it is not possible to discretely link a particular strategy with a particular component of the model. Rather, the strategies can affect multiple aspects of a person's life. For example, an environmental change, such as changing jobs, can affect one's predisposition to stress, decrease the amount of stress, change one's appraisal of the threat, and perhaps increase one's financial or social coping resources. This interactive effect can thus serve to justify the use of these prevention strategies for vulnerable groups.

Health education

This strategy of primary prevention in mental health involves the strengthening of individuals and groups through *competence building*. It is based on the assumption that many maladaptive responses are the result of a lack of competence, that is, a lack of perceived control over one's own life, of effective coping strategies, and the lowered self-esteem that results. Bloom[2] believes that competence building is perhaps the single, most persuasive preventive strategy for dealing with individual and social issues in most communities. A competent community is one that is aware of resources and alternatives, can make reasoned decisions about issues facing them, and can cope adaptively with problems. In this sense the concept of a competent community parallels the concept of positive mental health.[35]

Health education or competence building can be viewed as having four aspects. The first is increasing the individual's or group's awareness of issues and events related to health and illness. Awareness of normal developmental tasks and potential problems must be a foundational element. The second aspect is increasing one's understanding of the dimensions of potential stressors, possible outcomes (both adaptive and maladaptive), and alternative coping responses. A third element is increasing one's knowledge of where and how to acquire the needed resources. Many health professionals assume this is common knowledge, although for many

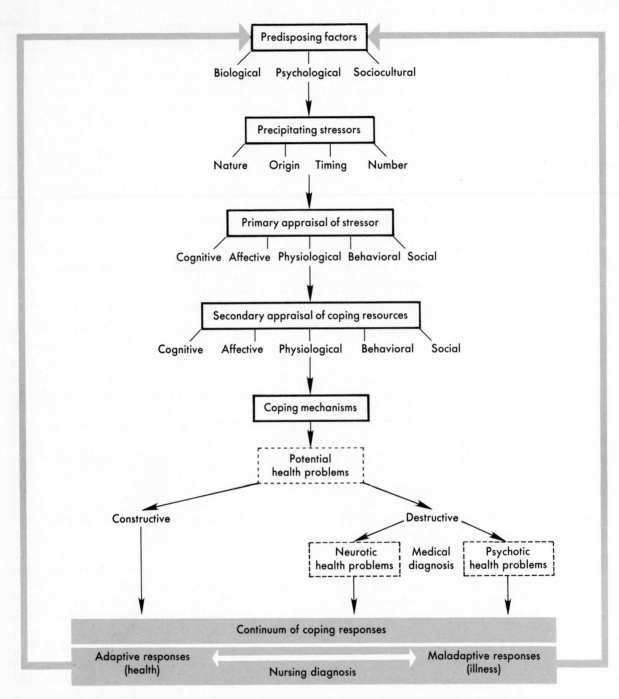

FIG. 5-1
Model of health-illness phenomena.

groups of individuals it is not. The fourth and final aspect of health education focuses on increasing the actual abilities of the individual or group. This means improving or maximizing one's coping skills, such as problem-solving skills or interpersonal skills, tolerance of stress and frustration, motivation, hope, self-esteem, and power. Ryan contends the following:

Self-esteem is to some extent an essential requirement to the very survival of the human organism . . . and is partially dependent on the inclusion of a sense of power within the self-concept. . . . A mentally healthy person must be able to perceive himself as at least minimally powerful, capable of influencing his environment to his own benefit, and further . . . this sense of minimal power has to be based on the actual experience and exercise of power.[67:50]

Health education has long been regarded by nurses as an essential part of nursing practice, yet it is difficult to quantify the degree or quality of mental health education actually implemented by nurses. It can take place in any setting, can assume a formal or informal structure, can be directed toward individuals or groups, and can be related to predisposing factors or potential stressors. Health education directed toward strengthening an individual's predisposition to stress can take various forms. Growth groups may be formed for parents that focus on parent-child relations, normal growth and development, or effective methods of child rearing. Groups of children or adolescents can discuss peer relationships, sexuality, or potential problem areas, such as drug abuse or promiscuity. Employee groups can be formed to discuss career burnout and related issues. Or a more activity-centered educational program can be initiated, such as Outward Bound, which helps the individual discover that step by step one can expand competence in mastering new, unexpected, and potentially stressful situations in an adaptive way.

Probably the most common type of health education program implemented at present is one that aids the individual in coping with a specific potential stressor. Consider, for example, the impending stressor or risk factor of marital separation. Families about to experience marital separation are vulnerable to emotional problems, physical complaints, and increased utilization of health care facilities.[3,77] Children and adults about to experience the event may be offered educational and supportive group intervention aimed at enhancing their ability to cope. Education groups can similarly be offered to those experiencing retirement, bereavement, or any other stressful event. Prepared childbirth classes are a well-known example of the type of anticipatory guidance that can be offered to high-risk groups.

Finally, health education activities can be directed to the larger community. One way to do this is by changing the attitudes and behavior of health care providers. This may involve activities related to dispelling myths and stereotypes associated with vulnerable groups, providing knowledge of normal parameters, increasing sensitivity to psychosocial factors affecting health and illness, and enhancing the ability to give sensitive, supportive, humanistic health care. Another community-level strategy requires public education on mental health issues and community resources. Misconceptions regarding vulnerable subgroups of the population need to be corrected. The stigma, misunderstanding, and fear surrounding mental illness is related to both the agencies providing mental health services and the people receiving these services who are often elderly, poor, or members of social minority groups. Unlike physical illness, which tends to evoke sympathy and the desire to help, mental disorders tend to disturb and repel people. Yet everyone encounters stress, and all people are subject to maladaptive coping responses. Mental health professionals can educate the public in the idea that health is a continuum, and illness is caused by a complex combination of factors. "In this way we may begin to understand that none of us is immune from mental illness or emotional problems, and that the fear, the anxiety, and even the anger we feel about people who suffer these problems may merely reflect some of our own deepest fears and anxieties."[61:57]

Environmental change

Activities in primary prevention involving environmental change have a social setting focus. They require the modification of an individual's or group's immediate environment or the larger social system. They are particularly appropriate actions when the environment has placed new demands on the person, when it is not responding to his developmental needs, and when it provides a diminished level of positive reinforcement for the individual. The nursing literature gives evidence that this is not an area of primary prevention in which nurses have been actively involved.

For the individual, various types of environmental changes may prove to promote one's mental health, including changes in one's economic, work, housing, neighborhood, or family situations. Economically, there may be the location of resources for financial aid or assistance obtained in the budgeting and managing of income. Work changes may include vocational testing, guidance, education, or retraining that can result in a change of jobs or careers. It may also mean that an adolescent, a housewife, or an older adult may be placed in a new career option. Changes in one's housing situation can involve moving to new quarters, which may mean leaving family and friends or returning to them, improvements in existing housing, or the addition or subtraction of co-inhabitants, whether they are family, friends, or roommates. Environmental changes that may benefit the family include attaining child care facilities, enrollment in a nursery school, grade school, or camp, or obtaining access to recreational, social, religious, or community facilities. The potential benefit of all of these changes should not be minimized or overlooked by mental health practitioners. They can promote mental health by increasing one's coping resources, modifying the nature of one's stressors, and possibly increasing one's positive, rewarding, and self-enhancing experiences.

Nurses can also affect environmental changes at a larger organizational and political level. One way is by influencing health care structures and procedures. Given the vulnerability of new parents, for example, nurses can work to implement birthing rooms and family suites in obstetrical settings. One might also become involved in the training of community, nonprofessional caregivers as one way of increasing the social supports available to vulnerable groups. Another approach would be to stimulate support for women's issues related to mental health, such as through studying the psychology of women; dispelling sex-role stereotypes; promoting feminist therapy[62]; sponsoring programs, conferences, and workshops on women's issues; and recruiting more women professionals into the mental health field. Obviously, if nurses believe they make a valuable contribution in promoting health, they should document the cost-effectiveness and quality of services they provide and lobby for greater patient access, adequate compensation, and greater participation in decision-making structures, such as hospital boards, advisory groups, or legislative bodies.

Within organizations, environmental change can be achieved through program consultation. Such consultation with a large corporation, for example, may lead to the formulation of more flexible retirement plans or a preretirement counseling program. Involvement in community planning and development can have an impact in many different areas. For instance, a community may be helped to meet the needs of the elderly for educational opportunities, recreational programs, and access to social support networks through telephone tie-lines or special transportation services. So too, the stress associated with environmental pollutants, such as chemicals and radiation, can be addressed.

Some environmental changes require involvement at the national level. It may be directed toward the media's portrayal of violence, laws on drunk driving, gun control legislation, access to family planning services, federal funding of abortion, the advocation of changes in child-rearing practices, including the provision of day-care centers, flex time and paternity leave, or the passage of equal rights legislation.

Of course many attitudes in and areas of the social system are in need of change, including racism, sexism, ageism, inadequate housing, poverty, and problems with the educational system. These could be examined by the Center for Prevention proposed by the President's Commission on Mental Health in 1978. The problem is that global problems such as these are too broad, too pervasive, and too diffuse to be adequately addressed, let alone resolved. Furthermore, the changes proposed under Reagan's program of the "New Federalism" will clearly mean that fewer governmental resources can be expected to aid such primary prevention efforts. For any prevention strategies to be successful in the future, it will be necessary to document the ways in which a particular group is vulnerable to a specific stressor, how the proposed prevention program will be beneficial and cost-effective, and the degree to which it succeeded or failed.

Supporting social systems

As a primary prevention strategy, supporting social systems is not an approach that attempts to remove or minimize the stressor or risk factor. Rather, its rationale is that of strengthening social supports as a way of buffering or cushioning the effects of a potentially stressful event. It is such an important concept for all levels of prevention—primary, secondary, and tertiary—that an entire section of the President's Commission on Mental Health was devoted to exploring ways to expand personal and social networks of families, neighbors, and community organizations to which people naturally turn to help them cope. It has implications for promoting health, helping people seek help earlier, supporting them in times of stress, and aiding the situation of the chronically mentally ill. Social support systems can be helpful in emphasizing the strengths of individuals and families and focusing on health rather than illness. For these reasons the commission recommended that "a major effort be developed in the area of personal and community supports which will":

1. Recognize and strengthen the natural networks to which people belong and on which they depend
2. Identify the potential social support that formal institutions within communities can provide
3. Improve the linkages between community support networks and formal mental health services
4. Initiate research to increase our knowledge of informal and formal community support systems and networks[61:15]

Given the goal that social support systems should be maximized, how does one go about achieving it? First, one needs to determine how much social support a high-risk group will need and then compare it to the amount of social support that is available. Although the question is straightforward, it is complicated by the fact that there are multiple determinants of each element. One's need for social support will be influenced by one's predisposing factors, the nature of the stressors, and the availability of other coping resources, such as economic assets, individual abilities and skills, and defensive techniques. The availability of social supports will similarly be influenced by one's predisposing factors, such as age, sex, or socioeconomic status, the nature of the stressor, and the characteristics of the environment. Acute episodic stressors tend to elicit more intense support, whereas in chronic problems, support resources tend to not persist. So too, changes or stressors viewed in a positive way by one's social network, such as the birth of a baby or a promotion, may elicit a great deal of support, whereas a negative event, such as a sudden death, may generate little support.

In addition, the quantity and type of social support that meets one need may not meet another. Research suggests that different characteristics of social support may be needed for different stresses. For example, in one study, family cohesiveness, family expressiveness, and spouse support were significant sources of support for the patient receiving dialysis, but the presence of a confidant was not.[15] However, Brown's study[5] found that an important factor in preventing depression was an intimate confiding relationship with a husband or boyfriend. Support from other relationships was not shown to be a specific factor. In Hirsch's study[33] of major life changes, he found that low-density, multidimensional support systems were more adaptive to the women he studied. Yet high-density support systems have commonly been regarded as the socially desirable, cultural ideal. Thus the match between the type and level of social support and the nature of the stressor is an important, but not entirely understood, one.

Even though many variables related to social support need further study, one can still use social support in designing and implementing interventions in primary prevention. Four particular types of interventions are possible. First, social support patterns can be used to assess communities and neighborhoods to identify problem areas and high-risk groups. Not only will this give information as to the quality of life, but the social isolation of a particular group might become apparent as well as central individuals whose aid may then be enlisted in developing community-based programs.

Another preventive intervention would be to improve linkages between community support systems and formal mental health services. Frequently mental health professionals are not aware of or comfortable with the existence or functioning of community support systems. To correct this, they should be taught the skills involved in utilizing and mobilizing community resources and social support systems. All types of health care providers need to be able to recognize when patients need social support and to provide them with access to appropriate community support systems.

The third type of intervention is to strengthen natural, existing caregiving networks. Health professionals can provide information and support to the variety of informal caregivers in the community who serve a very important and somewhat different function from more formalized and organized support systems. Gottlieb[23] notes that informal support systems provide (1) a natural training ground for the development of problem-solving skills, (2) a medium in which personal growth and development is based on repeated episodes of people learning to direct the process of change for themselves, and (3) a supportive milieu that capitalizes on the strength of existing ties among people in our communities, rather than fragmenting intact social units on the basis of diagnosed needs or specialized services.

Numerous such informal support groups exist. They may include church groups, civic organizations, clubs, women's groups, or work and neighborhood supports. Self-help groups are becoming more common as members organize themselves to solve their own problems. The members all share a common experience, work together toward a common goal, and use their own strengths to gain control over their lives. The processes involved in self-help groups are social affiliation, learning self-control, modeling methods to cope with stress, and acting to change the social environment.[48] They are familiar to the public through such groups as Alcoholics Anonymous, Weight Watchers, Parents Without Partners, and Parents Anonymous. They have also demonstrated their ability to help those people experiencing grief reactions, such as widows[10] and parents of children who died from the sudden infant death syndrome.

Working with natural, informal support systems should be done cautiously, however, so as to minimize undesirable consequences. One should attempt to create the least amount of disruption possible. Gottlieb[23] warns against the potentially damaging effects of well-intentioned consultation with informal caregivers by inadvertently suppressing their natural repertoire of helping behaviors. This might be an important point to remember in relation to all primary prevention strategies.

Finally, if an individual's social support is inadequate, interventions may need to be more direct. To determine what interventions are possible, Norbeck suggests that the following questions be asked*:

1. What is the capacity of the network to change?
    a. *Network structure.* Are there persons who can be brought into (or back into) the network?
    b. *Network functioning.* Can existing network members be assisted to provide the kind of support that is needed (e.g., allow talk about the pregnancy or about a loss)?

---

*Reprinted from Advances in Nursing Science, "Social support: a model for clinical research and application," by J. Norbeck by permission of Aspen Systems Corporation, © 1981.

    c. *Network disruption.* Can policies be changed or resources employed to minimize network disruption (e.g., due to hospitalization at a distant tertiary care facility)?
2. Does the individual have the interpersonal skills and attitudes required to establish and maintain contact with network members?
3. Is the individual receptive to using existing self-help or support groups or to having contact with a person who has coped with a similar experience?
4. If help from the indigenous social support system cannot be made available or acceptable, exactly what support does this individual require to cope with the current stressors or illness?
5. What long-term help would be required to assist the individual to establish and maintain an adequate social support network?[56;54]

One possible intervention may be to help the person or group develop, maintain, and use their network. The person may also be encouraged to consider expanding his network. This might require health education strategies with the goal of competence building. Alternatively, one can influence the network more directly. Network therapy involves assembling and mobilizing all the important members of the family's kin and friendship network. The focus is then on tightening social bonds within the network and breaking dysfunctional patterns.[71] For families who are isolated and whose networks are depleted, network members may not be available for such a strategy. In this case, arranging for the use of mutual support groups may be effective.

Finally, it should be noted that although supporting social supports is an effective intervention, it is not one that is limited to primary prevention activities. Rather, all nurses in all settings can utilize this strategy as a way of providing holistic care to maximize the health of individuals, families, and groups.

Working with groups

The nurse who is working in the area of primary prevention in mental health may be working with any level of the social hierarchy—individuals, families, communities, or even the larger society (Fig. 5-2). At this time she is likely to be working with groups of people as a way of maximizing the impact she can make and mobilizing the environment's potential to be supportive. A group approach, however, may not always be the most effective or efficient one. To decide if a group approach is indicated for a particular intervention, Loomis suggests that the nurse ask herself the following questions:

Biosphere

Society

Community

Group

Family

Individual

Body system

Organ

Tissue

Cell

FIG. 5-2
Levels of organization that make up the social hierarchy.

1. What are the client needs I am attempting to meet?
2. Can these needs be met in a group?
3. What are my own objectives for the proposed group?
4. What are the expectations of the system relative to the proposed group?
5. Is there any discrepancy or conflict between the answers to questions 1 through 4?[49:18-20]

Assuming that a group approach has been decided on, the next task of the nurse is to decide what type of group would be most appropriate. This may be accomplished by considering one's group goals, desired outcomes, and role of the nurse. It is particularly important to examine the role of the nurse, because different types of groups often have similar goals and even outcomes. For example, providing emotional support to members is usually a function of many groups—formal, informal, natural, and professional. So too, the imparting of new information to members can be a common outcome. A distinguishing characteristic, however, can be found in how the nurse functions in the group.

Marram describes three types of groups that the psychiatric nurse is particularly likely to be involved in.[51] The first is *group psychotherapy,* which uses the group process to treat people with existing mental disorders. They may vary in intensity and in the underlying theoretical framework used by the leaders. These groups can be distinguished by their overall emphasis on (1) personality reconstruction, (2) insight without reconstruction, (3) remotivation, (4) problem solving, (5) reeducation, or (6) support.[51] Nurses who lead such groups are actively and formally engaging patients in a therapeutic endeavor. However, the context is changed from that of a one-to-one relationship to that of a group relationship. Regardless, the responsibility for group psychotherapy resides with the nurse, and, for her to function in this role, she needs to have advanced education or extensive supervised experience. This type of group is associated with secondary and tertiary levels of prevention, and examples of it include inpatient groups, outpatient groups, special problem groups, family groups, therapy groups, and married couples groups.

The second type of group is commonly implemented in primary prevention strategies. This is the *therapeutic group,* which may be differentiated from group psychotherapy according to (1) how large a role emotional stress has played in the person's current level of health and (2) the primary goal or central objective of the group experience.[51] In group psychotherapy the emotional stress of the patient is of primary importance, and the group goal is one of treatment. In therapeutic groups, stress is the result of some change or life event that has the potential of producing a maladaptive response. One's goal, therefore, is that of prevention, education, and providing support. The individual in this group is on the healthy end of the health-illness continuum, although he may be experiencing a situational crisis of some type. The nurse still maintains responsibility for these groups, although her role may now be that of a health educator and facilitator. Examples of these groups can be found in general hospitals, clinics, nursing homes, industrial settings, business, schools, and penal institutions.

The third type of group is the *self-help,* or *mutual support, group,* which has been described under the strategy of supporting social systems. Their primary aims are to (1) control member behavior, (2) ameliorate stress due to common problems, and (3) maintain member self-esteem and social integration.[51] They do not focus on personality reconstruction or insight analysis. Although the goals of these groups may not necessarily differentiate them from other types of groups, they do differ in one very important criterion; they are led by the group members themselves. If a nurse is the leader with primary responsibility for the group, then it is not a self-help, or mutual support, group. In these groups, if professionals participate at all, they do so by invitation and usually only in an ancillary role.

Finally, the nurse who is utilizing a group approach should have an understanding of the development and processes that occur in groups to increase the therapeutic potential of the group for its members. These are described in Chapter 24.

 Evaluation

Throughout this chapter on primary prevention in mental health, mention has been made of the lack of clarity of concepts and assumptions, the lack of empirical studies identifying causal or predictive relationships, and the lack of understanding of the essential processes underlying preventive interventions. All of these problems are serious, and perhaps they all contribute to the lack of support for primary prevention as a public priority. Until we know more about an optimum fit between an individual and his social environment, it will be difficult to be able to help people define, select, create, and use environments that are growth producing for them.

There is a tendency when talking about primary prevention to think in terms of the total elimination of mental illness and stress. Yet these are not realistic goals, and maintaining them can only discourage any possible action. Perhaps it is possible to set goals of the reduction in suffering and the enhancement of the capacity to cope. But even these may be unattainable, given that the environment is constantly changing and adaptation to it is an ongoing challenge. Rather, if one focuses on the specific problems of a vulnerable group in our society, one's activity becomes more directed, and the chance of success increases.

Clearly there is a need for the evaluation of programs in primary prevention. In a world of shrinking resources, only those programs with proven effectiveness are likely to be supported in the future. It needs to be demonstrated that the prevention strategy used had both short-term and long-term effects which benefited the individual and society. One also needs to determine if the specific strategy implemented was the most effective, appropriate, and efficient one. Considering alternative approaches and comparing outcomes is an essential part of the evaluation process.

Although preventing all illness is not possible, preventing some particular problems is. But a number of barriers exist that make it difficult to expand primary prevention activities. When faced with a choice, the needs of the presently ill consistently take precedence over preventing problems in the future. This holds true for nurses, as well as for the larger society. Yet by being more farsighted both groups could benefit greatly. Nursing has long maintained its role in health education and supportive care. If it can document these actions and their effectiveness, it will demonstrate its value as a profession and its importance in promoting the well-being of society.

Suggested cross-references

The model of health-illness phenomena, including stressors, coping resources, social support systems, and family assessment, are discussed in Chapter 4. Chapter 19 describes prevention in relation to community mental health. Therapeutic aspects of groups are discussed in Chapter 24. Problems experienced by adolescents are discussed in Chapter 27, and problems of family violence and abuse are discussed in Chapter 28. Problems experienced by the elderly are discussed in Chapter 31.

SUMMARY

1. Caplan's three levels of preventive intervention were described. The major thrust in present psychiatric care is in secondary prevention, and primary prevention has yet to evolve as a major force in the mental health movement. Definitional problems related to primary prevention were identified.

2. Lack of consensus exists on the definition of mental health. Jahoda's conditions and criteria of mental health were discussed, including positive attitude toward self; growth, development, and self-actualization; integration; autonomy; reality perception; and environmental mastery. The concepts of cultural relativism, psychobiological resilience, and a health-illness continuum were related to mental health.

3. The idea of promoting mental health was critiqued, and it was suggested that primary prevention activities focus on illness prevention to be effective. Mental illness was conceptualized as having causative factors that are multiple, interactive, situational, and sociocultural, all of which result in maladaptive behaviorial responses. A paradigm for primary prevention was presented that attempts to reduce the incidence of particular stressful life events for vulnerable groups. The application of the nursing process with this view of primary prevention was described.

4. Developmental stages and tasks of the individual and family life cycles were identified. Assessment in primary prevention was presented as the identification of groups of people who are vulnerable to developing mental disorders or maladaptive coping responses to specific stressors or risk factors. The following vulnerable groups were described: adolescents, new parents, families, women, and mature adults.

5. Prevention strategies should be directed toward influencing predisposing factors, precipitating stressors, appraisal of stressors, and coping resources through the following interventions: health education, environmental change, and supporting social systems.
   a. Health education involves the strengthening of individuals and groups through competence building.
   b. Environmental change involves the modification of an individual's or group's immediate environment or the larger social system.
   c. Supporting social systems is a way of buffering or cushioning the effects of a potentially stressful event. Four strategies for supporting social systems were described.

6. Working with groups is useful to maximize the preventive impact of the nurse's actions and the environment's potential to be supportive. Three types and groups, group psychotherapy, therapeutic groups, and self-help groups, were described in relation to group goals, desired outcomes, and role of the nurse.

7. Evaluation of primary prevention activities is impeded by the lack of clarity of assumptions, empirical studies in the area, and essential processes underlying preventive interventions. In evaluating preventive strategies, one needs to demonstrate their effectiveness and efficiency in using resources.

References

1. Bieber, T., and Bieber, T.: Postpartum reactions in men and women, J. Am. Acad. Psychoan. 6(4):511, 1978.
2. Bloom, B.: Prevention of mental disorders: recent advances in theory and practice, Community Ment. Health J. 15(3):179, 1979.
3. Bloom, B., Asher, S., and White, S.: Marital disruptions as a stressor: a review of analysis, Psychol. Bull. 85:867, 1978.
4. Broverman, I., Broverman, D., and Clarkson, F.: Sex-role stereotypes and clinical judgments of mental health, J. Consult. Clin. Psychol. 34:1, 1970.
5. Brown, F., and Harris, T.: Social origins of depression, London, 1978, Tavistock Publications, Ltd.
6. Caplan, G.: Principles of preventive psychiatry, New York, 1964, Basic Books, Inc., Publishers.
7. Carmen, E., Russo, N., and Miller, J.: Inequality and women's mental health: an overview, Am. J. Psychiatry, 138:1319, 1981.
8. Chesler, P.: Women and madness, New York, 1972, Doubleday Publishing Co.
9. Cobb, S.: Social support as a moderator of life stress, Psychosom. Med. 38(5):306, 1976.
10. Conroy, R.C.: Widows and widowhood, N.Y. State J. Med. 77(3):357, 1977.
11. Cooperstock, R.: Sex differences in psychotropic drug use, Soc. Sci. Med. 12B:179, 1978.
12. Cronenwett, L., and Kunst-Wilson, W.: Stress, social support and the transition to fatherhood, Nurs. Res. 30(4):196, 1981.
13. Davidson, V.: Psychiatry's problem with no name: therapist-patient sex, Am. J. Psychoanal. 37:43, 1977.
14. Davis, A.: The woman as therapist and client, Nurs. Forum 16(34):250, 1977.
15. Diamond, M.: Social support and adaptation to chronic illness: the case of maintenance hemodialysis, Res. Nurs. Health 2:101, 1979.
16. Duvall, E.: Marriage and family development, ed. 5, Philadelphia, 1977, J.B. Lippincott Co.
17. Elkins, V.: The rights of the pregnant parent: two continents, New York, 1976, Schocken Books, Inc.
18. Erikson, E.: Childhood and society, ed. 2, New York, 1963, W.W. Norton & Co., Inc.
19. FDA Drug Bulletin, Feb. 1980, U.S. Government Printing Office.

20. Fishbein, E.: Fatherhood and disturbances of mental health: a review, J. Psychiatr. Nurs. **19**(7):24, 1981.

21. Forssman, H., and Thuwe, I.: One hundred and twenty children born after application for therapeutic abortion refused, Acta Psychiatr. Scand. **28**(1):21, 1974.

22. Goodstein, R.: Inextricable interaction: social, psychologic, and biologic stresses facing the elderly, Am. J. Orthopsychiatry **51**(2):219, 1981.

23. Gottlieb, B.: The primary group as supportive milieu: application to community psychology, Am. J. Community Psychol. **7**(5):469, 1979.

24. Gould, R.: The phases of adult life: a study in developmental psychology, Am. J. Psychiatry **129**:521, 1972.

25. Gray, J. et al.: Prediction and prevention of child abuse and neglect, Child Abuse Neglect **1**:45, 1977.

26. Greywold, E., Reese, M., and Belle, D.: Stressed mothers syndrome: how to short circuit the stress depression cycle, Behav. Med. **7**(11):12, 1980.

27. Guttentag, M., Salasin, S., and Belle, D., editors: The mental health of women, New York, 1980, Academic Press, Inc.

28. Guttentag, M., Salasin, S., and Legge, W.: Women's utilization of mental health services studied, Evaluation **3**:30, 1976.

29. Hefferin, E.: Life-cycle stressors: an overview of research, Fam. Community Health **2**(4):71, 1980.

30. Helper, M., et al.: Life-events and acceptance of pregnancy, J. Psychosom. Res. **12**:183, 1968.

31. Herman, J.: Father-daughter incest, Pro. Psychol. **12**(1):76, 1981.

32. Hilberman, E.: Overview: the "wife-beater's wife" reconsidered, Am. J. Psychiatry **137**:1336, 1980.

33. Hirsch, B.: Natural support systems and coping with major life changes, Am. J. Community Psychol. **8**:159, 1980.

34. Hollister, W.: Basic strategies in designing primary prevention programs. In Klein, D., and Goldston, S., editors: Primary prevention: an idea whose time has come, Department of Health, Education, and Welfare No. (ADM)77-447, Rockville, Md., 1977, National Institute of Mental Health.

35. Iscoe, I.: Community psychology and the competent community, Am. Psychol. **29**:607, 1974.

36. Jahoda, M.: Current concepts of positive mental health, New York, 1958, Basic Books, Inc., Publisher.

37. Jarrahi-Zadeh, I. et al.: Emotional and cognitive changes in pregnancy and early puerperium, Br. J. Psychiatry **115**:797, 1969.

38. Jonas, A.D., and Jonas, D.F.: The influence of early training on the varieties of stress responses: an ethological approach, J. Psychosom. Res. **19**(5-6):325, 1975.

39. Kennell, J., Voos, D., and Klaus, M.: Parent-infant bonding. In Heffer, R., and Kempe, C., editors: Child abuse and neglect: the family and the community, Cambridge, Mass., 1976, Ballinger Publishing Co.

40. Ketai, R., and Brandwin, M.: Childbirth-related psychosis and familial symbiotic conflict, Am. J. Psychiatry **136**(2):190, 1979.

41. Kessler, M., and Albee, G.: An overview of the literature of primary prevention. In Albee, G., and Jaffe, J., editors: Primary prevention of psychopathology, Hanover, N.H., 1977, University Press of New England.

42. Klein, C.: Coping patterns of parents of deaf-blind children, Am. Ann. Deaf **122**(3):310, 1977.

43. Lacoursiere, R.: Fatherhood and mental illness: a review and new material, Psychiatr. Q. **46**:109, 1972.

44. Lamb, H., and Zusman, J.: Primary prevention in perspective, Am. J. Psychiatry **136**(1):12, 1979.

45. Lederman, R.P. et al.: Relationship of psychological factors in pregnancy to progress in labor, Nurs. Res. **28**(2):94, 1979.

46. Lerner, H.: The taboo against female anger, Menninger Perspect. **5**:5, Winter, 1977.

47. Levenson, D., Darrow, C., and Kelin, E.: The seasons of a man's life, New York, 1978, Alfred A. Knopf, Inc.

48. Levy, L.: Self-help groups: types and psychological processes, J. Appl. Behav. Sci. **12**:310, 1976.

49. Loomis, M.E.: Group process for nurses, St. Louis, 1979, The C.V. Mosby Co.

50. Lynch, M.: Ill-health and child-abuse, Lancet, vol. 2, Aug. 16, 1975.

51. Marram, G.D.: The group approach in nursing practice, ed. 2, St. Louis, 1978, The C.V. Mosby Co.

52. Maslow, A.: Motivation and personality, New York, 1954, Harper & Row Publishers, Inc.

53. Mercer, R.: A theoretical framework for studying factors that impact on the maternal role, Nurs. Res. **30**(2):73, 1981.

54. Moulton, R.: Some effects of the new feminism, Am. J. Psychiatry **134**(1):1, 1977.

55. Neugarten, B., editor: Middle age and aging, Chicago, 1968, University of Chicago Press.

56. Norbeck, J.: Social support: a model for clinical research and application, Adv. Nurs. Sci. **3**(4):42, 1981.

57. Notman, M.: Midlife concerns of women: implications of the menopause, Am. J. Psychiatry **136**:1270, 1979.

58. Nuckolls, K.B., Cassel, J., and Kaplan, B.H.: Psychosocial assets, life crisis and the prognosis of pregnancy, Am. J. Epidemiol. **95**:431, 1972.

59. Pitt, B.: Atypical depression following childbirth, Br. J. Psychiatry **114**:1325, 1968.

60. Pratt, L.: Child-rearing methods and children's health behavior, J. Health Soc. Behav. **14**(3):61, 1973.

61. President's Commission on Mental Health, vols. 1 to 4, Washington, D.C., 1978, U.S. Government Printing Office.

62. Rawlings, E., and Carter, D.: Psychotherapy for women, Springfield, Ill., 1977, Charles C Thomas, Publisher.

63. Rogers, C.: On becoming a person, Boston, 1961, Houghton Mifflin Co.

64. Room, R.: The case for a problem prevention approach to alcohol, drug and mental problems, Public Health Rep. **96**(1):26, 1981.

65. Rosow, I.: Docs: ortho and para, Am. J. Orthopsychiatry, **51**(2):255, 1981.

66. Rutter, M.: Changing youth in a changing society, Cambridge, Mass., 1980, Harvard University Press.

67. Ryan, W.: Preventive services in the social context: power, pathology and prevention. In Bloom, B., and Buch, D., editors: Preventive services in mental health programs, Boulder, Colo., 1967, Western Interstate Commission for Higher Education.

68. Schaie, K.: Psychological changes from midlife to early old age: implications for the maintenance of mental health, Am. J. Orthopsychiatry **51**(2):199, 1981.

69. Sheehy, G.: Passages, New York, 1974, E.P. Dutton, Inc.

70. Sherman, J.: Therapist attitudes and sex-role stereotyping. In Brodsky, A., and Hare-Merstin, R., editors: Women and psychotherapy, New York, 1980, The Guilford Press.

71. Speck, R., and Rueveni, V.: Network therapy—a developing concept, Fam. Process **8:**182, 1969.
72. Streff, M.: Examining family growth and development: a theoretical model, Adv. Nurs. Sci. **3**(4):61, 1981.
73. Sundeen, S. et al.: Nurse-client interaction: implementing the nursing process, ed. 2, St. Louis, 1981, The C.V. Mosby Co.
74. "To . . . form a more perfect union . . .": Justice for American Women: Report of the National Commission on the Observance of International Women's Year, Washington, D.C., 1976, U.S. Government Printing Office.

75. U.S. Department of Labor: Twenty facts on women workers, Washington, D.C., 1980, Office of the Secretary, Women's Bureau.
76. Voysey, M.: Impression management by parents with disabled children, J. Health Soc. Beh. **13**(1):80, 1972.
77. Weiss, R.: Marital separation, New York, 1975, Basic Books, Inc., Publishers.

Annotated suggested readings

Cronenwett, L., and Kunst-Wilson, W.: Stress, social support and the transition to fatherhood, Nurs. Res. **30**(4):196, 1981.

The authors present a paradigm of variables that are involved in the transition to fatherhood. Such a paradigm can be used to generate theories, test hypotheses, and develop appropriate preventive interventions. Additional work of this type is greatly needed in nursing.

Delgado, M.: A model for mental health education in Hispanic communities, J. Psychiatr. Nurs. **18**(8):16, 1980.

This article describes a mental health education program specifically targeted to reach Hispanics. It discusses methods, settings, logistics, and recommendations for similar projects.

Eisenberg, L.: A research framework for evaluating the promotion of mental health and prevention of mental illness, Public Health Rep. **96**(1):3, 1981.

This excellent review article addresses specific topics and ways in which health may be promoted. Broad in scope and important in content.

Gammonley, J.: New directions for mental health education, J. Psychiatr. Nurs. **16**(12):40, 1978.

This is one of the few articles in the psychiatric nursing literature that focuses on mental health education. It is described in relation to both preventive and therapeutic programs.

Garbauno, J.: Changing hospital childbirth practices: a developmental perspective on prevention of child maltreatment, Am. J. Orthopsychiatry **50**(4):588, 1980.

A program to alter hospital policies and practices to promote more family-centered care is described in this article. It is a useful presentation of how to initiate change and problems that can arise in the process.

Guttentag, M., Salasin, S., and Belle, D., editors: The mental health of women, New York, 1980, Academic Press, Inc.

This edited book is a very good overview of issues related to women —a high-risk group for mental health problems.

Harman, D., and Brim, O.: Learning to be parents: principles, programs and methods, Beverly Hills, Calif., 1980, Sage Publications, Inc.

This is a major assessment of the field of parent education that includes the rationale and issues behind parent education and the methods, curriculum, and evaluation of parent education programs. Timely, practical, and thorough.

Hefferin, E.: Life-cycle stressors: an overview of research, Fam. Community Health **2**(4):71, 1980.

This article is precisely what the title describes —a review of research on life-cycle stressors that is very extensive, thorough, and well-organized. A valuable reference article.

Jacobson, A.: Melancholy in the 20th century: causes and prevention, J. Psychiatr. Nurs. **18**(7):11, 1980.

Depression among women is explored in this paper with a particular focus on primary prevention using support networks and anticipatory guidance for this high-risk population during critical developmental stages.

Johnson, S.: High-risk parenting, Philadelphia, 1979, J.B. Lippincott Co.

The nurse-author describes families who are at risk because of a variety of social, psychological and physiological stressors. This is an important book, which is recommended for all nurses working with families under stress.

Journal of Family Issues

This quarterly journal focuses on the family in contemporary society. It includes theoretical and applied research writing with special issues focusing on a particular topic in depth.

Kastenbaum, R.: Old age and the new scene, New York, 1981, Springer Publishing Co., Inc.

This is an anthology of psychosocial gerontology. The contributors are scholars and researchers whose viewpoints promote reevaluation of the elderly and greater awareness of the potential of later life.

Marram, G.D.: The group approach in nursing practice, ed. 2, St. Louis, 1978, The C.V. Mosby Co.

This text treats the scope, nature, and process of group work in nursing. Since all nurses work with and in groups, the content of this book should be essential knowledge.

Mercer, R.: A theoretical framework for studying factors that impact on the maternal role, Nurs. Res. **30**(2):73, 1981.

This article is recommended for its presentation of a theoretical framework useful in studying variables influencing the maternal role. This type of nursing theorizing and research can make a valuable contribution to the field.

Murray, R., and Zentner, J.: Nursing assessment and health promotion through the life span, ed. 2, Englewood Cliffs, N.J., 1979, Prentice-Hall, Inc.

The authors introduce the reader to the person and his family throughout the life span. The text is an excellent resource for nurses in teaching families normal development, how to deal positively with behaviors, and what changes to expect in the future.

Nix, H.: Why parents anonymous? J. Psychiatr. Nurs. **18**
(10):23, 1980.

*This article describes the formation of the self-help
group of Parents Anonymous to help with preventing
child abuse. The group's definition, structure, roles, and
processes are well described.*

Norbeck, J.: Social support: a model for clinical research
and application, Adv. Nurs. Sci. **3**(4):43, 1981.

*In this substantive article the author outlines the con-
cept of social support and discusses how it may be incorporated in nursing practice. An excellent bibliography
on the subject is also included.*

Norman, W., and Scaramella, T.: Midlife developmental
and clinical issues, New York, 1980, Brunner/Mazel, Inc.

*The authors focus beyond the losses and deprivations
of midlife to the potential for active fulfilling growth.
Addressed are social and intrapsychic factors that affect
perceptions of self and adaptational patterns, developmental challenges, options, and potentially problematic
areas that are critical in the clinical setting.*

Peterman, P.: Parenting and environmental considerations,
Am. J. Orthopsychiatry **51**(2):351, 1981.

*The efficacy of establishing a self-help group in a poor
urban area is described in this brief article. The effects
of environmental factors and their use as intervention
strategies to help promote positive parenting roles is discussed.*

Roberts, F.: A model for parent education, Image **13**:86,
Oct. 1981.

*This well-written article looks at why parent educa-
tion is often ineffective and presents a new model for
reconceptualizing its planning and delivery. The model
has applicability for preventive health education in
other areas as well.*

Robinson, K.: Working with a community action group, J.
Psychiatr. Nurs. **16**(8):38, 1978.

*This article describes the role of nurses working with a
community action group. The stages of group development
and related problems are analyzed.*

Rubington, E., and Weinberg, M.: Deviance: the interaction-
ist perspective, New York, 1981, Macmillan, Inc.

*This collection of papers is organized into four sec-
tions: the social deviant, the formal regulation of deviance, deviant subcultures, and the deviant identity. It
examines deviance as a social phenomena and the consequences of it.*

Rutter, M.: Changing youth in a changing society, Cambridge, Mass., 1980, Harvard University Press.

*This text is a contemporary review of the psychosocial
problems of adolescents in society. It addresses whether
there are definable problems specifically associated with
the adolescent age period, whether the problems are increasing or changing in character, and how the health
and social services should be geared to cope with them.*

Satir, V.: Peoplemaking, Palo Alto, Calif., 1972, Science &
Behavior Books.

*According to the author, the family is the "factory"
where human beings are made. This is a book written for
families about family process. It analyzes self-worth,
communication systems, and family rules in a most enjoyable way.*

Sedgwick, R.: Family mental health: theory and practice,
St. Louis, 1981, The C.V. Mosby Co.

*This excellent text on working with families is divided
into three sections: an overview of concepts and principles, a discussion of the clinical process, and clinical
application through case illustrations. This is one text
that should be read by all nurses.*

CHAPTER 6

REHABILITATIVE PSYCHIATRIC NURSING

Of equality—as if it harm'd me giving others the same chances and rights as myself—as if it were not indispensible to my own rights that others possess the same.

Walt Whitman, Thought

Learning objectives

After studying this chapter, the student will be able to:

- *define tertiary prevention and psychiatric rehabilitation.*

- *discuss concepts relative to an individual's rehabilitative nursing needs.*

- *describe the concepts of primary and secondary gain as they pertain to psychiatric rehabilitation.*

- *analyze the readiness of a patient for discharge from a treatment program.*

- *identify and discuss five factors relative to assessment of the family's resources for assisting the patient.*

- *describe and evaluate community resources relative to the needs of the recovering psychiatric patient.*

- *analyze the concept of stigma as it operates in the community.*

- *discuss the role of the nurse in interaction with the needs of the recovering patient.*

- *compare and contrast several models for the provision of rehabilitative psychiatric services.*

- *develop specific behavioral goals for rehabilitative psychiatric nursing care in conjunction with the patient and family.*

- *describe group interventions that are appropriate to tertiary prevention, including the nurse's role with self-help groups.*

- *discuss nursing interventions that are directed toward meeting the needs of families.*

■ *analyze the importance of nursing intervention at
a community level, including mental health education, membership in advocacy groups, networking, and political action.*

■ *describe the current status of tertiary prevention
program evaluation.*

■ *identify suggested readings for further study.*

The public health model of prevention specifies three levels of preventive health care activity: primary, secondary, and tertiary. Primary
prevention, as discussed in Chapter 5, is directed
toward decreasing the incidence of a health
problem by intervening before a potential disruption occurs. Secondary prevention is directed
toward intervention to decrease the prevalence
of a health problem by intervening promptly
when illness occurs to limit its severity and duration. This is the traditional area of concentration for psychiatric nurses and is the subject of
much of the content of this book. Tertiary prevention is the limitation of disability related to an
episode of illness. It is the subject of this chapter.

Any episode of illness involves potential lasting change in the individual's level of functioning. The more serious the health problem, the
greater is the possibility of a serious interference
with the individual's ability to function productively in the community. Episodes of illness that
involve hospitalization are generally more disruptive to the person's life-style and require a
greater readjustment as part of the recovery process. Nurses who are providers of care at the
secondary prevention level in institutional settings must maintain an awareness of the total
range of present and potential patient care
needs. Tertiary prevention usually begins prior
to discharge from the hospital.

Caplan[7] defines the goal of tertiary prevention
as one of reducing the rate in a community of
defective functioning resulting from mental
disorder. However this definition includes the
other levels of prevention. He adds that common
usage usually limits the meaning to reduction of
the rate of residual defect.[7] This is the sense in
which it will be used in this chapter.

Tertiary prevention is operationalized by the
performance of activities identified as *rehabilita-*

tion. Rehabilitation is the process of enabling
the individual to return to his highest possible
level of functioning. The goal is usually to match
or exceed the preillness functional level. This
may be achieved by capitalizing on strengths,
relearning old skills or learning new skills, depending on the effects of the health care problem and the person's response to it. Anthony
identifies the goal of psychiatric rehabilitation
as follows: "The goal of the psychiatrically disabled helpee is to perform the physical, intellectual and emotional skills needed to live, learn
and work in her or his particular community,
given the least amount of support necessary
from agents of the helping professions."[2:30]

Like primary prevention, the tertiary level of
prevention was largely ignored until the advent
of community mental health programs in the
1960s. The development of effective treatment
methodologies for psychosocial disruptions allowed mental health care providers to begin to
think about the future of former patients who
were able to reenter the community. Medication
and psychotherapy, in particular, were instrumental in assisting patients to develop positive
interpersonal relationships. Hospitalization was
avoided for some patients who were able to continue to function in the community with the help
of intensive intervention.

Psychiatric rehabilitation was given further
impetus as attention turned to the civil rights
of psychiatric patients. The right to treatment
in the least restrictive setting was established in
the courts and resulted in close scrutiny of people who had been hospitalized, in some cases
for many years. As people were returned to communities, it became obvious that many of them
lacked the skills they needed to function adequately. Scandals erupted in many areas as discharged psychiatric patients gravitated to shabby boarding houses, soup kitchens, and skid
row. Unaccustomed to managing their daily
affairs, many were victimized by people they
encountered on the streets. Many returned to
ths hospital for brief admissions, creating a "revolving door" between the hospital and the community. Others became inmates of other kinds
of institutions, especially jails and nursing
homes, as they demonstrated their inability to
cope.

The process of moving long-term hospital patients to the community is called *deinstitutionalization.* For this process to succeed, patients must be prepared to function at least minimally well in the community. This has become
an important focus of psychiatric rehabilitation.

However, all patients who have received treatment for a disruption in mental or emotional functioning are potentially in need of rehabilitative services. This chapter will focus on the nursing process as applied to psychiatric rehabilitation for any degree of residual impairment. The care of the chronically mentally ill person is discussed in greater depth in Chapter 30.

Bennett[6] discusses the conflict between the needs of society and the needs of the mentally ill person. Closing hospital wards leads to loss of jobs for hospital staff. Community living expenses must be met through tax revenues. Taxpayers may object to this use of their funds. Families may have been relieved by the decision to hospitalize a troubled member. They may not be eager to take him back. He recommends that the resolution to this dilemma may rest in study of the needs of patients and of the characteristics of hospital and community environments.[6] Therapeutic and damaging elements in both settings should be identified and this information used to develop more helpful patient care settings.

Rehabilitative psychiatric nursing must be studied in the context of the person and his social system. This requires a focus by the nurse on each of three elements: the individual, the family, and the community. This chapter has been designed to discuss each of these elements of the social system relative to the phases of the nursing process. Relevant nursing interventions will be identified at each phase.

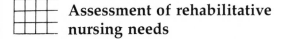

Assessment of rehabilitative nursing needs

The individual

Assessment of the person's need for rehabilitation begins at the time of the first contact between the nurse and the patient. A comprehensive psychiatric nursing assessment, as described in Chapters 4 and 17, is directed toward obtaining information that will enable the nurse to assist the patient to achieve his maximum possible level of functioning. This is, of course, the definition of rehabilitation. Nurses are expected to identify and reinforce the patient's strengths as one means of assisting him to cope with his weaknesses. This, too, is basic to the concept of rehabilitation. Thus good nursing care is really synonymous with rehabilitative nursing care.

When conducting the initial assessment of the patient, the nurse needs to think beyond the limits of her own patient care setting to try to anticipate the nature of the patient's other contacts with the health care system. In hospitals, this process is discharge planning and the need is obvious. However, nurses in community settings should also expect patients to progress to other levels of care. Although some people will need long-term maintenance outpatient care, many will be discharged from psychiatric care.

To assess the patient's readiness to move from one level of care to another, the nurse must understand the concepts of primary and secondary gain. *Primary gain* refers to the individual's efforts to cope with the predisposing and precipitating stressors. For instance, a person who feels compelled to wash his hands repetitively experiences a reduction in anxiety as a result of the behavior. The decrease in anxiety is the primary gain. Nursing care at the secondary prevention level focuses on interventions to assist the patient to develop healthier ways of accomplishing the primary gain.

Secondary gain refers to the other advantages that are associated with the sick role. In the American culture, sick people are expected to be incapacitated with limited ability to meet their own needs. Therefore they expect to receive help and attention from others. In return, they are expected to cooperate with a plan of care, indicating motivation to become well again. The extra attention and nurturing that is given to sick people can decrease the motivation to get better. Most people experience this even with a minor illness. A cold provides an excuse to stay home from school or work, sleep late, eat favorite foods, and indulge in relaxing activities. Even when one feels below par, there is pleasure associated with the release from daily responsibilities and a reluctance to resume them. The problem is magnified for the person who requires health care because of difficulties in coping with the stresses of daily life. Patient status can protect the person from the need to confront anxiety-provoking situations. Even when more effective coping mechanisms have been developed, it can be frightening to test them in a situation that was intolerable in the past. Bachmann[4] has described her experience as an expatient reentering the community. She discovered that it was difficult to relate to her old friends because of their difficulty understanding her experience. On the other hand, she lacked the self-confidence to reach out to new people. The greatest source of support for her was contact with other former patients. She comments that these significant relationships were discouraged by staff members who viewed them as a way of perpetuating illness. This emphasizes the need for the nurse to try to understand the patient's world and to respect his needs as he sees them. Bachmann also found the community boring compared to the hospital and began to develop a life pattern of working and sleeping. Nurses who are involved in busy community and family lives may fail to recognize the contrast that the patient experiences between the hospital and the community.

The resistance that is associated with secondary gain is sometimes thought to be a purposeful manipulation to avoid the resumption of responsibility. A punitive attitude toward the patient who is reluctant to move ahead is not

helpful. The person needs support and understanding. Helpful nursing interventions include the following:

1. Planning with the patient to resume activities one by one, starting with the least threatening
2. Role playing difficult situations before attempting to confront them
3. Accompanying the patient into the community to offer support if needed
4. Providing honest and timely feedback about the patient's attempts to become reengaged in his environment
5. Advocating for the patient's needs with family members and community agencies

Over an extended period of time, the reluctance to reenter the community tends to grow gradually. When a person is hospitalized for months or years, the handicap that Wing[28] has referred to as "institutionalism" develops. This is characterized by social withdrawal and resistance to leaving the hospital, even when the

TABLE 6-1. **Potential skilled activities needed to achieve the goal of psychiatric rehabilitation***

Physical	Emotional	Intellectual
Living skills		
Personal hygiene	Human relations	Money management
Physical fitness	Self-control	Use of community resources
Use of public transportation	Selective reward	Goal setting
Cooking	Stigma reduction	Problem development
Shopping	Problem solving	
Cleaning	Conversational skills	
Sports participation		
Using recreational facilities		
Learning skills		
Being quiet	Speech making	Reading
Paying attention	Question asking	Writing
Staying seated	Volunteering answers	Arithmetic
Observing	Following directions	Study skills
Punctuality	Asking for directions	Hobby activities
	Listening	Typing
Working skills		
Punctuality	Job interviewing	Job qualifying
Use of job tools	Job decision making	Job seeking
Job strength	Human relations	Specific job tasks
Job transportation	Self-control	
Specific job tasks	Job keeping	
	Specific job tasks	

*From Anthony, W.A.: Principles of psychiatric rehabilitation, © 1980, University Park Press, Baltimore.

surroundings are barely adequate. The institutional environment becomes comfortable because it is predictable and few demands are made. Some patients become angry or more symptomatic when they are being encouraged to move to the community. Some have hypothesized that this response of social withdrawal is a result of the lack of stimulation in the environment; others believe that it is a behavior related to severe mental illness, usually chronic schizophrenia. Although it is important that the cause be identified through research, in any case the nurse needs to work to assist the patient to develop trusting and caring relationships.

Discharge from an inpatient or partial hospitalization program should be based on careful interdisciplinary assessment of the patient's level of functioning. Gallagher[11] defines patient discharge as a process of social negotiation. He has reviewed the literature and identified other factors that frequently appear to determine readiness for discharge:

1. *Age.* Young patients are more likely to be discharged.
2. *Length of stay.* Potential for discharge decreases as the length of stay in the program increases.
3. *Life circumstances.* Housing and employment in the community increase the likelihood of discharge. Employment is a more important factor for men. Marriage, implying available housing, is more significant with women.
4. *Family wishes.* Family request facilitates release.
5. *Patient request for release.*

Although the success of the negotiation process and the influence of life factors may in reality determine discharge, nurses should strive to assess the patient's living skills and interpret this assessment to the patient, family, and interdisciplinary team. Anthony[2] has developed a matrix (Table 6-1) of the skills required for successful functioning in the community. He describes the physical, emotional, and intellectual components of the skills required for living, learning, and working. The nurse may use these examples in conjunction with the patient to identify the patient's strengths, establish goals, and set priorities for skill development. Use of such a model provides a rational basis for assessing the patient's readiness to function productively in the community. It also provides objective information that can be shared with the mental health care providers who will work with the patient in the agency to which he is transferred.

The family

The image of the isolated chronically mentally ill person who returns to a community where he has no connections has been widely publicized in recent years. However, the majority of mentally ill people are involved with their families and will have frequent contact with family members while they are in the community.[16] Therefore family resources must be assessed when a rehabilitation plan is being developed. Unfortunately, an adversary relationship frequently evolves between the patient's family and health care providers. The family may be viewed as the cause of the problem or as resistant to the treatment plan. Family members have a right to provide input to the treatment plan. They can identify potential problem areas. If their support is enlisted, they can be helpful in enhancing the patient's compliance with the plan. Hatfield[12] describes the needs of family members. She encourages mental health care providers to build alliances with families. She conducted a survey of 89 families of schizophrenic patients. She was able to identify the following patient behaviors or results of behaviors that are most disturbing to families:

1. Tension related to unpredictable behavior
2. Irregular sleep patterns that keep other family members awake as well
3. Mealtime disruptions
4. Argumentativeness
5. Negative relationships with siblings
6. Marital discord between parents

Although one might expect families to be angry at the patient for creating a disrupted family life or guilty for possibly playing a role in the problems, Hatfield elicited more feelings of grief and depression. If anger was present, it was usually directed at fate or the system rather than the patient.[12]

Doll[10] also conducted a survey of significant others of psychiatric patients. Whereas the Hatfield group was mostly upper middle class, the Doll group of 125 respondents was mostly lower middle and lower class. The findings of the two studies were quite consistent. The Doll group also denied shame or guilt connected to the patient's problem. These families were also able to accept some degree of deviant behavior, although there was a limit to their tolerance. High deviance did eventually lead to a decrease in acceptance of the patient. These families expressed the fear that there would be little or no change in the patient's condition. This was expressed as a feeling of being trapped.

Leavitt[17] interviewed the families of 16 patients who were being discharged from an inpatient psychiatric setting. They were all first-admission patients with an average length of stay of 1 month and 9 days. She found that the families were eager to discuss their responses to impending discharge with a receptive person. In general, the families were not prepared for the discharge of the hospitalized member. Leavitt identified several possible contributory factors relative to this response:

1. Pessimism about the future related to their opinion that the patient had not recovered
2. Lack of recognition of the hospital as a resource to the family
3. Lack of instruction and anticipatory guidance in how to respond to the patient's behavior
4. Failure to view themselves as a resource and as part of the treatment team
5. Limited communication with the staff concerning their perception of the patient's progress; inability to disagree with the staff's plan to discharge the patient
6. Absence of an empathic approach to the family by the staff

The nurse's assessment of the family should incorporate the growing body of knowledge about family responses to mental illness and about their needs. Supportive families need to be supported in turn so their resources are not depleted by the constant demands of the patient.

For some patients the emotional climate of the family to which they return can have a significant effect on their adjustment. Wing[27] has noted that schizophrenic patients have more problems when they are members of a hostile, critical, or overinvolved family. Vaughn and Leff[26] have found that schizophrenics have recurrences of their illnesses more frequently when there is a high level of expressed emotion in the family. These families need help to understand that intense emotion, either positive or negative, raises the patient's anxiety level. The emotional climate influences nonschizophrenic patients as well. Oversolicitousness reflects family members' insecurity and their concern that they might inadvertently cause a relapse. Protectiveness can be stifling to a patient who is striving to be independent and resume control of his own life.

On the other hand, rejection of the patient may also be a problem. Families sometimes view mental illness as a characterological weakness that can be overcome by their exertion of moral effort. This type of familial attitude may result in guilt on the part of the patient who believes that he has disappointed his significant others. Guilt leads to increased anxiety and decreased self-esteem. These are conditions that interfere with the achievement of a high level of functioning.

Reintegration of a patient into the family requires a readjustment of roles, particularly if a family member has been hospitalized for several weeks or months. In the normal family structure, functions are distributed among family members. The combination of functions assigned to a family member constitutes his role in the family. When a member is absent, others must perform his essential functions. If the absence is brief, the family structure readily reverts to its usual pattern when the missing member returns. However, if the member is away for a prolonged time, the family reorganization assumes an aspect of permanence. The members become emotionally attached to the new structure and may be reluctant to return to the earlier organization. Clinical example 6-1 illustrates this problem.

CLINICAL EXAMPLE 6-1

Ms. P was a 47-year-old woman who was hospitalized in the psychiatric ward of a general hospital following a suicide attempt. Her medical diagnosis was a major depressive episode. She gradually responded to interpersonal intervention and antidepressant medication and after 4 weeks felt well enough to return home.

The P family consisted of Mr. and Ms. P and their three children, a 16-year-old daughter and 12- and 10-year-old sons. The family was frightened and very concerned when Ms. P attempted suicide. The children worried about whether their behavior had caused their mother's depression. Mr. P spent a great deal of time reassuring them. He was more actively involved in the family than usual because he was the only available parent. He had to supervise the children's daily activities, assign chores, and referee their quarrels. He discovered that he liked getting to know his children better.

Lisa, the oldest child and only daughter, assumed

many of her mother's household responsibilities. She cooked, organized the cleaning, and supervised her brothers when her father was away. She enjoyed her new adult relationship with her father as they discussed household plans and problems with the younger children. During visits to the hospital, she became reluctant to tell her mother very much about what was happening at home.

When Ms. P returned home, everyone seemed happy and relieved. However, when she went into the kitchen to start dinner, Mr. P and Lisa insisted that she rest. She accepted this and was glad to see that Lisa was so capable. She also felt a bit guilty that her daughter had been required to take on so many extra duties. As Ms. P began to take over her household responsibilities, she found that she was frequently in conflict with Lisa, who would criticize her or her work. In addition, she felt shut out of the new relationship between Mr. P and the children. Because of her recent illness, she questioned whether her feelings were based in reality or if she was again becoming depressed. Fortunately, Ms. P discussed her dilemma with her nurse-therapist in the outpatient clinic who arranged for family counseling.

The P family situation is not an unusual one. The structure of the health care system with the discontinuity between home and hospital leads to problems such as theirs. Transitional services such as predischarge family counseling and postdischarge home visiting would have detected the potential problem and assisted the family to cope with the role changes that occurred. Family counseling assisted them to understand the reasons for their behavior. It only took a few sessions to help them reach a state of family equilibrium because the family was basically sound. Longer term intensive family therapy is often needed when the family system is seriously disturbed.

The nurse who is assessing the family as part of a rehabilitation plan should include the following areas:

1. Family structure, including developmental stage, roles, responsibilities, norms, and values
2. Family attitudes toward the mentally ill member
3. The emotional climate of the family
4. The social supports that are available to the family, including extended family, friends, financial support, religious involvement, and community contacts
5. The family's understanding of the patient's problem and the plan of care

Some of this information may be obtained by collaboration with the social worker. However, it is still a nursing responsibility to be available and accessible to the family. This includes regular planned contacts with the family and inclusion of the family as part of the treatment team.

The community

The community at large exerts a significant influence on the rehabilitation of its mentally ill members. Mental health professionals have a unique role in the community because they are simultaneously community members and advocates of the mentally ill. It can be difficult for patients and their families to demand that the community provide adequate services. Care providers, including nurses, can and should assume a leadership role in assessing the adequacy and effectiveness of existing community resources and in recommending changes.

Nurses in all treatment settings need to become familiar with the agencies in the community that provide services to patients. Most communities have a directory of social and medical services that can be consulted for basic information, such as location, type, and cost of the services provided. Most agencies serve a population that comes primarily from a particular geographical area, such as one part of a city, or in a rural area, perhaps one or several counties. As the nurse works with that population, she will become more familiar with other agencies that are involved with the same people. Nurses should pay attention to patients' evaluations of the agencies from which they receive services. This information helps to identify agencies that are responsive and helpful as opposed to those which are difficult for patients to approach. Personal contact with other community agencies can be very useful as part of a community assessment. This may be accomplished by arranging an appointment with an agency staff member. However, a more realistic picture of an agency's services can be obtained by accompanying a patient who is requesting services to the agency. This allows the nurse to see how the agency responds to the patient and how the patient handles his affairs in the community. The nurse can also provide emotional support to the patient if he is insecure about approaching a new situation. The nurse should identify herself to the staff of the agency and explain that she is accompanying the patient and also would like to learn more about the services that are offered.

Collaborative relationships between mental health care providers and community agencies are absolutely essential if rehabilitation is to succeed.

There are a wide range of services that need to be provided to patients as part of the tertiary prevention system. Those which are directed toward basic needs include provisions for shelter; food, clothing, and household management; income and financial support; meaningful activities; and mobility and transportation.[9] Other services provide for special needs that may differ from one patient to the next, such as general medical services, mental health services, habilitation and rehabilitation programs, vocational services, and social services.[9] A third group of services are integrative, with the purpose of coordinating the system. These include patient identification and outreach, individual

TABLE 6-2. Comprehensive array of services and opportunities for chronically mentally ill persons*

Basic needs/opportunities	Special needs/opportunities
Shelter	**General medical services**
Protected (with health, rehabilitative, or social services provided on site)	Physician assessment and care
Hospital	Nursing assessment and care
Nursing home	Dentist assessment and care
Intermediate-care facility	Physical/occupational therapy
Crisis facility	Speech hearing therapy
Semi-independent (linked to services)	Nutrition counseling
Family home	Medication counseling
Group home	Home health services
Cooperative apartment	
Foster care home	**Mental health services**
Emergency housing facility	Acute treatment services
Other board and care home	Crisis stabilization
Independent apartment/home (access to services)	Diagnosis and assessment
	Medication monitoring (psychoactive)
	Self-medication training
Food, clothing, and household management	Psychotherapies
Fully provided meals	Hospitalization: acute and long-term care
Food purchase/preparation assistance	
Access to food stamps	**Habilitation and rehabilitation**
Homemaker service	Social/recreational skills development
	Life skills development
	Leisure time activities
Income/financial support	
Access to entitlements	**Vocational**
Employment	Prevocational assessment counseling
	Sheltered work opportunities
	Transitional employment
Meaningful activities	Job development and placement
Work opportunities	
Recreation	**Social services**
Education	Family support
Religious/spiritual	Community support assistance
Human/social interaction	Housing and milieu management
	Legal services
Mobility/transportation	Entitlement assistance

Integrative services
Client identification and outreach
Individual assessment and service planning
Case service and resource management
Advocacy and community organization
Community information
Education and support

*From Department of Health and Human Services Steering Committee on the Chronically Mentally Ill: Toward a national plan for the chronically mentally ill, Pub. No. (ADM)81-1077, Washington, D.C., 1981, U.S. Government Printing Office.

assessment and service planning, case service and resource management, advocacy and community organization, community information, and education and support.[9] This overview of a community service system was developed by the Steering Committee on the Chronically Mentally Ill of the United States Department of Health and Human Services. It is described in greater detail in Table 6-2. Although the plan was developed with a focus on the chronically mentally ill, it is comprehensive and may be used to assess the range of services available to patients with all types of mental health care needs. These services may be provided in a variety of settings. Table 6-3 identifies the types of settings in which mental health care services might be provided according to the level of care that is needed.

It is important that an adequate number and type of services be available in the community. However, there is another aspect of community life that is more difficult to assess accurately and to deal with than that of service provision. This is the degree to which there is stigma attached to mental illness. According to Galla-

gher,[11] *stigma* was a term used by the Greeks to refer to body signs that indicated something negative about the person's worth. Today the stigma is attached to the behavior and does not relate to physical signs. A response to mental illness that is based on stigma is irrational and emotional. For this reason it is particularly difficult to change. Stigma is closely related to prejudice. Cumming and Cumming[8] found that student nurses tended to attribute mental illness to poor heredity or weak character. Although their landmark study of the effect of community education on attitudes toward the mentally ill was done in the 1950s, attitudes have changed little since then.

Gallagher[11] cites the contribution of the media to the perpetuation of stigma. Headlines always highlight the psychiatric history of a person who commits a crime. The positive achievements of rehabilitated formerly mentally ill people are seldom newsworthy. It would be rare, indeed, to see a headline stating "Child Saved from Burn-

TABLE 6-3. Typical settings for providing service clusters*

Acute treatment	Residential treatment	Rehabilitation	Psychosocial support
Housing setting			
Apartment/home (on site)	Public psychiatric hospital	Family	Family
Family (on site)	Nursing homes	Halfway house	Apartment
Foster family	Veterans hospital	Cooperative apartment (transitional)	Congregate housing (long term)
Crisis hostel	Forensic unit at public psychiatric hospital		Board and care home
Respite care home	Community forensic unit		Lodge
Emergency housing			Foster care home
General hospital			
Public psychiatric hospital			
Private psychiatric hospital			
Community mental health center inpatient unit			
Service setting			
Work		Social club	Social club
Telephone hotline		Psychosocial rehabilitation center	Psychosocial rehabilitation center
Other housing and hospital settings previously listed		Sheltered workshop	Sheltered workshop
		Industry setting	Community mental health center outpatient services
		Community college	Outpatient clinic
		Community mental health center outpatient services	Day treatment program
		Outpatient clinic	
		Day treatment program	

*From Department of Health and Human Services Steering Committee on the Chronically Mentally Ill: Toward a national plan for the chronically mentally ill, Pub. No. (ADM)81-1077, Washington, D.C., 1981, U.S. Government Printing Office.

ing House by Former Mental Patient." Television also contributes to the problem. Mental illness is portrayed as being a primary cause of violent behavior with the corollary that the mentally ill are always violent. This syllogistic message is destructive to the efforts of discharged patients to become productive community members.

Education is reported by Gallagher[11] to be the key factor in overcoming stigma. In general, more highly educated people have more realistic views of the range of behavior that may be associated with mental illness. However, this does not always correlate directly with complete acceptance. An individual might demonstrate intellectual understanding of mental illness and might be compassionate toward a friend or family member who receives psychiatric care. However, this same person might still oppose the establishment of a group home for the chronically mentally ill on his block or might refuse to ask a person with a history of psychiatric care to babysit for his children. These attitudes are as prevalent among nurses as they are among the general public. Consider this conversation between a head nurse and her supervisor:

NURSE: **Ms. T came back from sick leave today. She was in Riverview (a psychiatric hospital), you know.**

SUPERVISOR: **Yes, I know. How does she seem?**

NURSE: **All right, so far. I gave her a light assignment today, and I told her to come to me if she needs help.**

SUPERVISOR: **That's good. I hope she can handle things. She really *was* a good nurse.**

NURSE: **I do have one question for you. Should I let her have the medicine keys?**

On the surface, these two nurses seem concerned about the welfare of Ms. T and also seem to be appropriately planning for the care of the patients for whom they are responsible. However, they reflect some of the attitudes that can be most damaging toward people who are recovered from a mental illness. These include lack of confidence, an attitude of overprotectiveness and expectation of poor impulse control and unreliability.

Success in employment is a critical element of successful psychiatric rehabilitation. Prejudice toward mental illness can make it extremely difficult for an expatient to perform effectively in the work setting. Many employers are reluctant to hire people with a history of mental illness.

For this reason mental illness, including alcoholism and drug abuse, is included in the federal law prohibiting job discrimination on the basis of handicap. This means that to reject a job applicant because of a history of mental illness, an employer must prove that the person's disability will make it impossible for him to perform the job. This law is helpful in terms of enabling more people to become employed. However, it does not prevent the more subtle manifestations of discrimination, such as social isolation and devaluation of ability to do a good job.

Many patients and their families try to avoid stigma by keeping the nature of the person's illness a secret. The need for secrecy places additional stress on the family system, because there is always the fear that the truth will be revealed. Secrecy is also destructive because the family is essentially buying into the prevailing prejudice and conveying that there is something shameful about the patient's need for psychiatric treatment. Families are a part of society and as such, share the prejudices of other community members. Caplan[7] discusses the importance of assessing the family's prejudices, so they can be given assistance in recognizing and overcoming them. Otherwise, the patient may return to a setting where he is not trusted. This attitude may extend to relationships outside of the family. The whole family may decide to avoid talking about the illness of one member, because they perceive that others will blame the family for the problem.

Nurses who are also community members are in a position to monitor community attitudes. They can be helpful in interpreting the community to patients and also in modeling a realistic attitude toward the mentally ill members of the community. This requires awareness of one's own attitudes toward mental illness and the involvement of the mentally ill in society.

Planning and intervention

The individual

Treatment planning and intervention in rehabilitative psychiatric nursing focuses on fostering independence by maximizing the person's strengths. This is directly parallel to the nurse's role in physical rehabilitation. It differs from nursing care that is given to patients when they are acutely ill. During acute illness, whether physical or mental, people require a nurturing approach. The nurse must provide for all of the basic life functions that the person is unable to manage. However, the relationship gradually becomes less dependent as the patient grows stronger and better able to care for himself. Residual functional deficits may remain. The nurse and patient must then collaborate to devise ways for the patient to overcome any remaining impaired areas of functioning.

Peplau[22] described nursing roles relative to the patient's needs and ability to function. The unconditional mother-surrogate role related to the acutely ill phase and implied that the nurse would act in a maternal nurturing way. When the patient began to feel better, the nurse would assume a role characterized by some continuation of mother-surrogate functions with the addition of counseling, leadership, and resource person activities. The latter behaviors characterize the shift of responsibility from the nurse to the patient. People who choose nursing as a profession often have strong needs to nurture. It is important to be aware of this and not to let it interfere with the patient's need to develop self-care skills.

It may be difficult to alter traditional nurse-patient roles in a hospital or clinic setting. In recent years, there have been efforts to develop alternative settings for the delivery of mental health care, such as foster homes, halfway houses, and psychosocial rehabilitation centers. One such alternative treatment program is Soteria House.[21] In Greek, *soteria* means deliverance. Soteria House was developed as an alternative for psychotic patients to treatment programs based on the medical model. This avoids many of the problems associated with the need to assume the role of patient, including the implied dependency and lack of personal responsibility for behavior. Mosher and Menn[21] have compared the attitudes typical of Soteria House staff with those generally observed in a traditional mental health care setting (Table 6-4). Although it may appear that the Soteria approach fosters dependency, the ultimate objective is to help the person find meaning in his experience and to integrate it into his life. Staff acceptance of the patient and his right to his experience is critical for the patient's ultimate ability to accept himself. In addition, decision making and responsibility are controlled by patients unless they are absolutely unable to do so.

Another alternative intervention program has as its goal the maintenance of patients in their own homes in the community. This is the Training in Community Living program designed by Stein and Test.[25] In this model, when a person is

TABLE 6-4. A comparison of staff attitudes at Soteria House to those in a traditional mental health setting*

Soteria House	Traditional setting
Psychosis a valid experience	Psychosis an illness, therefore not an intimate part of person
"Being with" the individual	Maintain objectivity and distance
Important event, should be taken seriously	Getting over it most important
Understanding the experience important	Putting the experience behind important
Allow individual to experience his psychosis	Shore up defenses to suppress, repress, and abort psychosis
Regression allowed	Regression prevented or interrupted when possible
Containing, holding environment	"Moving on" environment
Growth and learning from psychosis valued	Getting over psychosis quickly valued
Minimal pressure to "get going"	Length of stay seen as critical

*From Mosher, L.R., and Menn, A.Z.: Lowered barriers in the community: the Soteria model. In Stein, L.A., and Test, M.A., editors: Alternatives to mental hospital treatment, New York, 1978, Plenum Press.

referred for hospital admission, the staff goes to the community with him rather than his going to the hospital to be with the staff. Nurses in this program accompany patients as they perform their usual activities, providing support and assistance when necessary. This real world experience with the patient enables the nurse to assess accurately the skills that the person needs to learn and to mutually agree on realistic goals. Staff contact is decreased as the patient demonstrates the ability to function independently. When the person is living with his family, they may also receive counseling and assistance in dealing with the patient's behaviors.

A third nonhospital intervention model is that developed by Polak et al.,[23] referred to as the Southwest Denver Model. They emphasize the need to consider and manipulate the social forces that influence the patient. This model also uses direct intervention in the social environment as the treatment approach. The major difference between this model and Training in Community Living is the focus. Whereas the latter model assists the patient to adjust to the environment, the Southwest Denver Model assists the environment to adjust to the needs of the patient. Intervention again takes place in the patient's social setting. If it is necessary for the patient to get away from his environment for a short time, foster care is arranged. Hospitalization is viewed as a last resort. If a patient is acutely psychotic or suicidal, an "intensive observation apartment" is available with close 24-hour supervision provided. A home day care program provides training in living skills in a home setting.

Foster home care is sometimes recommended for individuals who are discharged from the hospital, particularly those who have been hospitalized for a long time and have lost contact with relatives. There has been concern about foster home placement because lack of regulation of foster homes has resulted in situations where foster caregivers exploit the resident. However, well-run foster-care settings have been demonstrated to be effective.[18] Foster homes, of course, must be supplemented by treatment programs and provision for other psychosocial needs. Masnik, Olarte, and Rosen[19] describe a treatment program designed for patients with chronic mental illnesses. This was a "coffee group." Nonstructured group sessions were used to assess the condition and progress of patients and to encourage socialization. The social aspect was reinforced by the provision of coffee and cookies at each session.

These program examples are not meant to be an exhaustive catalogue of approaches to psychiatric rehabilitation. They demonstrate the application of creativity to a complicated problem. Nurses have been involved in most of these programs. There is a risk involved in challenging the traditional mental health care structures, but also a potential reward as people who have been excluded from society are reintegrated as productive members. It should be noted that comprehensive psychosocial rehabilitation programs, exemplified by the Fountain House model, are widely recommended for intervention with chronically mentally ill patients. These programs are discussed in Chapter 30.

Rehabilitative psychiatric nursing is directed toward maximizing the person's strengths and minimizing his weaknesses. The nursing care plan should be organized around very specific behavioral goals that are derived from a comprehensive assessment of the patient's living skills. These goals should be an extension of those which are developed as part of the secondary prevention process. Examples of such goals may be found in Chapters 7 to 14. This part of the nursing care plan may be labeled the discharge plan in an inpatient treatment setting. Discharge plans should also be developed in community settings to remind both the nurse and the patient that the ultimate goal is for independent functioning. Even patients who need long-term medications can usually receive maintenance prescriptions from their family physician as part of their general health care program. This helps to put the mental illness into perspective as a chronic health problem that is not so different from other chronic problems the patient might have.

Determination of a desired level of functioning must be an interactive process between the patient and the nurse. If the patient resists taking on activities that the nurse believes would be helpful, it is important to try to understand why this is so. Sometimes nurses try to push a patient ahead too rapidly. Behavior that has developed gradually over time and that has served a useful function for the patient cannot be changed quickly. Learning new behavior patterns and giving up old ones is frightening and anxiety provoking. The nurse must be sure that the patient's coping skills are adequate to deal with the stress of growth. Feedback must be solicited from the patient to be sure that the rehabilitation plan continues to be responsive to his needs. Sometimes the plan assumes greater importance than the patient. The nurse needs to guard against this.

Lamb et al.[15] have identified several guiding principles for the care of long-term psychiatric patients in the community. The first of these is that the patient must be given a sense of mastery over internal drives, symptoms, and environmental demands. To accomplish this, the care provider must use the second principle and work with the well part of the ego. "The goal is to expand the remaining well part of the person rather than to remove or cure pathology."[15:10] The third principle is that treatment should take place with the least possible envelopment of the patient and in a noninstitutional setting if possible. They advocate clear definition of goals

1/12/86

Dear Kathleen,

How are you? I'm fine. I have been meaning to write to you for a long time. How are the children. I saw the pictures that you sent for mommy Den. They, cedrick & Christine, grew so much. How about Didier? Did he get very tall? If I come to Haiti I know they won't recognize me. Tell them I said Hello anyway. How is the beauty salon, is everything going well. I don't think I will be coming to Haiti this year either because I need to make some money to pay to help pay for my school next year. But, Pierre-Michel will be coming in July for about a month. We are thinking about getting engaged in April for my birthday or for Easter. By the way, I have some bad news for you, Shilene broke-up her engagement with André. They don't want to say why the broke-ups. May be when I see you I'll give you all the details. Mommy Den had an operation on her foot and

been out of work for 2 months now.
She will be returning to work may
be of the 21st of January.

as another principle. The next is that work therapy should be a cornerstone of the program. They state that the change of status from mental patient to normal community resident is a crucial principle. The final principle states that normalization of the person's environment should always be a goal. These last two principles can be carried out by giving socialization goals high priority and by encouraging social activities in the community with community members.[16]

The nurse can perform the important role of advocacy for the patient. Significant others or community members may become impatient with the person as he struggles to regain control of his life. The nurse, with the patient's permission, can interpret the plan of care to others and enlist their support. She can also seek appropriate community services and assist the patient to make use of them. Human service systems are often not responsive to the needs of people who have problems dealing with stress. Role playing sometimes helps the patient practice the behaviors that he will need to use to find an apartment, obtain public assistance, or participate in a job interview. Group support may also be helpful. Small groups of people who are confronting similar challenges can provide a feeling of comradeship, as well as practical suggestions for handling specific situations. Nurses can organize and facilitate such groups.

Group support may also be found through involvement in self-help groups. These are groups of patients who meet to offer peer support and encouragement. Self-help groups do not solicit and frequently actively discourage involvement by mental health care providers. Providers may be viewed as representatives of an illness-focused system. Self-help groups emphasize the abilities of their members to serve as advocates for themselves and for others with similar problems. The nonthreatening experience of social support has been identified by Knight et al.[14] as the aspect of self-help groups that is most frequently described as helpful by members. Recovery, Inc., was the first self-help group formed by people with emotional problems. This group was modeled after Alcoholics Anonymous. More recently, other groups have organized to bring together chronically mentally ill people or those with a specific medical diagnosis, such as schizophrenia. Some self-help groups draw their membership from the families of mentally ill people who often feel caught between the demands of the patient on one hand and the health care providers on the other. Nurses can make patients aware of these groups and encourage them to attend. They can also offer themselves as resources to the group if the members identify a need with which a nurse could be helpful. Membership in a self-help group can be an important step toward independence by a person who is recovering from a mental illness.

The family

The involvement of a supportive family is tremendously important to the successful rehabilitation of a mentally ill person. The mental illness of a member is often a shock and a source of great stress to the family. Nurses are in a good position to assist families to cope with the stress and to adapt to related changes in the family structure. Hatfield[12] has described several needs of families related to the mental illness of a member. One important need is for knowledge. Families want to be able to understand the patient's behavior and how to respond helpfully to disturbed behavior. They would like a clear nontechnical explanation of the illness, as well as a prognosis that is as accurate as possible. Nurses can provide information, refer families to other health team members for further information, and provide suggestions on how to respond to disruptive behavior. One particularly perplexing problem for families is to be involved enough and interested enough without being intrusive on the one hand or distant on the other.[28] Nurses can offer assistance in this area by providing feedback to families about interactions that they have observed and by modeling effective communication skills. In some families, interaction will be disturbed to the extent that family therapy is required. Unless she has advanced preparation in this therapeutic modality, the nurse should refer the family to a qualified family therapist. Families also need to know about behaviors that could indicate a recurrence of the illness, so they can encourage the patient to seek help before hospitalization is required. Group education sessions for family members can be productive because participants can share experiences while they learn. This approach combines group support and education. Zelitch[29] has described a workshop series that was developed to meet the needs of patients' families with the following goals:

1. To educate families about mental illness
2. To engage the family's active participation in the patient's treatment
3. To facilitate self-help and support among families with similar concerns
4. To help families identify resources in the community
5. To assist relatives to assign priorities to their concerns
6. To teach relatives basic behavioral techniques that can be applied in dealing with the patient

Families also identified the need to be informed about available resources.[12] This enables them to assist the patient to utilize resources.

The second major need identified by the families in Hatfield's study[12] was to have someone with whom they could talk. Most of the people surveyed were self-help group members and had found that this peer support was helpful to them. The third need was for respite care resources. Respite care provides supervision for the patient in a community setting when the family needs relief from the demands of a mentally ill member. This service allows families to take a vacation or spend a short time away from the patient without feeling the guilt that they would if the patient was rehospitalized. The final need expressed was for crisis services, including home visiting. It can be very difficult for a family to persuade a disturbed member to go to a treatment facility, particularly if the patient has been hospitalized in the past and suspects that he will be again. Families are sometimes forced to wait until the situation becomes so bad that they must call the police to take the patient into custody. Crisis intervention in the home could avert this distressing situation.

Rubenstein[24] has described such a program. Treatment staff were alert to signs of an impending crisis, such as failure to keep appointments, failure to obtain prescriptions, and exceptional stress. If patients were unable to come to the clinic for treatment, nurses visited them at home. This enabled the treatment team to develop an accurate picture of the crisis as it occurred in the context of the family system. The nurse was able to help identify and eliminate the stressors in the situation, give prescribed medication if needed, and encourage the family to participate in treatment. Home visiting is an activity that is generally accepted by nurses, who are in turn usually well received in the community.

Helpful attitudes for professionals working with families of mentally ill patients have been identified.[28] Instead of approaching the family as an expert, which can lead to feelings of impotence resulting in anger, Wing and Olsen recommend a relationship of mutual learning. The nurse can then concentrate on empathizing with the family and participating with them in problem solving. Avoidance of the expert role also results in an attitude of accessibility that facilitates communication.

Anderson, Hogarty, and Reiss[1] have described a four-phase process for intervention with the families of schizophrenic patients. This model is summarized in Table 6-5. Phase I focuses on establishing a connection with the family. At first the therapist "joins" the family by engaging in social conversation and information sharing. This decreases anxiety by creating an atmosphere that is familiar to the family. Next the therapist assumes the role of "family ombudsman." This implies an alliance with the family and the avoidance of assigning blame for the patient's problems. The therapist shares information with the family and solicits their input for the treatment plan. The clinician's role is established as the family's representative and link with other parts of the health care system. The family's reactions to the illness are elicited, and their concern is mobilized in the patient's behalf. Finally, a treatment contract is agreed on. This includes the establishment of mutual goals.

Phase II is directed toward teaching survival skills for living with schizophrenia. This is done in the context of a day-long workshop. It is also hoped that a support network will be formed among the families who attend. In Phase III, the content from the workshop is applied to the individual family. There are generally two main themes during this phase: reinforcing family boundaries and the patient's gradually resuming responsibility. Respect for boundaries is communicated by allowing individuals to speak for themselves, allowing members to engage in separate activities, and by recognizing each member's area of vulnerability and limitation. Responsibility is gradually assumed by the patient by first helping with simple tasks, then functioning more independently as readiness develops. The family is encouraged to be patient because this can be a long slow process. Expectations must be realistic with one change made at a time. Phase IV begins when goals have been attained to the greatest possible extent. At this point, the family chooses between traditional family therapy or decreased involvement focus-

TABLE 6-5. Overview of the family intervention process*

Phases	Goals	Techniques
Phase I	Connect with the family and enlist cooperation with program	Joining
		Establishing treatment contract
	Decrease guilt, emotionality, and negative reactions to the illness	Discussion of crisis history and feelings about the patient and the illness
	Reduction of family stress	Empathy
		Specific practical suggestions that mobilize concerns into effective coping mechanisms
Phase II Survival skills workshop	Increased understanding of illness and patient's needs by family	Multiple family (education and discussion)
	Continued reduction of family stress	Concrete data on schizophrenia
		Concrete management suggestions
	Deisolation—enhancement of social networks	Basic communication skills
Phase III Reentry and application	Patient maintenance in community	Reinforcement of boundaries (generational and interpersonal)
	Strengthening of marital/parental coalition	
	Increased family tolerance for low-level dysfunctional behaviors	Task assignments
		Low-key problem solving
	Decreased and gradual resumption of responsibility by patient	
Phase IV Maintenance	Reintegration into normal roles in community systems (work, school)	Infrequent maintenance sessions
		Traditional or exploratory family therapy techniques
	Increased effectiveness of general family processes	

*From Anderson, C.M., Hogarty, G.E., and Reiss, D.J.: Schizophr. Bull. **6**:495, 1980.

ing on maintenance.[1] Although the model was developed for work with the families of schizophrenic patients, many of the principles apply to other families as well. Intervention utilizing the model should not be attempted without advanced education at the graduate level. However, understanding of family needs can facilitate the nurse's approach to relatives in her contacts with them. Nurses are often the most accessible members of the health care team, especially in inpatient settings. They can be very helpful if they try to understand family needs and reinforce family coping mechanisms.

The community

There are several ways in which nurses may intervene in the community to encourage the establishment of tertiary prevention programs. Among these are health education, membership in advocacy groups, networking, and political action. It has been noted that stigma decreases with increased formal education. Cumming and Cumming[8] hypothesized that community-based health education programs on the topic of mental health might have the same effect. They conducted a study based on this hypothesis in an attempt to change negative community attitudes toward the mentally ill. They failed in their efforts, but had some interesting observations related to the study. They believed that they should have found a way to motivate the community members to want to learn. They also assumed that they were aware of community attitudes, but later discovered that this was not so. They had used a psychiatrist as the educator in the project. They later decided that it might have been more effective to use community members, provided they were well-informed about the subject. The psychiatrist was a good teacher, but this was not the role expected of him by the community members. Finally, they came to believe that they should have stimulated direct involvement between community members and patients by encouraging volunteer activity as a part of the program.

Most nurses have a strong background and a firm belief in health education. Mental health education at the community level provides a real opportunity to have an impact on the experience of patients as community members. Greater understanding of the realities of the usual behaviors and the needs of the mentally ill could increase community acceptance, leading to the development of better services. People who refuse to allow group homes in their neighborhoods usually have irrational fears fueled by the media's distorted portrayal of mentally ill people. Education combined with direct contact with members of rehabilitation programs can be helpful in overcoming negative attitudes. Nurses should take advantage of opportunities to speak to community groups about mental health.

Membership by nurses in community advocacy groups can also be helpful. By this means, nurses can join forces with other professional and lay people who share concerns about the care of the mentally ill. The National Mental Health Association is the largest advocacy group that addresses mental health issues. Members of this organization have been instrumental in drawing attention to the needs of the mentally ill and in supporting positive legislation at the federal and state levels. They monitor the effectiveness of the mental health care system. Nurses can provide useful input to this part of their activities.

At a broader level, nurses can stimulate the development of collaborative relationships among advocacy groups, professional organizations, self-help groups, and concerned citizens. As fewer funds are available for the care of the mentally ill, the formation of coalitions is essential to lobby for the allocation of resources to mental health care. Coalition formation is also referred to as networking. Mitchell and Trickett[20] have identified functions served by social networks. They include "emotional support; task-oriented assistance; communication of expecta-

tions, evaluation, and a shared world view; and access to new and diverse information and social contacts."[20:30] These functions are also the factors that capture members' commitment to united action.

The activities of community-wide networks are frequently directed toward the political system. Aside from allocation of money and other resources, the nature of mental health care in a community is strongly influenced by the political structure of that community. As will be seen in Chapter 16, legal issues have a profound effect on mental health care delivery. Nurses need to be aware of and involved in the political process. They should communicate directly with their legislators at all levels, sharing their interests and concerns. Politicians are well aware of the need to be responsive to the priorities of their constituents. The number of nurses in the United States makes them a potentially powerful political force, but that power has seldom been exerted. If nurses are committed to positive health care, particularly at the primary and tertiary prevention levels, they must become visibly involved.

Nurses can also become more directly involved in the political system. They can run for office and support other nurses who are legislators. Nurses are often invaluable members of appointed boards and commissions having to do with health care. Their knowledge can be shared with others who are planning community health care systems. These voluntary activities are time consuming, but they can have great impact on the health care system. Community-level policies can either inhibit or facilitate direct care efforts. Active involvement in professional organizations often leads to productive and rewarding community activities. There is a great sense of satisfaction to be found in selling a community on a new idea and seeing it become a reality.

Evaluation

Many of the approaches to tertiary prevention that have been described are relatively new. Because of the long-term nature of many types of mental illness, the evaluation of these programs is in its early stages. Longitudinal studies will provide more valid and reliable measures of success or failure. Bachrach[5] has reviewed the literature on model programs for the care of chronically mentally ill people. She analyzed these programs at four levels. The first level is an evaluation of the success or failure of the individual program. The program may be measured according to a number of parameters. Externally determined criteria (e.g., cost-effectiveness or licensure standards), accomplishment of stated objectives, patient functioning, and patient or staff satisfaction are approaches to evaluation that have been used at the programmatic level. The second level is the assessment of commonalities among programs. Bachrach found the following eight common elements in successful programs[5]:

1. The targeting of a specific group of patients
2. Realistic linkages with other community resources
3. Provision of a full range of functions
4. Individualized treatment
5. Conformity with the local cultural system
6. Specialized training for staff
7. Liaison with a hospital for access to inpatient beds when needed
8. Presence of an internal evaluation system

The third level of evaluation relates to the reproducibility and generalizability of the program. This is identified as a problem by Bachrach for several reasons. One is that each program is developed in a cultural context that differs from others. Another is that model programs often have the advantage of special funding and other resources that are not available for duplicates. The very fact of being a model and therefore special can influence the outcome of a program. Another very important hindrance to reproducibility is the extent to which most successful programs depend on the leadership of one person or a small group of people who are extraordinarily committed to their program. There is frequently a charismatic leader associated with successful programs. Finally, the model programs are too new to tell whether they will stand the test of time.[5]

The fourth level of evaluation is that of relevance. This looks at the relationship of the program to the mental health care system. Bachrach[5] has named this impact evaluation. She questions whether model programs can really provide the answers to broader social problems. The model must be considered in the context of the system within which it exists.

Others have directed their efforts toward evaluating the effectiveness of rehabilitation programs by assessing the impact on the individual patient. Kelly et al.[13] looked for predictors of success in aftercare programs. They identified two, including involvement in occupational therapy and responsiveness to reinforcement in group therapy. Anthony et al.[3] have also recommended patient evaluation criteria. They settled on recidivism and posthospital employment as the most useful measures of community adjustment. However, they also recommend that evaluation efforts be extended and that rehabilitation programs take a closer look at their results. It is becoming obvious that if tertiary prevention efforts are to be supported in the future, it is necessary to prove that they are effective in both human and economic terms.

Suggested cross-references

The nursing process is discussed in Chapter 4. Intervention in social support systems is discussed in Chapters 4 and 5. Family assessment is discussed in Chapter 4, and identification of vulnerable families is discussed in Chapters 5 and 19. The care of the chronically mentally ill patient is discussed in Chapter 30.

SUMMARY

1. Tertiary prevention was defined as reduction of the rate of residual defect related to an episode of mental illness.

2. Psychiatric rehabilitation was identified as the process by which tertiary prevention is operationalized.

3. Concepts related to the assessment of the individual and rehabilitative nursing needs were described.

4. The concepts of primary and secondary gain were discussed as they relate to psychiatric rehabilitation.

5. Readiness for discharge from inpatient or partial hospitalization programs was analyzed in terms of patient characteristics and required skills.

6. Family assessment was discussed in the context of available resources for patient support. Important factors include family attitudes toward the patient, alterations in the roles of family members, the emotional climate of the family, the availability of social

support, and the family's understanding of the patient's illness.

7. Community assessment was described in terms of the nurse's responsibility to identify and evaluate community resources.

8. The phenomenon of stigma was presented as a representation of the resistance encountered by patients who attempt to reenter the social system.

9. The role of the nurse in planning and intervening in rehabilitative psychiatric care was related to responsiveness to the patient's readiness for increased independence.

10. Several model community programs for the provision of tertiary prevention services were described.

11. The development of specific mutual nurse-pa-

tient goals that are stated in behavioral terms was discussed relative to tertiary prevention.

12. Group intervention, including fostering self-help groups, was suggested as an appropriate activity for the nurse.

13. Strategies were presented for the support of the families of psychiatric patients. These included family education, involvement in a peer support group, provision for respite care, and crisis intervention, including home visiting.

14. Community interventions were proposed to encourage and support the development of tertiary prevention services. These include mental health education, membership in advocacy groups, networking, and political action.

15. Program evaluation was discussed in terms of the state of the art. Some criteria were identified, as were levels of evaluation. However, there is a need for more work in this area.

References

1. Anderson, C.M., Hogarty, G.E., and Reiss, D.J.: Family treatment of adult schizophrenic patients: a psycho-educational approach, Schizophr. Bull. **6**:490, 1980.
2. Anthony, W.A.: The principles of psychiatric rehabilitation, Baltimore, 1980, University Park Press.
3. Anthony, W.A. et al.: Efficacy of psychiatric rehabilitation, Psychol. Bull. **78**:447, 1972.
4. Bachmann, B.J.: Reentering the community: a former patient's view, Hosp. Community Psychiatry **22**:19, April 1971.
5. Bachrach, L.L.: Overview: model programs for chronic mental patients, Am. J. Psychiatry **137**:1023, 1980.
6. Bennett, D.: Deinstitutionalization in two cultures, Health Society **57**:516, 1979.
7. Caplan, G.: Principles of preventive psychiatry, New York, 1964, Basic Books, Inc., Publishers.
8. Cumming, E., and Cumming, J.: Closed ranks: an experiment in mental health education, Cambridge, Mass., 1957, Harvard University Press.
9. Department of Health and Human Services Steering Committee on the Chronically Mentally Ill: Toward a national plan for the chronically mentally ill, Pub. No. (ADM)81-1077, Washington, D.C., 1981, U.S. Government Printing Office.
10. Doll, W.: Family coping with the mentally ill patient: an unanticipated result of deinstitutionalization, Hosp. Community Psychiatry **27**:183, March 1976.
11. Gallagher, B.J., III: The sociology of mental illness, Englewood Cliffs, N.J., 1980, Prentice-Hall, Inc.
12. Hatfield, A.B.: The family as partner in the treatment of mental illness, Hosp. Community Psychiatry **30**:338, 1979.
13. Kelly, J.A. et al.: Objective evaluation and prediction of client improvement in mental health aftercare, Soc. Work Health Care **5**:187, Winter, 1979.
14. Knight, B. et al.: Self-help groups: the members' perspectives, Am. J. Community Psychology **8**:53, Jan. 1980.
15. Lamb, H.R. et al.: Community survival for long-term patients, Washington, D.C., 1976, Jossey-Bass, Inc., Publishers.
16. Lamb, H.R., and Goertzel, V.: The long-term patient in the era of community treatment, Arch. Gen. Psychiatry **34**:679, 1977.
17. Leavitt, M.: The discharge crisis: the experience of families of psychiatric patients, Nurs. Res. **24**:33, Jan.-Feb. 1975.
18. Linn, M.W. et al.: Hospital vs. community (foster) care for psychiatric patients, Arch. Gen. Psychiat. **34**:78, Jan. 1977.
19. Masnik, R., Olarte, S.W., and Rosen, A.: "Coffee groups": a nine-year follow-up study, Am. J. Psychiatry **137**:91, Jan. 1980.
20. Mitchell, R.E., and Trickett, E.J.: Task force report: social networks as mediators of social support, Community Mental Health J. **16**:27, Spring, 1980.
21. Mosher, L.R., and Menn, A.Z.: Lowered barriers in the community: the Soteria model. In Stein, L.I., and Test, M.A., editors: Alternatives to mental hospital treatment, New York, 1978, Plenum Press.
22. Peplau, H.E.: Interpersonal relations in nursing, New York, 1952, G.P. Putnam's Sons.
23. Polak, P.R.: A comprehensive system of alternatives to psychiatric hospitalization. In Stein, L.I., and Test, M.A., editors: Alternatives to mental hospital treatment, New York, 1978, Plenum Press.
24. Rubinstein, D.: Rehospitalization versus family crisis intervention, Am. J. Psychiatry **129**:715, 1972.
25. Stein, L.I., and Test, M.A.: An alternative to mental hospital treatment. In Stein, L.I., and Test, M.A., editors: Alternatives to mental hospital treatment, New York, 1978, Plenum Press.
26. Vaughn, C.E., and Leff, J.P.: The influence of family and social factors on the source of psychiatric illness, Br. J. Psychiatry **129**:125, 1976.
27. Wing, J.K.: Social psychiatry in the United Kingdom: the approach to schizophrenia, Schizophr. Bull. **6**:556, 1980.
28. Wing, J.K., and Olsen, R.: Community care for the mentally disabled, New York, 1979, Oxford University Press.
29. Zelitch, S.R.: Helping the family cope: workshops for families of schizophrenics, Health Soc. Work **5**:47, Nov. 1980.

Annotated suggested readings

Anderson, C.M., Hogarty, G.E., and Reiss, D.J.: Family treatment of adult schizophrenic patients: a psychoeducational approach, Schizophr. Bull. **6:**490, 1980.

The authors describe in detail an innovative approach to family intervention. Education is the focus until the family is ready to choose to deal with more psychodynamic issues. This article would be of interest to nurses with graduate level preparation who are involved in a family intervention program.

Anthony, W.A.: The principles of psychiatric rehabilitation, Baltimore, 1980, University Park Press.

This is an excellent book that describes a psychiatric rehabilitation program in great detail. It is clearly written and reflects the author's extensive experience in training mental health care providers to care for the seriously mentally ill.

Bachmann, B.J.: Reentering the community: a former patient's view, Hosp. Community Psychiatry **22:**19, April 1971.

In this article, a former patient describes her return to life outside the hospital. She shares the feelings that she experienced as she tried to cope with the demands of everyday life. She also reflects on the applicability to real-world situations of the values that she acquired in therapy. It is important for nurses to become aware of the experiences of discharged patients so that discharge planning can be relevant and helpful.

Bachrach, L.L.: Deinstitutionalization: an analytical review and sociological perspective, Department of Health, Education, and Welfare Pub. No. (ADM)79-351, Washington, D.C., 1979.

In this work the author attempts to pull together the many theories and opinions related to deinstitutionalization. It provides a good overview of the issues and includes a sociological analysis by the author. It is recommended for the advanced student or the nurse who is interested in performing research.

Bennett, D.: Deinstitutionalization in two cultures, Health Society **57:**516, 1979.

This article is an interesting exploration of the differences in the United States and United Kingdom approach to deinstitutionalization. The author conveys an understanding of the issues and events that have shaped these cultural differences. The contrast is fascinating.

Department of Health and Human Services, Steering Committee on the Chronically Mentally Ill: Toward a national plan for the chronically mentally ill, Pub. No. (ADM)81-1077, Washington, D.C., 1981, U.S. Government Printing Office.

This publication provides current and comprehensive information on the current status of the care of the chronically mentally ill in the United States. Mental health nurses should be familiar with its content and will find that it is a useful reference.

La Duke, D.L., et al.: Operation homeward bound—a military psychiatric transition program, J. Psychiatr. Nurs. **18:**22, July 1980.

The authors describe a psychiatric rehabilitation program that was implemented in a military setting. The primary interventions were educational in nature and focused on adaptation to the community, interpersonal skills, and job survival skills.

Langsley, D.G., Barter, J.T., and Yarvis, R.M.: Deinstitutionalization—the Sacramento story, Compr. Psychiatry **19:**749, 1978.

These authors demonstrate the effect of legislation on the provision of mental health care. They describe the changes that took place in Sacramento, California, in response to the passage of the Lanterman-Petris-Short Act, which reorganized the mental health care system in the state.

Leavitt, M.: The discharge crisis: the experience of families of psychiatric patients, Nurs. Res. **24:**33, Jan.-Feb. 1975.

This research report describes the results of interviews with the families of 16 psychiatric patients prior to discharge from the hospital. The investigator concluded that the families were not prepared to deal with the patient at home. She analyzes several reasons for this response.

Reid, L.: Approaches to the aftermath of schizophrenia, Perspect. Psychiatr. Care **17:**257, 1979.

The author discusses the reactions of the individual following hospitalization for psychotic behavior. A group approach focused on patient education is advocated, with encouragement of patients to ask questions and discuss their experiences. This is a good description of an effective nursing approach in a partial hospitalization setting.

Rubinstein, D.: Rehospitalization versus family crisis intervention, Am. J. Psychiatr. **129:**715, 1972.

This article describes a vigorous and responsive approach to crises as they arise with former inpatients. The intervention is family focused and directed toward keeping the patient in the community. The key role of the nurse is the maintenance of patient and family integrity by home visiting. Case studies illustrate the descriptive material.

Whitmer, G.L.: From hospitals to jails: the fate of California's deinstitutionalized mentally ill, Am. J. Orthopsychiatry **50:**65, Jan. 1980.

This is a presentation of the darker side of the deinstitutionalization experience as mandated by law in California. The author maintains that people who were forced out of state hospitals are now being found in state prisons. He criticizes the law in terms of the actual effect on people. It is a good demonstration of the impact of a political decision on human services.

.... The fears we know
Are of not knowing . . . It is getting late.
Shall we ever be asked for? Are we simply
Not wanted at all?

W.H. Auden, The Age of Anxiety

CHAPTER 7

ANXIETY

Learning objectives

*After studying this chapter, the student
should be able to:*

- *describe the characteristics of the concept of anxiety.*

- *compare and contrast the four levels of anxiety with regard to one's perceptual field, potential for learning, and continuum of coping responses.*

- *discuss the various theories that have been proposed on the origin of anxiety.*

- *analyze precipitating stressors that contribute to the development of anxiety.*

- *identify the physiological, behavioral, cognitive, and affective behaviors that are associated with anxiety.*

- *identify and describe the coping mechanisms associated with task-oriented reactions, ego-oriented reactions, psychological conversions, and physiological conversions.*

- *analyze the position of anxiety within the model of health-illness phenomena.*

- *formulate individualized nursing diagnoses for patients with varying levels of anxiety.*

- *assess the relationship between nursing diagnoses associated with anxiety and medical diagnoses of selected psychotic and neurotic disorders.*

- *develop long-term and short-term individualized nursing goals with patients who are experiencing anxiety.*

- *apply therapeutic nurse-patient relationship principles with appropriate rationale in planning the care of the patient who is experiencing anxiety.*

- *describe nursing interventions appropriate to the needs of the patient who is experiencing panic, severe, moderate, and mild levels of anxiety.*

- *analyze the indications for, techniques of, and problems associated with the relaxation interventions of systematic desensitization, meditation, and biofeedback.*

- *assess the importance of the evaluation of the nursing process when working with patients who experience anxiety.*

- *identify suggested readings for future study.*

During the past 20 years over 500 articles or books have been published on the topic of anxiety, which appears to be a pervasive aspect of contemporary life. It is created within the environment by threats of war, monetary inflation, the energy crisis, and political kidnappings. Anxiety is also created within the individual as one experiences inner confusion, conflicting values, role diffusion, and personal disenchantment. The seventeenth century was known as the Age of Enlightenment, the eighteenth as the Age of Reason, the nineteenth as the Age of Progress, and the twentieth as the Age of Anxiety. But anxiety is as old as human existence and belongs to no particular era or culture. It derives from the Greek root meaning "to press tight" or "to strangle"; the Latin term for "anxious" also denotes narrowness or constriction, usually with discomfort.

Although the concept of anxiety is timeless, its great impact on human life has been realized only in recent years. It is all-pervasive, and every corner of human endeavor is affected by anxiety. It is closely related to the terms "anger," when defined as "grief or trouble," and "anguish," which is described as "acute pain, suffering, or distress." Anxiety is a multidimensional concept, and it is manifested as a somatic, experiential, and interpersonal phenomenon. It therefore involves one's body, perceptions of self, and relationships with others. These elements make it a foundational concept in the study of psychiatric nursing and human behavior.

May defines anxiety as "diffuse apprehension that is vague in nature and associated with feelings of uncertainty and helplessness."[16:190] Feelings of isolation, alienation, and insecurity are also present as the person perceives that the core of his personality is being threatened. Experiences provoking anxiety begin in infancy and continue throughout life, concluding with the fear of the greatest unknown, death.

Understanding the concept of anxiety can be enhanced by exploring some of its characteristics. Anxiety is an emotion and a subjective experience of the individual. It is an energy, and as such cannot be observed directly. The perception of a nurse that a patient is anxious is an inference based on certain behaviors of the patient. As with all inferences, the nurse needs to validate this with the patient. Also, anxiety is an emotion without a specific object. It is provoked by the unknown and precedes all new experiences such as entering school, starting a new job, or giving birth to a child. This characteristic of anxiety differentiates it from fear, which is an ideation of the individual that has a specific source or object which the person can identify and describe. This distinction is evident in the phrases used in speaking of the two emotions; one speaks of *having* a fear but of *being* anxious. Another important characteristic of anxiety for the nurse is the fact that it is communicated interpersonally. This means that if a nurse is talking with a patient who is anxious, within a short time the nurse will also experience feelings of anxiety. Similarly, if a nurse is anxious in a particular situation, this will be readily communicated to the patient. The contagious nature of anxiety can therefore have positive and negative effects on the therapeutic relationship and must be diligently monitored by the nurse. It is also important to remember that anxiety is part of the fabric of everyday life. It is basic to the human condition and provides a valuable warning system to the individual. In fact, the capacity to be anxious is necessary for survival.

The balance between survival and death addresses the crux of anxiety—preservation of self. Anxiety occurs as a result of a threat to a person's selfhood, self-esteem, or identity. Tillich describes it as "the state in which a being is aware of its possible non-being."[27] It occurs when something central to one's personality, essential to one's existence and security, is being threatened. It may be connected with the fear of punishment and disapproval, withdrawal of love, disruption of a relationship, isolation, or loss of body functioning. Anxiety is experienced when the values a person identifies with his existence as a person are threatened. In this way culture is related to anxiety in that culture determines in part the values the individual holds as most important. These values include the physical, social, moral, and emotional elements of life. Underlying every fear is the anxiety of not being

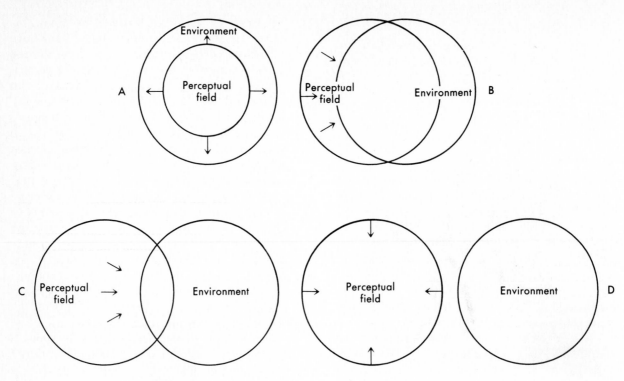

FIG. 7-1
Levels of anxiety. **A,** Mild. **B,** Moderate. **C,** Severe. **D,** Panic.

able to preserve one's own being, and this is the frightening element. However, a person can meet the anxiety and grow from it to the extent that his values are stronger than the threat.

All people therefore need a balance between courage and anxiety to preserve themselves, fulfill their beings, and affirm their existence. It is only by moving through anxiety-creating experiences that one achieves self-realization. Whenever a person moves through new possibilities, he enlarges his self-awareness, increases the scope of his activity, and expands his freedom. As May summarizes it, "the positive aspects of selfhood develop as the individual confronts, moves through and overcomes anxiety-creating experiences." [16:234]

Continuum of anxiety responses

In defining the concept of anxiety, Peplau[22] identified four levels of anxiety and described the effects of each on the individual (Fig. 7-1). The first is *mild anxiety,* which is associated with the tension of day-to-day living. During this stage the person is alert and his perceptual field is increased as he sees, hears, and grasps more

than previously. This kind of anxiety can motivate learning and can produce growth and creativity in the individual. The second level is *moderate anxiety,* in which the person focuses on immediate concerns and blocks out the periphery. His perceptual field is narrowed as he sees, hears, and grasps less. He thus experiences selective inattention but can attend to more if he is directed to do so. The third level is *severe anxiety,* in which the person's perceptual field is greatly reduced. He tends to focus on a specific detail and not think about anything else. All his behavior is aimed at getting relief and he needs much direction to focus on another area. The final level is *panic,* which is associated with awe, dread, and terror. At this time details are blown out of proportion. Because the individual is experiencing a loss of control, he is unable to do things even with direction. Panic involves the disorganization of the personality. It is a state in which a person can no longer function as an organized human being. With panic there is increased motor activity, decreased ability to relate to others, distorted perceptions, and loss of rational thought.[20] This is a frightening and paralyzing experience for the individual in which he

FIG. 7-2
Continuum of anxiety responses.

is unable to communicate or function effectively. This level of anxiety cannot persist indefinitely. It is incompatible with life, and, if it continued over a prolonged period, exhaustion and death would result.

The nurse working with a patient will be able to identify which level of anxiety is present on the basis of the behaviors she observes. The anxiety response may then be conceptualized on the continuum of coping responses described in the model of health-illness phenomena (Chapter 4). Fig. 7-2 characterizes the anxiety response as ranging from the most adaptive response of anticipation to the most maladaptive response of panic. The nurse's identification of the patient's level of anxiety and its position on the continuum of coping responses will be relevant to her nursing diagnosis and will subsequently affect the type of intervention she chooses to implement.

 Stressors

Anxiety is a prime factor in the development of the personality and formation of individual character traits. It is natural, then, that various theories of the origin of anxiety would exist. However, the present core of definitely established facts to support these theories is small.

Freud initiated the study of anxiety, and his position underwent a drastic change 30 years after he first formulated it. In the beginning Freud regarded anxiety as a purely physiological reaction to a person's chronic inability to reach an orgasm in sexual relations. He believed that if the sexual instincts were not allowed to express themselves directly, their energy would be converted into anxiety. Alleviation of anxiety therefore merely required the proper adjustments in the patient's sexual technique. Not un-

til much later did he see the importance of anxiety for a theory of personality development.[10]

His change in viewpoint led him to describe two types of anxiety—primary and subsequent. The essence of primary anxiety is the "traumatic" state, which originates in the infant as a result of the sudden stimulation and trauma of the birth process. The process of birth is the first experience attended by anxiety, and experiences of anxiety continue with the possibility that one's physical needs of hunger and thirst might not be met. Primary anxiety therefore was viewed as a state of tension or a drive produced originally by external causes. The environment was seen as being capable of threatening as well as satisfying, and this implicit threat predisposed the individual to anxiety in later life.

With increased age and ego development, a new kind of anxiety arises. Freud viewed this subsequent anxiety as the emotional conflict that takes place between two elements of the personality—the id and the superego. The id represents one's instinctual drives and primitive impulses, whereas the superego reflects one's conscience and culturally acquired restrictions. The ego, or I, serves as the battleground as it tries to mediate the demands of these two clashing elements. Freud therefore suggested that one major function of anxiety was to warn the person of impending danger. It was a signal to the ego that it was in danger of being overtaken.

Sullivan[26] disagreed with Freud in that he believed that anxiety could not arise until the ego reached a minimum stage of development in which the organism had some awareness of its environment. Sullivan viewed the fear of disapproval as central to his theory of anxiety. He looked to the origin of anxiety in the early bond between the infant and mothering one. Through this close emotional bond, anxiety is first conveyed by the mother to the infant, who responds as if he and his mothering person were one unit. As the child grows older, he sees this discomfort as related to what he himself does and conceives of his mother as approving or disapproving of his behavior. Sullivan believed anxiety in later life arises in interpersonal situations in which a person perceives he will be viewed unfavorably by another person whose opinion he values.

Sullivan identified two other aspects of anxiety that will be important in the nurse-patient relationship. The first is that a mild or moderate level of anxiety is frequently expressed as anger by the individual. The second is that areas in the personality marked by anxiety often become the areas of significant growth when, as in a therapeutic relationship, the individual can learn to deal with his anxiety constructively.

Will[28] believes that an individual's level of self-esteem is an important factor related to anxiety. A person with a high predisposition to anxiety is one who is easily threatened, has a low level of self-esteem, or has a poor opinion of himself. This is evident in a person with test anxiety. His anxiety is high because he doubts his ability to succeed. This may have nothing to do with his actual abilities, how prepared he is, or how much he studied; the anxiety is due only to his perception of his ability, which reflects his self-concept. He may, for instance, be well prepared for the examination, but his severe level of anxiety will reduce his perceptual field significantly and he may omit, misinterpret, or distort the meaning of the test items. He may even block out all his previous studying when handed the examination. The result will be a poor grade, and this will in turn reinforce his poor perception of self. Research supports the theory that individuals with high anxiety appear to have a greater discrepancy between their perceived self and ideal self.[25] Thus low self-esteem can be a cause of proneness to high anxiety.

Some behavioral theorists propose that anxiety is a product of frustration, which is anything that interferes with one's ability to attain a desired goal. The actual precipitating factor may be any of a number of internal or external stressors, but it acts to block the individual's attempt to obtain satisfaction and security. An example of an external frustration for a young man might be his factory's decision to lay off a certain number of employees, including himself.

In this instance, many of his goals may be potentially blocked, such as financial security, pride in work, and perception of self as family provider. An internal frustration is evidenced by the young college graduate who sets unrealistically high personal career goals and continues to be frustrated by job offers of a clerical or apprentice nature. In this case his view of self is being threatened by his unrealistic goals, and he is likely to experience feelings of failure, insignificance, and mounting anxiety.

Other experimental psychologists regard anxiety as a learned drive based on an innate desire to avoid pain. They believe that anxiety begins with the attachment of pain to a particular stimulus, and, if the reaction is strong enough, it may become extended or generalized to similar objects and situations. Learning theorists believe that individuals who have been exposed in early life to intense fears are more likely to demonstrate a high predisposition to anxiety in later life. In this respect, parental influences are important. The child who sees his parents respond with anxiety to every minor stress soon develops a similar pattern. This can also occur if the child's parents are completely unmoved by potentially stressful situations. In this case the child feels alone and lacks emotional support in family stress situations. It is the appropriate emotional response of parents that gives the child security and helps him learn constructive coping methods of his own.

Another way in which anxiety is theorized to arise is through conflict, which is defined as the clashing of two opposing interests. The person experiences two competing drives and must choose between them. A reciprocal relationship exists between conflict and anxiety; conflict produces anxiety and yet anxiety produces feelings of helplessness, which in turn increases one's perceived conflict. Dollard and Miller[8] conceptualize conflict as deriving from two tendencies: approach and avoidance. Approach is the tendency to do something or move toward something, whereas avoidance is the opposite tendency—not to do something or not to move toward something. The authors identify four kinds of conflict (Fig. 7-3). The first is the *approach-approach* conflict in which the individual is motivated to pursue two equally desirable but incompatible goals. This type of conflict seldom produces anxiety, which is more prevalent in conflicts involving avoidance. *Approach-avoidance* conflict occurs when the individual wishes both to obtain and avoid a goal at the same time.

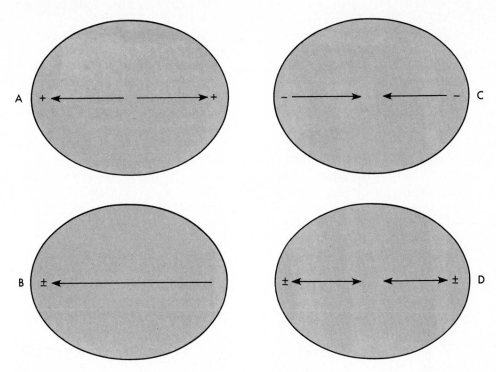

FIG. 7-3
Types of conflict. **A,** Approach-approach. **B,** Approach-avoidance. **C,** Avoidance-avoidance. **D,** Double approach-avoidance.

This can be evident in the patient who desires to express his anger but feels great anxiety and fear in doing so or in the business executive who wishes to be advanced within his company but to be promoted must compromise his values of honesty and loyalty. *Avoidance-avoidance* is a third kind of conflict in which the person must choose between two undesirable goals. This is a difficult choice, since neither alternative seems beneficial, and it is usually accompanied by much anxiety. The most common type of conflict situation is the *double approach-avoidance*. In this case the person can see both desirable and undesirable aspects of both alternatives. Frequently this is the kind of conflict experienced by a person who must choose between continuing to live with the pain of his social and emotional life and destructive coping patterns or expose himself to the threat and potential pain of the therapy process, should he seek psychiatric help. These kinds of double approach-avoidance conflict feelings are frequently described as ambivalence. In summarizing their theory, Dollard and Miller stress the importance of conditioning early in life but assert that still

little is known about how most complex learned drives are acquired or about those factors which permit one person to easily resolve a conflict while another is plunged into a tumultuous emotional state.

This same lack of scientific evidence is demonstrated in studies that attempt to identify a physiological cause for anxiety. Research attempts to discover endocrinological or metabolic causes continue, but nothing conclusive has yet been discovered. It has been determined, however, that the individual's general health does have a marked effect on his predisposition to anxiety. His coping mechanisms may be impaired by toxic influences, dietary deficiencies, reduced blood supply, hormonal changes, and other physical causes. In the presence of physical illness there is input from somatic sources that may reduce his capacity to cope with additional stressful inputs. In this way, too, fatigue increases irritability and feelings of anxiety. It appears that fatigue produced as a result of nervous factors predisposes the individual to a greater degree of anxiety than does fatigue that has resulted from purely physical causes. Thus fatigue may actually be an early symptom of anxiety, and patients complaining of nervous fatigue may already be suffering from a moderate anxiety state and be more susceptible to future stress situations.

Precipitating stressors

Given these numerous theories about the origin of anxiety, what kinds of events might precipitate feelings of anxiety within the individual? It is possible to group precipitating stressors into two categories: threats to one's physical integrity and threats to one's self-system. Threats to one's physical integrity suggest impending physiological disability or decreased capacity to perform the activities of daily living. They may include exposure to viral and bacterial infection or to environmental pollutants or safety hazards (external source); failure of one's own physiological mechanisms, such as the heart, immune system, or temperature regulator (internal source); lack of adequate housing, food, or clothing (external source); normal biological changes that might occur with pregnancy or aging (internal source); traumatic injury (external source); or failure to participate in preventive health practices in such areas as dental care, exercise, rest, or routine physical examinations (internal source). Pain is often the first indication that one's physical integrity is being threatened. It creates anxiety that often motivates the person to seek health care. Thus some preventive health programs try to generate mild anxiety. Because threats to one's physical integrity do produce anxiety, many of the patients nurses work with will experience these feelings.

Threats to one's self-system, the second category, are quite pervasive. Basically, they imply harm to one's identity, self-esteem, and integrated social functioning. They may include a variety of losses, such as a spouse, parent, or close friend through death, divorce, or relocation (external source); interpersonal difficulties at home, at work, or in the community (internal sources); change in job status (external source); assumption of a new role, such as parent, student, employee, or group leader (internal source); ethical dilemmas arising from one's religious, family, or work situation (external source); social or cultural group pressures (external source); and many of the threats to physical integrity previously mentioned, since the mind-body relationship is an intimate and overlapping one.

In fact, this distinction of categories is only theoretical, since the person responds to all stressors, whatever their nature and origin, as an integrated whole. Neither will any event be viewed as equally stressful to all individuals or even to the same individual at different times. The person's response will depend on the number and timing of the stressor and the predisposing factors previously described, as well as on the person's perception of the event and the resources he has available. By observing specific behaviors, the nurse will be able to assess the individual's level of anxiety, identify his coping responses, and then formulate an appropriate nursing diagnosis.

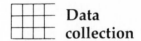 **Data collection**

Behaviors associated with anxiety

Anxiety can be expressed directly through physiological and behavioral changes. It can also be indirectly manifested through the formation of symptoms or coping mechanisms that attempt to defend one against anxiety. The nature of the behaviors displayed by the patient depends on his level of anxiety. The intensity of the behaviors will increase with the increasing level of anxiety.

In describing anxiety's effects on physiological functioning, it can be seen that mild and moderate anxiety heighten one's capacities, whereas severe and panic levels paralyze or overwork capacities and structures. The physiological responses associated with anxiety are primarily mediated through the autonomic nervous system. This involves the internal adjustment of the body without a conscious or voluntary effort by the individual. There are two kinds of autonomic responses: the sympathetic, which serve to activate body processes, and the parasympathetic, which act to conserve body responses.

Experimental studies support the predominance of the sympathetic reaction, which prepares the body to deal with an emergency situation by either a "fight" or "flight" reaction. When the cortex of the brain perceives a threat, it sends a stimulus down the sympathetic branch of the autonomic nervous system to the adrenal glands. Because of a release of epinephrine, respiration deepens, the heart beats more rapidly, and arterial pressure rises. Blood is shifted away from the stomach and intestines to the heart, central nervous system, and muscle. Glycogenolysis is accelerated, and the blood glucose level rises. For some individuals, however, the parasympathetic reaction may coexist or predominate and produce somewhat opposite effects. Other physiological reactions may also be evident. The variety of *physiological responses* to anxiety that the nurse may observe in patients can be summarized as follows:

Sympathetic responses

Increased heart rate and palpitations
Elevated blood pressure
Muscular tension, particularly of the chest, neck, and back
Difficulty breathing
Increased perspiration
Hyperventilation
Weakness and fatigability
Dilated pupils
Facial pallor
Constipation
Cold clammy skin
Dry mouth
Anorexia

Parasympathetic responses

Urinary frequency
Diarrhea
Lowered blood pressure
Slowed heart rate

Related responses

Headaches, blurring of vision
Nausea or vomiting
Sleep disturbances
Interference with sexual functioning
Abdominal discomfort

Psychomotor manifestations, or behavioral responses, will also be evident by the patient in the anxious state. Its effects have both personal and interpersonal aspects. High levels of anxiety affect one's coordination, involuntary movements, and responsiveness. They also act as disjunctive forces in human relationships. In an interpersonal situation, anxiety can be a warning that discomfort is to be anticipated and the person had best withdraw from the threatening situation. It is therefore common to see signs of withdrawal and decreased personal involvement with others displayed by the anxious patient. The possible *behavioral responses* the nurse might observe are as follows:

Restlessness (which may progress to agitation)
Physical tension
Tremors (varying from fine digital tremors to gross shaking of the entire body)

Startle reaction
Rapid speech
Lack of coordination of actions and movements
Accident proneness
Interpersonal withdrawal

Mental, or intellectual, functioning is also affected by anxiety. *Cognitive responses* the patient might display when experiencing moderate, severe, or panic levels of anxiety include the following:

Impaired attention
Poor concentration
Forgetfulness
Errors in judgment
Preoccupation
Blocking of thought
Decreased perceptual field
Reduced creativity
Diminished productivity
Confusion

Finally, the nurse will be able to assess a patient's emotional reactions, or *affective responses,* to anxiety by his subjective description of his personal experience. Frequently patients describe themselves as "tense, jittery, on edge, jumpy, worried, or restless." One patient attempted to describe his feelings in the following way: "I'm expecting something terribly bad to happen, but I don't know what. I'm afraid, but I don't know why. I guess you can call it a generalized bad feeling." All these phrases are expressions of a person's apprehension and overalertness. They convey the impression that all is not well, and it seems clear that the person interprets his anxiety as a kind of warning sign.

Anxiety is an unpleasant and uncomfortable experience that no one wants or will seek out. Most people will go to extremes to avoid it and frequently try to replace its awareness by some other feeling that is more tolerable. Pure anxiety is rarely seen, but it is usually observed in combination with other emotions. Patients might describe feelings of anger, boredom, contempt, depression, irritation, worthlessness, jealousy, self-depreciation, suspiciousness, sadness, or helplessness, which may be viewed as defenses to shield them from the distress of anxiety. This may present problems for the nurse who is trying to discriminate between anxiety and depression, for instance, because the content expressed by the patient may be similar.[18]

In fact, there are close ties between anxiety,

depression, guilt, and hostility, and these emotions often function in a reciprocal manner—one feeling acts to generate and reinforce the others. The relationship between anxiety and hostility is particularly close, since the pain one experiences with anxiety frequently gives rise to anger and resentment toward those perceived to be responsible, and these feelings of hostility then serve to increase one's level of anxiety. This cycle is evident in the case of a dependent and insecure wife who was very attached to her husband and who expressed numerous vague fears. In exploring her feelings, she also expressed great hostility toward him and their relationship, which symbolized her helplessness and increased her feelings of weakness. Verbalizing these angry feelings, however, served to further increase her anxiety and her unresolved conflict. Thus it is evident that anxiety frequently finds expression in anger, and a tense and anxious person is more likely to become angry.

Coping mechanisms

As the level of anxiety increases to the severe and panic levels, the behaviors displayed become more intense and injurious to the individual. It is obvious that these behaviors may be painful, uncomfortable, and unpleasant. It is also understandable, then, that people seek to avoid anxiety and the circumstances in which it arises. When experiencing anxiety, the individual uses various coping mechanisms to try to allay it, and the inability to cope with anxiety constructively is a primary causative factor in the creation of pathological behavior. In an attempt to neutralize, deny, or counteract anxiety the individual develops patterns of coping, and the pattern he uses to cope with mild anxiety tends to remain dominant when anxiety becomes more intense. It can be said that anxiety plays a major role in the psychogenesis of emotional illness, since many symptoms of illness develop as attempted defenses against anxiety. These symptoms also provide the outward but disguised symbolical expression of elements of the conflict.

It is beneficial for the nurse to be familiar with the coping mechanisms people use when experiencing the various levels of anxiety. The *mild level of anxiety* is the anxiety one experiences as the tension of day-to-day living. Menninger[19] identified a number of coping mechanisms people use to relieve this kind of tension. These include crying, sleeping, eating, yawning, laughing, cursing, physical exercise, daydreaming, and oral behavior, such as smoking and drinking. In interpersonal situations the individual copes with low levels of anxiety through superficiality, lack of eye contact, use of clichés, and limited self-disclosure. The person can also protect himself from anxiety by assuming roles he is comfortable in and limiting his close relationships to those with people having values similar to his own. Thus mild levels of anxiety are often handled without conscious thought and their effects can be minimized with little effort.

Moderate, severe, and panic levels of anxiety, however, pose greater threats to the ego and require the use of more energy to cope with the threat. It is possible to categorize these coping mechanisms as task-oriented reactions, ego-oriented reactions, psychological conversions, and physiological conversions. Each of these mechanisms will be explored.

TASK-ORIENTED REACTIONS. Task-oriented reactions involve one's cognitive abilities in an attempt to solve problems, resolve conflicts, and gratify one's needs. They are aimed at realistically meeting the demands of the stress situation, which has been objectively appraised. These are consciously directed and action oriented. These types of reactions can include attack, withdrawal, and compromise.

In *attack behavior* a person attempts to remove or overcome obstacles to satisfy a need. There are many possible ways of attacking problems, and this type of reaction may be destructive or constructive. Destructive patterns are usually accompanied by great feelings of anger and hostility, which may be discharged in negative or aggressive behavior that violates the rights, property, and well-being of others. Constructive patterns reflect a problem-solving approach and are evident in self-assertive behaviors that affirm one's own rights while also respecting the rights of others.

Withdrawal behavior may be expressed physically or psychologically. Physically, withdrawal involves removing oneself from the source of the threat. This can apply to biological stressors, such as smoke-filled rooms, exposure to irradiation, or contact with contagious diseases. An individual can also withdraw in various psychological ways, such as by admitting defeat, becoming apathetic, or lowering aspirations. As with attack, this type of reaction may be constructive or destructive. When it is used in a way that isolates the individual from others and interferes with his ability to work, the reaction begins to create additional problems for the individual and is often accompanied by the emotional states of fear, hostility, and guilt.

Because some situations cannot be resolved through either attack or withdrawal, *compromise* is frequently necessary. This involves changing one's usual way of operating, substituting goals, or sacrificing aspects of one's personal needs. Compromise reactions are usually constructive and are frequently employed in approach-approach and avoidance-avoidance situations. When the decision resolves the problem, the individual can then move on to other activities. Occasionally, however, the person realizes with time that the compromise is not acceptable, and he must then renegotiate a solution or adopt a different coping mechanism.

A person's capacity for task-oriented reactions and effective problem solving is greatly influenced by his expectation that he is likely to succeed in achieving at least a part of his goals. This, in turn, will depend on his remembering that he was successful in the past in situations of similar difficulty and that he was able to overcome the presenting obstacles. On this basis, he can go forward and attempt to do something about the stressful situation. Perseverance in problem solving also depends on the person's expectation that a certain level of pain and discomfort is likely to be involved and his belief that people like himself are capable of tolerating this. Herein lies the balance between courage and anxiety.

EGO-ORIENTED REACTIONS. Task-oriented reactions are not always successful in coping with stressful situations. Consequently, ego-oriented reactions are often used to protect the self. These reactions, also called *ego defense mechanisms*, serve as one's first line of psychic defense. Everyone uses defense mechanisms, and they frequently help one cope successfully with mild and moderate levels of anxiety. They function to protect the person from feelings of inadequacy and worthlessness and prevent awareness of anxiety. They can be used to such an extreme degree, however, that they distort reality, interfere with interpersonal relationships, limit one's ability to work productively, and promote ego disintegration instead of self-integrity. As coping mechanisms they have certain drawbacks. First, they operate on relatively unconscious levels so that the person has little awareness of what is happening and little control over events. Second, they involve a degree of self-

Ego defense mechanisms

Defense mechanism	Example
Repression: Involuntary exclusion of a painful or conflictual thought, impulse, or memory from awareness. It is the primary ego defense, and other mechanisms tend to reinforce it.	Mr. T does not recall hitting his wife when she was pregnant.
Suppression: A process often listed as a defense mechanism, but it is really a conscious analogue of repression. It is intentional exclusion of material from consciousness. At times, it may lead to subsequent repression.	A young man at work finds he is thinking so much about his date that evening that it is interfering with his work. He decides to put it out of his mind until he leaves the office for the day.
Identification: Process by which a person tries to become like someone he admires by taking on thoughts, mannerisms, or tastes of that individual.	Sally, 15-years-old, has her hair styled similarly to her young English teacher whom she admires.
Introjection: Intense type of identification in which a person incorporates qualities or values of another person or group into his own ego structure. It is one of the earliest mechanisms of the child; important in formation of conscience.	Eight-year-old Jimmy tells his 3-year-old sister, "Don't scribble in your book of nursery rhymes. Just look at the pretty pictures."
Displacement: Shift of emotion from a person or object toward which it was originally directed to another usually neutral or less dangerous person or object.	Timmy, a 4-year-old boy, is angry because he has just been punished by his mother for drawing on his bedroom walls. He begins to play "war" with his soldier toys and has them battle and fight with each other.
Projection: Attributing one's own thoughts or impulses to another person. Through this process one can attribute his own intolerable wishes, emotional feelings, or motivations to another person.	A young woman who denies she has sexual feelings about a co-worker accuses him without basis of being a "flirt" and says he is trying to seduce her.
Reaction formation: Development of conscious attitudes and behavior patterns that are opposite to what one really feels or would like to do.	A married woman who feels attracted to one of her husband's friends treats him rudely.

Ego defense mechanisms—cont'd

Defense mechanism	Example
Undoing: Act or communication that partially negates a previous one; primitive defense mechanism.	Larry makes a passionate declaration of love to Sue on a date. On their next meeting he treats her formally and distantly.
Regression: Retreat in face of stress to behavior characteristic of any earlier level of development.	Four-year-old Nicole who has been toilet trained for over a year begins to wet her pants again when her new baby brother is brought home from the hospital.
Sublimation: Acceptance of a socially approved substitute goal for a drive whose normal channel of expression is blocked.	Ed has an impulsive and physically aggressive nature. He tries out for the football team and becomes a star tackle.
Compensation: Process by which a person makes up for a deficiency in his image of himself by strongly emphasizing some other feature that he regards as an asset.	Mr. L, a 42-year-old businessman, perceives his small physical stature negatively. He tries to overcome this by being aggressive, forceful, and controlling in his business dealings.
Rationalization: Offering a socially acceptable or apparently logical explanation to justify or make acceptable otherwise unacceptable impulses, feelings, behaviors, and motives.	John fails an examination and complains that the lectures were not well organized or clearly presented.
Isolation: Splitting off of emotional components of a thought, which may be temporary or long term.	A second-year medical student dissects a cadaver for her anatomy course without being disturbed by thoughts of death.
Denial: Avoidance of disagreeable realities by ignoring or refusing to recognize them; probably simplest and most primitive of all defense mechanisms.	Mrs. P has just been told that her breast biopsy indicates a malignancy. When her husband visits her that evening, she tells him that no one has discussed the laboratory results with her.

deception and reality distortion. Therefore they are usually not adaptive in helping the individual to realistically cope with the problem.

Many defense mechanisms have been identified in the literature. Following is a description of some of the more common ones:

It is important to conclude a discussion of ego-oriented reactions, or defense mechanisms, with the observation that individuals frequently monitor their own level of emotional tolerance and consequent need for the employment of ego defenses. Caplan notes:

> I have learned to wait patiently, while exercising appropriate, direct and indirect surveillance, to see whether the person will feel strong enough after a while to begin to confront the loss, disappointment or threat and little by little to relax his defenses. This may sometimes take quite a long time.[6:416]

This idea is supported by Elliott,[9] who believes that one defense mechanism in particular, denial, may be used as an effective mechanism to actually allay anxiety immediately following a stressful event. She believes that if denial is gradually eliminated as the stress begins to subside, the person may better adapt to the new situation.

The evaluation of whether the patient's use of certain defense mechanisms is adaptive or maladaptive revolves around the consideration of the following four issues:

1. The accurate recognition of the patient's use of the defense mechanism by the nurse.
2. The degree to which the defense mechanism is used. Does it imply a high degree of personality disorganization? Is the person unresponsive to facts about his life situation?
3. The degree to which use of the defense mechanism impedes the patient's progress toward regained health.
4. The need underlying the patient's use of the ego defense mechanism.

A consideration of these areas by the nurse will enhance her understanding of the patient and her plan for his nursing care.

PSYCHOLOGICAL CONVERSIONS. If the ego defense mechanisms are not successful and the person's level of anxiety remains high, he is forced to use exaggerated and inappropriate coping mechanisms that may appear deviant or abnormal to others. These coping patterns can be described as psychological conversions and include the many hidden, unconscious, and devious pathways in which the effects of anxiety are converted psychologically. This group of coping mechanisms includes many patterns of behavior that may be classified as neurotic. A neurosis is a mental disorder characterized by anxiety but in which there is no distortion of reality.

One such pattern is a *phobic reaction,* which is a persistent fear of some object or situation that presents no actual danger to the patient or in which the danger is magnified out of proportion to its actual seriousness. The phobic object often symbolizes the original object or situation. The dynamics of this reaction include the exaggerated use of *displacement* to obtain relief from anxiety.

Although many clinicians describe the patient's type of phobia in ordinary language, there are names attached to specific phobias. These names are frequently derived from Greek words for the phobic object. The following list of common phobias and their objects will reflect the wide variety of situations and objects around which phobias may be centered:

Acraphobia—high places
Agoraphobia—open spaces
Algophobia—pain
Astraphobia—storms, thunder, and lightning
Claustrophobia—closed places
Hematophobia—blood
Monophobia—being alone
Mysophobia—germs and contamination
Nyctophobia—darkness
Ochlophobia—crowds
Pathophobia—disease
Pyrophobia—fire
Zoophobia—animals or a particular animal

Some of the feared objects are totally harmless from an objective view. Others are potentially dangerous, but the person's fears are out of proportion to the actual threat. Although the phobic object often symbolizes the underlying conflict, the nurse cannot identify this conflict immediately on knowing the object. Personal perceptions, life experiences, and cultural values all mesh to govern the meaning of the symbol for the patient. For example, a morbid fear of dogs might represent fear of aggressive impulses to one patient, fear of freedom of sexual expression for another patient, or fear and jealousy regarding close interpersonal relationships for still another. It is also true that phobias vary in degree of disability and discomfort. Mild fears require less psychic energy and can often be adapted to in everyday living, whereas some phobic reactions can become so severe that the person may be unable to leave home or is similarly handicapped.

Dissociative reactions are another type of psychological conversion in which the patient blocks off part of his life from conscious recognition due to the threat of overwhelming anx-

iety. The mildest dissociative manifestation is sleepwalking (somnambulism). Amnesia is another symptom that is sometimes present. It includes a loss of memory for a specific period of time or a loss of all past memories. In this type of amnesia the forgotten material is still present beneath the level of consciousness and is accessible to recall at a later time. A more unusual dissociative manifestation is the presence of multiple personalities. Although this reaction has received a great deal of attention in the media (e.g., *Three Faces of Eve, Sybil*), it is relatively rare. The patient displays two or more complete personality systems that are usually dramatically different. The defense mechanism of *repression* may be used in these reactions.

A final type of psychological conversion of overwhelming anxiety is the formation of *obsessions* and *compulsions*. These reactions may be experienced singularly or in combination. Several elements are usually present in obsessive-compulsive disorders, and they constitute the underlying psychodynamics of the disorder. They are as follows[24]:

1. Behavior or thoughts that persist beyond the need for and despite voluntary action
2. The presence of anxiety and possibly somatic distress because of the alien nature of such thoughts to the individual
3. Insight into the illogical and unreasonable nature of the thought or action that nevertheless fails to alter the behavior.

An *obsession* is a recurring thought that is unwanted but which cannot be voluntarily excluded from consciousness. Obsessive thoughts might center around a variety of topics from changing jobs to suicide, and they frequently concern fear of uncontrollable impulses (particularly harming another family member). The distinguishing element of these thoughts is that they are unwelcome and cannot be dismissed by the patient.

A *compulsion* is a recurring impulse to perform some act that cannot be resisted. It is, in a sense, an obsession in action. Mild examples of compulsive acts might include twirling one's hair or adjusting one's tie. Often, however, the compulsive behavior interrupts a person's normal daily behavior, as may be seen in the example of a person who feels compelled to wash his hands as much as 50 times a day. Compulsive behavior tends to relieve anxiety that would be overwhelming for the individual if he were restrained from performing the activity. The dynamics of this reaction include the exaggerated use of the defense mechanism of *undoing* by which the person undoes or annuls the possible effect of his unrecognized impulses.

These two behaviors may be combined in an obsessive-compulsive reaction. For example, the person who compulsively washes his hands might also experience obsessive thoughts relating to dirt and germs. Here again the repeated thought or act defends the person against experiencing severe anxiety. It may also reflect the exaggerated use of the defense mechanisms of *reaction formation* and *displacement*. Some cases of alcoholism, drug addiction, and obesity are basically compulsive. The important element with these reactions is that the person does not want to repeat the act, but he feels that he must. He does not enjoy his compulsions and rarely receives secondary gain from them. He views them as inappropriate and maladaptive.

PHYSIOLOGICAL CONVERSIONS. A fourth coping mechanism for high levels of anxiety is physiological conversion. Assessment of the linked psychological and physiological responses to anxiety-producing situations is essential in nursing practice. Continued anxiety imposes great demands on the individual's biological system. With time, it may not only cause disordered function of an organ, but it may also predispose a person to actual organic changes. These physiological changes which accompany anxiety serve no constructive purpose; they are not likely to help one cope with the danger. They can, however, form the basis for pathological changes in function that may progress to structural changes and lead to psychosomatic disorders and irreversible organic changes.

Psychosomatic disorders can affect any body part. Reactions are most commonly seen involving the following:

Skin (allergic eczema, hives, and acne)

Respiratory system (asthma, sinusitis, and bronchial spasms)

Cardiovascular system (hypertension and migraine headaches)

Musculoskeletal system (backaches and muscle cramps)

Gastrointestinal system (colitis, gastritis, constipation, hyperacidity, duodenal ulcer, and anorexia)

Genitourinary system (menstrual disturbances, impotence, and vaginismus)

The occurrence of symptoms seems to be related to the amount of tension the individual is experiencing, and patterns of remissions and exacerbations are common. With this kind of reaction the emotional tension is not discharged outwardly but is instead unconsciously channeled through the visceral organs. *Repression* is the dominant defense mechanism used. The nature of the organ affected depends on the constitutional makeup of the patient, as well as the nature of the stressful situation.

Another type of physiological conversion is *neurasthenia,* which is characterized by chronic mental and physical fatigue and a variety of vague aches and pains, including weakness, headaches, and back pain. This fatigue is selective in nature, however, in that the person will have energy for activities that interest him but complain of fatigue when faced with routine activities. This reaction is not due to overwork but is an attempt to reduce or mask areas of conflict.

A type of physiological conversion more disabling than neurasthenia has been described as *hysteria,* or *conversion reaction,* in which symptoms of some physical illness appear without an underlying organic pathological condition. It leads to the reduction of anxiety, and, as with phobias, the organic symptom usually symbolizes the conflict. For example, a patient who has an impulse to harm his domineering mother may develop paralysis of his arms and hands. The primary gain the patient receives from his symptom is that he is unable to carry out his impulse. He may also receive secondary gain in the form of attention, manipulation of others, freedom from responsibilities, and economic compensation. Although this kind of secondary gain was not part of the cause of the illness, it does complicate the treatment process. Conversion symptoms might include the following:

1. Sensory symptoms, such as areas of anesthesia, blindness, or deafness
2. Motor symptoms, such as paralysis, tremors, or mutism
3. Visceral symptoms, such as anorexia nervosa, headaches, or difficulty breathing

It is frequently difficult to diagnose this reaction. Other patient behaviors may be helpful in this regard. Often patients have a bland attitude toward the conversion symptom and the disability produced by it. They tend to display little anxiety or concern, and the classic term for describing this lack of concern is "la belle indifference." There is also a tendency for the patient to seek attention in a pervasive way not limited to the actual symptom. The basic dynamic pattern involves *regression* and the reduction of anxiety by getting sick. Thus the patient converts a conflict area into a more acceptable medical problem and places the responsibility for action on someone other than himself.

Hypochondriasis is another type of physiological conversion. It is characterized by an exaggerated concern with one's physical health that is not based on a real organic pathological condition. The person fears presumed diseases of various organs and is not helped by reassurance. This reaction differs from hysteria in that there is no actual loss or distortion of function. The patients appear worried and anxious about their symptoms. This concern may be based on physical sensations overlooked by normal persons or on symptoms associated with minor physical illness that the patient exaggerates out of proportion. This is frequently a chronic pattern for the individual, and it is often accompanied by a history of visits to numerous physicians.

These physiological coping mechanisms should be differentiated from malingering, which is a deliberate and fraudulent imitation or exaggeration of an illness. The person's conscious intent is to deceive the observer for a specific reason, such as for financial compensation following an automobile accident. The person exaggerates symptoms, is evasive, and often contradicts himself. He is feigning illness, and malingering is not a coping mechanism for anxiety.

Obviously, many coping mechanisms are available to the individual to use in minimizing anxiety. The use of some of these defense mechanisms appears to be essential for all human beings if they are to maintain emotional stability. The exact nature and number of the defenses used by the individual strongly influence his personality pattern. When these defenses are overused or used unsuccessfully, they are responsible for many physiological and psychological symptoms commonly associated with emotional illness. As Freud has said, "One thing is certain, that the problem of anxiety is a nodal point linking up all kinds of most important questions; a riddle, of which the solution must

cast a flood of light upon our whole mental life."[11:118]

 Nursing diagnosis

Formulating a nursing diagnosis depends on a clear understanding of the position of anxiety within the larger perspective of the model of health-illness phenomena (Fig. 7-4). First, it emerges as a "generalized anxiety reaction" to a person's primary appraisal of a stressor that is perceived to be threatening or harmful. Three aspects of anxiety are activated at this time: (1) the central nervous system is aroused; (2) anxiety is felt and is evident in various cognitive, affective, physiological, behavioral, and social changes; and (3) ways of coping with anxiety are brought into play. These coping mechanisms may be constructive or destructive in nature and may represent neurotic or psychotic health problems. Most of the behaviors and coping mechanisms described in this chapter in relation to anxiety could be classified as neurotic disorders or health problems. They are maladaptive anxiety responses associated with moderate and severe levels of anxiety (Fig. 7-4).

Psychosis, however, can emerge with the panic level of anxiety as the individual feels he is "breaking into pieces."[1] Unlike neurosis, the anxiety of psychosis is not just fear of failure or fear of being unable to cope with the threatening situation. It is the fear that the failure will reveal defeat in the "process of living" and failure in the "process of being." This can be seen in the woman who has just given birth to a baby and experiences a postpartum psychosis. In this case the fear manifests itself in connection with being a mother as the woman identifies with her own mother and with the child and experiences feelings of unfulfilled needs and personal inadequacies.

The nurse who has adequately assessed a patient and uses a conceptual model for understanding anxiety will be able to formulate a nursing diagnosis based on the patient's position on the continuum of anxiety responses. In doing so, she will review the objective data she has collected, as well as the subjective responses of the patient to her questions and statements. The patient's history will be important, as will be her own personal response to the patient, since anxiety is one experience that is readily communicated interpersonally. In formulating the nursing diagnosis in relation to anxiety, the research of Lagina[14] shows that nurses tend to refer more frequently to subjective observations than to objective behaviors. They appear to rely heavily on the patient's medical diagnosis of health problems, prognosis, and the therapy indicated. Lagina stresses the need for nurses to go beyond the patient's medical diagnosis to find out what behavior the patient is displaying and his pattern of responding to anxiety. She also suggests that nurses, in diagnosing their patients' anxiety, may be projecting some of their own anxiety, and she underscores the need to distinguish between the two.

The formulation of a nursing diagnosis re-

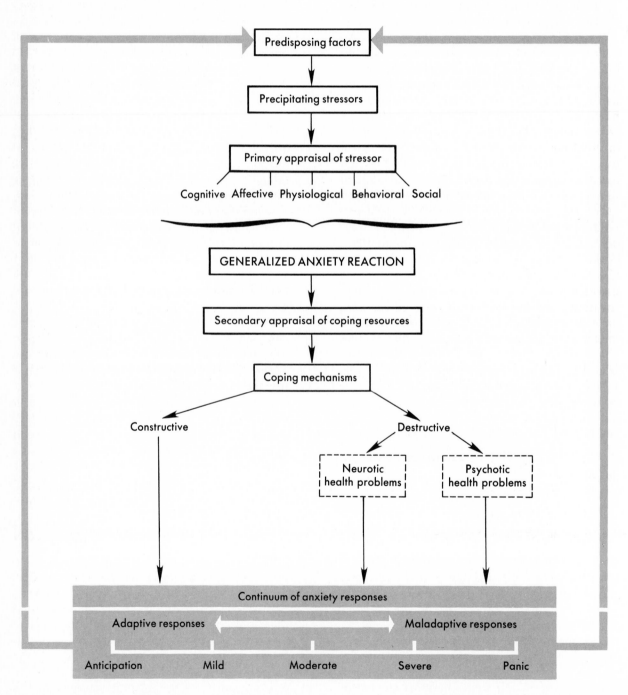

FIG. 7-4
Position of anxiety within the model of health-illness phenomena.

quires that the nurse determine the quality and quantity of the anxiety experienced by the patient and the constructive or destructive nature of the coping mechanism mobilized. In considering the quality of the anxiety, she might question the appropriateness of the patient's response to the perceived threat. Is it warranted, sensible, and adaptive or absurd and irrational? A problem may exist if the response is out of proportion to the threat. This would indicate that the patient's cognitive appraisal of the threat is unrealistic. The quantity of the reaction is her next consideration as she attempts to determine the degree or level of anxiety present. The escalation of the anxiety to the severe and panic levels indicates that the conflict is increasingly problematic and incapacitating for the patient. The nurse also needs to explore how the anxiety is being met or coped with. Constructive coping mechanisms are protective responses that confront the threat on the level of conscious awareness. Destructive coping mechanisms involve repression into the unconscious and tend to be ineffective, inadequate, disorganized, inappropriate, and exaggerated. They may be evident in bizarre behavior or symptom formation. Finally, the question may be posed as to the overall effect of the anxiety on the individual. Is it stimulating growth? Or is it interfering with effective living and life satisfaction? Is it enhancing one's sense of self? Or is it depersonalizing and despiritizing? Whenever possible, the patient should be included in identifying problem areas. This may not always be feasible, however, particularly if the patient's anxiety level is at the severe or panic level.

An appropriate nursing diagnosis would reflect these criteria. It should include the patient's problematic behavior pattern or nonproductive coping mechanism, the level of anxiety present and the related stressor. Nursing diagnoses can be formulated for any patient experiencing anxiety. It may be a coping response to a physical illness, a psychological illness, or a perceived threat to one's physical integrity or self-system. The patient may or may not also have been medically diagnosed. Some patients experiencing panic levels of anxiety may fall under the medical diagnostic category of psychotic. Patients experiencing severe and moderate levels of anxiety most commonly have neurotic disorders that fall under the affective, anxiety, somatoform, dissociative, and psychosexual disorder categories of the DSM-III.[7] However, many patients experiencing anxiety of a transient or less severe nature have no medically diagnosed health problem. Examples of possible nursing diagnoses associated with anxiety are given in Table 7-1. These are related to the diagnostic criteria for selected medical diagnoses associated with anxiety as described in the DSM-III. Obviously, a complete nursing assessment would include all problem areas of the patient, and many additional nursing problems would be identified in the way the patient's anxiety reciprocally influences his interpersonal relationships, self-concept, cognitive functioning, physiological status, and other aspects of his life. The identification of nurs-

TABLE 7-1. Comparative examples of nursing diagnoses and medical diagnoses associated with anxiety

Nursing diagnoses	Medical diagnoses as described in DSM-III*
Fear of leaving the house, indicating severe anxiety related to social role conflict	**Diagnostic criteria for AGORAPHOBIA** **A.** The individual has marked fear of and thus avoids being alone or in public places from which escape might be difficult or help not available in case of sudden incapacitation, e.g., crowds, tunnels, bridges, public transportation. **B.** There is increasing constriction of normal activities until the fears or avoidance behavior dominate the individual's life. **C.** Not due to a major depressive episode, obsessive-compulsive disorder, paranoid personality disorder, or schizophrenia.

*From American Psychiatric Association: Diagnostic and statistical manual of mental disorders, third edition, Washington, D.C., APA, 1980.

Continued.

TABLE 7-1. Comparative examples of nursing diagnoses and medical diagnoses associated with anxiety—cont'd

Nursing diagnoses	Medical diagnoses as described in DSM-III

Repeated attacks of immobilizing apprehension, indicating severe anxiety (related stressor or stimulus cannot be identified)	**Diagnostic criteria for PANIC DISORDER**
	
	A. At least three panic attacks within a 3-week period in circumstances other than during marked physical exertion or in a life-threatening situation. The attacks are not precipitated only by exposure to a circumscribed phobic stimulus.
	
	B. Panic attacks are manifested by discrete periods of apprehension or fear, and at least four of the following symptoms appear during each attack:
	
	   1. Dyspnea
	   2. Palpitations
	   3. Chest pain or discomfort
	   4. Choking or smothering sensations
	   5. Dizziness, vertigo, or unsteady feelings
	   6. Feelings of unreality
	   7. Paresthesias (tingling in hands or feet)
	   8. Hot and cold flashes
	   9. Sweating
	  10. Faintness
	  11. Trembling or shaking
	  12. Fear of dying, going crazy, or doing something uncontrolled during an attack
	
	C. Not due to a physical disorder or another mental disorder, such as major depression, somatization disorder, or schizophrenia.
	
	D. This disorder is not associated with agoraphobia.

Repetitive hand washing and recurring thoughts of dirt and germs, indicating severe anxiety related to sexual conflict	**Diagnostic criteria for OBSESSIVE-COMPULSIVE DISORDER** **A.** Either obsessions or compulsions: *Obsessions:* Recurrent, persistent ideas, thoughts, images, or impulses that are ego-dystonic, i.e., they are not experienced as voluntarily produced, but rather as thoughts that invade consciousness and are experienced as senseless or repugnant. Attempts are made to ignore or suppress them. *Compulsions:* Repetitive and seemingly purposeful behaviors that are performed according to certain rules or in a stereotyped fashion. The behavior is not an end in itself, but is designed to produce or prevent some future event or situation. However, either the activity is not connected in a realistic way with what it is designed to produce or prevent, or it may be clearly excessive. The act is performed with a sense of subjective compulsion coupled with a desire to resist the compulsion (at least initially). The individual generally recognizes the senselessness of the behavior (this may not be true for young children) and does not derive pleasure from carrying out the activity, although it provides a release of tension. **B.** The obsessions or compulsions are a significant source of distress to the individual or interfere with social or role functioning. **C.** Not due to another mental disorder, such as Tourette's disorder, schizophrenia, major depression, or organic mental disorder.

TABLE 7-1. Comparative examples of nursing diagnoses and medical diagnoses associated with anxiety—cont'd

Nursing diagnoses	Medical diagnoses as described in DSM-III

Paralysis of legs, indicating severe anxiety related to work conflict	**Diagnostic criteria for CONVERSION DISORDER**
	
	A. The predominant disturbance is a loss of or alteration in physical functioning suggesting a physical disorder.
	
	B. Psychological factors are judged to be etiologically involved in the symptom, as evidenced by one of the following:
	
	  1. There is a temporal relationship between an environmental stimulus that is apparently related to a psychological conflict or need and the initiation or exacerbation of the symptom
	  2. The symptom enables the individual to avoid some activity that is noxious to him or her
	  3. The symptom enables the individual to get support from the environment that otherwise might not be forthcoming
	
	C. It has been determined that the symptom is *not* under voluntary control.
	
	D. The symptom cannot, after appropriate investigation, be explained by a known physical disorder or pathophysiological mechanism.
	
	E. The symptom is not limited to pain or to a disturbance in sexual functioning.
	
	F. Not due to a somatization disorder or schizophrenia.

Inability to recall events pertaining to a car accident, indicating a panic level of anxiety related to the death of the patient's young daughter in the accident	**Diagnostic criteria for PSYCHOGENIC AMNESIA** **A.** Sudden inability to recall important personal information that is too extensive to be explained by ordinary forgetfulness. **B.** The disturbance is not due to an organic mental disorder (e.g., blackouts during alcohol intoxication).
Recurring episodes of colitis, indicating moderate anxiety related to financial pressures	**Diagnostic criteria for PSYCHOLOGICAL FACTORS AFFECTING PHYSICAL CONDITION** **A.** Psychologically meaningful environmental stimuli are temporally related to the initiation or exacerbation of a physical condition (recorded on axis III). **B.** The physical condition has either demonstrable organic pathology (e.g., rheumatoid arthritis) or a known pathophysiological process (e.g., migraine headache, vomiting). **C.** The condition is not due to a somatoform disorder.

Distorted visual and auditory perceptions, indicating a panic level of anxiety related to family rejection	**Diagnostic criteria for BRIEF REACTIVE PSYCHOSIS**
	
	A. Psychotic symptoms appear immediately following a recognizable psychosocial stressor that would evoke significant symptoms of distress in almost anyone.
	
	B. The clinical picture involves emotional turmoil and at least one of the following psychotic symptoms:
	
	  1. Incoherence or loosening of associations
	  2. Delusions
	  3. Hallucinations
	  4. Behavior that is grossly disorganized or catatonic

Continued.

TABLE 7-1. **Comparative examples of nursing diagnoses and medical diagnoses associated with anxiety—cont'd**

Nursing diagnoses	Medical diagnoses as described in DSM-III
	Diagnostic criteria for BRIEF REACTIVE PSYCHOSIS—cont'd **C.** The psychotic symptoms last more than a few hours but less than 2 weeks, and there is an eventual return to the premorbid level of functioning. (NOTE: The diagnosis can be made soon after the onset of the psychotic symptoms without waiting for the expected recovery. If the psychotic symptoms last more than 2 weeks, the diagnosis should be changed.) **D.** No period of increasing psychopathology immediately preceded the psychosocial stressor. **E.** The disturbance is not due to any other mental disorder, such as an organic mental disorder, manic episode, or factitious disorder with psychological symptoms.
Limited ability to concentrate and psychomotor agitation, indicating moderate anxiety related to child's illness	No related psychiatric diagnosis
Generalized hostility to staff and family, indicating moderate anxiety related to impending surgery	No related psychiatric diagnosis
Excessive use of denial and rationalization, indicating moderate anxiety related to poor school performance	No related psychiatric diagnosis

ing problems should be as complete as possible to ensure an adequate plan of care and intervention.

Planning and implementation of nursing interventions

Goal setting

The overall goal of the nurse working with an anxious patient is not to free him totally from anxiety but rather to help him develop the capacity to tolerate mild anxiety and to use it consciously and constructively. In this way his self will become stronger and more integrated and, as he uses these experiences as learning experiences, he will move on in his development. The patient will be able to meet anxiety constructively if he has sound, firm, and flexible values and if he is convinced that the values to

be gained in moving ahead are greater than those to be gained by escape. If one views anxiety as a war between the threat and the values a person identifies with his existence, then maladaptive behavior means that the struggle is won by the threat, whereas the constructive approach to anxiety means that the struggle is won by the person's values. Thus a general nursing goal is to help the patient evolve sound values. This does not mean that the patient assumes the nurse's values. Rather, the nurse works with the patient to sort out his own values, which transcend the present situation and extend toward the good of the community.

Anxiety can also be an important factor in the patient's decision to seek treatment. No one wants anxiety, but if it is present, then the lessening of it is desirable. If the patient's coping mechanism or symptom is not successful in minimizing his anxiety, his motivation for treatment will be increased. Conversely, anxiety about the therapeutic process can also contribute to its being delayed, impeded, or deterred.

The patient should be an active participant in the phases of planning and implementation. If the patient is actively involved in identifying relevant stressors and planning possible solutions, the success of the implementation phase will be maximized. Patients in extreme anxiety will not, initially, be able to participate in the problem-solving process. However, as soon as their anxiety is reduced, the nurse should incorporate them in her care to establish mutuality of approach and reinforce the fact that they are responsible for their own growth and personal development.

In formulating a plan of care for the patient the nurse first attends to the creation of nursing goals. Goals such as "decrease anxiety" and "minimize anxiety" lack specific behaviors and evaluation criteria, which minimizes their usefulness in guiding nursing care and evaluating its effectiveness. The long-term goals for the patient should relate to the nursing diagnosis. They should reflect the significant reduction or elimination of the problematic behavior identified in the nursing diagnosis as well as the learning of new, more constructive coping mechanisms. The short-term goals should break this down into discrete, more readily attainable steps. Short-term goals are important to provide smaller but significant progress toward the long-term goal accomplishment. Both these factors allow the nurse and patient to see progress throughout the relationship even if the ultimate goal still appears to be distant.

When the nursing diagnosis describes the patient's anxiety at the severe or panic levels, the highest priority short-term goals should address the lowering of the anxiety level. Only after this has been achieved can additional progress be made. The reduced level of anxiety should be evident in a reduction of behaviors associated with the severe or panic levels. The reduction of these behaviors, then, forms part of the content for the short-term goals. Following are examples of short-term goals for a particular patient.

After 10 days Mr. Jones will:

1. Attend and remain seated during all ward meetings
2. Participate at least three times during each meeting
3. Discuss one topic for a minimum of 10 minutes when meeting with his nurse
4. Attend all occupational therapy sessions
5. Sleep a minimum of 6 hours a night

When these goals are met, the nurse can assume and validate that her patient's level of anxiety has been reduced and she may then develop new short-germ goals that may be directed toward insight or relaxation therapy. Throughout the nursing process, it will be necessary for the nurse to continually reevaluate the level of her patient's anxiety. Kristic's study[13] of the anxiety level of hospitalized psychiatric patients throughout their total hospitalization found three specific crisis periods of increased anxiety. These were at the time of admission, after the fifth day of the hospitalization, and on discharge. She notes that not only is there need for intensive intervention at these times, but that nurses would have the greatest opportunity for implementing them. Studies such as these may provide a basis for prediction of periods of particular stress for patients that have direct implications for the planning and implementing of therapeutic nursing care.

Intervening in severe and panic levels of anxiety

The patient experiencing severe or panic levels of anxiety may be hospitalized. To reduce this patient's level of anxiety, most of the nursing actions will be supportive and protective. Initially, the nurse wishes to establish an open, trusting relationship. To accomplish this, she should actively listen to the patient and encourage him to discuss his feelings of anxiety, hostility, guilt, and frustration. She should answer his questions directly and offer unconditional acceptance of him. Both her verbal and nonverbal communications should convey awareness of the patient's feelings and acceptance of them. The patient might express himself in rapid, disjointed speech, hostile outbursts, or crying episodes. She should remain available to the patient and respect his use of personal space. In this regard research indicates that a 180-cm (6-foot) distance in a small room may create the optimum condition for openness and discussion of fears.[15] The more this distance is increased or decreased, the more anxious the patient may become.

The nurse's own feelings are of particular importance when working with a highly anxious patient. The nurse may find herself being unsympathetic to the patient, impatient with him, and frustrated by him. These are common feelings of reciprocal anxiety that the nurse should

be aware of and accepting of when they are
elicited. If the nurse is alert to the development
of anxiety in herself, she can learn from it and
use it therapeutically within the nurse-patient
relationship. It may, for example, be indicative
of some important emotional issue that the patient is unable to identify and verbalize. Or it
may reflect a conflict within the nurse that is
interfering with her ability to be therapeutic.
She should therefore be alert to the signs of
anxiety in herself, accept them, and attempt to
explore their cause. What is threatening her?
Is this patient a source of reflected esteem for
her? Has she failed to live up to what she imagines is the patient's ideal? Is she comparing herself to a peer or another health professional?
Is the patient's area of conflict one that she has
not resolved for herself? Is her anxiety related to
something that will or may happen in the future? Is her patient's conflict really one of her
own that she is projecting onto him?

If the nurse does not explore the reasons for
her own anxiety and instead denies it, it can
have detrimental effects on the nurse-patient relationship. Because of her own anxiety she may
be unable to differentiate between levels of
anxiety in others. She may also transfer her own
fears and frustrations to the patient, thus compounding his problem. Finally, her anxiety will
arouse defenses in other patients and staff that
will severely interfere with her therapeutic usefulness. She should strive to accept her patient's
anxiety without reciprocal anxiety by continually clarifying her own feelings and role.

CLINICAL EXAMPLE 7-1

Ms. R was a 35-year-old married woman and
mother of three children, ages 4, 6, and 9. She was
a full-time housewife and mother. Her husband was a
salesman and spent about 2 nights each week out of
town. She came to the clinic complaining of severe
headaches that "come upon me very suddenly and are
so terrible that I have to go to bed. The only thing
that helps is for me to lie down in a dark and absolutely quiet room." She said that these headaches
were becoming a real problem for everyone in the
family, and her husband told her that she "just had
to get over them and get things back to normal."

Mr. W, a psychiatric nurse, offered to see Ms. R in
therapy once a week. After 4 weeks, he was asked to
present his evaluation, treatment plans, and progress
report to the clinic staff at their regular weekly team
conference. Mr. W began his presentation by stating,

"This case is really a tough nut to crack. I'll start
with the progress report and say that there is none,
because I can't seem to get past all of the complaining
this patient does!" He then went on to discuss his
evaluation and treatment plan in depth. It became
obvious to the other members of the staff that Mr. W
saw his patient as a woman who was not living up to
her roles and responsibilities. He defended Ms. R's
husband even though the husband had refused to
come to the sessions with his wife. When the psychiatrist asked about the possibility of a medication
evaluation for Ms. R, the nurse replied, "Everyone
gets headaches. I don't think we should reward or reinforce this woman's complaints."

In reviewing this case, the staff noted that Mr. W
appeared to have problems relating empathically to
his patient because of her particular set of problems
and some of his own values and perceptions. Mr. W
agreed with this and said he had thought of asking
someone else to work with Ms. R. Mr. W's supervisor
observed that the nurse had problems with this type of
patient in the past, and a more constructive approach
would be to increase his supervision on this case,
focusing on the dynamics between the patient and
nurse that were blocking learning and growth for
both of them. Mr. W and his supervisor then set a time
when they could begin to meet with this purpose in
mind.

Another major area of intervention is providing for and reassuring the patient of his safety.
One way of decreasing his anxiety is by allowing the patient to determine what stress he can
handle at the time. The nurse should not force
or probe the severely anxious patient into situations he is not able to handle. She should not
attack his coping mechanism or attempt to strip
him of it. Rather, she should attempt to protect
his defenses. The coping mechanism or symptom is attempting to deal with an unconscious
conflict. The patient does not understand why
the symptom has developed nor what he is gaining from it. What he does believe is that the
symptom relieves some of the intolerable anxiety
and tension. If he is unable to release this anxiety, his tension will mount to the panic level and
he could lose control. It is also important to remember that the severely anxious patient has
not worked through his area of conflict and
therefore has no alternatives or substitutes for
his present coping mechanisms.

This principle of protecting the patient's defenses applies to whatever coping mechanism
the patient is utilizing. With physiological conversions, such as *psychosomatic illnesses* or
conversion reactions, the nurse should acknowledge the reality of the pain. Physiological

changes are occurring and do cause body discomfort. If medication is prescribed, it should be administered. While being supportive in this way the nurse may also attempt to give feedback to the patient by describing his behavior, identifying any precipitating factors she has observed, and reinforcing the idea that the cause of the illness is related to emotional factors that will eventually need to be analyzed to resolve the problem.

This principle also applies to severe levels of anxiety, as seen in psychological conversions such as *obsessive-compulsive reactions* and *phobias*. The nurse should not initially interfere with the repetitive act or force the patient to confront the phobic object. She should not ridicule the nature of his defense or attempt to argue with him about it or reason him out of it. He needs this coping mechanism to keep his anxiety within tolerable limits. With time, however, she can place some limits on his behavior and attempt to help him find satisfaction with other aspects of life. It is also important not to reinforce the phobia, ritual, or physical complaint by focusing attention on it and devoting a great deal of time to talking about it.

If the patient is hospitalized, the nurse can consult with other members of the health team to identify anxiety-producing situations for the patient and attempt to reduce them. She can set limits by assuming a quiet, calm manner, decreasing environmental stimulation, and limiting the patient's interaction with other patients to minimize the contagious aspects of anxiety. Supportive physical measures may also be helpful in decreasing a patient's anxiety, such as warm baths, massages, or whirlpool baths.

The nurse should also encourage the patient's interest in activity outside himself. Her rationale for doing this is to limit the time he has available for his destructive coping mechanisms and to increase his participation in and enjoyment of other aspects of life. Within the hospital setting he may become engaged in simple games, concrete tasks, or occupational or art therapy. It would be most beneficial if the nurse shared some of these activities with him to provide him with support and reinforce socially productive behavior. She might also schedule vigorous physical activities for him, such as walking, a sport, or an active hobby. This kind of physical exercise is helpful in the dissolution of anxiety because it provides an emotional release or discharge and directs the patient's attention outward. Similar interventions can be implemented with the severely anxious patient who is not hospitalized. The nurse and patient can plan a daily schedule or a list of activities that he can carry out in the community. Family members may be involved in the planning, since they can be very supportive in setting limits and stimulating outside activity.

Some nursing interventions can be detrimental and serve to increase the already high anxiety of severely anxious patients. These include pressuring the patient to change prematurely, being judgmental and verbally disapproving of the patient's behaviors, asking the patient a direct question that places him on the defensive, focusing in a critical way on the anxious feelings of the patient with other patients present, lacking awareness of her own behaviors and feelings, and withdrawing from the patient.

INTERVENING WITH MEDICATION. Another possible area for nursing intervention is in the administration of tranquilizing drugs to the highly anxious patient. Because anxiety is a pervasive problem, large portions of the population take tranquilizers. Americans are now spending over $500 million each year for drugs to relieve anxiety, and one out of every ten prescriptions written by physicians is for tranquilizing medication. It is essential to understand that the primary treatment of anxiety must not be based on drugs. Pharmacotherapy of anxiety should always be considered a secondary approach.

The major tranquilizers are frequently prescribed for patients experiencing a panic level of anxiety of psychotic proportions. The major actions of these drugs are to reduce anxiety and decrease psychotic symptoms. The minor tranquilizers such as diazepam (Valium), chlordiazepoxide (Librium), and meprobamate (Equanil) can also be effective in treating the symptoms of anxiety. However, they should be used only for temporary symptomatic treatment—either to give immediate relief under conditions of acute overwhelming stress or to stabilize the patient so that he may become more able to participate in the process of therapy. Use of these drugs for other than these reasons can be injurious for four reasons:

1. Drug therapy of anxiety states is not directed at the cause of the disorder, although it is the cause that should be determined and treated.

2. The drugs serve to mask the symptoms, yet the problem can continue to develop and increasingly incapacitate the patient.

TABLE 7-2. **Summary of nursing interventions in severe and panic
levels of anxiety**
*Goal—Support and protect the patient and reduce his anxiety to a
moderate-mild level*

Principle	Rationale	Nursing actions
Establish an open trusting relationship	Reduce the threat that the nurse poses to the highly anxious patient	Listen to the patient Encourage the patient's discussion of feelings Answer questions directly Offer unconditional acceptance Be available to the patient Respect his use of personal space
Awareness and control of nurse's own feelings	Anxiety is communicated interpersonally; reciprocal anxiety in the nurse can interfere with her ability to be therapeutic	Openness to one's own feelings Acceptance of both positive and negative feelings, including the development of anxiety Explore the cause of one's feelings Use this understanding of one's feelings in a therapeutic way
Reassure the patient of his safety and protect his defenses and coping mechanisms but do not focus on or reinforce the presenting maladaptive behaviors	Severe and panic levels of anxiety can be reduced by initially allowing the patient to determine what stress he can handle If the patient is unable to release his anxiety, his tension may mount to the panic level and he may lose control; at this time, he has no alternatives for his present coping mechanisms	Initially accept and support, rather than attack, the patient's defenses Acknowledge the reality of the pain associated with the patient's present coping mechanisms but do not focus on the phobia, ritual, or physical complaint itself Administer treatments or medications that will/may help to reduce the patient's discomfort Give feedback to the patient about his behavior, stressors, appraisal of stressors, and coping resources Reinforce the idea that one's physical health is related to one's emotional health and that this is an area which will need exploration in the future In time, begin to place limits on the patient's maladaptive behavior in a supportive way

TABLE 7-2. Summary of nursing interventions in severe and panic levels of anxiety—cont'd

Goal—Support and protect the patient and reduce his anxiety to a moderate-mild level

Principle	Rationale	Nursing actions
Identify and attempt to reduce anxiety-provoking situations for the patient	The patient's behavior may be modified by altering his environment and his interaction with it	Assume a calm manner with the patient
		Decrease environmental stimulation
		Limit the patient's interaction with other patients to minimize the contagious aspects of anxiety
		Identify and modify anxiety-provoking situations for the patient
		Administer supportive physical measures, such as warm baths and massages
Encourage the patient's interest in activity outside himself	By encouraging outside activities, the nurse acts to limit the time the patient has available for his destructive coping mechanisms, while increasing his participation in and enjoyment of other aspects of life	Initially share an activity with him to provide support and reinforce socially productive behavior
		Provide for physical exercise of some type
		Plan a schedule or list of activities that can be carried out daily
		Involve family members and other support systems as much as possible

3. Symptomatic use of drugs robs the patient of his motivation for self-understanding and growth.

4. Users of minor tranquilizers often develop a tolerance to their effects and require a higher dosage, making possible the development of physical and psychological dependence and addiction.

Also, use of these drugs in combination with alcohol may result in a serious or even fatal sedative reaction. For further information on these drugs refer to Chapter 15. Table 7-2 summarizes the principles, rationale, and nursing actions in severe and panic levels of anxiety.

Intervening in a moderate level of anxiety

All the nursing interventions previously mentioned are supportive interventions and are directed toward the general short-term goal of reducing the anxiety of a severely anxious or panicky patient. When the patient's anxiety is reduced to a moderate level, the nurse can develop additional goals to aid the patient in his problem-solving efforts to cope with the stress. Long-term goals that are directed toward helping the patient understand the cause of his anxiety and learn new ways of controlling it are insight oriented or reeducative in nature. The interventions used by the nurse were originally described by Peplau[21] and Burd[5] and reflect the problem-solving process. Short-term goals may be written for each step of this process, including recognition of anxiety, insight into the anxiety, and coping with the threat. These interventions can be implemented in any setting—psychiatric, community, or general hospital.

RECOGNITION OF ANXIETY. After analyzing the patient's behaviors and determining his level of anxiety, the nurse helps the patient to recognize he is anxious. She helps him explore his underlying feelings with such questions as "Are you feeling anxious now?" or "Are you uncomfortable?" It is also helpful for the nurse to identify the patient's behavior and link it to the feeling of anxiety (e.g., "I noticed you smoked three cigarettes since we started talking about your sister. Are you feeling anxious?"). In this way the nurse acknowledges the patient's feeling, attempts to label it for the patient, encourages the patient to describe it further, and relates it to a specific behavioral pattern. She is also validating her inferences and assumptions with the patient.

The patient's goal, however, is often to avoid or negate his anxiety. He therefore might use any of the following resistive approaches described by Meares[17]:

1. *Screen symptoms.* In this case the patient focuses his attention on minor physical ailments. The purpose of these apparently unrelated complaints is to avoid acknowledging his anxiety and conflict areas.

2. *Superior status position.* The patient attempts to control the interview by questioning the nurse's abilities or asserting the superiority of his own knowledge or experiences. It is important that the nurse not respond emotionally to this approach. She should not accept the patient's challenge and compete with him, since a conflict of this kind would serve only to further avoid the issue of anxiety.

3. *Emotional seduction.* By means of this technique the patient attempts to manipulate the nurse and to elicit feelings of pity or sympathy from her.

4. *Superficiality.* The patient relates on an obvious level and resists any attempts by the nurse to explore underlying feelings or analyze issues.

5. *Circumlocution.* In this case the patient gives the pretense of answering questions asked of him, but he succeeds instead in talking around the topic and actually avoiding it.

6. *Amnesia.* This is a type of purposeful "forgetting" of a certain incident or event to avoid confronting and exploring it with the nurse.

7. *Denial.* The patient may use this approach only when discussing significant issues with the nurse or may generalize his denial to all others including himself. His purpose is often to avoid humiliation.

8. *Intellectualization.* The patient who utilizes this technique usually has some knowledge of psychology or medicine. He is able to verbalize appropriate insights and analysis yet lacks personal involvement in the problem he describes. He is not actually participating in the problem-solving process.

9. *Hostility.* The patient believes that offense is the best defense. He therefore relates to others in an aggressive defiant manner. The greatest danger in this situation is that the nurse will take his behavior personally and respond, in turn, with anger. This serves to reinforce the patient in avoiding the exploring of his anxiety.

10. *Withdrawal.* The patient may resist the nurse by replying in vague, diffuse, indefinite, and remote ways.

All these resistive approaches may create feelings of frustration, irritation, or reciprocal anxiety in the nurse. It will be important for her to recognize her own feelings and identify the behavior pattern of the patient that might be causing them.

CLINICAL EXAMPLE 7-2

Mr. T was a 28-year-old male who was transferred from the neurological unit to the psychiatric unit where Ms. P was assigned to be his primary nurse. Ms. P was 24 years old and had been working on the unit for 3 years. In completing her nursing assessment of Mr. T, the nurse noted that he was experiencing a paralysis of his legs, which began gradually approximately 4 weeks previously. All neurological tests were negative, and he was transferred to the psychiatric unit for evaluation and treatment. He was an only child, unmarried, and had been living at home with his parents. He had completed college and was employed in the postal service. He had been dating one girl for 2 years and had recently proposed to her. She had told him that she was not ready to get married yet but she did want to continue seeing him. Mr. T had a small group of close friends, males and females, and they visited him often in the hospital, as did his family.

Ms. P had established a good relationship with her patient and spent much time with him. She found his friends to be kind and jovial and noted that one of Mr. T's strengths was his sense of humor and "ready smile." She observed, however, that his girl friend never visited with him alone. Mr. T, meanwhile, had many cards, gifts, and visitors and appeared to be most appreciative of everything done for him.

A physical therapist came to work with Mr. T on a regular basis, and this was a very difficult time of the day for him. While watching them work together one day, Ms. P remarked how impersonal and brusque the physical therapist was in relating to her patient. In discussing this observation in nursing rounds the next day, Ms. P began to realize that some of her actions were being influenced by her feelings of sympathy and pity for the patient and blame she had been unconsciously projecting onto his girl friend. She wondered if his joviality, agreeable nature, and professed signs of gratitude were not indications of his manipulation of her and emotional seduction of her feelings toward him. The more she thought about this possibility, the more likely it seemed. At the end of the nursing rounds that morning, she requested that she be able to present his case in the staff treatment meeting the next day. Other staff were also feeling frustrated in their care for him and agreed that the conference would be most valuable.

In attempting to deal with these patient defenses and intervene successfully, the importance of a trusting relationship becomes evident. If the nurse establishes herself as a warm and responsive listener, gives the patient adequate time to respond, and is supportive of his self-expressions, she will become less threatening to him. In helping him recognize his anxiety, the nurse should use open questions that move from nonthreatening topics to central issues of conflict. It may be helpful to vary the amount of anxiety to enhance the patient's motivation. In time, supportive confrontation may be used in reflecting back to the patient his repeated use of a particular resistive pattern. If, however, the patient's level of anxiety begins to rapidly rise, the nurse might choose to refocus the patient to a previous discussion topic.

INSIGHT INTO THE ANXIETY. Once the patient is able to recognize his anxiety, the subsequent nursing interventions strive to expand the present context of the patient. The patient may be asked to describe the situations and interactions that immediately precede the increase in anxiety. Together the nurse and patient make inferences about the precipitating causes or biopsychosocial stressors.

The nurse then helps the patient see which of his values are being threatened. It is possible to link the threat with underlying causes and to analyze how the conflict developed. To do this, the patient's present experiences are related to his past ones. The depth of this analysis depends on the nurse's educational and professional experiences. It is also important to explore how the patient reduced anxiety in the past. How did he handle anxiety, and what kinds of actions produced relief?

COPING WITH THE THREAT. If previous coping responses have been adaptive and constructive, the patient should be encouraged to utilize them. If not, the nurse can point out their maladaptive or destructive effects. She can share her perception with the patient that his present way of life is apparently unsatisfactory and distressing to him and does not attempt to change things for the better. The patient needs to assume responsibility for his own actions and realize that he has placed limitations on himself;

other people are not doing it to him. In this phase of intervention the nurse assumes an active role as she interprets, analyzes, confronts, and correlates cause and effect relationships. She should proceed clearly so that the patient can follow while maintaining his anxiety within appropriate limits. If his anxiety becomes too severe, she may change topics temporarily.

There are various ways the nurse can help the patient in his problem-solving efforts. One way of helping the patient cope is to reevaluate the nature of the threat or stressor. Is it as bad as the patient perceives it? Is his cognitive appraisal realistic? Together they might discuss his fears and feelings of inadequacy and analyze his projective identification. Does he fear others are as critical, perfectionistic, and rejecting of him as he is of others? Is his conflict based in reality, or is it the result of unvalidated, isolated, and perhaps distorted thinking? By sharing his fears with family members, peers, and staff, the patient frequently sees his own misperceptions, and with their support he can validate his ideas, values, and goals.

Another approach is to help the patient modify his behavior and learn new ways of coping with stress. He may decide to restructure his goals or evolve different values based on feedback from those around him. Or he might consider alternatives to mastering the situation. The nurse may act as a role model in this regard or engage the patient in role playing to decrease his anxiety about new responses to problematical situations. One nursing function therefore is to educate the patient in aspects of mild anxiety that can be constructive and growth producing. Physical activity should be encouraged as a way to discharge anxiety. Interpersonal resources such as family members or close friends should be incorporated into the nursing plan of care to provide the patient with support.

Frequently the cause for the anxiety will arise from an interpersonal conflict. In this case, analyzing the situation with the patient by himself is significantly less helpful than including the involved persons and opening communication between them. In this way cause and effect relationships are more open to examination, and coping patterns can be examined in light of their effect on others as well as the patient himself.

Working through this problem-solving or reeducative process with the patient will take time. He has to accept it on an intellectual and an

TABLE 7-3. Summary of nursing interventions in a moderate level of anxiety
Goal — Help the patient in his problem-solving efforts to cope with stress

Principle	Rationale	Nursing actions
Establish and maintain a trusting relationship	Reduce the threat the nurse poses to the patient	Be a warm and responsive listener Give the patient adequate time to respond Be supportive of the patient's self-expressions.
Awareness and control of the nurse's own feelings	Resistance by the patient may produce negative feelings in the nurse that can block future progress	Recognize own feelings Identify the behavior pattern or resistive approach of the patient that might be causing them Explore the patient's behavior and the nurse's response to them with the patient to learn and grow from them
Help the patient recognize his anxiety	To adopt new coping responses the patient first needs to be aware of his feelings and to overcome his conscious or unconscious denial and resistance	Help the patient to identify and describe his underlying feelings Link the patient's behavior with his feeling Validate all inferences and assumptions with the patient Use open questions to move from non-threatening topics to issues of conflict Vary the amount of anxiety to enhance the patient's motivation In time, supportive confrontation may be used judiciously
Expand the patient's insight into the development of his anxiety	Once the patient recognizes his feelings of anxiety, he needs to be helped to understand its development, including precipitating stressors, appraisal of the stressor, and resources available to him	Help the patient describe the situations and interactions that immediately precede his anxiety Review with the patient his appraisal of the stressor, which of his values are being threatened, and the way in which the conflict developed Relate his present experiences with relevant ones from the past
Help the patient learn new adaptive coping responses	New adaptive coping responses can be learned through analyzing coping mechanisms used in the past, reappraising the stressor, utilizing available resources, and accepting responsibility for change	Explore how the patient reduced anxiety in the past and what kinds of actions produced relief Point out the maladaptive and destructive effects of present coping responses Encourage the patient to use adaptive coping responses that have been effective in the past Focus responsibility for change on the patient

TABLE 7-3. Summary of nursing interventions in a moderate level of anxiety—cont'd
Goal — Help the patient in his problem-solving efforts to cope with stress

Principle	Rationale	Nursing actions
		Assume an active role with the patient correlating cause and effect relationships while maintaining his anxiety within appropriate limits
		Assist the patient in reappraising the value, nature, and meaning of the stressor when appropriate
		Help the patient identify ways he can restructure goals, modify behavior, utilize resources, and test out new coping responses
		Utilize role playing if appropriate
		Educate the patient in the growth-producing aspects of mild anxiety
		Encourage physical activity to discharge energy
		Include significant others as resources and social supports in helping the patient learn new coping responses
		Allow the patient time to implement new adaptive coping responses

emotional level, and breaking previous behavioral patterns can be difficult. Throughout the implementation phase the nurse needs to be patient and consistent in her approach and continually reappraise her own anxiety. Table 7-3 summarizes the nursing interventions that help the moderately anxious patient in his problem-solving efforts to cope with stress.

Relaxation interventions

In addition to the problem-solving function of coping addressed previously, one can also cope with stress by regulating the emotional distress associated with it. Long-term goals that are directed toward helping the patient regulate emotional distress are supportive or palliative. Although distress can be regulated in maladaptive ways, such as taking drugs, denying the facts, or withdrawing, only the adaptive responses will be described in this chapter. These include the relaxation techniques of systematic desensitization, meditation, and the use of biofeedback. All human beings have a natural and protective mechanism against "overstress,"

which Benson calls the "relaxation response."[2] This response brings about a decreased heart rate, lower metabolism, and decreased respiratory rate. Relaxation, therefore, is the ultimate stress management technique because the relaxation response is the physiological opposite of the fight or flight, or anxiety, response.

Relaxation techniques are useful nursing interventions when the patient's level of stress interferes with his ability to function and be productive. They have long been used in helping women deal with childbirth because they form the basis for childbirth education. However, new ways are presently being discovered of using relaxation techniques with all kinds of people in various stress situations. These include helping patients handle pain; overcome test anxiety; sleep better; overcome side effects related to chemotherapy, surgery, or myocardial infarctions; handle various medical, nursing, and dental procedures; monitor the emotional triggers associated with chronic illnesses, such as asthma, muscle tension, ulcers, hypertension, tension headaches, or colitis; and deal with anger more constructively.

Relaxation can be taught in many ways, individually, in small groups, or even in larger group settings. It is within the scope of nursing practice and, as a group of interventions, requires no special equipment, does not need a physician's supervision, and can be implemented in a variety of settings. A major benefit of relaxation interventions for the patient is that after a number of training sessions, the patient can practice the techniques on his own. This puts the control in the patient's hands and increases his self-reliance.

In 1929, relaxation training was originated by a physiologist named Edmunt Jacobson[12] who developed a method of combating tension and anxiety by instructing patients to tense and relax various muscle groups in the body systematically. The philosophy of the method is that it is physically impossible to be "nervous" in a part of the body if in that part the person is completely relaxed. The aim of the training was not for people to be devoid of stress, but rather to feel comfortable with themselves and alert to their internal and external environment. Relaxation did not become popular in psychiatric circles until the late 1950s when Wolpe[29] developed the procedure called "systematic desensitization" and produced research evidence demonstrating its effectiveness in treating phobic patients.

The various relaxation procedures are very similar, and they all require a thorough assessment of oneself and one's patient. It is essential that the nurse learn how to relax herself because it is impossible for one tense person to teach another tense person to relax. The nurse should also remember that relaxation is a learned skill that develops over time. Trying "too hard" is a deterrent and can actually create tension, whereas an open willingness to relax is most growth producing. A complete assessment of the patient must also be done with particular focus given to where the patient experiences anxiety in his body. Relevant muscle groups should be identified and given emphasis in the relaxation interventions.

The goal of systematic desensitization is to help the patient change his response to the threatening stimulus. To be successful, the person must have sufficient skills for coping with whatever he fears. For example, a person may be afraid of driving, but he can, in fact, drive and is limited only by his fear. This is different from the person who fears heterosexual contacts, but actually lacks the social skills in this regard. This technique involves the pairing of deep muscle relaxation with imagined scenes depicting situations that cause the patient to feel anxious. The assumption is that if the person is taught relaxation rather than anxiety while imagining such scenes, the real-life situation that the scene depicted will cause much less anxiety.

One of the important parts of systematic desensitization is deep muscle relaxation. As a therapeutic tool it is very effective and can be utilized by itself to decrease tension and anxiety. It can also be combined with other types of interventions such as supportive or insight therapy. The basic premise is that muscle tension is related to anxiety, and if tense muscles can be made to relax, the person will experience a reduction in anxiety. The method used for relaxing the muscles involves the tensing and relaxing of voluntary muscles in an orderly sequence until the body, as a whole, is helped.

Rimm and Masters[23] describe the procedure. The patient should be seated in a comfortable chair in an open and unrestricted manner. The environment may contain soft music or pleasant visual cues. Before beginning the exercises, a brief explanation should be given that relates anxiety to muscle tension and describes the relaxation procedure about to be begun. The patient should take a deep breath and exhale slowly. A sequence of tension-relaxation exercises is then initiated. The patient is instructed to tense each muscle group for about 10 seconds while the nurse describes how tense and uncomfortable this body part feels. He then is asked to relax this muscle group as the nurse comments, "Notice how all the hardness and tension is draining from your hands. Now notice how they feel warm, soft, and calm. Compare this feeling to when they were tense and see how much better they feel now." The patient should be reminded to tense only the muscle group named and not other muscles.

The patient then proceeds to the next muscle group in the following sequence:

1. *Hands.* First the fists are tensed and relaxed. Then the fingers are extended and relaxed.

2. *Biceps and triceps.* These are tensed and relaxed.

3. *Shoulders.* They are pulled back and relaxed and then pushed forward and relaxed.

4. *Neck.* The head is turned slowly as far to the right as possible and relaxed, turned to the

left and relaxed, and then brought forward until the chin touches the chest and relaxed.

5. *Mouth*. The mouth is opened as wide as possible and relaxed. The lips form a pout and then relax. The tongue is extended out as far as possible and relaxed and is then retracted into the throat and relaxed. It is pressed hard into the roof of the mouth and relaxed and then is pressed hard into the floor of the mouth and relaxed.

6. *Eyes*. They are opened as wide as possible and relaxed and then closed as hard as possible and relaxed.

7. *Breathing*. The patient inhales as deeply as possible and relaxes. He then exhales as much as possible and relaxes.

8. *Back*. The trunk of the body is pushed forward so the entire back is arched, and then it is relaxed.

9. *Midsection*. The buttock muscles are tensed and relaxed.

10. *Thighs*. The legs are extended and raised about 6 inches off the floor and then relaxed. The backs of the feet are pressed into the floor and relaxed.

11. *Stomach*. It is pulled in as much as possible and relaxed and is then extended and relaxed.

12. *Calves and feet*. With legs supported, the feet are bent with the toes pointing toward the head and then relaxed. Feet are then bent in the opposite direction and relaxed.

13. *Toes*. The toes are pressed into the bottom of the shoes and relaxed. They are then bent to touch the top inside of the shoes and relaxed.

The final exercise asks the patient to become *completely* relaxed, beginning with his toes and following the sensation up through his body to his eyes and forehead. When the patient learns the procedure, he can eliminate some of the exercises and employ them only on the muscles that usually become tense. This is individual for each person and may include the shoulders, forehead, back, or neck. He may also eliminate the tensing exercises and perform only the relaxation ones.

This procedure may be followed or replaced by another approach to evoke the relaxation response—meditation. The basic components for meditation include the following[2]:

1. A quiet environment
2. A passive attitude
3. A comfortable position
4. A word or scene to focus on

The first three components are necessary elements for any relaxation procedure. The fourth component in meditation refers to the process in which the patient is asked to select a cue word or scene with pleasant connotations. He is then instructed to close his eyes, relax each of the major muscle groups, and then begin repeating the word silently to himself each time he exhales.

Another method of tension reduction is the use of biofeedback. During a biofeedback training session small electrodes connected to the biofeedback equipment are attached to the patient's forehead. The patient is then instructed to concentrate on relaxing, which will reduce the pitch of the biofeedback tone created by his tension. The higher the pitch, the more muscle tension. Once he has developed the ability to relax, the patient is then encouraged to apply the technique in stressful situations.

If systematic desensitization is employed, the patient must be able to attain muscle relaxation. Additional steps are then undertaken. A hierarchy, or graded series, of situations or scenes is identified. They must be realistic, concrete situations created by the patient. They are then ranked from 1 to 10, with a rating of 1 evoking little or no anxiety and a rating of 10 evoking intense or severe anxiety. The patient is asked to imagine the scenes, beginning with the first and employing his ability to relax. If he experiences no anxiety, he continues on to the next scene. If he experiences anxiety, he stops and restores himself to the state of relaxation. This procedure is implemented repeatedly until the hierarchy is completed. The success of this method of intervention appears to be because it indirectly encourages patients to expose themselves to objects or situations that are actually feared, and it is most effective in the treatment of phobias.

Additional steps may also be taken. The patient may role play the stressful situation with the nurse or other patients. While role playing, he is asked to identify the location and level of his anxiety and practice relaxing it away. The patient can practice relaxing while at home, as well as when in proximity to feared situations. These exercises teach the practical use of relaxation and allow the patient to rehearse them with some safety. Ideally, he will learn to recognize when and how his body responds to stress and will initiate relaxation exercises accordingly. The final step is to regulate one's response

TABLE 7-4. Common problems and solutions associated with relaxation training*

Problem	Solution	Problem	Solution
Muscle cramps	Ask the patient to generate less tension in these areas for shorter periods of time and to tense and relax the muscles more slowly; if cramps do occur, let the patient manipulate the cramped muscle, wait a few minutes, and then continue	Inability to relax certain muscle groups	Work with the patient to evaluate the technique and develop an alternate tensing strategy
Movement, such as stretching, yawning, or shifting position	Sometimes this is to help the patient assume a more relaxed position and should be encouraged; if it is disruptive, review the specific relaxation technique being used and evaluate its effectiveness	Strange or unfamiliar feelings, such as floating, lack of body perception, etc.	This is a common occurrence if relaxation techniques are new to the patient; convey this to him, ask him to open his eyes and look around and become oriented; encourage the patient to respond to relaxation as an enjoyable, rather than fearful, experience
Laughter or talking	Initially this may indicate embarrassment or nervousness over a new situation; since doing the facial exercises may create "funny-looking" expressions, it may be helpful for the nurse to do them with the patient	Sense of "losing control"	Sometimes these exercises focus directly on issues of control that may be problematic in themselves for the patient; if so, spend more time discussing his subjective experience, introduce the exercises more gradually, and spend more time ensuring that the positive expectancies established earlier are fulfilled
Noise	Initially a quiet room is best, which minimizes the disruptions associated with phones ringing, clocks ticking, and doors slamming; gradually, the patient should be helped to relax with some background noise, since the everyday world is filled with sounds	Sense of "internal arousal" or inside tension despite external relaxation	Explain to the patient that these exercises effect voluntary muscle control, whereas internal tension results from involuntary muscles also; however, voluntary and involuntary control are interrelated and, with practice, the patient should feel decreased internal tension
Intrusive thoughts	If intrusive thoughts result in anxiety or discomfort for the patient, the nurse can either increase her dialogue or help the patient select a new group of thoughts or images; if the intrusive thoughts involve sexual arousal, the nurse can note that this is not unusual and continue to focus on other images	Failure to follow instructions	Identify and analyze the underlying cause, has the patient forgotten or misunderstood the directions, or is he trying to control the nurse and therapy situation
Sleep	This is *not* a desired outcome; the nurse should be careful not to use the word sleep, but rather "relaxed but very awake"; the patient can also be asked to focus on the sound of her voice	Problems with practicing	Assist the patient in arranging his work and home schedules to allow for two 20-minute sessions per day; if a problem continues, the patient's lack of cooperation and resistance should be discussed
Coughing and sneezing	This is usually only a problem with heavy smokers; in this case, the nurse should not encourage very deep breaths because they might cause the smoker to cough	Words and phrases to avoid	Assess the patient before and during the exercises for phrases that appear to be annoying or tension producing for him; these should be avoided in the first few sessions

*Data from Bernstein, D., and Borkovec, T.: Progressive relaxation training, Champaign, Ill., 1973, Research Press.

when actually coping with the stressor and to maintain these new relaxation skills. This will require nursing care feedback and follow-up and perhaps the development of personalized stress management programs for the patient.

As with any other nursing intervention, problems can arise in the teaching, learning, and practicing of these relaxation techniques. If a little is good, it should not be assumed that a lot is even better. It has been observed that when the response was elicited for two limited daily periods of 20 to 30 minutes, no adverse side effects resulted. However, when elicited more frequently, some patients might experience a "withdrawal from life" that can complicate or compound previous psychiatric problems.[3] Furthermore, relaxation techniques should not be used to insulate oneself from the outside world. Mild levels of anxiety are growth producing and the fight or flight response is often appropriate and essential for survival. Other common problems specific to relaxation training are summarized in Table 7-4.

Evaluation

Evaluation is an ongoing process engaged in by the nurse and patient that is part of each phase of the nursing process. Even before she begins to formulate the nursing diagnosis, the nurse should ask herself: "Did I critically observe my patient's physiological and psychomotor behaviors? Did I listen to his subjective description of his experience? Did I fail to see the relationships between his expressed hostility or guilt and his underlying anxiety? Did I assess his intellectual and social functioning?" In concluding her collection of data, the nurse should analyze the data she has collected. Was she able to identify the precipitating stressor for the patient? What was his perception of the threat? How was this influenced by his physical health, past experiences, and present feelings and needs? Did she correctly identify the patient's level of anxiety and try to validate it with him? Was she able to identify the patient's coping mechanisms and determine if they were constructive or destructive in nature? The diagnosis itself should be stated clearly and precisely. It should include the patient's problematical behavior pattern and his level of anxiety.

Nursing goals should be mutually determined and should describe what the nurse wishes to accomplish within a designated time span. Her

plan of action explains how and why. When using the criteria of adequacy, effectiveness, appropriateness, efficiency, and flexibility in judging the nursing goals and actions, the following questions can be raised:

■ Was the planning and implementation a mutual process as much as possible?
■ Were my goals and actions adequate in number and sufficiently specific to minimize my patient's level of anxiety?
■ Did I work through all the stages of the problem-solving process with my patient?
■ Were his maladaptive responses reduced?
■ Did he learn new adaptive coping responses?
■ Was the care plan reasonable in terms of our mutual constraints of time, energy, and expense?
■ Were my many inferences, such as anxiety level, stressors, and coping patterns, appropriately validated with the patient and other staff members?
■ Was I accepting of the patient and did I critically monitor my own anxiety level throughout the relationship?
■ Was I able to modify my interventions on the basis of the patient's changing needs and feelings?
■ Did I include the patient in the evaluation process?

Answering these questions will allow the nurse to review the total care she provided. Additional patient needs may become evident at this time. The nurse will also identify personal strengths and limitations in working with the anxious patient. Plans may then be made for overcoming the areas of limitation and further improving the quality of the nursing care provided. Throughout this process the nurse supports the belief that the "clarification of anxiety makes possible expanded awareness and an expansion of the self, which means the achieving of emotional health."[16:150]

Suggested cross-references

Therapeutic relationship skills, including self-awareness of the nurse, are discussed in Chapter 3. The model of health-illness phenomena, with a detailed discussion of precipitating stressors, and the phases of the nursing process are discussed in Chapter 4. Nursing intervention in psychotic panic states is discussed in Chapter 11. Somatic therapies are discussed in Chapter 15.

SUMMARY

1. Anxiety was defined as diffuse apprehension that is vague in nature and is associated with feelings of uncertainty and helplessness. It occurs as a result of a threat to one's self-esteem or identity. It is an emotion without an object that is subjective in nature and communicated interpersonally. The capacity to be anxious is necessary for survival, and the positive aspects of selfhood develop as the individual confronts, moves through, and overcomes anxiety-creating experiences. Four levels of anxiety were identified and described: mild, moderate, severe, and panic. Mild anxiety increases one's perceptual field, motivates learning, and can produce growth and creativity in the individual.

2. Many theories of the origin of anxiety have been proposed, but the present core of definitely established facts to support these theories is small. Predisposing factors may be related to the threat of deprivation, the emotional conflict between the id and superego, the fear of interpersonal disapproval and rejection, low self-esteem, frustration, a learned response to avoid pain, conflict situations involving avoidance, and the person's general health status. There are two major types of precipitating factors: threats to one's physical integrity and threats to one's self-system.

3. Data collection by the nurse should include both behavioral responses and coping mechanisms. Physiological responses associated with anxiety are primarily mediated through the autonomic nervous system. They are predominantly sympathetic in nature and serve to activate body processes in a "fight or flight" reaction. Behavioral responses reflect increased activity and restlessness. Withdrawal and decreased personal involvement are common social manifestations of high levels of anxiety. Affective responses convey apprehension and vague fears and may also include feelings of anger, boredom, depression, worthlessness, and helplessness. As anxiety increases, cognitive functioning is characterized by a decreased perceptual field, poor concentration, and errors in judgment.

4. The individual uses various coping mechanisms to deny or allay his anxiety. These defenses against anxiety are reflected in pathological behavior or symptoms of emotional illness that provide the outward but disguised symbolical expression of elements of the conflict. Mild levels of anxiety are often handled without conscious thought, and their effects can be minimized with little effort. Task-oriented reactions, ego-oriented reactions, psychological conversions, and physiological conversions are coping mechanisms used with moderate and severe levels of anxiety.

a. Task-oriented reactions are conscious attempts to realistically meet the demands of the stress situation. They are action-oriented responses and include *attack, withdrawal,* and *compromise.*

b. Ego-oriented reactions, or *defense mechanisms,* serve as one's first line of psychic defense, since they protect the person from feelings of inadequacy and anxiety. Thirteen specific defense mechanisms were defined and described.

c. Psychological conversions include phobic reactions, dissociative reactions, obsessions, and compulsions. A *phobia* is a persistent fear of an object or situation that presents no actual danger or whose danger is magnified out of proportion. In *dissociative reactions* the patient blocks off part of his life from conscious recognition due to the threat of overwhelming anxiety. These reactions include somnambulism, amnesia, and multiple personalities. An *obsession* is an unwanted recurring thought. A *compulsion* is a recurring impulse to perform some act that cannot be resisted.

d. Physiological conversions are changes in the biological system that accompany anxiety.

5. The position of anxiety within the larger perspective of the model of health-illness phenomena was described. Constructive coping mechanisms lead to adaptive responses, whereas destructive coping mechanisms lead to maladaptive responses and can be expressed as either neurotic or psychotic health problems. Formulating a nursing diagnosis requires that the nurse determine the quality (appropriateness) of the patient's response, the quantity (level) of his anxiety, and the nature of the coping mechanism mobilized. The diagnosis when stated should include the patient's problematical behavior pattern or nonproductive coping mechanism and his level of anxiety.

6. Possible nursing diagnoses and selected medical diagnoses were related. The overall goal of the nursing intervention is to help the patient develop the capacity to tolerate mild anxiety and use it consciously and constructively.

7. The highest priority nursing goals should address lowering the patient's severe or panic levels of anxiety, and related nursing interventions should be supportive and protective. The development of a therapeutic relationship is necessary in which the nurse critically monitors her own anxiety level. The patient's needs are met through the protection of his defenses and providing for the discharge of anxiety through physical activity. Supportive chemotherapy may also be administered.

8. When the patient's anxiety is reduced to the mild or moderate level, insight-oriented or reeducative nursing interventions may be implemented. This involves the patient in a problem-solving process that includes the following steps: recognition of anxiety, insight into the anxiety, and coping with the threat.

9. Nursing interventions that help the patient cope with stress by regulating the emotional distress associated with it were also described. These included the relaxation techniques of systematic desensitization, meditation, and the use of biofeedback. A major benefit of these interventions for the patient is that they place the control in the patient's hands and increase his self-reliance.

10. In evaluating the nursing care given, the nurse reviews and analyzes each phase of the nursing process. By examining her effectiveness in working with an anxious patient, the nurse enlarges her own self-awareness and increases her therapeutic potential.

References

1. Arieti, S.: Anxiety and beyond in schizophrenia and psychotic depression, Nurs. Digest **2:**70, March 1974.
2. Benson, H.: The relaxation response, New York, 1975, William Morrow & Co., Inc.
3. Benson, H., et al.: The relaxation response, Psychiatry **37:**37, Feb. 1974.
4. Bernstein, D., and Borkovec, T.: Progressive relaxation training, Champaign, Ill., 1973, Research Press.
5. Burd, S.: Effects of nursing intervention in anxiety of patients. In Burd, S.F., and Marshall, M.A., editors: Some clinical approaches to psychiatric nursing, New York, 1963, Macmillan, Inc.
6. Caplan, G.: Mastery of stress: psychosocial aspects, Am. J. Psychiatry **138**(4):413, 1981.
7. Diagnostic and statistical manual of mental disorders, ed. 3, Washington, D.C., 1980, The American Psychiatric Association.
8. Dollard, J., and Miller, N.: Personality and psychotherapy, New York, 1950, McGraw-Hill Book Co.
9. Elliott, S.: Denial as an effective mechanism to allay anxiety following a stressful event, J. Psychiatr. Nurs. **18**(10):11, 1980.
10. Freud, S.: Problem of anxiety, New York, 1936, W.W. Norton & Co., Inc.
11. Freud, S.: A general introduction to psychoanalysis, New York, 1969, Pocket Books.
12. Jacobson, E.: Progressive relaxation, ed. 3, Chicago, 1974, University of Chicago Press.
13. Kristic, J.: Anxiety levels of hospitalized psychiatric patients throughout total hospitalization, J. Psychiatr. Nurs. **17**(7):33, 1979.
14. Lagina, S.: A computer program to diagnose anxiety level, Nurs. Res. **20:**491, 1971.
15. Lassen, C.: The effect of proximity in the psychiatric interview, J. Abnorm. Psychol. **82:**226, June 1973.
16. May, R.: The meaning of anxiety, New York, 1950, Ronald Press Co.
17. Meares, A.: The management of the anxious patient, Philadelphia, 1963, W.B. Saunders Co.
18. Mendels, J., Weinstein, N., and Cochrane, C.: The relationship between depression and anxiety, Arch. Gen. Psychiatry **27:**649, 1972.
19. Menninger, K., Maymann, M., and Rugyser, P.: The vital balance, New York, 1963, The Viking Press.
20. Oden, G.: Individual panic: elements and patterns. In Burd, S., and Marshall, M., editors: Some clinical approaches to psychiatric nursing, New York, 1963, Macmillan, Inc.
21. Peplau, H.: Interpersonal techniques: the crux of psychiatric nursing, Am. J. Nurs. **62:**53, June 1962.
22. Peplau, H.: A working definition of anxiety. In Burd, S., and Marshall, M., editors: Some clinical approaches to psychiatric nursing, New York, 1963, Macmillan, Inc.
23. Rimm, D., and Masters, J.: Behavior therapy, New York, 1974, Academic Press, Inc.
24. Salzman, L., and Thaler, F.: Obsessive-compulsive disorders: a review of the literature, Am. J. Psychiatry **138**(3):286, 1981.
25. Shand, J., and Grau, B.: Perceived self and ideal self ratings in relation to high and low levels of anxiety in college women, J. Psychol. **87:**55, Jan. 1977.
26. Sullivan, H.S.: The interpersonal theory of psychiatry, New York, 1953, W.W. Norton & Co., Inc.
27. Tillich, P.: The courage to be, New Haven, Conn., 1952, Yale University Press.
28. Will, O.: Psychotherapy in reference to the schizophrenic reaction. In Stein, M., editor: Contemporary psychotherapies, New York, 1961, The Free Press of Glencoe.
29. Wolpe, J.: The practice of behavior therapy, New York, 1973, Pergamon Press, Inc.

Annotated suggested readings

Aadalen, S.P., and Stroebel-Kahn, F.: Coping with quadriplegia, Am. J. Nurs. **81:**1471, 1981.
This is a case study of the physical and emotional trauma experienced by the author after an accident that left her a quadriplegic. She discusses the adaptive mechanisms she and her family used as they coped with this event and which kinds of professional support could have aided in their adjustment.
American Psychiatric Association: Diagnostic and statistical manual of mental disorders, ed. 3, Washington, D.C., 1980, The Association.

This required reference text for all psychiatric nurses contains the categories and codes of axes I and II and the complete text and criteria related to each of the diagnostic categories associated with medically diagnosed psychiatric health problems.
Bell, J.: Stressful life events and coping methods in mental illness and wellness behaviors, Nurs. Res. **26:**136, March-April, 1977.
This descriptive comparative study examines not only the relationship between stressful life events and mental illness and wellness behaviors but also the coping methods

used by individuals exhibiting each behavior. Data collection included the use of the Holmes and Rahe Social Readjustment Rating Scale. The author summarizes her study with implications for nursing and health care.

Breeden, S., and Kondo, C.: Using biofeedback to reduce tension, Am. J. Nurs. **75:**2010, 1975.

This brief article supports the use of biofeedback training to reduce stress and relieve stress-related illness. It describes how biofeedback works and briefly reviews three clinical experiences in biofeedback training sessions.

Burd, S.: Effects of nursing intervention in anxiety of patients. In Burd, S.F., and Marshall, M.A., editors: Some clinical approaches to psychiatric nursing, New York, 1963, Macmillan, Inc.

Following the approach outlined by Peplau, the author uses the problem-solving and learning process to develop a framework for intervening with anxious patients. The article reports the results of a small study conducted to examine the framework; principles as well as techniques are described.

Fischer, W.: Theories of anxiety, New York, 1970, Harper & Row, Publishers, Inc.

Freudian, neo-Freudian, learning theory, physiological, and existential formulations of anxiety are clearly synthesized and impartially described. An attempt is also made to integrate the theories based on common experiential phenomena. This is a good source book for a more detailed comparison of the various theories of anxiety.

Garrison, J., and Scott, P.: A group self-care approach to stress management, J. Psychiatr. Nurs. **17**(6):9, 1979.

A procedure is described for teaching patients the use of relaxation as a coping skill. Each of the three components of this group training is clearly defined in the article, including progressive relaxation and clinical meditation.

Hawkrigg, J.J.: Agoraphobia. I and II, Nurs. Times **71:**1280, 1337, 1975.

Agoraphobia is defined and pertinent clinical features are described. The article reports the results of a research project on treating agoraphobia and compares the treatment modalities of relaxation, systematic desensitization, behavioral counseling, reinforced graded practice, and stress inoculation.

Hays, D.: Teaching a concept of anxiety, Nurs. Res. **10:**108, Spring 1961.

This article summarizes a small study that involved teaching patients about anxiety. It relates levels of anxiety, perceptual and behavioral changes, and learning tasks of the anxious person.

Kerr, N.: Anxiety: theoretical considerations, Perspect. Psychiatr. Care **16:**36, Jan.-March 1978.

The author describes the theoretical formulations about anxiety by Freud, Horney, and Kierkegaard. Her presentation is clear and concise.

Kjervik, D.: Dual personality: assessment and reintegration, J. Psychiatr. Nurs. **17**(7):28, 1979.

This is one of the few articles in the nursing literature that discusses the relatively rare phenomenon of dissociation, or multiple personalities. Theoretical considerations are presented; then practical application of the theory is made to a case of dual personality.

Kristic, J.: Anxiety levels of hospitalized psychiatric patients throughout total hospitalization, J. Psychiatr. Nurs. **17**(7):33, 1979.

Nurses interested in conducting research in psychiatric nursing will benefit from reading the report of this clinical study for the research process it describes, the findings it reveals, and the implications for nursing care it discusses.

May, R.: The meaning of anxiety, New York, 1950, Ronald Press Co.

This book brings together various theories of anxiety, synthesizes common elements of these theories, and suggests some constructive methods for dealing with anxiety. It incorporates philosophy, culture, biology, and psychology in its discussion and supports its analysis of anxiety with pertinent clinical studies. It is an excellent text and a "classic" in the field.

Oden, G.: Individual panic: elements and patterns. In Burd, S.F., and Marshall, M.A., editors: Some clinical approaches to psychiatric nursing, New York, 1963, Macmillan, Inc.

The author explores the questions "What is panic?" and "What happens during a panic episode?" She reviews the literature on both individual and group panic and presents the results of her research study related to the identification of the elements and patterns of individual panic. Seven case studies are described.

Olson, L.: Intervention in a pathological cycle of anxiety, J. Psychiatr. Nurs. **12:**21, March 1974.

This is a case presentation of a 13-year-old girl hospitalized with myasthenia gravis and experiencing high levels of anxiety. The plan of care developed with the aid of a nursing consultant is described, and it includes problems, goals, and nursing approaches.

Rimm, D., and Masters, J.: Behavior therapy, New York, 1974, Academic Press, Inc.

This text addresses two basic questions—"How does one do behavior therapy?" and "What is the evidence demonstrating that behavior therapy is truly effective?" It provides detailed accounts of a variety of behavior therapy techniques including desensitization, assertiveness training, and operant procedures, as well as the rational-emotive therapy of Ellis. It also describes the empirical findings that demonstrate the effectiveness of the techniques in various settings. It is a thorough and clear text on this subject.

Roncoli, M.: Bantering: a therapeutic strategy with obsessional patients, Perspect. Psychiatr. Care **12:**171, Oct.-Dec. 1974.

The author explores the strategy of the therapist as a psychological humorist who assists the obsessional patient to gain insight through the use of bantering. Bantering is defined as ridiculing lightly and good naturedly. The purpose is to release the patient's aggression and anger and the therapist's feelings of exasperation.

Salzman, L., and Thaler, F.: Obsessive-compulsive disorders: a review of the literature, Am. J. Psychiatr **138**(3):286, 1981.

The authors reviewed the studies on obsessive-compulsive disorders published from 1953 to 1978. They report on various theories of the etiology of the disorders and treatment modalities used and conclude that, although the disorders are prevalent, there are little new data concerning their treatment, and serious questions about the effectiveness of the various treatment approaches remain.

Sheer, B.: The effects of relaxation training on psychiatric inpatients, Issues Mental Health Nurs. **2**(4):1, 1980.

The purpose of the author's research was to determine if psychiatric inpatients who receive relaxation training as a part of their nursing care show a decrease between pretest and posttest scores on an anxiety scale. Although the results of the data did not support this hypothesis, this article is worth reading for the research process it describes.

Sutterly, D., and Donnelly, G., editors: Coping with stress: a nursing perspective, Germantown, Md., 1981, Aspen Systems Corp.

This text is a collection of articles about stress and nursing organized around the following areas: models of stress, stress and life events, stress of illness, self-regulation of stress, and stress and the caregiver.

Tillich, P.: The courage to be, New Haven, Conn., 1952, Yale University Press.

This book is concerned with anxiety, its conquest, and the meaning of courage. Tillich believes anxiety comes from the loss of the meaning of life, whereas the "courage to be" involves participation as well as individualization. This distinguished book is a classic in the field.

Trygstad, L.: Simple new way to help anxious patients, R.N. **43**(12):28, 1980.

This brief article is useful for the relaxation techniques and model scripts described by the author.

White, R., and Gilliland, R.: Elements of psychopathology, New York, 1975, Grune & Stratton, Inc.

All the basic information needed to understand the mechanisms of defense is brought together in a readable form from a psychoanalytical frame of reference. Each defense mechanism is organized into general comments, definition, clinical examples, clinical syndromes that illustrate the mechanism, and examples of the use of the mechanisms in normal behavior. This book is of value to the student and is also an excellent review for the clinician.

To venture causes anxiety,
but not to venture, is to lose one's self.
And to venture in the highest sense
is precisely to be conscious of one's self.

Sören Kierkegaard

CHAPTER 8

ALTERATIONS IN
SELF-CONCEPT

Learning objectives

*After studying this chapter, the student
should be able to:*

- *define the following terms: self-concept, body
  image, self-ideal, self-esteem, role, and identity.*

- *discuss factors and experiences throughout the life
  cycle that influence each of the above concepts.*

- *describe the characteristics of a healthy personality structure.*

- *analyze the stressors affecting self-esteem, role,
  body image, and identity.*

- *identify and describe behaviors that are associated
  with low self-esteem, role strain, disturbed body
  image, negative identity, identity confusion, and
  depersonalization.*

- *formulate individualized nursing diagnoses for patients with alterations in self-concept.*

- *assess the relationship between nursing diagnoses
  associated with alterations in self-concept and
  medical diagnoses of selected psychotic and neurotic disorders.*

- *develop long-term and short-term individualized
  nursing goals for patients who are experiencing
  alterations in self-concept.*

- *apply therapeutic nurse-patient relationship principles with appropriate rationale in planning the
  care of the patient who is experiencing an alteration in self-concept.*

- *describe the progressive levels of nursing interventions appropriate to the needs of the patient who
  is experiencing an alteration in self-concept.*

- *assess the importance of the evaluation of the nursing process when working with patients with alterations in self-concept.*

- *identify suggested readings for future study.*

242

O f all man's atttributes, the self appears to be the most complex and most intangible. One can neither see nor touch a self-concept, yet it has been a topic of concern to behavioral scientists since the late 1800s. The concept of self is not clearly defined, has various meanings, and is used in many different ways. But the self is the most real thing in one's experience and it is the frame of reference through which a person perceives, conceives, and evaluates the world around him. Self-concept can be defined as all the notions, beliefs, and convictions that constitute an individual's knowledge of himself and influence his relationships with others. It includes the perceptions of one's characteristics and abilities, one's interaction with other people and the environment, one's values associated with experiences and objects, and one's goals and ideals.

Helping professionals of all backgrounds have increasingly come to view the self-concept as a critical and central element for the understanding of people and their behavior, and it is now the subject of an enormous body of theory and research. This inquiry has given rise to a theoretical school known as "self theory," which is based on the principle that man's behavior is always meaningful and that a person reacts to the world in terms of the way he perceives it. No two people have identical self-concepts. The self-concept emerges or is learned as a result of each person's unique experiences within himself, with other people, and with the realities of the world. Because it is the frame of reference through which the person interacts with the world, it is a powerful influence on human behavior. Self theorists believe it is impossible to understand a person fully or to accurately predict his behavior without understanding his internal frame of reference. This involves sharing his own private perceptual world and his views of himself. Thus understanding a patient's self-concept is a necessary component of all nursing care.

Continuum of self-concept responses

Although theories of self-concept development vary considerably, there is general agreement that the self-concept does not exist at birth. The self develops gradually as the infant recognizes and distinguishes others and vaguely begins to differentiate himself as a separate individual. The boundaries of the self are defined as a result of exploratory activity and experience with his own body as the infant interacts with his environment. At first, the process of self-differentiation is slow, but with the development of language, the process becomes accelerated. Language helps to clarify the concept of the self, and the child's own name is a major linguistic aid. The use of a proper name helps the child identify himself and perceive himself as someone special, unique, and independent. In general, the ability to use language enables the child to make clear distinctions between himself and the rest of the world and to symbolize and understand his experiences. Once the infant has begun to differentiate himself from other people and the environment, the continued process of self-concept development is greatly benefited by the following:

- Interpersonal and cultural experiences that generate positive feelings and a sense of value and worth
- Perceived competence in areas that are valued by the individual and society
- Self-actualization, or the implementation and realization of one's true potential

The self-concept is learned in part through accumulated social contacts and experiences with other people. Sullivan[40] called this development "learning about self from the mirror of other people." What a person believes about himself is a function of his interpretation of how others see him, which he infers from their behavior toward him. His concept of self therefore rests in part on what he thinks others think of him. "Significant others" in the life of a child particularly affect the development of self-concept, and, for a young child, the most significant others in his life are his parents. How they help him grow and react to his experiences has a tremendous influence on him. According to Combs and Snygg:

No experience in the development of the child's concepts of self is quite so important or far-reaching as his earliest experiences in his family. It is the family which introduces a child to life, which provides him with his earliest and most permanent self definitions. Here it is that he first discovers those basic concepts of self which will guide his behavior for the rest of his life.[10:134-135]

They believe that the family provides the individual with his earliest experiences of (1) feelings of adequacy or inadequacy, (2) feelings of acceptance or rejection, (3) opportunities for identification, and (4) expectancies concerning acceptable goals, values, and behaviors. Studies indicate that parental influence is strongest during early childhood and continues to have a significant impact through adolescence and young adulthood.[14] However, with age, the power and influence of friends and other adults increases, and they now become significant others to the individual. Parents and immediate family therefore are crucial to the initial development of the self-concept, and the continuing development and change in self-perceptions are influenced by countless experiences with many other people.

Culture and socialization practices also affect self-concept and personality development. An understanding of the dominant cultural patterns of the individual's environment gives important clues to the sources of personality formation. General culture patterns as well as cultural subdivisions, such as social class membership, have formative influences on the individual's view of self. According to Combs and Snygg:

> The culture in which we move is so completely a part of our experience as to overshadow almost all else in determining the nature of the self. Even our definitions and values are not left entirely to our own experience but are colored, interpreted and valued one way or another by the culture into which we are born, as they are interpreted to us by the acts of the people who surround us.[10.86]

A person's view of himself is not exclusively a collection of the views, expectations, and desires of others. Each person can observe his own behavior the same way that others do and form opinions about himself. One's perception of reality is selective, however, according to whether the experience is consistent with one's current concept of self. The way a person behaves is a result of how he perceives the situation, and it is not the event itself that elicits a specific response but rather the individual's subjective experience of the event. An individual's needs, values, and beliefs strongly influence his perceptions. One more readily perceives that which is meaningful and consistent with present needs and personal values. Similarly, people behave in a manner that is consistent with what they believe to be true. In this case, a fact is not what is but what one believes to be true. Once perceptions are acquired and incorporated into one's self-system, they can be difficult to change. There are ways, nonetheless, to change or modify one's perceptions, and these can include modification of cognitive processes, exposure to drugs, sensory deprivation, and biochemical changes within the body.

As the self-concept develops, it brings with it a unique perspective in viewing one's relationship with the world. What a person perceives and how he interprets what he perceives are conditioned by his concepts of self. A person with a weak or negative self-concept and who is unsure of himself is likely to have a narrowed or distorted perceptual field. Because he feels easily threatened, his anxiety level will rise quickly and he will become preoccupied with defending himself. In contrast, a person with a strong or positive self-concept can explore his world openly and honestly because he has a background of actual experiences of acceptance and success. Positive self-concepts are the result of actual positive experiences that lead to perceived competence.

In conclusion, it can be stated that self-concept is a critical and central variable in human behavior. Individuals with positive self-concepts function more effectively, which is evident in interpersonal competence, intellectual efficiency, and environmental mastery. In contrast, negative self-concept is correlated with personal and social maladjustment. Like the other nursing problems described in this text, it is possible to view one's self-concept responses along

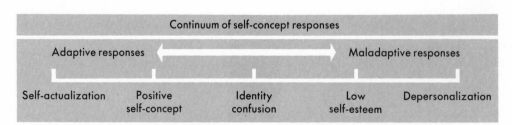

FIG. 8-1
Continuum of self-concept responses.

the health-illness continuum of coping responses described in Chapter 4. Fig. 8-1 describes the range of self-concept responses from the most adaptive state of self-actualization to the most maladaptive response of depersonalization.

Precisely because one's self-concept pervades every aspect of life, therapeutic interventions related to self-concept are a core element in psychiatric nursing practice. This requires an understanding of the various components of the self, including the concepts of body image, self-ideal, self-esteem, role, and identity, which will now be briefly discussed. The chapter will then focus on the use of the nursing therapeutic process model for maladaptive responses related to self-concept.

Body image

The concept of one's body is central to the concept of self. The body can be thought of as a capsule in which one is permanently enclosed and through which one interacts with the world. One lives with his body 24 hours a day from birth until death. It is the most material and visible part of the self, and, although it alone never accounts for one's entire sense of self, it remains a life-long anchor for self-awareness. An individual's attitude toward his body may mirror important aspects of his identity. A person's feelings that his body is big or small, attractive or unattractive, or weak or strong also reveal something about his self-concept.

Body image can be defined as the sum of the conscious and unconscious attitudes the individual has toward his body. It includes present and past perceptions as well as feelings about size, function, appearances, and potential. Body image is a dynamic entity because it is continually being modified by new perceptions and experiences. It serves as a target or screen on which the person projects significant personal feelings, anxieties, and values.

One is not born with a body image. The infant receives input from his body but reacts to it in a global, undifferentiated way. As he gradually explores parts of his body, receives sensory stimulation from others, and begins to manipulate the environment, he becomes aware of the separateness of his own body from others. In the development of body awareness, the external body, that is, the body that can be seen and felt to the touch, is easier to learn about and is discovered earlier than the inner body. This recognition grows out of pleasurable and painful experiences. Actually, pain becomes the more dominant learning experience because pain sensory endings are distributed over the total surface of the body while sensations of pleasure are concentrated in a few erotic zones. For the preschooler the exploration of genitals and the discovery of anatomical differences between the sexes becomes especially important. The body occupies a middle position between the external world and the self as the agent of one's perceiving, thinking, and acting. The body can be viewed more externally and objectively than one's inner tensions, thoughts, and feelings. With increasing age there is a further differentiation of the self as a body and the self as a mind that can solve problems, make decisions, and experience feelings.

During the age of adolescence the physical self is of more concern than during any other period of life except, perhaps, old age. Basic physical changes force the body into the adolescent's awareness. He has lost the security of a familiar body. New sensations, features, and body proportions have emerged. Height, weight, and physical strength increase, and the growth of secondary sex characteristics may be troublesome or embarrassing. The development of breasts, menarche, growth of pubic and facial hair, and voice changes must be integrated into the individual's evolving body image. Physical changes at adolescence also symbolize the end of childhood; maturity is just over the horizon. Adult proportions begin to emerge, although it is impossible to be certain of the nature, extent, or duration of changes still to come. Soon the outline of mature features will be complete. So the adolescent is anxious—will his mature physical self become reasonably close to his ideal? One's body image during adolescence is a crucial element in shaping his self-concept and in facilitating or retarding his attainment of status and adequate social relations.

Early adulthood sees some stability of body change. For the healthy adult, the body experience is a moment-to-moment, highly flexible aspect of his daily life pattern. As he has grown older, his view of the importance of his body experience has changed. It can be truly said that the child "lives in his body," as compared to the adult who lives in his mind. To the child, eating, crawling, walking, and defecating can be all consuming, as can coughing and being febrile, congested, or constipated. They can occupy his sense of reality totally. The intensity of the child's involvement with his body, however, must be diminished in the course of his developing into an adult with a broadening sense of what is real. The diminution must be selective, since the emerging adult needs to retain a flexible potential fullness of awareness of direct body sensation and a blending in of body awareness into all aspects of his life. Many parts of his body experience must achieve the autonomy of automatic responses, such as walking and breathing. Other aspects of the body experience must emerge as flexibly adjusted pleasures, such as eating, orgasm, and exercise.

Middle age brings new challenges as different body parts age at different rates. The individual realizes his body is not functioning as well as it previously had. The later years of life accelerate the decline in physical abilities and can severely influence one's life-style and self-concept. As one's body image develops, extensions of the body become important, and anything that extends the effectiveness or control of one's body function can be called one's own. Clothes become indentified closely with the body, and in the same way toys, tools, and possessions serve as extensions of the body and help to widen one's sense of self. Still later, position and wealth serve similar functions.

When the individual values his body and acts to preserve and protect it, the body image becomes the basis of sympathy through which the bodies and possessions of others are also valued. Body image, appearance, and positive self-concept are related. Studies have indicated that the more a person accepts and likes his body, the more secure and free from anxiety he feels.[23] It has also been shown that people who accept their bodies are more likely to manifest high self-esteem than people who dislike their bodies.[18] Thus the concept of body-image is a central one to understanding self theory, and the relationship between the two will have implications for developing and implementing nursing care.

Self-ideal

The self-ideal is the individual's perception of how he should behave based on certain personal standards. The standard may be either a carefully constructed image of the kind of person one would like to be or merely a number of aspirations, goals, or values that one would like

to achieve. The self-ideal creates self-expectations that are based in part on society's norms and to which the person tries to conform. The formation of the self-ideal begins in childhood and is influenced by significant others who place certain demands or expectations on the child. With time, the child internalizes these expectations, and they form the basis of his own self-ideal. New self-ideals that may persist throughout life are taken on during adolescence, and they are formed from identification with parents, teachers, clergy, and age contemporaries. In old age additional adjustments must be made that reflect diminishing physical strength and changing roles and responsibilities.

There are a number of factors that influence one's self-ideal. The first is that a person tends to set goals within a range determined by his abilities. One does not ordinarily set a goal that is accomplished without any effort nor one that would be entirely beyond one's abilities. Self-ideals are also influenced by cultural factors as the person compares his self-standards with those of his peers so that his behavior will be consistent with his culture. Other influencing factors would include one's ambitions and the desire to excel and succeed, the need to be realistic, the desire to avoid failure, and the presence of feelings of anxiety and inferiority. Based on these factors, one's self-ideal may be clear and realistic and thus facilitate personal growth and relations with others, or it may be vague, unrealistic, and demanding. The adequately functioning individual, however, demonstrates congruence between his perception of self and his self-ideal. That is, he sees himself as being very much like the person he would like to be.

In summary, self-ideals are important in maintaining mental health and balance. They serve as internal regulators and help a person maintain an even course in the face of conflicting or confusing circumstances. For mental health the self-ideal must not be too high and too demanding nor too vague and shadowy, and yet it must be high enough to give continuous support to self-respect.

Self-esteem

Self-esteem is the individual's personal judgment of his own worth obtained by analyzing how well his behavior conforms to his self-ideal. The frequency with which his goals are achieved will directly result in the development of feelings of superiority (high self-esteem) or inferiority (low self-esteem) (Fig. 8-2). If a person is

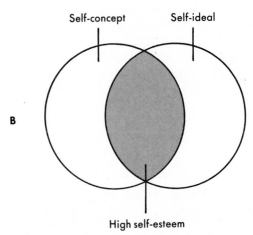

FIG. 8-2

A, Individual with a low level of self-esteem due to a large discrepancy between self-concept and self-ideal. **B,** Person with greater conformity of self-concept and self-ideal and therefore a person with a high level of self-esteem. (From Sundeen, S.J. et al.: Nurse-client interaction: implementing the nursing process, ed. 2, St. Louis, 1981, The C.V. Mosby Co.)

repeatedly successful, he tends to feel superior, but if he fails to live up to his expectations, he feels inferior. High self-esteem is a feeling rooted in unconditional acceptance of self, despite mistakes, defeats, and failures, as an innately worthy and important being. It involves accepting complete responsibility for one's own life.

Self-esteem is derived from two primary sources: the self and others. It is first of all a function of being loved and of gaining the respect of others. Self-esteem is lowered when love is lost and when one fails to receive approval from others. Conversely, it is raised when love is regained and when one is applauded and praised. The origins of self-esteem can be traced to childhood and are based on acceptance, praise, and respect. Coopersmith[11] described the four best ways to promote a child's self-esteem as follows:

1. Providing him with success
2. Instilling ideals
3. Encouraging his aspirations
4. Helping him build defenses against attacks of his self-perceptions

This should provide him with a feeling of significance—success in being accepted and approved of by others, a feeling of competence—ability to cope effectively with life, and a feeling of power—control over one's own destiny.

Self-esteem increases with age, although it is most threatened during adolescence. At this time, concepts of self are being modified and many self-decisions need to be made. The adolescent has to make an occupational choice and decide if he is good enough to succeed in a given career. He has to decide whether he is able to participate or is accepted in various social activities. Heterosexually, is he attractive enough to interest and attract a desirable member of the opposite sex? Will he succeed in marriage? Does he have the courage to carry out his convictions? Is he capable of performing the roles assigned to him?

With adulthood the self-concept stabilizes, and maturity provides a clearer picture of self. The adult tends to be more self-accepting and less idealistic than the adolescent. He has learned to cope with many of his self-deficiencies and maximize his self-strengths. Of course, not all adults attain maturity, and some continue to function as adolescents for many of their adult years. In later life, self-esteem problems again arise due to the new challenges posed by menopause, retirement, loss of spouse, and physical disability.

High self-esteem has been correlated with low anxiety, effective group functioning, and acceptance of others. It is also a prerequisite to self-actualization according to Maslow; once self-esteem is achieved, the individual is free to concentrate on achieving his potential.[30] Low self-esteem has been correlated with poor interpersonal relations, and a sense of low self-worth is particularly prominent in schizophrenia and depressive disorders.

Role

Roles are sets of socially expected behavior patterns associated with an individual's function in various social groups. Identity emerges from self-concept and is evident in the form of role behavior.[21] Roles can provide a means for social participation and a way to test out identities for consensual validation by significant others. The individual assumes various roles that he attempts to integrate into one functional pattern. Because these roles overlap and intertwine, an understanding of the person requires the nurse to see him in the context of the several roles he occupies. On the basis of his perception of role adequacy in the most "ego-involved" roles, the individual develops a level of self-esteem. High self-esteem results from roles that meet our needs and are congruent with our self-ideal. Many factors, including the following, influence an individual's adjustment to the role he occupies:

1. The clarity of the behaviors appropriate to the role and his knowledge of specific role expectations
2. The consistency of the response of significant others to his role
3. The compatibility and complementarity of his various roles
4. The congruency of cultural and his own expectations for role behavior
5. The segregation of situations that would create incompatible role behaviors

There are two basic types of roles. The first is an ascribed role over which the individual has no choice. Examples of ascribed roles include age and sex. The second is an assumed role that the individual selects or achieves by choice. These roles include occupation and marital or family roles.

Sex roles are important roles that affect one's performance in other roles. They are particularly significant for the performance of family roles, but they permeate most other roles as well and are frequently the cause of role conflict or disturbance. Another difficult role problem faced by the individual growing up in contemporary society is that of emancipation from one's parents and the establishment of an independent life. This primarily occurs during adolescence and early adulthood when there is marked ambiguity in role definitions. The social roles of child and adolescent make it difficult to prepare oneself for adulthood. The child is not expected to be responsible; the adult is. The child is expected to be submissive; the adult dominant. The child is expected to be asexual; the adult is expected to

be sexually mature and maintain intimate sexual relationships. Yet there are few transitional procedures or "rites of passage" to help the adolescent shift his role behavior. A final crisis is faced during old age when role behavior must again be changed by aging parents who rely on their children and yet strive to balance their lives by maintaining a sense of independence and a high level of self-esteem. It is obvious that role behavior is intimately related to self-concept and identity, and role disturbances frequently involve conflicts between independent and dependent functioning.

Identity

The word identity is derived from the Latin root *idem,* meaning the same. It is the organizing principle of the personality system that accounts for both the unity and continuity of the personality. Identity is the awareness of the process of "being oneself," which is derived from self-observation and judgment. It is the synthesis of all self-representations into an organized whole, and it is not associated with any one accomplishment, object, attribute, or role assumed by the individual. It is different from self-concept in that it refers to a feeling of distinctness from others. It implies consciousness of oneself as an individual with a definite place in the general scheme of things. The person with a sense of identity feels integrated, not diffuse. When a person acts in accordance with his self-concept, his sense of identity is reinforced; when he acts in ways contrary to his self-concept, he experiences anxiety and apprehension. Behavior that conforms with the self-concept may thus be viewed as behavior that preserves one's sense of identity.

The person with a strong sense of identity sees himself as a unique individual. Indeed, the very word individual, as a synonym for person, implies a universal need to perceive oneself as separate from others. This depends in part on a sense of self-perceived consistency, not only at a particular moment, but also over time. One needs to perceive the person he is today as, if not the same person he was yesterday, at least similar to and having links with the person he was yesterday. This does not imply, however, that one attains a stable, fixed identity. Rather, as Bugenthal says, "to be human is . . . to be incomplete, needing; for life to be ever open, uncertain. Only as I allow full awareness of my needs and wants can I approach real wholeness."[8:276]

Identity combines many conscious and unconscious elements. It connotes autonomy as a person, based on understanding of, and confidence in, self. In this sense autonomy arises from feelings of self-respect, competency, and mastery over one's destiny. Autonomy implies self-government and self-acceptance with a tendency toward self-assertion and self-expansion. Identity also includes a person's body image, his own perceptions of his role performance, and the definitions of self contained in these roles.

The concept of ego identity was developed by Erikson[13] and built within his formulation of the eight stages of development in the human life cycle. For each stage, Erikson describes a "psychosocial crisis" that must be resolved for further growth and personality development. It is in adolescence that the crisis of "identity versus identity diffusion" occurs. The process of identity formation, however, does not begin in adolescence. Rather, the groundwork is laid in infancy and evolves through the steps of introjection and identification. Introjection, or incorporation, depends on a mutually satisfying relationship between the infant and the mothering one. The safety of this relationship allows the child to reach out for his first "love objects." Through the process of identification the child further broadens and expands his sense of self as he identifies with parents, peers, teachers, and folk heroes. But identity is more than the process of successive identifications. It is, rather, the capacity to synthesize successive identifications into a coherent, consistent, and unique whole.

Identity formation begins where the usefulness of identification ends and is the major task of the adolescent period. At no other phase of the life cycle are the promise of finding oneself and the threat of losing oneself so closely aligned. The adolescent's task is one of self-definition as he strives to integrate significant identifications and previous roles into a unique and reasonably consistent sense of self. Just as the process of identity formation did not begin in adolescence, neither does it end there. It is an evolving configuration, and the circumstances in later periods of life greatly influence one's sense of identity.

An important aspect in achieving identity is the issue of one's sexuality. Sexual identity is the image one has of oneself as a male or a female and convictions about what membership in that group implies. "What does it feel like to be a girl?" "Do I like being a boy?" The answers to these questions are built up gradually from in-

fancy as the result of learned conceptions about males and females. Society's ideals of masculinity and femininity provide important standards for judging oneself as good, bad, inferior, superior, desirable, or undesirable. These ideals are passed down from generation to generation and become an important part of the culture that transmits expectations to males and females. If males in a soceity are defined as superior, this idea becomes part of the self-image of both males and females. If passivity and obedience are feminine ideals in a society, most little girls will be taught and expected to be unassertive and obedient.

It is recognized that men and women differ from each other anatomically, hormonally, and genetically. Anatomical differences involving strength, ratio of muscle to fat, and reproductive organs are obvious. Hormone and chromosome differences between the sexes are less obvious. The question of the relationship of these differences to personality, sexual behavior, and conceptions of masculinity and femininity is controversial and still open for question. How much weight do chromosomal and hormonal factors have versus environment and learning? One psychologist, John Money,[33] who has done extensive research into sexual behavior, has concluded that sexual identity and sex-typed behavior are established primarily by learning experiences in the first 3 years of life. This area merits further research, which will hopefully yield greater freedom and experimentation in the expression of sexuality in society. This is an important element of the personality because the security of one's sexual identity is a cardinal factor in the achievement of a stable ego identity.

In addition, much of one's identity is expressed in relationships with others. How a person relates to other people is a central personality characteristic. This presents a paradox in that everyone is a part of humanity and yet each person is also separate from all others, and the achievement of identity is both the precursor to and partial prerequisite for the establishment of an intimate interpersonal relationship. Research has shown that only after a stable sense of identity has been established can one engage in genuinely intimate, mature, and successful relationships.[35]

Meier identified the following six attributes of ego identity, which can serve to summarize this discussion:

1. The individual recognizes himself as an intact body organism, separate from other organisms.
2. The individual acknowledges his sexuality.
3. The individual regards the various aspects of himself, such as roles, values, and actions, as compatible.
4. The individual's regard for himself is congruent with the way in which he is regarded by society.
5. The individual is aware of the relationships between past, present, and future.
6. The individual has goals of value that can be realized.[31:65]

Meier notes that not all these attributes are of equal importance nor are they always present to the same degree. Rather, the individual's quest for identity is an evolving one, whereby new elements of identity are in the process of being added or changed as one attempts to answer the question "Who am I?"

The healthy personality

It is possible to describe the healthy personality according to developmental theory and the dynamics of the self. This description may help to give perspective to the many aspects of the self previously discussed. An individual with a healthy personality would experience the following:

1. *A positive and accurate body image.* Body image is the sum of the conscious and unconscious attitudes the individual has toward his body. It includes present and past perceptions, as well as his feelings about size, function, appearance, and potential. A healthy body awareness would be based on self-observation and appropriate concern for one's physical well-being.

2. *A realistic self-ideal.* Self-ideal is the individual's perception of how he should behave or the standard by which he appraises his behavior. An individual with a realistic self-ideal would have attainable life goals that are valuable and worth striving for.

3. *A positive self-concept.* Self-concept consists of all the aspects of the individual of which he is aware. It includes all of his self-perceptions, which direct and influence his behavior. A positive self-concept implies that the individual expects to be successful in life. It includes the acceptance of the negative aspects of the self as part of the individual's personality. Such a person believes he can master his environment.

He does not fear rejection but feels secure and accepted. He faces life openly and realistically and affirms his own existence.

4. *A high self-esteem.* Self-esteem is the individual's personal judgment of his own worth, obtained by analyzing how well he matches up to his own standards and how well his performance compares with others. It is evolved through the comparison of the individual's self-ideal and self-concept. A person with high self-esteem views himself as someone worthy of respect and dignity. He believes in his own self-worth, and he approaches life with aggressiveness and zest. The individual with a healthy personality is one who sees himself to be very much like the person he would like to be.

5. *A clear sense of identity.* Identity is the integration of inner and outer demands in the individual's discovery of who he is and what he can become. It is the realization of personal consistency. The individual with a clear sense of identity experiences a unity of personality and perceives himself to be a unique individual. His "sense of self" gives his life direction and purpose.

6. *An openness to people.* The individual with a healthy personality has the ability to relate to others intimately. Through open and honest communication he can trust others and enter into mutual and interdependent relationships. His capacity for sharing enables him to enter into a relationship with another person and experience love, freedom, and interdependence.

An individual with these qualities is able to perceive himself and his world accurately. His insight into himself creates a feeling of harmony and inner peace.

 Stressors

Stressors affecting self-esteem

Problems with self-concept can be contributed to by predisposing factors that originate in early childhood experiences. Because the infant initially views himself as an extension of his parent, he is very responsive to both his parents' own self-hate and any perceived feelings of hatred toward himself. Parental rejection is an important factor in that it causes the child to be uncertain of himself and other human relationships. As a result of his failure to be loved, the child fails to love himself and is unable to reach out with love to others. As he grows older, the child may experience lack of recognition and appreciation by parents and significant others as an intrinsically valuable and important individual. He may learn to feel inadequate because he is not encouraged and motivated to be independent, to think for himself, and to take responsibility for his own needs and actions. Overpossessiveness, overpermissiveness, or overcontrol, exercised by one or both parents, can nurture a feeling of unimportance and lack of esteem in the child. Harsh and demanding parents can set unreasonable standards, often raising them before the child has developed the ability to meet them. Parents may also subject their children to unreasonable harsh criticism and inconsistent punishment. These actions can cause early frustration, defeatism, and a destructive sense of inadequacy and inferiority. Another factor in creating such feelings may be the rivalry or unsuccessful emulation of an extremely bright sibling or of a prominent parent, which can often generate a sense of hopelessness and inferiority. In addition, repeated defeats and failures can also destroy one's sense of self-worth. In such an instance the failure, in itself, does not produce a sense of helplessness but the internalization of the failure as proof of personal incompetency does.

With age, additional factors emerge that can both cause and perpetuate feelings of low self-esteem. The individual who lacks a sense of meaning and purpose in life also fails to accept responsibility for his own well-being. He becomes dependent on others and self-indulgent and fails to develop his inherent capabilities and innate potential. He denies himself the freedom to full expression, including the right to make mistakes and fail, and becomes impatient, harsh, and demanding with himself. He sets standards that cannot be met. Examinations are constructed that cannot be passed. Self-consciousness and observation then turn to self-contempt and an underlying sense of self-defeat. This results in a further loss of self-trust.

These self-ideals or goals are often silent assumptions and the person may not be immediately aware of them. They reflect high expectations for oneself and are unrealistic in relation to one's proved capacities. When the individual judges his performance by these unreasonable and inflexible standards, he cannot live up to his ideals and, as a result, experiences feelings of guilt and low self-esteem. Horney[20] has described these inner dictates as the "tyranny of the shoulds" and has identified some of the common ones:

1. I should be the utmost of generosity, considerateness, dignity, courage, unselfishness.

2. I should be the perfect lover, friend, parent, teacher, student, spouse. Everyone should love me.

3. I should be able to endure any hardship with equanimity.

4. I should be able to find a quick solution to every problem.

5. I should never feel hurt; I should always be happy and serene.

6. I should know, understand, and foresee everything. I should be competent in all ways.

7. I should always be spontaneous; I should always control my feelings.

8. I should assert myself; I should never hurt anybody else.

8. I should never be tired or get sick.

10. I should always be at peak efficiency. I should not make mistakes.

The person who overemphasizes these rules or ideals often makes the following series of deductions: "Everyone should love me . . . If he doesn't love me, I have failed . . . I have lost the only thing that really matters . . . I am unlovable . . . There is no point in going on . . . I am worthless." This inner punishment results in feelings of depression and despair because the demands on self are those no human being could fulfill, and they reflect a disloyalty to what one can feel or do as he is at present. Obviously, slavishly striving for these ideals frequently interferes with other activities, such as living a reasonably healthy, tranquil life and having satisfying relationships with other people.

These predisposing factors lay the groundwork for potential feelings of low self-esteem. Specific problems are initiated or precipitated by almost any difficult or stressful situation for which the person does not have the capacity to adjust. Loss of one's job, failure of a love relationship, and the breakup of a marriage are a few of the many life events that can pose a threat to one's self-esteem. When the self is threatened and the concepts of the self become inconsistent, anxiety is aroused and discomfort is produced. This process is described in greater detail in Chapter 7.

Stressors affecting role

During his lifetime the individual is faced with numerous role transitions or changes in role relationships, expectations, or abilities. These role transitions may require the person to incorporate new knowledge and alter his behavior. Meleis[32] has identified three categories of role transitions: (1) developmental, (2) situational, and (3) health-illness. *Developmental transitions* are normative changes associated with growth. *Situational transitions* involve the addition or subtraction of significant others, which may occur through birth or death. An example of this transition is the change from nonparental to parental status. *Health-illness transitions* result from moving from a well state to an illness state. Each of these role transitions can precipitate a threat to the individual's self-concept and can result in role conflict.

People who experience stress associated with expected roles or positions are said to experience *role strain*.[16] Role strain is experienced as frustration, since the person may feel torn in opposite directions or feel inadequate or unsuited to performing certain roles. Over time, role strain places a considerable burden on the person, and the individual will tend to act to alleviate role strain and heighten the gratification of high role adequacy. Role strain, as a general term, incorporates the concepts of role conflict, role ambiguity, and role overload.[4]

Role conflict is said to occur when a person is subjected to two or more contradictory expectations that the person cannot simultaneously meet in behavior. Conflict can arise because two internal needs, drives, or motives are incompatible, or because an internal need, drive, or motive opposes an external demand. For example, role conflict can occur because there are cultural expectations that certain attributes go with certain roles. In this case the role conflict is caused by the incongruency between the individual's and society's expectations for specific role behavior. This is evident in a society's sex-role stereotyping and may be experienced by the woman who enters a traditionally male occupation or vice versa. Another source of conflict is different perceptions of appropriate role-related behavior among individuals. An example of this is evident in family roles. Each adult brings to a marriage a set of perceived family roles that have been greatly influenced by their own upbringing. Often the individuals' perceptions may be contradictory and pose problems within the marriage.

Role ambiguity appears when shared specifications set for an expected role are incomplete or insufficient to tell the involved individual what is desired or how to do it. This lack of knowledge of specific role expectations and confusion regarding appropriate role behavior can be very stressful for the individual. This is particularly evident among adolescents, since society's demands have become stronger, more diversified, and more immediate and often produce feelings of confusion, frustration, alienation, and violence. Adolescents are pressured to play different roles by their parents, the mass media, and their peers. They are expected to "earn their own keep," yet are unable to find jobs in times of high unemployment and economic inflation. They are confused by the discrepancy they see between the reality of the practiced morality of society and the morality they learned as a child and accepted as reality. Some young people turn to violence as a way of asserting themselves, whereas others become apathetic and alienated in response to their perceived role ambiguity.

A final type of role strain is *role overload*, which occurs when a person is faced with a role set that is too complex. The person lacks the adequate or appropriate resources that may be physical, intellectual, emotional, or economic for performing the necessary role requirements. Each of the roles undertaken by the individual may be making legitimate discreet demands, but together the expectations are overwhelming and perhaps impossible to carry out. An example of this is the numerous roles of the contemporary woman—wife, cook, mother, employee, chauffeur, maid, lover, etc.

A particularly relevant source of role strain in contemporary American society is evident in the values, beliefs, and behaviors related to sex roles. The differences between male and female body structures have given rise to a number of theories or propositions. Freud gave a great deal of weight to biological factors in the determination of both male and female sexuality. Erikson supported his belief that anatomy predestined the individual to certain types of behavior. These psychoanalytical views have come under attack in recent years for their theories of femininity and masculinity, and for the effects these theories are believed to have had on sexuality and role behavior. They largely ignore the influence of culture and learning on one's self-perceptions.

Despite this, research demonstrates the continued existence of clearly defined sex-role stereotypes for men and women. Broverman's work[7] indicates that women are perceived as relatively less competent, less independent, less objective, and less logical than men. Men are perceived as lacking interpersonal sensitivity, warmth, and expressiveness in comparison to women. Moreover, stereotyped masculine traits are more often perceived to be desirable than stereotyped feminine characteristics.

To the extent that these results reflect societal standards of sex-role behavior, both women and men are put in role conflict by the difference in the standards. If a woman adopts the behaviors specified as desirable for a man, she risks censure for her failure to be appropriately feminine; if she adopts the behaviors designated as feminine, she is deficient in the valued behaviors associated with masculinity. So, too, if a man adopts the behaviors specified as desirable for a woman, his masculinity and sexuality may be questioned and his contributions may be devalued or ignored; if he adopts the behaviors associated with masculinity, he risks alienating attributes of his personality associated with warmth, tenderness, and responsiveness. Thus when a woman steps out of her home, where her sex role has traditionally been defined and confined, and enters the world of work, she may expect to experience heightened role strain. Similarly, the man who arrives home from work in the evening may feel uncertain or conflicted about how he should relate to his school-age son, infant daughter, or working wife.

Most important, both men and women incorporate both the positive and negative traits of the appropriate stereotype into their self-concepts. Since more feminine traits are negatively valued than are masculine traits, women tend to have more negative self-concepts than do men. Women also have higher rates of mental illness than men and are more likely to become depressed. Grove and Tudor[17] suggest a number of possible reasons for this. First, many women are restricted to a single, major social role as housewife, whereas most men have two roles—household and work—and therefore two sources of gratification. Second, some women find their role expectations regarding raising children and keeping house to be limiting and frustrating and wish to work but are unable to, whereas other women are forced to work for financial reasons at jobs that are not gratifying and would rather remain at home caring for their house and children. In either situation one's role preferences are not being met. Third, the housewife role is unstructured and invisible and often perceived to be of low status, particularly with the current value and status placed on "career women." Fourth, even when a married woman works, she is often in a less satisfying position than a man because of discrimination and limited oppor-

tunity. Fifth, expectations confronting women are unclear and diffuse and may result in an unclear female identity.

Role conflict and role ambiguity therefore arise from the biological factors and social expectations set for men and women. Role overload can also occur for the woman who has numerous, often conflicting, roles imposed on her. The existence of a women's movement in many countries of the world can be viewed as an attempt by women to examine their own identities and determine appropriate role behavior. According to a Labor Department survey, "The old-fashioned 'typical American family' with a breadwinner husband, a homemaker wife, and two children, now makes up only 7 percent of the nation's families."[5] Thus the interaction of marriage, parenting, and employment emerges as a likely source of role strain for women.

Work does not imply, however, a singular social role. It is possible to distinguish between women who perceive their employment as careers and those who view their work as a job. Women are still in the minority of most high-status occupations. Only 9.2% of physicians, 4.7% of lawyers, 1.6% of engineers, and 28.7% of college and university teachers were women according to the 1970 census. Most of the women in these fields, moreover, are clustered near the bottom in terms of professional status and financial reward. Holahan and Gilbert[19] conducted a study that compared role conflict experienced by career and noncareer (job) women in relationship to the roles of worker, spouse, parent, and self as a self-actualizing person. Greater role conflict was reported by the job vs. career group, particularly involving the parent vs. self and spouse vs. self roles. The career group reported receiving significantly more life satisfaction from both work and self roles than the job group.

This and other studies suggest that work which is viewed as desirable, valuable, and adequately compensated for by the woman can bring greater life satisfaction. Hunt has listed the needs of women that may be met by work as those for "money, identity, achievement, status, personal pride, inner joy, and for many a woman, whether she realizes it or not, a means of achieving a lasting peace rather than a cease-fire within marriage."[36] Furthermore, a large scale study conducted by the Department of Health, Education, and Welfare found housewives had higher symptom rates than employed women, and professionally employed women had lower symptom rates than those in other occupational categories.

The problem appears to be the lack of support received by women who are performing multiple roles. This lack of support is reflected in amount of payment received, willingness by other family members to share family tasks, and encouragement for the woman pursuing her own life goals. At present, in American society, women are being socialized to seek an ideal that includes marriage, children, higher education, and satisfying work outside the home, and they are increasingly being expected to perform in both the "feminine" and "masculine" spheres. This potentially has both positive and negative aspects. First, it can be argued that it merely replaces the traditional woman's role with another equally confining one. By valuing the new role, the traditional role of wife and mother assumed by women becomes devalued. Second, although women are expected to assume more "masculine" qualities, a corresponding trend for men to assume more "feminine" role behaviors is not obvious. Third, the woman who wishes to seek such an expanded role is faced with the task of reconciling the often conflicting goals of work, marriage, homemaking, and parenting. Yet there is little organized support by society to aid the woman, and thus her task can be formidable or overwhelming.

Despite social and economic changes, there is often little sharing of tasks when men and women are both gainfully employed. Rather, most industrial societies have witnessed a gradual change in the obligations of women, who now perform a double, or "dual," role—outside employment and continued responsibility for home and children. The expectation exists that the woman will make the adjustments needed both at home and in her career, including housekeeping and managing; arranging meals, lessons, and appointments; entertaining; caring for the sick; and communicating with the family. There is also the traditional expectation that the wife will be the primary caretaker of the child and will subsume other activities to this end. Johnson and Johnson[22] report that the wives and mothers of dual-career families with young children experience difficulties in respect to the proliferation of role demands in both home and job situations. The greatest strain was in the mater-

nal role, in which both guilt and anxiety predominated.

Although it may appear that attitudes toward sex roles are changing, the division of household labor within the family is not. In Berk's study[3] wives reported that they did 86% of the kitchen cleaning, 92% of the laundry tasks, 88% of the meal preparation, 89% of the straightening tasks, 74% of the outside errands, and 76% of "other" household tasks. Even the stereotypically husbandly duties of taking out the garbage and paying the bills were generally done by wives (60% and 62%, respectively). Furthermore, married women employed outside the home were not found to do a significantly smaller proportion of household work. Neither did the presence of preschool children affect the division of labor. They conclude that women with small children at home just work harder.

Given these factors, it is understandable that Weissman[41] found that the search for work by the young educated housewife is associated with a moderate degree of stress and mild depressive symptoms. On the one hand they wanted to find self-expression through work outside the home, and, on the other hand, they held traditional values about marriage and children; thus career adaptations had to be made to fit personal and family needs. One attempted solution to this role strain is for the woman to try to become "superwoman" and do everything well. Not only is this virtually impossible, but the attempt is exhausting and self-defeating.

Bailyn[2] compares this situation to that of a man. He too is faced with different values in his work and family, and some degree of conflict along the same lines also exists for him. His situation is eased, however, by the existence in his environment of a hierarchy of values that precludes the necessity of conscious decision. Unless family needs reach crisis proportions, the demands of his work come first. Very little is written about paternal role strain, accommodation, or the career and homemaking changes made by men in a dual career family. Comparatively, the role set of women appears far more complex, and, in light of these findings, the increased susceptibility of women to the stress of role strain seems hardly surprising at all.

One might conclude, therefore, that sex roles will continue to be a source of role strain until care of one's children, home, and career are viewed as equally valuable and important by both sexes and until gender is regarded as irrelevant to the abilities, personalities, and activities of the individuals involved. Such a change in attitude should begin with nurses and other mental health clinicians who, by accepting the stereotyped views of society, indirectly serve to increase role strain. Broverman's research[6] shows that clinicians have different concepts of health for men and women and that these differences parallel the sex-role stereotypes prevalent in our society. The cause of mental health may be better served if both men and women were encouraged by psychiatric clinicians toward maximum realization of individual potential, rather than to an adjustment to existing restrictive sex roles.

Stressors affecting body image

There are some specific stressors that can cause disturbances in body image and related changes in self-concept. One threat is the loss of a major body part, such as an eye, breast, or leg. Disturbances also may occur following a surgical procedure in which the relationship of body parts is disturbed. The results of the surgical intervention may be either visible, as with a colostomy or gastrotomy, or invisible, as with a hysterectomy or gallbladder removal. Changes in body size, shape, and appearance can threaten one's self-perceptions. These changes can be the result of a rapid weight gain or loss, a skin infection, or even plastic surgery. Threats to body image can occur because of a pathological process that causes changes in the structure or function of one's body, such as arthritis, multiple sclerosis, Parkinson's disease, cancer, pneumonia, and heart disease. The failure of a body part to function, as experienced by the paraplegic or the patient recovering from a stroke, is particularly difficult to integrate into one's self-perceptions. The physical changes associated with normal growth and development may pose problems for the individual, as might some potentially threatening medical or nursing procedures, such as enemas, catheterizations, suctioning, radiation therapy, dilation and curettage, and organ transplantation.

All of these stressors can pose a threat to one's body image with resultant changes in levels of self-esteem and role perception. In fact, any threat to body integrity is interpreted as a threat to self and increases one's anxiety level. How the individual perceives the seriousness of the threat determines the type of coping mechanism called into play. Factors that influence the degree of threat to one's body image have been identified by Norris[34]:

1. The meaning of the stressor for the individual. Does it threaten his ideal of youth and wholeness and act to decrease his self-esteem?
2. The degree to which his pattern of adaptation is interrupted. Does it jeopardize his security and self-control?
3. The coping capacities and resources available to him. What response is elicited from significant others, and what help is offered him?
4. The nature of the threat, extent of change, and rate at which it occurs. Is the change one of many small adjustments over time or a great and sudden readjustment?

Stressors affecting identity

Various developmental stages can precipitate threats to one's identity. Adolescence is perhaps the most critical, since it is a time of upheaval, change, anxiety, and insecurity. Adolescents are modifying their concepts of self, and they are more analytical about not only themselves but also the world in general. Adolescents are faced with many important decisions. They have to make an occupational choice and decide if they are good enough to succeed in a given career. They must determine if they have the ability to participate in various social activities. Are they attractive enough heterosexually to interest and succeed with a member of the opposite sex? Will they succeed in marriage? Do they have the courage to carry out their convictions as an individual apart from the crowd while remaining a member of the crowd? Are they a leader, follower, or coward? Are they satisfied with their roles and can they implement them comfortably?

Constant parental intervention interferes with adolescent choices. In our culture this is related to the fact that there is no cutoff point and no fixed limit to parental intervention. Parental distrust leads a child to wonder whether his own choices are correct and to feel guilty if he goes against parental ideas. Parental distrust implies belittlement of the child because it devalues the child's opinions, and belittlement leads inevitability to indecisiveness, feelings of nothingness, exasperated impulsiveness, and acting out in an attempt to achieve some identity. When the parent does not trust the child, the child ultimately loses respect for the parent. It has been found that parents and children do not disagree on significant issues, such as war, peace, race, or religion. Instead, personal and narrow con-concerns—fads, dating, a party, the car, cur-fews, doing homework—create the conflict be-tween parents and youth. Here parental inter-vention interferes with option choices and iden-tity.

Peers also add to the problems of identity. The adolescent wants to belong, to feel needed and wanted. The peer group, with its rigid standards of behavior, gives him this feeling. It provides a bridge between childhood and adulthood. The adolescent loses himself in the fads and the lan-guage of the group. However, because all the members of the peer group are searching to de-fine their identity and are beset by the pressures and frustrations of a complex society, the peer group is often a cruel testing ground that hurts as much as it helps. Taught to be competitive, the young person competes with his friends, "putting them down" to bring himself up. Mem-bership in the peer group is bought at a high price; the adolescent must surrender much of his identity to get in. Often there is open destruc-tion of self-esteem and ferocious insistence on conformity. In sexual relationships, adolescents introduce further uncertainty into their lives, which can interfere with the development of a stable self-concept.

An adult's problems of identity are simpler than those of an adolescent. Maturity stabilizes self-concept and provides a firmer picture of self. A serious threat to identity in adulthood is cul-tural discontinuity. This occurs when a person moves from one type of cultural setting to an-other and experiences the emotional upheaval that accompanies the change to a new cultural milieu. When faced with differing cultural stan-dards, many people have difficulty maintaining their self-system. In addition, problems within the social structure, such as political upheavals, economic depression, and high unemployment, can pose threats to the identity of individuals.

Cultural stressors confront a person in chal-lenging personal values: conforming vs. indi-viduality, cowardice vs. bravery, winning vs. losing, career vs. marriage, equality vs. superior-ity, cooperation vs. competition, dependence vs. independence, intelligence vs. feeling. Although these values are not necessarily opposite nor mutually exclusive, they raise fundamental questions that the individual must resolve and integrate into his personality structure. One's sexual identity can also be influenced by cul-tural pressures, which can control both the way in which one expresses sexuality and the way in which it is a part of one's self-system. Defini-tions of acceptable approaches to the opposite sex, the values placed on virility, the necessity for procreation as proof of virility, the definitions of suitable sex partners, and the values concern-ing marital fidelity may all be culturally deter-mined.

In late maturity and in old age, identity prob-lems again arise. New problems and roles result from the process of aging and from the view of the elderly held by the more youthful members of society. Menopause, retirement, and increas-ing physical disability are problems for which the aging person, as he enters his declining years, must work out adaptive coping behavior.

Finally, there may also be physiological factors that disturb one's sense of reality, interfere with an accurate perception of the world, and threat-en the maintenance of one's ego boundaries and identity. Such stressors include oxygen depriva-tion, hyperventilation, biochemical imbalances, severe fatigue, and sensory and emotional isola-tion. Alcohol, drugs, and other toxic substances may also produce self-concept distortions. Usu-ally these stressors produce only temporary changes within the individual.

Whether the problem in self-concept is precip-itated by psychological or sociological stressors, the critical element is the patient's perception of the threat. As the nurse assesses pertinent be-haviors and formulates a nursing diagnosis, she must continue to validate her observations and inferences to establish a mutual and therapeu-tic relationship with the patient.

Data collection

Assessing the various components of a pa-tient's self-concept will present a challenge to the nurse. Because self-concept is the corner-stone of the personality, it is intimately related to states of anxiety and depression, problems in interpersonal relationships, and acting out and self-destructive behavior. All behavior is moti-vated by a desire to enhance, maintain, or de-fend the self; so the nurse will have a wealth of information to evaluate. There is a need, how-ever, for the nurse to delve beyond the objective and observable behaviors to the subjective and internal world of the patient. Only when the nurse explores this realm will the patient's ac-tions be given meaning.

The nurse can begin the assessment by ob-serving the patient's appearance. The person's posture, cleanliness, makeup, and clothing all provide data. She might discuss his appearance with him to determine his values and ideals related to his body image. Observing or inquiring about his eating, sleeping, and hygiene patterns gives clues to his biological gratifications and tendencies toward self-preservation. These initial observations should lead the nurse to ask, "What does my patient think about himself as a person?" She might ask him to describe himself or how he feels about himself. What strengths does he think he has? What does he see as his areas of weakness? What is his self-ideal? Does he conform to it? Does fulfillment of his self-ideal bring him satisfaction? Does he value his strengths? Does he view his weaknesses as important personality deficits or are they relatively unimportant to his self-concept? What are his priorities? Is he a participant in life or an observer? Does he feel unified and self-directed or diffuse and other directed?

The nurse can then compare the patient's responses to his behavior, looking for inconsistencies or contradictions. How does he relate to other people? How does he respond to compliments and criticisms? She can also examine her affective response to the patient. Is it one of hopelessness, despair, anger, or anxiety? The nurse's own response to the patient is often a good indication of the quality and depth of the patient's pain.

Behaviors associated with low self-esteem, role strain, and disturbed body image

Low self-esteem is a major problem for many people, and it can be expressed in moderate and severe levels of anxiety. It involves negative self-evaluations and is associated with feelings of being weak, helpless, hopeless, frightened, vulnerable, fragile, incomplete, worthless, and inadequate. Low self-esteem is a major component of depression, which acts as a kind of punishment and anesthesia for the individual. Low self-esteem indicates self-rejection and self-hate, which may be a conscious or unconscious process and may be expressed in direct or indirect ways.

Direct expressions of self-hate or low self-esteem may include any of the following behaviors:

1. *Self-derision and criticism.* The patient has a negative cognitive set and believes he is doomed to failure. Although the expressed purpose of the criticism may be self-improvement, there is no constructive value to it and the underlying goal is to demoralize oneself. This oc-

curs when the individual places himself in a situation he cannot handle and then subjects himself to ridicule. He might describe himself as "stupid," "no good," or "a born loser." He views the normal stressors of life as impossible barriers and becomes preoccupied with self-pity.

2. *Self-diminution.* The minimizing of one's ability, which is accomplished by avoiding, neglecting, or refusing to recognize one's real assets and strengths.

3. *Guilt and worrying.* A destructive activity by which the individual terrorizes and punishes himself. It may be expressed through nightmares, phobias, obsessions, or the reliving of painful memories and indiscretions. It indicates self-rejection.

4. *Physical manifestations.* These might include hypertension, psychosomatic illnesses, and the abuse of various substances, such as alcohol, drugs, tobacco, or food.

5. *Postponing decisions.* A high level of ambivalence or procrastination produces an increased sense of insecurity.

6. *Denying oneself pleasure.* The self-rejecting person feels the need to punish himself and expresses this through denying himself the things he finds desirable or pleasurable. This might be a career opportunity, a material object, or a desired interpersonal relationship.

7. *Disturbed interpersonal relationships.* The person may be cruel, demeaning, or exploitive with other people. This may be an overt process, or he might develop a passive-dependent pattern of relating, which indirectly exploits others. Another behavior included in this category is withdrawal or social isolation, which arises from his feelings of worthlessness.

8. *Withdrawal from reality.* When the anxiety resulting from self-rejection reaches the severe or panic levels, the individual may dissociate and experience hallucinations, delusions, and feelings of suspicion, jealousy, or paranoia. Such withdrawal from reality may be a temporary coping mechanism or a long-term behavior pattern, indicating a profound problem of identity confusion.

9. *Self-destructiveness.* Self-hatred can be expressed through accident proneness or attempting dangerous feats. Extremely low levels of self-esteem can lead to the ultimate act of rejection, which is suicide.

10. *Other destructiveness.* People who have overwhelming consciences may choose to act out against society. This activity serves to para-

lyze their own self-hate and displaces or projects it on victims in their environment.

There are also indirect forms of self-hate that complement and supplement the direct forms. They may be chronic patterns for the individual and difficult to change in therapy:

1. *Illusions and unrealistic goals.* Self-deception is the core element; the individual refuses to accept a limited here and now. Illusions increase the possibility of disappointment and further self-hate. The illusions or goals frequently involve money, love, power, prestige, marriage, sex, children, family, success, and parenthood. Examples of illusions are "If I were married, I would be happy" and "Money brings fulfillment." This indirect form of low self-esteem may make the person sensitive to criticism or overresponsive to flattery. It may also be evident in the defensive mechanisms of blaming others for one's failures and becoming hypercritical with others to create the illusion of superiority.

The individual may also attempt to compensate by expressing an exaggerated opinion of his ability. He may continually boast, brag of his prowess and exploits, or claim possession of extraordinary talents. An extreme compensatory behavior for low esteem is gradiose thinking and related delusions.

Yet another example of unrealistic goals is evident in the perfectionist whose standards are high beyond reach or reason. Such individuals strain compulsively and unremittingly toward impossible goals and measure their own worth entirely in terms of productivity and accomplishment. The result of such striving, however, is often vulnerability to emotional turmoil and impaired productivity. This tendency may further serve as a predisposing factor toward the development or recurrence of depressive illnesses.[9]

2. *Boredom.* This involves the rejection of one's possibilities and capabilities. The individual may neglect or reject aspects of himself that have great potential for future growth.

3. *Polarizing view of life.* In this case the individual has a simplistic view of life in which everything is worst or best, wrong or right. He tends to have a closed belief system that acts as a defense against a threatening world. Ultimately this view of life will lead to confusion and disappointment.

The behaviors associated with low self-esteem are described in Clinical example 8-1 and at above right.

BEHAVIORS ASSOCIATED WITH LOW SELF-ESTEEM

Criticism of self and/or others
Denying oneself pleasure
Disturbed interpersonal relationships
Exaggerated sense of self-importance
Guilt
Illusions and unrealistic goals
Other destructiveness
Physical complaints
Polarizing view of life
Procrastination
Rejection of personal capabilities
Self-derision
Self-destructiveness
Self-diminution
Substance abuse
Withdrawal from reality
Worrying

CLINICAL EXAMPLE 8-1

Mrs. G was a 66-year-old woman who was admitted to the psychiatric hospital with the diagnosis of major depression, single episode, with melancholia. She told the admitting nurse that "things have been building up for some time now" and she had been seeing a private psychiatrist for the past 6 months who suggested she enter the hospital. Mrs. G slowly recounted an extensive medical history with numerous gastrointestinal problems. These did not, however, significantly interfere with her functioning. She had been employed in a community college as a librarian until 18 months previously when she was forced to retire. Mrs. G said she had been married for 39 years and had two grown children who were married and lived out of state. Her husband worked as an accountant but had retired a month previously. She said that since her retirement she had felt "useless and lost and closed in by their apartment." She seldom left the apartment, however, and had lost contact with many of her friends. She said she worried a great deal about their financial situation, especially now that her husband was also retired. He has repeatedly reassured her that they have sufficient funds, but she cannot stop worrying about it. She said her children called her weekly, but she thought they did this only out of duty and were not "really interested" in her or her husband. She thought that if they did love her and were concerned about her, they would never have moved out of state.

Mrs. G said that she liked her job very much and thought she was good at it. A younger woman took her place at the library, and Mrs. G was very bitter when talking about her. She said that, little by little, this woman took over duties Mrs. G was responsible for and one day even cleaned out Mrs. G's desk and took it as her own. Since her retirement, she said "things have been going downhill steadily." She said she is not a good housewife and she dislikes cooking. These tasks had become even more difficult since her husband retired because he is "always underfoot and criticizing what I do." In the past couple of weeks, she had had great difficulty sleeping, a decreased appetite, fatigue, and little interest in her personal appearance. She said that it seemed to her that all she had to do was to "wait around to die."

In this clinical example, Mrs. G's favorable perception of self was closely related to her ability to work. Her retirement created role changes for her, and she found it difficult to adapt to them. This example points out the close relationship that exists between feelings of *low self-esteem* and *role strain*. The situation was further compounded by her husband's retirement. Mrs. G's feelings of low self-esteem were evident in her self-criticism, refusal to recognize her own strengths, worrying, physical complaints, reduced social contacts, and unrealistic expectations of her family. Her diagnosis of major depressive episode, with melancholia, was based on the severity of her feelings of self-depreciation, somatic problems, saddened emotional tone, history of losses, and absence of a manic episode.

Low self-esteem is also a major dynamic element occurring with problems of *disturbed body image*. Clinical example 8-2 illustrates the effect of the loss of a body part on a person's self-concept.

CLINICAL EXAMPLE 8-2

Mrs. M was a 29-year-old married woman who was admitted to the general hospital for a total hysterectomy. Her history was presented in a nursing care conference because she was making many demands on the nursing staff and the head nurse noticed that many of the staff were avoiding caring for her. Mrs. M had been married for 2 years and did not have any children. It was observed that Mr. M seldom visited his wife, although the staff noticed that she spoke to him over the phone almost daily. Mrs. M complained that she was unable to sleep at night and often rang for the nurses with apparently minor requests. She appeared to have established a relationship with one of the evening nurses who was able to describe some of Mrs. M's concerns.

Mrs. M appeared to have a severe level of anxiety

about her hysterectomy. She feared the effect of the operation on her sexual desires, sexual attractiveness, ability to have intercourse, and ability to respond to her husband. Without her reproductive organs she said she felt "inadequate and no longer like a woman." She said that she and her husband always planned on having children and she wondered if her husband might leave her in the future. She also feared that she would look older and that having the hysterectomy would cause her to lose her beauty and youth.

When the nursing staff became aware of Mrs. M's many fears and concerns, they were better able to understand her behavior and plan appropriate nursing care. They discussed with her the physiological implications of a hysterectomy and encouraged her to openly verbalize her feelings. Mr. M was not aware of his wife's concerns, and the nursing staff supported open discussions between them. As the staff were able to identify Mrs. M's specific concerns, they realized that some of their previous avoidance behavior was due to their own fears and discomfort. The female nurses had identified with her as a patient, and the hysterectomy, in some ways, threatened their own concepts of self, body integrity, and sexual identity.

Behaviors associated with problems in identity

Erikson[12] identified a common alteration of self-concept in the syndrome of *identity confusion*. He believed it to be a normative crisis, however, because it occurred during adolescence—a normal phase of increased conflict that is characterized by a high growth potential. The transitory stage of acute identity confusion poses the possible failure to achieve integration and continuity of one's self-images. Adolescents may appear excessively self-conscious because of their extreme self-doubt. They may also display a diffused time perspective, which consists of a sense of great urgency and yet also of a loss of consideration for time as a dimension of living. They may feel very young and very old simultaneously and ambivalently hope and fear that change will come with time. These contradictory feelings may be displayed in a general slowing of activities, which reflects an underlying sense of despair. A diffused sense of industry is also often present, which is evident in inability to concentrate on the work they are supposed to be doing. This may be accompanied by a distaste for competition. Although they may be intelligent and previously successful in office work, schoolwork, and sports, adolescents may lose the capacity for work, exercise, and sociability.

The identity crisis of adolescence is a transitory one and may be resolved in a number of ways. It is possible to view these resolutions as either short-term or long-term ego-oriented coping mechanisms to ward off the anxiety and uncertainty of identity confusion. Logan[28] has described the following four broad categories of short-term defenses:

- Activities that provide temporary escape from the identity crisis
- Activities that provide temporary substitute identities
- Activities that serve temporarily to strengthen or heighten a diffuse sense of self
- Activities that represent short-term attempts to make an identity out of the fact of meaningless and identity diffusion itself—that try to assert that the meaning of life is meaningless itself

The first category of temporary escape includes any of a number of activities that seem to provide intense immediate experiences, experiences which so overwhelm the senses that when one is involved in them, the issue of identity literally does not exist because one's entire being is taken up with "right now" sensations. Examples of this might include drug experiences, loud rock concerts, fast car and motorcycle riding, some forms of hard physical labor, exercise, or sports, and even obsessive television watching.

The category of temporary substitute identity is derived from being a "joiner"; the identity of a club, group, team, movement, or gang may function as one's basis for self-definition. The individual temporarily adopts the group definition as his own identity, in a kind of totalistic devotion to the larger entity. The adolescent's need to join and "belong" makes him particularly vulnerable to being manipulated by various religious groups and political sects. Being a devoted "follower" and imitator of an idolized figure, such as a guru, rock star, sect leader, or life-style rebel, can also provide a temporary substitute identity for those who may not actually "join" a group. Temporary substitute identities can also be obtained by playing a certain role within a group, such as clown, bully, or chauffeur, or by purchasing objects that are marketed with ready-made identities. Thus a certain type of cologne, make of car, or article of dress imply

built-in personalities that the person can adopt as his own.

The third category of defenses involves the idea of "putting oneself up against something" to feel more intensely alive. This is evident in risk taking for its own sake, which creates a feeling of heroic bravado and notoriety. Engaging in competitive activities, such as sports, academic achievement, and popularity contests can also fit into this category. The idea here is that competition and comparison with an outsider more sharply define one's own sense of self. Another example of this is the use of bigotry and prejudice. By adopting a bigoted stance toward some outgroup or scapegoat one can temporarily strengthen one's own sense of esteem or ego integrity. Superpatriots, youth gangs, and cliques are all examples of this temporary defense.

The final category helps to explain the fads adolescents indulge in with such fervor and that seem so meaningless to others. It is suggested that the sheer force of commitment to the fads is an attempt to transform them into something meaningful. It is obvious, however, that all of these categories of short-term coping mechanisms do overlap and can be used to compound the overall effect. Logan emphasizes this point in analyzing the problem of drug abuse and the powerful hold it has on some adolescents:

One may take drugs for the intense, immediate experience and the escape from worldly concerns into heightened sensations that they provide. The very acts of procuring, smuggling, selling, and taking drugs provide challenging risks of harm, arrest, and illness that may make one feel more daringly and rebelliously alive. The taking of drugs may also be the initiation ceremony for "joining," and the badge of membership for belonging to the group and life-style from which one derives a temporary identity. A sense of identity may also be derived from the role of freak, head, or pusher that one plays within the drug culture. The drug culture may also be a vehicle for bigotry and prejudice—the contemptuous "put-down" of the "straight" world for its narrow-minded rejection of drugs helping to boost the self-esteem of drug users. One might speculate that a kind of identity might be derived from the kind of "stuff" one habitually purchases and uses. Finally, one even might argue that drugs may be taken because of the faddish meaninglessness of the act—as a kind of final affirmation and flinging in the face of society that, yes, life is meaningless, so meaningless, in fact, that the drug-taker makes a career of meaninglessness.[28:506-507]

Any of these short-term defenses may develop into a long-term one that will be evident in maladaptive behavior. Other resolutions or long-term defenses are also possible for the adolescent. A positive resolution or adaptive response is one that produces an integrated ego identity and unified self, as has previously been described. Another type of long-term resolution has been identified as that of *identity foreclosure*.[29] This occurs when a young person adopts "ready made" the kind of identity desired by his elders without really coming to terms with his own desires, aspirations, or potential. This is a less desirable long-term resolution as is that of adopting a deviant, or *negative, identity*.

A negative identity is one that is at odds with the values and expectations of society. This choice of delinquent roles may be caused by pressing demands made on the adolescent by parents or significant others to adopt a particular self-definition. The individual may think his autonomy is in jeopardy or he may not value social norms. He then attempts to define the self in a nonprescribed or antisocial manner. The choice of a negative identity represents an attempt to retain some mastery in a situation in which a positive identity does not seem possible or desirable. It is like saying, "I would rather be somebody bad than nobody at all." Clinical example 8-3 describes the negative identity assumed by an adolescent with a medical diagnosis of conduct disorder—undersocialized, aggressive.

CLINICAL EXAMPLE 8-3

Ken was a 17-year-old boy who was referred to the local community mental health center by his high school nurse. She made the referral after attending a team conference at school concerning Ken's repeated behavioral problems. He had a history of aggressive and destructive behavior in school, poor peer relationships, and low academic performance. The school had suspended him on three occasions previously, and the result of the team conference was to expel him for the remainder of the school year.

Mr. P, a psychiatric nurse at the mental health center, established a contract to work with Ken and his family. He noted that Ken was an obese young man (112.5 kg [250 pounds]) who took little interest in his appearance. His dress was sloppy, his complexion unclean, and his hair oily. He sat slumped in the chair in a disinterested and slightly defiant posture.

As Ken talked about himself, he complained of many pressures he experienced in his part-time job at a local hardware store. He thought the work was too difficult and tiring and that he was qualified for better and more prestigious work. When asked for specifics, he could not identify another job in particular. He also expressed a great deal of harrassment from his family. His mother and father had been married for 31 years, and he was the only child of the marriage. His mother

worked part time at a bakery, and his father was recently retired from his job as a supervisor at a local utility company where he was highly regarded.

Ken said that his father "always had things for me to do." He described how his father signed him up for various team sports—baseball, basketball, football—without acknowledging how much Ken hated sports and how uncoordinated he was. His father also stressed good grades and "the necessity of college" for success in life. Ken described his mother as passive and polite and said he had little respect for her. He said his aggressive outbursts occurred both at home and at school—whenever he was frustrated. People reacted by staying out of his way. He said he never hurt anyone with his temper. He mostly destroyed property and objects.

Ken avoided the subject of peers but, when asked about friends, said that there were a couple of boys in the neighborhood he "hung out with." They were older than he was. Most had dropped out of high school and were employed in odd jobs. He denied drug use but said they drank heavily, especially on the weekends. He said he had no girl friends and "wasn't interested in complicating my life with some broad."

Ken displays many of the behaviors characteristic of a negative identity. His actions seem to challenge the accepted activities of youth. The nurse working with Ken explored with him his underlying feelings and self-perceptions. Great anger with his father began to surface and Ken was able to verbalize about it. Because he was the only son, he felt like he was competing with his father and had to live up to his father's ideals. Ken feared failing in trying to adopt a positive identity, and he resented the identity his father was trying to impose on him. He thought he had no part in defining it and it did not represent his real self.

This example demonstrates that although identity confusion is a normative crisis of adolescence, the adoption of a negative identity can establish a maladaptive coping response which continues throughout life. So, too, problems of identity confusion may emerge at any point during one's adult years.

In general, the following are characteristics of a person experiencing *identity confusion*:

■ Lack of a sense of continuity between past and present
■ A high degree of anxiety
■ Less certainty about characteristics of self
■ Fluctuations in feelings about self

Such a person may be confused about standards by which to evaluate himself and fluctuate between unbending resistance and overeasy compliance.

An important group of behaviors that relate to a negative self-concept include disruptions in interpersonal relationships or problems of intimacy. The presenting behavior may be one of withdrawal or distancing. If a person is experiencing an undefined identity, he may wish to ignore or destroy those people who threaten him. The problem is one of gaining intimacy, but it is reflected in the behaviors of isolation, denial, and withdrawl from others.

A contrasting behavior that may be evident is one of personality fusing. Erikson has pointed out that true intimacy involves a sense of mutuality, which implies a firm self-delineation of the partners and not a diffused merger of two people. If a person is struggling to cope with a weak or undefined identity, however, he may try to establish his sense of self by fusing or belonging to someone else. This may occur in formal relationships, intense friendships, or brief affairs, since each can be seen as a desperate attempt to outline one's own identity. This nonautonomous fusion, however, leads to a further loss of identity. Some of these behaviors will be evident in Clinical example 8-4.

CLINICAL EXAMPLE 8-4

Mrs. P was seen by a psychiatric nurse in the psychiatric outpatient department of a general hospital. She was a well-dressed 24-year-old woman who had numerous somatic complaints, including decreased appetite, frequent headaches, fatigue, and difficulty falling asleep. She reported she had no energy or interest in doing anything or being with people. She said she dreaded each new day and felt abandoned and all alone.

She was married at the age of 17 to the only boy she ever dated in high school. He was 19 at the time and she "looked up to him tremendously." He established a successful career in the insurance business and she stayed at home to care for the house. She described herself as "centering my whole world around him." Three months previously he had told her that he wanted a separation and suggested she begin making a new life for herself. He said he intended to move out of the house at the end of the present month, but Mrs. P said that she hoped he would not do that when he saw how much she loved and needed him.

Mrs. P also described feelings of being unloved and

unlovable. She said she "felt empty inside" and "didn't really know who she was." She complained about her appearance and expressed much fear about living alone, finding a job, and getting along with people, especially men.

Many of the behaviors displayed by Mrs. P reflect the problem of *identity confusion*. She married at an early age before defining her own sense of self as an autonomous individual. Her only experience in a close relationship was with her husband, and she attempted to establish her own identity by living through his. Within the security of the marriage she managed to avoid any self-analysis, but the reality of the impending separation brought forth her fears and self-doubts. She displayed a low level of self-esteem and an unresolved conflict between dependency and independency.

Personality fusion and problems with identity have serious implications also for the larger family system. Dysfunctional families are frequently characterized by a fusion of ego mass that may be evident in severe symptomatology by one or more family members. This may be expressed in some form of family violence or abuse described in Chapter 28 or in the scapegoating of one family member who may become the "diagnosed" or "symptomatic" psychiatric patient as described in Chapter 25.

Identity confusion can also be expressed as pathological narcissism in which the individual has an exaggerated sense of self-importance manifested as extreme self-absorption. The person has an unrealistic idealized self that is based in illusion rather than reality. He believes he has solved his search for identity, but his idealized notion of self reflects a kind of alienation of his own being. In narcissism, according to Kernberg, "The normal tension between actual and ideal self . . . is eliminated by the building up of an inflated self-concept in which the actual self and ideal self . . . are confused."[25:238] Thus unlike the person with low self-esteem who keenly perceives the discrepancy between his actual self and self-ideal, the narcissist rejects the reality of who he really is by subscribing to an idealized self. His resulting state of identity confusion may be characterized by fantasies of unlimited success, an insatiable need for attention and admiration, exploitative interpersonal relationships, feelings of entitlement, and the lack of empathy for others.

A more maladaptive response to problems in identity involving withdrawal from reality occurs when the individual experiences panic levels of anxiety. This panic state produces a blocking off of awareness, a collapse in reality testing, and feelings of depersonalization. *Depersonalization* is a feeling of unreality in which one is unable to distinguish between inner and outer stimuli. It is, in essence, a true alienation from oneself. The individual has great difficulty distinguishing self from others, and one's body has an unreal or strange quality about it. It is the subjective experience of the partial or total disruption of one's ego and the disintegration and disorganization of one's self-concept. Because of this, it is the most frightening of human experiences. It develops as an outcome of uncertainties in human relationships. The individual has a not-loved feeling and, as a result of his failure to be loved, he fails to love himself. Depersonalization serves as a defense, but it is destructive in nature because it masks and immobilizes anxiety without in any way diminishing its intensity. It can occur in a variety of clinical illnesses, including depression, schizophrenia, manic states, and organic brain syndromes, and it represents the advanced stage of ego breakdown associated with psychotic states.

There are many behaviors associated with depersonalization. The primary one is that the patient experiences feelings of estrangement as though he were hiding something from himself. He experiences of lack of inner continuity and sameness and feels as if life is happening *to* him rather than his living by his own initiative. The patient may say that the world appears queer, dreamlike, or frightening. He may experience a loss of identity and express confusion regarding his own sexuality. He may describe related feelings of insecurity, inferiority, frustration, fear, hate, shame, and a loss of self-respect and be unable to derive a sense of accomplishment from any activity.

In depersonalization there may be a loss of impulse control and an absence of feeling and emotion that is manifested in impersonality, stiffness, formality, and rigidity in social situations. The individual may become lifeless and lack spontaneity and animation. He may plod through each day in a state of numbness and may respond to situations ordinarily eliciting emotion without characteristic love, hate, anxiety, or guilt. A heightened sense of isolation may mark his interpersonal relationships. He may become increasingly passive, as shown by withdrawing from social contacts, failing to assert himself, losing interest in his surroundings, and allowing others to make decisions for him.

Another sign of depersonalization is a disturbance in the individual's perception of time and space. He may become disoriented with regard to time and be unable to correctly recognize events as pertaining to yesterday or tomorrow or to plan his activities with reference to a time schedule. There may be a disturbance of memory characterized by aphasia, amnesia, or memory distortion. His thinking and judgment may be impaired and reflect great confusion and distortion or focus on trivial details. Problems in information processing can be evident in visual hallucinations, and disturbed interpersonal relationships may be reflected in delusions, auditory hallucinations, and incongruent or idiosyncratic communication.

A final common behavior associated with depersonalization is a confused or *disturbed body image*. The person may have a feeling of unreality about parts of his body. He may describe the feeling that his limbs are detached, the size of his body parts is changed, or he is unable to tell where his body leaves off and the rest of the world begins. Some patients describe the feeling that they had stepped outside their bodies and were observing themselves as detached and foreign objects. The many behaviors associated with depersonalization are summarized in Table 8-1. Clinical example 8-5 may further help to clarify the problem of depersonalization.

CLINICAL EXAMPLE 8-5

Mr. S was a 40-year-old man who had no previous history of psychiatric hospitalizations. Two months before his present admission, he was severely burned while on the job as an employee of a steel-making plant. He received second- and third-degree burns over his face, hands, chest, and back, and was treated in the burn center of a large university hospital. Three days before he was to be discharged from the burn unit, he experienced a psychotic episode. He reported hearing voices telling him to kill himself, and he was unable to recall any events surrounding the accident that produced his burns. He said he "felt his arms were withering away and his eyes were falling into his skull." He was unable to change the dressing on his burns even though he had been able to do this previously. When looking at his arms or chest, his face remained impassive and he showed no emotion. He began to talk continuously about returning to work but was unable to identify how long he had been out on sick leave or the amount of time recommended by his doctor for recovery.

TABLE 8-1. Behaviors associated with depersonalization

Affective	Perceptual	Cognitive	Behavioral
Experiences loss of identity	Auditory and visual hallucinations	Confusion	Blunting of affect
Feelings of alienation from self		Disoriented to time	Emotional passivity and nonresponsiveness
Feelings of insecurity, inferiority, fear, shame	Confusion regarding one's sexuality	Distorted thinking	
Feelings of unreality	Difficulty distinguishing self from others	Disturbance of memory	Incongruent or idiosyncratic communication
Heightened sense of isolation		Impaired judgment	Lack of spontaneity and animation
Lack of sense of inner continuity	Disturbed body image		Loss of impulse control
Unable to derive pleasure or a sense of accomplishment	Experiences the world as dreamlike		Loss of initiative and decision-making ability
			Social withdrawal

With the onset of these symptoms he was transferred from the burn unit to the psychiatric unit of the hospital. He remained socially isolated on the unit and refused to participate in ward meetings and group activities. At times he would wander into other patients' rooms and take pieces of their clothing. He would later be seen wearing this clothing on the unit and the staff would intervene to return it to its owner.

It is obvious from this example and the previous discussion that the various feelings and perceptions associated with depersonalization represent extreme defenses against threats to self that do not serve to alleviate the anxiety and, in fact, may add to it by the frightening nature of the experience. The patient views his own behavior as foreign, and he sees himself as a strong, unknown, and unpredictable being whom he does not recognize. As both a participant and a spectator, he observes himself with great fear, since he is unable to control his own impulses. He cannot completely escape the pain of self-awareness. He therefore disowns his behavior, feelings, thoughts, and body and becomes alienated from his true self and personal identity.

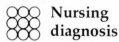 ## Nursing diagnosis

The nature of an individual's self-concept is a critical aspect of his overall personality adjustment. Problems with self-concept are associated with feelings of anxiety, hostility, and guilt. These often create a circular and self-propagat-

ing process for the individual that ultimately results in maladaptive coping responses (Fig. 8-3).

Most individuals who express dissatisfaction with life, display deviant behavior, or have difficulty functioning in social or work situations have problems related to self-concept. The nature of the patient's problem, the degree of disruption, and his level of anxiety will be determined by the patient and nurse together on the basis of the behavioral or objective data the nurse has collected, as well as the subjective responses and description of the patient. In completing an assessment the nurse attempts to identify relevant stressors and link these to the problem the patient is experiencing related to self-concept.

The formulation of a nursing diagnosis should specify the nature of the patient's maladaptive coping response and any relevant stressors. Six alterations in self-concept described in this chapter include low self-esteem, role strain, disturbed body image, identity confusion, negative identity, and depersonalization. When these problems are related to appropriate stressors, a nursing diagnosis is formulated.

In practice, maladaptive responses indicating alterations in self-concept can be seen in a wide variety of people experiencing threats to their physical integrity or self-system. It is an area of nursing diagnoses that is by no means limited to the psychiatric setting, and it does not have a discreet category of medical diagnoses associated with it. Because it pertains to one's basic personality structure and feelings about oneself, it is a group of nursing diagnoses that can emerge with a number of neurotic and psychotic

Text continued on p. 269.

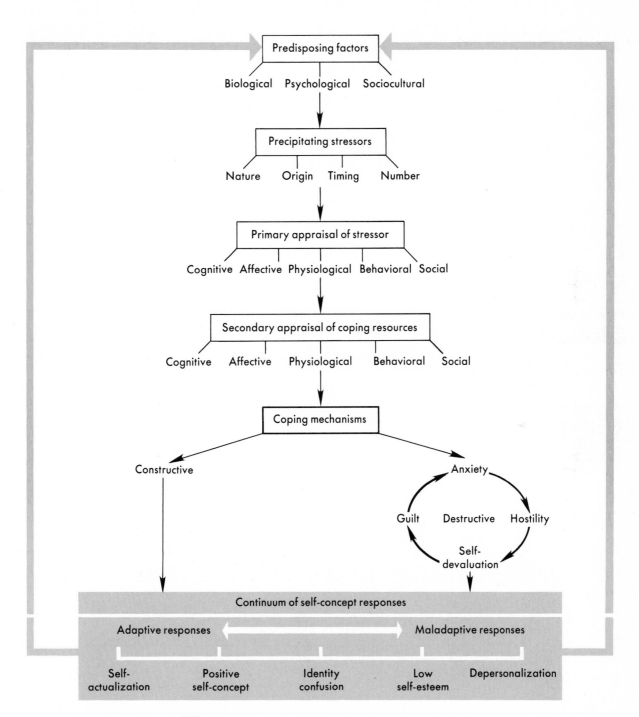

FIG. 8-3
Model of health-illness phenomena with self-concept
responses.

TABLE 8-2. Comparative examples of nursing diagnoses and medical diagnoses associated with alterations in self-concept

Nursing diagnoses	Medical diagnoses as described in DSM-III*

Identity confusion related to developmental crisis of adolescence	**Diagnostic criteria for IDENTITY DISORDER**
	
	A. Severe subjective distress regarding uncertainty about a variety of issues relating to identity, including three or more of the following:
	
	    1. Long-term goals
	    2. Career choice
	    3. Friendship patterns
	    4. Sexual orientation and behavior
	    5. Religious identification
	    6. Moral value systems
	    7. Group loyalties
	
	B. Impairment in social or occupational (including academic) functioning as a result of the symptoms in **A**
	
	C. Duration of the disturbance of at least 3 months
	
	D. Not due to another mental disorder, such as affective disorder, schizophrenia, or schizophreniform disorder
	
	E. If 18 or older, does not meet the criteria for borderline personality disorder

Low self-esteem related to death of spouse	**No mental disorder—UNCOMPLICATED BEREAVEMENT**
Disturbed body image related to fear of becoming obese	**Diagnostic criteria for ANOREXIA NERVOSA** **A.** Intense fear of becoming obese, which does not diminish as weight loss progresses **B.** Disturbance of body image, e.g., claiming to "feel fat" even when emaciated **C.** Weight loss of at least 25% of original body weight or, if under 18 years of age, weight loss from original body weight plus projected weight gain expected from growth charts may be combined to make the 25% **D.** Refusal to maintain body weight over a minimal normal weight for age and height **E.** No known physical illness that would account for the weight loss
Depersonalization and panic response related to rejection by boyfriend	**Diagnostic criteria for SCHIZOPHRENIFORM DISORDER** **A.** Meets all of the criteria for schizophrenia (p. 372) except for duration **B.** The illness (including prodromal, active, and residual phases) lasts more than 2 weeks but less than 6 months
Low self-esteem related to fear of public speaking	**Diagnostic criteria for SOCIAL PHOBIA** **A.** A persistent, irrational fear of, and compelling desire to avoid, a situation in which the individual is exposed to possible scrutiny by others and fears that he or she may act in a way that will be humiliating or embarrassing **B.** Significant distress because of the disturbance and recognition by the individual that his or her fear is excessive or unreasonable **C.** Not due to another mental disorder, such as major depression or avoidant personality disorder

*From American Psychiatric Association: Diagnostic and statistical manual of mental disorders, third edition, Washington, D.C., APA, 1980.

TABLE 8-2. Comparative examples of nursing diagnoses and medical diagnoses associated with alterations in self-concept—cont'd

Nursing diagnoses	Medical diagnoses as described in DSM-III
Role conflict related to incompatibility of newly assumed work and family roles	**Diagnostic criteria for ADJUSTMENT DISORDER** **A.** A maladaptive reaction to an identifiable psychosocial stressor that occurs within 3 months of the onset of the stressor **B.** The maladaptive nature of the reaction is indicated by either of the following: 　1. Impairment in social or occupational functioning 　2. Systems that are in excess of a normal and expectable reaction to the stressor **C.** The disturbance is not merely one of a pattern of overreaction to stress or an exacerbation of one of the mental disorders previously described
Negative identity related to unrealistic parental expectations	**Diagnostic criteria for CONDUCT DISORDER, socialized, nonaggressive** **A.** A repetitive and persistent pattern of nonaggressive conduct in which either the basic rights of others or major age-appropriate societal norms or rules are violated, as manifested by any of the following: 　1. Chronic violations of a variety of important rules (that are reasonable and age appropriate for the child) at home or at school (e.g., persistent truancy, substance abuse) 　2. Repeated running away from home overnight 　3. Persistent serious lying in and out of the home 　4. Stealing not involving confrontation with a victim **B.** Evidence of social attachment to others as indicated by at least two of the following behavior patterns: 　1. Has one or more peer-group friendships that have lasted over 6 months 　2. Extends himself or herself for others even when no immediate advantage is likely 　3. Apparently feels guilt or remorse when such a reaction is appropriate (not just when caught or in difficulty) 　4. Avoid blaming or informing on companions 　5. Shows concern for the welfare of friends or companions **C.** Duration of pattern of aggressive conduct of at least 6 months **D.** If 18 or older, does not meet the criteria for antisocial personality disorder
Low self-esteem related to overly high self-ideals	**Diagnostic criteria for DYSTHYMIC DISORDER** **A.** During the past 2 years (or 1 year for children and adolescents) the individual has been bothered most or all of the time by symptoms characteristic of the depressive syndrome but that are not of sufficient severity and duration to meet the criteria for a major depressive episode **B.** The manifestations of the depressive syndrome may be relatively persistent or separated by periods of normal mood lasting a few days to a few weeks, but no more than a few months at a time **C.** During the depressive periods there is either prominent depressed mood (e.g., sad, blue, down in the dumps, low) or marked loss of interest or pleasure in all, or almost all, usual activities and pastimes

Continued.

TABLE 8-2. **Comparative examples of nursing diagnoses and medical diagnoses associated with alterations in self-concept—cont'd**

Nursing diagnoses	Medical diagnoses as described in DSM-III
	D. During the depressive periods at least three of the following symptoms are present: 1. Insomnia or hypersomnia 2. Low energy level or chronic tiredness 3. Feelings of inadequacy, loss of self-esteem, or self-deprecation 4. Decreased effectiveness of productivity at school, work, or home 5. Decreased attention, concentration, or ability to think clearly 6. Social withdrawal 7. Loss of interest in or enjoyment of pleasurable activities 8. Irritability or excessive anger (in children, expressed toward parents or caretakers) 9. Inability to respond with apparent pleasure to praise or rewards 10. Less active or talkative than usual or feels slowed down or restless 11. Pessimistic attitude toward the future, brooding about past events, or feeling sorry for self 12. Tearfulness or crying 13. Recurrent thoughts of death or suicide **E.** Absence of psychotic features, such as delusions, hallucinations, or incoherence, or loosening of associations **F.** If the disturbance is superimposed on a preexisting mental disorder, such as obsessive-compulsive disorder or alcohol dependence, the depressed mood, by virtue of its intensity or effect on functioning, can be clearly distinguished from the individual's usual mood
Role strain related to incongruency of cultural and self-role expectations about aging	No mental disorder—PHASE OF LIFE PROBLEM
Depersonalization related to drug toxicity	No related psychiatric diagnosis
Disturbed body image related to cerebral vascular accident	No related psychiatric diagnosis
Depersonalization related to sensory deprivation	No related psychiatric diagnosis
Disturbed body image related to leukemia chemotherapy	No related psychiatric diagnosis

disorders. In fact, it is a group of nursing diagnoses that potentially could be related to all of the 16 diagnostic categories identified in the DSM-III,[1] since the psychodynamics of all of these disorders ultimately reflect on one's view of self. Table 8-2 presents some of the many possible nursing diagnoses that pertain to alterations in self-concept. Each of these nursing diagnoses is then related to the diagnostic criteria for a selected medical diagnosis as described in DSM-III.[1]

Planning and implementation of nursing intervention

Goal setting

Research indicates that patients with negative self-concepts believe their illnesses have a greater negative effect on their lives, have less hope and optimism about the future, and are more anxious about their illnesses.[38] These findings support the need for effective nursing intervention related to problems with self-concept.

The general goal of the nursing intervention is to facilitate the person's self-actualization by helping him grow, develop, and realize his potential while compensating for his impairments. The nurse's focus is to help the individual understand himself more fully and accurately so he can direct his own life in a more satisfying way. In a sense, nursing intervention concerns all that is involved in promoting the patient's self-realization. This means helping him strive toward a clearer and deeper experience of his feelings, wishes, and beliefs; toward a greater ability to tap his resources and to use them for constructive ends; and toward a clearer perception of his direction in life with the assumption of responsibility for himself and his decisions. It involves replacing repression with consciousness and unreality with reality. Sustaining, protecting, and enhancing the self results in increased self-esteem and self-acceptance, which is the essence of personality integration. A positive therapeutic outcome results in greater self-direction, tolerance, flexibility, and risk taking. A reorganization of the self will result in a change in behavior, and changes in behavior are outcomes of changes in the concept of the self.

Self-awareness is a crucial aspect in bringing about changes in self-concept, but people usually spend little time in introspection. Certain conditions or events, however, do stimulate self-awareness. This may occur when stimuli from the body are intensified, as in states of pain, fatigue, or anger, or when stimuli from the environment are decreased, as in sensory deprivation or states of isolation. Self-awareness may be triggered when something unexpected or extraordinary takes place, when the person has succeeded well or failed miserably, or when the person is confronted with himself by looking in a mirror, listening to his voice on a tape recorder, or reading an old letter. Special occasions, such as birthdays, anniversaries, New Year's Eve, or a death may stimulate introspection, and it may also be initiated when others direct their attention to the person through conversation or touch.

Once the person begins to look at and analyze himself, changes in the self become possible. Frequently they are the result of feelings of failure, unhappiness, anxiety, inadequacy, doubt or perplexity, or perceived discrepancies between one's concept of self and the demands of the environment or the expectations of others. Usually changes in the self occur only as a result of experiences and they take place gradually. Occasionally, however, a change may take place suddenly when a person has a traumatic experience that forces him to face the fact that he is inadequate or out of step with his peers and that something drastic must be done to remedy the situation.

The nurse should take all these factors into consideration when planning nursing care. Since the goal is to increase the patient's self-realization and acceptance, he must be an active participant in the formulation and implementation of specific plans. The nurse therefore must move with the patient and assess his readiness for growth within the therapeutic relationship. Together they formulate long-term goals that should reflect a positive resolution of the problem and the stressor identified in the nursing diagnosis. Short-term goals should be as clear and explicit as possible. They should identify realistic steps that the patient can accomplish. In this way the patient's self-confidence will increase, and this will directly affect his feelings of self-esteem. These goals should emphasize his strengths instead of his pathological condition, and, if they are mutually identified, they will serve to motivate him and help him assume increased responsibility for his own behavior. Following are examples of goals related to role conflict:

Long-term

Mrs. P will resolve role conflict by achieving greater congruency between work and family roles.

Short-term

After 1 week:
1. Mrs. P will describe her responsibilities in both her work and home roles.
2. She will identify aspects of these roles that provide her with satisfaction.
3. She will identify areas of role incompatibility.

After 2 weeks:
1. She will describe three alternative ways of increasing the complementarity of the roles.
2. She will discuss the advantages and disadvantages of each alternative.

After 3 weeks:
1. Mrs. P will take the necessary measures to implement one of the above alternatives.

Following are examples of goals related to disturbed body-image:

Long-term

Mr. B will accept his modified body image after treatment with chemotherapy for leukemia.

Short-term

After the first phase of chemotherapy:
1. Mr. B will identify the medications he is receiving.
2. He will describe the effect they have on his illness and related body systems.
3. He will express his feelings (e.g., anger, sadness) about his illness and therapy.
4. He will identify three positive aspects of his modified body image.

Intervening in alterations in self-concept

The mutually identified goals can be accomplished by a problem-solving approach that focuses primarily on the present, removes much of the responsibility from the nurse, and actively engages the patient in working on his difficulties. This approach increases the patient's self-confidence and self-esteem. It requires that the patient first develop *insight* into his problems and life situation and then take *action* to effect lasting behavioral change. The nurse must thus incorporate both the responsive dimensions (insight oriented) and the action dimensions (action oriented) of the therapeutic relationship as described in Chapter 3 in implementing her nursing care.

The focus of this approach is on the patient's cognitive appraisal of his life, which may contain faulty perceptions, beliefs, and convictions. The patient's awareness of his feelings and emotions is also important, since they may be subject to misconceptions that arise from the acceptance of his cognitive analysis. Often the patient's display of affect is a clue to significant problem areas. Only after examining his cognitive appraisal of the situation and related feelings can he gain insight into the problem and bring about behavioral change. Adaptive behavior is based both on insight and on actually carrying out an appropriate solution to the presenting problem.

It is possible therefore to describe principles of nursing care that are applicable to the various problems with self-concept. These principles will be incorporated within a problem-solving approach and will be presented as progressive levels in the sequence in which they occur. It should also be noted that these principles focus primarily on the level of the individual. They may, however, be implemented in conjunction with group- or family-level interventions, and it is expected that the nurse would include the patient's family, significant others, and community supports whenever possible. Such a mobilization of the patient's possible coping resources can have both preventive and curative effects.

LEVEL 1—EXPANDED SELF-AWARENESS. A consistent picture of the self is necessary for security, and most people, to avoid anxiety, resist change. The ego resists change because any change becomes a threat to its stability and integration. Furthermore, the closer a deviant perception of the self is to the core of the self-concept, the more difficult it is to change. In general, change in the self is easier when there is an absence of threat. Threat forces a person to defend himself, and under threat, perceptions are narrowed and it becomes difficult for the person to form new perceptions of himself.

To expand the patient's self-awareness and reduce the element of threat, the nurse should adopt an accepting attitude toward the patient. Acceptance by the nurse allows the patient the security and freedom to examine all aspects of himself as a total human being with both positive and negative qualities. The basis of a therapeutic relationship will be established by listening to the patient with understanding, responding nonjudgmentally to him, expressing genuine interest in him, and conveying a sense of caring and sincerity. Creating a climate of acceptance allows previously denied experiences to be brought into consciousness and explored. This broadens the patient's concept of self and helps him to accept all aspects of his personality. It also indicates to him that he is a valued individual who is responsible for himself and able to help himself. This is important because the nurse must work through whatever ego strength the patient possesses. To the extent that a person has certain elements of ego strength—the capacity for self-control, some adeptness at reality testing, and a degree of ego integration—there is a foundation on which to build.

Most patients seen in clinics, the general hospital, and the community setting will possess a fair amount of ego strength. Hospitalized individuals, however, might have limited ego resources with which to work. Psychotic patients who are experiencing feelings of depersonalization and identity confusion are often difficult challenges for the nurse. They tend to isolate themselves and withdraw from reality so that there is little ego strength available for problem solving. For this type of patient, expanding self-awareness means first confirming the patient's identity. The nurse should attempt to provide supportive measures to decrease the panic level of anxiety experienced by this fragile and vulnerable patient. Her nursing actions will be more active while they exert less pressure on the patient. Additional interventions related to anxiety and psychotic states are described in Chapters 7 and 11.

The nurse can spend time with the patient in an undemanding way and approach him in a nonaggressive manner. Initially she may accept his need to remain nonverbal and attempt to clarify and understand his verbal communication even though it may be distorted or lacking in apparent logic. She should prevent him from isolating himself from others and establish a simple routine for him. If the patient displays bizarre behavior, such as inappropriate laughing or mannerisms, she can provide control for him and set limits on his behavior. It is important to orient him frequently to reality and reinforce appropriate behavior. The patient should be helped to increase the activities that provide positive experiences for him. This may involve the use of occupational therapy, recreational therapy, or activity groups. It has been shown that success at tasks and increased involvement with objects can increase self-esteem.[27] Movement therapy or body ego technique provides a special goal-directed way to facilitate the development of identity, body image, and ego structure and bring about changes in experiences that are necessary for ego growth. It is predominantly a nonverbal therapy because the emphasis is on movement and not on what the person says.[37]

The patient experiencing depersonalization often exhibits poor hygiene and an unkempt personal appearance. The nurse who is aware of her own value system regarding cleanliness and grooming can assist the patient who is unable to care for himself. She can use patience and repetition to establish health routines and kindly but firmly encourage the patient to care for himself. By her verbal and nonverbal messages she can encourage the patient to take pride in his appearance and reinforce any progress made in this area. Another possible nursing intervention in the area of body image is to use photographic self-image confrontation. This involves taking photographs of the patient and discussing them with him. Spire[39] found that this intervention produced positive behavioral changes with schizophrenic patients and provided a means for establishing a nurse-patient relationship and mutually exploring some aspects of the self.

Mutuality is often difficult to establish with a patient experiencing depersonalization. Initially the nurse will determine appropriate activities and incorporate the patient into them without asking for a response. Gradually, however, the nurse can expect greater participation and involve the patient in decision making that affects his care. Table 8-3 summarizes the nursing interventions appropriate to level 1.

Sometimes the attitude or behavior of the nurse can actually block or prevent the patient from expanding his self-awareness. This can be done in the form of criticism, belittlement, condemnation, condescension, indifference, or insincerity. If the nurse has an impersonal attitude or ignores the patient, it can decrease his self-esteem. Excessive demands on the patient or direct challenges to his self-concept at this time can result in his further withdrawal. The nurse should not allow him to remain alone or inactive, attempt to shame him into improving his habits, or assume total care for him. If the nurse avoids these attitudes and behaviors and strives for acceptance, she removes herself as a source of threat and encourages the patient to lower his defenses. He is then prepared to undertake the next step in the problem-solving approach.

LEVEL 2—SELF-EXPLORATION. At this level of intervention the nurse encourages the patient to examine his feelings, behavior, beliefs, and

TABLE 8-3. **Summary of nursing interventions in alterations in self-concept at level 1**
Goal—Expand the patient's self-awareness

Principle	Rationale	Nursing actions
Establish an open trusting relationship	Reduces the threat that the nurse poses to the patient and helps him to broaden and accept all aspects of his personality	Offer unconditional acceptance Listen to the patient Encourage discussion of his thoughts and feelings Respond nonjudgmentally Convey to the individual that he is a valued person who is responsible for himself and able to help himself
Work with whatever ego strength the patient possesses	Some degree of ego strength, such as the capacity for reality testing, self-control, or a degree of ego integration, is needed as a foundation for later nursing care	Identify the ego strength possessed by the patient Guidelines for the patient with limited ego resources are as follows: 1. Begin by confirming his identity 2. Provide support measures to reduce his panic level of anxiety 3. Approach him in an undemanding way 4. Accept and attempt to clarify any verbal or nonverbal communication 5. Prevent him from isolating himself 6. Establish a simple routine for him 7. Set limits on inappropriate behavior 8. Orient him to reality 9. Reinforce appropriate behavior 10. Gradually increase activities and tasks that provide positive experiences for him 11. Assist him in personal hygiene and grooming 12. Encourage the patient to care for himself
Maximize the patient's participation in the therapeutic relationship	Mutuality is necessary for the patient to assume ultimate responsibility for his own behavior and maladaptive coping responses	Gradually increase the patient's participation in decisions that affect his care Convey to the patient that he is a responsible individual

thoughts, particularly in relationship to the current stressful situation. The patient's feelings may be expressed verbally, nonverbally, symbolically, or directly. Acceptance continues to be important in this level because when the nurse accepts the patient's feelings and thoughts, she is helping him to accept them also. The nurse should facilitate the expression of strong emotions, such as anger, sadness, and guilt. In a sense, the patient's emotions or affect serve as clues to the exploration of inner thoughts and the examination of current behavior.

As the patient is helped to focus his attention on the meaning that experiences have for him, he is clarifying his perceptions and concept of himself and his relationship to the people and events around him. The nurse can elicit his perception of self-strengths and weaknesses and have him describe his self-ideal. He can be made aware of his self-criticisms. Frequently recognition in itself is a powerful therapeutic tool that motivates the patient to change. Jourard[24] has noted that many patients will experience a reduction in anxiety following the experience of full self-disclosure to an interested nurse. He believes patients withhold self-disclosure because of anxiety and the belief that no one is really interested in them.

It is important for the nurse to accept and deal with her own feelings before involving herself in the self-exploration of others. Her self-awareness will limit the potential negative effects of countertransference in the relationship. It will also allow her the freedom to manifest authentic behavior, which she, in turn, can elicit and reinforce in the patient. Often patients will experience great difficulty in discussing or describing their feelings. This might be because society tends to discourage self-revelation or because the patient is honestly out of touch with his own inner self. In this case the nurse can use herself therapeutically by sharing her own feelings with the patient, verbalizing how she might feel in the situation or mirroring her perception of the patient's feelings.

The nurse can facilitate the patient's thinking by using reflection to paraphrase and sharpen the meanings in the patient's discussion. Validation and empathic responses are essential to guide the patient to the next level of nursing intervention. In all these ways the nurse provides encouragement, since most patients have strong tendencies to avoid thinking and talking about disturbing aspects of their problems. In addition, the nurse's reflections or clarifications of meaning help the patient to perceive more precisely what he has been discussing. Verbalized thoughts that have been responded to by the nurse often become more concrete and tangible. Reflected responses can also provide subtle guides for the patient because they often emphasize particular verbal content whose significance may have escaped the patient's attention.

In implementing these actions the nurse must be careful not to reinforce the patient's self-pity by responding with sympathy. Patients frequently disclaim any personal responsibility for their "plight," and they fail to see how their own behavior precipitates the very things about which they complain. Examples of this are patients who seek treatment because of things that happened *to* them, such as their wife left them, their husband beats them, or their boss fired them, and patients who seek help because of things that have *not* happened, such as not being happy or having friends. These patients fail to see that they have a choice in life and that personal growth and satisfaction involve both risk and responsibility. The nurse can clarify with the patient that he is not helpless or powerless in the face of difficulties. He is power-

less when he sees himself as such and gives up control and responsibility for his behavior. Each person is responsible for his own behavior, including the things he decides to do and those which he decides not to do. One must also accept the responsibility for the logical consequences of those behaviors which one selects. Only if a patient fully understands the implications of his actions and the scope of his choices can he proceed to set goals, explore alternatives, and effect change.

In stressing the importance of behavior, the nurse helps the patient see that he chooses to behave in certain ways. If the patient projects his problems onto the environment, she can discuss with him the difficulty in changing situations and other people and instead explore the possibilities of changing his own self. This means helping the patient realize that when he says "I can't" he really means "I don't want to." The nurse should not give the impression that she has the power to change a patient's life. That power lies with him alone. She can, however, help him to maximize his strengths, utilize available resources, and see that there is more to life than being involved with misery and pain.

Self-exploration need not take place solely within the one-to-one relationship. Family sessions and group meetings can be helpful to clarify how the individual appears to others. These meetings can supplement the individual sessions with the patient, or similar nursing interventions can be applied within a regular family therapy or group therapy situation. Regardless, the nurse will be collecting information on the patient's thinking about himself, his use of logical or illogical reasoning, and his reported or observed emotional reactions. Interventions at this level should see the patient progress from denying or attributing contradictory feelings to the external situation, to realizing his own conflict in the particular situation, to recognizing a major conflict within himself (Table 8-4).

LEVEL 3—SELF-EVALUATION. This level involves hard work for the patient as he critically examines his own behavior, accepts the consequences for it, and judges it on the basis of whether it is his best possible choice. At this point, the problem should be clearly defined, and the patient should be helped to understand that his beliefs influence both his feelings and his behavior. It is only by actively and system-

TABLE 8-4. **Summary of nursing interventions in alterations in self-concept at level 2**
Goal—Encourage the patient's self-exploration

Principle	Rationale	Nursing actions
Assist the patient to accept his own feelings and thoughts	When the nurse shows interest in and accepts the patient's feelings and thoughts, she is helping him to do so also	Attend to and encourage the patient's expression of his emotions, beliefs, behavior, and thoughts—verbally, nonverbally, symbolically, or directly Utilize therapeutic communication skills and empathic responses Note his use of logical and illogical thinking and his reported and observed emotional responses
Help the patient to clarify his concept of self and his relationship to others through self-disclosure	Self-disclosure and understanding one's self-perceptions are prerequisites to bringing about future change; this may, in itself, produce a reduction in anxiety	Elicit his perception of self-strengths and weaknesses Assist him to describe his self-ideal Identify his self-criticisms Help him to describe how he believes he relates to other people and events
Be aware and have control of your own feelings	Self-awareness allows the nurse to model authentic behavior and limits the potential negative effects of countertransference in the relationship	Openness to one's own feelings Acceptance of both positive and negative feelings Therapeutic use of self by: 1. Sharing one's own feelings with the patient 2. Verbalizing how another might have felt 3. Mirroring her perception of the patient's feelings
Respond empathically, not sympathetically, emphasizing that the power to change lies with the patient	Sympathy can reinforce the patient's self-pity; rather, the nurse should communicate that the patient's life situation is subject to his own control	Use empathic responses and monitor oneself for feelings of sympathy or pity Reaffirm to the patient that he is not helpless or powerless in the face of his problems Convey verbally and behaviorally that the patient is responsible for his own behavior, including his choice of maladaptive or adaptive coping responses Discuss with him the scope of his choices, his areas of ego strength, and coping resources that are available to him. Utilize the support systems of family and groups to facilitate the patient's self exploration Assist the patient in recognizing the nature of his conflict and the maladaptive ways in which he tries to cope with it

atically challenging his faulty beliefs and perceptions that he can hope to alter his feelings and change his behavior. Previously identified misperceptions and distortions should be evaluated. Irrational beliefs, such as the following, should be brought to light and analyzed:

- Everyone must love me.
- I must be competent and adequate in all ways.
- I am unable to control my own happiness and destiny.
- I should condemn myself for making mistakes.
- I am better off if I avoid responsibilities rather than trying to face them.
- I am controlled by my past and can never break free of it.
- If I worry about potential problems, my anxiety will prevent their occurrence.
- My life is a disaster if it doesn't work out exactly as I had planned.

The patient's hopelessness should be countered by exploring areas of realistic hope. It is important to point out the mature part of the patient's personality and contrast it to the childhood part that causes problems. The behaviors that interfere with effective functioning have to be put in perspective so that the patient can clearly see that his maladaptive behavior is only a small part of his total personality. Sometimes the patient is unable to identify any areas of strengths and few may be readily obvious to the nurse. This requires additional thinking on her part. All people, no matter how disturbed their behavior, have some areas of personal strength. The nurse should examine the following areas:

1. Hobbies
2. Skills
3. School
4. Work
5. Character traits
6. Interpersonal skills
7. Personal qualities, such as loyalty and honesty
8. Appearance

As she is able to see positive aspects of the individual, she should share them with him to expand his own awareness.

The concepts of success and failure need to be placed in proper perspective. Failures occur every moment of every day, and they are a natural consequence of human activity. As long as people strive to achieve, they will frequently not reach their goals. The only way to avoid failure is to do absolutely nothing. Failure may be caused by one's own mistakes; it may be a result of lack of motivation; or it may be due to cir-

cumstances beyond one's control. But failure is the unavoidable outcome of human effort. The problem arises when individuals are labeled or label themselves as failures merely because they fail. This is illogical and potentially destructive. As an inherent aspect of life, failure should be viewed as a neutral concept rather than a negative one. If misperceptions such as this and unrealistic goals can be changed in the direction of greater accuracy where reality is concerned, maladaptive behavior and feelings of self-depreciation are likely to be reduced.

Unrealistic self-ideals, dependency patterns, and denial are all potential areas that can be analyzed. The patient can be helped to realize that all behavior and coping responses have both positive and negative consequences. Contrasts can be drawn between behavior that is destructive, inhibitory, or sabotaging, and that which is productive, enhancing, and growth producing. It is important for the patient to see that he acts in self-defeating ways because there is some "payoff" or personal gain in it for him. The drawbacks or disadvantages to the patient's maladaptive coping responses will probably be well known to him. The payoffs, or secondary gains, may be more obscure and well repressed. Following are some commonly experienced payoffs[26]:

- Procrastination
- Avoiding risks
- Retreating from the present
- Not having to accept responsibility for one's actions
- Avoiding working or having to change

More specific payoffs should be identified by the nurse and patient together, relative to his particular problem. For example, possible secondary gains that can be derived from being obese include having people feel sorry for you, having an excuse for not dating or being married, being the focus of dieting attention, or being easily recognized and noticed when with other people. Possible secondary gains for an adult remaining dependent on his parents might include not having to make one's own decisions, having someone else to blame if things go wrong, being protected from having to take risks and venture out in the world on one's own, having an excuse for not establishing lasting intimate relationships with one's peers, or not having to establish one's own identity, but rather adopting the values and goals of others. Such payoffs can be identified for each nursing diagnosis formulated by the nurse.

The nurse becomes more active in this level of intervention. She begins confronting, interpreting, persuading, and challenging the patient. Her goal is to increase the patient's objectivity in dealing with the stressors he perceives. She may utilize a number of techniques at this time. In interpretation and confrontation, the nurse offers information that the patient may not have or does not recognize as relevant. Supportive confrontation may be particularly effective in calling to the patient's attention inconsistencies in words and actions that he has not seen. The climate of acceptance established by the nurse in level 1 and the empathic communication developed in level 2 provide a basis for confrontation in level 3. This groundwork is necessary to prevent premature confrontation, which can be destructive.

The use of reflection allows the nurse to restate the meaning or emphasize the significance of the patient's revelations. It functions to inform the patient that the nurse understands what is being said, and it encourages him to continue his self-evaluation. Reflections and confrontations are often phrased in the form of questions, and the use of questions can also encourage the patient to search for additional information. In this regard the questions should be specific and not vague or overwhelming, which occurs when one repeatedly asks "Why?" Suggestion can be used to introduce alternative ways of thinking or behaving.

The nurse may use various aspects of role theory during this level of intervention. She may assist the patient in role clarification, which is the gaining of knowledge, information, and cues needed to perform a role. It involves the identification of appropriate behaviors, clarification of expectations, and specification of goals relative to the role, taking into consideration the influence of significant others and the context of the situation. Role clarification therefore reduces the potential for, or existence of, role strain. The nurse can also encourage the patient to participate in any activity in which he can observe his own behavior. The use of role playing may be particularly effective in providing the patient with feedback and increasing his insight. Through it, he may be able to gain objectivity toward the irrationality and self-destructiveness of his self-criticisms.

The nurse-patient relationship provides a rich source of information for the patient. Within this relationship he is enacting and experiencing many of his problem areas and the nurse can use this as a "study in miniature." The nurse can assist the patient in observing how he reacts in the one-to-one situation. She can share her reactions with him to give him feedback on how he affects others and openly disclose some of her own feelings about the patient's behavior. The analysis and use of transference and countertransference reactions comprises the nurse's "therapeutic use of self." When a block arises within the relationship or the nurse experiences increased anxiety, she should use this opportunity to explore its meaning with the patient. She should confront the problem and openly discuss it with him. This can also be done in family therapy or group therapy sessions.

Psychodrama, a special form of group therapy, provides the patient with an additional opportunity to gain self-insight. In psychodrama the therapist organizes the events so that the patient has an audience to whom he plays a role structured for him by the therapist. In this therapy modality the audience acts as a standard against which the patient can obtain evidence for the social adequacy of his own reactions and behavior.

During this level of intervention the patient and nurse critically evaluate his behavior (Table 8-5). Misperceptions, unrealistic goals, and distortions of reality are explored. This provides the patient with sufficient knowledge to progress to the next level of the problem-solving process.

LEVEL 4—REALISTIC PLANNING. The nurse and patient are now ready to formulate possible solutions or alternatives. This begins by investigating what solutions were attempted in the past and evaluating their effectiveness. When inconsistent perceptions are held by the individual, he is faced with a number of choices. He can change his perceptions and beliefs to bring them closer to the reality that cannot be changed. Or he may seek to change his environment to bring it in line with what he believes. When his behavior is not consistent with his self-concept, he can change his behavior to conform to his self-concept, change the beliefs underlying his self-concept so that they include his behavior, or change his self-ideal while leaving his self-concept intact.

At this time, all possible solutions should be openly discussed with the patient. The nurse must be careful not to use her influence to persuade the patient to do anything that represents her own values rather than the patient's. She

TABLE 8-5. Summary of nursing interventions in alterations in self-concept at level 3
Goal —Assist the patient's self-evaluation

Principle	Rationale	Nursing actions
Help the patient to clearly define the problem	Only after the problem is accurately defined can alternative choices be proposed	Identify relevant stressors with the patient and his appraisal of them Clarify to the patient that his beliefs influence both his feelings and behaviors Mutually identify faulty beliefs, misperceptions, distortions, illusions, and unrealistic goals Mutually identify areas of strength Place the concepts of success and failure in proper perspective Explore with the patient his use of coping resources
Explore the patient's adaptive and maladaptive coping responses to his problem	It is then necessary to examine the coping choices the patient has made and evaluate both the positive and negative consequences of them	Describe to the patient how all coping responses are freely chosen and have both positive and negative consequences Contrast adaptive and maladaptive responses Mutually identify the disadvantages of the patient's maladaptive coping responses Mutually identify the advantages or "payoffs" of the patient's maladaptive coping responses Discuss how these payoffs have perpetuated the maladaptive response Utilize a variety of therapeutic skills, such as the following: 1. Facilitative communication 2. Supportive confrontation 3. Role clarification 4. The transference and countertransference reactions occurring in the one-to-one relationship 5. Psychodrama

should help him conceptualize his goals. If they are within his reach, she can support his efforts to reach them. If the patient has conflicting goals, she helps him identify which ones are more realistic or obtainable by discussing the emotional and practical consequences of each goal.

The nurse can work with the patient in various ways. He may be encouraged to give up superhuman standards by which he judges his behavior. These standards may set him up for failure and create a pathological cyclical pattern that will need to be broken. Together they may work at destroying illusions that are not part of his authentic self. Perhaps the patient will need to lower his self-ideal and limit his personal goals to make them consistent with what is humanly possible. He should be encouraged to renew involvement with life and enter new experiences for their growth potential.

The techniques of role rehearsal, role modeling, and role playing may be employed. In role rehearsal the person imagines how a particular situation might take place and how his role might evolve. He mentally enacts his role and tries to anticipate the responses of significant

TABLE 8-6. Summary of nursing interventions in alterations in self-concept at level 4
Goal —Assist the patient in formulating a realistic plan of action

Principle	Rationale	Nursing actions
Help the patient identify alternative solutions	Only when all possible alternatives have been evaluated can change be affected	Help the patient understand that he can only change himself, not others
		If the patient holds inconsistent perceptions, help him to see that he can change the following:
		1. His beliefs or ideals to bring them closer to reality
		2. His environment to make it consistent with his beliefs
		If his self-concept is not consistent with his behavior, he can change the following:
		1. His behavior to conform to his self-concept
		2. The beliefs underlying his self-concept to include his behavior
		3. His self-ideal
		Mutually review how coping resources may be better utilized by the patient
Help the patient conceptualize his own realistic goals	Goal setting that includes a clear definition of the expected change is necessary	Encourage the patient to formulate his own (not the nurse's) goals
		Mutually discuss the emotional, practical, and reality-based consequences of each goal
		Help the patient clearly define the concrete change to be made
		Encourage the patient to enter new experiences for their growth potential
		Utilize role rehearsal, role modeling, and role playing when appropriate

others. Role rehearsal is important in anticipating and planning the course of future action. Role modeling occurs when the individual observes someone else playing a certain role so that he is able to understand and emulate the behaviors in that role. The person he observes may be the nurse, a family member, a group member, or peer. The nurse can be important in assisting the patient in his role learning. She can model behavior that may be posing problems for the patient, such as the appropriate expression of feelings, specific socialization skills, or realistic self-expectations. Proceeding one step further, the nurse and patient may role play certain situations to conceptualize alternative solutions. Nursing actions appropriate to this level of intervention are summarized in Table 8-6. Ultimately, the patient should decide on a plan of action that includes a clear definition of the concrete change to be achieved. Converting a "talking decision" into an "action decision" is the final, but obviously most important, step.

LEVEL 5—COMMITMENT TO ACTION. The nurse assists the patient to become committed to his decision and then achieve his own goals. The patient's development of self-awareness, self-understanding, and insight is not the ultimate desired outcome of the nursing therapeutic process. Insight alone does not make problems disappear or transform one's world in magical ways. Although a patient may have obtained a high level of insight, he may nevertheless continue to function at a minimal level. Such a patient may be able to intellectually discuss with great ease the nature of his problem and the in-

TABLE 8-7. Summary of nursing interventions in alterations in self-concept at level 5
Goal —Assist the patient to become committed to his decision and achieve his own goals

Principle	Rationale	Nursing actions
Help the patient take the necessary action to change maladaptive coping responses and maintain adaptive ones	The ultimate objective in promoting the patient's insight is to have him replace the maladapative coping responses with more adaptive ones	Provide opportunity for the patient to experience success
		Reinforce the strengths, skills, and healthy aspects of the patient's personality
		Assist the patient in gaining the assistance he might need (vocational, financial, and social services)
		Utilize family and groups to enhance the patient's self-esteem
		Allow the patient sufficient time to change
		Provide the appropriate amount of support and positive reinforcement for the patient to help him maintain his progress

fluences contributing to it. But the problem itself continues to be unresolved. Some patients actually use their insights to resist moving forward and avoid the hard work involved in making behavioral changes. The value of having the patient gain insight and increase his self-understanding is so that he can gain perspective on why he behaves the way he does and what must be done to break the maladaptive coping pattern.

Providing opportunity for the patient to experience success becomes essential at this time. To help him commit himself to his goal, the nurse can relate to the patient how she sees him, correcting his own poor self-image. In this mirroring technique she can openly and honestly describe to the patient the normal healthy parts of his personality and how by using these parts he can achieve his goal. She should reinforce his strengths or skills and provide him with opportunities to use them whenever possible.

Sometimes the lack of vocational or social skills may be a causative factor for low self-esteem. If so, nursing intervention can be directed toward gaining vocational assistance for the patient. Group involvement may be instrumental in raising self-esteem.[15] The experience of being accepted by others, the sense of belonging and being important to others, and the opportunity to develop interpersonal competence can all enhance self-esteem.

At this point the individual needs a great deal of support and positive reinforcement in affecting and maintaining change. For many patients this will mean breaking chronic behavior patterns and exposing themselves to real risk. A person must actively maintain the processes learned to avoid slipping back to the old behavior. Doing this is difficult and requires that the patient build on the progress he has made in the other levels. Successful change is a continuing process of modifying not only one's behavior but one's environment to help ensure that the change to new ways of behaving is permanent. Otherwise there will be a relapse.

The nurse serves as a transition between the pain of the past and the positive gratification the future holds. It is important that both the nurse and patient allow sufficient time for change. A significant amount of time may be required for patterns that developed over months or years to be broken and new ones established. The nurse's role now becomes less an active and directive one, but rather one of confirming the value, potential, and accomplishments of the patient (Table 8-7).

 Evaluation

Problems with self-concept are prominent in many psychological disorders. Changes in self-concept are accompanied by greater self-realization and self-acceptance and lead to behavioral changes and improved personality adjustment. To evaluate the success or failure of the nursing care given in this area, each phase of the nursing process should be reviewed and analyzed by the nurse and patient.

The nurse's assessment should include both the objective and observable behaviors as well as the subjective perceptions of the patient. Did she explore his areas of strengths and weaknesses and elicit his self-ideal? Was information obtained on his body image, feelings of self-esteem, role satisfaction, and sense of identity? Did she compare his responses to his behavior, and were any inconsistencies or contradictions identified? Was she aware of her own affective response to the patient, and how did this affect her ability to be therapeutic?

Before formulating a nursing diagnosis, the nurse should have discussed with the patient his appraisal of stressful life events and the nature of the threat they posed to him. Did they determine his level of anxiety and was he able to express related feelings, such as hostility, sadness, or guilt? Were the therapeutic goals realistic, explicit, adequate, and efficient? Were the patient's coping resources adequately assessed and utilized?

The nurse should have adopted a problem-solving approach that placed responsibility for growth on the patient. The most fundamental nursing action should have been to create a climate of acceptance that confirmed the patient's identity and conveyed a sense of value or worth. In expanding the patient's self-awareness, how effective was the nurse in promoting the patient's full and pertinent self-disclosure? Was he able to listen more fully to himself and others? What behaviors or attitudes did the nurse display that prevented the patient from expanding his self-awareness? Was the nurse able to manifest authentic behavior in the relationship and share her thoughts and reactions with the patient? What interventions were used and which ones proved to be beneficial—validation, reflection, confrontation, suggestion, role clarification, or role playing? Did the nurse progress on the basis of her patient's readiness and motivation?

What was the outcome of the patient's cognitive analysis and exploration of feelings? Was he able to transfer his new perceptions into possible solutions or alternative behavior? How did the nurse help him implement his plans? What success did he experience? Did they both allow sufficient time for changes to occur? The degree of overall success achieved through nursing care can be determined by eliciting the patient's perception of his own growth and comparing his behavior to the characteristics of the healthy personality as described in this chapter. Not everyone will achieve all these characteristics, but success has been achieved if the patient's potential has been maximized.

Suggested cross-references

Definitions of mental health are discussed in Chapters 2 and 5. Therapeutic relationship skills are discussed in Chapter 3. The model of health-illness phenomena and the phases of the nursing process are discussed in Chapter 4. Interventions with family and group support systems and other coping resources are discussed in Chapters 5 and 6. Interventions related to anxiety are discussed in Chapter 7. The relationship of role strain and low self-esteem to depression is discussed in Chapter 9. Self-destructive behaviors, including anorexia, obesity, and suicide are discussed in Chapter 10. Nursing intervention in psychotic panic states is discussed in Chapter 11. Family therapy is discussed in Chapter 25. The family dysfunctions of violence and abuse are discussed in Chapter 28.

SUMMARY

1. Self-concept is a critical and central element for the understanding of people and their behavior. It is defined as all the notions, beliefs, and convictions that constitute an individual's knowledge of himself and influence his relationships with others. One's self-concept does not exist at birth but is learned as a result of a person's unique experiences within himself, with significant others, and with the realities of the world.

2. Body image is the sum of the conscious and unconscious attitudes the individual has toward his body. It includes present and past perceptions, as well as feelings about size, function, appearance, and potential. It is continually modified by new perceptions and experiences.

3. Self-ideal is the individual's perception of how he should behave based on certain personal standards, aspirations, goals, or values. Mental health is associated with a clear, realistic self-ideal and congruence between one's perception of self and his self-ideal.

4. Self-esteem is the individual's personal judgment of his own worth obtained by analyzing how well his behavior conforms to his self-ideal. High self-esteem is a feeling rooted in unconditional acceptance of self, despite mistakes, defeats, and failures, as an innately worthy and important being.

5. Roles are sets of socially expected behavior patterns associated with an individual's function in various social groups. Ascribed roles are assigned roles over which the person has no choice. Assumed roles are those selected or chosen by the person.

6. Identity is the organizing principle of the personality that accounts for the unity, continuity, consistency, and uniqueness of the individual. It connotes autonomy and includes perceptions of one's sexuality. Identity formation begins in infancy and proceeds throughout life but is the major task of the adolescent period.

7. Individuals with positive self-concepts function more effectively, which is evident in interpersonal competence, intellectual efficiency, and environmental mastery. Because negative self-concept is correlated with personal and social maladjustment, self-concept change is a core element in psychiatric nursing practice.

8. Stressors related to alterations in self-concept were identified and briefly described.

a. Stressors affecting self-esteem include parental rejection, unrealistic parental expectations, repeated failures, lack of personal responsibility, dependency on others, and unrealistic self-ideals.

b. Stressors affecting role include incongruent role expectations or incompatible role demands (role conflict), lack of knowledge of specific role expectations (role ambiguity), and lack of adequate resources for performance of a complex role set (role overload).

c. Stressors affecting body image include loss of a body part; changes in body size, shape, appearance, or function; physical changes associated with normal growth and development; and medical and nursing procedures.

d. Stressors affecting identity include the tasks associated with various developmental stages, particularly adolescence, peer pressure, cultural discontinuity, and changes in the social structure. Physiological factors such as oxygen deprivation, biochemical imbalance, fatigue, isolation, sensory deprivation, and toxic drugs may also produce self-concept distortions.

9. Data collection by the nurse should include objective and observable behaviors as well as the subjective and internal world of the patient. Behaviors relative to problems with self-concept were identified and described in clinical examples.

10. The formulation of a nursing diagnosis should specify the nature of the patient's maladaptive coping response and any relevant stressors. Six problems with self-concept described in this chapter include low self-esteem, disturbed body image, role strain, negative identity, identity confusion, and depersonalization. Nursing diagnoses associated with alterations in self-concept were presented and related to the diagnostic criteria for selected medical diagnoses.

11. The goal of nursing intervention is to facilitate the person's self-actualization by helping him grow, develop, and realize his potential while compensating for his impairments. Changes in the self occur only as a result of experiences and they take place gradually. If the goals are clear, realistic, and mutually identified, they will serve to motivate the patient and help him assume increased responsibility for his own behavior.

12. Nursing intervention helps the patient examine his cognitive appraisal of the situation and his related feelings to help him gain insight, and then take action to bring about behavioral change. This problem-solving approach includes the following levels of intervention: (a) expanded self-awareness, (b) self-exploration, (c) self-evaluation, (d) realistic planning, and (e) commitment to action. it can be used with individuals, families, or groups.

13. A climate of acceptance was noted to be of particular importance in broadening the patient's concept of himself, helping him to accept all aspects of his personality, and conveying to him that he is a valued individual who is responsible for himself and able to help himself. Confirming the patient's identity is particularly important with problems of identity confusion and depersonalization.

14. The nurse and patient together evaluate the success of the nursing care in each step of the nursing process. The degree of overall success can be determined by eliciting the patient's perception of his own growth and comparing his behavior to the characteristics of the healthy personality as described in this chapter.

References

1. American Psychiatric Association: Diagnostic and statistical manual of mental disorders, ed. 3, Washington, D.C., 1980, The Association.
2. Bailyn, L.: Notes on the role of choice in the psychology of professional women. In Lifton, R., editor: The woman in America, Boston, 1967, Beacon Press.
3. Berk, S., Berk, R., and Berheide, C.: The non-division of household labor. In Fisher, A., editor: Women's worlds, NIMH Supported Research on Women, Rockville, Md., 1978, National Institute of Mental Health.
4. Biddle, B.: Role theory: expectations, identities, and behaviors, New York, 1979, Academic Press, Inc.
5. Boston Globe, March 8, 1977.
6. Broverman, I., et al.: Sex-role stereotypes and clinical judgments of mental health, J. Consult. Clin. Psychol. **24:**1, Jan. 1970.
7. Broverman, I., et al.: Sex-role stereotypes: a current appraisal, J. Soc. Issues **28:**59, Feb. 1972.
8. Bugenthal, J.: The search for existential identity, San Francisco, 1976, Jossey-Bass, Inc., Publishers.
9. Burns, D.: The perfectionist's script for self-defeat, Psychol. Today **14**(11):34, 1980.
10. Combs, A., and Snygg, D.: Individual behavior: a perceptual approach, New York, 1959, Harper & Row, Publishers, Inc.
11. Coopersmith, S.: The antecedents of self-esteem, San Francisco, 1967, W.H. Freeman & Co., Publishers.
12. Erikson, E.: The problem of ego-identity, J. Am. Psychoanal. Assoc. **4:**56, Jan. 1956.
13. Erikson, E.: Childhood and society, New York, 1963, W.W. Norton & Co., Inc.
14. Fitts, W.: The self concept and self actualization, Nashville, Tenn., 1971, Dede Wallace Center Monograph No. 3.
15. Goldberg, C., and Stanitis, M.A.: The enhancement of self-esteem through communication in group therapy, J. Psychiatr. Nurs. **15**(12):5, 1977.
16. Goode, W.: A theory of role strain, Am. Sociol. Rev. **25:**438, 1960.
17. Grove, W., and Tudor, J.: Adult sex roles and mental illness, Am. J. Sociol. **78:**812, 1973.
18. Hamachek, D.: Encounters with the self, New York, 1971, Holt, Rinehart & Winston, Inc.
19. Holahan, C., and Gilbert, L.: Interrole conflict for working women: careers versus jobs, J. Appl. Psychol. **64:**86, 1979.
20. Horney, K.: Neurosis and human growth, New York, 1950, W.W. Norton & Co., Inc.
21. Horrocks, J., and Jackson, D.: Self and role: a theory of self-process and role behavior, Boston, 1972, Houghton Mifflin Co.
22. Johnson, C., and Johnson, F.: Attitudes toward parenting in dual-career families, Am. J. Psychiatry **134:**391, 1977.
23. Jourard, S.: Personal adjustment: an approach through the study of the healthy personality, New York, 1963, Macmillan, Inc.
24. Jourard, S.: The transparent self, New York, 1971, Litton Educational Publishing, Inc.
25. Kernberg, O.: Borderline conditions and pathological narcissism, New York, 1975, Jason Aronson, Inc.
26. Kottler, J.: Promoting self-understanding in counseling: a compromise between the insight and action-oriented approaches, J. Psychiatr. Nurs. **17**(12):18, 1979.
27. Lancaster, J.: Activity groups as therapy, Am. J. Nurs. **76:**947, 1976.
28. Logan, R.: Identity diffusion and psychosocial defense mechanisms, Adolescence **13**(51):503, 1978.
29. Marcia, J.: Development and validation of ego-identity status, J. Pers. Soc. Psychol. **3:**551, 1966.
30. Maslow, A.: Motivation and personality, New York, 1954, Harper & Row, Publishers, Inc.
31. Meier, E.: An inquiry into the concepts of ego identity and identity diffusion, Soc. Casework **13:**63, Feb. 1964.
32. Meleis, A.: Role insufficiency and role supplementation: a conceptual framework, Nurs. R. **24:**264, 1975.
33. Money, J., and Ehrhardt, A.: Man & woman, boy & girl, Baltimore, 1972, Johns Hopkins University Press.
34. Norris, C.: The professional nurse and body image. In Carlson, C., editor: Behavioral concepts and nursing intervention, Philadelphia, 1970, J.B. Lippincott Co.
35. Orlofsky, J., Marcia, J., and Lesser, I.: Intimacy vs. isolation: crisis of young adulthood, J. Pers. Soc. Psychol. **27:**211, 1973.
36. Rostow, E.: Conflict and accommodation. In Lifton, R., editor: The woman in America, Boston, 1967, Beacon Press.
37. Salkin, J.: Body ego technique, Springfield, Ill., 1973, Charles C Thomas, Publisher.
38. Schwab, J., Clemmons, R., and Morder, L.: The self-concept: psychosomatic applications, Psychosomatics **7:**1, Jan.-Feb. 1966.
39. Spire, R.: Photographic self-image confrontation, Am. J. Nurs. **73:**1207, 1973.
40. Sullivan, H.S.: The interpersonal theory of psychiatry, New York, 1963, W.W. Norton & Co., Inc.
41. Weissman, M. et al.: The educated housewife: mild depression and the search for work, Am. J. Orthopsychiatry **43:**565, 1973.

Annotated suggested readings

American Psychiatric Association: Diagnostic and statistical manual of mental disorders, ed. 3, Washington, D.C., 1980, The Association.

This required reference text for all psychiatric nurses contains the categories and codes of axes I and II and the complete text and criteria related to each of the diagnostic categories associated with medically diagnosed psychiatric health problems.

Berne, E.: Games people play, New York, 1964, Grove Press, Inc.

This well-known book is divided into three sections. In Part I the theory behind transactional analysis is presented. Part II contains descriptions of various interpersonal games, and Part III explores the possibility of being game free. Berne's theory of TA has implications for problems with self-concept and is recommended reading for all nurses.

Burns, D.: The perfectionist's script for self-defeat, Psychol. Today **14**(11):34, 1980.

This article describes the price perfectionists pay in the compulsive striving toward impossible goals. A treatment approach, which uses cognitive therapy or thought reform, is also discussed.

Dellas, M., and Gaier, E.: The self and adolescent identity in women: options and implications, Adolescence **10**:399, 1975.

In light of the changing sex role standards and the reassessment of the status of women in society, the authors explore three possible female identity patterns —traditional role and stereotype, achievement and role success, and bimodal. Problems related to each are also discussed.

Ellis, A.: Humanistic psychotherapy: the rational-emotive approach, New York, 1974, McGraw-Hill Book Co.

This text introduces the idea of rational-emotive therapy (RET). It is a cognitive therapeutic approach in which Ellis works with patients to change their irrational belief systems.

Erikson, E.: Identity: youth and crisis, New York, 1968, W.W. Norton & Co., Inc.

Erikson's extensive formulations on the adolescent crisis of identity are presented in this text. His stages of the life cycle are briefly reviewed, and the pathology of identity confusion is explored through theory and case history. This is an important work on a previously unexplored developmental stage.

Glasser, W.: Reality therapy, New York, 1965, Harper & Row, Publishers, Inc.

This text introduces the reader to a therapeutic approach called reality therapy. It is based on three elements: reality, responsibility, and right and wrong. The author presents the basic formulations of his theory and applies them in specific clinical examples.

Gruendemann, B.: The impact of surgery on body-image, Nurs. Clin. North Am. **10**:635, 1975.

This article summarizes the impact of surgery on the patient's view of himself and his body. It presents aids to a nursing assessment, guides to formulating nursing goals, and methods for nursing intervention.

Hauser, M.: Cognitive commands change, J. Psychiatr. Nurs. **19**(2):19, 1981.

A nurse therapist reviews three specific techniques for working with parent-child interpersonal and behavioral problems: (1) Ellis' restructuring beliefs, (2) Meichenbaum's coping via internal speech, and (3) Gordon's problem solving. All of these are cognitive techniques that are aligned with social learning theory.

Kanfer, F., and Goldstein, A., editors: Helping people change, New York, 1975, Pergamon Press, Inc.

A number of authors contributed excellent articles that deal with such topics as cognitive change, self-management, modeling, and role play.

Kerr, N.: Pathological narcissism, Perspect. Psychiatr. Care **18**(1):29, 1980.

The author reviews the many facets of narcissism including its development, psychodynamics, and interpersonal aspects. It includes a good bibliography for further reading on the problem.

Meier, E.: An inquiry into the concepts of ego integrity and identity diffusion, Soc. Casework **13**:63, Feb. 1964.

This article is recommended for its description of the attributes and behaviors associated with ego identity. Those associated with identity diffusion as a result of the stress of cultural changes are also presented.

Meleis, A.: Role insufficiency and role supplementation: a conceptual framework, Nurs. Res. **24**:264, 1975.

This article offers a theoretical basis for the diagnosis of nursing problems related to role insufficiency. The basis for nursing intervention is role supplementation, and appropriate strategies are described. The role of the nurse is discussed, and a predictive and prescriptive paradigm is presented.

Money, J., and Ehrhardt, A.: Man & woman, boy & girl, Baltimore, 1972, Johns Hopkins University Press.

One of the authors, John Money, is a significant researcher in the field of sex behavior. This text describes how sex roles are learned, how boys become masculine and girls feminine, and what the results of the failure to learn the role are. Also included is a discussion of some of the findings in hormonal research.

Moscato, B.: Sex-role stereotyping. In Kneisl, C.R., and Wilson, H.S., editors: Current perspectives in psychiatric nursing, vol. 2, St. Louis, 1978, The C.V. Mosby Co.

Various aspects of sex-role stereotyping are presented —historical considerations, stereotypical patterns, implications for the mental health care delivery system, and behaviors evidenced by nurses. This is a highly recommended reading.

Raimy, V.: Misunderstandings of the self, San Francisco, 1975, Jossey-Bass, Inc., Publishers.

The premise of this book is that misunderstandings of the self may be major hindrances to personal and social adjustment. The author presents an approach to psychotherapy that is an application of self-concept theory and describes faulty beliefs or misconceptions as responsible for psychological disturbances. The text is easy to read and integrates sophisticated features of various psychotherapies that involve cognitive change. It is also provocative for the advanced reader.

Rogers, C.: On becoming a person, Boston, 1961, Houghton Mifflin Co.

Personal growth is the focus of this text, and Rogers discusses it from the point of view of the individual as well as the therapist in a helping relationship. The text is a compilation of important papers that are addressed to a variety of mental health disciplines. It is a highly recommended reading.

Rubin, T.: Compassion and self-hate, New York, 1975, David McKay Co., Inc.

Two opposing forces are explored in this text—compassion and self-hate. The author believes that a therapeutic relationship that reduces self-hate and enhances compassion contributes to human growth and the enhancement of inner peace. The text is written in a conversational manner but is provocative and stimulating in content.

Salkin, J.: Body ego technique, Springfield, Ill., 1973, Charles C Thomas, Publisher.

Body ego technique represents an educational and therapeutic approach to the normal development of body image and self-identity. The author gives an in-depth account of procedures, materials, and technique and describes how to use the elements of movement, rhythm, space, and force to facilitate the development of ego strength. The text is explicit and is a useful reference for interventions related to dance and body movement.

Searles, H.: Anxiety concerning change, as seen in the psychotherapy of schizophrenic patients—with particular reference to the sense of personal identity, Int. J. Psychoanal. **42:**74, Feb. 1961.

The author proposes that change for the schizophrenic patient threatens his sense of identity, which is tenuous and precarious. Developmental factors are explored, and implications for therapy are presented. It is advanced reading for the nurse therapist.

Stein, M., Vidich, A., and White, D., editors: Identity and anxiety, New York, 1960, The Free Press of Glencoe.

This book explores contemporary threats to authentic identity. Part I defines and examines identity and anxiety. Part II traces the threats to stable identity imposed by political and social upheavals. Part III explores the challenge of evolving a personal style within a mass society. This is substantial reading for the advanced student or practitioner.

Yorburg, B.: Sexual identity, New York, 1974, John Wiley & Sons, Inc.

The author draws on biology, anthropology, history, psychology, and sociology to explore the conceptions of ideal masculine and feminine behavior and emotions. Her belief is that in any particular society these learned, sex-typed role definitions and expectations result in differing basic self-images or sexual identities for men and women. The particular ramifications of the contemporary sexual identity of women are analyzed.

CHAPTER 9

DISTURBANCES
OF MOOD

Lying awake, calculating the future,
Trying to unweave, unwind, unravel
And piece together the past and the future,
Between midnight and dawn, when the
past is all deception,
The future futureless . . .

T.S. Eliot

Learning objectives

*After studying this chapter, the student
should be able to:*

- *define mood, its four adaptive functions, and the continuum of emotional responses.*

- *identify the characteristics that lead to the recognition of severe disturbances of mood.*

- *describe the concepts of grief, mourning, and the delayed grief reaction.*

- *discuss the clinical entities of depression and mania, including their prevalence and classification in DSM-III.*

- *analyze stressors affecting the grief reaction and the factors that place a person at high risk.*

- *evaluate the various theories that have been proposed on the causation of severe disturbances of mood.*

- *state the value of an integrated multicausal model of severe disturbances of mood.*

- *identify and describe behaviors that are associated with uncomplicated grief reactions, delayed grief reactions, depression, and mania.*

- *formulate individualized nursing diagnoses for patients with disturbances of mood.*

- *assess the relationship between nursing diagnoses associated with disturbances of mood and medical diagnoses of selected psychotic and neurotic disorders.*

- *develop long-term and short-term individualized nursing goals for patients who are experiencing disturbances of mood.*

285

■ *apply therapeutic nurse-patient relationship principles with appropriate rationale in planning the care of a patient who is experiencing a disturbance of mood.*

■ *describe nursing interventions appropriate to the needs of the patient who is experiencing an uncomplicated grief reaction, depression, or mania.*

■ *assess the importance of the evaluation of the nursing process when working with patients with disturbances of mood.*

■ *identify suggested readings for future study.*

Variations or fluctuations in mood are a dominant feature of human existence. They indicate that a person is perceiving his world about him and responding to it on some level. Extremes in mood have also been linked with extremes in the human experience, such as creativity, madness, despair, ecstasy, romanticism, personal charisma, and interpersonal destructiveness. These extremes in mood appear to have captured the interest, fascination, and curiosity of scientists, philosophers, and novelists alike, who romanticize, study, and exaggerate the possible alliance between mood, deep emotional experience, and talent.

In this text, *mood* refers to a prolonged emotional state that influences one's whole personality and life functioning. It pertains to one's prevailing and pervading emotion and is synonymous with the terms of affect, feeling state, and emotion. As with other aspects of the personality, emotions or moods serve an adaptive role for the individual.

The four adaptive functions of emotions have been identified as social communication, physiological arousal, subjective awareness, and psychodynamic defense.[36] The components of affective communication, such as crying, posture, facial expression, and touch, promote early mother-child attachment and the later formation of other interpersonal bonds. Depressive mood states also initiate physiological arousal involving the central nervous system, biogenic amines, and neuroendocrine systems. Theories regarding the protective function of the resulting conservation-withdrawal response with decreased activity have been postulated. The subjective components of human emotions are believed to play important functions in goal setting and in the monitoring of current behavior, particularly in judging personal reality against internalized values and goals. Finally, the fourth adaptive function of emotions is in aiding in psychodynamic defense on both the conscious and unconscious levels.

Continuum of emotional responses

The variety of emotions one can experience, such as fear, joy, anxiety, love, anger, sadness, and surprise, are all normal accompaniments of the human condition. The problem arises in trying to evaluate when a person's mood or emotional state is maladaptive, abnormal, or unhealthy. Grief, for example, is a healthy adaptive separative process that attempts to overcome the stress of a loss. Grief work, or mourning, therefore is not a pathological process. It is an adaptive response to a real stressor. The absence of grieving in the face of a loss is suggestive of maladaptation.

If one views the expression of emotions on a continuum of health and illness, some relevant parameters become apparent (Fig. 9-1). At the adaptive, or healthy, end is emotional responsiveness. This involves being affected by, and being an active participant in, one's internal and external worlds. It implies being open to one's feelings and aware of them. If used in such a way, feelings provide us with valuable learning

FIG. 9-1
Continuum of emotional responses.

experiences. They are barometers that give a person feedback about himself and his relationships with others, and they help a person function more effectively in his world. Also adaptive in the face of stress is an uncomplicated grief reaction. Such a reaction implies that the person is facing the reality of his loss and is immersed in the work of grieving.

A maladaptive response would be the suppression of emotions. This may be evident as a denial of one's feelings, a detachment from them, or an internalization of all aspects of one's affective world. Although a transient suppression of feelings may, at times, be necessary to cope, such as in an initial response to a death or tragedy, prolonged suppression of emotions, such as in delayed grief reaction, will ultimately interfere with effective functioning.

The most maladaptive emotional responses or severe mood disturbances can be recognized by their intensity, pervasiveness, persistence, and interference with usual social and physiological functioning. These characteristics apply to the severe emotional states of depression and mania, which complete the maladaptive end of the continuum of emotional responses.

Nursing intervention in disturbances of mood requires an understanding of a range of emotional states. To assist in this process, the phenomena of grief, the delayed grief reaction, depression, and mania will now be briefly described.

Grief

Grief is the subjective state that follows loss. It is one of the most powerful emotional states experienced by an individual and it affects all aspects of one's life. It forces the person to stop his normal activities and to focus on his present feelings and needs. Most commonly, it is the response to loss of a loved person through death or separation, but it also occurs following the loss of something tangible or intangible that is highly regarded. It may be a valued object, a cherished possession, an ideal, a job, or status. As a response to the loss of a loved one, grief is a universal reaction experienced by everyone at some time in life. As one's interdependence on others grows, there is an increased chance that one must face loss, separation, and death, which elicits intense feelings of grief. The capacity to form warm satisfying relationships with others also makes one vulnerable to sadness, despair, and grief when those relationships are terminated.

As a natural reaction to a life experience, grief is universal. It involves stress, pain, and suffering and an impairment of the capacity to function that can last for days, weeks, or months. The understanding of grief and its manifestations has become of great practical importance. As Noyes commented:

With research linking bereavement to increased morbidity and mortality, grief has emerged as a model of psychosocial stress to be understood in terms of its impact on physical and emotional health.[47:137]

The ability to experience grief is gradually formed in the course of normal development and is closely related to the acquisition of the capacity for developing meaningful object relationships. The process of growth and development is a series of goal attainments marked by emotional withdrawals from previous positions and reinvestment in new prospects that are thought to offer increased security. Progress is stimulated by physiological growth, which provides new abilities, strengths, and skills, as well as by encouragement and reinforcement from parents and significant others. Goals become more complex, and conflicts in life's choices create inner stress, turmoil, pressure, and unrest. Energies previously turned inward are projected to external objects. If the gratification obtained from the external object is relatively complete and fulfilling, the external object is valued as necessary to the self and is loved. If there is a change in the object, gratification ceases and readjustment is necessary. The person may withdraw within himself, feel isolated, and become preoccupied with his own person and feelings. This is a part of the grieving process. It is resolved only when the lost object is internalized, bonds of attachment are loosened, and new object relationships are established.

Grief responses may be either uncomplicated and adaptive or morbid and pathological. Uncomplicated grief runs a consistent course that is modified by the abruptness of the loss, one's preparation for the event, and the significance of the lost object. It is a self-limited process of realization, that is, it makes real the fact of the loss. Uncomplicated reactions can be considered to be the process of normal mourning or simple bereavement. Mourning includes all the psychological processes set in motion within the individual by the loss. The psychological symptom of increased preoccupation with all the detailed memories of the lost object is the work of mourning. Freud[25] described it as the painful and necessary work of readjustment to the loss. As mourning is extended over time, there is a "working through" of an affect that, if released in its full strength, would overwhelm the ego.

The mourning process begins with the introjection of the lost object. When a person grieves, his feelings are directed to the mental image he possesses of the loved one. Thus the mechanism of introjection serves as a buffering mechanism. Through reality testing, the individual realizes that the love object no longer exists, and he withdraws his emotional investment from it. This is accompanied by an internal struggle because the individual does not willingly abandon a source of personal gratification. The ultimate, productive outcome is that reality wins out, but this is accomplished slowly over time. When the mourning work is completed, the ego becomes more free and uninhibited to invest in new objects.

Although the specific reactions to grief may vary, it has to be worked out. If not, the person will continue to experience emotional conflict. Hodge has explained it as follows:

> The problem must be brought into the open and confronted, no matter how unpleasant it may be for the patient. *The grief work must be done.* There is no healthy escape from this. We might even add that the grief work *will* be done. Sooner or later, correctly or incorrectly, completely or incompletely, in a clear or a distorted manner, *it will be done.* People have a natural protective tendency to avoid the unpleasantness of the grief work, but it is necessary and the more actively it is done, the shorter will be the period of grief. If the grief work is not actively pursued, the process may be fixated or aborted or delayed, with the patient feeling that he may have escaped it. However, almost certainly a distorted form of the grief work will appear at some time in the future.[28:230]

Delayed grief reaction

A maladaptive, or pathological, response to loss implies that something has prevented it from running its normal course. Two types of pathological grief reactions have been identified by Lindemann—the delayed reaction and the distorted reaction.[42] Depression is one type of a distorted grief reaction.

Persistent absence of any emotion may signal an undue delay in the work of mourning, or a *delayed grief reaction.* The delay may occur in the beginning of the mourning process or become evident in a retarding of the process once it has begun or both. This reaction reflects the exaggerated use of the defense mechanisms of denial and suppression in an attempt to avoid the intense distress associated with grief. The delay and rejection of grief may occasionally involve many years.

The underlying emotions associated with the loss may be triggered by a deliberate recall of circumstances surrounding the loss or by a spontaneous occurrence in the patient's life. A classic example of this is the anniversary reaction in which the person experiences incomplete or abnormal mourning at the time of the loss only to have the grieving response recur at anniversaries of the original loss.

Depression

The individual who does not engage in the process of mourning can experience a pathological grief reaction known as *depression,* or melancholia. It is an abnormal extension or overelaboration of sadness and grief. Depression is the oldest and most frequently described psychiatric illness. It has been recognized and described since as early as 1500 BC, and it appears to be part of the human condition that is familiar to all and yet mysterious to many. The term "depression" is used in a variety of ways. It can refer to a sign, symptom, syndrome, emotional state, reaction, disease, or clinical entity. In this chapter it will be viewed as a clinical entity that is severe, abnormal, maladaptive, and incapacitating in nature.

The Wall Street Journal called depression the disease of the 1970s, and some mental health workers consider it to cause more total suffering and anguish in the world than any other single medical or psychiatric illness. Depression may range from mild and moderate states to severe states with psychotic features. Psychotic depression is relatively uncommon, however, accounting for less than 10% of all depressions. It is estimated that 15% to 30% of adults experience clinical depressive episodes, most often of moderate severity, at some point in their lives, with the onset of depressive illness peaking in the 40s and 50s. However, only 25% of persons with depressive symptoms seek mental health professional attention. Furthermore, 50% to 80% of all suicides are attributed to depression, and perhaps as much as 75% of all psychiatric hospitalizations.[60] There is also an almost universal trend, independent of country, of the greater prevalence of depression among women than among men in a fairly consistent female-to-male ratio of $2:1$.[69]

Research has also revealed the high incidence of depression among patients hospitalized for medical illnesses, as well as the fact that these depressions are largely unrecognized and hence untreated by health care personnel. Depression is found in all severities of medical illness, although its intensity and frequency were higher in patients who were more severely ill. Certain types of diseases are frequently associated with depression, especially gastrointestinal (35%), neurological (21%), and respiratory (20%).[60] This research suggests that depression is undoubtedly a common accompaniment of any major medical illness.

At first glance, the grieving person and the depressed person may seem indistinguishable. Both are in despair. Both are unable to be interested in the world around them. Neither can believe the pain and sadness will ever cease. Both may feel life is finished or wish it were, and for both, time is meaningless.

However, there are differences between the states of mourning and depression. Drake and Price[22] believe the difference is the quality of the individual's attachment to the loved object. The degree and nature of the attachment determines the nature of the loss phenomenon and the extent of the depressive reaction to the loss. The disruption of a "normal" attachment results in a sense of loss and grief that is resolved in simple mourning and bereavement. In contrast, disruption of an "inordinate" attachment results in a grieving process that leads into a cycle of depression, since the person is unable to cope with life and function effectively.

Freud made the following distinction between mourning and melancholia:

> The distinguishing mental features of melancholia are profoundly painful rejection, abrogation of interest in the outside world, loss of capacity to love, inhibition of all activity, and a lowering of self-regarding to a degree that finds utterances in self reproaches and culminates in a delusional expectation of punishment. . . . with one exception, the same traits are met with in grief. The fall in self-esteem is absent in grief.[25:246]

Many theorists disagree with Freud's position and believe the lowering of self-esteem and ambivalence toward the loved object are present in both reactions. A difference is acknowledged, however, in the level of regression experienced in both reactions as the depressed individual regresses more deeply and fully in response to the loss.

A final difference is apparent in the acknowledgment of the loss. The mourner attends to all things that are connected in any way with the person he mourns. Although his pain is heightened, it is not meaningless; rather, it is an acknowledgment of the loss, and positive feelings toward the lost object predominate. The depressed individual wishes to deny the loss and separation. Even though his affective responses express sorrow, he continues to deny his need to mourn or even that a need to mourn exists. Depression is, in a sense, abortive grieving. The specific defenses that are used to block the mourning process are repression, suppression, denial, and dissociation. There may even be the unconscious wish to be rewarded for suffering by the restoration of the lost object. Because this is impossible, the depressed person's hopelessness takes on an added dimension. The denial of the loss in depression results in profound feelings of guilt, anger, and despair that focus on one's own unworthiness.

Mania

In addition to the severely depressed disturbance of mood, one may also experience manic episodes. These episodes, like those of depression, can vary in intensity and accompanying level of anxiety from moderate manic states to severe and panic states with psychotic features. Basically, *mania* is characterized by a mood that is elevated, expansive, or irritable. The term, *hypomania*, is used to describe a clinical syndrome that is similar to, but not as severe as, that described by the term mania or manic episode.

In DSM-III, both manic episodes and depressive episodes are contained under the category of major affective disorders. Mania, however, is not given a separate category of classification as is depression. Rather, the major affective disorders are separated into two subgroups—major depression and bipolar disorders—based on whether or not manic and depressive episodes are involved longitudinally (Table 9-1).[4] In this classification, major depression may involve either a simple episode or a recurrent depressive illness, but without manic episodes. When there

TABLE 9-1. Classification of major affective disorders (DSM-III) relative to depressive and manic episodes

| | Major depression | | Bipolar disorders | | |
	Simple	Recurrent	Manic	Depressed	Mixed
Depressive episode	Yes	Yes	—	Yes-present	Yes-present
Manic episode	No	No	Yes-present	Yes-past	Yes-present

has been one or more manic episodes, with or without a major depressive episode, the category of bipolar disorder is used. Bipolar disorders are subdivided according to the symptoms of the current episode as manic, depressed, or mixed.

Thus if one experiences a depressive episode with no manic episodes, it would be classified as a major depression. If one experiences a depressive episode with a history of manic episodes in the past or at present, it would be classified as a bipolar disorder.

Although a bipolar affective disorder is far less common than a major depressive illness, it has been estimated that 0.4% to 1.2% of the adult population has the disorder. The onset of bipolar illness peaks below age 30, and it appears to be equally common in women as in men.

 ## Stressors

Stressors affecting the grief reaction

The individual is constantly experiencing losses and thus continually struggling with the tasks of integrating them. The intensity of a person's grief reaction only becomes meaningful when one understands his earlier losses and separations. A person who is reacting to a recent loss is behaving as he did in previous separations. The intensity of the present reaction therefore becomes more understandable when one realizes that the reaction is not only to the present loss but to earlier losses as well. Loss by definition is negative, a deprivation. But the ability to sustain, integrate, and recover from loss is a sign of personal maturity and growth.

Uncomplicated grief reactions can be considered to be the process of normal mourning or simple bereavement. Mourning includes a com-

plex sequence of psychological processes and their behavioral manifestations. It is accompanied by the subjective experiences of anxiety, anger, pain, despair, and hope. The sequence is not a smooth unvarying course, however. It is filled with turmoil, regressions, and potential problems. Certain factors have been identified that influence the outcome of the mourning process[49]:

Childhood experiences (especially the loss of significant others)
Losses experienced later in life
Previous history of psychiatric illness (especially depression)
Life crises prior to the bereavement
Nature of the relationship with the lost person or object, including kinship, strength of attachment, security of attachment, dependency-independency bonds, and intensity of ambivalence
Process of dying (when applicable), including age of deceased, timeliness, previous warnings, preparation for bereavement, expression of feelings, and preventability of the death
Social support systems
Secondary stresses
Emergent life opportunities

These should be assessed by the nurse for each person experiencing a loss. Two of the factors—the nature of the relationship with the lost person and the mourner's perception of the preventability of the death—have been identified as prime predictors of the intensity and duration of the bereavement.[17] Concurrent crises, the circumstances of the death, and a pathological relationship with the deceased are all factors that contribute to a failure to successfully resolve grief.[43]

Loss of a loved one has been identified as a major precipitating stressor for grief reactions. Most individuals resolve this loss through simple bereavement and do not experience pathological grief reactions or depression. A number of external and internal factors, however, can inhibit the process of mourning. An external factor may be the immersion of the mourner in practical, necessary tasks that accompany the loss but which are not directly connected to the emotional fact of the loss. These tasks may include funeral arrangements, completing the unfinished business of the deceased, or being forced to search for immediate employment and sources of support. All these tasks foster denial of the loss, which also may be encouraged by cultural norms that minimize or negate the finality of the loss. The American norm of "courage in the face of adversity" can prevent the mourner from any open display of grief.

Mourning may also be inhibited when the bereaved does not receive support from his social network or support systems. Nonsupportiveness that suppresses grieving can be evident when significant others inhibit the mourner's expression of sadness, anger, and guilt, block his review of the lost relationship, and attempt to orient him too quickly to the future. Finally, the widespread use of tranquilizers and antidepressant medications may serve to suppress normal grief and encourage the development of pathological grief reactions.

Internal factors that inhibit mourning are often fostered by social learning that encourages the control and hiding of feelings. Crying, for example, may be seen as a sign of weakness and something to be avoided, especially in men. Two emotions are particularly repressed and suppressed in our society—grief and anger— and this may create many emotional problems for the individual. Another inhibiting factor is the belief that the quantity and quality of emotion is so unique that it cannot be effectively communicated through verbal or nonverbal channels. Both these factors lead to suppression of the mourning process and rely heavily on the intellectual concepts of behavior.

Stressors affecting depression and mania

The existence of severe disturbances of mood, such as in depressive and manic episodes, has been accounted for by numerous theories or models of causation. These models identify a variety of stressors that may affect the individual's coping response and adjustment. Some of the theories are in conflict with each other, some are not supported by research, and certainly all of them are not applicable to each person. Rather, they present the range of causative factors that may be operative in severe disturbances of mood.

GENETIC FACTORS. The first theory addresses *genetic* aspects of depression. There is wide agreement that both heredity and environmental factors play an important role in depressive illness.[71] Genetic factors related to severe mood disturbances have been investigated in Scandinavia, Germany, Great Britain, and the United States. Four basic techniques of genetic investigation are used: (1) familial aggregation studies, comparing illness rates within and between generations of a particular family; (2) twin studies comparing illness rates in monozygotic and dizygotic twins; (3) general population surveys, comparing illness rates of relatives of depressed patients with those of the general population; and (4) linkage studies, using known genetic markers, such as blood type or color blindness.[36]

Studies using only familial aggregations do not necessarily demonstrate the role of genetics, since the resulting disturbances may be the result of nutritional, infectious, or psychological factors. However, studies using genetic markers, such as blood type or color blindness, provide more compelling evidence that bipolar affective disorder is transmitted by an X-linked dominant gene. Among patients with major depression, no genetic marker has yet been found.

Other evidence from investigations supporting genetic transmission includes an increased frequency of the illness in relatives of the patient compared with the population, a greater concordance rate for the disease in monozygotic twins than in dizygotic twins, an increased frequency of psychiatric abnormalities in relatives of the affective disorder patient than in the general population, and onset of the illness at a characteristic age without any evidence of a precipitating event. One might conclude by saying that good evidence exists for the role of a genetic factor in affective disturbances. Additional studies continue to be made in this important area of psychiatric research.

OBJECT LOSS THEORY. The *object loss* theory of depression has been advanced by Bowlby,[13,14] Robertson,[55] and Spitz,[63] and it refers to the traumatic separation of the person from significant objects of attachment. Two interrelated issues are important to this theory: loss during childhood as a predisposing factor for the occurrence of adult depressions and separation, in adult life as a precipitating stress for depression.

The first issue proposes that a child has ordinarily formed a tie to a mother figure by 6 months of age, and once that tie is ruptured, the child experiences separation anxiety, grief, and the process of mourning. Furthermore, this mourning process of the early years of life frequently affects future personality development and predisposes the child to psychiatric illness. As Bowlby states:

Unfavorable personality development is often to be attributed to one or more of the less satisfactory responses to loss having been provoked during the years of infancy and childhood in such degree, over such length of time, or with such frequency, that a disposition is established to respond to all subsequent losses in a similar way.[14:22]

Evidence for this model was reported by Spitz[63] in 1942 when he described a deprivational reaction in infants separated from their mothers in the second half of the first year of life. The reaction was characterized by apprehension, crying, withdrawal, psychomotor slowing, dejection, stupor, insomnia, anorexia, and gross retardation in growth and development. This syndrome is called anaclitic depression, and it has been questioned whether it is caused by the separation or the adverse effects of institutionalization in an orphanage. A similar separation reaction was described by Robertson and Bowlby[13] in older children. They identified three stages of response:

1. A "protest" stage in which the child appeared restless and tearful and searched for his mother
2. A "despair" stage of apathetic withdrawal
3. A "detachment" stage seen in some children who rejected their mothers on reunion

From a research point of view, the connection between early object loss and adult depression can be considered to be unproved. More recent work by Robertson[55] casts doubt on the universality of the behavioral responses he described and suggests that appropriate mothering during the separation period can prevent their occurrence. Although studies indicate that, as a group, depressive patients seem to experience more parental loss from death, separation, and other causes than do normal and other diagnostic groups, that factor alone does not seem sufficiently universal to account for all forms of depression. There is even speculation about the beneficial or immunizing effects of having successfully coped with a loss early in development.

The second issue relative to this theory views loss in adult life as a precipitating stressor for depression. The loss may be real or imagined and may include the loss of love, a person, physical functioning, status, or self-esteem. Many losses take on importance because of their symbolical meaning, which makes the reactions to them appear to be out of proportion to reality. In this sense, even an apparently pleasurable event, such as moving to a new home, may involve the loss of old friends, warm memories, and neighborhood associations. Loss of hope is another significant loss that is often overlooked. Because of the actual and symbolical elements involved in the concept of loss, the patient's perception takes on primary importance.

In concluding this discussion of the object loss theory, it is necessary to place this model in proper perspective based on research in this area. Some studies have failed to demonstrate a relationship between separation and depression.[18] Other studies support the relationship but suggest that depression may be the cause of alienation and object loss and not vice versa.[31] Thus the following conclusions may be proposed:

1. Loss and separation events are prominent among the possible precipitating stressors of depression.
2. Loss and separation are not universal in all depressions.
3. Not all people who experience loss and separation will develop depressions.
4. Loss and separation are not specific to depression but may serve as precipitating events for a wide variety of psychiatric and medical illnesses.
5. Loss and separation may result from depression.

AGGRESSION-TURNED-INWARD THEORY. The *anger-turned-inward* theory of Freud[25] views depression as the inward turning of the aggressive instinct, which for some reason is not directed at the appropriate object, with accompanying feelings of guilt. The process is initiated by the loss of an ambivalently loved object. The person feels both angry and loving toward the object at the same time, but he is unable to express his angry feelings because he may be suppressing them, think they are inappropriate or irrational, or have developed a pattern throughout life of containing feelings, especially ones he views in a negative way. He then directs his angry feelings inward and turns them toward himself. Freud believed that if one went so far as to commit suicide, the self-destructive act was a strike against the hated and loved object as well as against the self.

This theory does not lend itself to empirical verification. Even though it is one of the most widely quoted theories of depression, there is little systematic evidence to substantiate it. Some researchers have identified patients suffering from depression who outwardly express their anger and hostility. Furthermore, the redirection of hostility at outside objects has not been consistently correlated with clinical improvement. In some instances it may actually have negative effects on the patient's view of self and problem resolution. It should therefore be viewed as one possible theory of causation that is not applicable to all people experiencing disturbances of mood.

PERSONALITY ORGANIZATION THEORY. Another psychodynamic view of depression focuses on the major psychosocial variable of low self-esteem. The patient's problem of self-concept is an underlying issue, regardless of whether this is expressed as dejection and depression, or overcompensated with an air of supreme competence as displayed in manic and hypomanic episodes. Threats to self-esteem arise for the individual from poor role performance, perceived low-level everyday functioning, and the absence of a clear self-identity.[65]

Three forms of personality organization that could lead to depression have been identified by Arieti.[5] One form of depression, that based on the "dominant other," occurs because the patient has relied on an esteemed other for self-esteem. Satisfaction is experienced only through an intermediary. Clinging, passivity, manipulativeness, and avoidance of anger characterize the person with this type of depression. There is a noticeable lack of personal goals and a predominant focus on problems.

Another form results when a person realizes he may never be able to accomplish a desired, but unrealistic, goal. This is the "dominant goal" type of depression. This person is usually seclusive, arrogant, and often obsessive. He has set unrealistic goals for himself and evaluates them with an all-or-nothing standard. He spends an inordinate amount of time engaged in wishful thinking and introverted searches for meaning.

The third type of depression is manifested as a constant mode of feeling. These patients "inhibit any form of gratification because of strongly held taboos." They experience emptiness, "hypochondriasis, pettiness in interpersonal relationships, and a harsh critical attitude toward themselves and others."[5]

This view of depression looks at the patients' belief systems in relation to their experiences. Even in the absence of an apparent precipitating stressor, their depression appears to be preceded by a severe blow to their self-esteem. It emphasizes the crucial position of one's self-concept in determining adaptation or maladaptation and the importance of the patient's appraisal of his life situation.

COGNITIVE MODEL. The *cognitive* model of Beck[7,8,10] proposes that people experience symptoms of depression because their thinking is disturbed. He proposes that depression is a cognitive problem that is dominated by the patient's negative evaluation of himself, his world, and his future. This theory is in contrast to other theories that propose that the depressive affect is primary and the negative cognitive set is secondary. Beck suggests that in the course of his development certain experiences sensitize the individual and make him vulnerable to depression. He also acquires a tendency to make extreme, absolute judgments; loss is viewed as irrevocable and indifference as total rejection.

The depression-prone person, according to this theory, is likely to explain an adverse event as a personal shortcoming. For example, the deserted husband believes "She left me because I'm unlovable," instead of considering the other possible alternatives, such as personality incompatibility, the wife's own problems, or her change in feelings toward him. As he focuses on his personal deficiencies, they expand to the point where they completely dominate his self-concept. He can think of himself only in a negative way and is unable to acknowledge his other abilities, achievements, and attributes. This negative set is reinforced when he interprets ambiguous or neutral experiences as additional proof of his deficiencies. Comparisons with other people further lower his self-esteem, and thus every encounter with others becomes a negative experience. His self-criticisms increase as he views himself as deserving of blame.

Depressed patients become dominated by pessimism; they expect future adversities and experience them as though they were happening in the present or had already occurred. Their predictions tend to be overgeneralized and extreme. Since they view the future as an extension of the present, they expect their failure to continue permanently. Thus pessimism dominates their activities, wishes, and future expectations.

Beck proposes that the constellation of negative thoughts which characterize depression remains relatively dormant until a person becomes depressed. Depressed individuals are capable of logical self-evaluation when not in a depressed mood or when only mildly depressed. When depression does occur, after some precipitating life stressors, the long-dormant negative cognitive set makes its appearance. As depression develops and increases, the negative idiosyncratic thinking increasingly replaces objective thinking.

Although the onset of the depression may appear to be sudden, Beck suggests it develops over weeks as each experience is interpreted as further evidence of failure. As a result of this "tunnel vision," the individual becomes hypersensitive to experiences of loss and defeat and oblivious to experiences of success and pleasure. He has difficulty acknowledging anger, since he thinks he is responsible for, and deserving of, insults from others and problems in living. Along with low self-esteem, he experiences feelings of apathy and indifference. He is drawn to a state of inactivity and withdraws from life. He lacks all spontaneous desire and only wishes to remain passive. Because he expects failure, he lacks the ordinary mobilization of energy to make an effort to achieve.

Suicidal wishes can be viewed as an extreme expression of the desire to escape. The patient sees his life as filled with suffering with no chance of improvement. Given this negative set, suicide seems to be a rational solution. It promises to end his misery and relieve his family of a burden, and he begins to believe that everyone would be better off if he were dead. The more he considers the alternative of suicide, the more desirable it may seem, and as his life becomes more hopeless and painful, the stronger his desires become to end his life.

Naturalistic, clinical, and experimental studies have provided substantial support for this model of depression.[9] The nurse, using this theoretical model in her practice, will find it useful in understanding the personal world of the depressed person and organizing her observations regarding the depressed person's idiosyncratic logic and thinking.

LEARNED HELPLESSNESS MODEL. The *learned helplessness* model evolved from Seligman's research with dogs, from which he postulated a theory of human depression. He defines helplessness as a "belief that no one will do anything to aid you and hopelessness a belief that neither you nor anyone else can do anything."[61] His theory proposes that it is not trauma per se that produces depression, but the belief that one has no control over the important outcomes in one's life and therefore the person refrains from making adaptive responses. Learned helplessness is both a behavioral state and a personality trait of a person who believes that he has lost control over the reinforcers in his environment. These negative expectations lead to hopelessness, passivity, and an inability to assert oneself.

Seligman suggests that people resistant to depression have experienced mastery in life. Their childhood experiences proved that their actions were effective in producing gratification and removing annoyances. In contrast, those susceptible to depression have had lives devoid of mastery. Their experiences proved that they were helpless to influence their sources of suffering and gratification or they controlled too many reinforcers that did not allow for the development and use of their coping responses against failure.

Abramson, Seligman, and Teasdale[1] proposed an attributional reformulation of the learned helplessness hypothesis. According to the attributional reformulation, the kinds of causal attributions people make for lack of control influence whether or not their helplessness will entail low self-esteem and whether or not their symptoms of helplessness will generalize across situations and time. According to the reformulation, three attributional dimensions are crucial for explaining human helplessness and depression: internal-external, stable-unstable, and global-specific.

In brief, the reformulated model postulates that attributing lack of control to internal factors leads to lowered self-esteem, whereas attributing lack of control to external factors does not. Attributing lack of control to stable factors should lead to an expectation of uncontrollability in future situations and, consequently, helplessness deficits extended across time. Similarly, attributing lack of control to global factors should lead to an expectation of uncontrollability in other situations and, consequently, helplessness deficits extended across situations. Alternatively, attributing lack of control to unstable specific factors should lead to short-lived situation-specific helplessness deficits.

Abramson, Seligman, and Teasdale summarized the implications of the attributional reformulation for the helplessness model of depression:

1. Depression consists of four classes of deficits: motivational, cognitive, self-esteem, and affective.
2. When highly desired outcomes are believed improbable or highly aversive outcomes are believed probable, and the individual expects that no response in his repertoire will change their likelihood (helplessness), depression results.
3. The generality of depressive deficits will depend on the globality of the attribution for helplessness, the chronicity of the depression deficits will depend on the stability of the attribution for helplessness, and whether self-esteem is lowered will depend on the internality of the attribution for helplessness.
4. The intensity of the deficits depends on the strength, or certainty, of the expectation of uncontrollability and, in the case of the affective and self-esteem deficits, on the importance of the outcome.[1:68]

In concluding a discussion of this model, three points are worth noting. The first is that the attributional reformulation of helplessness and depression bears a significant similarity to Beck's cognitive model of depression previously described. The second point is that this model is proposed as a sufficient, but not necessary, condition for depression, which means that other physiological and psychological factors can produce the symptoms of depression in the absence of an expectation of uncontrollability. Finally, it must be emphasized that the reformulation model is still in the process of being empirically validated.

BEHAVIORAL MODEL. The behavioral model studied by Lewinsohn[41] is derived from a social learning theory framework in which the cause of depression is assumed to reside in the person-behavior-environment interaction. Social learning theory assumes that psychological functioning can best be understood in terms of continuous reciprocal interactions among personal factors, such as cognitive processes, behavioral factors, and environmental factors, all operating as interdependent determinants of one another. The relative influences exerted by these interdependent factors differ in various settings and for different behaviors.

This theory views people as being capable of exercising considerable control over their own behavior. They do not merely react to external influences. They select, organize, and transform incoming stimuli. Thus people are not viewed as powerless objects controlled by their environments, but neither are they absolutely free to do whatever they choose. Rather, people and their environment are reciprocal determinants of one another.

The concept of reinforcement is crucial to this view of depression. Reinforcement is defined in terms of the quality of one's interactions with one's environment. Person-environment interactions with positive outcomes constitute positive reinforcement. Such interactions strengthen the person's behavior. The experience of little or no rewarding interaction with the environment causes the person to feel sad or blue. Thus the key assumption in this model is that a low rate of positive reinforcement is the historical antecedent of depressive behaviors.

Two particular variables are important in this regard. One is that the individual may fail to provide the appropriate responses to initiate positive reinforcement. The other is that the environment may fail to provide the reinforcement and thus worsen the patient's condition. These variables are often apparent, since depressed patients have been shown to be deficient in the social skills needed to interact effectively with others. In turn, other people find the behavior of the depressed person to be distancing, negative, or offensive and avoid him as much as possible.

Depression is likely to occur if certain positively reinforcing events are absent; particularly those which fall into the following categories[40]:

Positive sexual experiences
Rewarding social interaction
Enjoyable outdoor activities
Solitude
Competence experiences

These may be described as "being sexually attractive," "being with friends," "being relaxed," "doing my job well," and "doing things my own way." It also occurs in the presence of certain punishing events, particularly those which fall into three categories:

Marital discord

Work hassles

Receiving negative reactions from others

This model of depression emphasizes an active, rather than passive, approach to the person and relies heavily on an interactional view of personality. Within this model, social interpersonal behavior, cognitive factors, and self-regulatory mechanisms play important roles, and treatment is aimed at assisting the person to increase the quantity and quality of positively reinforcing interactions with the environment and decrease aversive interactions.

BIOCHEMICAL MODEL. Another major area of research on depression involves a *biochemical* model, which explores chemical changes in the body that take place during depressed states. Whether these chemical changes cause depression or are a result of the depression is not yet clearly understood. However, significant abnormalities can be demonstrated in the functioning of many body systems during a depressive illness. These include electrolyte disturbances, especially of sodium and potassium; neurophysiological alterations based on findings from electrophysiological studies using electroencephalography and evoked potential methods; dysfunction and faulty regulation of autonomic nervous system activity; adrenocortical, thyroid, and gonadal changes; and neurochemical alterations in the neurotransmitters, especially in the biogenic amines, which serve as central nervous system and peripheral neurotransmitters, including norepinephrine, serotonin, dopamine, and acetylcholine.

The possibility of hormonal causes of depression was generated by the increased prevalence of depression among women as compared to men. Thus interest was stimulated in the relation of depression to female sex hormones. However, despite evidence suggesting that depression may be linked to the menstrual cycle, research has not succeeded in relating depression to any specific hormone, and the situation remains unresolved.

Disturbances in both classes of biogenic amines, the catecholamines (dopamine and noradrenaline) and the indolamines (serotonin and tryptamine), have also been hypothesized to cause affective disorders.[6] The catecholamine hypothesis states that depression is associated with a deficiency of catecholamines, particularly norepinephrine, in the central nervous system, and mania is associated with an excess of catecholamine. A consensus appears to be developing on the possible role of lowered serotonin levels in both depression and mania and elevation of catecholamines in the switch process from depression to mania.

The research in support of this hypothesis has been extensive and of high quality. The discovery of neuropharmacological abnormalities is not surprising, nor does it preclude psychological causes as well. Furthermore, a biochemical model based on one amine is undoubtedly an oversimplification.[68] According to Akiskal and McKinney, "biochemical statements that propose a causal relationship between a chemical event in the brain and a set of observable behaviors or subjective experiences present serious philosophical problems,"[3] since neurobiology has dismissed the possibility of such a direct one-to-one relationship.

Although the research in this model of depression is conflicting at times, there is sufficient evidence to suggest that a variety of precipitating stressors can induce changes in biogenic amines, and the neuropharmacological mechanisms that have been investigated might form final common pathways for both psychological and biological causes. Some depressions might be due primarily to neuropharmacological dysfunctions, resulting in reduced norepinephrine; others might be due to events whose psychological effect would presumably have parallel neurophysiological phenomena resulting in reduced release of norepinephrine. In other cases both effects might apply, the life event tipping the balance more easily into depression because activity of the norepinephrine-producing system was already reduced.

LIFE STRESSORS. Disturbances of mood are a specific response to stress. Although this statement is undoubtably true, its simplicity tends to mask the full implications of it. For example, there are two major types of stress that a person may experience. The first is the stress of major life events that are evident to others. The second type of stress may not be obvious at all to others, but it is the minor stress or irritations of daily life. These are the small disappointments, frustrations, criticisms, and arguments that, when accumulated over time, and in the absence of compensating positive events produce a major and chronic negative impact. McLean notes:

> Nondepressed persons also report high rates for these kinds of stressors, but the critical difference is that, on the average, nondepressed persons experience compensating numbers of positive events and outcomes within the same time period that effectively offset the negative impact of the routine stressors. It is the ratio between negative and positive events and outcomes that is decisive for mood determination.[45:186]

It is appropriate, therefore, to examine in more detail some of the sources of life stressors that may produce disturbances of mood. Four such sources include major life events, roles, coping resources, and physiological changes.

Major life events. Holmes and Rahe[29] did the pioneering work in this area with the development of the Social Readjustment Rating Scale described in Chapter 4. Subsequently, others have used this approach for measurement of stress concentrations experienced by people who have become depressed shortly thereafter.

Research conducted by Paykel et al.[51] on life events and depression reveals that, on the average, depressed patients reported the occurrence of nearly three times as many important life events during the 6 months before the onset of their clinical depressive episode as did normal subjects. The events included loss of self-esteem, interpersonal discord, socially undesirable occurrences, and major disruptions of life patterns. The authors found that those events perceived as undesirable were most often the precipitants of depression. He further categorized the events into "exit" events, which involved separation and interpersonal losses, and "entrance" events, which involved the introduction of a new person into the social sphere of the subject. Analysis of the data showed that exit events more frequently than entrance events were followed by worsening of psychiatric symptoms, physical health changes, impairment of social role performance, and depressive illnesses in particular. The concept of exit events in his study overlaps with the psychiatric concept of loss.

Most psychiatric clinicians are convinced that a relationship does exist between stressful life events and depression. Some believe that life events play the primary or major role in depression; others are more conservative, limiting the role of life events to that of contributing to the onset and timing of the acute episode. Any definitive conclusions, however, should be made with caution. The fact is that all people experience stressful life events, but not all people become depressed. This suggests that specific events can contribute only partially to the onset or the development of depression. Wender[70] noted that, when the incidence of a single event to account for the disease is low, as with affective disorders, the power of a single event to account for the disease is relatively limited. Thus, in an analysis of loss in relation to depression, exits from the social field occurred in 25% of depressives and 5% of controls. Exits preceded depression in only a small, although substantial, number of depressive cases. Furthermore, less than 20% of the population experiencing exits became clinically depressed. This evidence suggests that other factors must also be significant in the development of disturbances of mood.

Roles. The relationship between role strain and depression has gained popularity with the emergence of the women's movement in American society. Women have higher rates of depression, and various theories have been proposed linking depression with various aspects of women's lives. For example, Beck[11] examined learned helplessness and prejudice as possible explanations for depression in women. Very few research studies, however, have explored the relationship between role strain and depression. The most notable work in this area has been done by Ilfeld who developed nine scales to measure current social stressors defined as "those circumstances or conditions of daily social roles which are generally considered to be problematic or undesirable."[32] These scales measure ongoing stressful experiences instead of single "events" that occurred in the past. They include stressors from the social role areas of neighborhood, job, financial affairs, homemaking, parenting, marriage, singlehood, unemployment, and retirement. The survey population was divided into five subgroups to compare the relative potency of different social stressors and the differential effects of any one stressor across each population. He found that current social stressors are significantly related to depressive symptoms for each of the five groups. Table 9-2 presents a summary of the five subgroups and a ranking of the stressors for each group in order of magnitude of stress from the greatest to the least.[33] These findings indicate that current marital/singlehood stressors have the highest correlation for all groups except single employed women. Parenting, job, and financial stressors were intermediate in association. The parenting scale, however, was constructed only for parents who had a child 6 years or older. Therefore they did not assess the role strain associated with parenting children under 6 years of age. Also, homemaking was not assessed for men, only women.

It is possible to analyze each social role stressor in more detail. It becomes obvious in doing so that much of the literature focuses on women. This is a reflection of the predominance of depression among women as compared to men and the increasing interest in women's changing roles in contemporary society. Role strain associated with marriage emerges as a major stressor related to depression for both men and women. Jacob et al.[34] studied role expectation and role performance in distressed and nondistressed couples and found that nondistressed couples reported (1) greater satisfaction, pleasure, and fidelity in sexual relationships with spouses, (2) more shared activities and positive emotional interchanges, and (3) greater wife influence in various areas of family decision making. Gove[27] studied the rates of mental illness among married men and women. He found higher rates of mental illness for married women, whereas single, divorced, and widowed women have lower rates than men. From this, he concludes that being married has a protective effect for males but a detrimental effect for females.

Another explanation for differences in rates of mental illness, particularly depression, between men and women may be the role strain inherent in parenting. LeMasters[38] and Dyer[23] found an "extreme crisis reaction" to the birth of the first child in many young mothers, particularly those with extensive professional training or work experience. Cohen[20] found more pregnancy-related emotional problems in multiparas than in primiparas, commenting that it looked as though these mothers had realized that pregnancy and parenting were sources of conflict and dissatisfaction.

An interesting finding in this regard reported by Ilfeld[33] is the relatively low position of parenting as a social role stressor for employed married men and unemployed married women as compared to its primary ranking along with marriage as a social role stressor for employed married women (Table 9-2). This finding is interesting, especially since it includes only those individuals with children over 6 years of age. It suggests an interaction and possible role strain between parenting and employment for women.

Additional research also shows that married career women have, or need, supportive husbands.[52,53] The nature of this support, however, is not clearly described in the literature. Much of the literature on two-career families directly documents the additive nature of the mother's role, that is, the assumption of a career role in addition to her domestic role.[30] Ilfeld[33] did not even include homemaking as a social role for men. Division of household labor did emerge as an important aspect of Rosenfield's study.[58] She examined the relationship between depressive symptoms and traditional and nontraditional sex-role relationships in the family in terms of division of labor. In nontraditional relationships, males were found to have higher levels of depressive symptoms than females. She suggests that this gives further support to a sex-role basis

TABLE 9-2. **Summary of Ilfeld's findings on social role stressors and depression***

	Employed married fathers	Employed married mothers		Unemployed married mothers	Employed single men	Employed single women
Stressors (in degree of magnitude)	Marriage	Marriage	} equal	Marriage	Singlehood	Financial
	Job	Parental		Homemaking	Financial	Singlehood
	Financial	Financial	} equal	Parental	Neighborhood	
	Parental	Neighborhood		Financial	Job	
	Neighborhood	Job		Neighborhood		
		Homemaking				

*Data from Ilfeld, F.: Am. J. Psychiatry **134:**161, Feb. 1977.

for sex differences in depressive symptoms.

Clearly, the relationship between role strain and depression merits further exploration. Research in this area, however, must take into account the complexity of factors involved in causal or interactive relationships. Stuart has identified these as follows[64]:

1. *Predisposing factors*. Important variables include sex, marital status, income, age, education, type of occupation, social position, level of social integration, past experiences (particularly history of disturbances of mood), and a sense of mastery over one's own fate or locus of control.

2. *Role strain as a precipitating stress*. Measurements should provide for identification of roles; type of role strain experienced (role conflict, ambiguity, discontinuity, or overload); magnitude, intensity, and unpredictability of strain; degree of control over roles; duration of role strain (short term vs. habitual pattern or personality characteristic); and interaction among roles.

3. *Affective significance of role strain*. The meaning or significance of the role strain experienced should be placed within the context of the need-value system of the individual.

4. *Coping-defensive patterns available*. Focus should be placed on the individual's social support systems that might act as buffers, including family members and a community of significant others who express shared values. The marital relationship merits particular emphasis through examining the supportiveness of the spouse, ways in which this support is expressed, power relationships within the marriage, and levels of marital satisfaction and intimacy.

5. *Illness outcome*. In addition to depressive symptoms, one might assess the length and intensity of disability, areas of impaired functioning, and long-term consequences of the depression (i.e., role strain that induces depression might serve to legitimize future role failure).

6. *Adaptive outcome*. Research in this area would assess specific coping strategies used by individuals to handle role strain, including division and delegation of responsibilities, changing expectations, clarifying goals, and use of social resources. Research of this nature would have direct implications for planning and implementing preventive and therapeutic interventions in the future.

Coping resources. Life stress may also take the form of inadequate coping resources. Personal resources available to individuals include their socioeconomic status (income, occupation, social position, and education), families (nuclear and extended), interpersonal networks, and the secondary organizations provided by the broader social environment. The far-ranging effects of poverty, discrimination, inadequate housing, and social isolation cannot be ignored or taken lightly. The results of three studies are relevant in this regard.

In the first study Myers, Lindenthal, and Pepper[46] report that the level of social integration is associated with the relationship between life events and psychiatric symptoms and changes in that relationship over 2 years. In particular, those who report few life events but significant symptoms are less well integrated than those who report few symptoms but many events. Three particular deficiencies in social networks or support systems serve to increase the individual's vulnerability to stress—social isolation, social marginality, and status inconsistency.

The second study, which takes into consideration these issues, was reported by Brown and Harris.[15] Using data collected from a community survey in London, they examined the relationship between psychosocial stress and subsequent affective disorders among women. They found that working-class married women with young children at home had the highest rates of depression. They were five times more likely to become depressed than middle-class women given equal levels of stress. Four factors were found to be significant in this regard: loss of a mother in childhood, three or more children under age 14 living at home, absence of an intimate and confiding relationship with a husband or boyfriend, and lack of full- or part-time employment outside the home. The first three factors were more frequent among working-class women. Confidants other than a spouse or boyfriend did not have a protective effect. Rather, an important factor in preventing depression in the presence of stress was the amount of emotional support the husband or boyfriend gave the woman and the general levels of satisfaction and intimacy inherent in the relationship. Employment outside the home was seen to provide a protective effect by alleviating boredom, increasing self-esteem, improving financial affairs, and increasing social contacts. This is the type of research needed to answer etiological questions regarding life stress and illness.

A final and most important study was conducted by Warheit[67] on the relationship between life-event losses, coping resources, and depressive symptoms. The major findings of the research can be summarized as follows:

1. Persons having high life-event loss scores had higher depression scores than those with low to moderate loss scores.

2. The presence of a spouse was significantly correlated with lower depression scores for all groups. The presence of relatives nearby was not significant. The availability of friends was significantly correlated with lower depression scores for the high-loss group.

3. Low socioeconomic status (SES) was significantly correlated with higher depression scores. It was also found that 64.8% of those in the low SES group were in the high-loss group, compared with 31.1% of those in the high SES group. The data suggest that low SES places persons in double jeopardy; they have fewer resources with which to cope and experience more losses.

4. A series of regression equations showed that losses, absence of resources, and preexisting depressive symptoms were powerful predictors of depression scores. Of these variables, the most powerful predictor was preexisting depressive symptoms, followed by absence of resources (including personal, familial, social, cultural, and socioeconomic status). Life-event loss scores had the lowest predictive value.

The author concludes that these data illustrate the complex nature of the interrelationships between life events, coping resources, and depressive symptoms:

> The findings suggest that while life-event losses and the absence of personal and social resources are related to high depression scale scores, other factors are statistically (and probably theoretically) more important sources of explanation of depressive symptomatology. The findings also suggest that for some persons, at least, depressive symptomatology is a trait condition that may predispose them to life events which in turn exacerbate their preevent levels of psychiatric distress. The data also indicate that life-event losses are mitigated somewhat by the availability of personal, familial, interpersonal, and other resources; this finding has implications for early therapeutic intervention designed to assist those experiencing significant life-event losses.[67:507]

Physiological changes. Disturbances in mood may also occur as a response to physiological changes produced by drugs or a wide variety of physical illnesses. Drug-induced depressions have been noted to occur following treatment with various antihypertensive drugs and the abuse of addictive substances, such as amphetamines and barbiturates.

Depression may also occur secondary to a wide variety of medical illnesses, for example, viral infections, nutritional deficiencies, endocrine disorders, anemias, and central nervous system disorders, such as multiple sclerosis, tumors, and cerebral vascular disease. The depressions of the elderly are particularly complex because the differential diagnosis often involves organic brain damage and clinical depression. The diagnostic differentiation is complicated by the fact that persons with early signs of senile brain changes, vascular disease, or other neurological diseases associated with age may be more at risk for depression than is the general population. In the United States there has been a tendency to overdiagnose arteriosclerosis and senility in persons over 65, without recognizing that depression may manifest itself by a slowing of psychomotor activity, a reduction of intellectual functioning, a decrease in concentrating ability, and a loss of interest in sex, hobbies, and activities, changes that may be taken as signs of brain damage.[36]

Mania has also been found to occur secondary to drugs, infections, neoplasms, epilepsy, and metabolic disturbances. The evidence that mania can result from a variety of pharmacological, structural, and metabolic disturbances suggests that mania, like depression, is a clinical syndrome with multiple causes. The diversity of causes probably involves more than one pathophysiological pathway and challenges any unitary model of causation, whether the proposed factor of causation be biochemical, psychological, genetic, or structural.

INTEGRATIVE MODEL. There is continuing debate throughout psychiatry over the nature of depression—that is, whether depression is a single illness with different signs and symptoms or whether there are several different diseases. This discussion of the various models or theories of causation of severe mood disturbances also suggests the controversies in psychiatric research and practice. Each of these theories contributes to an understanding of mood disturbances. It is obvious that many of them overlap and interrelate. It is also clear from recent research that there are multiple causes for mood disturbances involving an interactive effect among predisposing and precipitating factors that are biological and psychosocial in ori-

TABLE 9-3. Summary of models of causation of severe mood disturbances

Model	Mechanism
Genetic	Transmission through heredity and family history
Object loss	Separation from loved one and disruption of attachment bond
Aggression turned inward	Turning of angry feelings inward against oneself
Personality organization	Negative self-concept and low self-esteem influence one's belief system and appraisal of stressors
Cognitive	Hopelessness experienced because of negative cognitive set
Learned helplessness	Belief that one's responses are ineffectual, and reinforcers in the environment cannot be controlled
Behavioral	Loss of positive reinforcement in life
Biochemical	Impaired monoaminergic neurotransmission
Life stressors	Response to life stress from four possible sources: major life events, roles, coping resources, and physiological changes
Integrated	Interaction of chemical, experiential, and behavioral variables acting on the diencephalon

gin. Thus a unitary theory is not possible, but perhaps a unified theory is. Table 9-3 summarizes these major theories on causation.

Akiskal and McKinney[2,3] have presented a unified model of depression that attempts to integrate the various conceptual models which now exist. They view depression as the feedback interaction of three sets of variables at the chemical, experiential, and behavioral levels, with the diencephalon serving as the field of action. They propose that impairment in one of the variables affects the other two. Thus any one of the three variables can contribute to a depression and produce changes in the other two areas. For example, a chemical imbalance can result in distorted perceptions, or a major life change can cause a chemical imbalance. In their model, depressive illness is the culmination of various processes that converge in those areas of the di-

encephalon which modulate arousal, mood, motivation, and psychomotor functions. The specific form the illness will take depends on the interaction of the following factors:

1. Genetic vulnerability—important particularly in recurrent and manic-depressive illnesses
2. Developmental events—early object loss that may sensitize the individual to future stress, create negative cognitive sets, and originate experiences resulting in learned helplessness
3. Physiological stressors—stimuli such as viral infections and childbirth that induce physiochemical changes
4. Psychosocial stressors—stressful life events that overwhelm the coping mechanisms of the individual

This integrative multicausal model presents a useful frame of reference for the nurse because it is holistic in nature and encourages the assessment of behavior in developing appropriate nursing interventions. It also presents a variety of causative factors and stresses the interrelationship of them in explaining present behavior. Obviously predisposing factors are important, and the way in which they interact with the precipitating event is crucial in determining whether a severe mood disturbance will result. Such an integrated model is most valuable for the nurse to utilize when completing a patient assessment and implementing nursing care.

 Data collection

Behaviors associated with uncomplicated grief reactions

The successful resolution of uncomplicated grief reactions follows, to some degree, a sequence of phases or steps by which the nurse can determine if healing is occurring. Knowledge of behaviors associated with the normal process of mourning allows the nurse to provide supportive interventions, as well as identify maladaptive responses, if they should occur. Various theorists have identified stages of grief and mourning, including Bowlby,[14] Kübler-Ross,[37] and Engel,[24] and there are many similarities among these stages.

A cross-cultural study of grief and mourning in 78 cultures indicated that the mourning process and the accompanying state of grief represent a universal human response.[57] The specific form of emotional expression varies from culture to culture, but an emotionless reaction to the loss of a loved person is rare. Bowlby's phases present a comprehensive review of the process of mourning and they can be applied to losses of any type. These phases of mourning are (1) the urge to recover the lost object, (2) disorganization, and (3) reorganization. Each phase will be briefly described with the emotional component of mourning that accompanies it.

Phase 1 is characterized by disequilibrium. Initially the survivor experiences feelings of shock and disbelief. This reaction is followed by a numbed sensation in which the survivor does not acknowledge the reality of the death and hopes to recover his loss. Two of the major affective components of this phase are weeping and anger. Tears are evoked by loss, and crying fulfills an important function in the work of mourning. Crying involves both an acknowledgment of the loss and a regression to a more childlike state. Tears among the survivors are generally accepted, and they elicit certain kinds of support and help from the group, although this varies greatly from culture to culture.

Anger is the other major component of this stage. It may erupt toward nurses or other health care personnel whom the survivor associates with the death. The mourner may also turn this anger on himself, particularly if he feels the death was his responsibility in any way. Guilt is a related emotion as the survivor berates himself for failing to do right by the lost one. The greater the survivor's ambivalence toward the deceased, the greater will be his sense of guilt.

Phase 2 is characterized by disorganization. When the survivor realizes the loss is permanent, despair sets in and his behavior becomes increasingly disorganized and restless. He experiences a loss of self-esteem, and profound feelings of loneliness, fear, and helplessness overwhelm him. This phase is a painful and alarming one for the individual, and he might use the mechanism of denial to protect himself. Symptoms of somatic stress might appear. Lindemann[42] identified the most common ones: (1) the tendency to sighing respirations, (2) the complaint of lack of strength and exhaustion, and (3) the occurrence of digestive difficulties, such as loss of appetite and feeling of emptiness in the stomach. There may be the reactivation of old conflicts such as dependence vs. independence and trust vs. mistrust.

The sensorium is generally altered, and there is a slight feeling of unreality, emotional distance from others, and a preoccupation with the image of the deceased. There may be a recurrent experience of tearful longing for the deceased associated with thoughts, memories, or mental images of him. They may be triggered by any reminder of the lost one and may be especially intense and painful at night. Many survivors have illusions of seeing or feeling the presence of the dead person. In extreme cases this experience takes the form of frank but transient hallucinations. There may be much random activity but an inability to organize and complete specific tasks. Life is devoid of enthusiasm and daily activities proceed in an automatic manner. Social interaction is greatly reduced, and feelings of helplessness may complicate the process of mourning in two ways: there is a sense of powerlessness over restoring the lost person and a helplessness in the face of continuing life without the companionship of the deceased.

Phase 3 is one of reorganization. The survivor no longer lives in the past and begins to break his attachment to the lost person. He establishes new goals and interpersonal relationships. He may incorporate the values, behaviors, and goals of the deceased in an appropriate and satisfying way. He tests out new behavior and expands his own sense of identity.

The successful work of mourning takes 6 months to a year, with the intensity of the initial reaction subsiding after a couple of weeks. Like any other process, it can take one of several courses. Those which enable the individual ultimately to relate to new objects and to find satisfaction in them are commonly judged to be adaptive, or healthy. Those which fail in this outcome are believed to be maladaptive, or pathological.

In recent years attention has been focused on the development of somatic illness and increased mortality as a consequence of the death of or separation from a loved object. The loss of a loved person has been identified as a precipitating factor in the onset or the identification of such diverse diseases as asthma, pulmonary tuberculosis, peptic ulcer, ulcerative colitis, diabetes, coronary occlusion, myocardial infarction, cardiac failure, thyrotoxicosis, pernicious anemia, leukemia, and multiple sclerosis.[48]

Psychiatric illness can also be a sequel to loss. Parkes,[50] in an investigation of the relationship between bereavement and mental illness, found that 2.9% of 3245 admissions to psychiatric hospitals took place within 6 months of the death of a close relative. The frequency of admission after the death of a spouse was six times greater than would be expected by chance alone. Although the bereaved patients proved to have a variety of psychiatric illnesses, the most common diagnosis was depression. Although the evidence relating object loss to somatic symptom formation does not prove a cause-and-effect relationship, it strongly suggests that grief related to object loss may contribute to a number of diverse somatic reactions.

Behaviors associated with delayed grief reactions

The designation of grief as pathological indicates that something has prevented it from running its normal course. The defenses that were used successfully in the uncomplicated grief reaction become exaggerated or maladaptive in the pathological reaction. The result may be a delayed grief reaction or a distorted reaction, such as in depression or mania. Delayed grief reactions may be indicated by excessive hostility and grief, prolonged feelings of emptiness and numbness, an inability to weep or express emotions, low self-esteem, use of the present tense instead of the past when speaking of the loss, persistent dreams about the loss, retention of the clothing of the deceased, an inability to visit the grave of the deceased, and the projection of living memories into an object that is held in place of the lost one. Clinical example 9-1 illustrates some of the behaviors associated with a delayed grief reaction.

CLINICAL EXAMPLE 9-1

Mrs. G was a 38-year-old married woman who had no history of previous depression. She came to the local community mental health center complaining of "severe throbbing headaches, difficulty falling asleep, fitful and disturbing dreams when asleep, and poor appetite." She said she felt "disgusted" with herself and "useless" to her family. At present she was living alone with her husband.

Her family history revealed that she had three children—two boys and a girl. Her eldest son, age 20, was attending college out of state, and her daughter, 19 years of age, was living with a girl friend in an apartment in the same city. Her youngest son was killed in an automobile accident 2 years ago when he was 15 years old. She described him as her "baby" and expressed much guilt for contributing to her son's death. She scolded herself for allowing him to drive to the shore for the weekend with friends, and said she now worries a great deal about her other two children. She said she was trying to protect them from the dangers of the world, but they resented her advice and concern. On questioning by the nurse, Mrs. G reported that these feelings of sadness and guilt had emerged in the last month and seemed to be triggered by the graduation of her son's high school class.

In this example Mrs. G was experiencing a delayed grief reaction that was precipitated by the emotionally invested event of her deceased son's would-be graduation. She had failed to progress through the process of mourning at the time of her son's death and was beginning to engage in the "grief work" at the present time. The behaviors she displayed were consistent with the state of depression she was experiencing.

Because feelings of sadness, disappointment, and frustration are normal accompaniments of human life, the boundary between normal and abnormal mood is often difficult to define. Basically, behaviors associated with severe mood disturbances or affective disorders reflect an increase in the intensity or the duration of otherwise normal emotions. They may range from behaviors associated with moderate anxiety (and indicative of neurotic health problems) to those associated with panic levels of anxiety (and indicative of psychotic health problems). In severe forms, disturbances of mood can be recognized as being maladaptive because of their intensity, pervasiveness, persistence, and interference with effective daily functioning. This may be reflected in impaired body functioning; the inability to perform expected social roles, such as at work, in the family, or at school; suicidal thoughts; and interference with reality testing, such as delusions, hallucinations, or confusion.

Behaviors associated with depression

The behaviors associated with depression are varied. Sadness and slowness may predominate, or there may be states of agitation. The key element to a behavioral assessment is change—the individual changes his usual behavioral patterns and responses. Research indicates that the individual working through the normal mourning process responds to his loss with a set of psychological symptoms that are often indistin-

TABLE 9-4. Behaviors associated with depression

Affective	Physiological	Cognitive	Behavioral
Anger	Abdominal pain	Ambivalence	Aggressiveness
Anxiety	Anorexia	Confusion	Agitation
Apathy	Backache	Inability to concentrate	Alcoholism
Bitterness	Chest pain	Indecisiveness	Altered activity level
Denial of feelings	Constipation	Loss of interest and motivation	Drug addiction
Despondency	Dizziness	Self-blame	Intolerance
Dejection	Fatigue	Self-depreciation	Irritability
Guilt	Headache	Self-destructive thoughts	Lack of spontaneity
Helplessness	Impotence	Pessimism	Overdependency
Hopelessness	Indigestion	Uncertainty	Poor personal hygiene
Loneliness	Insomnia		Psychomotor retardation
Low self-esteem	Lassitude		Social isolation
Sadness	Menstrual changes		Tearfulness
Sense of personal worthlessness	Nausea		Underachievement
	Overeating		Withdrawal
	Sexual nonresponsiveness		
	Sleep disturbances		
	Vomiting		
	Weight change		

guishable from depression but are accepted by him and by his environment as normal. In contrast, patients with depression experience their condition as a "change" unlike their usual self, which often leads them to seek help.[19]

A number of behaviors are associated with states of depression. These may be divided into affective, physiological, cognitive, and behavioral manifestations (Table 9-4). Obviously, some of these behaviors are contradictory and incompatible. The lists are intended to describe the spectrum of possible behaviors, acknowledging that not all individuals experience all of them.

The most common and central behavior is that of the depressive mood. This is not necessarily described by the patient as "depression" but as feeling sad, blue, down in the dumps, unhappy, or unable to enjoy life. Crying commonly occurs. On the other hand, some depressed persons do not cry, and describe themselves as "beyond tears." The mood disturbance of the depressed patient resembles that of normal unhappiness multiplied in intensity and pervasiveness. Another mood that often accompanies depression is anxiety—a sense of fear and intense worry. Both depression and anxiety may show diurnal variation, that is, a pattern of change whereby certain times of the day, such as morning or evening, are consistently worse or better.

In the literature there is a lack of agreement on which behaviors typically reflect depression and which are most significant for assessment, treatment, and prognosis. Neither are the identified behaviors exclusive to depression; they may also appear in other kinds of health problems. Levitt and Lubin[39] reviewed the literature and listed the symptoms of depression cited in at least 2 of 13 selected sources published between 1961 and 1969. They also reviewed the symptoms of depression appearing in at least 2 of 16 depression measurement instruments. Of the 24 self-rating measures of depression, the following four are most commonly used: the Minnesota Multiphasic Personality Inventory (MMPI) depression scale, the Beck Depression Inventory, the Zung Self-Rating Depression Scale, and the Depression Adjective Checklist. Beck[7] provided further data by reviewing the proportions of depressed patients manifesting various symptoms. Table 9-5 selectively summarizes the findings of Levitt and Lubin and Beck. Using patient reporting as the criterion reference (Beck's data on severely depressed patients), the cardinal symptoms of a depressive syndrome, as defined by their presence in at least 75% of cases, include feelings of inadequacy and helplessness, loss of motivation, psychomotor retardation, indecisiveness, crying spells, loss of interest and enjoyment, fatigability, sleep disturbance, pessimism, dejected mood, and self-devaluation.

TABLE 9-5. **Symptoms of depression and their prevalence**

Symptom	Sources using symptom[39] (%)	Measurement instruments monitoring symptom[39] (%)	Severely depressed patients showing symptom[8] (%)
Self-devaluation	54	100	81
Dejected mood	92	87	88
Suicidal thoughts	100	81	74
Pessimism, feelings of hopelessness	77	81	87
Loss of appetite	77	75	72
Sleep disturbance	77	75	87
Loss of libido	84	44	61
Fatigability	46	81	78
Loss of interest, enjoyment	46	62	92
Guilt feelings	70	62	60
Social withdrawal	38	69	64
Crying spells	38	44	83
Indecisiveness	30	50	76
Constipation	30	44	52
Psychomotor retardation	30	81	87
Loss of motivation	46	62	86
Diurnal mood variation	40	20	37
Feelings of inadequacy, helplessness	30	20	90

Finally, the potential for suicide should always be assessed in severe mood disturbances. Suicide and other self-destructive behaviors are discussed in detail in Chapter 10. The intensity of the feelings of anger, guilt, and worthlessness may precipitate suicidal thoughts, feelings, or gestures, as illustrated in Clinical example 9-2.

CLINICAL EXAMPLE 9-2

Mr. W was a 60-year-old man who lived alone. His son and daughter were married and lived in the same state. His wife died 2 years ago, and since that time his children had often asked him to move in with either of them. He had consistently refused to do this, believing that both he and his children needed privacy in their lives. Six months ago he was diagnosed as having advanced prostatic cancer with metastasis. After the diagnosis was made and because of increasing disability, he left his job and began to receive disability compensation. He visited his children and their families on the average of twice a month and kept his regularly scheduled visits with the medical clinic. The nurses and physicians at the clinic noted he was "despondent and withdrawn" but viewed this as a normal reaction to his diagnosis and family history. No interventions were implemented based on his emotional needs. A week after attending the clinic for a routine, follow-up visit, he went to the cemetery where his wife was buried and at her gravestone shot himself in the head. A grounds keeper of the cemetery heard the shot, discovered what had happened, and called an ambulance. Mr. W was taken to the emergency room of the nearest hospital and, with prompt medical care, survived the suicide attempt.

This example dramatically emphasizes three important points. First, the experience of a medical illness frequently involves a loss of some type for the individual—loss of function, body part, or appearance. Therefore all patients should be assessed for the presence of depression. Second, all people experiencing states of depression and despair have the potential for suicide. Third, nurses can intervene in a variety of ways to support the grieving and mourning process whether it is of an uncomplicated or pathological nature. Nursing actions can be preventive, curative, or rehabilitative, based on the nursing assessment and diagnosis.

Behaviors associated with mania

Mania and hypomania occur more rarely than depressive states. Some believe that mania is a mirror image of depression and that even though the behaviors are dissimilar, the dynamics are related. According to this view manic behavior is a defense against depression as the individual attempts to deny his feelings of worthlessness and helplessness. His elation and hyperactivity are an appeal for love and a protection from depression.

The essential feature of mania is a distinct period of intense psychophysiological activation. Some of the behaviors associated with it are given in Table 9-6. In this state the predominant mood is either elevated or irritable accompanied by one or more of the following symptoms: hyperactivity, the undertaking of too many activities, lack of judgment of the consequences of actions, pressure of speech, flight of ideas, distractibility, inflated self-esteem, and hypersexuality.

If the mood is elevated or euphoric, it is often infectious in nature. Patients report feeling happy, unconcerned, carefree, and devoid of problems. Although such experiences would seem enviable, these affects are exhibited without any concern for reality or the feelings of others. Mood is often expansive, and some patients have extraordinary delusional notions about their power and importance. They characteristically involve themselves in various seemingly senseless and risky enterprises.

Alternately, the mood may be irritable, especially when the patient's plans are thwarted. In such a case they can be contentious and readily provoked by seemingly harmless remarks. Self-esteem is inflated during a manic episode, and, as the activity level increases, the feelings about the self become increasingly disturbed. Delusional grandiose symptoms are in evidence, and the patient is willing to undertake any project possible.

In contrast to depressed patients, manic patients are extremely self-confident, with an ego that knows no bounds; they are "on top of the world." Accompanying this magical omnipotence and supreme self-esteem is an equally inordinate lack of guilt and shame. Often there is a denial of realistic danger. The patient's boundless energy, cunning, planning, schem-

TABLE 9-6. Behaviors associated with mania

Affective	Physiological	Cognitive	Behavioral
Elation or euphoria	Dehydration	Ambitious	Aggressive
Expansive	Inadequate nutrition	Denial of realistic danger	Excessive spending of money
Humorous	Needs little sleep	Distractibility	Grandoise acts
Inflated self-esteem	Weight loss	Flight of ideas	Hyperactivity
Intolerable of criticism		Grandiosity	Increased motor activity
Lack of shame or guilt		Illusions	Irresponsible
		Lack of judgment	Irritable or argumentative
		Loose associations	Poor personal grooming
			Provocative
			Sexually overactive
			Socially active
			Verbose

ing, and inability to forecast resulting consequences frequently lead to irresponsible enterprises and excessive spending, as well as to misdemeanors of a sexual, aggressive, or possessive nature. In contrast to the depressed state, patients in the manic state have heightened libidinal drives, with abounding energy and a heightened sexual appetite. Characteristic physical changes can be related to the basic affect: inadequate nutrition, partly because manic patients have no time to eat, and serious loss of weight in conjunction with their insomnia and overactivity. In severe cases, there may be dehydration, which requires prompt attention.

In addition to mood disturbance, speech is often disturbed. As the mania gets more intense, formal and logical speech is displaced, and speech becomes loud, rapid, and difficult to interpret. As the activated state increases, speech becomes full of plays on words and irrelevancies that can increase to loosened associations and flight of ideas. Some of these behaviors are evident in Clinical example 9-3.

CLINICAL EXAMPLE 9-3

Mr. B was a 30-year-old single man who was admitted to the psychiatric unit of the local community hospital. He had been hospitalized 2 years ago for problems related to alcoholism. He was accompanied to the hospital by a friend who lived with him. His friend said that for the past 2 months Mr. B had been "running on ten cylinders instead of four." He slept and ate little and talked constantly, sometimes so fast that no one could understand what he was trying to say. He had redecorated his bedroom in the apartment twice and had gone into debt buying a new "mod" wardrobe. His friend brought him in because his behavior was becoming more erotic and his physical condition was failing.

The nurse who admitted Mr. B asked about his social relationships. He revealed that his girl friend of 7 years had left him 6 months ago for another man. He said that initially he thought she would "see the light," but she had refused to see him since then. Mr. B said this "upset" him a little at the time, but he was sure it was "for the best and there were plenty other women out there just waiting for him."

Associated behaviors found in mania include lability of mood with rapid shifts to brief depression. Such behavior accounts for those patients who have loosened associations and alternately laugh and cry. In addition, hallucinations of any type, ideas of reference, and frank delusions may be present with predominant feelings of guilt and thoughts of suicide. Manic episodes have a high tendency toward recurrence, only about 25% of manic patients have only one episode, and almost all individuals with manic episodes also have depressive episodes. However, there is variation in the duration and severity of the manic episode and in the intervals between relapses and recurrences.

All of these clinical examples illustrate the interrelatedness of disturbances of mood with the problem of self-esteem and disrupted interpersonal relationships. Because of the intensity of the reaction, multiple aspects of the individual's life are affected. This may also include his physical health, as reflected in the lists of physiological behaviors. Another effect on physical functioning is the possible onset of psychosomatic illness. Hypertensive crises, irritable bowel syndromes, coronary occlusions, rheumatoid arthritis, migraine headaches, and various dermatological conditions can occur in conjunction with severe mood disturbances.

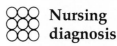 **Nursing
diagnosis**

The diagnosis of disturbances of mood depends on an understanding of many interrelated concepts, including anxiety, self-concept, and hostility. One task of the nurse in formulating a diagnosis is to decide if the patient is experiencing primarily a state of anxiety or depression. It is often difficult to distinguish between them because they may coexist in one patient and present similar behaviors. Crary and Crary[21] suggest some comparative observations that may be helpful to the nurse. They note that the depressed patient is often slowed down in speech and movements, whereas the anxious patient often responds normally or more actively. The depressed patient is reluctant to discuss his problems or symptoms, while the anxious patient is more likely to discuss his symptoms and related topics. The depressed patient has decreased his outside interests, whereas the anxious patient usually retains interest in some things. The depressed patient has difficulty enjoying things, but the anxious patient can enjoy some activities. The depressed patient usually feels worse in the morning or after sleep, whereas the anxious patient usually feels worse in the evening and better after sleep or rest; and the depressed patient usually has a decreased appe-

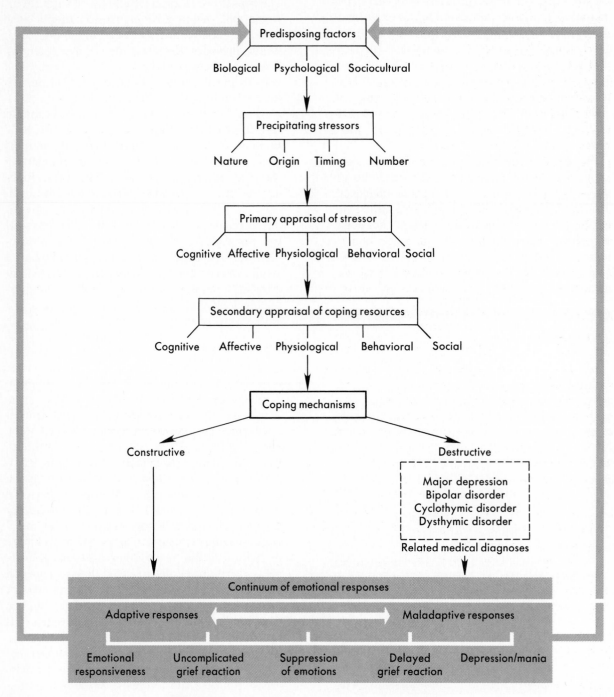

FIG. 9-2
Model of health-illness phenomena with continuum
of emotional responses.

tite and enjoyment of food, while the anxious patient usually eats intermittently and generally enjoys at least some foods.

An appropriate nursing diagnosis should include the patient's maladaptive coping response and related stressor. Fig. 9-2 presents the model of health-illness phenomena with the continuum of emotional responses. The maladaptive responses are a result of feelings of anxiety, hostility, self-devaluation, and guilt. This model suggests that nursing care will be centered around increasing self-esteem and encouraging the appropriate expression of emotions.

The model also identifies some medical diagnoses that are appropriate to disturbances of mood or affective disorders. The psychiatric classification of affective disorders has reflected, to a large extent, the controversies surrounding the nature, cause, and treatment of these disorders. Although these traditional labels are no longer used in the revised DSM-III, nurses should be familiar with them because they may continue to have some research and clinical value.

One traditional distinction has been to separate patients into psychotic vs. neurotic affective states. Unfortunately these terms have acquired multiple meanings and have lost their precision in defining clinical or research practice. Another traditional distinction has been between endogenous vs. reactive, or exogenous, types of depression. Endogenous depressions were believed to have resulted from early personality development and intrinsic biological processes, whereas exogenous, or reactive, types were believed to have occurred in response to external environmental stress, such as recent loss or disappointment. Research, however, has failed to verify the existence of these traditional distinctions. Thus the psychotic-neurotic distinction and the endogenous-reactive dichotomy are better regarded as continuums along which patients may be placed. Most patients are intermediate on the continuum and few are at the extremes. Neither classification is used in DSM-III.

Another classification system developed by Robins and Guze[56] avoids the controversial endogenous-reactive and psychotic-neurotic dichotomies. They propose a distinction between primary and secondary affective disorders based on two criteria, chronology and the presence of associated illnesses. "Primary" affective disorders are the disorders in patients who have been well or whose only previous episodes of psychiatric disease were mania or depression. "Secondary" affective disorders include feelings of sadness, inadequacy, and hopelessness that occur with another preexisting psychiatric disorder, such as anxiety reactions. It also includes symptoms secondary to medical illnesses.

A final distinction is the bipolar-unipolar one. It proposes the separation of depressed patients with a history of manic episodes (the bipolar group) from those patients who have had only recurrent episodes of depression (the unipolar group). Among the newer approaches, the bipolar-unipolar distinction has achieved considerable rapid acceptance. DSM-III accepts the evidence pointing to the importance of the distinction between unipolar and bipolar forms of affective disorder.

DSM-III distinguishes three categories of "primary" affective disorders or disturbances of mood not due to any other physical or mental disorder[4]:

1. Major affective disorders
2. Other specific affective disorders
3. Atypical affective disorders

Major affective disorders include the subcategories of bipolar disorder and major depression. These are distinguished by whether or not there has ever been a manic episode. When there has been one or more manic episodes, with or without a history of depression, the category of bipolar disorder is used. Bipolar disorder is subclassified as mixed, manic, or depressed. Major depression is subclassified as single episode or recurrent and with or without psychotic features and the presence of melancholia.

Other specific affective disorders include cyclothymic disorder and dysthymic disorder. In cyclothymic disorder there are symptoms characteristic of both the manic and depressive states but not of sufficient severity and duration to meet the criteria for a major affective disorder. In dysthymic disorder the symptoms are not of sufficient severity and duration to meet the criteria for a major affective disorder, and there have been no manic periods. Atypical affective disorders are a residual category for individuals who do not meet the criteria for the other two major categories.

Based on this discussion of dynamics, criteria, and diagnostic categorization, it is now possible to present some nursing diagnoses related to disturbances in mood. In Table 9-7, selected nursing diagnoses are related to appropriate medical

TABLE 9-7. **Comparative examples of nursing diagnoses and medical diagnoses associated with disturbances in mood**

Nursing diagnoses	Medical diagnoses (as described in DSM-III)*
Simple bereavement related to death of mother	No mental disorder—UNCOMPLICATED BEREAVEMENT
Depression related to hyperthyroidism	**Diagnostic criteria for ORGANIC AFFECTIVE SYNDROME** A. The predominant disturbance is a disturbance in mood, with at least two of the associated symptoms listed in criterion B for manic or major depressive episode B. No clouding of consciousness, as in delirium; no significant loss of intellectual abilities, as in dementia; no predominant delusions or hallucinations, as in organic delusional syndrome or organic hallucinosis C. Evidence, from the history, physical examination, or laboratory tests, of a specific organic factor that is judged to be etiologically related to the disturbance

Manic state related to discovery of spouse's extramarital affair	**Diagnostic criteria for BIPOLAR DISORDER, MANIC**
	
	Currently (or most recently) in a manic episode (if there has been a previous manic episode, the current episode need not meet the full criteria for a manic episode)
	
	Diagnostic criteria for a MANIC EPISODE
	
	A. One or more distinct periods with a predominantly elevated, expansive, or irritable mood; the elevated or irritable mood must be a prominent part of the illness and relatively persistent, although it may alternate or intermingle with depressive mood
	
	B. Duration of at least 1 week (or any duration if hospitalization is necessary), during which, for most of the time, at least three of the following symptoms have persisted (four if the mood is only irritable) and have been present to a significant degree:
	
	  1. Increase in activity (either socially, at work, or sexually) or physical restlessness
	  2. More talkative than usual or pressure to keep talking
	  3. Flight of ideas or subjective experience that thoughts are racing
	  4. Inflated self-esteem (grandiosity, which may be delusional)
	  5. Decreased need for sleep
	  6. Distractibility, i.e., attention is too easily drawn to unimportant or irrelevant external stimuli
	  7. Excessive involvement in activities that have a high potential for painful consequences which is not recognized, e.g., buying sprees, sexual indiscretions, foolish business investments, reckless driving
	
	C. Neither of the following dominate the clinical picture when an affective syndrome (i.e., criteria A and B above) is not present, that is, before it developed or after it has remitted:
	
	  1. Preoccupation with a mood-incongruent delusion or hallucination (see definition below)
	  2. Bizarre behavior
	
	D. Not superimposed on either schizophrenia, schizophreniform disorder, or a paranoid disorder
	
	E. Not due to any organic mental disorder, such as substance intoxication

*From American Psychiatric Association: Diagnostic and statistical manual of mental disorders, third edition, Washington, D.C., APA, 1980.

TABLE 9-7. **Comparative examples of nursing diagnoses and medical diagnoses associated with disturbances in mood—cont'd**

Nursing diagnoses	Medical diagnoses (as described in DSM-III)

Postpartum depression related to new role as parent	**Diagnostic criteria for ADJUSTMENT DISORDER**
	
	A. A maladaptive reaction to an identifiable psychosocial stressor, that occurs within 3 months of the onset of the stressor
	
	B. The maladaptive nature of the reaction is indicated by either of the following:
	
	    1. Impairment in social or occupational functioning
	    2. Symptoms that are in excess of a normal and expectable reaction to the stressor
	C. The disturbance is not merely one instance of a pattern of overreaction to stress or an exacerbation of one of the mental disorders previously described
	
	D. It is assumed that the disturbance will eventually remit after the stressor ceases or, if the stressor persists, when a new level of adaptation is achieved
	
	E. The disturbance does not meet the criteria for any of the specific disorders listed previously or for uncomplicated bereavement

Attempted suicide related to loss of child in utero	**Diagnostic criteria for MAJOR DEPRESSIVE EPISODE**
	
	A. One or more major depressive episodes
	
	B. Has never had a manic episode or hypomanic episode
	
	Diagnostic criteria for MAJOR DEPRESSIVE EPISODE
	
	A. Dysphoric mood or loss of interest or pleasure in all or almost all usual activities and pastimes; the dysphoric mood is characterized by symptoms such as the following: depressed, sad, blue, hopeless, low, down in the dumps, irritable; the mood disturbance must be prominent and relatively persistent, but not necessarily the most dominant symptom, and does not include momentary shifts from one dysphoric mood to another dysphoric mood, e.g., anxiety to depression to anger, such as are seen in states of acute psychotic turmoil; (for children under 6, dysphoric mood may have to be inferred from a persistently sad facial expression)
	
	B. At least four of the following symptoms have each been present nearly every day for a period of at least 2 weeks (in children under 6, at least three of the first four)
	
	    1. Poor appetite or significant weight loss (when not dieting) or increased appetite or significant weight gain (in children under 6, consider failure to make expected weight gains)
	    2. Insomnia or hypersomnia
	    3. Psychomotor agitation or retardation (but not merely subjective feelings of restlessness or being slowed down) (in children under 6, hypoactivity)
	    4. Loss of interest or pleasure in usual activities, or decrease in sexual drive not limited to a period when delusional or hallucinating (in children under 6, signs of apathy)
	    5. Loss of energy; fatigue
	    6. Feelings of worthlessness, self-reproach, or excessive or inappropriate guilt (either may be delusional)
	    7. Complaints or evidence of diminished ability to think or concentrate, such as slowed thinking, or indecisiveness not associated with marked loosening of associations or incoherence
	    8. Recurrent thoughts of death, suicidal ideation, wishes to be dead, or suicide attempt

Continued.

TABLE 9-7. Comparative examples of nursing diagnoses and medical diagnoses associated with disturbances in mood—cont'd

Nursing diagnoses	Medical diagnoses (as described in DSM-III)*
Attempted suicide related to loss of child in utero—cont'd	**C.** Neither of the following dominate the clinical picture when an affective syndrome (i.e., criteria A and B above) is not present, that is, before it developed or after it has remitted: 1. Preoccupation with a mood-incongruent delusion or hallucination (see definition below) 2. Bizarre behavior **D.** Not superimposed on either schizophrenia, schizophreniform disorder, or a paranoid disorder **E.** Not due to any organic mental disorder or uncomplicated bereavement
Depression related to son's departure from home to college	No mental disorder—**PHASE OF LIFE PROBLEM**
Development of ulcerative colitis related to suppression of grief	Diagnostic criteria for **PSYCHOLOGICAL FACTORS AFFECTING PHYSICAL CONDITION** **A.** Psychologically meaningful environmental stimuli are temporally related to the initiation or exacerbation of a physical condition (recorded on axis III) **B.** The physical condition has either demonstrable organic pathology (e.g., rheumatoid arthritis) or a known pathophysiological process (e.g., migraine headache, vomiting) **C.** The condition is not due to a somatoform disorder
Process of normal mourning related to mastectomy	No related psychiatric diagnosis

diagnoses from DSM-III. Although these are not intended to be all inclusive, they do reflect the complementary, yet distinctive, nature of the nursing and medical diagnosis.

 Planning and implementation of nursing interventions

Goal setting

The general goal of the nurse working with a patient who is experiencing an uncomplicated grief reaction is to support the patient in the subjective experience of his grief work or to help the person mourn. This means helping the person know what has been lost, that his pain is worthy of his own respect, and that real hope lies in acknowledging rather than denying his

loss. He needs to extricate himself from his bondage to the lost object and find new patterns of rewarding interaction. In this way he copes with the loss, integrates it into his past, and grows from the experience. The content of the mutual long-term goals will therefore refer to the patient's completing the process of grieving, mourning, or bereavement. This may take 6 months to a year or possibly longer, since the duration of the grieving process varies considerably among different cultural groups. Short-term goals are necessary to identify specific realistic steps the patient can take as he works through the mourning process. They should reflect progression through Bowlby's[14] phases: (1) the urge to recover the lost object, (2) disorganization, and (3) reorganization. Possible short-term goals may include the following:

The patient will:
1. Express feelings of sorrow caused by the loss of her husband within 10 days
2. Describe her ambivalence (love and anger) toward her husband by the end of 1 month
3. Review her relationship with her husband, including shared pleasures, regrets, etc.

When the patient is experiencing a maladaptive disturbance of mood, the long-term goals may be directed toward reinitiating a delayed grief reaction or exploring areas of conflict underlying a depressive or manic state. When nursing intervention is planned, psychotherapeutic, sociotherapeutic, and somatotherapeutic factors should be considered collectively and conjointly. The long-term goals of nursing care for the patient with a severe mood disturbance have the following aims:
1. To allow for the recognition and continuous expression of feelings, including denial, hopelessness, anger, guilt, blame, helplessness, regret, hope, and relief within a supportive therapeutic atmosphere
2. To allow for the gradual analysis of the stressors the individual is experiencing while strengthening his self-esteem
3. To increase the patient's sense of identity, control, awareness of choices, and responsibility for behavior
4. To encourage the establishment of healthy interpersonal ties with others
5. To promote the understanding of the nature of one's maladaptive emotional responses and acquire more adaptive coping responses to life stressors

Specific short-term goals should be generated from the behaviors displayed by the patient, present areas of difficulty, and relevant stressors. Goal setting should involve a holistic view of the patient and his world. It is probable that goals will need to be developed regarding the patient's self-concept, physical status, behavioral performance, expression of emotions, and interpersonal relationships. All these areas can directly relate to the disturbance of mood displayed by the patient. The participation of the patient in setting these goals can be a significant first step in regaining mastery over his own life.

Intervening in uncomplicated grief reactions

The overall goal of the nurse is to assist the patient who has experienced a loss to work through the process of grieving or mourning and to prevent maladaptive emotional responses. The grieving process is resolved when the lost object is internalized, bonds of attachment are loosened, and new object relationships are established. Grief reactions most commonly occur as a response to separation. They may also occur, however, following the loss of something tangible or intangible that is highly regarded. Thus loss of a body part or function, job, opportunity, relationship, family possessions through an accident, or status and regard among one's peers can all precipitate grief reactions.

Nurses frequently care for patients who have experienced losses related to the body and its parts and functions. Such losses include body parts (amputation and mastectomy), internal organs, sensory loss (vision and hearing), sexual function (impotence and menopause), and aging (mental functioning and physical strength). More than 40,000 limb amputations are performed annually in the United States. Breast amputation is a major approach to the treatment of mammary cancer, a disease that accounts for 25% of all malignancies in women. Such partial loss of the body is an increasingly common experience, and it often results, at least temporarily, in a disturbance in body image (Chapter 8). The precise nature of the patient's reaction to a loss of body part and is unconsciously comparable to the loss of a significant person. Consequently, a process of mourning is initiated and grief is the normal emotional response.

In a larger sense, loss and separation are the recurrent themes of human life, and all change can be regarded as loss—the loss of the past in the movement to something new. This new area can be anticipated or feared, valued or dreaded. It can also be a normal developmental change, such as entering school or getting married. Even if society regards the event as a positive one, the significance of it for the individual may be quite different. Thus both the nature of the change or loss, as well as the significance of it, needs to be appropriately assessed by the nurse. The principles underlying therapeutic nursing interventions in complicated grief reactions are the same, however, regardless of the exact nature of the loss.

Interventions in this area can be initiated through anticipatory guidance even before the loss occurs. This involves talking about the impending loss with the individual and his family, if appropriate. Past losses may be reviewed and analyzed to clarify the meaning of the present loss. Since losses are present in all aspects of life and in all settings, any nurse may implement these interventions. For example, the industrial nurse may discuss the impending retirement of an employee; an office nurse may discuss the implications of a scheduled hysterectomy for a young woman; or a public health nurse may focus on a mother's feelings about her youngest child starting school. Many opportunities for interventions in this area are overlooked by nurses and yet their preventive potential is immeasurable.

Engel[24] identifies a number of preventive actions the nurse can implement in working with a dying patient and his family. He suggests that news of death or impending death should be communicated to a family group, rather than an individual alone, in a private setting. The nurse should be prepared for the possibility of staying with and comforting the bereaved at least until a friend or clergyman arrives. The survivor's need to see the dying or dead patient should be met whenever possible because this is helpful in facing the reality of death.

When the nurse is confronted with an angry hostile reaction from the survivor, two considerations should be kept in mind. First, the person could be justified, but, if not, he may be trying to deal with his own anger and guilt toward the dying person. In this case the reaction is not directed toward the nurse as a person, but it serves as an important coping mechanism in the initial stage of mourning. Another defense that may be displayed by the survivor after hearing the news is disbelief and distraught behavior. The nurse should find a place for the survivors to cry and express their feelings, since this is an important need of the bereaved. The nurse should also be considerate of the cultural, religious, and social customs of the mourners, regardless of how different they may be from her own. Finally, Engel stresses the importance of the need for the patient to grieve for himself. This point is emphasized by Kübler-Ross[37] in her work with dying patients.

The principal task of the nurse is to support the process of normal mourning, and her effectiveness will be increased if she is able to identify those individuals who are likely to experience difficulty in this task. The factors used in the nursing assessment will be helpful in this re-

gard. Childhood experiences and later losses provide information about early separations that predispose the individual to renewed conflicts and unresolved feelings which may surface in the present loss or disruption. Previous history of psychiatric illness alerts the nurse to recurrent depressive episodes or decreased coping abilities. Information about life crises prior to the bereavement reveals the amount of stress previously experienced and the quantity of adaptive resources available at present. The nature of the relationship with the lost person or object is a critical factor. A close interpersonal relationship, a strong attachment, a high degree of dependency, and great ambivalence are all factors that will make the mourning process more complex and painful. As Bugen states, "Individuals who believe that they now have no life of their own or who cling to symbolic vestiges of the deceased will perceive their world only through grief-colored glasses."[17:205]

When the separation occurs through death, the process of dying is also crucial. A sudden death poses greater problems for the bereaved, as do a denial of emotions in the early mourning phase, the death of a child or young adult, and a belief that the death was preventable. Bugen asserts that the belief that the death was preventable is the "single most influential factor contributing to the prolongation of the human grief response."[17:202] The bereaved's support systems, secondary stresses, and future opportunities are relevant factors in planning interventions and promoting future growth.

Before the nurse becomes actively involved with the bereaved, she must have an understanding of her own feelings and reactions to loss. Time should be spent recalling previous losses in her own life, examining related feelings, and resolving areas of conflicts. If she is uncomfortable or ambivalent about death or has delayed the grief work involved in a personal loss, she will be unable to be therapeutic with the bereaved she hopes to help. Hope is an essential quality for the nurse to possess. Her hope and commitment in the future can be transmitted to the bereaved. Hope also involves sharing and a sense of partnership. These are demonstrated in the nurse-patient relationship as the nurse shares the grief work of the bereaved. Finally, nurses working with patients in the process of mourning need support systems of their own. Nursing peers, supervisors, and other professionals can provide formal or informal opportunities for ventilation and rejuvenation. This is essential because assisting the bereaved in the process of mourning can be psychologically draining and interpersonally painful at times.

The core nursing interventions are directed toward helping the patient go through the "grief work" by helping him experience the feelings and emotions connected with the loss and eventually find new patterns of rewarding interaction. He needs to accept the reality of the loss and realize that grieving is appropriate and sharing it makes it less painful. In establishing a contract, the nurse can explain that she would like to help the bereaved talk over any feelings and difficulties he might have related to the loss. Many people find it is easier to talk to an impartial "outsider" about painful memories, ambivalent feelings, and problems that threaten self-esteem. With the nurse the bereaved does not have to fear alienation from the family. In addition, it is important for the nurse, in establishing the contract, to convey her belief in the person's recovery and future coping ability.

Initially the person may be in a dazed or numbed condition. If so, he will need help in making even simple decisions. He will also need time to organize his ideas and take in what has happened. After the initial reaction has subsided, it will be possible to explore the loss, related memories, and affect of the bereaved. A useful beginning point is a discussion of the circumstances and nature of the loss. This often mobilizes the expression of significant and related feelings and reveals those which are absent or inappropriately expressed, such as sadness or anger. Many bereaved people are surprised and frightened by the intensity of their emotions. They may ask, "Is this normal?" or "Am I going mad?" Distractability, difficulty remembering, and a sense of unreality may cause worry and concern. Reassurance that they are not going mad and that such feelings are normal is helpful, particularly if the nurse does not seem frightened or alarmed by them. Nurses can show by their willingness to reveal their own feelings that they are not ashamed of them or rendered useless by them.

Guilt, anger, and sadness are all important emotions to be explored. Crying is an effective emotional release that can communicate strong feelings and drain off immobilizing energy or tension. At times, the values of the nurse or society may negate crying as an emotional outlet because it is viewed as a sign of weakness or causes discomfort in others. Nurses need to guard against these prejudices and encourage crying as an acceptable emotional release. In these instances silence and companionship are often the most therapeutic responses. The appropriateness of sadness and the common occurrence of anger and guilt need to be communicated to allow the free expression of these emotions. Asking how the person feels about a certain event, suggesting the way the person may have felt ("that must have made you feel angry"), or describing how another person would feel in the situation ("that would make me feel isolated and forgotten") may help the bereaved person explore his emotions. In the beginning the bereaved may test out the nurse for the clichés of reassurance used by others. The person may be exploring whether the nurse can confront the loss. If the nurse does not respond in a stereotyped and superficial way, the bereaved may begin to express "bad" memories as well as "good."

Initially, defenses need to be supported, but with time they should be analyzed and released. Denial needs to be changed to developing awareness. Reaction formation may lead to idealization of the lost one and may have to be dealt with by releasing the negative emotions involved. In projective identification the anger and guilt are acknowledged in another but not as part of oneself, and the concern is with the other. With this defense the nurse needs to promote more direct expression of feeling. The goal is to place the loss in perspective and loosen the bonds of attachment.

A number of resistances may appear. Early resistance shows as attempts to concentrate on the practical or financial problems rather than the emotional. The bereaved may ask help in getting a job or collecting the insurance. The nurse can offer appropriate assistance or referral in these areas while also encouraging the expression of grief and promoting the mourning. The nurse must not join with the bereaved in avoiding the grief. Another resistance occurs when the person shuts out the nurse through such statements as "No one really knows what I'm going through" or "You're so young, how can you possibly understand what it's like?" Other resistances occur when the person focuses on the nurse's losses as a way of escaping his own or when he claims that his grief is resolved, although the nurse realizes it is a premature resolution.

It may be necessary for the nurse to work directly or indirectly to promote an appropriate social network support, that is, support that will

TABLE 9-8. Summary of nursing interventions in uncomplicated grief reactions

*Goal—Assist the patient who has experienced a loss to work through the process of grieving
or mourning and prevent maladaptive emotional responses*

Principle	Rationale	Nursing actions
Grieving can be facilitated by anticipating losses and their consequences	Anticipatory guidance by the nurse can be an effective intervention in primary prevention	Discuss impending losses and their significance with the patient and family Review past losses
Support the patient and family at the time of the loss	Therapeutic interventions at the time of the loss can prevent future maladaptive responses	Be prepared to stay with and comfort the bereaved until others arrive Use the family group or significant others as a coping resource to provide initial support for those experiencing the loss Provide the bereaved a place to express their feelings Unconditionally accept the emotional responses of those grieving Incorporate the cultural, religious, and social customs of those grieving in one's nursing care
Identify those persons at high risk for maladaptive responses	Nursing interventions will be more effective if adapted to a person's unique needs	Individuals at high risk for maladaptive responses should be identified by assessing factors that significantly influence the outcome of the mourning process
Awareness and control of nurse's own feelings	Self-awareness is a prerequisite for the "therapeutic use of self" in working with those experiencing loss	Understand one's own feelings and reactions to loss Recall previous losses and resolve areas of conflict Communicate hope in the future and commitment to the work of grieving in the nurse-patient relationship Utilize one's own personal and professional support systems for ventilation and rejuvenation

promote the expression of grief. The nurse may modify the bereaved's support system or may mobilize various significant others, such as the clergy. The nurse may hold a conjoint interview with the family to open up channels of communication and break the conspiracy of silence that frequently blocks grief.

The use of daytime sedatives and tranquilizers should be avoided. They may help the person maintain a calm appearance and avoid crying, but they artificially extend the period of denial and suppress the normal process of mourning. With the suppression of these emotions the balance of normal ambivalence may be tipped to its extreme, producing depression instead of mourning with its greater degree of maladapta-

tion. They can also encourage the development of patterns of drug dependence, sedation, and inhibition of grief in response to stress.

As the grief process is resolved, the person will be seen investing himself in new situations and relationships. The loss is placed in perspective, the attachment bonds are released, and energy is directed back out into the world. New patterns of rewarding interaction should be encouraged and reinforced.

It is important that in terminating the nurse-patient relationship, sufficient time is allowed for dealing with the loss termination imposes. The person may wish to continue the relationship as a substitute for the previous loss. Awareness of these issues will allow the nurse to con-

TABLE 9-8. Summary of nursing interventions in uncomplicated grief reactions—cont'd

Goal—Assist the patient who has experienced a loss to work through the process of grieving or mourning and prevent maladaptive emotional responses

Principle	Rationale	Nursing actions
Help the patient go through the "grief work"	This will help him accept the reality of the loss and realize that grieving is an appropriate and healthy response	Convey belief in the person's recovery and future coping ability
		Initially assist the patient in immediate decision making if necessary
		Explore the circumstances and nature of the loss
		Facilitate the patient's expression of feelings, including guilt, anger, and sadness
		Offer acceptance and assurance of the appropriateness and commonality of the patient's positive and negative emotions
		Initially support the patient's ego defense mechanisms; with time, encourage his analysis and release of them by placing the loss in perspective and loosening bonds of attachment
		Work through any resistances that may occur in the nurse-patient relationship
		New patterns of rewarding interactions should be encouraged and reinforced
		Deal with the loss imposed by the termination of the nurse-patient relationship
Promote social network support as a coping resource	The positive role social support plays in dealing with loss has been well established in both research and clinical practice	Mobilize a social support system for the patient that is appropriate to his needs (i.e., family, clergy, and community agency)
		Facilitate the formation and growth of organizations that act as support groups to others

front them and encourage the independence of the bereaved.

Other therapeutic nursing interventions look to society in general. The nurse can work to encourage others in her community to accept the open expression of grief and the display of emotions. If these are accepted and supported, one type of stress can be avoided. In addition to changing attitudes, the nurse can facilitate the growth of organizations for the bereaved. The effectiveness of widow-to-widow groups, colostomy associations, and single-parent groups has been well established. Support groups play a significant role in preventing maladaptive emotional responses and are an appropriate area for nursing intervention. These interventions related to uncomplicated grief reactions are summarized in Table 9-8.

Intervening in depression and mania

Maladaptive emotional responses may emerge at unpredicted moments, can vary in intensity from mild to severe, and can be transitory, recurrent, or more stable trait conditions. Episodes of depression and mania can occur in any setting and can arise in conjunction with existing medical problems. So too, the treatment of mood disturbances can take place in various settings—at home, at an outpatient department, or in a hospital. The choice of where the patient can be best treated depends on the severity of the illness, available support systems, and resources of the treatment center. In timing one's intervention the nurse should remember that help given when maladaptive patterns of thought and behavior are developing is likely to be more acceptable and effective than help given a long time after these maladaptive patterns have been established. Thus early diagnosis and treatment are associated with more positive outcomes.

The nursing interventions that will be described relative to severe mood disturbances are based on a unified, multicausal, and interactive model of affective disorders. Such a model dismisses the notion of either one cause or one cure modality for the range of maladaptive emotional responses. Rather, it proposes that affective problems have many determinations and many dimensions that affect all aspects of a person's life. Thus a single approach to nursing care would be inadequate. Nursing interventions must instead reflect the complex nature of the model and address all maladaptive aspects of a person's life. Intervening in as many areas as possible should have the maximum effect in modifying maladaptive responses and alleviating severe mood disturbances. The ultimate aim of these nursing interventions is to teach the patient adaptive coping responses and increase the satisfaction and pleasure he receives from his world.

These nursing actions can be implemented in any setting. They are described on the basis of patients' needs in the following areas:

1. Environmental
2. Nurse-patient relationship
3. Affective
4. Cognitive
5. Behavioral
6. Social
7. Physiological

The specific interventions that will now be described are derived from an integration of the models of the causation of severe mood disturbances presented earlier in this chapter.

ENVIRONMENTAL INTERVENTIONS. Environmental interventions are useful when the patient's environment is highly dangerous, impoverished, aversive, or lacking in personal resources. In caring for the patient with a severe mood disorder, high priority should be given to the potential for suicide. Hospitalization is definitely indicated when there is a suicidal risk.

In the presence of a history of rapidly progressing symptoms and the absence or rupture of the usual support systems in the environment, hospitalization is strongly indicated. Nursing care in this case means protection and assuring the patient he will not be allowed to harm himself. Specific interventions related to the suicidal patient are described in Chapter 10.

The depressed patient must always be assessed for possible suicide. The patient is at particular risk for suicide when he appears to be coming out of his depression because he may then have the energy and opportunity to kill himself. Acute manic states are also life threatening. These patients show poor judgment, excessive risk taking, and an inability to evaluate realistic danger and the consequences of their actions. In an acute manic episode immediate environmental measures must be instituted to prevent a fatal outcome.

Another kind of environmental intervention involves changing the physical or social setting by assisting the patient to move to a new environment. Sometimes a change in the patient's general pattern of living is indicated, such as a leave of absence from work, a change of jobs, a new peer group, or leaving one's family setting. Environmental changes such as these serve to decrease the immediate stress and mobilize additional support systems.

NURSE-PATIENT RELATIONSHIP. Both depressed and manic patients present unique challenges to the nurse who wishes to engage them in a therapeutic alliance. Depressed patients resist involvement through the defenses of withdrawal and nonresponsiveness. Because of their negative view of life they tend to remain isolated, verbalize little, feel they are unworthy of help, and form dependent attachments to others.

In working with depressed patients, the nurse's approach should be a quiet, warm, and accepting one. She should demonstrate the qualities of honesty, empathy, and compassion. Admittedly, it is not always easy to give warm, personal care to a person who is unresponsive and detached. The nurse may feel angry or resentful of his helplessness or fear rejection by him. The nurse needs patience and a belief in the potential of each person to grow and change. If this is calmly communicated to the patient, both verbally and nonverbally, in time he may begin to respond to the nurse's perceptions.

The nurse should avoid assuming an over-aggressive or lighthearted approach with the depressed individual. Comments such as "You have so much to live for," "Cheer up—things are sure to get better," or "You shouldn't feel so depressed" convey little understanding of and respect for the patient's feelings. They will create more distance between the nurse and patient and block the formation of a potential relationship. Neither should the nurse sympathize with the patient. Subjective overidentification by the nurse can cause her to experience similar feelings of hopelessness and helplessness and seriously limit her ability to be therapeutic.

Rapport is best established with the depressed patient through shared time, even if the patient talks little, and supportive companionship. The very presence of the nurse indicates that she believes the patient is a valuable person. The nurse should adjust to the depressed patient's pace by speaking more slowly and allowing him sufficient time to respond. She should address him by name, talk to him, and listen to him. By studying the life and interests of the patient, the nurse might select topics that can serve as points of entry and lay the foundation for more meaningful discussions.

In contrast, elated patients may be very talkative and need simple explanations and concise truthful answers to questions. Although the manic patient might appear to be very willing to talk, he resists involvement through the defenses of manipulation, testing limits, and superficiality. His hyperactivity, short attention span, flight of ideas, poor judgment, lack of insight, and rapid mood swings all present special problems to the nursing staff.

Manic patients can be very disruptive to a unit and resist engagement in the work of therapy. They may dominate group meetings or therapy sessions by their excessive talking and manipulate the nursing and medical staff or patient group. By identifying a vulnerable area of another person or a group's area of conflict, manic patients are able to exploit and manipulate others. This provokes defensive and angry responses in others. Nurses are particularly susceptible to these feelings, since they often have the most contact with patients and the responsibility for coordinating and maintaining the psychiatric unit. When anger is generated, there is a breakdown of coordinated therapeutic care. Thus the maneuvers of manic patients serve as diversionary tactics. By alienating themselves they can avoid exploring their own problems.

It is important for nurses to understand how manic patients are able to manipulate others and their reasons for doing so. The treatment plan for these patients should be thorough, well coordinated, and consistently implemented. Constructive limit setting on manic patients' behavior is an essential part of the therapeutic plan. The entire treatment team must be consistent in their expectations of these patients and progressive limits set as situations arise. Other patients may also be encouraged to carry out the limits decided on. Pressure applied by peers can sometimes be more effective than pressure applied by the staff. Frequent staff meetings are recommended to reduce faulty communication, share in understanding the manic patient's behavior, and assure steady progress toward therapeutic goals.

One goal of nursing care is to ultimately increase the patient's self-control, and this should be kept in mind when setting limits with manic patients. They need to see that they have the ability to monitor their own behavior and that the staff is there to help them in this area. Also, it should be pointed out that there are many positive aspects to their behavior. The ability to be outgoing, expressive, and energetic are coping strengths that can be maximized in the therapeutic process.

AFFECTIVE INTERVENTIONS. Affective interventions are necessary because patients with mood disturbances have difficulty identifying and expressing feelings. Feelings that are particularly problematic are hopelessness, sadness, anger, guilt, and anxiety. A range of interventions are available to the nurse in meeting the patient's need in this area.

Intervening in the area of emotions requires self-understanding in the nurse. Whether or not the nurse's interventions will be therapeutic depends greatly on her values regarding the various emotions, her own emotional responsiveness, and her ability to offer genuine respect and nonjudgmental acceptance. The nurse must be able to experience feelings and express them herself if she expects to help her patient in this important aspect of his life.

Initially, the nurse must hope for depressed patients. They have a genuine need for repeated reassurance. The nurse can reinforce the fact that depression is a self-limiting disorder and things will be better in the future. The nurse can express this calmly and simply. Her intent is not to cheer the patient but to reassure him that, although recovery is a slow process involving weeks or months to complete, he will feel progressively better and will not remain at his current level of depression. Related to this, the nurse may acknowledge the patient's inability to take comfort from this reassurance. For him, only the depression is real; past or future happiness is an illusion. However, by affirming her belief, she may make his existence more tolerable.

This initial reassurance is a way of acknowledging the patient's pain and despair, while also conveying to him the nurse's sense of hope in his recovery. It is not the premature reassurance of "Don't worry—everything's going to be just fine." It is an openness to his feelings and acknowledgment of them. This is a very important first step. It also tells him that his present state is not permanent but is changeable. For the depressed patient who lacks a perspective of time, it directs his thoughts beyond the present time and into the future with genuine hopes for tomorrow.

Nursing actions in this area should convey that expressing feelings is normal and necessary. Blocking or repressing emotions is partly responsible for his present pain. She can help him to realize that his overwhelming feelings of dejection and worthlessness are defenses that serve to prevent him from dealing with his problems. Encouraging a patient to express his unpleasant or painful emotions through verbalizing them can reduce their intensity and make the person feel more alive and masterful. Thus the nursing actions should be directed toward first helping the patient experience his feelings and then express them. These actions are prerequisite to implementing interventions in the cognitive, behavioral, or social areas.

When the nurse accepts without criticism the anger, despair, or anxiety expressed by the patient, he sees that expressing feelings is not destructive or a sign of weakness. Sometimes, however, the expression of anger by the patient changes his cognitive set from self-blaming to other blaming. It may allow him to see himself as more effective because it connotes power, superiority, and mastery. How this anger is expressed is important because aggressive behavior can be destructive and serve to further isolate him interpersonally. Many patients experiencing both depressive and manic emotional states have problems with the expression of anger and need to learn effective assertive behavior. This important area of nursing intervention is explored in more depth in Chapter 12.

Relaxation techniques may also be useful in helping both manic and depressed patients deal with their anxiety and tension and obtain more pleasure from life. Reducing anxiety to tolerable levels broadens the individual's perceptual field and allows the nurse to introduce interventions in the cognitive and behavioral areas. Nursing actions to reduce anxiety are described in Chapter 7.

To successfully implement any of these nursing actions related to the patient's affective needs, she must utilize the variety of facilitative communication skills and responsive and action dimensions in the therapeutic nurse-patient relationship. These are described in Chapter 3. Particularly important among these are empathy skills, reflection of feeling, open-ended feeling-oriented questions, validation, self-disclosure, and confrontation. Feelings are the essence of empathy and, as such, make empathy an essential therapeutic quality. The various other communication skills must also be used to focus on feelings rather than facts. The patient with a severe mood disturbance will challenge the nurse's therapeutic skills and stringently test the level of her caring and commitment.

COGNITIVE INTERVENTIONS. When intervening in the cognitive area, the nurse has three major aims, which require that the nurse begin with the patient's conceptualization or definition of his problem:

1. To increase the patient's sense of control over his goals and behavior
2. To increase the patient's self-esteem
3. To assist the patient in modifying his negative expectations

Depressed patients usually see themselves as victims of their moods and environment. They do not view their behavior and their interpretation of events as possible causes of depression. They assume a passive stance and wait for someone or something to come along that will lift their mood. One task of the nurse, therefore, is to move the patient beyond his limiting preoccupation with his mood to a recognition of other aspects of his world that are related to it. To do this, the nurse will progress gradually with the patient. The first step is to help him explore his feelings. This is followed by eliciting his view of the problem. In so doing the nurse accepts the patient's perceptions but need not accept his conclusions. Together they need to define the problem so as to give the patient a sense of control, a feeling of hope, and a realization that change may indeed be possible.

Nursing actions may then be focused on

*supportive
allowed the client
time to express
his feelings*

modifying the patient's thinking. Depressed patients are noticeably dominated by negative thoughts. The effect of this is that often, despite a successful performance, the patient will view it negatively because of his pessimistic world view. Cognitive changes may be brought about in a number of ways. Frequently, negative thinking is an automatic process of which the patient is not even aware. The nurse can therefore assist him in identifying his negative thoughts and decreasing them through thought interruption or substitution. Concurrently, the patient can be encouraged to increase his positive thinking by reviewing his personal assets, strengths, accomplishments, and opportunities. Next the patient can be assisted in examining the accuracy of his perceptions, logic, and conclusions. In so doing, misperceptions, distortions, and irrational beliefs become evident. The patient should be helped to move from unrealistic to realistic goals and attempt to decrease the importance of unattainable goals. All of these actions serve to enhance the patient's self-understanding and increase his level of self-esteem. More detailed interventions in this area are explored in Chapter 8, which addresses alterations in self-concept—a problem inherent in disturbances of mood.

Also, because the depressed patient tends to be overwhelmed by his despair, it is important to limit the amount of negative personal evaluations he engages in. One way this can be accomplished is by involving the patient in productive tasks or activities; another way is to increase his level of socialization. These benefit the patient in two complementary ways: they limit the time he can spend on brooding and self-criticism, and they provide positive reinforcement in themselves.

A final consideration in this area is that the nurse needs to realize the meaning, nature, and value the patient places on his behavior and mood change. Most research has been focused on the psychopathologic nature of affective disorders. One study that explored the positive aspects of them found that patients with bipolar illnesses receive pronounced short- and long-term positive effects from their manic-depressive illness.[35] The patients reported short- and long-term increases in productivity, creativity, sensitivity, social outgoingness, and sexual intensity. It is important for the nurse to understand these attributions because they suggest that disturbances of mood can produce powerful reinforcers of a maladaptive response and thus make change more difficult. It would appear that for some patients, the positive consequences of an illness may outweigh their perception of negative outcomes.

BEHAVIORAL INTERVENTIONS. Successful behavior is a powerful antidepressant. This idea, however, seldom occurs to depressed patients who use their despondent mood as a rationalization for inactivity. They believe, instead, that once their mood lifts, they will be able to be productive once again. Such an idea is consistent with a negative cognitive set and a sense of helplessness over one's life. But inactivity prevents the patient from obtaining satisfaction and receiving social recognition. So, in actuality, it serves to reinforce one's depressive state.

Nursing interventions in this area therefore focus on activating the patient in a realistic, goal-directed way to move the patient in the direction of adaptive coping responses. The assignment of therapeutic tasks can be viewed as directed activities, strategies, or homework assignments mutually determined by the nurse and patient based on their long-term treatment goals. They are action-oriented and behavior focused and allow the patient to explore alternative coping responses. Some of the benefits derived from assigning therapeutic tasks as identified by Goldberg include the following:

1. The client continues to be involved with the therapist even when not in therapy, thus strengthening the therapeutic relationship.
2. The responsibility for change is the client's.
3. The implication is that the client can change, which instills hope.
4. If successfully completed, therapeutic tasks tend to enhance the client's self-esteem.
5. They help restructure a system.
6. They teach problem-solving skills by providing the client an opportunity for experiential learning.
7. They test the flexibility of a person or system and reveal areas of resistance to change.
8. They encourage the generalization of therapeutic gains beyond the therapy session.[26:157]

Many depressed patients benefit from nursing actions that encourage them to redirect their self-preoccupation to interests in the outside world. The timing of these interventions is crucial. The patient should not be forced into activities initially. Neither will he benefit from coming into contact with too many people too soon. Rather, the nurse should encourage activities gradually and suggest escalating involvement on the basis of the mobilization of his energy.

For severely depressed hospitalized patients a structured daily program of activities can be beneficial. Because these patients lack motivation and direction, they are reticent to initiate actions. In this case the nurse should provide a tangible structure for activities, taking into consideration the patient's tolerance to stress and probability of succeeding. The particular task should not be too difficult nor too time consuming. Success tends to increase the patient's expectations and the possibility of future success. Failure tends to increase his feelings of worthlessness and hopelessness.

The elated patient usually needs little encouragement to become involved with others. Because of his short attention span and restless energy, however, he cannot deal with complicated projects. He needs tasks that are simple and that can be completed quickly. In his environment he needs room to move about and furnishings that do not overstimulate him.

The patient's ability to accomplish tasks and be productive will depend on a number of factors. First, expectations and goals for him should be small enough to ensure successful performance, relevant to his needs, and focused on positive activities. Following is a positive activities list* that contains categories of rewarding or potentially rewarding activities[54].

---

1. Planning something you will enjoy
2. Going on an outing (e.g., a walk, a shopping trip downtown, a picnic)
3. Going out for entertainment
4. Going on a trip
5. Going to meetings, lectures, classes
6. Attending a social gathering
7. Playing a sport or game
8. Spending time on a hobby or project
9. Entertaining yourself at home (e.g., reading, listening to music, watching TV)
10. Doing something just for yourself (e.g., buying something, cooking something, dressing comfortably)
11. Spending time just relaxing (e.g., thinking, sitting, napping, daydreaming)
12. Caring for yourself, making yourself attractive
13. Persisting at a difficult task
14. Completing a routine task or unpleasant task
15. Doing a job well

---

*From Rehm, L.: A self-control therapy program for treatment of depression. In Clarkin, J., and Glazer, H., editors: Depression: behavioral and directive intervention strategies, New York, 1981, Garland Publishing, Inc.

16. Cooperating with someone else on a common task
17. Doing something special for someone else, being generous, going out of your way
18. Seeking out people (e.g., calling, stopping by, making a date or appointment, going to a meeting)
19. Initiating conversation (e.g., at a store, party, or class)
20. Discussing an interesting or amusing topic
21. Expressing yourself openly, clearly, or frankly e.g., opinion, criticism, anger)
22. Playing with children or animals
23. Complimenting or praising someone
24. Physically showing affection or love
25. Receiving praise, compliments, attention

Next, attention should be focused on the task at hand, not what has yet to be done or was done incorrectly in the past. Finally, positive reinforcement should be based on actual preformance. If such an approach is used consistently over time, the nurse can expect the patient to demonstrate increasing amounts of productive behavior.

When considering possible activities for the patient, occupational and recreational ones are usually easily identified by the nurse. These can be most valuable and are well represented in the positive activities list. Another source of accomplishment is in the area of movement and physical exercise. Brown[16] has made the following observations about the relationship between mood and movement:

■ Physical fitness is often associated with a feeling of well-being and reduced depression and anxiety.
■ Fitness appears to be associated with physical and psychological benefits regardless of the subject's age.
■ The biological benefits of exercise may be associated in part with changes produced among brain amines, salt metabolism, muscle neuronal activity, and striatal functions.
■ A comprehensive history of the depressed patient's motor activity is useful in prescribing an exercise regimen of maximum benefit.

Jogging, walking, swimming, bicycling, and aerobics are popular forms of exercise that may be incorporated in a regular program of physical activity for the patient. They are beneficial because they improve the patient's physical condition and provide a release of emotions and tensions.[59,62]

SOCIAL INTERVENTIONS. Evidence from diverse sources indicates that social factors play a major role in the causation, maintenance, and resolution of affective disorders, particularly depression. Socialization serves to moderate the experience of depression by providing an experience that is incompatible with depressive withdrawal and by providing a source of increased self-esteem through the social reinforcers of approval, acceptance, recognition, and support.

A major problem in the social area is that patients with maladaptive emotional responses have fewer interpersonal skills and are less accomplished in social interaction. In addition, they may be avoided by others because of their self-absorption, pessimism, or elation. One nursing action to counteract this problem is to help the patient improve his interpersonal style and increase his social skills. This can be accomplished in a sequential learning process that includes the following:

1. Assessing the patient's social skills, supports, and interests
2. Reviewing existing and potential social resources available to the patient
3. Instruction and modeling of effective social skills
4. Role playing and rehearsal of troublesome social situations and interactions
5. Feedback and positive reinforcement of effective interpersonal skills
6. Encouraging the initiation of socialization in an expanded social arena

This final accomplishment often proves to be difficult for depressed patients who report they are unable to meet new people and engage in an active social life. Thus increasing a patient's social activities is another area of nursing intervention. Involvement with others often is a result of shared activities. The nurse can work with the patient to identify recreational, career, cultural, religious, and personal interests and how to best pursue these interests through community groups, organizations, and clubs. Women's groups, single parents groups, jogging clubs, church groups, and neighborhood associations are all possible opportunities for expanding one's social network. Although this may appear to be a relatively simple nursing intervention, it is often one that taxes the nurse's knowledge of resources and creativity.

In addition to a one-to-one relationship, patients with maladaptive emotional responses can also benefit from family and group therapy. In the context of family therapy the behaviors of depression can be interpreted as signs of dependency, which is contributed to and supported by other family members. The patient's sense of powerlessness in human relationships is examined in light of family patterns, and all family members are expected to take responsibility for their share of the continuing pattern.

The notion that friends and partners often reinforce and support the patient's depression has been well documented. When a person gets depressed, he usually receives a lot of attention and secondary gain from others who respond by being helpful, nurturing, or annoyed. But when the patient acts in a nondepressed way, there is little attention paid to him. Therefore one goal of family therapy is to have the family reinforce adaptive nondepressed behavior and ignore his maladaptive depressive responses.

There is also a need for family interventions with manic patients. In one study that followed the families of patients with bipolar manic-depressive illness, the authors noted the following:

> The recurring psychopathology of manic-depressive patients has significant effects on the psychosocial adaptation of their spouse and children. Not only is the genetic predisposition handed down over generations, but the environment may have long-term detrimental effects on the children's personality.[44:1537]

The "wavering capacity for interpersonal relatedness" on the part of the patient and other family members is a clear indication for nursing interventions at the family level of care.

Group therapy can also provide multiple benefits. Knowledge that others have ambivalence and the sharing of guilt concerning this, as well as the realistic sympathy and support of the group members, enable the depressed patient to lessen his guilt, give up his maladaptive behavior patterns, and develop more satisfying relationships with others in the group. Van Servellen and Dull developed a format for group treatment of women with major depressive illness. The overall aim is to increase self-worth and self-esteem through identification with the group and awareness of personal strengths. The depressed women in Van Servellen and Dull's group[66] identified several general goals:

1. Learning more about their individual behavior and relationships with others based on feedback from members and group process.
2. Increasing social support through group relatedness.
3. Gaining a heightened sense of identity, self-understanding, and control over their own lives.

4. Realizing that other people have problems similar to their own, which helps to reduce their sense of loneliness and isolation, thereby also decreasing feelings of hopelessness, helplessness, and powerlessness.
5. Learning new ways to cope with stress from others in the group.
6. More realistically modifying their perceptions and expectations of self and others.
7. Allowing for the expression of feelings of hopelessness and frustration within the supportive context of the group.

An essential part of any therapeutic intervention is the evaluation of its effectiveness. The authors also present a format for evaluation that can be used to measure change in the specific patients in group treatment. Research in comparing and evaluating various therapeutic modalities used by nurses continues to be a high priority in the future.

PHYSIOLOGICAL INTERVENTIONS. Interventions in this area include both physical care and somatic therapies. They begin with a thorough physical examination and health history to determine present health status, past and present health problems, and the presence of current treatments or medications that may be affecting the patient's mood state.

In depression, physical well-being may be forgotten or the patient may not be capable of caring for himself. The more severe the depression, the more important is the physical care.

The anorexic patient may need to have his diet monitored. Staying with the patient when he is eating, arranging for preferred foods, and encouraging frequent small meals may be helpful. Recording his intake and output and weighing him daily will help in evaluating this need.

Sleep disturbances are common. It is best to plan activities according to each patient's energy levels; some feel best in the morning and others in the evening. A scheduled rest period may be helpful, but patients should not be encouraged to take frequent naps or remain in bed all day.

The patient's appearance may be neglected and all his movements slowed. If it is necessary to assist the hospitalized patient with bathing or dressing, it should be done matter of factly with the explanation that he is being helped because he is unable to do it for himself at the present time. Cleanliness and interest in appearance can be noticed and praised. It is important for the nurse to allow the patient to help himself whenever possible. Often the nurse might rush the patient or do a task herself to save time, but these do not facilitate the patient's recovery and should be avoided.

The manic patient primarily needs protection from himself. He may be too busy to eat or take care of himself. Eating problems can be handled in the same way as with the depressed patient. Sleep is scarce; so rest periods should be provided along with supportive interventions, such as baths, soft music, and whirlpools. The manic patient may also need help in selecting appropriate clothes and carrying out hygiene activities. Setting limits and firm decisive actions are effective approaches to the physical care of the patient with a severe mood disturbance.

Antidepressant medications are frequently administered to elevate the mood of the depressed patient. At this time no single drug has been found to be effective for all kinds of depressions. Of the two types of antidepressants—tricyclics and monoamine oxidase (MAO) inhibitors—the former are used more commonly. Tricyclic drugs appear to be the most effective class of antidepressants. They pose a smaller risk of side effects than the MAO inhibitors and appear to be useful against relapses of depression. Lithium carbonate is considered by many to be the drug of choice in the treatment of mania. Some believe that it not only produces a remission of symptoms but also actually prevents a recurrence of the manic state. The overall success rate of drugs for the treatment of depression is 70% to 90%. Electroconvulsive therapy (ECT) is also used with depressed patients, particularly those with recurrent depressions and those who are resistant to drug therapy. ECT is regarded by many as a specific therapy for those severe depressions characterized by somatic delusions and delusional guilt, accompanied by a lack of interest in the world, suicidal ideation, and weight loss. A more detailed discussion of antidepressant medication and electroconvulsive therapy is presented in Chapter 15.

A recent development in this area is a laboratory test for somatically treatable depression—the dexamethasone suppression test (DST). The test is easy, relatively inexpensive, and of minimal risk to the patient. The DST is most useful in identifying patients who do not display the typical behaviors of depression but who are likely to respond to somatic treatments, such as antidepressant therapy or ECT. It may also be useful in monitoring recovery from depression and assist in the decision about when to stop maintenance antidepressant therapy safely.

Sleep deprivation therapy may also be effec-

TABLE 9-9. Summary of nursing interventions in depression and mania

Goal—Teach the patient adaptive emotional responses and increase the satisfaction and pleasure he receives from his world

Principle	Rationale	Nursing action
Modify the patient's environment if it is dangerous, impoverished, aversive, or lacking in personal resources	All patients with severe mood disturbances are at high risk for suicide; environmental changes can protect the patient, decrease the immediate stress, and mobilize additional resources	Continually evaluate the patient's potential for suicide Hospitalize the patient when there is a suicidal risk Assist the patient to move to a new environment when appropriate (i.e., new job, peer group, family setting)
Establish and maintain a therapeutic nurse-patient relationship	Both depressed and manic patients resist becoming involved in a therapeutic alliance; acceptance, persistence, and limit setting are necessary	Utilize a warm, accepting, empathic approach Be aware of and in control of one's own feelings and reactions (i.e., anger, frustration, sympathy) With the depressed patient: 1. Establish rapport through shared time and supportive companionship 2. Allow the patient time to respond 3. Personalize his care as a way of indicating his value as a human being With the manic patient: 1. Give simple truthful responses 2. Be alert to possible manipulation 3. Set constructive limits on negative behavior 4. Use a consistent approach by all health team members 5. Maintain open communication and sharing of perceptions among team members 6. Reinforce the patient's self-control and positive aspects of his behavior
Assist in the patient's recognition and expression of emotions	Patients with severe mood disturbances have difficulty identifying and expressing feelings	Demonstrate emotional responsiveness and acceptance Utilize facilitative communication skills and the responsive and action dimensions described in Chapter 3 Respond empathically with a focus on feelings rather than facts Acknowledge the patient's pain and convey a sense of hope in his recovery Help the patient experience his feelings and then express them Assist the patient in the appropriate expression of anger Reduce the patient's anxiety to mild-moderate levels
Aid the patient in modifying his negative cognitive set	This will help to increase his sense of control over his goals and behaviors, enhance his self-esteem, and modify his negative expectations	Review with the patient his conceptualization of the problem but do not necessarily accept his conclusions Identify the patient's negative thoughts and help him to decrease them through thought interruption or substitution Help him increase his positive thinking Examine the accuracy of his perceptions, logic, and conclusions

Continued.

TABLE 9-9. Summary of nursing interventions in depression and mania—cont'd

Goal—Teach the patient adaptive emotional responses and increase the satisfaction and pleasure he receives from his world

Principle	Rationale	Nursing action
Aid the patient in modifying his negative cognitive set—cont'd		Identify misperceptions, distortions, and irrational beliefs
		Help him move from unrealistic to realistic goals
		Decrease the importance of unattainable goals
		Limit the amount of negative personal evaluations he engages in
		Realize the meaning, nature, and value the patient places on his behavior and mood change
Activate the patient in a realistic goal-directed way	Successful behavioral performance counteracts feelings of helplessness and hopelessness	Assign appropriate action-oriented therapeutic tasks
		Encourage activities gradually, escalating them as the patient's energy is mobilized
		Provide a tangible structured program when appropriate
		Set goals that are realistic, relevant to the patient's needs and interests, and focused on positive activities
		Focus on present activities, not past or future activities
		Positively reinforce successful performance
		Attain mutuality whenever possible
		Incorporate physical exercise in the patient's plan of care
Enhance the patient's establishment of interpersonal relationships	Socialization is an experience that is incompatible with withdrawal and increases self-esteem through the social reinforcers of approval, acceptance, recognition, and support	Assess the patient's social skills, supports, and interests
		Review existing and potential social resources
		Instruct and model effective social skills
		Use role playing and rehearsal of social interactions
		Give feedback and positive reinforcement of effective interpersonal skills
		Encourage increasing socialization in an expanded social arena
		Intervene with families to have them reinforce adaptive emotional responses of the patient
		Support or engage in family and group therapy when appropriate
Promote the patient's physical health and well-being	Physiological changes occur in disturbances of mood; physical care and somatic therapies are required to overcome problems in this area	Complete a nursing assessment of the patient's physiological health status
		Assist the patient to meet his self-care needs, particularly in the areas of nutrition, sleep, and personal hygiene
		Encourage the patient's independence whenever possible
		Administer prescribed medications and treatments

tive in the treatment of depression. Research indicates that depriving some depressed patients of a night's sleep will bring about an improvement in their clinical condition.[12] The means by which sleep deprivation works is not known, and the duration of the improvement varies greatly. Further developments in somatic therapies will have direct implications for nursing care.

All of the previously described nursing interventions in depression and mania are summarized in Table 9-9. It appropriately reflects the holistic nature of the nursing care given to patients with disturbances of mood.

 Evaluation

The effectiveness of nursing care is determined by changes in the patient's maladaptive emotional responses and the effect they have on his present functioning. Problems related to self-concept and interpersonal relationships merge and overlap. Since all individuals experience life stress and related losses, one of the fundamental questions the nurse can ask related to evaluation is "Did I assess my patient for problems in this area?"

Of particular significance with this problem are the many special aspects of transference and countertransference that may occur. The patient's heightened attachment and dependency behaviors and his lowered defensiveness can lead to intense transference reactions that should be worked through. Themes of loss and fear of loss, control of emotions and lack of control, and ambivalence predominate. Termination of the nurse-patient relationship may be difficult, since the patient experiences it as another loss that requires mourning and integration.

Countertransference issues can be related to the nurse's own bereavements, her attitudes about anger, guilt, sadness, and despair, her ability to confront these emotions openly and objectively, and, most important, her own conflicts about death and loss. Difficulties related to any of these issues can be evident in avoidance behavior, preoccupation with fantasies, blocking of feelings, or shortening of sessions. The nurse can expect to review and perhaps rework her feelings about personal bereavement. Her nursing care will be more appropriate and effective if she is aware of these issues and sensitive to her own feelings and conflicts regarding loss. Supervision and peer support groups can be of great help to her in this area.

Suggested cross-references

Therapeutic relationship skills and self-awareness of the nurse are discussed in Chapter 3. The model of health-illness phenomena, including precipitating life stressors and the phases of the nursing process are described in Chapter 4. Strengthening coping resources through health education, environmental change, and supporting social systems is presented in Chapters 5 and 6. Interventions related to self-concept and cognitive therapy are discussed in Chapter 8. Interventions with the suicidal patient are discussed in Chapter 10. Disruptions in interpersonal relationships are discussed in Chapter 11. Problems with anger and limit setting are discussed in Chapter 12. Somatic therapy is discussed in Chapter 15. Group therapy is discussed in Chapter 24. Family therapy is discussed in Chapter 25. Care of the dying and their family is discussed in Chapter 32.

SUMMARY

1. Mood refers to a prolonged emotional state that influences one's whole personality and life functioning. It pertains to one's prevailing and pervading emotion and is synonymous with the terms affect, feeling state, and emotion. Four adaptive functions of mood and a continuum of emotional responses were described. Severe mood disturbances can be recognized by their intensity, prevasiveness, persistence, and interference with usual social and physiological functioning.

a. Grief is an individual's subjective response to the loss of a person, object, or concept that is highly valued. Uncomplicated grief is a healthy, adaptive, reparative response that is closely related to the acquisition of the capacity for developing meaningful object relationships. An uncomplicated grief reaction is the process of normal mourning. Mourning is resolved only when the lost object is internalized, bonds of attachment are loosened, and new object relationships are established. The work of mourning may take 6 months to a year. If grief is not worked through, delayed grief reactions and depression can occur.

b. Depression was distinguished from grief by the attachment to the loved object, degree of regression, acknowledgment of the loss, and intensity of emotions over time.

c. Mania is characterized by a mood that is elevated, expansive, or irritable. Hypomania is similar to mania but less severe. The prevalence of depression and mania was described, as well as their classification in DMS-III.

2. Stressors affecting the grief reaction and factors that place a person at high risk for maladaptive responses were identified. Ten models of causation of severe mood disturbances were discussed. These included the genetic, object loss, aggression turned inward, personality organization, cognitive, learned helplessness, behavioral, biochemical, life stressors, and integrated models. An integrated multicausal model is the most valuable for the nurse to use when implementing nursing care.

3. The phases associated with the process of mourning as described by Bowlby were presented. These are the urge to recover the lost object, disorganization, and reorganization. They can be applied to losses of any kind. Behaviors associated with delayed reactions, depression, and mania, were identified. The key element of a behavioral assessment is change in the person's usual patterns and responses.

4. Maladaptive emotional responses were related to feelings of anxiety, hostility, self-devaluation, and guilt. The psychiatric classification of affective disorders was discussed. Selected nursing diagnoses were related to appropriate medical diagnoses from DSM-III.

5. The general goal of the nurse when working with a patient who has experienced loss is to support the patient in the subjective experience of his grief work. He needs to extricate himself from his bondage to the lost object and find new patterns of rewarding interaction. When the patient is experiencing a maladaptive disturbance of mood, the long-term goals may be directed toward reinitiating a delayed grief reaction or exploring areas of conflict underlying a depressive or manic state. Psychotherapeutic, sociotherapeutic, and somatotherapeutic factors should be considered collectively and conjointly. More specific short-term goals should be identified with the patient based on his behavior, present area of difficulty, and relevant stressors.

6. Interventions in uncomplicated grief reactions were described as anticipatory guidance, supporting the process of normal mourning, and social system intervention. Interventions in depression and mania were presented in the environment, nurse-patient relationship, affective, cognitive, behavioral, social, and physiological areas. Intervening in as many areas as possible should have the maximum effect in modifying maladaptive responses and alleviating severe mood disturbances.

7. When evaluating the nursing care, the nurse should pay particular importance to problems with transference and countertransference. Supervision and peer support groups can be helpful to the nurse in working with patients experiencing grief reactions.

References

1. Abramson, L., Seligman, M., and Teasdale, J.: Learned helplessness in humans: critique and reformulation, J. Abnormal Psychol. **87**:49, 1978.
2. Akiskal, H., and McKinney, W.: Depressive disorders: toward a unified hypothesis, Science **182**:20, Oct. 5, 1973.
3. Akiskal, H., and McKinney, W.: Overview of recent research in depression, Arch. Gen. Psychiatry **32**:285, 1975.
4. American Psychiatric Association: Diagnostic and statistical manual of mental disorders, ed. 3, Washington, D.C., 1980, The Association.
5. Arieti, S., and Bemporad, J.: The psychological organization of depression, Am. J. Psychiatry **137**:1360, 1980.
6. Baldessarini, R.: Biogenic amine: hypotheses in affective disorders. In Flach, F., and Draghi, S., editors: The nature and treatment of depression, New York, 1975, John Wiley & Sons, Inc.
7. Beck, A.: The diagnosis and management of depression. Philadelphia, 1973, University of Pennsylvania Press.
8. Beck, A.: Cognitive therapy and emotional disorders, New York, 1976, International Universities Press.
9. Beck, A., and Rush, A.: Cognitive approaches to depression and suicide. In Servan, G., editor: Cognitive defects in development of mental illness, New York, 1977, Brunner/Mazel, Inc.
10. Beck, A. et al.: Cognitive therapy of depression, New York, 1979, The Guilford Press.
11. Beck, C.: The occurrence of depression in women and the effect of the women's movement, J. Psychiatr. Nurs. **17**(11):14, 1979.
12. Bhanji, S.: Treatment of depression by sleep deprivation, Nurs. Times, **73**:540, 1977.
13. Bowlby, J.: Grief and mourning in infancy and early childhood, Psychoanal. Study Child **15**:9, 1960.
14. Bowlby, J.: Processes of mourning, Int. J. Psychoanal. **42**:22, 1961.
15. Brown, G., and Harris, T.: Social origins of depression, London, 1978, Tavistock Publications, Ltd.
16. Brown, R., Ramirez, D., and Taub, J.: The prescription of exercise for depression, Physician Sports Med. **6**(12):34, 1978.
17. Bugen, L.: Human grief: a model for prediction and intervention, Am. J. Orthopsychiatry **47**:196, April 1972.
18. Cadoret, R. et al.: Depressive disease: life events and onset of illness, Arch. Gen. Psychiatry **26**:133, 1972.

19. Clayton, P. et al.: Mourning and depression: their similarities and differences, Can. Psychiatr. Assoc. **19**:309, 1974.

20. Cohen, M.: Personal identity and sexual identity, Psychiatry **29**:1, 1966.

21. Crary, W., and Crary, G.: Depression, Am. J. Nurs. **73**:472, 1973.

22. Drake, R., and Price, J.: Depression: adaptation to distuption and loss, Perspect. Psychiatr. Care **13**:163, Oct.-Dec. 1975.

23. Dyer, E.: Parenthood as crisis: a restudy, Marriage Family Living **25**:196, 1963.

24. Engel, G.: Grief and grieving, Am. J. Nurs. **64**:93, Sept. 1964.

25. Freud, S.: Mourning and melancholia. Standard edition of the complete psychological works of Sigmund Freud, vol. 14, London, 1957, Hogarth Press.

26. Goldberg, C.: Therapeutic tasks: strategies for changes, Perspect. Psychiatr. Care **18**(4):156, 1980.

27. Gove, W.: The relationship between sex roles, marital status, and mental illness, Soc. Forces **51**:34, Sept. 1972.

28. Hodge, J.: They that mourn, J. Relig. Health **11**:229, 1972.

29. Holmes, T., and Rahe, R.: The social readjustment rating scale, J. Psychosom. Res. **2**:213, 1967.

30. Holmstrom, L.: The two-career family, Cambridge, Mass., 1972, Schenkman Publishing Co., Inc.

31. Hudgens, R., Morrison, J., and Barchha, R.: Life events and onset of primary affective disorders, Arch. Gen. Psychiatry **16**:134, 1967.

32. Ilfeld, F.: Characteristics of current social stressors, Psychol. Rep. **39**:1231, 1976.

33. Ilfield, F.: Current social stressors and symptoms of depression, Am. J. Psychiatry **134**:161, Feb. 1977.

34. Jacob, T. et al.: Role expectation and role performance in distressed and normal couples, Abnormal Psychol. **87**:286, 1978.

35. Jamison, K. et al.: Clouds and silver linings: positive experiences associated with primary affective disorders, Am. J. Psychiatry **137**(2):198, Feb. 1980.

36. Klerman, G.: Overview of affective disorders. In Freedman, A., Kaplan, H., and Sadock, B., editors: Comprehensive textbook of psychiatry, vol. 2, Baltimore, 1980, The Williams & Wilkins Co.

37. Kübler-Ross, E.: On death and dying, New York, 1969, The Macmillan Publishing Co., Inc.

38. LeMasters, E.: Parenthood as crisis, Marriage Family Living **19**:352, 1957.

39. Levitt, E., and Lubin, B.: Depression: concepts, controversies, and some new facts, New York, 1975, Springer Publishing Co., Inc.

40. Lewinsohn, P., and Amenson, C.: Some relations between pleasant and unpleasant mood related activities and depression, J. Abnormal Psychol. **87**:644, 1978.

41. Lewinsohn, P., Youngren, M., and Grosscup, S.: Reinforcement and depression. In Depue, R., editor: The psychobiology of the depressive disorders, New York, 1979, Academic Press, Inc.

42. Lindemann, E.: Symptomatology and management of acute grief, Am. J. Psychiatry **101**:141, Sept. 1944.

43. Maddison, D., and Walker, W.: Factors affecting the outcome of conjugal bereavement, Br. J. Psychiatry **113**:1057, 1967.

44. Mayo, J., O'Connell, R., and O'Brien, J.: Families of manic-depressive patients: effect of treatment, Am. J. Psychiatry **136**:1535, 1979.

45. McLean, P.: Remediation of skills and performance deficits in depression. In Clarkin, J., and Glazer, H., editors: Depression: behavioral and directive intervention strategies, New York, 1981, Garland Publishing, Inc.

46. Myers, J., Lindenthal, J., and Pepper, M.: Life events, social integration, and psychiatric symptomatology, J. Health and Soc. Behav. **16**:421, 1975.

47. Noyes, R.: Book review of grief and mourning in cross-cultural perspective, Am. J. Psychiatry **135**:137, 1978.

48. Parens, H., McConville, B., and Kaplan, S.: Prediction of frequency of illness from the response to separation, Psychosom. Med. **28**:162, 1966.

49. Parkes, C.: Bereavement: studies of grief in adult life, New York, 1972, International Universities Press.

50. Parkes, C., and Brown, R.: Health after bereavement: a controlled study of young Boston widows and widowers, Psychosom. Med. **34**:449, 1972.

51. Paykel, E. et al.: Life events and depression, Arch. Gen. Psychiatry **21**:753, 1969.

52. Rapoport, R., and Rapoport, R.: Dual career families, London, 1971, Penguin Books, Ltd.

53. Rapoport, R., and Rapoport, R.: Early and later experiences as determinants of adult behavior: married women's family and career patterns, Br. J. Sociol. **22**:16, March 1971.

54. Rehm, L.: A self-control therapy program for treatment of depression. In Clarkin, J., and Glazer, H., editors: Depression: behavioral and directive intervention strategies, New York, 1981, Garland Publishing, Inc.

55. Robertson, J., and Robertson, J.: Young children in brief separation: a fresh look, Psychoanal. Study Child **26**:264, 1971.

56. Robins, E., and Guze, S.: Establishment of diagnostic validity in psychiatric illness, Am. J. Psychiatry **126**:983, 1970.

57. Rosenblatt, P., Walsh, R., and Jackson, D.: Grief and mourning in cross-cultured perspective, New Haven, Conn., 1976, HRAF Press.

58. Rosenfield, S.: Sex differences in depression: do women always have higher rates? J. Health Soc. Behav. **21**:33, March 1980.

59. Sachs, M.: Running therapy for the depressed client, Topics Clin. Nurs. **3**(2):77, 1981.

60. Secunda, S., editor: The depressive disorders, special report 1973, U.S. Department of Health, Education, and Welfare, National Institute of Mental Health.

61. Seligman, M.: Helplessness: on depression, development and death, San Francisco, 1975, W.H. Freeman and Co., Publishers.

62. Smith, A., and Brandt, S.: Physical activity: a tool in promoting mental health, J. Psychiatr. Nurs. **17**(11):24, 1979.

63. Spitz, R.: Anaclitic depression, Psychoanal. Study Child **2**:313, 1942.

64. Stuart, G.W.: Role strain and depression: a causal inquiry, J. Psychosoc. Nurs. **19**(12):20, 1981.

65. Van Servellen, G.: Women treating women for depression, J. Psychosoc. Nurs. **19**(8):22, 1981.

66. Van Servellen, G., and Dull, L.: Group psychotherapy for depressed women: a model, J. Psychosoc. Nurs. **19**(8):25, 1981.

67. Warheit, G.: Life events, coping stress, and depressive symptomatology, Am. J. Psychiatry **136**(4B):502, 1979.
68. Weiss, J. et al.: Neurotransmitters and helplessness: a chemical bridge to depression, Psychol. Today, **7**:57, Dec., 1974.
69. Weissman, M., and Klerman, G.: Sex differences and the epidemiology of depression, Arch. Gen. Psychiatry **34**:98, Jan. 1977.
70. Wender, P.: On necessary and sufficient conditions in psychiatric exploration, Arch. Gen. Psychiatry **16**:41, 1967.
71. Winokur, G.: Heredity in the affective disorders. In Anthony, E., and Benedek, T., editors: Depression and human existence, Boston, 1975, Little, Brown & Co.

Annotated suggested readings

Akiskal, H., and McKinney, W.: Overview of recent research in depression, Arch. Gen. Psychiatry **32**:285, 1975.

This article translates data from psychodynamic, sociobehavioral, and neurobiological research into a clinically meaningful framework. Ten models of depression are described and an integrated model is presented that incorporates and synthesizes findings from different schools. This is advanced reading with an extensive bibliography for the interested nurse.

American Psychiatric Association: Diagnostic and statistical manual of mental disorders, ed. 3, Washington, D.C., 1980, The Association.

This is a required reference text for all psychiatric nurses. It contains the categories and codes of axes I and II and the complete text and criteria related to each of the categories associated with medically diagnosed psychiatric health problems.

Authier, J., Authier, K., and Lutey, B.: Clinical management of the tearfully depressed patient: communication skills for the nurse practitioner, J. Psychiatr. Nurs. **17**(2):34, 1979.

The first section of this article deals with the management of the patient who has a legitimate reason to be depressed, followed by a discussion of the more complex management of "illegitimate" tears in a categorization of personality types.

Baker, B., and Lynn, M.: Psychiatric nursing consultation: the use of an inservice model to assist nurses in the grief process, J. Psychiatr. Nurs. **17**(5):15, 1979.

The authors relate an account of their consultation with medical-surgical nurses in relation to their feelings of caring for the dying via the development, implementation, and evaluation of an inservice model.

Beck, A., Rush, A., Shaw, B., and Emery, G.: Cognitive therapy of depression, New York, 1979, The Guilford Press.

This primary reference describes cognitive therapy and combines both theory and clinical practice. It is necessary reading for nurses who wish to utilize this approach.

Belmaker, R., and von Praag, H.: Mania: an evolving concept.

This text surveys the rapidly developing area of primary affective disorders. Good reference source.

Bowlby, J.: Processes of mourning, Int. J. Psychoanal. **42**:317, 1961.

Bowlby describes the object loss model of depression and his stages of mourning in this important article. This is a "classic" in the field and highly recommended as a primary reference.

Clarkin, J., and Glazer, H.: Depression: behavioral and directive intervention strategies, New York, 1981, Garland Publishing, Inc.

This highly recommended text is quite comprehensive in behavioral intervention in depression. Its four parts include assessment of depression, major behavioral models, clinical treatment strategies (including suicide and somatic treatments), and special groups (such as children and the elderly).

Cohen, S.: Helping depressed patients in general nursing practice, Am. J. Nurs. **77**:1007, 1977.

This is a programmed instruction unit included in this listing because of its focus on the general nursing setting and its use of numerous clinical examples. It is recommended for the beginning student or practitioner.

Dealing with death, Am. J. Nurs. **76**:1486, 1976.

This is a series of three articles discussing adaptation to death. Two are particularly good—"The Grieving Patient and Family" and "The Grieving Nurse." The last article contends that nurses who work with the dying also go through a grieving process and explains this process within the stages of dying described by Kübler-Ross.

Engel, G.: Grief and grieving, Am. J. Nurs. **64**:93, Sept. 1964.

This article is a recommended reading because in it the author describes his stages of grieving in some detail.

Freihofer, P., and Felton, G.: Nursing behaviors in bereavement: an exploratory study, Nurs. Res. **25**:332, Sept.-Oct. 1976.

Terminally ill patients and their families were studied to determine nursing behaviors that offer greatest support, comfort, and ease of suffering to loved ones. The behaviors were categorized and have implications for nursing care.

Gaylin, W.: Feelings: our vital signs, New York, 1979, Harper & Row, Publishers, Inc.

This text attempts to analyze and describe feelings. The author contends that feelings are important and serve a purpose; they provide for our survival both as individuals and as a species.

Goldberg, C.: Therapeutic tasks: strategies for change, Perspect. Psychiatr. Care **18**(4):156, 1980.

The value of therapeutic action-focused tasks is well described in this article through the effective use of clinical examples. Practical, pertinent, and clearly written by the nurse author.

Gordon, M.: Final payments, New York, 1978, Random House, Inc.

This recent novel describes the reaction of a young woman to the death of her father. It explores the nature of loss, guilt, love, and friendship in a perceptive and honest way.

Guest, J.: Ordinary people, New York, 1976, Ballantine Books, Inc.

This popular novel, which was later made into a movie, describes the moving story of a family's response to the death of a son. The issues of depression, self-concept, and family relationships are woven throughout this sensitive story.

Harris, E.: The dexamethasone suppression test, Am. J. Nurs. **82**:784, 1982.

This brief article describes the indications and procedures related to this recently developed test for somatically treatable depression.

Hauser, M., and Feinberg, D.: An operational approach to the delayed grief and mourning process, J. Psychiatr. Nurs., **14**:29, July, 1976.

The authors describe Bowlby's phases of mourning and identify psychological components related to each phase. They identify appropriate nursing interventions based on their model. It is a well-written article with direct clinical application.

Jackson, P.: Chronic grief, Am. J. Nurs. **74**:1288, 1974.

This article describes the role of the nurse in working with parents who give birth to a defective child. In the case presentation the parents are helped to work through the stages of grief over an extended period of time.

Jacobson, A.: Melancholy in the 20th century: causes and prevention, J. Psychiatr. Nurs. **18**(7):11, 1980.

The nurse author examines the detrimental aspects of depression for both individuals and society. Her unique contribution, however, is her focus on primary prevention activities that may be implemented by nurses. Well researched, well conceived, and well written.

Kiev, A.: Somatic manifestations of depressive disorders, Princeton, N.J., 1974, Excerpta Medica Foundation.

This brief text reviews the various physical behaviors associated with depression. Individual chapters discuss the gastrointestinal tract, sleep, sexual dysfunction, and pain.

Lamperelli, P., and Smith, J.: The grieving process of adoption: an application of principles and techniques, J. Psychiatr. Nurs. **17**(10):24, 1979.

This clinical article focuses on the grief process at work in surrendering a baby for adoption, along with some of the problems that are encountered and what can be done to help the unmarried mother in her grief work. Good application of theory.

Lindemann, E.: Symptomatology and management of acute grief, Am. J. Psychiatry **101**:141, Sept. 1944.

In this "classic" article Lindemann describes the course and management of normal and abnormal grief reactions on the basis of his observations of 101 patients. It is an important work in the study of grieving.

Mandel, H.: Nurses' feelings about working with dying, Am. J. Nurs. **81**:1194, 1981.

The value of this brief article is in the elaboration of feelings and attitudes expressed by nurses who are working with the chronically and terminally ill. These feelings can serve as a good starting point for increasing one's self-awareness and in stimulating the need for support systems for nurses working with the dying.

Parkes, C.: Bereavement, New York, 1972, International Universities Press.

This book describes the effect of bereavement on health, common reactions to bereavement, actions used to postpone grief, the function of anger, one's search for a new identity, and abnormal forms that grief may take. It views bereavement as a transition and considers some factors that affect the course of grief. It is easy reading and clinical examples are described throughout.

Rankin, N.: Name that feeling! An innovative teaching tool, J. Psychosoc. Nurs. **19**(12):37, 1981.

This article describes a simple but innovative teaching strategy for promoting awareness of different kinds of feelings to beginning nursing students.

Scarf, M.: Unfinished business: pressure points in the lives of women, New York, 1980, Doubleday and Co., Inc.

Using 10 case studies, the journalist author describes the causes and consequences of female depression. Readable and provocative.

Schneider, J.: Hopelessness and helplessness, J. Psychiatr. Nurs. **18**(3):12, 1980

The concepts of hopelessness and helplessness are thoroughly described in this article along with the effect of the concepts on patients in a general hospital setting. Valuable suggestions for nursing intervention are proposed and demonstrated in case examples.

Schoenberg, B. et al., editors: Bereavement: its psychosocial aspects, New York, 1975, Columbia University Press.

This is an excellent collection of essays that uses a multidisciplinary approach. Bereavement is examined in light of sociological research, clinical studies, and theoretical designs. Support systems, the role of health professionals, and therapeutic interventions are also described. It is a useful reference for nurses.

Stotland, E.: The psychology of hope, San Francisco, 1969, Jossey-Bass, Inc., Publishers.

This text presents a theory of motivation and hope. It explores the relationship of hope to action, anxiety, and psychosis and outlines a form of therapy using the element of hope.

Van Servellen, G., and Dull, L.: Group psychotherapy for depressed women: a model, J. Psychosoc. Nurs. **19**(8):25, 1981.

The authors present a useful format for group treatment of depressed women along with a research design to evaluate the effectiveness of therapy.

Walker, K. et al.: Social support networks and the crisis of bereavement, Soc. Sci. Med. **11**:35, 1977.

Selected social network and urban community literature is reviewed, and various models of support structure are assessed in terms of their adequacy in meeting the diverse needs of the bereaved.

CHAPTER 10

SELF-DESTRUCTIVE BEHAVIOR

Out, out brief candle!
Life's but a walking shadow, a poor player
That struts and frets his hour upon the stage
And then is heard no more. It is a tale
Told by an idiot, full of sound and fury,
Signifying nothing.

William Shakespeare, Macbeth, Act V

Learning objectives

After studying this chapter, the student
will be able to:

- compare and contrast indirect and direct self-destructive behavior.

- identify individuals who represent a high suicide risk.

- assess the behaviors of an individual that are indicative of direct or indirect self-destructive activity.

- describe the continuum of coping responses related to self-enhancing/self-destructive behavior.

- analyze the role of anxiety and depression in the development of self-destructive behavior.

- identify biopsychosocial stressors that predispose the individual to or precipitate the initiation of self-destructive behavior.

- differentiate suicide threats and attempts as related to the concepts of ambivalence and hostility.

- discuss behaviors characteristic of the indirect self-destructive behaviors of obesity, anorexia nervosa, and noncompliance with a prescribed health care plan.

- analyze coping mechanisms related to indirect and attempted direct self-destructive behavior.

- formulate nursing diagnoses relative to direct and indirect self-destructive behavior.

- mutually establish long- and short-term nursing care goals that take into account the need to protect the patient from self-destructive impulses and promote self-enhancing behavior.

- *intervene with self-destructive patients to protect the patient, increase self-esteem, reinforce healthy coping mechanisms, promote insight into the underlying problem, mobilize environmental resources, and teach the patient and significant others about the identified problem and recommended health care plan.*

- *utilize supervision to analyze her own feelings relative to self-destructive behavior.*

- *evaluate the effectiveness of nursing interventions and modify the plan of care.*

- *identify suggested readings for further study.*

Continuum of self-enhancing to self-destructive responses

Many daily activities involve an element of risk. For instance, riding in an automobile exposes a person to the risk of physical injury if the car is involved in an accident. Even if no accident occurs, there is increased stress from exposure to hazardous situations that creates anxiety and requires the use of coping mechanisms. As another example, choice of diet may indicate a willingness to take risks. A family that lives on a farm and uses organic methods to raise most of their food is exposed to a much lower level of potentially harmful chemicals than the family that usually eats commercially prepared foods.

Since life is characterized by a pervasive element of risk, each individual must choose the amount of potential danger to which he is willing to expose himself. Sometimes these choices are conscious and rational. For instance, the elderly person who decides to stay in the house on an icy day has chosen not to risk falling and possibly fracturing a bone. Other risk-taking behavior is unconsciously determined. The soldier who volunteers for a suicide mission is probably unaware of his motivation, although if asked, he would be likely to cite patriotism or concern for his comrades. Most people go through life accepting some risks as part of their daily routine, while carefully avoiding others. The person who constantly takes chances while driving may refuse to fly in an airplane because he feels unsafe.

Even though life is risky, there is a norm in most societies that defines the degree of danger to which the person may expose himself. This norm varies according to the age, sex, socioeconomic status, and occupation of the individual. For instance, there is great reluctance in contemporary American society to allow women to participate in "contact" sports with men. Although this attitude is undoubtedly determined by many factors, the reason that is usually given is that women are not strong enough to compete with men and would get hurt. In general, the very young, the old, and women are viewed as needing to be protected from harm.

There is great ambivalence toward those who engage in potentially self-destructive behavior. Some risk takers are greatly admired, particularly athletes, members of the military services, those with dangerous occupations, and those who place themselves in danger to help others. At the same time, feelings of admiration may be accompanied by fear and perplexity about the danger-seeking behavior. The varying attitudes toward cigarette smoking provide another example of cultural ambivalence. On one hand, smoking is viewed as mature behavior, denoting sophistication and social acceptability; on the other, it is seen as socially alienating, immature, and inconsiderate of the needs of others.

Indirect self-destructive behavior

Although there has been an awareness of the range of self-destructive behavior from subtle to overt, until recently, there has been little systematic attention given to the covert and generally long-term end of the continuum. Farberow[8] has differentiated indirect from direct self-destructive behavior. Direct self-destructive behavior (DSDB) includes any form of suicidal activity. The intent of this behavior is death and the individual is aware of this as the desired outcome. Indirect self-destructive behavior (ISDB) is any activity that is detrimental to the physical well-being of the person and potentially has the outcome of death. However, the person is unaware of this potential and will generally deny it if confronted. Examples of ISDB that will be used in this chapter include eating disorders, such as obesity, anorexia nervosa, and bulimia, and noncompliance with medical treatment. Abuse of alcohol and drugs is also self-destructive in nature. This behavioral disruption is discussed in detail in Chapter 14. Other ISDBs identified by Farberow[8] include cigarette smoking, automobile accidents, self-mutilation, gambling, criminal activity and socially deviant behavior, stress-seeking behavior, and participation in high-risk sports.

ISDB may be differentiated from DSDB, or suicidal behavior, by its duration and by the individual's awareness of the purpose of the behavior. ISDB is usually long term and repetitive, whereas suicidal behavior, if not interrupted, leads rapidly to death. This distinction differentiates between the individual who is involved in numerous traffic accidents as the result of drinking and driving (ISDB) and the person who is killed while sober by driving his car into a wall at a high rate of speed (DSDB). Although the latter situation is usually classified as accidental, it may be assumed that many one-car accidental deaths are really suicidal in nature.

The other cardinal feature of ISDB is the person's use of the mechanism of denial, frequently accompanied by rationalization. If the dangerous nature of the behavior is recognized intellectually, it is not taken seriously. For instance, a hypertensive person may avoid salting food and adding salt while cooking, but eat potato chips, cured meats, and processed foods with a high sodium content. The patient may respond to confrontation about this behavior by saying, "I know I shouldn't eat those foods, but I feel good. A little bit once in a while can't hurt me." Another example is the anorexic person who is a student of nutrition but refuses to acknowledge her own starvation. This recognition of potential harmfulness without any change in behavior or actual denial of any danger is typical of the indirectly self-destructive person. It should also be recognized that denial can help the individual to function. Everyone engages in risky activities on a daily basis. Denial controls the anxiety that would interfere with activities of daily living if there was complete awareness of the dangers of everyday life. The failure of this mechanism may lead to maladaptive neurotic behaviors, such as phobias. The nurse must assess whether the individual is using denial in a healthy adaptive manner, or if it is interfering with adaptation and healthier coping mechanisms must be explored.

Nurses are frequently involved in caring for patients who are resistant to recommended self-care activities. It has been estimated that at least 50% of patients do not comply with health care providers' recommendations.[13] Since our society is characterized by an increasing elderly population, there is also an increase in the incidence of chronic diseases, such as cardiovascular disease, cancer, cerebrovascular accident, renal disease, and diabetes mellitus. The medical and nursing care of all these conditions requires self-care activities on the part of the patient. Diet, activity, and medications must be controlled. Good health practices are necessary to prevent complications or the development of additional illnesses. To support the patient in performing self-care, the nurse must understand the underlying emotional issues and assist the patient to deal with them.

Anorexia nervosa is a condition that occurs almost exclusively among young women. It has been described by Bruch as "the relentless pursuit of excessive thinness."[3] The incidence of anorexia nervosa in the United States has been increasing for the last 20 years. Prior to 1960, it was rarely seen. Recent estimates of prevalence are 1.3 to 2.4 per 100,000 total population. However, there have been reports of a prevalence of one in 250 in white females who are in the high-risk age group of 12 to 18 years old.[17] Most anorexic young women are members of upper or upper middle class families. It is extremely rare in situations where food is scarce and is also rarely seen in blacks.[17]

Another eating disorder that is similar in some respects to anorexia nervosa is *bulimia*. The bulimic patient experiences episodes of binge eating, frequently followed by vomiting. Binge eating is compulsive intake of food that is stopped only when the person vomits, experiences pain, runs out of food, or is interrupted. This disorder is also almost exclusively one of adolescent, white, socioeconomically secure, young women. It is differentiated from anorexia nervosa by the fact that severe weight loss is not generally seen and the individual is well aware that her behavior is abnormal.[17] Bulimic patients are usually able to maintain a more normal weight by alternating binging and vomiting or by eating very little between binges.

The third eating disorder that is indirectly self-destructive is *obesity*. There is no generally accepted definition of obesity. A guideline is that obesity is considered to be present when the person weighs more than 20% over his ideal weight; overweight is defined as 10% above the ideal weight. The problems with this criterion are that height and weight charts have not been developed scientifically, and individual characteristics, such as proportion of muscle mass to total body weight are not considered. When it is performed correctly, measurement of skinfold thickness over the midtriceps area is a more accurate way to determine the presence of obesity.[17] It has been estimated that one third of

FIG. 10-1
Prevalence of overweight in males and females from infancy to age 69.

the population of the United States is overweight. Obesity is sometimes described as a disorder that is characteristic of an affluent society. In reality, there is a higher prevalence of overweight and obesity among the poor in affluent *(wealthy)* societies. Low-calorie foods, such as meat, seafood, fruits, and vegetables, are expensive. Poor people tend to eat diets that are high in carbohydrates, leading to weight gain. Obesity is also related to low activity levels. Fig. 10-1 illustrates the prevalence of overweight and obesity by age and sex in the United States.[16] No definite correlation has been found between obesity and educational level. However, there is a lower prevalence among people who achieve a higher socioeconomic status than that of their parents. The inverse is also true. In terms of the major religious groups, prevalence is highest among Jews, followed by Roman Catholics, and lowest among Protestants. Obesity is clearly a major public

TABLE 10-1. Risk factors for suicidal behavior*

Factor	High risk	Low risk
Age	Over 45 years or adolescent	25 to 45 years or under 12 years
Sex	Male	Female
Marital status	Divorced, separated, or widowed	Married
Socialization	Isolated	Socially active
Occupation	Professional workers (medicine, dentistry, or law) or student	Blue collar workers
Employment	Unemployed	Employed
Physical illness	Chronically or terminally ill	No serious medical problems
Mental illness	Depression, delusions, or hallucinations	Personality disorder
Drug and alcohol use	Intoxicated and/or addicted	Neither intoxicated nor addicted
Previous attempts	At least one	None
Plan	Definite plan specified	Vague plan
Method	Violent means: shooting, hanging, or jumping	Nonviolent means: drugs, poison, or carbon monoxide
Availability of means	Readily available	Not yet obtained

*Risk factors are relative and intended as a guide to assessment. *Low* risk never means *no* risk.

health problem that is a significant risk factor for the development of other serious health problems, including heart disease, hypertension, some forms of cancer, and diabetes mellitus.

Direct self-destructive behavior

The ultimate level of self-destructiveness is suicidal behavior. The stigma attached to suicide makes it difficult to determine the magnitude of the problem. The reported suicide rate in the United States in 1975 was 12.6 per 100,000 population. The rate for males was 18 per 100,000 and that for females was 6.6.[20] The United States ranks fifteenth of thirty developed nations that collect statistics on cause of death. In 1970, the countries with the highest rates were as follows: Hungary (33.1), Czechoslovakia (23.9), Austria (22.3), Finland (21.6), and Sweden (21.5). The five lowest were Greece (3.5), Italy (5.4), Israel (6.4), The Netherlands (7.4), and Norway (8.1).[20]

Many deaths that appear to be accidental may in reality be suicidal. Inferences about the motivation for accidental death can sometimes be made based on a "psychological autopsy." This is a retrospective review of the individual's be-

havior for the time preceding his death and is accomplished by tracing the person's activities and interviewing those with whom the dead person had contact just prior to death.

Suicidology has become an important subspecialty in psychiatry. Specialists in this field have done much work in an effort to identify groups of people who are at risk for suicide. It has been possible to develop profiles of high-risk groups. In general, males commit suicide more frequently than females (a ratio of about 3:1), and women attempt suicide more frequently than men (also about 3:1).[19] Suicide rates also vary with age. For example, the rate for white men increases steadily with age. In contrast, the rate for white women peaks at age 45 to 54 and then declines. In general, married people have the lowest rates, those never married are next, and divorced or widowed people have the highest rate, with the exception of older, never-married white men.[15] Table 10-1 summarizes the risk factors associated with suicidal behavior.

Theories of self-destructive behavior are intertwined with those of self-concept and alterations in mood. Understanding of the behaviors to be discussed in this chapter will be enhanced by careful study of Chapters 8 and 9. To con-

FIG. 10-2
Continuum of self-enhancing to self-destructive behaviors.

template or initiate destruction of the self, one must have low regard for the self. Low self-esteem leads to depression, which is always present to some extent in self-destructive behavior. The range of behaviors related to the self that includes self-destructive behavior is illustrated in Fig. 10-2.

It should be noted that the levels of behavior in the continuum overlap. This indicates that growth-promoting risk-taking behavior may be self-enhancing. For instance, the young girl who learns and excels at gymnastics is building her self-esteem and projecting a positive self-concept. However, if she attempts to do stunts for which she is not prepared and does not take safety precautions, her behavior becomes indirectly self-destructive. Similarly, there are times when ISDB may merge into DSDB. For instance, a diabetic who has never complied completely with his prescribed diet and medication regimen may become very discouraged and intentionally take an overdose of insulin. The nurse must be aware of this tendency and be alert to subtle shifts in the mood and behavior of self-destructive patients.

 Stressors

Self-destructive behavior may result from almost any stress that is experienced by the individual as overwhelming. Therefore stressors are to some extent individualized, as is the person's ability to tolerate stress. All self-destructive behaviors may be viewed as attempts to escape from life situations that have become uncomfortable or intolerable. Anxiety is therefore central to the cause of self-destructive behavior.

The anxiety that is associated with a deliberate attempt at self-destruction is overwhelming. It

is difficult to imagine if it has not been experienced. Most people cringe from contemplating their own deaths, much less initiating the destruction of the self. In fact, Shneidman[19] believes that self-death is experienced differently from the death of another, since self-death literally cannot be experienced. Therefore, in a sense, the person who destroys himself actually destroys everything else *but* himself.

In contrast, people who are engaged in gradually self-destructive behavior tend to deny their eventual deaths, usually believing that they can assume control at any time. This fantasy of being able to control, although it alleviates anxiety, also helps to perpetuate the behavior. Such activities as overeating may also decrease anxiety and thus are difficult to change. The anxiety that leads to self-destructive behavior may evolve from a variety of sources: physiological, psychological, and sociocultural.

Stressors affecting indirect self-destructive behavior

PHYSIOLOGICAL STRESSORS. There is no definitive research indicating a direct relationship between a biological factor and most forms of ISDB. Some forms of obesity do seem to be biologically determined. Endocrine disorders, such as hypothyroidism, hypercortisolism (Cushing's syndrome), the Stein-Leventhal syndrome, and hypogonadism[6] result in obesity. The latter three disorders are quite rare, and known physiological stressors account for very few instances of obesity. Endocrinological disorders have been explored in conjunction with anorexia nervosa. However, most studies have been done after the condition is well advanced and may be the result, rather than the cause, of starvation. There is some suggestion that dopamine may play a role in the development of this disorder. Dopamine is known to be an appetite depressant, so elevated dopamine levels could contribute to anorexia nervosa.[17] However, the fact that most anorexics experience extreme hunger would tend to negate this theory.

Familial tendencies toward obesity and overweight have been identified. However, it is premature to assume that this is due to heredity. It may be more related to sociocultural dietary patterns. It is difficult to identify a familial tendency for anorexia nervosa because the disorder has been so rare in the past that there are few longitudinal data on the children of anorexic women.

Research has revealed that overweight and obese people tend to have more fat cells than thin people. Fat cells develop during the last trimester of intrauterine life, the first 6 to 8 months after birth, and again during the adolescent growth spurt.[17] Children who gain weight at these critical times are at greater risk for obesity as adults. These data have implications for health education and primary prevention, particularly for nurses working in community health settings or schools. It has also been determined that there is a relationship between weight and activity level. Overweight people have been observed to be less active, even when engaged in sports, than people of normal weight.[17]

PSYCHOLOGICAL STRESSORS. Psychologically, one of the antecedents of self-destructive behavior is depression. Filstead[10] has identified that despair is usually present when ISDB occurs. He describes despair as "a psychosocial state that people experience when they are trying to resolve what has become a serious personal problem . . . and realize that there does not appear to be any way to resolve it."[10] The ISDB may be serving as a defense against underlying despair. For instance, a person who is obese may overeat to overcome anxiety related to an inadequate self-concept. However, the behavior is self-defeating and does not resolve the problem. As self-dissatisfaction increases, despair may break through into awareness. If this happens, the person is at high risk for suicidal behavior.

Low self-esteem and depression contribute to the development of anorexia nervosa. This problem occurs at a point in psychosexual development that is characterized by emotional upheaval. Adolescents must establish a personal identity and become independent of parental control. Bruch[3] believes that anorexic behavior may follow a new experience that is viewed as threatening or may even be precipitated by a casual remark that is perceived as being critical of the patient's weight. She observes that, "they act as if no one had ever told them that developing curves and roundness is part of normal puberty."[3] Young women who are anorexic reject their growing feminine body configuration and strive for a childlike smallness. This lack of acceptance of the self leads to low self-esteem and depression that contributes to the continuation of the problem. It is interesting that obese young people may reflect the opposite pole of the same problem. They avoid the threat of growing sexuality by becoming unattractive and maintain a regressive childlike role by relating to the world through food. Parents may perpetuate the problems of children who have eating disorders by reinforcing dependency through their involvement in trying to persuade the child to eat or not to eat.

Adult obese persons are also frequently dependent people who feel insecure. Food may represent the security they felt during infancy. Comparisons have been made to alcoholism and the alcoholic's use of alcohol to protect him from the stresses of life. Alienation of others from the obese person often results in loneliness, adding to insecurity and depression, which leads to continued overeating.

Another issue that is prominent in relationship to ISDB is one of control. Whatever the risky behavior that is being performed, it is under the control of the actor. In addition, there are frequently power struggles between the person who is performing the behavior and significant others who recognize the perilous nature of the behavior and try to change it. For instance, the parents of anorexic patients become very worried as their daughter becomes more and more emaciated. As they try to persuade or force her to eat, she becomes more and more determined to circumvent their efforts. If forced to eat, the anorexic will induce vomiting, take laxatives or diuretics, or exercise frantically, thus continuing to maintain control. The control issue is clearly reflected in this statement by Annie Ciseaux, the pseudonym of a nurse who is also anorexic: "The moment I surrendered myself to my parents' wishes that I eat—in other words when I refused to be responsible any more for what I was to become: a fat powerless person—I felt my self-esteem evaporate."[5]

Obese people again reflect the opposite side of the same behavioral pattern. As others try to persuade them to lose weight, they control the situation by sneaking food. This behavior leads to remorse, which causes anxiety, resulting in further eating. The motivation for dieting must come from within the dieter if weight loss is to occur.

Control is also a theme that is relevant to noncompliant behavior. The person who has a chronic illness often feels betrayed by his body, which, in the past, has been under his control. Compliance with a therapeutic regimen may be perceived as an admission that a problem exists and that the person cannot manage the problem without help. Refusal to perform required self-care activities returns a sense of control. As long as overt symptoms do not occur or can be ignored, the person maintains an illusion of health. As in the situations described, significant others may become concerned about the implications of noncompliant behavior. However, if they try to intervene, the sense of loss of control is increased and the person may become even more resistant. Powerful emotions, including anger, fear, and depression, underlie the overt behavior of self-control. If the person is not assisted to cope with these feelings, the ISDB will continue, or it may progress to more directly suicidal behavior.

SOCIOCULTURAL STRESSORS. Sociocultural factors are believed to play an important role in the development of eating disorders. Family eating patterns are transmitted to children beginning even before birth. The nutritional status of the mother has a direct effect on the health of the infant. Sociocultural factors influence dietary patterns. Ethnic background may affect a mother's decision to breast feed or bottle feed. It has been demonstrated that bottle fed babies have a higher tendency to be overweight. Ethnicity also has an influence on food preferences. People of Italian descent become accustomed to high carbohydrate diets, whereas people with Oriental backgrounds tend to consume more seafood and vegetables. Economic status also affects diet. In affluent societies, obesity tends to be more prevalent among the poor. Anorexia nervosa, on the other hand, occurs more frequently in the upper middle and upper classes.

Powers[17] has applied Minuchin's description of psychosomatogenic families to the understanding of the eating disorders. The characteristics of this type of family include a special configuration and functioning, child involvement in parental conflicts, and the presence of a physiological vulnerability in the child. There are four characteristics of the family configuration. The first is enmeshment. This means that individuality is lost within the identity of the family group. Autonomy is not encouraged. Role confusion results from lack of clear boundaries among family members. Emotionally, there is overinvolvement and intrusion on the thoughts and feelings of other members. The second characteristic is overprotectiveness and the third is rigidity. Finally, there is conflict avoidance, which results in a lack of resolution of conflicts. Conflict may be denied, or there may be continuous fighting without addressing the real problem. Family conflicts are focused on the problematic member, thus avoiding confrontation with the real issue. The true conflict may really lie between the parents, but is acted out by the physiologically vulnerable child.[17]

Disorders of eating are also influenced by the cultural definition of ideal body image. In the contemporary United States, thinness is valued, particularly for women. Pubertal girls who begin to develop rounded body contours may interpret this as fatness and attempt to counteract the effects of normal growth and development by dieting. This behavior sometimes leads to anorexia nervosa. The idealization of slimness can also assist the anorexic girl to justify her behavior by entering modeling, the theater, or the dance.

Sociocultural factors also influence the occurrence of noncompliance with treatment. Leventhal[14] points out that most people develop their concept of the experience of illness through childhood episodes of acute infectious diseases. Treatment is instituted to cure the illness and when the symptoms disappear the treatment is discontinued. This conceptualization is not applicable to chronic illness, but is still the expectation of many patients. Many chronic diseases are characterized by episodic exacerbations of overt symptoms during a long-term covert disease process. If the acute illness model is applied, the patient assumes that the periods of time when no symptoms are experienced are times of wellness. Therefore, treatment is unnecessary. Leventhal[14] and others have also found that patients have difficulty identifying symptoms of chronic health problems, such as hypertension, except when they are severe. These findings have serious implications for the health care of the chronically ill.

Chronic illness also does not fit the pattern of sick role behavior that is acceptable in our society. The sick person is expected to acknowledge his illness, comply with treatment, and then recover. When recovery does not take place, the lack of conformity with cultural norms regarding sickness can lead to guilt and contribute to reluctance to comply with health care needs. Patient education programs must provide adequate information about the nature of the health problem, but must also recognize and attend to the patient's emotional responses to the illness experience.

Stressors affecting direct self-destructive behavior

When the sense of self-worth is extremely low, self-destructive behavior reaches its peak. It is at this point that suicidal behavior is likely to take place. Suicide implies a loss of the ability to value the self at all. This, in turn, may be related to unresolved grief, a perceived failure in life, or anger at the self.

Unexpressed anger at others may also lead a person to vent these feelings on himself. The individual may feel that his anger is not justified and then become guilty or may not be able to direct appropriate feelings outward. Since feelings must be attended to, the direction may be changed, with the self bearing the brunt of the attack. Some people with this problem may exhibit masochistic behavior. Masochism relates to the need to inflict pain on the self. Others may derogate the self or may underachieve. Still others may be so angry that they try to kill themselves.

Freudian theorists have viewed self-destructive behavior as the direction of hostile feelings toward an internalized love object. Ambivalence was an important component of the theory. More recently additional emphasis has been placed on the importance of the feelings of helplessness, hopelessness, and dependency in self-destructive behavior.

These feelings will be recognized as characteristics of depression. Individuals who are severely depressed are always suicidal risks. The extreme outcome of the self-directed anger that is believed to be present in depression is suicide. This is also the ultimate way of expressing hostility toward significant others. However, it is believed that there is always a kernel of hope that help will arrive, and someone will rescue the suicidal person by demonstrating that they really do care.

Bahra[2] has identified four psychological mechanisms that lead to suicide: ego destruction, ego withdrawal, displaced hostility, and response to hallucinations or delusions. Ego destruction refers to loss of self-esteem resulting in self-condemnation and guilt. This becomes a vicious circle that strikes at the integrity of the ego. Ego withdrawal occurs as the result of a buildup of stress. Withdrawal is difficult to maintain. Frequently the stress is a major loss, leading to a feeling of isolation. Displaced hostility is manifest in two different patterns: the first is a need to punish a significant other and the second is a hostile response to a real or imagined threat.

Another precursor to self-destructive behavior may be extreme confusion or personality disorganization.[2] This may be related to organic mental disorder, psychosis, or ingestion of hallucinogenic drugs. Many times, self-destructive behavior that is caused by one of these problems occurs inadvertently. The young person who is under the influence of PCP (phencyclidine) may feel invincible and walk in front of a truck or jump out a window. The psychotic person may harm himself because he is hearing voices that tell him to do so. The person may be quite unaware of the ultimate implications of his behavior.

Self-destructive behavior may also be related to a multiplicity of social and cultural factors. Durkheim,[7] in his pioneer study of suicidal behavior, identified three subcategories of suicide, based on the individual's motivation:

1. *Egoistic suicide* results from the individual's being poorly integrated into society.
2. *Altruistic suicide* results from obedience to customs and habit.
3. *Anomic suicide* results when society is unable to regulate the individual.

It is clear that in Durkheim's opinion the structure of society has a great influence on the individual and may either help to sustain him or lead him to destroy himself.

Choron[4] points out the importance of loneliness as a stressor related to suicide. This may refer either to the existential loneliness experienced by the psychotic individual or the loneliness that results from the loss of a loved one or self-esteem. He adds that interpersonal conflicts may also be stressors. Therefore the mere existence of relatedness is not sufficient to prevent suicides. The quality of the relationship must also be considered.

A related concept is the interpersonal frustration theory of suicide developed by Krauss.[13] This theorist agrees that interpersonal relationships are influential on suicidal behavior. He identified several propositions based on this belief:

1. Some people are more vulnerable to interpersonal frustration. These people tend to direct aggression inward and have a history of problems with interpersonal relationships.
2. The more meaningful the frustration is to the person, the more intense the feelings and the more serious the consequences.
3. Some cultures seem to produce greater occurrence of interpersonal frustration and thus have higher suicide rates.
4. Cultures that support positive interpersonal relationships tend to have lower suicide rates.

Patients with chronic, painful, or life-threatening illnesses may engage in self-destructive behavior. Frequently these people consciously choose to kill themselves. Quality of life becomes an issue that does, at times, supersede quantity of life. There may be an ethical dilemma for the nurse if she becomes aware of the patient's choice to engage in one of these behaviors. There are no easy answers to the question of how to resolve this conflict. Each nurse must do so according to her own belief system.

At this time it seems likely that self-destructive behavior is determined by a variety of factors, probably differing from one person to the next. For this reason it is extremely important to completely assess the patient's medical, psychological, and social history. Identification of probable causative factors leads to individualized planning for nursing care.

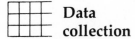

Data collection

Behaviors associated with indirect self-destructive behavior

The common characteristics of all varieties of ISDB are that it is progressively or potentially detrimental to the individual, the individual is intellectually aware that his behavior is risky, and he denies that he will suffer significant negative consequences from his behavior. This complex of behaviors will be examined for the examples of eating disorders, including overweight/obesity and anorexia nervosa/bulimia, and noncompliance with prescribed health care practices.

Overweight and *obesity* generally result from an imbalance between calories consumed and energy expended. The exception to this rule occurs when a disruption in endocrine functioning causes disordered metabolism. It has been theorized that people who have a larger number of fat cells have a greater tendency to obesity than those with fewer fat cells. Longitudinal research is in progress to validate this theory.[17] However, it has been established that fat babies have a greater tendency to be fat children, and fat children tend to become fat adolescents and adults. Hence good nutrition and encouragement of activity in infancy and childhood leads to a tendency for normal weight in adulthood.

Some obese people experience a body image distortion. This is more frequently a problem for people who have had early onset of overweight problems. The body image disturbance takes the form of an inaccurate perception of body appearance combined with a feeling of dislike for the self. An interesting feature of this behavior is that it tends to persist even after weight has been lost. Many formerly obese people continue to view themselves as fat, even though they are cognitively aware that their weight is normal.

Contributing to the negative self-concept of overweight people is the commonly encountered belief that overweight is evidence of a moral defect related to the sin of gluttony. It may be viewed as a controllable problem, by the patient as well as others, resulting in guilt that compounds the problem. Guilt and self-dislike may lead to sporadic self-denial interspersed with episodes of binge eating. Some people become night eaters.[17] These people are able to control their eating all day, but then consume huge numbers of calories during the evening or night. A similar pattern is that of stringent dieting alternating with overeating, leading to a fluctuating weight pattern. People who fall into this category are susceptible to fad diets that promise quick weight loss with minimum deprivation. They are also vulnerable to using drugs to aid weight loss. Fad diets and diet pills do not assist the person to change basic eating patterns. Thus future weight gain is inevitable because the person returns to old habits as soon as a few pounds have been lost.

Food has multiple meanings for people. To assist an obese individual, it is necessary to discover the meaning of food for that person. For some, food represents love, particularly the unconditional love of infancy. Giving up food is then experienced as a severe deprivation. For these people, eating may also serve as consolation and is indulged in when stress is increased.

Food also represents a cultural identity. People with strong ethnic ties find it hard to follow a diet that does not consider their cultural dietary patterns. There are also status implications associated with food and eating. The upper class places a great value on thinness, but also values indulgence, including appreciation of gourmet foods. The behavior that is seen relative to eating patterns and weight reflect the individual's perception of food and eating.

Perception is also an important aspect of the behavior of young women with *anorexia nervosa*. These people perceive that they are fat and literally starve themselves to achieve their goal of being thin. However, because of the distortion in body image that they experience, the goal is unattainable. Even when emaciated to the point that their appearance is skeletal, they will maintain that they are fat and persist in their attempt to lose weight.

Bruch[3] describes the typical anorexic process as beginning with a diet. Initially, the dieter experiences a sense of deprivation and difficulty in maintaining the restrictions. However, she then enters a stage of pride in her accomplishment and this perpetuates the behavior. At the same time, biological effects of starvation cause distortions in perception of body sensations. There is a heightening of sensory experience and a feeling that has been compared to intoxication. As the condition progresses, the patient begins to feel special and different because of her superhuman effort and extraordinary accomplishment. This results in her alienation and isolation from others who fail to understand her behavior and its meaning to her. She then becomes increasingly absorbed in her own world and her behavior assumes even greater importance to her.[3]

Anorexia nervosa is really a misnomer. Anorexia means lack of appetite. People with anorexia nervosa do experience hunger, and it is the victory over hunger that provides their reward. Anorexics are often fascinated with food and cooking, becoming students of nutrition. They may compulsively loiter in places where food is sold or served and watch other people eat. Their life becomes centered around food and the avoidance of eating. Anorexics go to extremes to avoid weight gain. They will induce vomiting, take diuretics and laxatives, and exercise strenuously. If they are forced to eat, these associated behaviors are exacerbated. Ciseaux described her discovery of vomiting to compensate for eating and her compulsion to vomit as soon as she had eaten.

In addition to the disturbance in body image, Bruch[3] describes decreased internal awareness and a sense of ineffectiveness as characteristics of anorexia nervosa. Decreased internal awareness refers to both emotional awareness and recognition of body sensations. Bruch believes that this results from the parents' failure to respond to the patient's needs during infancy. Since feeding was not directly related to hunger when she was an infant, the adolescent is also less aware of the relationship. The sense of ineffectiveness leads to the great need of anorexics to control at least one aspect of their lives. Hence, they focus all their attention on mastery of their weight and eating.[3]

As the disorder continues, signs of starvation become more evident. Amenorrhea occurs early in the course of the illness. It is now believed that the menarche is triggered by body size. Frisch[11] has identified that the mean body weight at menarche is 48 kg, and the weight range for 50% of girls is 43 to 51 kg. This research is being validated by the study of recovering anorexics. It was believed that amenorrhea

TABLE 10-2. Comparison of Feighner and DSM-III criteria for the diagnosis of anorexia nervosa

Feighner[9]	DSM-III*
Onset before 25 years old	Unrelenting fear of obesity
Loss of at least 25% of pre-illness weight	Disturbed body image
Distorted attitude toward food, eating, or weight	Loss of at least 25% of pre-illness weight; if under 18, expected weight gain from height and weight charts may be considered in calculating the 25%
No known medical illness causing weight loss	
No known psychiatric illness causing anorexia	Refusal to maintain weight within norms for age and height
At least two of the following:	No known physical illness
1. Amenorrhea	
2. Lanugo	
3. Bradycardia	
4. Episodic overactivity	
5. Episodic bulimia	
6. Vomiting (may be self-induced)	

*From American Psychiatric Association: Diagnostic and statistical manual of mental disorders, third edition, Washington, D.C., APA, 1980.

was a symptom of anorexia nervosa. It is now believed that it is secondary to weight loss. Early symptoms of anorexia nervosa are difficult to identify because the problem is usually not recognized until a significant weight loss has already occurred. Therefore initial assessment reveals symptoms of starvation as well as those of the anorexia itself.

Feighner[9] is another theorist who has described behaviors characteristic of anorexia nervosa. The six criteria include onset prior to age 25; weight loss of at least 25% of preillness weight; a distorted attitude toward food, eating, or weight, despite attempts to change this behavior; no known medical illness that would cause weight loss; no known psychiatric illness, such as depression, that would result in anorexia; and at least two of the behaviors of amenorrhea, lanugo, bradycardia, episodes of overactivity, episodes of bulimia, and vomiting (including self-induced). The behaviors identified by Feighner[9] are compared to those recommended for diagnosis of anorexia nervosa by DSM-III[1] in Table 10-2. The Feighner criteria are widely used in settings where anorexia nervosa research is taking place. Clinical example 10-1 illustrates behaviors that are characteristic of anorexia nervosa.

CLINICAL EXAMPLE 10-1

Ms. L was a 17-year-old, white unmarried woman who was admitted to a general hospital medical unit with a diagnosis of malnutrition. On admission, she was 5 feet, 5 inches (162.5 cm) tall and weighed 92 pounds (40.4 kg). She told Ms. B, her primary nurse, that she was on a special diet. She ate no breakfast, a carrot for lunch, and an apple for dinner. She also said that she would be jogging in the halls twice a day. It was very important that she maintain her exercise routine of running 10 miles daily. Physical assessment revealed the presence of lanugo, especially on the arms and buttocks, amenorrhea of 8 months' duration, and dry skin and mucous membranes. At lunchtime, Ms. L offered her tray to another patient, and then watched her while she ate. Soon after this, she began to jog up and down the hall.

Ms. B tried to communicate to Ms. L her concern that she was starving and could die. Ms. L said, "You sound just like my parents. You want me to be fat just like they do. You're jealous that I can control my body." When her parents visited, they were observed to be a well-dressed, upper middle class couple. They gave Ms. L a box of candy. She became furious, throwing the candy on the floor and demanding that they tell the nurses to give her the carrots and apples that she had requested. The parents told Ms. B that they were frustrated and frightened. They recognized that their daughter's irrational behavior could be fatal.

They said that she began to diet after her physical education teacher told her she was getting too large to compete in gymnastics. She had always been athletic and had won several prizes for her gymnastic ability. The L's were unconcerned at first, but then realized that she had nearly stopped eating. Coercion did not persuade her to eat. After many family arguments, they forced her to see the family physician who recommended hospitalization.

A diagnosis of anorexia nervosa was made, and Ms. L was transferred to the psychiatric unit for treatment.

The prognosis for anorexia nervosa is unclear at the present time. Powers reports a mortality of 10% to 20%.[17] Bruch believes that psychotherapists must identify the patient's concerns and avoid dealing exclusively with eating patterns if there is to be any long-term change.[3] Longitudinal studies are clearly needed to determine whether the body image distortions and disordered eating patterns are overcome when weight is gained.

People who are *noncompliant* with recommended health care activities are generally aware that they have chosen not to care for themselves. They usually have a reason for noncompliance, such as being asymptomatic, not being able to afford the treatment they need, not understanding the activity they are to perform, or not having time. These are rationalizations and help to alleviate the underlying anxiety that is really causing the noncompliance. Patients may also minimize the seriousness of their problems. Many chronic illnesses are characterized by long periods of stability, during which the person may not be aware of discomfort. This reinforces the noncompliant behavior.

Patients with chronic illnesses frequently hunt for health care providers who will prescribe other, less disruptive, treatment plans than the ones they are trying to avoid. They are susceptible to questionable practices such as miracle cures and faith healing in their search for the return of complete health. Patients who are receiving chemotherapy or radiation for cancer become frustrated with the side effects of the treatment. They are easily victimized by those who promote "cures" that involve no discomfort, but have no scientifically proven effectiveness. The popular literature is constantly reporting miraculous new treatments for chronic diseases. Most of these are invalid and lead to more suffering for those who become hopeful and are then disappointed.

The most prominent behavior associated with

noncompliance is refusal to acknowledge the seriousness of the health problem. This denial interferes with acceptance of treatment. However, at the same time, it protects the ego from the anxiety that recognition of impaired health will create. The greater the threat imposed by the illness, the greater will be the tenacity of resistance to treatment. Many chronic illnesses are associated with advancing age. Anxiety is increased because admission of illness also implies recognition that one is growing older. In a society that values youth, this behavior is not surprising. If one considers the resistance of middle-aged people to admitting that they need bifocals, refusal to acknowledge hypertension or diabetes mellitus should be anticipated. Societal attitudes reinforce the behavior of the noncompliant individual.

An unfortunate aspect of noncompliance is that guilt about not following health care recommendations may also interfere with obtaining regular care. The hypertensive person who has not been taking his medication will be reluctant to have his blood pressure checked because an elevated reading will undermine his defensive system. If the medical system treats these people like children and chastises them for their behavior, they feel even guiltier and are more reluctant to seek routine health care.

Noncompliant people are also struggling for control. Serious illness is often perceived as an attack on the person and a betrayal by his body. The patient needs to reassert his control and prove that he is still the master of his fate. The diabetic who cheats on his diet is gambling that he still has control over his body and can resist his problem by will. Most chronically ill people need to test the limits of their control and the validity of the prescribed self-care regimen. Clinical example 10-2 illustrates the problem of noncompliance with a prescribed health care regimen.

CLINICAL EXAMPLE 10-2

Ms. C was a 61-year-old, white married woman who had been in good health most of her life. She had three grown children who had left home and established their own families. She had been a homemaker since her marriage at age 19. She and her husband were both looking forward to his retirement in 6 months. They planned to buy a recreational vehicle and travel around the United States.

Ms. C visited the gynecologist regularly. She was very concerned about having annual Pap smears. Since she was receiving no other regular health care, the nurse practitioner who worked with this physician did a complete physical examination each time Ms. C was seen. On her most recent visit, laboratory studies revealed an elevated blood glucose level. She was then referred to an internist for a more thorough examination. The new physician hospitalized her for a short time. Her diagnosis was diabetes mellitus, adult onset. Ms. C was told that her condition was not serious and could be controlled by diet. She was 20 pounds (9 kg) overweight and was advised that she needed to lose the excess weight. Before discharge, she was instructed about her diet, how to test her urine, and about possible complications of diabetes. A public health nursing referral was made.

Ms. C was frightened about her condition but did not mention this because no one else seemed very concerned. When she first arrived home, she was conscientious about following her diet and testing her urine. She felt very well and was proud when she lost 5 pounds. When the public health nurse visited, she congratulated Ms. C on how well she was doing. As time went on, Ms. C began to wonder if she was really so sick. She had never felt ill. On her husband's birthday, she fixed a special dinner and baked a cake. She decided she deserved a reward for "being good" and did not follow her diet. She anxiously tested her urine at bedtime and it was negative. Then her son and his family visited the C's for a week. She fixed all their favorite foods and ate with them. She still felt fine and decided she did not need to test her urine. When it was time for her next checkup, she postponed calling the physician. She was very busy preparing for retirement travel.

The public health nurse contacted the physician's office to find out about the results of Ms. C's visit. When she discovered that Ms. C had not been seen, she made a home visit. Ms. C talked with her, but was not very receptive to her expressed concern. Ms. C said she would try to diet, but emphasized that she really felt well and was not sure if the diet was realistic in view of her travel plans. She agreed that she would see her physician immediately if she developed any signs of illness and that she would make an appointment for a physical examination at her convenience. The public health nurse's plan was to visit Ms. C again in a month. However, she noted that it was unlikely that Ms. C would observe her treatment plan until she experienced overt behavioral disruption related to her illness.

Behaviors associated with suicide (direct self-destructive behaviors)

Suicidal behavior is usually broken down into the categories of suicide threats, suicide attempts, and successful suicide. In addition, certain suicide attempts may be referred to as suicide gestures. The gesture is described as a suicide attempt that is primarily directed toward the goal of receiving attention rather than actual destruction of the self. Use of this term is questionable because it has acquired a pejorative connotation. The implication is often that it is *only* an attention-seeking behavior and should not be taken seriously. All suicidal behavior is serious, whatever the intent, and deserves the serious consideration of the nurse. Therefore suicide gestures will be included in the general category of suicide attempts.

The suicide threat may be veiled but usually occurs before overt suicidal activity takes place. Verbally, the suicidal person may make a statement such as "Will you remember me when I'm gone?" or "Take care of my family for me." If taken in the context of recent stressors and the person's life situation, statements such as these may be ominous. Nonverbal communication is frequently the vehicle for the suicide threat. The person may give away prized possessions, make a will or funeral arrangements, or systematically withdraw from all friendships and social activities. Sometimes a person may make a direct verbal suicidal threat, but this is less common. The threat is an indication of the ambivalence that is usually present in the suicidal behavior. It represents the hope that someone will recognize the danger and rescue the person from his self-destructive impulses. It may also represent an effort to discover whether anyone cares enough to prevent the individual from harming himself.

Jourard[12] has presented an interesting analysis of suicidal behavior related to the wish for rescue. He believes that suicide is sometimes the result of an "invitation to die" extended by significant others. The invitation may be communicated by failure to respond to a suicide threat or, at times, even more directly. For instance, a woman was admitted to the hospital following the ingestion of iodine. She was severely depressed and highly suicidal. After a course of electroconvulsive therapy she recovered and went home. The social history revealed that her husband's occupation was tombstone carver. He reportedly had prepared a tombstone for the patient with only the date of death missing and kept it in a back room of their house. A few months after discharge the patient successfully committed suicide.

Suicide attempts include any actions taken by the individual toward himself that will lead to death if not interrupted. In the assessment of suicidal behavior much emphasis is placed on the lethality of the suicidal method that is threatened or used. Although all suicide threats and attempts are to be taken seriously, more vigorous and vigilant attention is indicated when the person is planning or tries a highly lethal means such as gunshot, hanging, or jumping. Less lethal means include carbon monoxide and drug overdose, which allow time for discovery once the suicidal action has been initiated. Assessment of the suicidal person also includes the factors of whether the person has made a specific plan and whether the means to carry out the plan are available. The most suicidal person would be one who plans a violent death (e.g., gunshot to the head), has a specific plan (e.g., as soon as his wife goes shopping), and has the means readily available (e.g., a loaded gun in a desk drawer). This person is exhibiting little ambivalence about his plan. On the other hand, the person who thinks he might take a bottle of aspirin if the situation at work does not improve soon is communicating an element of hope and is really asking for help in coping with his work situation.

Several assessment tools, or lethality scales, have been developed by staff members at suicide prevention centers. One good example was developed by the Los Angeles Suicide Prevention Center (pp. 346 and 347). It takes into consideration risk factors, stressors, the lethality of the method, coping mechanisms, and support systems to arrive at an overall rating of suicide potential.

Clinical example 10-3 illustrates the behavior of a suicidal person. It may be used in conjunction with the Assessment of Suicidal Potentiality if the student wishes to practice assessment skills as related to the suidical patient.

CLINICAL EXAMPLE 10-3

Mr. Y was a 52-year-old black man who was employed in the foundry of a large steel mill. He had worked for the company for 20 years. He lived in a rented room in a blue collar neighborhood near the mill. Most of his neighbors were Appalachian white and southern black families who had moved to the community to work at the mill. There was an undercurrent of racial tension in the neighborhood, but Mr. Y was not involved in conflicts with his neighbors. He had separated from his wife before moving to the community and had no close friends or family. The separation resulted from his violent behavior related to drinking binges.

ASSESSMENT OF SUICIDAL POTENTIALITY*

Name _____ Age _____ Sex _____ Date _____

Rater _____ Evaluation _____

	1 2	3 4 5 6	7 8 (9)
	Low	Medium	High

Suicide potential

Age and sex	_____	Resources	_____	Total	_____
Symptoms	_____	Prior suicidal behavior	_____		
Stress	_____	Medical status	_____	Number of categories rated	_____
Acute vs. chronic	_____	Communication aspects	_____		
Suicidal plan	_____	Reaction of significant other	_____	Average	_____

Rating for category

1. Age and sex (1-9) ( )

Male
- 50 plus (7-9) ( )
- 35-49 (4-6) ( )
- 15-34 (1-3) ( )

Female
- 50 plus (5-7) ( )
- 35-49 (3-5) ( )
- 15-34 (1-3) ( )

2. Symptoms (1-9) ( )

Severe depression: sleep ( )
disorder, anorexia, weight
loss, withdrawal, de-
spondent, loss of interest,
apathy (7-9)

Feelings of hopelessness, ( )
helplessness, exhaustion
(7-9)

Delusions, hallucination, loss ( )
of contact, disorientation
(6-8)

Compulsive gambler (6-8) ( )

Disorganization, confusion, ( )
chaos (5-7)

Alcoholism, drug addiction, ( )
homosexuality (4-7)

Agitation, tension, anxiety ( )
(4-6)

Guilt, shame, embarrass- ( )
ment (4-6)

Feelings of rage, anger, hos- ( )
tility, revenge (4-6)

Poor impulse control, poor ( )
judgment (4-6)

Frustrated dependency (4-6) ( )

Other (describe): ( )

Rating for category

3. Stress (1-9) ( )

Loss of loved person by ( )
death, divorce, separation
(5-9)

Loss of job, money, prestige, ( )
status (4-8)

Sickness, serious illness, sur- ( )
gery, accident, loss of
limb (3-7)

Threat of prosecution, crimi- ( )
nal involvement, exposure
(4-6)

Change(s) in life, environ- ( )
ment, setting (4-6)

Success, promotion, in- ( )
creased responsibilities
(2-5)

No significant stress (1-3) ( )

Other (describe): ( )

4. Acute versus chronic (1-9) ( )

Sharp, noticeable, and sud- ( )
den onset of specific symptoms (1-9)

Recurrent outbreak of similar ( )
symptoms (4-9)

Recent increase in long- ( )
standing traits (4-7)

No specific recent change ( )
(1-4)

Other (describe): ( )

5. Suicidal plan (1-9) ( )

Lethality of proposed meth- ( )
od—gun, jump, hanging,
drowning, knife, poison,
pills, aspirin (1-9)

*From Los Angeles Suicide Prevention Center: Assessment of suicidal potentiality, Los Angeles, The Center.

	Rating for category
Availability of means in proposed method (1-9)	( )
Specific detail and clarity in organization of plan (1-9)	( )
Specificity in time planned (1-9)	( )
Bizarre plans (4-6)	( )
Rating of previous suicide attempt(s) (1-9)	( )
No plans (1-3)	( )
Other (describe):	( )

6. **Resources (1-9)**   ( )

No sources of support (family, friends, agencies, employment) (7-9)	( )
Family and friends available, unwilling to help (4-7)	( )
Financial problem (4-7)	( )
Available professional help, agency, or therapist (2-4)	( )
Family and/or friends willing to help (1-3)	( )
Stable life history (1-3)	( )
Physician or clergy available (1-3)	( )
Employed (1-3)	( )
Finances no problem (1-3)	( )
Other (describe):	( )

7. **Prior suicidal behavior (1-7)**   ( )

One or more prior attempts of high lethality (6-7)	( )
One or more prior attempts of low lethality (4-5)	( )
History of repeated threats and depression (3-5)	( )
No prior suicidal or depressed history (1-3)	( )
Other (describe):	( )

8. **Medical status (1-7)**   ( )

Chronic debilitating illness (5-7)	( )
Pattern of failure in previous therapy (4-6)	( )
Many repeated unsuccessful experiences with doctors (4-6)	( )

	Rating for category
Psychosomatic illness, e.g., asthma, ulcer, etc. (2-4)	( )
Chronic minor illness complaints, hypochondria (1-3)	( )
No medical problems (1-2)	( )
Other (describe):	( )

9. **Communication aspects (1-7)**

Communication broken with rejection of efforts to reestablish by both patient and others (5-7)	( )
Communications have internalized goal, e.g., declaration of guilt, feelings of worthlessness, blame, shame (4-7)	( )
Communications have interpersonalized goal, e.g., to cause guilt in others, to force behavior, etc. (2-4)	( )
Communications directed toward world and people in general (3-5)	( )
Communications directed toward one or more specific persons (1-3)	( )
Other (describe):	( )

10. **Reaction of significant other (1-7)**   ( )

Defensive, paranoid, rejected, punishing attitude (5-7)	( )
Denial of own or patient's need for help (5-7)	( )
No feelings of concern about the patient; does not understand the patient (4-6)	( )
Indecisiveness, feelings of helplessness (3-5)	( )
Alternation between feelings of anger and rejection and feelings of responsibility and desire to help (2-4)	( )
Sympathy and concern plus admission of need for help (1-3)	( )
Other (describe):	( )

Mr. Y was seen by the occupational health nurse, Ms. G, when he came to the employee health clinic following a 6-week absence from work. He had been hospitalized for broken ribs and a concussion after he had been beaten and robbed by a gang of adolescents in an alley behind his home. Ms. G was familiar with this employee because he had been a participant in the company's Employee Assistance Program for alcoholics. When she saw him in the clinic, she immediately noted that he appeared depressed. His face was expressionless, his posture slumped, and he had lost weight. He appeared disheveled, which was a change from his usual neat appearance. He said he did not feel ready to return to work, but had received a letter from the personnel office requesting that his condition be evaluated by the company's physician. His speech was slow and halting and so soft that he could barely be heard. He told Ms. G that he had a request to make of her. He knew from past conversations that she was an animal lover. He wanted her to take his pet dog because he did not feel able to care for it adequately and the neighbors who kept it while he was in the hospital had neglected it.

Ms. G was very concerned about Mr. Y and asked him how he was spending his time. He said he kept the television on and he thought a lot. When asked, he said he felt "too shaky" to go outside unless he absolutely had to. He thought the boys who attacked him were still in the neighborhood. Ms. G asked if he had thought about harming himself. Mr. Y looked startled, then admitted that he saw no other solution to his problem. "It makes sense. I don't have anybody. If you take Rover, I can go." With further questioning, he admitted that he had a loaded revolver at home and planned to use it after he left the clinic. Ms. G realized that Mr. Y needed help immediately. She asked the clinic secretary to sit with him while she discussed his situation with the physician.

Completed suicide may take place after warning signs have been missed or ignored. Some people do not reveal any easily recognizable warning signs. Research that has been done on completed suicide has of necessity been retrospective. However, it can be informative to interview survivors. This procedure is referred to as the psychological autopsy. The information obtained from these inquiries can be used to better understand suicidal behavior and to enhance the effectiveness of primary prevention activities.

Significant others of suicidal people, including survivors, have many feelings about this behavior. There is a significant element of hostility inherent in suicidal behavior. Frequently the message to significant others, stated or implied, is "You should have cared more." At times, when the person survives the attempt, this message may be transmitted in a manipulative way. An example is the adolescent girl who discovers that her boyfriend is dating someone else and takes an overdose of over-the-counter sleeping pills. If she sets the scene so she will almost inevitably be discovered and makes sure that her boyfriend hears of her behavior, she is behaving in a hostile manipulative way. A remorseful response by the boyfriend would be reinforcing and increase the likelihood that the behavior will be repeated in the future. It is important to treat these attempts seriously and help the patient develop healthier communication patterns. Persons who do not really intend to die may do so if they are not discovered in time.

When suicide is successful, the survivors are left with many feelings that they cannot communicate to the involved object, the dead person. This may lead to an unresolved grief reaction and depression. Some suicide prevention centers have become involved in what Shneidman[19] refers to as postvention to assist people to deal with this dilemma. Survivors are assisted either individually or in groups to express their feelings and work through their grief.

Coping mechanisms

The most prominent coping mechanism relative to ISDB is denial. Even though the individual may verbalize that his behavior is potentially harmful, direct injury to the self is denied. For instance, the overweight person will remark, "I shouldn't do this—but I will" as he cuts a large slice of cake. Most obese people can recite all the risks associated with obesity, but there is no sense of immediate personal threat.

Other people who engage in risk-seeking behavior enjoy the feeling of challenging fate and gambling that they will overcome danger. Daredevils, soldiers, and people who participate in dangerous sports deny the importance of the risk involved. The sense of mastery they feel when they win the gamble reinforces future repetition of the behavior.

Rationalization is another coping mechanism that is often present with ISDB. The noncompliant patient may give numerous reasons for his inability to comply with his health care plan. These explanations are really ways of decreasing the anxiety and fear that are related to recognition of a serious illness.

Many patients also use intellectual defenses. Anorexics and overweight people may become students of nutrition, thus gaining a sense of mastery over their behaviors. Noncompliant patients may seek out information about their illness and then use conflicts among the experts to justify their reluctance to accept treatment.

Regression is another characteristic of these patients. Eating disorders frequently have a relationship to the feeding patterns that the person experienced during infancy. Overeating may be pleasurable because having a good appetite was rewarded during childhood. Anorexic patients often begin dieting when confronted with the need to behave in a more adult manner. It is as if maintaining a childlike appearance will allow the continuation of childlike behavior. The occurrence of amenorrhea reinforces this perception. ISDB also invites parental interaction from significant others who try to persuade the person to behave in a self-enhancing way.

It must be remembered that these coping mechanisms may be standing between the person and self-destruction. They are defending him from strong emotional responses to life events that are a serious threat to the ego. If challenged too strongly without provision of other means of coping, underlying depression will become overt and may lead to suicidal behavior.

Suicidal behavior indicates the imminent failure of the coping mechanisms. A suicidal threat may be a last-ditch effort to get enough help to be able to cope. Completed suicide represents the failure of the coping and adaptive mechanisms.

 Nursing diagnosis

When considering the nursing diagnosis of self-destructive behavior, the nurse must incorporate information about the seriousness and immediacy of the patient's harmful activity. Nursing diagnoses for these patients will generally also refer to other behavioral problems that have been discussed in other sections of this book, including anxiety, communication, unresolved grief, self-concept disorders, and anger. Self-destructive behavior generally evolves from other behavioral problems. Following are nursing diagnoses related to suicidal behaviors as described in the case of Mr. Y on p. 345:

■ Suicidal threat, including a specific, very lethal plan, with the means at hand, related to anxiety aroused by a recent assault and robbery
■ Social isolation related to lack of friends and estrangement from family
■ Depression related to isolation and feelings of insecurity

Table 10-3 describes nursing diagnoses related to the case study of Ms. L on p. 343 and the

TABLE 10-3. Comparative examples of nursing diagnoses and the medical diagnosis associated with anorexia nervosa

Nursing diagnoses	Medical diagnosis as described in DSM-III*
Starvation related to refusal to eat	**DIAGNOSTIC CRITERIA FOR ANOREXIA NERVOSA**
Compulsive physical activity related to need to maintain control of self, represented by losing weight	**A.** Intense fear of becoming obese, which does not diminish as weight loss progresses
Refusal to eat related to need to demonstrate control and a distorted body image	**B.** Disturbance of body image, e.g., claiming to "feel fat" even when emaciated
Amenorrhea related to starvation	**C.** Weight loss of at least 25% of original body weight or, if under 18 years of age, weight loss from original body weight plus projected weight gain expected from growth charts may be combined to make the 25%
Distorted body image related to anxiety over assuming an adult role	**D.** Refusal to maintain body weight over a minimal normal weight for age and height
	E. No known physical illness that would account for the weight loss

*From American Psychiatric Association: Diagnostic and statistical manual of mental disorders, third edition, Washington, D.C., APA, 1980.

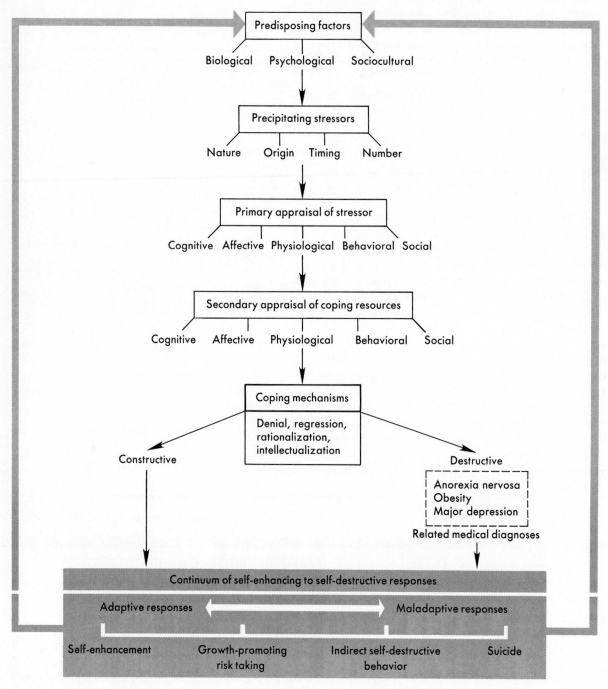

FIG. 10-3
Model of health-illness phenomena related to self-destructive behavior.

DSM-III criteria for the medical diagnosis of anorexia nervosa.

The following are nursing diagnoses related to the case study of Ms. C on p. 344:

■ Noncompliance with the diabetic diet (1800 calories a day as recommended by the American Dietetic Association) related to a moderate level of anxiety resulting from fear of aging
■ Lack of acceptance of the medical diagnosis of diabetes mellitus related to the defense of intellectualization to cope with the threat of chronic illness

Fig. 10-3 relates self-destructive behavior to the model of health-illness phenomena.

Planning and implementation of nursing interventions

Goal setting

Careful attention must be given to the assignment of priorities in setting goals with the self-destructive patient. Highest priority should be given to goals that are relevant to the preservation of life. In terms of this constellation of behaviors, further consideration must be given to first identifying goals related to immediately life-threatening behavior. For example, the actively suicidal person must first be prevented from acting on his impulses. At a later time attention can be given to the development of insight into the suicidal behavior and substitution of healthy coping mechanisms. The anorexic person must be prevented from starving to death as the highest priority goal.

ISDBs also serve as coping mechanisms. Therefore there is great resistance to changing these behaviors. Goals must incorporate the development of new ways of coping that will replace the old self-destructive ones.

In dealing with self-destructive behavior, it may appear that the nurse and the patient are pursuing incompatible goals. Suicidal patients may resist attempts to protect them and may actively try to evade their observers. However, most of these patients have some ambivalence. The nurse, in setting positive, life-preserving goals, is appealing to the healthy part of the person's self that wants to survive and be better able to cope with life. The very act of seeking help is an expression of this healthy aspect of the personality. The positive attitude of the nurse in setting constructive goals conveys a sense of hope to a patient who may be feeling hopeless.

Following are examples of goals related to DSDB:

Long-term
By 2 weeks before discharge from the hospital, the patient will refrain from attempts to inflict physical harm on himself.
Short-term
1. In 3 days the patient will voluntarily remain within the view of a staff member.
2. In 1 week the patient will inform a staff member when he feels like hurting himself.
3. In 2 weeks the patient will state two reasons why he does not want to hurt himself.
4. In 3 weeks the patient will list three good things about himself.

Following are examples of goals related to ISDB:

Long-term
The patient will take prescribed medications and perform self-care activities independently as recommended by the health care team.
Short-term
1. In 2 weeks, the patient will verbalize feelings related to his medical diagnosis.
2. In 4 weeks, the patient will describe the relationship between the medical diagnosis and the recommended self-care activities.
3. In 4 weeks, the patient will describe the consequences of failure to carry out self-care activities.
4. In 6 weeks, the patient will verbally accept responsibility for his health care behavior and will participate in self-care activities on his own initiative.
5. In 6 weeks, the patient will have stable biopsychosocial functioning based on compliance with an individualized self-care treatment plan.

If the patient is made aware of a treatment plan of this type, he can actively engage in evaluating his progress and modifying the plan. This again reinforces the message of confidence that the patient will be able to change his behavior and find more satisfaction in life.

Intervening in self-destructive behavior

There are common elements in nursing intervention with all patients who exhibit self-destructive behavior. The first important matter for the nurse to consider is her own response to people who are trying to destroy themselves. It can be difficult for a person who is happy and involved in life to imagine the depth of despair that leads to suicidal impulses or the lack of caring for the self that results in behavior which is physically, psychologically, and socially damaging, even if it is not immediately lethal. On the other hand, a nurse who is depressed and dissatisfied with her own life may be threatened by interacting with patients who are more upset because she may fear similar consequences for herself. The latter nurse may also overidentify with the patient. This limits one's ability to help the patient because of the tendency to assume that the patient's situation and one's own are exactly alike, whereas in reality this is probably not so. It is therefore crucial that the nurse examine her own feelings. A therapeutic approach is empathic and nonjudgmental, with limitation of subjective responses through awareness of one's own attitudes.

The highest priority nursing activity with the self-destructive patient is to protect him from inflicting further harm on himself and, if suicidal, from killing himself. The message of protection is conveyed to the patient verbally and nonverbally. Verbally, the patient is informed of the nurse's intention not to allow harm to come to the patient.

To the anorexic patient, she might say, "We will not allow you to starve yourself to death. You may choose whether to eat voluntarily or to be fed by us, but you will be prevented from starving to death." To the suicidal patient she might say, "I understand that you are feeling impulses to harm yourself. I will be here with you to help you control those impulses and I will do whatever is necessary to protect you. I'd like to talk with you about how you are feeling whenever you feel able to share that with me." The nonverbal communications should reinforce and be congruent with the verbal. Obviously, dangerous objects such as belts, sharp implements, glass, and matches should be taken from the suicidal patient. It is recognized that it is impossible to render an environment perfectly safe. Even walls and floors can inflict injury if the patient throws himself against them. However, the removal of dangerous objects gives a message of concern. One-to-one observation of the extremely suicidal individual also communicates caring. This observation should be carried out with sensitivity, the nurse neither hovering over the patient nor remaining aloof from him. The patient's nonverbal cues can guide the one-to-one interaction. It is important to remain alert until the mental health team and the patient agree that the self-destructive crisis is over. Suicidal patients may appear to be feeling much better immediately prior to making an attempt. This is attributed to the feeling of relief that is experienced when the decision has been made and the plans have been finalized. Nurses have been fooled by this behavior pattern, relaxing their vigilance, only to have the patient kill himself when he is allowed to be alone for a moment.

If anorexic patients are being forced to eat, they must be observed carefully following a meal to prevent induced vomiting. Vigilance during meals is necessary because anorexic patients are usually very accomplished at hiding food in napkins, giving it to other patients, burying it in plants, and other means of disposing of it without eating it. They also require limits on activity and close observation of bowel and bladder functioning to be sure that they are not secretly taking laxatives or diuretics.

Self-destructive people have low self-esteem. The nurse may intervene in this area by treating the patient as someone who is deserving of her attention and concern. Positive attributes of the patient should be recognized with genuine praise. An attempt to manufacture reasons to praise the patient is usually recognized as artificial and has the effect of lowering the patient's self-esteem. The message is that the patient is so bad that one has to search for positive characteristics.

Overweight people frequently have low self-esteem. They perceive their inability to achieve a normal weight as a character flaw and feel shame about their size. The nurse can help them identify their positive attributes. Recognition for success in weight loss is also helpful and provides motivation for continued dieting and exercise.

As the nurse gets to know the patient, she should be alert to strengths that can be built on to provide the patient with positive experiences, as illustrated in Clinical example 10-4.

CLINICAL EXAMPLE 10-4

Ms. P was an extremely suicidal woman who was very depressed. She spoke little and spent much of her time pacing in an agitated manner. Her husband was distressed about her condition and was willing to share with the nurse a description of Ms. P when she was well. He revealed that Ms. P loved to bake and had never bought anything from a bakery. The nurse arranged to get the ingredients for Ms. P to show her how to bake bread. Ms P did so reluctantly but put a great deal of energy into beating and kneading the dough. As she did so, she explained her activity to the nurse. She received sincere praise for the completed bread from the nurse and from other patients with whom it was shared. The nurse incorporated the baking activity as a regular part of her intervention with Ms. P.

━━━━━━━━━━━━━━━━

Closely related to the building of self-esteem is the reinforcement of healthy coping mechanisms. Ms. P's bread making was a way for her to express her anger more productively than by pacing. If past healthy coping mechanisms can be identified, these may be reinforced. In addition, growth may take place through the learning and practice of new adaptive behaviors.

Behavior modification programs may be initiated to teach new coping patterns. Eating disorders are often approached in this way. Many of the popular weight loss groups are built around behavior modification principles. Public weighing in results in group approval for weight loss and disapproval for failure to lose. Other diet plans recommend techniques, such as saving a dollar for each pound lost and buying a (nonfood) treat when the goal is reached, or buying an article of clothing in a smaller size that will fit when excess weight is lost. Posting an unflattering photograph on the refrigerator door deters the obese person from eating. Changes in eating habits are also recommended. These include eating slowly and chewing food well, eating only in a designated place, putting the fork down between bites, and refraining from other activities while eating.

Principles of behavior modification are also recommended by some anorexia nervosa treatment programs. Privileges may be granted for pounds gained. For instance, a patient may be confined to her room until she gains 2 pounds, restricted from visitors until 5 pounds have been gained, and so on. Some programs use feeding by nasogastric intubation as a type of aversive stimulus. Tube feeding is initiated if the patient fails to consume the required number of calories in a specified period of time or if weight declines by a predetermined amount. Other programs avoid tube feeding except in emergency situations. These health care providers feel that the insertion of a feeding tube reinforces the patient's low self-esteem and may be interpreted as punishment for misbehavior rather than an effort to be helpful. Activity limitations and constant observation by staff are also unpleasant conditions that the patient can change only by altering her behavior. Some treatment teams also advocate refusing to inform the patient of either her present or her goal weight. This avoids end-less arguments about desirable weight and decreases to some extent the anxiety the patient feels about increasing weight. Behavior modification programs are structured to allow the patient to assume more responsibility for her behavior as she demonstrates her ability to behave responsibly. Group interaction and peer support are encouraged.

For noncompliant patients, healthy coping implies the assumption of responsibility for self-care. Interventions must be directed toward the development of understanding of the meaning of the illness experience to the patient.

It may be helpful to assist the patient to explore the predisposing and precipitating factors influencing his behavior. Once the acute crisis is over, understanding the underlying feelings and realizing how they developed and got out of control may help the person to change his behavior in the future. The nurse without advanced preparation in psychiatric nursing should not probe for feelings that the patient is reluctant to discuss and should avoid making interpretations of behavior. These approaches can be very stressful and have the potential to precipitate a new crisis, which the inexperienced nurse may be unable to handle.

If the self-destructive behavior represents a response to other behavioral disruptions, appropriate nursing interventions should be directed toward these problems. The angry patient must be helped to deal constructively with his anger. The patient who has physiological needs must be helped to meet those needs. For example, the anorexic patient who is in a state of starvation is unable to think rationally and interpret her sensations correctly until she has been stabilized metabolically. Attempts to help her develop insight during the period of starvation are certain to fail. When she is physiologically stable, psychotherapy may be initiated.

Issues of control are usually present when self-destructive behavior occurs. A person may be so determined to demonstrate control of his life that he participates in harmful behavior because it is discouraged by others. Bruch[3] has observed that this is a characteristic of anorexic patients. Schlemmer and Barnett[18] describe the manipulative behavior that they have experienced in their work with anorexia nervosa patients. They note that manipulation seems to occur in response to limits. For instance, self-induced vomiting, which is a common behavior of anorexics, occurred in only one patient. The treatment program had no limits specified relative to vomiting. Patients who were being treated with behavior modification were more manipulative than those who were not. The behavior modification treatment plan was very structured and initially involved strict limits. The authors advise that nurses respond to manipulation with consistent enforcement of limits. They observed that as patients grew to trust the reliable response of the staff, manipulation decreased. They also made it clear to the patients that they retained control of their weight gain or loss. It was recommended that nursing staff meet together regularly to express their feelings and provide group support. The constant limit testing of a self-destructive patient can be frustrating to nursing staff.[18] All forms of self-destructive behavior are controlling in nature. In effect, the patient challenges others to try to stop him from harming himself, although in reality everyone knows that the patient retains the right to choose growth-promoting or harmful behavior.

Frequently, self-destructive behavior reflects a lack of both internal and external resources. Mobilization of social support systems is an important aspect of nursing intervention. Significant others probably have many feelings about the self-destructive behavior of the patient. They need an opportunity to express their feelings and to make realistic plans for the future. Family members need to be made aware of control issues and helped to encourage self-control of the behavior by the patient. Both the patient and the family may need assistance in seeing that caring can be expressed by fostering self-care, as well as by providing care. Families of suicidal patients may be frightened of future suicidal activity. They need to be aware of behavioral clues to suicide and of community resources that can assist with crises. In reality, suicidal behavior frequently recurs. False reassurance should be avoided. A better approach is to foster improved communication patterns and an ability to cope in the family. The nurse may help people sort out their feelings and frequently may want to refer significant others for social work intervention or initiate a referral for family therapy.

Community resources may also be important for the long-term care of the self-destructive person. Self-help groups such as Weight Watchers, Diet Workshop, TOPS, and Recovery, Inc. may provide the recovering patient with needed peer support. Family therapy may assist in the reintegration of a family group that has been disrupted by the patient's recent experiences. Public health nurses, clergy, and other community-based helping people can be helpful in providing the patient and family with day-to-day support. The nurse may be active in explaining resources to the patient and in initiating referrals to other agencies.

Patient education is another important aspect of nursing intervention. The nutritional knowledge of patients with eating disorders should be assessed. Dieters, in particular, may be helped by learning about the nutritional values of various foods. Meal planning based on a food exchange system or on calorie counting gives the patient a feeling of control. Others respond better to following a diet pattern that has been designed by someone else. In either case, referral to a nutritionist for diet teaching is advisable. Questions about fad diets should be answered honestly. Analysis of the nutritional value of the diet by the nurse or nutritionist and the patient may help the patient assess diet plans more accurately in the future. Health teaching for overweight patients should also emphasize the importance of exercise as a way of improving general health and maximizing weight loss. Community resources for exercise, such as adult education classes, YWCA and YMCA exercise programs, and aerobic dance programs can be identified and information provided to the patient. Patients who are noncompliant with prescribed health care regimens may not understand the nature of their problem. Knowledge should be assessed and appropriate teaching initiated. Many patients are willing to participate in self-care if it makes sense to them. Teaching ways to monitor health status may also be helpful. For instance, if a hypertensive patient can check his own blood pressure, he can learn to associate his health care activities with his physiological response. Patients who are on medication regimens, such as psychotropic medication for the previously suicidal patient, should know the prescribed dosage, frequency, and side effects of the medication. Information about how to handle any future crises should be provided to the patient. If there has been an explanation of the possible reason for the patient's behavior, this may be reinforced with him at termination to help him integrate his experience into his self-concept. Helping a patient to work through his self-destructive behavior can be an extremely rewarding aspect of psychiatric nursing. Table 10-4 summarizes nursing interventions for patients with self-destructive behavior.

TABLE 10-4. Summary of nursing interventions for patients with self-destructive behavior

Principle	Rationale	Nursing action
Goal: Prevention of infliction of physical harm to the self		
The patient must be protected from harming himself	Highest priority is given to life-saving patient care activities The patient's behavior must be supervised until self-control is adequate for safety	Close observation Removal of harmful objects Provision of a safe environment Provision for basic physiological needs
Increase self-esteem	Self-destructive behavior reflects underlying depression related to low self-esteem and anger directed inward	Identify patient strengths Encourage patient to participate in activities that he likes and does well Encourage good hygiene and grooming Foster healthy interpersonal relationships
Reinforcement of healthy coping mechanisms	Maladaptive coping mechanisms must be replaced with healthy ones to manage stress and anxiety	Assist the patient to recognize unhealthy coping mechanisms Identify alternative means of coping Reward healthy coping behaviors
Goal: Acceptance of help from family and community support systems		
Mobilization of social support systems	Social isolation leads to low self-esteem and depression, perpetuating self-destructive behavior	Assist significant others to communicate constructively with the patient Promote healthy family relationships Identify relevant community resources Initiate referrals to community resources
Patients and significant others should receive education about identified health care needs	Understanding of and participation in health care planning enhances compliance	Involve patient and significant others in care planning Explain characteristics of identified health care need, nursing care needs, medical diagnosis, and recommended treatment and medications Elicit response to nursing care plan Modify plan based on patient feedback

Evaluation

Evaluation of the nursing care of the self-destructive patient requires careful monitoring of the patient's behavioral status on a daily basis. Involvement of the patient in evaluation of his progress can provide reinforcement and an incentive to work toward a goal. Modifications of the plan of care are frequently necessary as the patient reveals more of himself and his needs to the nurse. As soon as possible, the patient should become a participant in the planning, evaluation, and modification process.

Unfortunately, self-destructive behavior has a tendency to recur. Nurses sometimes become discouraged and angry with patients who return again and again with the same behavior. When this occurs, the nurse may be caught in the trap of feeling responsible for the patient's behavior. Once the nurse has given the best nursing care she knows how to give, she has done as much as she can for the patient. It is impossible to change a patient's total life situation for him. The nurse can only help to identify alternative behaviors and provide encouragement for change. If the patient returns, the nursing process must be reinitiated with an attitude of hope that this time the patient will learn and grow more and be better able to live a satisfying life.

Suggested cross-references

Therapeutic relationship skills are discussed in Chapter 3. The model of health-illness phenomena and the phases of the nursing process are discussed in Chapter 4. Mobilization of social support systems and health education are discussed in Chapters 5 and 6. Interventions related to low self-esteem are discussed in Chapter 8. Depression is discussed in Chapter 9. Substance abuse is discussed in Chapter 14. Behavior modification approaches are discussed in Chapter 21.

SUMMARY

1. Self-destructive behavior varies in degree from slow and insidious (overeating) to immediate and dangerous (suicide attempts).

2. Stereotypes of self-destructive people are usually misleading. The majority of people engage in some form of self-destructive behavior.

3. Descriptive information was presented about indirect self-destructive behavior. The examples of this behavior that were used throughout the chapter were obesity, anorexia nervosa, and noncompliance with a prescribed health care plan.

4. Data were presented about identification of groups at high risk for suicide.

5. The continuum of coping responses from self-enhancing behavior to suicide was presented. Anxiety and the attempt to escape from it are central to the occurrence of self-destructive behavior.

6. Other behavioral disruptions, including psychosis, may lead to self-destructive behavior.

7. Depression related to low self-esteem and unexpressed anger is intimately related to self-destructive behavior.

8. Issues of control are prominent relative to self-destructive behavior.

9. Social factors, such as loneliness, interpersonal frustration, family communication patterns, cultural changes, and patterns of a subculture may lead to self-destructive behavior.

10. Behaviors characteristic of indirect self-destructive behavior, including anorexia nervosa, obesity, and noncompliance were discussed, including the core behavior of denial of potential personal harm.

11. Characteristics of suicidal threats, attempts, and completed suicide were discussed, including warning signs, assessment of suicidal risk, and the necessity to understand ambivalence as it relates to suicidal behavior. The function of hostility in suicidal behavior was discussed.

12. Coping mechanisms related to indirect self-destructive behavior include denial, rationalization, intellectualization, and regression. Suicide represents the failure of all coping attempts.

13. Examples of nursing diagnoses related to self-destructive behavior were presented.

14. Initially, it may be necessary to set goals for self-destructive patients, but they should be encouraged to participate as soon as possible. Highest priority is given goals that preserve the person's life. An ex-

ample of long- and short-term goals was presented.

15. Nursing interventions should focus on protecting the patient, increasing self-esteem, reinforcing healthy coping mechanisms, understanding the underlying problem, mobilization of environmental resources, and patient education.

16. The nurse must explore her own feelings relative to the self-destructive behavior of patients.

17. Evaluation is based on the patient's increasing ability to behave in a self-enhancing manner. An attitude of hopefulness is necessary even when patients revert to their self-destructive behaviors and require readmission.

References

1. American Psychiatric Association: Diagnostic and statistical manual of mental disorders, ed. 3, Washington, D.C., 1980, The Association.
2. Bahra, R.J.: The potential for suicide, Am. J. Nurs. **75:**1782, 1975.
3. Bruch, H.: The golden cage: the enigma of anorexia nervosa, Cambridge, Mass., 1978, Harvard University Press.
4. Choron, J.: Suicide, New York, 1972, Charles Scribner's Sons.
5. Ciseaux, A.: Anorexia nervosa: a view from the mirror, Am. J. Nurs. **80:**1468, 1980.
6. Douglass: Endocrinology and other uncommon causes of obesity. In Powers, P.S.: Obesity: the regulation of weight, Baltimore, 1980, The Williams & Wilkins Co.
7. Durkheim, E.: Suicide, New York, 1951, The Free Press. (Translated by J.A. Spaulding and G. Simpson.)
8. Farberow, N.L., editor: The many faces of suicide: indirect self-destructive behavior, New York, 1980, McGraw-Hill Book Co.
9. Feighner, J.P. et al.: Diagnostic criteria for use in psychiatric research, Arch. Gen. Psychiatry **26:**57, 1972.
10. Filstead, W.J.: Despair and its relationship to indirect self-destructive behavior. In Farberow, N.L., editor: The many faces of suicide: indirect self-destructive behavior, New York, 1980, McGraw-Hill Book Co.
11. Frisch, R.E.: Critical weight at menarche, initiation of adolescent growth spurt, and control of puberty. In Grumbach, M.M., Grave, G.D., and Mayer, F.E., editors: Control of the onset of puberty, New York, 1974, John Wiley & Sons, Inc.
12. Jourard, S.: Suicide: an invitation to die, Am. J. Nurs. **70:**269, 1980.
13. Krauss, H.H.: Suicide: a psychosocial phenomenon. In Wolman, B.B., editor: Between survival and suicide, New York, 1976, Gardner Press, Inc.
14. Leventhal, H.: Wrongheaded ideas about illness, Psychol. Today **16:**48, 1982.
15. Linden, L.L., and Breed, W.: The demographic epidemiology of suicide. In Shneidman, E.S., editor: Suicidology: contemporary developments, New York, 1976, Grune & Stratton, Inc.
16. Los Angeles Suicide Prevention Center: Assessment of suicidal potentiality, Los Angeles, The Center.
17. Powers, P.S.: Obesity: the regulation of weight, Baltimore, 1980, The Williams & Wilkins Co.
18. Schlemmer, J.K., and Barnett, P.A.: Management of manipulative behavior in anorexia nervosa patients, J. Psychiatr. Nurs. **15:**35, Nov. 1977.
19. Shneidman, E.S., editor: Suicidology: contemporary developments, New York, 1976, Grune & Stratton, Inc.
20. Wekstein, L.: Handbook of suicidology: principles, problems and practice, New York, 1979, Brunner/Mazel, Inc.

Annotated suggested readings

Alvarez, A.: The savage god, New York, 1971, Bantam Books.

This is a well-written book that presents suicide against a historical and literary background. The author was acquainted with Sylvia Plath, a writer who committed suicide. He writes about his experiences with her and his observations of her behavior.

Anderson, N.P.: Suicide in schizophrenia, Perspect. Psychiatr. Care **11:**106, 1973.

This article identifies the characteristics of suicidal behavior in schizophrenic patients, including interpretation of psychotic communication and the existence of depression in schizophrenics. A case illustration is presented.

Bahra, R.J.: The potential for suicide, Am. J. Nurs. **75:**1782, 1975.

The author approaches suicidal behavior from a psychoanalytical base. He identifies typical assaults on self-esteem and discusses in depth four mental mechanisms that lead to true suicide attempts.

Ciseaux, A.: Anorexia nervosa: a view from the mirror, Am. J. Nurs. **80:**1468, 1980.

This author, using a pseudonym, describes her personal experience with anorexia nervosa. She provides insight into the anorexic person's view of her behavior and her interpretations of the responses of others to her. The article is illustrated with a fascinating self-portrait accompanied by the author's explanation of the meaning of the picture.

Cohen, F., and Lazarus, R.S.: Coping with the stress of illness. In Stone, G., editor: Health psychology: a handbook, San Francisco, 1979, Jossey-Bass, Inc., Publishers.

The authors present an analysis of coping and adaptation behaviors related to the experience of serious physical illness. They discuss the complexity of coping processes and review current research. They conclude by making recommendations for future study. Many of the issues that they delineate have implications for patient compliance with health care regimens. This work is appropriate for graduate level study.

Durkheim, E.: Suicide, New York, 1951, The Free Press. (Translated by J.A. Spaulding and G. Simpson.)

This is a classic that identified demographic factors which apply to suicidal behavior. Durkheim also described types of suicidal behavior that are still discussed in contemporary literature. This study is also of note because it was one of the first attempts to apply research techniques to a sociological study.

Farberow, N.L., editor: The many faces of suicide: indirect self-destructive behavior, New York, 1980, McGraw-Hill Book Co.

This book is highly recommended as a resource on a variety of indirectly self-destructive behaviors. The contributors are knowledgeable about their topics and discuss them in relationship to the characteristics of this behavioral pattern. Included are the problems of noncompliance with therapeutic plans, drug abuse, alcohol abuse, hyperobesity, cigarette smoking, self-mutilation, automobile accidents, gambling, criminal and deviant activity, stress-seeking behaviors, and high-risk sports.

Frederick, C.J.: The role of the nurse in crisis intervention and suicide prevention, J. Psychiatr. Nurs. 11:27, Jan.-Feb. 1973.

The author applies crisis intervention principles to the treatment of suicidal patients. He includes a helpful list of interventions and discusses the management of the hospitalized suicidal person.

Hafen, B., and Faux, E., editors: Self-destructive behavior, Minneapolis, 1972, Burgess Publishing Co.

This book is an excellent resource both for the neophyte and the experienced psychiatric nurse. The various articles present research findings and good general information about self-destruction.

Jourard, S.: Suicide: an invitation to die, Am. J. Nurs. 70:269, 1970.

This is a provocative article that connects family process to suicidal behavior. It leads the reader to consider the broader social system, which usually affects the behavior of the identified patient.

Mahan, L.K.: A sensible approach to the obese patient, Nurs. Clin. North Am. 14:229, June 1979.

This is a thorough review of contemporary views of obesity. A convenient table describes various treatments for obesity. There is a good description of the behavior modification approach to treatment. The author also discusses the importance of activity and the components of a healthy reducing diet.

Menninger, K.: Man against himself, New York, 1938, Harcourt, Brace & World, Inc.

This classic work investigated self-destructive behavior long before it was fashionable to do so. Menninger took a psychoanalytical approach to suicidal behavior and identified several levels of attempts at self-destruction.

Moore, J.A., and Coulman, M.V.: Anorexia nervosa: the patient, her family and key family therapy interventions, J. Psychiatric Nurs. 19:9, May 1981.

In this article, anorexia nervosa is discussed in the context of family dynamics. The presentation is based on the theoretical framework of structural family therapy. Concepts are illustrated with clinical vignettes. This is a clear presentation of the involvement of the family in the anorexic patient's illness.

Morgan, H.G.: Death wishes? The understanding and management of deliberate self-harm, New York, 1979, John Wiley & Sons, Inc.

This book provides an excellent comparison of the characteristics of suicide and nonfatal deliberate self-harm. Reports of recent research are included. Studies cited address such issues as epidemiological factors, treatment, and implications for prevention. The author clarifies the need for further study of this phenomenon. This book is particularly recommended for readers who have an interest in research.

Niswander, G.D., Casey, T.M., and Humphrey, J.A.: A panorama of suicide, Springfield, Ill., 1973, Charles C Thomas, Publisher.

A fascinating collection of psychological autopsies is presented here. Reading them adds depth to one's understanding of the many facets of suicidal behavior.

Powers, P.S.: Obesity: The regulation of weight, Baltimore, 1980, The Williams & Wilkins Co.

The author has included a wealth of information on obesity and other eating disorders in this volume. A particular strength is the inclusion of reports of relevant research with critical evaluation of the results. Extensive bibliographies are also an asset.

Pretzel, P.W.: Understanding and counseling the suicidal person, New York, 1972, Abingdon Press.

This author takes a philosophical approach to the problem of suicide in this deeply humanistic view of the subject. Although intended for clergy, there are approaches to counseling that are equally applicable to nursing.

Price, J.H., and Pritts, C.: Overweight and obesity in the elderly, J. Gerontol. Nurs. 6:341, 1980.

This article focuses on factors related to obesity in the elderly. However, the principles that are included are applicable to the understanding and treatment of overweight individuals in all age groups. This is a readable article that covers the topic quite thoroughly.

Schlemmer, J.K., and Barnett, P.A.: Management of manipulative behavior of anorexia nervosa patients, J. Psychiatr. Nurs. 15:35, Nov. 1977.

This article describes the nursing care of anorexia nervosa patients in a research setting. It includes a description of a behavior modification approach to this disorder. The authors describe the applicability of research findings to nursing practice. Unfortunately, the research protocol and data analysis are not included.

Shneidman, E.S., editor: Suicidology: contemporary developments, New York, 1976, Grune & Stratton, Inc.

This anthology is edited by one of the United States' most respected suicidologists. The information included is well selected and may be particularly useful to the experienced practitioner who may want to gain more depth in knowledge of suicidal behavior.

Stanitis, M.A., and Ryan, J.: Noncompliance: an unacceptable diagnosis? Am. J. Nurs. 82:941, June 1982.

The authors challenge the acceptability of the nursing diagnosis of noncompliance. They point out that this is a value-laden term which may result in the development of negative attitudes toward the patient. They also question whether compliance with a medical regimen is always a positive behavior. This article could be assigned as a stimulus for group discussion.

Wekstein, L.: Handbook of suicidology: principles, problems and practice, New York, 1979, Brunner/Mazel, Inc.

This well-written book provides an extensive examination of suicidal behavior. The author is knowledgeable about the use of psychotherapy with suicidal patients. He includes some suggested experiential learning activities and illustrates theory with case histories. He also includes current research in suicidology. This is a useful reference for both the student and the practitioner of psychiatric nursing.

Wolman, B.B., editor: Between survival and suicide, New York, 1976, Gardner Press, Inc.

This anthology includes chapters by several of the more controversial psychiatric theorists. The volume is stimulating and thought provoking, since many of the writers take unique approaches to their subject matter.

CHAPTER 11

DISRUPTIONS IN
RELATEDNESS

*The emptiness caused by dissatisfaction
with mere achievement and the helplessness
that results when the channels of relation
break down have brought forth a loneliness
of soul such as never existed before.*

Karl Jaspers, Existenzphilosophie*

Learning objectives

*After studying this chapter, the student
should be able to:*

- *describe the characteristics of a healthy interpersonal relationship.*

- *discuss the development of relatedness throughout the life cycle.*

- *identify five possible disruptions that can occur in the process of relatedness.*

- *compare and contrast the states of aloneness and existential loneliness.*

- *analyze the developmental, sociocultural, biochemical, genetic, and psychodynamic stressors that contribute to the development of disruptions in relatedness.*

- *identify and describe behaviors that are associated with disruptions in relatedness, including impaired communication, withdrawal, suspicion, dependency, and manipulation.*

- *discuss the manifestation of impaired relationship behaviors in patients with medical diagnoses of paranoid schizophrenia, catatonic schizophrenia, dependent personality disorder, and antisocial personality disorder.*

- *formulate individualized nursing diagnoses for patients with disrupted relationship patterns.*

- *assess the relationship between the nursing and medical diagnoses of individual patients.*

- *identify the individual's attempts to cope with the anxiety created by the inability to establish healthy interpersonal relationships.*

- *develop long-term and short-term individualized nursing goals with patients who are experiencing disruptions in relatedness.*

*Translated by Kaufmann, F. In Kaufmann, W., editor: Existentialism from Dostoevsky to Sartre, New York, 1956, Meridian Books.

■ *apply therapeutic nurse-patient relationship principles with an appropriate rationale to the care of the patient who is unable to establish healthy relationships.*

■ *analyze nursing interventions appropriate to the needs of the patient who is suspicious, dependent, withdrawn, manipulative, or who is unable to communicate effectively.*

■ *assess the importance of the evaluation of the nursing process when working with patients who experience disrupted interpersonal relationships.*

■ *identify suggested readings for future study.*

Continuum of social responses

Human beings are socially oriented and to achieve satisfaction with life, they must be able to establish positive interpersonal relationships. A healthy interpersonal relationship is one in which the individuals involved experience intimacy with each other while maintaining separate identities. According to Sullivan,[29] intimacy is characterized by sensitivity to the needs of the other person and mutual validation of personal worth. There may or may not be a sexual component to the intimate relationship. Other characteristics of healthy relatedness as delineated by Rogers[24] include open communication of feelings, acceptance of the other as a valued separate person, and deep empathic understanding. To achieve this depth of involvement with another person, there must be willingness to take the risk of self-revelation. This can be a frightening experience, particularly if either individual has been more reserved about expressing feelings. Fear of exposure of the self frequently inhibits people from developing intimate relationships.

Issues of control are also involved when people relate to each other. There are times when it is necessary to subordinate individual needs to the needs of the other individual or to the demands of the relationship itself. At other times it may be more important to the individual to be self-assertive and to set aside the needs of others. The mature person must be able to sort out priorities of needs and to share with others the rationale for his behavior. Within the context of any relationship there is a continuum of dependent to independent behavior on the part of

each participant. Ideally, there should be some balance between these behaviors within the relationship. This balance can be described as interdependence. The interdependent person identifies areas where there is a need to rely on others and experience the caring aspects of dependency. There are also times when it is appropriate and gratifying to self-esteem to function independently. In addition to behaving in this flexible way, the interdependent person can allow another to be dependent on him or independent of him, according to the other person's need. In this case each individual assumes responsibility for control of his own behavior but also receives support and assistance from significant others when it is needed.

Every person has the potential to be involved in relationships at many levels, from the intimacy just described to superficial transient contacts. Intimate and interdependent relationships provide a secure base from which the person derives self-confidence in coping with the various demands of day-to-day life. A lack of intimacy with family members and friends leaves only a series of superficial encounters, depriving the person of many of life's most meaningful experiences. The support of significant others frees energy for involvement with social groups, work groups, and the community. The mature adult is able to maintain involvement at all these levels and feel satisfied with the quality of his relationships with others.

Learning to relate to others in a mature way is a growth process that takes place throughout the developmental cycle. The infant is by necessity dependent on others for meeting all its biological and psychosocial needs. A consistent reliable relationship with a mothering person resulting in the establishment of trust is essential at this stage of the growth process. People who fail to accomplish the task of establishing basic trust are handicapped in relating to others as they continue to grow and develop.

As a child grows older and develops motor skills, independence becomes a possibility and he strives to establish himself as an individual, separate from the mothering person who has been meeting all his needs. This leads to conflict as more powerful adults set limits on behavior, often frustrating the child's efforts toward independence. Loving, consistent limit setting, however, communicates caring and provides the beginning of the development of a capacity for interdependence. As the child grows older, the parents' guidelines for behavior are internalized, and a value system begins to emerge.

At this point the child enters school and begins to learn interdependent concepts of cooperation, competition, and compromise. Peer relationships become important, as does the approval of adults from outside the family group, such as teachers, scout leaders, and parents of friends.

By preadolescence, the individual becomes involved in an intimate relationship with a friend of the same sex, a "best friend." This relationship is characterized by sharing and offers another opportunity for clarification of values and recognition of individual differences. This is usually also a very dependent relationship and intrusions by others are actively resisted. However, as adolescence develops, the dependence on a close friend of the same sex usually yields to a heterosexual relationship, also very dependent in nature. Simultaneous with these dependent relationships with peers, the individual vigorously asserts independence from parents. This striving for independence, often marked by rebellious behavior, is supported by peers who are engaged in the same struggle. Parents can facilitate growth by consistent limit setting and a caring tolerance of the adolescent's rebellious outbursts. As the individual learns to balance parental demands and peer group pressures, another step toward mature interdependence is taken.

The adolescent period ends when the person is able to be self-sufficient, maintaining an interdependent relationship with parents and peers. Decisions are now made independently, with the advice and opinions of others taken into account. The individual may marry and begin a new family unit. Occupational plans are made and implemented. The mature person will demonstrate self-awareness by balancing dependent and independent behavior and by allowing others to be dependent or independent as appropriate. Sensitivity to and acceptance of the feelings and needs of oneself and of others is critical to this level of mature functioning. Interpersonal relationships are characterized by mutuality.

Parenting and adult friendships will test the person's ability to foster independence in others. This involves a need to give up some dependence on the other person so he may grow. Children gradually separate from parents as they grow and friends may move away or drift apart. The mature person must then be self-reliant and find other supports to augment those which have diminished or been lost. Pleasure can be found in the development of an interdependent relationship with children as they grow. The freedom that results from decreased dependent demands by children can be used for new activities which promote self-growth.

As adulthood continues, change continues to occur. There are losses, such as the physical changes of aging, the death of parents, loss of occupation through retirement, and later the deaths of friends and of one's spouse. The need for relatedness must still be satisfied. The mature person grieves over these losses and recognizes that others can help resolve the grief. However, there are also new possibilities even in the face of loss. Old friends and relatives cannot be replaced, but new relationships can develop. Grandchildren may become important to the grandparent, who may delight in spending time with them that was never available for children. The aging person may also find a sense of relatedness to the culture as a whole. Life assumes deeper meaning in relation to the individual's perception of his accomplishments and contributions to the welfare of the whole. The mature older person can accept whatever increase in dependence is necessary but also retain as much independence as possible. Even loss of physical health need not necessarily force the person to give up all independence. Self-esteem is enhanced by the ability to maintain mature relatedness throughout life.

Disruptions can occur in the development of mature interdependent interpersonal relationships. Some individuals find it difficult to establish or maintain close relationships. They may *withdraw* from other people, sometimes to the point where they are unable to maintain themselves in the community. A similar situation can occur when a person is isolated by others. In other cases individuals may experience excessive *dependency* on other people, draining the resources of those to whom they relate and potentially inviting rejection by friends and relatives. A third disruption in relatedness is *manipulation* of other people. In this case closeness is not established and other people are treated as objects to be maneuvered to meet the needs of the manipulator. Individuals who are experiencing problems in the area of relatedness are likely to have difficulty in experiencing basic trust in others. Therefore there is generally some degree of *suspicion* present along with any of the behaviors described. Another behavior that frequently accompanies disruptions in relatedness is *impaired communication*. Verbal and nonverbal communication patterns may be distorted or incongruent, thus keeping others at a safe distance and preventing the development of intimacy.

In addition, loneliness is likely to be a component of the lives of these people. The loneliness of lack of intimacy with others is pervasive and painful. This is difficult to imagine if it has not been experienced. The pain of loneliness can be shared empathically to some extent and often arouses anxiety in the person with whom it is shared. Biographical accounts of experiences of a psychiatric patient, such as *I Never Promised You a Rose Garden* by Joanne Greenberg or *The Bell Jar* by Sylvia Plath, also communicate some of the character of this existential pain. Frieda Fromm-Reichman conceptualized extreme loneliness as she worked with many withdrawn patients. She hypothesized that it should be differentiated from anxiety and that perhaps it is an even more frightening experience than anxiety. She describes loneliness as a state in which past relationships are for the most part forgotten and there is little hope of any future relationship.[13] It is a difficult concept to study because the person who is lonely is unable to communicate about it, the person who has been lonely does not usually want to remember what it was like, and the person who is studying it becomes anxious when he tries to understand it. Loneliness of this kind must be differentiated from aloneness and solitude. The latter conditions may be sought out by individuals from time to time and may be conducive to contemplation, creativity, and the growth of self-awareness.

Behaviors that are related to interpersonal relationships may be represented on a continuum that ranges from healthy interdependent interactions to those which involve no real contact with other people. This continuum of coping responses is illustrated in Fig. 11-1.

Stressors

Disruptions in relatedness evolve as the result of various experiences that influence the growth of the individual. In most instances a series of life events predisposes the individual to difficulty with interpersonal relationships. Many people cope with their interpersonal problems and describe themselves as reasonably satisfied with this aspect of life. However, additional stress can cause a marginally satisfying interpersonal life to become grossly disrupted. Response to various stressors is highly individualized. However, the factors to be discussed are likely to cause some degree of interpersonal disruption for most people. It is also essential to remember that an increase in the level of stress is experienced by the individual as anxiety, which is at the root of the behavioral disruptions that occur.

Since the capacity for relatedness is the result of a *developmental process,* anything that inhibits the accomplishment of relevant developmental tasks will also decrease the individual's ability to develop healthy interpersonal relationships. The family is the unit within which the first experiences with closeness to others take place. Lack of maternal stimulation or attention deprives the infant of a sense of security and there is failure to establish basic trust. This can lead to a suspicious attitude toward others that may continue throughout life. The quality of mothering attention is also important. A child may be adequately fed and receive impeccable physical care but without any communication of maternal caring. A child who is treated like an object may well become an adult who treats others like objects. Rather than responding to

FIG. 11-1
Continuum of social responses.

personal expressions of caring, the person may rely on material possessions to feel secure. Early experiences of maternal deprivation also frequently lead to severe depression in the child, as demonstrated in the studies of Spitz.[29] Without corrective experiences, and provided he survives, the child will probably develop into a withdrawn and chronically depressed adult. Early experiences such as these can lead to the most serious of psychiatric disorders and frequently to chronic institutionalization.

Another group of potential problems arises as the child begins to strive for independence. Inhibition of the toddler's efforts to develop autonomy can result in excessive dependency that may continue into adulthood, resulting in a fearful clinging person. Inconsistent limit setting or lack of limits can interfere with the person's ability to perceive the needs and rights of others, thus blocking the ability to achieve intimacy in relationships.

The value system that is held by the parents is communicated to the preschool and school-aged child. In addition, the exposure to other ideas that comes about as school begins and the child's world expands to include parts of the community broadens his developing value system. Congruency between parental and community values facilitates this process for the child. Lack of clarity about values may result in confusion in adulthood, with vulnerability to compliance with the ideas of others rather than a healthy personal decision-making ability. It is also possible that value confusion may lead to antisocial behavior by a person who has a flexible value system that encompasses a variety of possible behaviors based on the individual's self-interest.

Family communication patterns may also be stressors leading to disruptions in relationships. Patients with a medical diagnosis of schizophrenia are frequently members of families with identifiably disturbed communication patterns. In a survey of current family research relative to schizophrenia, Wynne, Toohey, and Doane[40] identify the following three types of family communication patterns that are being investigated by schizophrenia researchers: communication deviance studies, initiated by Wynne and his associates[39,40]; the expressed emotion studies of Brown, Vaughn, and Leff[32,40]; and the family relationship test investigated by Scott and colleagues.[40] The communication deviance studies use projective tests, such as the Rorschach and the Thematic Apperception Test (TAT), to study the communication patterns of identified schizo-

phrenic patients and their immediate family members. These studies have demonstrated that deviant patterns of communication exist in families in which a child becomes schizophrenic. The expressed emotion studies[32] analyze interviews with family members of schizophrenic patients in terms of the frequency of critical comments about the patient, as well as assigning a global rating for the amount of hostility, warmth, or overinvolvement expressed by the relative. These characteristics were related to the future course of the illness. It was found that a high amount of expressed emotion by relatives is associated with a higher frequency of relapses. The Family Relationship Test[40] measures family members' perceptions of interpersonal relationships by use of an adjective checklist. It was found that patients who view their parents as "well" have a better prognosis than those who perceive their parents as "ill."

The role of the family in producing impaired interpersonal relationships has been studied extensively by Bateson and his associates.[4,5] These theorists state that basic intrafamilial relationship problems frequently become manifest in the symptomatic behavior of one family member. This deviant behavior develops when the family is subjected to intolerable levels of stress. Satir[25] notes that a family member who acts "crazy" may serve the function of keeping the family system intact. This is further supported by the frequent observation that, as the "family symptom bearer" gets better, other family problems get worse.[25] Satir further states that the family system operates within a set of rules that concern communication and "it is the rigidity or restrictions of these rules and the consequent distortions which ultimately create the need for symptoms."[25] For example, if there is a family rule that hostility is never expressed directly between family members, and the parents are involved in a conflict which they may not confront, tension will build up within the family system. One of the children may respond to this tension by "acting crazy" and performing destructive acts in the home. Family tension is then kept in control by identifying the symptom bearer as the cause of the problem and justifying his behavior as the result of his "illness," whereas in reality he is expressing the conflict between the parents.

Another family communication pattern that has been linked to the development of psychotic behavior is the double-bind theory developed by Bateson and associates.[5] The components of the double bind are described as follows:

1. The presence of two or more persons, one of whom is the "victim"
2. Repeated experience with the process so that it becomes the expected pattern of communication
3. A "primary negative injunction" that promises punishment either for performance of a given action or for failure to perform a given action; punishment being described as "withdrawal of love. . . . expression of hate or anger—or most devastating—the kind of abandonment that results from the parent's expression of extreme helplessness"[5]
4. A "secondary injunction" that conflicts with the primary injunction at a more abstract level, with similar threats of punishment; usually transmitted nonverbally and may negate any or all parts of the message in the primary injunction
5. A "tertiary negative injunction" that forbids the victim to escape[5]

In the following example of communication that follows the double-bind pattern, a hospitalized schizophrenic man in his early twenties is being visited by his parents. As they arrive, the mother says, "Aren't you glad to see us, dear?" As the son says, "Yes, I am" and moves forward to embrace his mother, she turns away to her husband and remarks about the dreariness of the hospital. The son then withdraws and waits passively for his parents to continue the interaction. In this case the primary injunction was to be glad to have a parental visit. However, when the son tried to demonstrate his gladness, the mother's nonverbal communication of turning away communicated her displeasure at his action and a secondary injunction not to initiate closeness. This nonverbal message was enhanced by her remark about the dreariness of the setting, which at another level could be interpreted as a rebuke to her son whose illness brought her there. Also coexisting in this scene is the double message "You should be glad to see me, but I'm not glad to see you." It should also be noted that a lack of response to the first statement, "Aren't you glad to see us, dear?" would not be a solution to the problem because this directly challenges the primary injunction and will also be dealt with by punishment. Therefore the young man, who has no way of

being rewarded for his behavior, protects himself by withdrawing from the situation.

Although the mother in this scene seems like a villain, complementing the son's role of victim, any family member can be cast in any role and multiple victimizers may exist. Unfortunately, the mother is sometimes stereotyped as the one who always creates double binds for psychotic children. The other misconception that can occur easily is that this behavior is intentional and maliciously directed toward the defenseless child. Parents are not usually aware of doublebinding behavior and when confronted about it tend to respond defensively. The problem lies within the family system and the total communication process which occurs within that system. For instance, the father in the example, who stood by while his wife set up the double bind, is equally responsible for doing nothing to clarify the confused communication.

Social relationships outside of the family may also be disrupted and have a lasting effect on behavior. Failure to develop intimacy with peers, first of the same sex and later of the opposite sex, leads to social isolation in adulthood. Such an individual may appear cool and aloof and is likely to become involved in superficial relationships. There is likely to be a romanticized idea of heterosexual relationships and disappointment when this does not materialize. This person may also become depressed as an adult because of a vague sense of what an intimate relationship could be like compared to the reality of what the person is experiencing. Involvements with others may be transient and characterized by approach-avoidance behavior as the person tries to pursue closeness. The individual who has difficulty establishing intimacy may also be extremely dependent, clinging to any relationship that may potentially bring fulfillment but frightened to take the risk of self-disclosure, which would lead to a truly mature involvement.

The person who reaches maturity with a capacity for healthy interpersonal relationships is still vulnerable to psychological stressors that may interfere with his success. Either a series of losses or a single significant loss may lead to difficulty in establishing future intimate relationships. The pain of a loss can be so great that the individual will withdraw from future involvements, rather than risking a repetition of pain. This response is of course enhanced if the person had difficulty during any of the developmental tasks pertinent to relatedness. Losses of significant others may cause difficulty with future relationships, but so may other kinds of losses. The loss of a job is a blow to the individual's self-esteem and can also result in future withdrawal and problems with relatedness unless the person has a well-established interpersonal support system.

Sociocultural factors can also be stressors relative to the person's ability to establish and maintain relatedness. In contemporary culture there are many forces that tend to make the individual feel isolated and lonely. Cultural mores discourage reaching out to casual acquaintances. Friendships are often transient because of the mobility involved in many occupations. Packard[23] studied transient populations and found higher rates of mental hospital admissions, more aggressive behavior, and more marital discord in this group. Even family relationships acquire an ephemeral quality as children move from place to place, frequently seeing parents only occasionally. Friends are often closer than siblings, at times creating a vague discomfort and a cultural nostalgia for the "good old days" of the close-knit extended family.

Certain groups within the culture are particularly vulnerable to isolation. The elderly are frequently ignored in our production-oriented culture. Older people are takers of material goods and the young must be the givers. We have little tolerance as a society for those who are not actively involved in the economic system. Paradoxically, even if older people have the ability to be active, they are pushed out of the system to make room for the young.

Involuntary social isolation also happens to the handicapped and chronically ill of any age. People with terminal illnesses or disfiguring disorders are frequently avoided by others. This is also true for people with long-term psychiatric problems. Although there has been an effort to decrease chronic institutionalization, there is great resistance to integration of the disabled into the community. This externally imposed isolation may result in withdrawal, depression, dependency, suspicion, impaired communication, manipulative behavior, or any combination of these as the individual tries to cope with loneliness.

Nurses frequently encounter patients with behaviors related to disrupted interpersonal relationships in the general hospital setting. Even a reasonably well-adjusted person may have difficulty maintaining a satisfactory level of intimacy while hospitalized. The hospital environment tends to be impersonal, which enhances the patient's sense of isolation. Patients who must be isolated because of concern about infection or, in the psychiatric setting, to control behavior are susceptible to the effects of sensory deprivation and need creative nursing care to intervene in this problem. On the other hand, patients in critical care areas may experience sensory overload, also leading to a feeling of loneliness and separation from others.

Other sociocultural stressors are related to the cultural norms present in contemporary society. For instance, there is an idealized expectation that people will be involved in "meaningful" relationships, which is constantly reinforced through the media. Heterosexual relationships in particular are romanticized, which is perhaps reflected in the increasing numbers of adolescent out-of-wedlock pregnancies and early marriages leading to divorce. This cultural attitude leads to the experience of loneliness as described by Gordon: "the sense of deprivation that comes when certain *expected* human relationships are absent."[14:26] For the purpose of this discussion, the term "aloneness" will be utilized to differentiate this degree of loneliness from the existential kind of loneliness described earlier. The dynamics of aloneness as experienced by many Americans include the following[14]:

1. Feelings of hopelessness
2. Escape into unsatisfying relationships
3. Fear of experiencing lonely feelings
4. Denial of loneliness
5. Feelings of worthlessness and failure

A spiral of repetitive behavior often results, with feelings of helplessness, hopelessness, and worthlessness accumulating until the person in desperation often resorts to self-destructive behavior. This behavioral pattern has been graphically described by Judith Rossner in her book *Looking for Mr. Goodbar.*

Some groups in society prey on the alone and the lonely. In recent years there has been a flood of various planned group experiences that are advertised as therapeutic. Most of them promise a degree of intimate human experience. Encounter groups, when under the direction of a skilled therapist, often can be helpful to the isolated person. However, there is danger that the group leader may be untrained and unsophisticated in dealing with emotional problems. Another cultural development that attracts those who are lonely, particularly the young, is the various religious cults, which offer the attraction of a close-knit community and a sense of commonality of belief and effort. This sense of belonging is so important that cult members may sever all ties with family and friends and behave in compliance with the demands of the group, even if this is in conflict with a previous value system.

Although closeness is an ideal that is viewed as positive in this culture, a different message is given at the same time. This message is that it is acceptable to be selectively intimate, but most people should not be trusted and it is important to be careful in interpersonal contacts. This attitude can create confusion and a sense of insecurity. In a relatively short period of time, people have gone from leaving houses unlocked all the time to installing several locks on each door, burglar alarms, and guard dogs. Rising crime rates cause fear and more reluctance on the part of many people to risk closeness or contact with strangers. Some urban residents, particularly the elderly, become virtual prisoners in their homes and experience loneliness and all the associated behaviors.

Compounding these problems is another sociocultural stressor. There are indications that the family unit is becoming less stable. The divorce rate has been rising. Mobility has broken up the extended family, depriving people of all ages of an important support system. This has resulted in less contact between the generations, with young people losing the wise advice of grandparents and older people missing the stimulation of youth. Tradition, which provides a powerful link with the past and a sense of identity, is also less observed when the family is fragmented. The current resurgence of interest in ethnicity and "roots" may reflect the striving of isolated people to associate themselves with a specific identity. The many stresses on the family system have made it more difficult for family members to accomplish the developmental tasks relevant to intimacy.

There is a strong probability that there are *biochemical stressors* associated with difficulty in establishing and maintaining effective interpersonal relationships. For instance, people with a medical diagnosis of one or another form of schizophrenia are generally withdrawn, dependent, exhibit unusual communication patterns, and may be suspicious of other people. A great deal of research is presently being directed toward discovering a biochemical disorder associated with at least some of the schizophrenic disorders. This research tends to be con-

fusing because various studies frequently contradict each other. It should also be noted that even if a particular biochemical disruption is discovered, it will not explain the origin of schizophrenia, but will be evidence of some other, more basic, problem which may still be unidentified. For example, knowing that a person who exhibits the behaviors associated with diabetes mellitus has hypoglycemia does not define the real cause of the problem, which is a deficit in insulin production by the pancreas related to heredity, diet, or some other basic stressor.

At the present time, there seems to be a rapidly growing amount of evidence that at least some cases of schizophrenia are related to an excess of dopamine in key areas of the brain, probably the mesocortical and mesolimbic nerve tracts. The dopamine hypothesis[21,33] has been supported by (1) noting that the administration of dopaminergic agents (amphetamines, L-dopa, or apomorphine) leads to initiation or exacerbation of psychotic behavior and (2) ascertaining that neuroleptic drugs (phenothiazine) act at the synapse by binding dopamine receptor sites. This theory is viewed as the most promising one and is being studied intensively by biochemical researchers.

Another biochemical theory that continues to be investigated is the platelet monoamine oxidase (MAO) theory,[21] which hypothesizes that schizophrenics have lower levels of MAO in the bloodstream than do others. This theory is related to the amine theory, in that MAO is an enzyme that deactivates brain cell amines, including dopamine. Low levels of MAO, then, would lead to high levels of dopamine. However, there have been many methodological problems associated with the platelet MAO research.

Another theory is the indolamine hypothesis. This theory suggests that a defect in the metabolism of the indolamine serotonin results in the production of the hallucinogenic substances bufotenine and dimethyltryptamine (DMT). Evidence that supports this hypothesis includes the presence of bufotenine in the urine of schizophrenic patients. Researchers have also induced an excited state in normal persons or recurrence of psychosis in schizophrenics by producing an excess of substrate through administration of the amino acids tryptophan and methionine. Methyl groups combine with the substrate to produce bufotenine and DMT.[17]

The transmethylation hypothesis links schizophrenia to an abnormality in the transmethylation of catecholamines, resulting in the production of dimethoxyphenylethylamine (DMPEA), which is similar to mescaline. Findings in terms of this theory are equivocal at this point, but the possibility is still under consideration.[17,21]

Biochemical research is important not only because it may reveal clues to the cause or, more likely, causes of schizophrenia but also because understanding of biochemical processes may provide important guidelines to treatment. In addition, the identification of measurable biochemical imbalances, such as low platelet MAO, could lead to simple tests to identify at-risk populations, ultimately leading to methods of preventing the onset of some types of schizophrenia.

Another group of studies directed toward the identification of populations at risk for schizophrenia are those which focus on genetic tendencies for similar behavioral disturbances. In general, it has been found that monozygotic twins, even when adopted at birth by different parents and raised separately, show greater concordance for the occurrence of schizophrenia than do dizygotic twins.[8] Other studies have demonstrated that first-degree relatives (parents, siblings, and children) of schizophrenic patients also are at greater risk than the general population, but less so than monozygotic twins. Because these results are found even when environmental influences are controlled, as in the twin-separation studies, there is strong evidence for a genetic aspect to at least some forms of schizophrenia.[8]

Modern day researchers emphasize that genetic and biochemical studies constantly reinforce the assumption that interaction between the individual and his environment is necessary for the manifestation of schizophrenic behavior. For instance, not all monozygotic twins are concordant for schizophrenia. The expectation is that biochemical and genetic research will yield information about a stress threshold which, when low, predisposes the individual to the development of schizophrenic behavior. However, other factors, such as disturbed family communication patterns and lack of social support systems, will probably continue to be important to an understanding of the "schizophrenic syndrome."

Many *psychological theories* have been advocated as causes of disturbances in the ability to establish and maintain satisfying relationships. Psychologically, it is known that high anxiety levels result in an impaired ability to relate to others. As has been described in the chapter on anxiety, the level of anxiety experienced determines the degree of difficulty that may occur. Prolonged and/or extremely intense anxiety, together with a limited ability to cope, is

believed to be the cause of relationship difficulties of psychotic proportions. This theory will be further explored from the psychoanalytical and interpersonal points of view.

Psychoanalytical theory states that schizophrenic behavior results when the ego can no longer withstand the pressures emanating from the id and from external reality. The ego of the psychotic person has limited ability to cope with stress because of serious deficiencies in the symbiotic mother-child relationship that inhibited psychological development. The initial response to high levels of stress and anxiety is to employ ego defense mechanisms pathologically in an effort to control unacceptable impulses and thoughts. An example of this is the development of paranoid delusions, a pathological manifestation of the mechanism of projection. So much libido (psychic energy) is invested in the maintenance of repression that there is little left to invest in the performance of activities of daily living. Therefore the person withdraws from usual activities and has difficulty maintaining basic physiological needs such as nutrition and hygiene. If stress continues and the anxiety level is unabated, ego functioning may deteriorate further. The person then has difficulty maintaining repression and may be flooded with frightening and primitive thoughts and impulses. There is also difficulty differentiating self from environment as ego identity disintegrates. Communication at this point is confused, garbled, and highly symbolical, reflecting primary process thought, which is usually kept unconscious. There is little capacity for relatedness with others.

Will states the interpersonal view of schizophrenia as, "the expression of complicated patterns of behavior adopted by the organism in an effort to deal with a gross inadequacy in relating to other humans."[36] Will further states that the behavior is a response to stress, demonstrates a disordered personality structure, involves communication, and provides some degree of security and comfort.

The mother-infant relationship sets the stage for later behavioral problems. The mother's extreme anxiety is communicated empathically to her child. Confusing and conflicting messages are received from significant others before the child has developed enough skill in communication to clarify meanings. There is lack of a feeling of continuity in the relationship with significant

others, leading to incorporation of behavior that
seems to be unacceptable into the "not-me"
component of the self-system. This results in a
distorted view of reality. Anxious family members
teach the child a distorted perception of the
culture. Fear of people also develops, which inhibits
learning and restricts the use of consensual
validation. Adolescence brings many anxiety-provoking
experiences related to the need to
develop a firm sense of identity. Normal developmental
experiences lead to extreme anxiety and
loneliness. The person is then trapped in a conflict
between a longing for intimacy and a fear of
the loss of the limited human contact he has.[36]

Five categories of stressors that may lead to
impairments in interpersonal relationships have
been discussed: developmental, sociocultural,
biochemical, genetic, and psychological. The
interplay among these factors leads to the behavior
that the nurse observes while relating to
an individual, family, or group. It is essential
to consider each of these areas when performing
a thorough nursing assessment.

 **Data
collection**

The behaviors that are observed in response to
disruptions in relatedness are representative of
the individual's attempt to cope with the anxiety
arising from the feeling of loneliness and the
related feelings of fear, anger, shame, guilt, and
insecurity. Frequently occurring behaviors include
impaired communication, withdrawal,
suspicion, dependency, and manipulation.

Behaviors associated with schizophrenia

Disruptions in communication accompanied
by withdrawal and suspicion are evident in the
thought process and interaction patterns of patients
who have the medical diagnosis of schizophrenia,
paranoid type.[2] Clinical example 11-1
illustrates this disruption.

CLINICAL EXAMPLE 11-1

Mr. D is a 24-year-old single man who was admitted
for the third time to the psychiatric unit of an acute
general hospital. His diagnosis was chronic schizophrenia,
paranoid type. His other admissions had been
at ages 19 and 22 and had each lasted a month. His
outpatient treatment since the last admission had

consisted of individual supportive therapy provided by
the clinical nurse specialist, chemotherapy, and family
therapy provided by the social worker. He had also
been referred to the vocational rehabilitation counselor
and was about to start a job training program.

Mr. D was brought to the hospital by his parents.
They expressed great disappointment in his readmission
because they had hoped that he was "finally
going to lick this thing." They thought that the recurrence
of his psychotic behavior was probably related
to his impending involvement in the job training
program. They could identify no other recent stressors
that might have upset him.

Mr. D's nurse therapist, Ms. T, evaluated his condition
soon after his admission to the hospital. He appeared
frightened and was curled up in a chair when
she approached him. He did not look at her when she
greeted him and seemed preoccupied with his own
thoughts. Ms. T was not sure that he was aware she
was there. She sat down a few feet away from him
and again stated his name. He looked at her blankly
for a brief moment, said, "hello," and then went back
to staring into space. When asked what brought him
to the hospital, he replied, "My father's car." Ms. T observed
that Mr. D seemed rather upset and asked if
something was bothering him. He told her nothing
could bother him because God had told him that he
was invincible. He knew many people were jealous
of his powers and were trying to destroy him, but he
had special protection. He then showed her a rabbit's
foot that was sent to him by God to protect him from
"evil forces." As Ms. T reached out to touch the rabbit's
foot, Mr. D pulled it away and shouted angrily,
"Don't touch that! It's mine! They want you to take it
away to destroy my powers, but I won't let you!" Ms. T
assured Mr. D that she would not take away his rabbit's
foot, since it had great importance for him. He
gradually relaxed. She asked if he could say more
about the contact he thought he had had with God. He
replied that God had spoken to him and told him about
the evil forces. He knew these forces existed because
they put bad thoughts in his head. He also heard people
talking about him and commenting on his behavior.
There were several voices, and he thought he
recognized the voices of his father and Dr. M, who
saw him once a month to evaluate his medications.
He denied any visual hallucinations. His speech was
disjointed and at times difficult to follow because of
loose associations. For instance, he said, "Mother
brought me here . . . birth . . . rebirth . . . deliverance
. . . didn't like that movie." As Ms. T attempted to
explore his feelings about his parents' returning him
to the hospital, he turned away and angrily told her
to leave him alone because she was "one of them,
those g ___ d ___ f ___ liars." Ms. T responded that
she would continue to work with him to help him
regain control of his life while he was in the hospital.
However, she added that she could see he was tired
and upset so she would leave and see him again later.

For his first 3 days in the hospital, Mr. D continued
to be hostile, refusing to eat or drink and not sleeping

except when under the influence of medication, which he took reluctantly when presented with the clear alternative of state hospital commitment. The content of his speech revolved around the messages he received from God and the evil forces who were trying to destroy him. He would tolerate only brief interactions with his therapist and other staff members. He did not interact at all with other patients, whom he believed to be staff members and "undercover agents" who were supposed to report on his behavior. He totally refused to see his parents, consistently referring to his mother as "That b _____."

With the assistance of consistent interpersonal support and medication, Mr. D gradually began to gain control over his thoughts. There was a steady decline in the amount of delusional speech, and although the auditory hallucinations continued, he was able to ignore them or block them out by talking with someone. He revealed to Ms. T that he became upset after his parents had a violent argument and threatened to divorce each other. They pulled him into their conflict by demanding to know with whom he would choose to live and he was unable to respond to that demand except by becoming psychotic. He was disappointed that he had missed the beginning of his job training program and was hopeful that he would still be able to start vocational rehabilitation soon. Ms. T gently helped Mr. D to look at his feelings toward his parents and also informed the family therapist of the events preceding his admission. His discharge plan was for referral to a day treatment program for a short stay until the vocational rehabilitation referral was again available. Individual therapy, pharmacotherapy, and family therapy were all to continue.

From the description of Mr. D's hospitalization experience, it is apparent how disrupted communication can interfere with the ability to function. Mr. D was placed in an impossible communication situation by his parents when forced to choose between them. The timing of this family upheaval could well have been related to Mr. D's recent improvement and his move toward more independent behavior by entering the vocational rehabilitation program. If the family equilibrium depended on Mr. D's being the symptom bearer, the pressure from his parents was that he should continue in his role. Their perception of the reason for Mr. D's becoming upset further supports this hypothesis. They attributed his problem to the vocational rehabilitation plan, which was moving him away from the family, and not their argument, which essentially pulled him back in.

Mr. D, in his distress, most likely experienced *ambivalent feelings* toward his parents. He was very dependent on them so feared angering them and risking rejection. At the same time, he became very angry because of the demands they made on him but was blocked in expressing his anger by his need for them. He was able to resolve this problem only by withdrawing and, at an unconscious level, by relying on repression, regression, and projection to handle the unacceptable impulses aroused by the conflict situation.

Hallucinations, such as Mr. D's experiences of hearing God and of hearing people talk about him, frequently occur in schizophrenic patients. A hallucination is a sensory perception that takes place without external stimuli. The biochemical theorists suspect that hallucinatory experiences result from a metabolic response to stress that results in the release of hallucinogenic neurochemicals, such as bufotenine and DMT. Psychoanalytical theorists view hallucinations as an attempt by the ego to defend against alien impulses that have been repressed but are threatening to enter awareness. The mechanism of projection allows the ego to deal with the impulses as threats from the outside, thus alleviating some of the anxiety. Stated in the framework of interpersonal psychiatry, the hallucination is the autonomous expression of a specific zone of interaction, usually auditory, which symbolically represents the dissociated processes of the person's personality.[22] These dissociated experiences are included in the "not-me" component of the personality, which includes those experiences arousing such great anxiety that they were not integrated into awareness within the self-system. When the self-system is flooded with anxiety, as it is during an acute schizophrenic episode, the usual security operations are not adequate. The dissociated thoughts that come into awareness are then dealt with by means of projecting them as the verbalizations of others.[22]

Both psychodynamic theories relate hallucinatory experiences to efforts to alleviate panic levels of anxiety and both identify projection as the mechanism that is used to accomplish this goal. *Delusions* may be explained in a similar way. A delusion is a fixed false belief. Some delusions are suspicious in nature, or *paranoid,* such as Mr. D's belief that evil forces wanted to destroy him. In this instance, unacceptable (egoalien) aggressive impulses are projected outside the individual and perceived as being directed toward him. Paranoid delusions may also include a sexual component if the ego defense is directed toward sexual impulses. For instance, a woman who believes that the man next door wants to break into her house and rape her may be projecting her own unconscious sexual feelings for him. Paranoid delusions with homosexual content also occur with schizophrenic patients. This indicates a defense against an onslaught of homosexual impulses that are very frightening to the patient. If the patient is confronted with unavoidable close contact with a member of the same sex, homosexual panic can occur. When this happens, the patient enters a panic state with lack of impulse control and frequently very aggressive behavior.

Other delusions are *grandiose* in nature. Mr. D's belief that God had singled him out and given him special powers was a grandiose delusion. Grandiosity occurs in schizophrenic patients but is particularly marked in patients with a diagnosis of manic episode; bipolar disorder, mixed; or bipolar disorder, manic. Delusions of grandeur may endow the person with a special power or talent or may identify him with a famous or powerful person, such as God, a political leader, or a sports hero. This is an example of the pathological use of the mechanism of identification. It usually reflects a low self-esteem and a poorly formed ego identity. In this case increased anxiety brings about a sense of powerlessness. Idenfication with a powerful entity such as God allows the ego to acquire some of the power that is lacking within the personality structure. It is also a means of dealing with extreme fear. People with grandiose delusions may feel invincible and involve themselves in dangerous situations. It is important to keep in mind that the identification process takes place at an unconscious level and that the patient really believes he is God or the president of the United States.

Somatic delusions focus on the body and usually include the conviction that the person is the victim of a frightening disease. The person may believe that he is becoming incapacitated or that parts of his body are dead or rotting away. A variation of the somatic delusion is the belief that all or part of the body is distorted or misshapen. An attractive young male patient with this type of delusion refused to turn on the light when he used the bathroom because he feared what he might see in the mirror. Bizarre somatic delusions are associated with schizophrenia.

Delusions of fatal or debilitating illness are frequently associated with depression, as are *delusions of poverty*. The person is convinced that he is penniless and is responsible for the downfall of his family. This is a reflection of a pervasive sense of guilt and low self-esteem. These patients may make remarks such as "Everything I touch turns to ashes."

The nature of delusional thinking is such that it defies conventional logic. Its function is a protective one in helping the person cope with anxiety that would otherwise be overwhelming.

Clinical example 11-2, in contrast with that of Mr. D, deals with Ms. W, who is psychotically withdrawn and has a medical diagnosis of schizophrenia, catatonic type.[2]

CLINICAL EXAMPLE 11-2

Ms. W is a 26-year-old single childless woman who lives with her parents. She was brought by ambulance to the emergency room of a large university hospital and referred to the psychiatric service for evaluation. The evaluator, a psychiatric nurse, observed Ms. W immobile, lying propped up in a hospital bed. She was totally mute and kept her eyes fixed straight ahead. She did not move voluntarily, and when moved by the examiner, offered some resistance. However, when she had been moved, she would maintain the new position. For instance, the nurse raised Ms. W's right arm 6 inches above the bed. When she let go of the arm, the patient did not move it for 5 minutes, at which time the nurse moved it back to a resting position on the bed.

Ms. W had been accompanied to the hospital by her parents, who gave the following history. Mr. and Mrs. W had been married for 20 years before their daughter was born and they had despaired of ever having a child. They had lavished her with anything she wanted and had also set high standards for her behavior. She had always been a well-behaved child, rarely requiring punishment by her parents. In fact, she was very sensitive to criticism and would burst into tears at a harsh word. She had had few friends, sharing the family feeling that most other people did not have their high standards for behavior. She was particularly uncomfortable around young men, although she spoke of wanting to marry someday. She had attended an exclusive women's college, majoring in biology. At the time of her hospitalization, she was working as a research assistant in a cancer research laboratory. She was responsible for the care of laboratory rats being used for a study of the effects of suspected carcinogenic agents. She was a steady worker and apparently had performed adequately on the job, since she had recently received a merit raise.

About a month prior to admission Ms. W had mentioned that a new laboratory assistant had been hired.

This was a young man who began asking her to have lunch with him. She had told her parents that she mistrusted his motives, and she started to find reasons not to eat lunch. The quality of her work began to deteriorate. She attempted to avoid this man at work, but he persisted in his attentions and the day before admission asked her out to dinner and a movie the following weekend. She refused. That evening she seemed preoccupied and spent the evening reading. Her parents noticed that she rarely turned a page. The next morning she did not get up when called for work. When her parents entered her room, they found her much as she was on admission, immobile and mute. They tried throughout the day to arouse her but finally called their family physician, who advised them to take her to the emergency room.

Ms. W was a rigid, inhibited young woman who had built her personal security around her relationship to her parents, assuming the role of a perfect daughter. Any threat to that relationship threatened the foundation of her security as well, giving rise to extreme anxiety. This dependency on her parents interfered with Ms. W's ability to develop an adult level of relatedness. She was unable to establish intimacy with anyone outside her own family circle. Intellectually, she was aware of this problem and had rationalized that she owed a great deal to her aging parents and should repay them by continuing to share her life with them. She therefore placed plans for marriage and a family far into the future. The intrapsychic conflict between her wish for closeness and her wish not to displease her parents by leaving them created a large amount of anger, which was not compatible with her self-concept of the dutiful and obedient daughter. She defended against the anxiety this aroused by using repression and reaction formation. However, when an attractive young man began to exhibit interest in her, her usual defenses crumbled and she was overwhelmed by anxiety and primitive anger. She then resorted to extreme withdrawal as a way of controlling her frightening feelings. At an unconscious level she feared that any voluntary movement whatsoever would lead to uncontrolled eruption of all her feelings, which she viewed as exceedingly destructive. Her behavior therefore was self-protective.

Ms. W represents the kind of disruption in relatedness that is described by Fochtman.[12] The schizophrenic patient has difficulty with differentiation of himself as separate from significant others. At the same time, he must incorporate the other person, resisting any separation initiated by the other. There is also difficulty integrating experiences, causing fragmentation of perceptions.

All of these factors result in a conflict that Burnham, Gladstone, and Gibson have termed the *need-fear dilemma*.[7] Ms. W is strongly drawn toward wanting intimacy and dependency on others (the need), but is ambivalent because she also fears being engulfed and losing her own identity. This is an example of the approach-avoidance type of conflict described in Chapter 7. This dilemma is one of the most common characteristics of most types of schizophrenia.

Many theorists have attempted to identify patterns of behavior that would be diagnostic of schizophrenia. However, these efforts have been confounded by the identification of a variety of types of schizophrenia. In DSM-III,[2] the American Psychiatric Association has divided schizophrenia into the following types:

1. Disorganized, formerly hebephrenic, characterized by frequent incoherence, no systemized delusions, and disturbances in affect of a blunted, inappropriate, or silly nature
2. Catatonic, characterized by stupor, negativism, rigidity, excitement, and/or posturing
3. Paranoid, characterized by persecutory delusions, grandiose delusions, jealousy of delusional proportion, and/or persecutory or grandiose hallucinations
4. Undifferentiated, characterized by delusions, hallucinations, incoherence, or gross disorganization, but not meeting the criteria for more than one
5. Residual, characterized by a history of previous episode(s), lack of current prominent psychotic symptoms, continuing behavioral evidence of the illness[1]

In addition to these criteria for each type of schizophrenia, the American Psychiatric Association has also developed criteria for a schizophrenic disorder that apply to all types (Table 11-1). To be classified as schizophrenia, at least one episode of the illness must last more than 6 months. Conditions with episodes that last less than 6 months are referred to as schizophreniform disorders.[2]

The behaviors that have been described as criteria for the medical diagnosis of schizophrenia have evolved over the course of many years and will continue to evolve as more is learned

TABLE 11-1. Diagnostic criteria for a schizophrenic disorder*

A. At least one of the following during a phase of the illness:
1. Bizarre delusions (content is patently absurd and has *no* possible basis in fact), such as delusions of being controlled, thought broadcasting, thought insertion, or thought withdrawal
2. Somatic, grandiose, religious, nihilistic, or other delusions without persecutory or jealous content
3. Delusions with persecutory or jealous content if accompanied by hallucinations of any type
4. Auditory hallucinations in which either a voice keeps up a running commentary on the individual's behavior or thoughts, or two or more voices converse with each other
5. Auditory hallucinations on several occasions with content of more than one or two words, having no apparent relation to depression or elation
6. Incoherence, marked loosening of associations, markedly illogical thinking, or marked poverty of content of speech if associated with at least one of the following:
   a. Blunted, flat, or inappropriate affect
   b. Delusions or hallucinations
   c. Catatonic or other grossly disorganized behavior

B. Deterioration from a previous level of functioning in such areas as work, social relations, and self-care

C. Duration: Continuous signs of the illness for at least 6 months at some time during the person's life, with some signs of the illness at present; the 6-month period must include an active phase during which there were symptoms from A, with or without a prodromal or residual phase, as defined below
   Prodromal phase: A clear deterioration in functioning before the active phase of the illness not due to a disturbance in mood or to a substance use disorder and involving at least *two* of the symptoms noted below
   Residual phase: Persistence, following the active phase of the illness, of at least *two* of the symptoms noted below, not due to a disturbance in mood or to a substance use disorder
   Prodromal or residual symptoms
   1. Social isolation or withdrawal
   2. Marked impairment in role functioning as wage earner, student, or homemaker
   3. Markedly peculiar behavior (e.g., collecting garbage, talking to self in public, or hoarding food)
   4. Marked impairment in personal hygiene and grooming
   5. Blunted, flat, or inappropriate affect
   6. Digressive, vague, overelaborate, circumstantial, or metaphorical speech
   7. Odd or bizarre ideation, or magical thinking, e.g., superstitiousness, clairvoyance, telepathy, "sixth sense," "others can feel my feelings," overvalued ideas, ideas of reference
   8. Unusual perceptual experiences, e.g., recurrent illusions, sensing the presence of a force or person not actually present
   Examples: 6 months of prodromal symptoms with 1 week of symptoms from A; no prodromal symptoms with 6 months of symptoms from A; no prodromal symptoms with 2 weeks of symptoms from A and 6 months of residual symptoms; 6 months of symptoms from A, apparently followed by several years of complete remission, with 1 week of symptoms in A in current episode

D. The full depressive or manic syndrome (criteria A and B of major depressive or manic episode), if present, developed after any psychotic symptoms, or was brief in duration relative to the duration of the psychotic symptoms in A

E. Onset of prodromal or active phase of the illness before age 45

F. Not due to any organic mental disorder or mental retardation

*From American Psychiatric Association: Diagnostic and statistical manual of mental disorders, third edition, Washington, D.C., APA, 1980.

about this syndrome. Because of this evolutionary process, nurses will hear discussions of other classifications of behavior. Some with historical or current significance include Bleuler's primary (the four A's) and secondary symptoms of schizophrenia, Schneider's first- and second-rank symptoms, and the diagnostic criteria developed by the International Pilot Study of Schizophrenia.

The first effort to identify a group of behaviors typical of schizophrenia was that of Eugen Bleuler, who also renamed the disorder from its previous designation "dementia praecox." Bleuler identified primary and secondary symptoms of schizophrenia. Primary symptoms, frequently called the "four A's," include an *a*ffective disturbance, disordered *a*ssociation of thought, *a*utism, and *a*mbivalence.[20] One disturbance in affect is a "blunting" or shallowness of affective expression, demonstrated by minimal change in facial expression and a monotonous tone of voice. Hostility may be expressed if the patient feels threatened. This may be directly or symbolically expressed and may seem out of proportion to the situation. Some patients use cursing or obscene language as a means of expressing hostile feelings. Another affective disturbance is the expression of affect inappropriate to the subject being discussed. For instance, a patient describing her impulse to murder her children begins to giggle.

Associations between thoughts are often disrupted in schizophrenic patients. Sometimes *blocking of thoughts* occurs. In this case the patient begins to speak but then stops and loses track of the meaning of the statement. *Looseness of association* is revealed when the patient makes a statement that sounds jumbled, such as in the following example:

NURSE: **How can we improve your nursing care, Mr. J?**
MR. J: **Improve? Can't improve. Can't prove a thing. Got me in this jail, but can't prove anything.**

Mr. J. seems to drift away from the topic, but reveals that he views the hospital as a jail and suspects he is there because he has been accused of something. It is up to the nurse at this point to explore further the meaning of his statement. This loosely connected speech is frequently highly symbolical. Although the patient's own speech may be highly symbolical, he tends to interpret the speech of others very literally. An example follows:

NURSE: **How are you feeling, Mr. J?**
MR. J: **(Touches various parts of his body) I guess I feel OK.**

This is often referred to as *concrete* thought and speech. Speech may also be lacking in goal direction, as in *tangential speech* when the person begins to respond to a question but follows with a series of related topics, never really getting to the point of the original statement. *Circumstantial speech* is an instance in which the person does get to the point but only after adding many unnecessary details to the response. *Perseveration* is a pattern of speech in which the person repeats the same word or phrase over and over again. The word or phrase chosen may have symbolical significance to the patient. There are other speech patterns in which it is more difficult to grasp the patient's meaning. Sometimes patients respond by rhyming, which is called *clang association.* A patient might say, "Play ball, call, fall, tall, etc." Another disrupted attempt at communication is *echolalia,* in which the patient repeats whatever he hears. The following is an example of echolalia:

NURSE: **How are you today, Mr. J?**
MR. J.: **How are you today, Mr. J?**

A related behavior is *echopraxia,* in which the patient mimics the body position of another person. In *word salad* the patient expresses a random jumble of words, apparently aimless and meaningless.

Autism refers to a preoccupation with the self and with inner experience. The person may withdraw from any voluntary contact with others and seem to go inside a shell. Speech is highly personalized and may include *neologisms,* which are made-up words understood only by the patient. Some patients create and populate whole imaginary worlds. An example of this is Yr, created by Debbie in *I Never Promised You a Rose Garden.* As Debbie became more involved in the real world, she found that she had to give up Yr and its people. Nonverbal behaviors associated with autism include rocking, head banging, stroking or fondling the self, and sometimes curling up in a fetal position.

Ambivalence results in difficulty with decision making. Schizophrenics may debate endlessly about the alternatives in a situation that requires making a choice. They may also have strong simultaneous positive and negative feelings about a situation, which can be confusing and frightening. This may be reflected particularly in their response to significant others, who may be loved and hated with equal intensity at the same time.

All these behaviors are reflective of the degree of disruption of ego function being experienced by the patient. Problems of affect demonstrate compromised ability of the ego to inhibit impulses unless the control is absolute, resulting in no expression of feeling. Problems in association indicate the intrusion of primary process thinking from the id, which results in much use of symbolism and in difficulty in maintaining a logical thought sequence. Autism reveals a disturbance of ego boundaries with decreased ability to distinguish between reality and fantasy and need to identify the self in concrete ways, by touching and feeling. It also represents an effort to decrease stimuli by withdrawing into the self. Ambivalence represents an inability to use secondary process thought for logical decision-making purposes. It also indicates confusion and fear about strong conflicting feelings, which may give rise to frightening impulses.

In a relationship context this complex of

behaviors may serve a protective function. The schizophrenic person has difficulty controlling impulsive behavior. This is easier when others are not around. He also has trouble differentiating himself from others and may not be sure where he ends and the other person begins. He is usually not able to trust others and becomes frightened that he will be harmed in some way when others are around. Communication patterns that are hard to understand and sometimes threatening in content tend to drive people away. The inherent problem in this for the ambivalent schizophrenic is that he feels less threatened with people at a distance but abandoned if they get too far away.

Bleuler also listed secondary symptoms of schizophrenia that he considered to be less specific to the condition and less essential for making the diagnosis. They include such behaviors as delusions, hallucinations, stupor, and negativism.[20]

Another description of behaviors typical of schizophrenia has been developed by Kurt Schneider. He has divided them into first- and second-rank symptoms. Schneiderian first-rank symptoms include hearing one's thoughts spoken aloud, auditory hallucinations commenting on one's behavior, somatic hallucinations,

the belief that one's thoughts are controlled, the belief that one's thoughts can be spread to others, delusions, and outside control or influence of one's actions.[19]

Second-rank symptoms include other hallucinations, depression, euphoria, perplexity, and emotional blunting.[19] Schneider has emphasized that none of the behaviors he has identified are absolutely indicative of schizophrenia but that the presence of a number of them in the absence of any other identifiable pathological condition makes the diagnosis of schizophrenia probable. The clinical and family history must also be considered. It seems unlikely that specific behavioral criteria for schizophrenia will be developed until more is understood about the stressors that cause this disruption in behavior.

The International Pilot Study of Schizophrenia (IPSS) was initiated by the World Health Organization[37,38] as an effort to obtain new knowledge about the epidemiology of schizophrenia. The countries involved included Denmark, India, Colombia, Nigeria, England, the Soviet Union, Taiwan, the United States, and Czechoslovakia. A major problem in the cross-cultural interpretation of epidemiological studies has been doubt as to whether diagnosticians in various settings have used the same diagnostic criteria. For instance, schizophrenia is diagnosed far more frequently in the United States than it is in Great Britain. Therefore one of the major objectives of

TABLE 11-2. Behaviors characteristic of schizophrenia according to Bleuler, Schneider, and the IPSS

Bleuler[20]	Schneider[19]	IPSS[3]
Primary behaviors	**First rank behaviors**	
Affective disturbance	Auditory hallucinations commenting on behavior	Bizarre delusions
Ambivalence	Belief that actions are controlled or influenced from outside	Hearing thoughts spoken aloud
Autism		Incoherent speech
Disordered thought association	Belief that one's thoughts are controlled	Nihilistic delusions
	Belief that one's thoughts can spread to others	No depressed facies
Secondary behaviors	Delusions	No early waking
Delusions	Hearing thoughts spoken aloud	No elation
Hallucinations	**Second rank behaviors**	Poor insight
Negativism	Depression	Poor rapport
Stupor	Emotional blunting	Restricted affect
	Euphoria	Unreliable information given
	Other hallucinations	Widespread delusions
	Perplexity	

the IPSS was to develop and standardize diagnostic criteria that could be used in all nine countries participating in the study and have as high a degree of reliability and validity as possible. Bartko[3] reports a 12-point diagnostic system that was derived from the work of the IPSS. The twelve signs and symptoms include restricted affect, poor insight, hearing one's thoughts spoken aloud, absence of early waking, poor rapport, lack of depressed facies, lack of elation, widespread delusions, incoherent speech, unreliable information given, bizarre delusions, and nihilistic delusions. Carpenter[9] points out that use of a diagnostic system such as that presented by Bartko does not preclude the necessity for the clinician to learn to know the patient as a person. Knowledge of strengths, as well as symptoms, is essential for the clinician to be of assistance to the individual who seeks therapy. Table 11-2 summarizes the criteria cited by Bartko in comparison with those of Bleuler and Schneider.

The IPSS[37,38] represents a major step forward in the epidemiological study of mental illnesses. The study included a 2-year follow-up of the patients who were included in the initial study population. A high percentage of patients were interviewed a second time, providing valuable information about the course of the illness in the nine cultures. Interestingly, subjects who live in developing nations seemed to fare better than those from the more highly developed societies. This study has laid the foundation for future important epidemiological studies.

Behaviors associated with suspicion

Schizophrenia is a severe mental disorder. Many people experience disruptions in interpersonal relationships that are less severe. Sometimes these disruptions are characterized by suspiciousness. A suspicious person is exhibiting a problem with the ability to trust. This may derive from the earliest life experiences as related to the basic sense of trust described by Erikson or may be the result of disruptive experiences later in life, as will be demonstrated in Clinical example 11-3.

CLINICAL EXAMPLE 11-3

Mr. J is an 80-year-old man who lives by himself in the ghetto of a large city. He was referred to a community health nurse following a 2-week hospitalization. He was admitted to the hospital after being arrested for "intoxication" when he was found unconscious on the street. Fortunately, he was taken to a hospital where they discovered that he was comatose because of diabetic acidosis. An attempt was made to refer Mr. J to a nursing home, but he vehemently insisted on returning to his own home. The purpose of the community health nursing referral was to evaluate his ability to cope at home and to assess his ability to manage his American Dietetic Association diet and oral hypoglycemic medication.

Ms. B, the community health nurse, made her first visit the day following Mr. J's discharge from the hospital. When she knocked at his door, there was a long pause and then a feeble voice asked who was there. When she identified herself, the door opened a crack and Mr. J peeked out at her. He said he recognized her blue uniform and would let her in his apartment. There was another pause punctuated with the sound of several locks being undone. At last Ms. B was face-to-face with a withered old man. His apartment was sparsely furnished but neat. The one comfortable chair faced a battered black and white television set. The shades at the window were drawn, leaving most of the room in shadows. A brief inspection of the kitchen revealed sparsely stocked cupboards. There was no evidence of insects or rats. A scrawny cat rubbed against the nurse's leg. Mr. J introduced him as "Tiger."

Ms. B sat down to talk with Mr. J and learn more about his perception of his condition. He knew about his diabetes and seemed to understand his diet but doubted that he could comply with it. He said that he usually ate sweet rolls and coffee for breakfast, soup for lunch, and cereal with milk for dinner. He shopped at a small corner grocery store and bought only what he could carry home. Meats were expensive and he had little money left for food after he paid his rent and utility bills. He was also hesitant to go out very often because he had been knocked down and robbed earlier in the year.

Mr. J said he had lived in the neighborhood many years and stayed there because of his memories of happier times. However, he thought the area had gone downhill. Most of his friends had died or moved away. His children lived in the suburbs, and were "too busy" to see him often, although they had asked at times for him to live with them. He doubted their motives, saying that he thought they probably wanted control of his Social Security checks, his only income.

Ms. B asked if he knew about the senior citizens center two blocks away where they served a hot meal daily and had many activities. He said he had heard about it but had no desire to socialize with the people who went there, since the others in the neighborhood were "not his kind." He also suspected that they would not serve foods that he liked. He again expressed his feelings about the lack of safety in the neighborhood and said that was the reason for his many locks. He watched the news on television every day and there were always stories about thefts and muggings of elderly people. He then confided that he also kept a gun near his bed so if "they" came in at night he would be able to defend himself.

Ms. B spent a little more time on diabetic teaching, trying to help Mr. J find ways to manage his diet within his real social and economic limitations. She planned eventually to introduce the idea of "Meals on Wheels" but realized that she needed to gain his trust first. As she left, she promised to return in 2 days to see how he was doing. Mr. J's response was, "That's up to you. I don't know why you should bother. Nothing will change much."

■■■■■■■■■■■

Mr. J is a person who has become suspicious primarily in response to sociocultural and environmental stressors. His own personal experience of being mugged and the reinforcement he receives from the television news lead him to believe that he lives in a basically hostile environment. Most of his suspiciousness is probably also based on reality. The nurse, of course, will validate as much of the information he gave as possible so that her assessment will be accurate. Mr. J's feelings of vulnerability are probably also related to the frailty associated with aging, which was reinforced by his recent experience of illness and hospitalization. His suspiciousness is functional for him in that it protects him from the dangers in his environment and reduces the anxiety arising from his feeling of vulnerability. It is not functional insofar as it is extending to his children, who probably could be more supportive if they knew he was in need and could possibly persuade him that they wanted him to live with one of them because they cared for him and his safety. His possession of a gun is also potentially harmful to him, since a young intruder could probably overpower Mr. J and would be more likely to harm him if he were armed.

Many people in this society, young and elderly, are isolated from others and know little of their neighbors. Isolation from others can lead to fear and misunderstanding, resulting in an attitude of suspicion. It is obvious how this can develop into a vicious circle, thus leading to a major social problem.

Suspiciousness may be considered in terms of a continuum from completely trusting to completely distrusting. Of course, most people fall somewhere between the extremes. Behavior at either extreme can be problematical. Complete

naiveté can result in others taking advantage of the individual. Such people are usually described as gullible and are ineffectual in influencing others. Extreme suspiciousness, on the other hand, results in behavior that is usually described as paranoid and is of psychotic proportions. Aaronson[1] describes a relationship between alienation and paranoid behavior. The paranoid person often disclaims any power or control over his life. He does not seek a link between his behavior and the outcomes of that behavior. He may, then, become involved in behavior that is not socially acceptable, resulting in isolation. It seems conceivable that the cycle could begin with a sense of powerlessness or could begin with alienation leading to a feeling of a lack of control of one's destiny. In any case, this is a severe disruption in relatedness, requiring therapeutic intervention. The paranoid person uses the mechanism of projection to attribute his own unacceptable impulses to other real or imaginary people and feels that he is being persecuted.

Behaviors associated with dependency

Behaviors of withdrawal and suspiciousness alleviate anxiety by decreasing interpersonal contacts. Sometimes people who have disrupted intimate relationships deal with their anxiety by behaving in an excessively dependent way. This type of behavior is demonstrated by Clinical example 11-4 of a patient with a medical diagnosis of dependent personality disorder and panic disorder.

■■■■■■■■■■■

CLINICAL EXAMPLE 11-4

Ms. R, the psychiatric liaison nurse, was called to see Ms. J, a patient on the medical service of a general hospital. Ms. J had been admitted to the hospital complaining of attacks of dizziness, tremulousness, dyspnea, and diaphoresis. She stated the fear that she was "losing her mind." The nurses on the medical unit had called Ms. R because, although the medical workup was almost completed and the results were entirely negative, the patient continued to complain of the same symptoms. The nurses were frustrated because Ms. J was constantly asking to have her bed adjusted, her water refreshed, her bedroom slippers found, and similar requests. In addition, she would have attacks of panic with hyperventilation during which she needed close nursing observation and help rebreathing into a paper bag to prevent loss of consciousness. Through careful nursing observation, the nurses were able to identify that the panic attacks occurred most frequently during visits from family members and often when her demands of the hospital staff were not complied with readily. The nurses were also aware that their frustration with Ms. J's constant demands and lack of response to their nursing intervention was interfering with their ability to give her good nursing care.

When Ms. R interviewed Ms. J, she observed that the patient lay curled on the bed and spoke in a soft, barely audible tone. She teared frequently during the conversation. She spoke readily of her past when questioned but quickly refocused the discussion to her present complaints. Ms. J revealed that she was 45 years old, married, and the mother of a daughter, age 23. She said that she felt very close to her daughter who had married and moved away from home 3 months ago. The attacks began soon after she left. Her daughter now lived about a mile from Ms. J and was described as devoted to her mother. Mr. J was employed as a pharmacist and was required to work some evenings. Ms. J said she had not minded this until her daughter had left home. She then began to find the evenings that her husband worked to be difficult because she felt lonely and did not want to bother her daughter with visits or phone calls. She said that her family was her whole life. Ms. R asked Ms. J about other interests that she might have. She said that her main diversion was watching television, although she also read a few magazines and did a little sewing. She enjoyed cooking for others but not herself, and usually did not eat when her husband was working. She was on speaking terms with her neighbors but not really friendly with them. Because of her husband's objections, she had never worked outside of the home.

As she spoke with the nurse, Ms. J began to appear more and more anxious. She became tremulous and started to breathe rapidly. Ms. R helped her to rebreathe and comforted her by talking soothingly and patting her on the shoulder. After Ms. J seemed calmer, Ms. R asked if she thought her behavior was related to the topics that they had been discussing. Ms. J said that she could see no connection and stated that her symptoms were real to her, not just in her head, which was what people kept telling her. Ms. R assured her that she could see that she was indeed uncomfortable but that very nervous people sometimes showed their nervousness in physical ways. Soon after this Ms. R had to leave. As she left the room, Ms. J asked her if she would be back.

Ms. R later discussed Ms. J with the nursing staff. She explained that the patient was a very dependent woman who had for many years lived vicariously through her family, especially her daughter. When her daughter married, Ms. J felt abandoned but could not express her feelings directly. Her dependent style of relating blocked her from assertively reaching out for other activities to gratify her need for relatedness. Her frustration and loneliness caused anxiety. Her coping response took the form of a physiological conversion. This behavior was reinforced when she received a great deal of attention focused on her illness. Thus her hospitalization was providing her with not only the primary psychological gain of knowing that her symptoms were being explored and treated but also the secondary gain of the renewed attention and consideration from her family. Her symptoms were not conscious behaviors on her part but were her response to her anxiety. Therefore she could not understand why people kept suggesting that there was really no physical basis for her illness. Any increase in her anxiety level, then, caused an increase in her symptoms and in her dependent behavior. Ms. J needed help with this problem because, although people were initially sympathetic to her need for dependency gratification, they would soon become frustrated with her, as is demonstrated by the response of the nursing staff.

Behaviors associated with manipulation

The disruptions in relatedness discussed so far have involved either too much distance from other people or the need for too much closeness to others. Another disruption in relatedness focuses on individuals who are superficially involved with others. These are people who use manipulative behaviors, treating others as objects. The patient who demonstrates this in Clinical example 11-5 has a history of multiple drug abuse and a medical diagnosis of antisocial personality.

CLINICAL EXAMPLE 11-5

Mr. Y is a 20-year-old single man who was committed to an inpatient psychiatric unit by a judge for a psychiatric evaluation. He had been charged with sale of illicit drugs, statutory rape of his 15-year-old pregnant girl friend, and contributing to the delinquency of a minor. He had been arrested on the grounds of a junior high school where he was selling PCP and barbiturates to a group of young teenagers.

In jail, Mr. Y had been observed to be "crazy" by the guards. He paced his cell, chanted, and threw his food on the floor. On the basis of this behavior, the judge was requested to order a psychiatric evaluation and did so. On arrival at the psychiatric unit, Mr. Y continued to behave in the same manner. However, his behavior did not seem typical of psychosis. There was no evidence of hallucinations or disorders of thought or affect. When unaware that he was observed, Mr. Y seemed relaxed and was noted at one time to be conversing with another patient. By the day after admission he seemed to be free of his symptomatic behavior. At this point the staff began to describe him as a "nice guy." He complimented female staff members and behaved toward them in a pleasantly seductive manner. He was deferential to the physicians and readily agreed to abide by all the rules. He was helpful with other patients. In group meetings he admitted that he had behaved badly in the past and described how he had been led astray by his friends. He said he became involved in drugs because he wanted to be "one of the gang" and he "needed the bread" so he "had to" start selling drugs. By the end of his first week in the hospital he had elicited the sympathy of all the other patients and of the staff. However, an interview with his parents revealed that he had had a stormy adolescence, including arrests for vandalism and expulsion from school at age 14 for drug use and fighting. They said he had become involved with friends who were a bad influence. His family was glad he was getting help, because they had always known he was "sick."

Nine days after admission, following visiting hours, it was noted that Mr. Y and two other patients looked lethargic. Their speech was slurred, and their gaits were ataxic. The nursing staff immediately collected urine and blood specimens for toxicological analysis. The unit was searched for hidden drugs, but none were found. The results of the toxicology screening tests, however, were positive for barbiturates. Suspicion was immediately focused on Mr. Y, since the other patients involved were young adolescents with no history of drug abuse. When confronted, he seemed amazed that he could be suspected and pointed out his past behavior as a model patient. He acknowledged that he had behaved strangely and said he had wondered if someone had "slipped" him some drugs. He was convincing but was warned that if he was seen to be involved in any way with drugs, he would be sent directly back to jail.

As part of the evaluation, the social worker had been working with Mr. Y's pregnant girl friend. As the girl began to trust the social worker, she confided that she was not sure that Mr. Y had fathered her child, since she had had to turn to prostitution to help support them. Mr. Y, who had been unemployed for a year, had been angry when told of her pregnancy because it meant a reduction in his income, and he had pressured her to have an abortion. She had refused because she hoped it was his baby and that he would decide to marry her once he saw the child. However, when she told him that her decision to have the baby was final, he assaulted her and then told her he did not want to see her again.

Mr. Y began to pressure the physicians for their decision on his ability to be held responsible for his actions. He seemed to be actively engaged in therapy and promised to continue with outpatient treatment if recommended for probation. He also convinced his family of his good intentions and they agreed to allow him to move into their house. On the basis of these indications of positive behavioral change, Mr. Y did receive a recommendation for probation, which was carried out by the judge.

Three months after discharge from the hospital Mr. Y and a friend were arrested for operating a PCP-manufacturing lab in the friend's garage.

The manipulative person presents a particularly difficult nursing problem. There is frequently little motivation for change because, as is demonstrated in the case of Mr. Y, manipulative behavior has inherent rewards. It helps the individual accomplish a desired goal. The manipulator is goal oriented or self-oriented, not other oriented. However, this person is skilled at giving the impression of involvement with others and may be charming to gain the confidence of the other. Mr. Y was able to gain the confidence of the staff and knew that he needed to do so to have the support he needed in court. Another prominent characteristic of the manipulator is an absence of awareness of the lack of relatedness to others and the assumption that all interpersonal relationships are opportunistic in nature. This person cannot imagine an intimate, sharing relationship because he assumes that if he does not maintain control, the other person will take advantage of or control him. Shostrom[28] sees this issue of controlling or being controlled as central to manipulative behavior. He adds that these same issues are primary in actualizing behavior, but the actualizer expresses manipulative behavior creatively, whereas the manipulator is self-defeating.

The major behaviors representative of disruptions in relatedness have been presented. Individual patients frequently experience combinations of these behaviors and the nurse must be able to identify the complex spectrum of behavior that any person may exhibit when confronted with high levels of stress and anxiety. In some cases a usual mode of behavior, such as manipulation, may be exaggerated or combined with a change in behavior. For instance, a manipulative person may withdraw when confronted by his manipulations and may be rejected by those he has been trying to manipulate. In other instances the behavior that appears in response to stress may be different from the individual's usual style of relatedness. A person who is usually gregarious may withdraw when under great stress. It is helpful to include in the nursing assessment a description of the patient's usual interpersonal relationships to provide a baseline of normal behavior for that individual. This helps to avoid measuring the patient's progress against the nurse's rather than the patient's norm.

Coping mechanisms

The behaviors associated with disruptions in relatedness are in themselves attempts to cope with the anxiety that is associated with threatened or actual existential loneliness. Unfortunately, as demonstrated by the case studies presented in this chapter, these attempts to cope may lead to a marginal adjustment and may, at times, serve to drive people even farther away. Thus the person is always caught in the approach-avoidance conflict of the need-fear dilemma,[7] seeking some degree of human contact on the one hand and pushing people away on the other.

The dependent person copes by clutching others and refusing to let go, inviting rejection when others feel smothered by clinging behavior. This person has no faith at all in his ability to rely on himself. Dependent behavior is often reciprocal with the dominant behavior of a partner. Reaction formation may be a coping mechanism that is used to avoid confrontation of the anger that results from feeling unable to become involved in self-actualizing activities. The manipulator, on the other hand, copes by dehumanizing others and, in the process, himself. Feeling is so threatening that its very existence is denied. The withdrawn person craves interpersonal contact but fears rejection even more. Retreat into a shell is protective but is also a deprivation and therefore not rewarding. Extremely withdrawn people are using the mechanism of regression. Suspicious people keep others at arm's length by refusing to believe that they are to be trusted. This is frequently a defense against confronting the lack of a more basic trust in the self. Such a confrontation would result in intolerable anxiety and ego disintegration. Projection is the coping mechanism underlying suspicious behavior.

People with schizophrenia rely on coping mechanisms that tend to be primitive and sometimes only marginally effective in controlling their interpersonal anxiety. Searles[27] has delineated several aspects of schizophrenic communication that are used as coping mechanisms.

The first mechanism described by Searles is displacement. This results in the direction of the communication toward an object that is not the real stimulus for the response. There may also be a temporal discrepancy between the conscious and unconscious objects. For example, a patient who is angry at the nurse may talk about a past quarrel with a close friend. Searles[27] relates this to the person's poor differentiation of "perceptual-conceptual" experience, which leads him to perceive similar objects as identical.

Projection is a mechanism discussed earlier as it relates to the development of paranoid delusions and auditory hallucinations. Aside from projective verbalizations, schizophrenic patients frequently also project meaning to the nonverbal communication of others, which reflects the meaning attached to the person's own nonverbal behavior. Projection can reveal a great deal about a person's world view and about which aspects of existence are difficult for him to handle.

Another coping mechanism used by schizophrenic patients is introjection. Searles believes that this mechanism is at the root of the patient's feeling he is controlled or influenced by others. The behavior and even sometimes the unconscious impulses of the other person are experienced by the patient as his own and reflected in his behavior. For instance, the patient may act out an unconscious wish of a significant other person that is transmitted nonverbally.

Condensation entails the concentration of several thoughts and feelings into a relatively simple verbal or nonverbal message. This may be expressed as a repetitive statement or gesture, which may assume a variety of meanings, as if the person has very limited resources of communication. Searles believes that this is related to a lack of differentiation of concrete figurative meanings. For example, a statement that seems to be clear and straightforward may also be highly complex and symbolical.[27] The patient may be unaware of the hidden meanings, and the nurse may need supervisory help to interpret the communication.

Patients may unconsciously protect themselves from experiencing overwhelming emotion by means of isolation. Much of this may be related to ambivalent feelings and helps the individual cope with the anxiety aroused by these conflicting feelings.[27]

As can be seen from this discussion, many coping mechanisms may be reflected in impaired communication patterns. Behavior that is symptomatic of a high level of anxiety may also be reflective of the person's attempt to cope with the anxiety. The nurse must understand this complex interrelationship between anxiety, coping, and observable behavior to plan appropriate nursing interventions.

TABLE 11-3. **Comparative examples of nursing diagnoses and medical diagnoses associated with paranoid schizophrenia**

Nursing diagnoses	Medical diagnoses as described in DSM-III*
Use of disordered communication (loose association, concreteness) related to fear of intimate human contact	Diagnostic criteria for SCHIZOPHRENIA, PARANOID TYPE
Paranoid delusions related to severe anxiety, leading to the projection of threatening aggressive impulses	A type of schizophrenia dominated by one or more of the following:
Auditory hallucinations related to severe anxiety due to fear of loss of control	1. Persecutory delusions 2. Grandiose delusions 3. Delusional jealousy 4. Hallucinations with persecutory or grandiose content
Inability to continue with rehabilitation plan related to impending disintegration of family support system	
Isolation of self from others related to impaired ability to trust based on disrupted family situation	

*From American Psychiatric Association: Diagnostic and statistical manual of mental disorders, third edition, Washington, D.C., APA, 1980.

TABLE 11-4. **Comparative examples of nursing diagnoses and medical diagnoses associated with catatonic schizophrenia**

Nursing diagnoses	Medical diagnoses as described in DSM-III*
Refusal to move or speak related to fear of loss of control of sexual and aggressive impulses	Diagnostic criteria for SCHIZOPHRENIA, CATATONIC TYPE
Avoidance of heterosexual relationships related to ambivalence about own sexuality	A type of schizophrenia dominated by any of the following: 1. Catatonic stupor (marked decrease in reactivity to environment and/or reduction of spontaneous movements and activity) or mutism 2. Catatonic negativism (an apparently motiveless resistance to all instructions or attempts to be moved) 3. Catatonic rigidity (maintenance of a rigid posture against efforts to be moved) 4. Catatonic excitement (excited motor activity, apparently purposeless and not influenced by external stimuli) 5. Catatonic posturing (voluntary assumption of inappropriate or bizarre posture)
Deterioration in job performance related to moderate anxiety based on fear of closeness	

*From American Psychiatric Association: Diagnostic and statistical manual of mental disorders, third edition, Washington, D.C., APA, 1980.

TABLE 11-5. **Comparative examples of nursing diagnoses and medical diagnoses associated with dependent personality disorder and panic disorder**

Nursing diagnoses	Medical diagnoses as described in DSM-III*

Inability to express feelings of loneliness, anger, and depression related to daughter's leaving home and husband's frequent absences

Attacks of dizziness, tremulousness, dyspnea, and sweating related to panic level of anxiety from perceived threat of abandonment by significant others

Concern that she is "losing her mind" related to panic level of anxiety from perceived loss of control of self and others

Diagnostic criteria for DEPENDENT PERSONALITY DISORDER

The following are characteristic of the individual's current and long-term functioning, are not limited to episodes of illness, and cause either significant impairment in social or occupational functioning or subjective distress

A. Passively allows others to assume responsibility for major areas of life because of inability to function independently (e.g., lets spouse decide what kind of job he or she should have)

B. Subordinates own needs to those of persons on whom he or she depends in order to avoid any possibility of having to rely on self (e.g., tolerates abusive spouse)

C. Lacks self-confidence (e.g., sees self as helpless, stupid)

Diagnostic criteria for PANIC DISORDER

A. At least three panic attacks within a 3-week period in circumstances other than during marked physical exertion or in a life-threatening situation. The attacks are not precipitated only by exposure to a circumscribed phobic stimulus.

B. Panic attacks are manifested by discrete periods of apprehension or fear, and at least four of the following symptoms appear during each attack:

1. Dyspnea
2. Palpitations
3. Chest pain or discomfort
4. Choking or smothering sensations
5. Dizziness, vertigo, or unsteady feelings
6. Feelings of unreality
7. Paresthesias (tingling in hands or feet)
8. Hot and cold flashes
9. Sweating
10. Faintness
11. Trembling or shaking
12. Fear of dying, going crazy, or doing something uncontrolled during an attack

C. Not due to a physical disorder or another mental disorder, such as major depression, somatization disorder, or schizophrenia.

D. The disorder is not associated with agoraphobia.

*From American Psychiatric Association: Diagnostic and statistical manual of mental disorders, third edition, Washington, D.C., APA, 1980.

TABLE 11-6. Comparative examples of nursing diagnoses and medical diagnoses associated with antisocial personality disorder

Nursing diagnoses	Medical diagnoses as described in DSM-III

Nursing diagnoses

Feigned psychotic behavior related to preference for hospital over jail setting

Provision of illicit drugs to others and drug abuse related to resistance to social controls

Desertion of pregnant girl friend related to lack of perception of needs of others

Repeated violations of rules and laws related to inadequately developed superego (conscience)

Medical diagnoses as described in DSM-III

Diagnostic criteria for ANTISOCIAL PERSONALITY DISORDER

A. Current age at least 18

B. Onset before age 15 as indicated by a history of three or more of the following before that age:

1. Truancy (positive if it amounted to at least 5 days per year for at least 2 years, not including the last year of school)
2. Expulsion or suspension from school for misbehavior
3. Delinquency (arrested or referred to juvenile court because of behavior)
4. Running away from home overnight at least twice while living in parental or parental surrogate home
5. Persistent lying
6. Repeated sexual intercourse in a casual relationship
7. Repeated drunkenness or substance abuse
8. Thefts
9. Vandalism
10. School grades markedly below expectations in relation to estimated or known IQ (may have resulted in repeating a year)
11. Chronic violations of rules at home and/or at school (other than truancy)
12. Initiation of fights

C. At least four of the following manifestations of the disorder since age 18:

1. Inability to sustain consistent work behavior, as indicated by any of the following: (a) too frequent job changes (e.g., three or more jobs in 5 years not accounted for by nature of job or economic or seasonal fluctuation), (b) significant unemployment (e.g., 6 months or more in 5 years when expected to work), (c) serious absenteeism from work (e.g., average 3 days or more of lateness or absence per month), (d) walking off several jobs without other jobs in sight (NOTE: similar behavior in an academic setting during the last few years of school may substitute for this criterion in individuals who by reason of their age or circumstances have not had an opportunity to demonstrate occupational adjustment)
2. Lack of ability to function as a responsible parent as evidenced by one or more of the following: (a) child's malnutrition, (b) child's illness resulting from lack of minimal hygiene standards, (c) failure to obtain medical care for a seriously ill child, (d) child's dependence on neighbors or nonresident relatives for food or shelter, (e) failure to arrange for a caretaker for a child under 6 when parent is away from home, (f) repeated squandering, on personal items, of money required for household necessities
3. Failure to accept social norms with respect to lawful behavior, as indicated by any of the following: repeated thefts, illegal occupation (pimping, prostitution, fencing, selling drugs), multiple arrests, a felony conviction
4. Inability to maintain enduring attachment to a sexual partner as indicated by two or more divorces and/or separations (whether legally married or not), desertion of spouse, promiscuity (ten or more sexual partners within 1 year)
5. Irritability and aggressiveness as indicated by repeated physical fights or assault (not required by one's job or to defend someone or oneself), including spouse or child beating

TABLE 11-6. Comparative examples of nursing diagnoses and medical diagnoses associated with antisocial personality disorder—cont'd

Nursing diagnoses	Medical diagnoses as described in DSM-III
	6. Failure to honor financial obligations, as indicated by repeated defaulting on debts, failure to provide child support, failure to support other dependents on a regular basis
	7. Failure to plan ahead, or impulsivity, as indicated by traveling from place to place without a prearranged job or clear goal for the period of travel or clear idea about when the travel would terminate, or lack of a fixed address for a month or more
	8. Disregard for the truth as indicated by repeated lying, use of aliases, "conning" others for personal profit
	9. Recklessness, as indicated by driving while intoxicated or recurrent speeding
	D. A pattern of continuous antisocial behavior in which the rights of others are violated, with no intervening period of at least 5 years without antisocial behavior between age 15 and the present time (except when the individual was bedridden or confined in a hospital or penal institution)
	E. Antisocial behavior is not due to either severe mental retardation, schizophrenia, or manic episodes

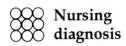 **Nursing diagnosis**

When diagnosing a disruption in an individual's relatedness, the nurse should take into account the degree of disruption experienced by the patient, the behaviors that demonstrate the presence of the disruption, and the stressors that are leading to the disruption. Generally, there are multiple patient problems that must be considered when one is planning nursing care; so the diagnosis should be thorough and should reflect depth in understanding the patient's life situation.

Table 11-3 illustrates nursing diagnoses related to the case study of Mr. D (p. 368) as compared to the DSM-III[2] criteria for the diagnosis of schizophrenia, paranoid type. The latter set of criteria must be combined with the general criteria for the diagnosis of schizophrenia (Table 11-1).

Table 11-4 identifies nursing diagnoses related to the case study of Ms. W (p. 370) in comparison to the DSM-III[2] criteria for the diagnosis of schizophrenia, catatonic type. Again, the general criteria for the diagnosis of schizophrenia (Table 11-1) must be considered as well.

The following nursing diagnoses relate to the case study of Mr. J (p. 375) and demonstrate the nursing needs of a patient with a less severe level of suspicion than that demonstrated by Mr. D. There is no corresponding psychiatric medical diagnosis in this case.

■ Social isolation related to fear of leaving his apartment
■ Failure to follow American Dietetic Association diet related to difficulty carrying and affording the required foods
■ Weakened family ties related to distance from children
■ Possession of a gun related to lack of trust in the safety of his environment

The nursing diagnoses illustrated in Table 11-5 relate to the case of Ms. R (p. 376) and demonstrate the nursing care needs of a dependent patient. The nursing diagnoses may be compared with the DSM-III[2] criteria for the diagnoses of dependent personality disorder and panic disorder.

The nursing diagnoses relating to the case study of Mr. Y (p. 377) demonstrate the nursing care needs of a manipulative patient. They are compared to the DSM-III[2] criteria for the diagnosis of antisocial personality disorder given in Table 11-6.

Fig. 11-2 illustrates the model of health-illness phenomena related to disruptions in interpersonal relationships.

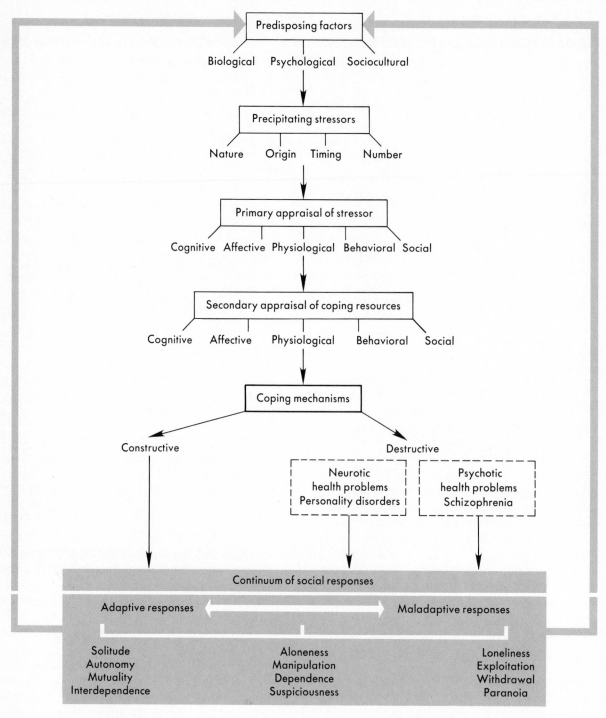

FIG. 11-2
Model of health-illness phenomena applied to interpersonal relationships.

Planning and implementation of nursing intervention

Goal setting

It can be difficult to set mutual goals with a patient in the area of relatedness. This is in part because mutuality must be based on a strong nurse-patient relationship, and it is, of course, difficult to develop a strong relationship with a patient who has problems establishing intimacy. In addition, the setting of a goal implies a commitment to change. Many patients who have disruptions in human relationships are reluctant to commit themselves to change. Since most of these behavioral disruptions are also serving as coping mechanisms, there is additional resistance to change.

For these reasons, even though it is desirable to have the patient's full participation in goal setting, it may be necessary for the nurse to set initial goals. This must be done with consideration to all the data collected in the nursing assessment and should be based on the nursing diagnosis. Environmental constraints also need to be considered, especially since to overcome a problem with relatedness, the person must be involved with others. At first, the other person may be the nurse, but eventually the behaviors learned in the nurse-patient relationships should be transferred to other interpersonal relationships.

Long-term goals should be directed toward alleviation of the patient's particular problem with relatedness. For instance, a goal for a withdrawn patient might be to inquire about the activities of other family members. For a suspicious patient, it might be to initiate a new relationship with a coworker. A goal for a dependent person could be to join a new social activity group in an area of interest, such as a sport or a craft and attend regularly. A long-term goal for a manipulative patient might be to spontaneously ask about the welfare of another person. For a person who exhibits impaired communication, a goal might be to use logical and coherent speech when relating to others. Each of these long-term goals must be approached by a series of short-term goals. For instance, the long-term goal for the dependent person to join an activity group might be broken down as follows:

1. After 1 week of contact with the nurse the patient will attend an activity group accompanied by the nurse and observe the group meeting.
2. After observing two group sessions with the nurse the patient will participate in one simple individual activity within the group setting.
3. After two individual activity sessions the patient will attend the group session with the nurse and participate in an activity with one other group member.
4. After two sessions of participating in an activity with one other member the patient will attend with the nurse and join in an activity involving the whole group.
5. After two sessions of whole-group activity the patient will attend the group accompanied by another member and join in whole-group activity.
6. After two sessions accompanied by another member the patient will attend the group alone and participate fully in activities.
7. The patient will join a new social activity group in an area of interest and attend regularly (original long-term goal).

This kind of stepwise progression gradually exposes the patient to more complex interactions and decreases the involvement of the nurse. The timing may require modification depending on the patient's response, but a time sequence should be included to stimulate progress.

Goals that are developed with patients who have impaired relationships may take a long time to accomplish. These patients frequently use bizarre communication patterns to avoid intimate relationships, so are usually reluctant to take the risk of communicating more directly. However, it is still possible to develop goals directed toward modification in disrupted communication patterns. Grosicki and Harmonson[15] demonstrate this in their nursing action guide for dealing with hallucinating patients. The long-term goals they developed focus on involvement in satisfying interpersonal relationships and on learning more effective methods of coping with anxiety. The short-term goals focus on relating first to an individual and later to groups and on verbalizing the occurrence and content of the hallucination. Goals with these patients may also focus on the modification of specific communication patterns. For example, the patient will use nonverbal communication that is congruent with the verbal content of his speech. Another example of a goal for a patient with impaired communication is "The patient will verbally identify angry feelings when they occur during a one-to-one interaction." These goals need to be developed with the active participation of the patient and must be congruent with his ability to tolerate anxiety, since learning to relate more directly and openly is an anxiety-provoking experience. Increasing the anxiety level before the patient has increased coping ability and environmental supports may only reinforce the patient's use of dysfunctional coping behaviors.

Intervening in withdrawal

The interpersonal relationship between the nurse and the patient is central to the practice of psychiatric nursing. In the case of a patient who has a disruption in the area of relatedness, it is even more complicated than it is with other patients to establish and maintain a therapeutic relationship. The disrupted behavior will also be experienced in the context of the therapeutic nursing relationship. The nurse therefore has the additional challenge of establishing a relationship with a patient who already has problems relating to others. It takes a great deal of sensitivity and self-awareness to do this successfully. One of the most frustrating, but also one of the most potentially rewarding, experiences for the psychiatric nurse is that of intervening therapeutically with a withdrawn patient, particularly one who is psychotic. Withdrawn patients do not often respond quickly to nursing intervention. They usually need consistent, repeated approaches by the nurse to convince them of her sincere concern.

The extremely withdrawn patient may be mute and immobile, challenging the nurse's ingenuity in giving nursing care that attends to all the biological, psychological, and social needs. In her classic article on the nursing care of the withdrawn patient, Will[35] cites three general focuses for nursing intervention. These include the fulfillment of the patient's needs, the facilitation of communication, and the facilitation of social participation. Frequently the highest priority must first be given to the fulfillment of biological needs. Food and fluid intake must be carefully monitored to maintain adequate nutrition and hydration. If the patient is relatively immobile, intravenous or gavage feeding may be necessary. This should be explained to the patient in terms of the need to maintain his health, as opposed to it being seen as a punitive measure. It is equally important to record urinary

output and frequency of defecation. Urinary retention with bladder distention and fecal impaction are complications that can be avoided by good nursing care. If the patient refuses to move voluntarily, positioning and skin care are other nursing concerns. Even if the patient will respond to direction from the nurse, reminders to attend to personal hygiene will probably be required. Although withdrawn people may appear indifferent to others, it must be remembered that this apparent lack of concern is probably a defense. Even people who seem completely oblivious to their surroundings are likely to be aware of everything that happens. Frequently a patient who has recovered from a state of catatonic stupor is able to describe in detail conversations and events that occurred during the stupor. Empathy can help the nurse to understand how the patient may feel about being fed, bathed, and dressed. These activities are best carried out in a matter-of-fact way and with the attitude conveyed that the nurse is sensitive to the patient's needs and feelings. Patients who do not perform self-care should still be given the opportunity to do so by being instructed to perform simple tasks. The patient who is being bathed can be given a soaped washcloth and asked to wash himself. In this way the nurse may assess the patient's progress. As the patient can perform one task, another should be introduced, with the nurse developing a hierarchy of successively more complex tasks for the patient to master with the ultimate goal of achieving maximum possible responsibility for meeting his own biological needs.

Communicating with the withdrawn patient demands great patience on the part of the nurse. It can be uncomfortable to sit in silence with a mute person if one is accustomed to the more usual action-oriented role of the nurse. There may be a temptation to chatter aimlessly, to make trite remarks, or to fidget. As always, the nurse needs to analyze her own response to the situation and be sure that her nursing interventions are goal directed. For instance, if the nurse has assessed the patient's baseline interests and knows that he is a football fan, telling him about a big game can be a way of stimulating his interest in his environment. However, if she tells the patient the details of her date the night before, she is more likely trying to make herself less anxious by filling up the silence. Constant chatter also conveys to the patient the message that there is no expectation for him to verbalize. It is much more therapeutic to make open-ended statements followed by pauses so the patient may respond if he feels inclined to do so. Direct questions may be experienced as intimidating or intrusive by the patient and should be used judiciously. Questions giving a choice should be used only if there is a choice to be made. Asking a patient if he wants his medication when he should definitely take it is not a clear message and should be avoided. Statements should be clear and concise but not infantilizing. Information from the nursing assessment can guide the nurse in selecting language appropriate to the sociocultural background of the patient.

Awareness of nonverbal communication is particularly important in interacting with a withdrawn patient. Even a totally silent patient may communicate a great deal through body language and gestures. Feelings may be communicated nonverbally, sometimes more accurately than by verbalization. For instance, a tense person who holds his body rigidly and glares at the nurse may be angry but may not feel able to tell her this. Depressed people often communicate the depth of their despair by a body position that looks tired, droopy, and bent as if to ward off unexpected assaults. Anxiety is communicated nonverbally and may contribute to the nurse's discomfort when interacting with a withdrawn patient.

The withdrawn person may also indicate increased accessibility to others nonverbally. The establishment of eye contact by a person who has usually avoided it may signal the beginning of a relationship. Reaching out or the acceptance of a touch may have the same meaning. Relaxation of a usually tense body posture can be the first sign of increased comfort with the nurse. Other nonverbal signs of decreasing withdrawal include attention to personal appearance and initiation of interpersonal contacts in other activity.

The nurse's own nonverbal activity is also an integral part of the relationship. Many times, gestures and grimaces may be automatic, but they convey a message to the other person. Since the withdrawn patient is usually still very sensitive to events in the environment, the nurse needs to develop an awareness of habitual body language. Feedback from colleagues and supervisors can be helpful in this respect and should be encouraged by the nurse. If videotape is available, it can provide immediate input about nonverbal and verbal communication and can be a helpful tool in supervision. If videotaping is done with a patient, it should, of course, be carefully planned and done only with the patient's informed consent. Role play with other professionals can often be equally useful and eliminate the concern about adversely influencing the therapeutic relationship.

Nonverbal means of communicating can be therapeutic in the nursing care of the withdrawn patient. Looking directly at a patient when greeting him may convey concern. A gentle touch can establish contact with a withdrawn depressed person. Leaning toward a patient but maintaining a comfortable distance screens out other people and transmits the message that the nurse is focusing attention on the patient only. Caring for physiological needs is a powerful means of expressing caring. An attitude of concerned, but not intrusive, interest allows the patient to control the pace of the development of closeness. The process of relating to a withdrawn patient requires much sensitivity of the nurse.

The initial intervention with a person who is socially isolated or withdrawn is generally most effective as a one-to-one relationship between the nurse and the patient. However, the ultimate goal is to facilitate the patient's ability to establish healthy interpersonal relationships with a variety of other people to experience a fulfilling life. As the nurse and patient begin to relate more comfortably, others should gradually be included in the patient's social sphere. The nurse can help the patient try to relate to others. Another person can be invited to join a card game or to share in a discussion. In the hospital setting the nurse is often in a good position to introduce the patient to others with whom he might have something in common, since she has knowledge of others in the environment. In the community the nurse can utilize her knowledge of community resources and refer the patient to a social group that is likely to be compatible with his needs and interests. As the process of expanding the patient's sphere of relationships is taking place, the nurse must be careful not to give the impression that the goal is to reject the patient. Time for individual interaction should still be scheduled on a regular basis so the therapeutic relationship can continue to grow.

Brown, Cornwell, and Weist[6] describe the ways that the elderly in institutions are depersonalized, leading to their alienation from the social system. These staff behaviors include impersonal communication, such as not using the correct name; material depersonalization, such as not allowing personal objects to be kept; routinization of life activities; and deprivation of protection, exemplified by leaving the windows open in cold weather. In contrast, Carter and Galliano[10] describe a personalizing intervention with a group of elderly nursing home residents who were isolating themselves as a protection from the pain of potential losses.

For many patients the family is the focus of much of the interpersonal difficulty. Frequently family therapy is indicated and should be undertaken only by a therapist who is especially trained for this modality. However, the nurse who is working with the patient can assist the family to understand the patient's needs. If the patient does not want to visit with the family, the nurse may help them to maintain the relationship by demonstrating her concern for the family members and by suggesting things they can do for the patient, such as bringing favorite foods or taking care of errands. Sometimes a family needs help in seeing small signs of progress. Often family members have questions about the patient's care. The nurse can be helpful by educating the family about the treatment process. Of course, the patient should be included in this teaching and should be informed about contacts between the nurse and the family.

Nursing intervention with the withdrawn patient should be directed toward the accomplishment of reasonable goals. A shy person should not be expected to become a gregarious one. Knowledge of the person's usual personality is helpful in setting expectations. However, the patient is the best source of information about goal accomplishment. The individual's comfort or discomfort with his life-style and interpersonal relationships should always be the primary criterion for therapeutic progress.

Terminating a relationship with a withdrawn patient may be difficult for the nurse. The patient is likely to resist termination from a person to whom he has become close after a time of loneliness and isolation. He may be frightened that he will not be able to maintain the ability to form healthier relationships. New problems are often brought up at termination and usually indicate an attempt to prolong an important relationship. The nurse, too, will have many feelings about terminating with a patient with whom she worked so hard to build a relationship. Even the satisfaction of contributing to the growth of another person cannot erase the pain of severing the relationship. However, the experience of a well-handled termination can be the culmination of the therapeutic relationship by helping the patient learn to deal with a loss in a healthy, mature way.

Intervening in suspiciousness

Nursing interventions with a suspicious patient are in many respects similar to those with the withdrawn patient. The primary long-term goal with the suspicious patient is that the patient will demonstrate trust in the nurse. The patient will then, hopefully, also develop the ability to trust others who are deserving of being trusted. People demonstrate trust by making themselves accessible to others, both physically and emotionally. Thus the trusting patient will not evade contact with the nurse and will also share thoughts and feelings with her. This process develops gradually in any relationship but may be particularly slow when the patient has difficulty trusting other people.

Reliability is one factor that helps to foster trust. The nurse must follow through on commitments made to the patient. When working with a suspicious or paranoid patient, the nurse can make a point of informing the patient of when they will be talking and then follow through with the schedule as a means of demonstrating reliability. Very suspicious people may not tolerate prolonged contacts, since this tends to raise the anxiety level as the person tries to defend himself from what he perceives as a potential attack from another person. In this instance the nurse may plan several brief contacts spaced throughout the day, thus also repeatedly reinforcing her reliability.

Suspicious patients also at times may have difficulty in maintaining their physiological well-being. Fear may interfere with sleep. A light in the room at night may be helpful. Sleeping medication may be offered, but if the paranoid patient refuses to take it, insistence by the nurse will only increase the insomnia by further agitating the patient. Priority in this case should probably be given to persuading the patient to take prescribed antipsychotic medications, which will usually also cause some drowsiness. Refusal to eat and/or drink may be another problem encountered with the suspicious patient. Attempts to force oral intake usually meet with failure and are frustrating to both nurse and patient. Sometimes a suspicious patient will eat food brought by his family, food he prepares himself, or packaged food. Whenever possible these preferences should be respected. As the patient learns to trust the nurse and the hospital, he will begin to eat and drink. If the patient is in danger from dehydration or malnutrition, the physician may take drastic action and prescribe gavage feeding or intravenous therapy. If this does occur, careful explanations should be given as the treatment takes place. Treatment will be experienced by the patient as an intrusive assault on his physical being, and much supportive nursing care will be required.

Since suspicious people do fear intrusion from others and question the motives of those who approach them, care must be taken to respect the patient's right to privacy. The patient may appreciate intervals of solitude that can be worked into the daily schedule. Warning should be given of the approach of another person so as to avoid startling the suspicious patient. The patient should be allowed to control the amount of self-revelation that takes place in the interaction with the nurse. A probing approach will only alienate the patient and retard the development of trust. As trust grows, anxiety will decrease and the patient will have less need of his suspicious defenses. The growth of the patient's ability to confide in the nurse is one way to measure the success of nursing intervention with the suspicious patient.

Most people interact with a variety of therapeutic team members, especially in the hospital setting. When the patient has difficulty establishing trust, it is best if one or two people are designated as those who will work consistently and closely with him. However, other staff members should be aware of the treatment plan, and their approach to the patient should be consistent with that of the primary caregivers. Significant others should also be made aware of the care plan and should be encouraged to participate in it. Consistency among those who have close contact with the patient also promotes the development of trust.

Openness and honesty on the part of the nurse demonstrate to the patient that she can be trusted. For instance, if the nurse plans to meet with the patient's family, she should inform the patient of this plan. She should then discuss the issue of confidentiality of information with both the patient and family. Families of suspicious patients often abound with family secrets, and the nurse should not become involved in this communication pattern. The best way to avoid this problem is to include the patient in family meetings. If the patient refuses to attend or if the family attempts to exclude the patient by telephoning or intercepting the nurse during a visit, it is best to have a plan of action prepared. In most instances the nurse should inform the patient and the family that information shared between the nurse and family members will also be shared with the patient. This approach reinforces the value of openness in communication that is a characteristic of a trusting relationship. Families often try to keep information from the member who is the identified patient to protect him. In reality, the patient usually learns the hidden information and then feels justified in his lack of trust of those who did not include him.

The nurse should also strive to be honest with the patient who asks questions about the plan of care. The patient has a right to participate in the care planning and should know the rationale for any treatment. For example, the paranoid person who is receiving antipsychotic medication should never be tricked into taking it by being given the liquid preparation in juice. Medication should always be identified to the patient and questions about it should be answered by the nurse or referred to the physician if she does not know the answer. If an attempt is made to trick the patient into taking medicine and the patient discovers this, the unfortunate results may be a refusal by the patient to eat or drink anything and a reality-based inability to trust health team members.

As with a withdrawn patient, the nurse must help the suspicious person who has learned to trust her to be able to trust others as well. The nurse can help the patient identify behaviors that are characteristic of trusting and trustworthy people. The ultimate goal is for the patient to be able to differentiate trustworthy from untrustworthy people and to experience trust appropriately—not to trust everyone. Thomas[31] has described the trusting person as comfortable with growing self-awareness and able to share this awareness with others, accepting of others without needing to change them, open to new experiences, consistent in words and actions over time, and able to delay gratification. By sharing these characteristics with the patient, the nurse can teach a more rational basis for deciding who to trust. In addition, discussion of these criteria with reference to the patient will help to identify his progress toward the goal of becoming a trusting person.

Intervening in impaired communication

Good communication skills, empathy, and creativity are necessary for providing good nursing care to patients with impaired communication. In addition to the concepts presented here, the relationship principles discussed in Chapter 3 are also applicable. One effect that impaired communication has on interpersonal relationships is to maintain distance between the participants. This can be done by not revealing feelings or by transmitting unclear messages. In either case the receiver is allowed to perceive only a portion of the information that is available to the sender. At other times, inadequate or inaccurate perception and evaluation may interfere with clear communication.

To understand the unclear messages of a schizophrenic patient, the nurse must listen carefully and observe the patient, in addition to being aware of the communication context. Much of the patient's speech may be symbolical. For example, a patient who was feeling pressured by a nurse's persistent efforts to persuade him to accept a visit from his wife remarked, "It sure looks hot outside." This was interpreted to mean that the patient was feeling "hot" (angry) because of the nurse's pressure. The nurse chose not to share the interpretation with the patient, who had difficulty handling anger, but responded to his message by easing the pressure she was placing on him. Interpretation to the patient of the meaning of symbolical communication must be done cautiously. The patient is speaking indirectly for a reason. The symbolism may screen thoughts and feelings that would be difficult to handle if stated directly. The patient is usually not consciously aware of the symbolical meaning of his speech. At best, the response to an ill-considered interpretation could be denial of the correctness of the interpretation. At worst, the patient could lose control of his behavior and enter a panic state because of the anxiety aroused by bringing unconscious material into awareness. The responsible nurse will try not to bring forth behavior that neither she nor the patient can handle.

A supportive approach often works well with patients who exhibit impaired communication. Many of these patients distrust the meaning of words because they have had past experiences with incongruent communications. They are very sensitive to nonverbal behavior and its meanings and immediately perceive whether the nonverbal behavior supports the verbal message. The nurse therefore needs to be self-aware and to use both verbal and nonverbal communication purposefully in the nursing intervention. Open-ness can be supportive to the patient. Real people become angry, sad, happy, contented, and fearful. The nurse can be a model for the patient of how to acknowledge feelings and, more important, how to express them appropriately. Feelings are part of human relationships. Consider Clinical example 11-6.

CLINICAL EXAMPLE 11-6

Ms. S was a nursing student who had been relating to Ms. A, a patient in a psychiatric unit, for 6 weeks. The relationship would terminate in 2 more weeks, when Ms. S's clinical experience in psychiatric nursing was to end. Ms. S arrived on time for her appointment with Ms. A and went to their usual meeting place. Ms. A was across the room watching television. Ms. S waited 10 minutes and then approached Ms. A, who agreed to talk with her. Ms. S was aware that she was annoyed because she had been looking forward to talking with Ms. A. She was also aware of the possible effect of the termination process on Ms. A's behavior.

Contrast these two possible approaches that Ms. S could choose to take with Ms. A:

EXAMPLE 1

MS. S: **Ms. A, you seemed to be ignoring me.**
MS. A: **I was just interested in my story.**
MS. S: **Well, that's all right. I know your story's important to you—and we just have 2 weeks left.**
MS. A: **Uh-hum. I won't be here much longer myself.**

EXAMPLE 2

MS. S: **It seemed hard for us to get together today.**
MS. A: **I was just interested in my story.**
MS. S: **I know. I was feeling impatient with you because you seemed to be avoiding me. Then I realized that I'll be leaving in 2 weeks. That's really very frustrating to me.**
MS. A: **Every time I get so I can talk to somebody, they leave.**
MS. S: **Sounds like you're frustrated too.**

In the first example Ms. S maintains a you-me focus throughout the interaction sample. She implies her annoyance but does not validate this for Ms. A, who then indirectly expresses her annoyance. Ms. S also gives a double message when she says, "That's all right" and then clearly indicates why it is not all right, "We just have 2 weeks left." Ms. A is likely to be confused at this point. In the second example Ms. S puts the interaction into an "us" context. She shared her analysis of the reason for her behavior and for the patient's behavior and shared her thoughts with the patient. She expressed her frustration in a nonthreatening way and indicated that she could understand that Ms. A might have similar feelings. She has set the stage for a productive discussion of termination.

Some patients, particularly schizophrenics, take time to reach a level of trust where they can tolerate feelings directed from the nurse toward them. The nurse can, however, model expression of feelings by interacting with other staff members in the presence of the patient and then discussing the situation with the patient. People who are frightened of feelings need to see that they can be verbalized without causing the devastation that the patient may have been fantasizing. When patients do take a risk and make a feeling statement to another person, they need feedback about how the other person was affected. The expression of caring can be even more difficult than anger because caring leaves one vulnerable to rejection. Patients often need to experience socially acceptable ways of giving and receiving both positive and negative feelings.

The threat of closeness can result in many behaviors that are indicative of the patient's resistance. Wildman[34] cites such behaviors of the schizophrenic patient as "physical withdrawal, psychological withdrawal, verbal threats or rejections, physical attack, symbolic derogations or gestures" as examples of resistance to closeness. She states that the nurse must be sensitive to the meaning of these communications and direct nursing intervention toward reducing the interpersonal anxiety, thereby reducing the patient's resistance to involvement. This means that the nurse may at times overlook behaviors that would, in another context, be unacceptable. For instance, a patient may use grossly obscene language in an effort to drive the nurse away. Inexperienced nurses may take the patient's remarks personally and respond with indignation or a moralistic lecture. To be successful, the nurse needs to respond at the level of the patient's anxiety and assure him that she will not demand more than he can tolerate. It is also important that the nurse continue to exhibit interest in the patient. If she is driven away, his negative self-concept will be reinforced, as will the antisocial behavior. When the patient has gained some trust in the nurse, feedback can be given about the effect of his behavior on other people, later coupled with the concept that the patient is responsible for his behavior and its consequences.

Because of the schizophrenic patient's fear of closeness, touch should be used judiciously. Touch is a powerful communicative tool. Patients who are sensitive to issues of closeness may experience a casual touch as an invasion or as an invitation to intimacy, which may be even more frightening. Physical contact with a person of the same sex may be experienced by the patient as a homosexual advance and may precipitate a panic reaction. If procedures requiring physical contact must be carried out, careful explanations should be given both before and during the procedure. An efficient impersonal approach to physical nursing care may be least threatening to a patient experiencing interpersonal anxiety.

Touch may also have significance for patients with poorly defined ego boundaries. Sometimes these patients touch other people to identify for themselves their separateness from the other. However, other patients, when touched, find it difficult to be aware of their individuality and experience a sense of fusion with the other. Very regressed patients may seek out cuddling and rocking as if they are trying to recreate the symbiosis of infancy. Some therapists, such as Laing, use this reparenting approach with schizophrenic patients who are severely interpersonally incapacitated. Ego boundaries may also be reinforced by clearly separating self from other in communication. Statements such as "It's time for us to take our bath" are extremely confusing to a patient who does not know where his self ends and the nurse's self begins. The use of "I" and "you" helps the patient clarify this issue.

Confusion about ego boundaries is one example of the problem that schizophrenic patients often have with reality orientation. The healthy ego can identify between fantasy and reality most of the time by using logical thinking, comparison with past experience, and consensual validation with other people. When the ego is overwhelmed with anxiety, the ability to reality test is seriously compromised. Another behavior representative of this problem is delusional thinking. The delusional patient is absolutely convinced of the reality of his beliefs even when they are contradicted by logical thought and by the perception of others. Nursing intervention with a delusional patient requires great sensitivity. Communication channels must be kept open while the nurse avoids supporting and reinforcing the delusion. Stripping the patient of his delusion is removing his desperate attempt to defend himself from overwhelming anxiety and could result in an outburst of uncontrolled assaultive behavior. A direct attack on the delusion usually results in an angry response and a feeling of alienation on the part of the patient. An expression of doubt, tactfully phrased, is generally more acceptable. A patient who expresses fear that gangsters are planning to kill him may be able to accept the response, "You are safe here in the hospital and I would like to help you learn more about what makes you so afraid." This shifts the focus from the imaginary gangsters to the patient's fear, which is real. Consistent acceptance of the patient and supporting the growth of a therapeutic nurse-patient relationship will gradually alleviate the patient's anxiety, allowing him to relinquish his delusions. This is accomplished most easily when there is no loss of face involved. The nurse can help the patient explain the delusion and the purpose it served, saying, for example, "When you first came here you were very frightened and you did not understand what was happening to you. Your idea about the gangsters was a way of explaining your feelings. Now you are beginning to learn more about yourself and you are finding other explanations." Some patients have well-entrenched delusional systems and are not able to give them up. These patients are sometimes able to function well if they can learn not to talk about their delusions except in therapeutic sessions or with significant others who can tolerate such a discussion.

Auditory hallucinations are another type of disruption in reality testing. Like delusions, they represent a high level of interpersonal anxiety and a projection of repressed ideation to objects outside of the self and originate at an unconscious level. Field and Ruelke[11] identify seven phases of hallucinatory behavior, the understanding of which can help to guide nursing intervention. The first phase is a recollection of interactions with a person who has been helpful to the patient in the past. This recollection results in a decrease of anxiety. The second phase is a repetition of the first-phase experience, establishing a pattern. During the third phase, the person begins to worry that the anxiety-relieving experience will not continue, which leads to more frequent repetition of the experience and a decreased ability to distinguish fantasy from reality. This requires withdrawal from inter-

action with real people. Other people notice and comment on the person's behavior at phase 4. This causes increased anxiety and more need for the hallucinated reassurance. At phase 5 the experience becomes less pleasant. Derogatory aspects of the person's self-system are introduced. As the voice (or voices) becomes accusatory and makes threats, the anxiety level begins to increase again. The person may be inclined to agree with the voice or may try to convince himself that it is wrong. Phase 6 is the point at which others usually intervene because interference with the patient's ability to function becomes severe, resulting in extreme withdrawal and preoccupation. At this point the patient also rejects responsibility for his behavior and feels under the control of outside forces. An attempt at compromise takes place at phase 7. The patient tries to bargain for a return to the earlier anxiety-relieving experience. According to this explanation of the hallucination process, the patient's objective is relief of anxiety. This principle must be kept in mind when nursing intervention is planned. As with the delusional patient, a vigorous effort at invalidating the hallucination could cause increased anxiety and result in an even greater need for the hallucination.

Schwartzman[26] has enumerated several principles for nursing intervention with the hallucinating patient. Before intervening, the nurse should assess the need that is being met by the hallucination. In the context of the process just described, the need would be related to the cause of the underlying anxiety. As the assessment proceeds, the nurse will also be establishing a trusting nurse-patient relationship. It is important to recognize and acknowledge the affective component of the hallucinated experience. Alertness to nonverbal communication can facilitate this recognition. Nonverbal cues can also help the nurse identify when the patient is hallucinating and thus be able to intervene. The nurse may then function as the patient's link with reality, telling the patient that the hallucination is not real to the nurse. The reality of the experience to the patient should not be negated; rather, the nurse tries to cast doubt on the experience by presenting her perception of reality. Encouraging the patient to talk about reality-based issues is also helpful. Many patients report that their auditory hallucinations are most bothersome when they are alone and there are no competing stimuli. Field and Ruelke[11] even suggest teaching the patient to set up competing stimuli by singing when hallucinations are present. It may take some time before the patient is able to gain enough ego strength to reality test independently. Some patients continue to hallucinate indefinitely, but learn to live and function with the voices in the background.

In addition to reality testing, patients who have difficulty sorting out messages need help with organization. Schizophrenic patients are frequently disorganized. Sometimes behavior is so fragmented that nursing help is needed to accomplish even familiar tasks, such as eating and dressing. Instructions should be given step by step and in clear simple language, such as "Put your right arm in the right sleeve; put your left arm in the left sleeve" until the person is fully dressed. It may be tempting to perform the task for the patient because structuring activity in this way can be time consuming. However, helping the patient to perform whatever activities he can helps to maintain his self-esteem. Another way of assisting the patient to structure his day is to provide him with a schedule of planned activities. He then knows what to expect and can prepare for events before they occur. Nursing contacts should be included in the schedule. Regular brief contacts are less threatening to the patient who fears closeness than a single long interaction with the nurse. The length of nurse-patient interactions can be increased as the patient is able to tolerate increased interpersonal intimacy.

Decision making is another problem for patients who have difficulty processing complex messages, resulting in ambivalence. The nurse can be helpful by minimizing the need for the patient to make choices. Even filling out a selective menu can be overwhelming to a patient who is being bombarded by thoughts and feelings, as well as environmental stimuli. Family members can provide information about the patient's likes and dislikes and his usual routine so that nursing care can be individualized. As the patient's anxiety level decreases, choices can be offered, beginning with two alternatives such as "Do you want a ham sandwich or a roast beef sandwich?" As decision-making ability grows, the nurse can help the patient to identify and evaluate alternatives. Patients may try to persuade the nurse to make major life decisions for them. It should be kept in mind that decision making also entails responsibility for the outcome of the decision. A more appropriate role for the nurse is to assist the patient to assess all the facets of a decision and then to support the strength that he demonstrates by making his own choice.

Nursing intervention with a patient who is experiencing an impairment of his ability to communicate is challenging. The nurse must devise ways to circumvent the communication barriers erected by the patient. This requires alertness, keen observation, and openness to the subtle messages the patient transmits. The nurse's communication skills become her most important tools in engaging the patient in a helping relationship.

Intervening in dependency

At first the dependent patient may appear to be too trusting. However, this person also lacks confidence in the willingness of others to be available to him and to meet his needs. In addition, he lacks confidence in his own ability to be self-sufficient. Therefore he clings to others, fearing that if they are allowed any distance, they will not return.

Hill[16] has identified four therapeutic goals in her work with dependent women: (1) to express real feelings and ideas, (2) to make decisions comfortably, (3) to accept pleasurable experiences, and (4) to be able to control panic. She also points out that unless the patient has threatened or attempted suicide, it is best to help him remain out of the hospital, since the secondary gain of being cared for impedes progress toward these goals.

To help the patient express feelings and ideas and accept them as his own, the nurse first has to help the person identify feelings. Attention to nonverbal communication may provide clues as to the patient's feelings. It can be helpful to draw the patient's attention to gestures, body posture, and facial expression. The nurse should listen for undercurrents of thought and recurring themes in the patient's conversation and attempt to articulate these. Another approach is to consistently ask the patient, "What do you think about . . . ?" or "How do you feel about . . . ?" thus conveying the expectation that the patient does have opinions and feelings to share. Role modeling can also help. The nurse can share her own feelings with the patient if they have had an experience that aroused an emotional response. For instance, the nurse might say, "I was annoyed when the head nurse called me away just as we were getting into a good discussion."

Dependent people try to place the nurse in the parental role, which is also a comfortable role for most nurses to assume. Therefore the nurse must take care to relate to the patient as an adult, conveying the assumption that he is a mature person, perfectly capable of managing his own life. The patient will probably resist this and try to prove his helplessness to the nurse, who must resist the urge to act like a parent. This part of the nursing care of the dependent patient can be frustrating, since the patient becomes demanding and attention seeking. Reasonable requests should be consistently met, and limits of acceptable behavior should be discussed with the patient. Active involvement of the patient in developing the plan of care may greatly improve the chances for successful goal accomplishment.

The use of a type of behavior modification approach can be therapeutic when caring for a dependent patient. Appropriate behavior such as making decisions, helping others, or caring for the person's own needs is rewarded by attention and warm praise. Attention-seeking, dependent, or infantile behavior is ignored, and inappropriate requests meet with no response. In time, the incidence of mature behavior should increase as the patient realizes that dependent behavior results in little need gratification.

There is often a tendency on the part of nurses to avoid contact with dependent patients because of the expectation that they will be clinging and demanding. Unfortunately, this attitude tends to reinforce the patient's expectation that people will not seek him out and will not spontaneously meet his needs. His anxiety level then rises and he becomes even more demanding of attention, which reinforces the nurse's frustration with him. This cycle must be broken by the nurse. If the patient is given attention by the nurse without having to make demands, the anxiety level is alleviated and gradually the patient will begin to make fewer demands. If the nurse then begins to respond less to the patient's high anxiety level, the patient will also begin to learn to control his panic, thus beginning to learn to function as a mature adult. As this occurs, significant others must also be included so they can also learn new ways of interacting with the patient. This is another instance in which family therapy is often an important component of the overall therapeutic plan.

Intervening in manipulation

Significant others must also be involved in the plan of care for the manipulative patient. This is particularly true because manipulative people frequently achieve their ends by setting others at odds. For instance, the patient may complain to his family about his treatment, encouraging the family to confront the staff about the poor nursing care their family member is receiving. At the same time the patient may be telling the staff about his mistreatment at the hands of his family. The staff therefore is tempted to interpret the family's complaint as an indication of guilt arising from past mistreatment of the patient. Staff and family are then in conflict, and attention is distracted from the patient, who thus can avoid the discomfort of looking at his own behavior. When the staff finally realizes what is happening, the result is usually anger at the patient. There should be awareness of this tendency so that a punitive response can be avoided. Often when manipulative patients are hospitalized, this scenario is played out over and over until the patient is sent home still successfully relating to others as objects.

Manipulative patients must be held responsible for their own behavior. They are adept at attributing responsibility to others. Staff members must communicate effectively with each other so that consistent messages are given. These patients alertly recognize any inconsistency and use it to again focus attention on others. They usually are resistive to rules and must have clear limits that are consistently enforced by all staff members and, whenever possible, by family members as well.

These patients frequently have real strengths as leaders within the patient group. One constructive nursing approach is to encourage them to identify and capitalize on their strengths. They may be given responsibilities within the patient care unit and can be encouraged to help other patients with hygiene, eating, and other activities. They are often intelligent and respond well to being challenged to participate actively in planning their own care. However, they are extremely resistant to recognizing or dealing with feelings and need consistent encouragement to attempt this. Nurses become frustrated with manipulative patients because they seem to be so aware of what is happening and so in control of most situations, yet so unaware of the needs of others. It must be remembered that they have little tolerance for intimacy and that their maneuvering of others is an effective way of keeping them at a safe distance. Manipulative people are often charming, and it is easy to get involved with them. However, as soon as the other person begins to make demands or show signs of emotional closeness, the patient will dilute the relationship by withdrawing, by frustrating the other, or by distracting attention from himself.

Behavior modification techniques may be helpful in decreasing manipulative behavior. The patient is usually impatient with delays in gratification and relies on material, rather than emotional, means of gratification. Reinforcers used in a behavior modification program should therefore be concrete and readily available, such as points that may be accumulated to qualify for privileges, such as a weekend at home or a trip to the canteen. Other reinforcers might be a visit or a favorite food. Cigarettes are frequently used as reinforcers, but this should be weighed against the adverse effects of cigarette smoking and the seeming endorsement of the habit when cigarettes are provided by health professionals. Lack of response to undesirable behavior is the least reinforcing but is not always possible. If

behavior is disruptive and there must be a response, it should be matter of fact and one that is not desired by the patient. For instance, removal from contact with others for a predetermined period of time may discourage undesirable behavior, whereas a lecture that entails a great deal of attention may in reality be a reinforcer.

No matter what type of disruption in relatedness the patient is experiencing, the core concept on which nursing care is based is that of accessibility. The nurse must be physically accessible to the patient on a regular basis so that there is an opportunity for interaction. In addition, there must be psychological accessibility, meaning that the nurse exhibits interest in the

TABLE 11-7. Summary of nursing interventions with disruptions in relatedness

Goal — Growth toward achieving maximum interpersonal satisfaction by establishing and maintaining self-enhancing relationships with others

Principle	Rationale	Nursing interventions
Establish a trusting relationship	An atmosphere of trust facilitates open expression of thoughts and feelings; risk-taking is necessary when sharing thoughts and feelings; basic trust offers the patient the support needed to take interpersonal risks; support is also important when attempting new behaviors	Initiate a nurse-patient relationship contract that is mutually agreed on by nurse and patient Develop mutual, behaviorally stated goals for nursing intervention Maintain consistent behavior by all nursing staff members Demonstrate honest communication of responses to the patient's behavior Provide honest and immediate feedback to the patient concerning behavioral change Provide for privacy and comfort during interactions Maintain confidentiality Demonstrate accessibility
Identify and support the patient's strengths	Success in self-care, interpersonal relationships and activities promote enhanced self-esteem; recognition of strengths by trusted people helps the patient recognize his positive attributes; attention that is given to positive behavior is a reward and reinforces the behavioral pattern	Assess the patient's constructive coping behaviors Encourage the patient to perform self-care and make decisions to the extent of his ability Maintain the patient's dignity while providing needed assistance with activities of daily living Offer genuine praise for the patient's accomplishments Initiate activities that allow the patient to experience success Educate the patient and significant others about health care needs and treatment

Continued.

TABLE 11-7. Summary of nursing interventions with disruptions in relatedness—cont'd

*Goal —Growth toward achieving maximum interpersonal satisfaction by establishing and maintaining
self-enhancing relationships with others*

Principle	Rationale	Nursing interventions
Promote clear, consistent, and open communication	Healthy interpersonal relationships require open communication; patients with disordered thinking need assistance in identifying and understanding reality. Close relationships are often frightening at first and must be encouraged by a supportive environment; clear and consistent limits on behavior reduce the successful use of manipulative behavior	Individualize communication based on the patient's educational level, cultural background, and mental state Use congruent verbal and nonverbal communications Validate the meaning of communications with the patient Recognize the symbolic content of communication Act as a role model by sharing here-and-now feelings, perceptions, and reactions with the patient Give empathic encouragement of self-exploration by the patient Set limits as required in a clear and consistent manner
Alleviate high levels of interpersonal anxiety	Severe and panic levels of anxiety result in thought fragmentation, self-absorption, difficulty interpreting internal and external stimuli, impaired judgment, and a shortened attention span; these behaviors interfere with interpersonal relationships; a structured predictable environment and minimal interpersonal pressure alleviate anxiety	Whenever possible, respond to the patient's stated needs Maintain a calm supportive approach Minimize environmental stimuli Explain procedures and other events Recognize defensive behaviors utilized by the patient (e.g., delusions, hallucinations, and ego defense mechanisms) Assist the patient to use healthier coping responses, but avoid premature challenge of less healthy ways of coping Teach anxiety-relieving techniques (e.g., relaxation techniques and physical activities) Provide external controls when necessary Provide prescribed medications Promote structure by providing a schedule of activities, giving specific step-by-step instructions, minimizing the need to make choices, and having frequent brief contact with the patient Encourage self-control, but protect the patient from impulsive destructive behavior Respect the patient's need for control of his personal space

TABLE 11-7. **Summary of nursing interventions with disruptions in relatedness—cont'd**

Goal —Growth toward achieving maximum interpersonal satisfaction by establishing and maintaining self-enhancing relationships with others

Principle	Rationale	Nursing interventions
Maintain biological integrity	Use of the mechanisms of regression or projection may result in lack of attention to basic biological needs; lack of adequate rest and nutrients can endanger the patient; deficiencies in personal hygiene interfere with the development of interpersonal relationships; psychotropic medications may cause alterations in blood pressure and pulse, sometimes resulting in syncope; these medications also are associated with a number of side effects that are distressing, but usually reversible if appropriate intervention occurs	Assess the patient's eating, sleeping, elimination, and hygiene habits Ascertain food and fluid preferences If necessary, offer food and fluids at regular intervals Assist patient with eating and drinking if necessary Ascertain usual elimination patterns Assist to bathroom if necessary Record intake and output if a disruption is suspected or identified Record bowel movements and offer prescribed laxatives if needed Monitor vital signs Encourage bathing when needed; assist if necessary Ensure the availability of clean clothing; preferably the patient's own street clothing Ensure the availability of toiletries and cosmetics Encourage appropriate care of hair and teeth Facilitate shaving as desired Provide a restful environment for sleep Initiate sleep-promoting nursing measures Offer prescribed sedation if required Observe for medication side effects and initiate relevant health teaching

patient and strives to understand him and to clarify communication and demonstrate an empathic attitude. If the nurse-patient relationship is a healthy one, the patient can learn how to find satisfaction in other human relationships. Table 11-7 summarizes some nursing interventions relevant to the care of the patient who is experiencing disruptions in relatedness.

 Evaluation

Evaluation of the degree of success or failure of nursing intervention when that intervention focuses on the therapeutic relationship can be a difficult process. Since the relationship is central to effective delivery of nursing care, it is threatening for many nurses to scrutinize their ability to relate to others. This kind of evaluation must take place at two levels. One level is directed toward the nurse and her participation in the relationship. Introspection may be of some value in accomplishing this, particularly if a nurse stops to review an interaction immediately after it takes place. Blind spots about one's own feelings that may be present while one is involved with the patient may become clearer in retrospect. However, self-evaluation is colored by one's self-perceptions. Supervision from an experienced nurse-therapist can be extremely helpful in identifying some of the nuances of the relationship that may be less obvious to the nurse herself. Constructive supervision can help the nurse to identify the dynamics of the relationship and can help her deal with the resistance to change that often occurs on the part of the patient. No matter how experienced a nurse becomes, her own perception of her participation in a relationship is affected by her self-concept, and the need for supervision is never lost.

At another level, evaluation of nursing care considers the patient's behavior and the behavioral changes that the nurse works to facilitate. Input about these changes is collected from several sources. The patient is the primary source. He should be encouraged to verbally explore experiences with relationships, past and present. Changes in behavior should be validated with the patient to determine if he is also aware of change. When the nurse and patient discuss their respective views of their relationship, the patient is again participating in an evaluation of the usefulness of the relationship to him. Sharing feelings and intimate thoughts denotes increased trust and a willingness to risk self-revelation. Nonverbally, the patient also reveals responses to the therapeutic relationship. Accessibility to the nurse for prearranged interactions indicates trust and involvement in the relationship. Eye contact usually takes place more often when one person is comfortable with another. Touching may communicate closeness. Initiation of activities with others indicates more openness to relatedness. Increased decision making and assumption of leadership roles imply an improved self-esteem and increasing self-confidence. Such behaviors can be observed and documented and also validated with other staff members. Therefore these are useful evaluation criteria.

Significant others may also contribute to the evaluation process. They have known the patient prior to the occurrence of any behavioral disruption and can provide information about the patient's behavioral norms. They can also assist in validating behavioral changes, particularly in terms of whether the changes continue in the patient's usual environment. For the hospitalized patient, change may be seen in the protected hospital setting, but the patient may have a great deal of difficulty in transferring this behavioral change to the community setting. Involving families in this kind of assessment helps to teach the family the behaviors that have been learned by the patient and gives them an idea of what is reasonable to expect from the patient. This may help to avoid some of the turmoil described by Leavitt[18] in her study of the families of discharged psychiatric patients. She found that most of the family members she surveyed found help and support outside the hospital and that they had little idea of what to expect of the patient after discharge. This emphasizes the need to involve families in the total nursing care plan, including evaluation of the results of the care that has been given.

Evaluation is, of course, continually taking place throughout the course of the relationship. The nurse must review the assessment and add more information as gaps become apparent. Knowledge of past relationship experiences can explain much about present behavior and should be progressively explored as the relationship grows. Observation of the patient's interaction with significant others may also reveal areas that require further exploration. As new behaviors are observed, the nursing diagnosis will be refined. Evaluation of the nursing diagnosis should lead the nurse to revision of the goals. Also, as the nurse and patient become more involved in a mutual relationship, the patient will become more active in participating in identification of nursing needs and goal setting. Nursing actions need constant revision based on feedback from the patient, the patient's family, peers, the clinical supervisor, and self. The nursing approach must be modified as the nurse-patient relationship grows and as the patient moves toward autonomy and the ability to establish and maintain a variety of mature interpersonal relationships.

Suggested cross-references

Therapeutic relationship skills are discussed in Chapter 3. The model of health-illness phenomena and the phases of the nursing process are discussed in Chapter 4. Nursing interventions related to severe and panic levels of anxiety are described in Chapter 7. Building social skills is described in Chapter 9. Working with dysfunctional families is discussed in Chapter 25.

SUMMARY

1. A healthy interpersonal relationship was defined as one in which the individuals involved experience intimacy with each other while maintaining separate identities. There should also be a balance between dependent and independent behavior, described as interdependence.

2. The capacity for relatedness develops throughout the life cycle. The normal process of the development of relatedness was described.

3. Possible disruptions that can occur in the process of relatedness included impaired communication, withdrawal, suspicion, dependency, and manipulation.

4. The concept of loneliness was presented as an existential experience involving profound emotional pain and a feeling of total alienation from human relationships. This was differentiated from aloneness and solitude, which may be sought out by those who also are able to relate to others.

5. Stressors that lead to disruptions in relatedness were described. They include any disruption in the normal interpersonal developmental process; sociocultural factors, including value conflicts, isolation of certain societal groups, and fragmentation of family systems; biochemical formulations, particularly the dopamine hypothesis of schizophrenia; genetic theories; and psychodynamic processes, including the psychoanalytic, interpersonal, and family process models.

6. The behaviors associated with disruptions in relatedness were presented. Behavioral responses were identified as impaired communication, withdrawal, suspicion, dependency, and manipulation. These were related through presentation of case studies to the medical diagnoses of paranoid schizophrenia, catatonic schizophrenia, dependent personality disorder, panic disorder, and antisocial personality disorder. An additional case example was provided of an isolated elderly man. Each of these behavioral disruptions involved an inability to establish and maintain healthy interpersonal relationships.

7. Examples were presented of nursing diagnoses for each of the case studies, and these were compared to medical diagnostic criteria.

8. Coping mechanisms were discussed as they apply to disruptions in the ability to maintain relatedness. It was emphasized that the behaviors of impaired communication, withdrawal, suspicion, dependency, and manipulation function as coping mechanisms.

9. Long- and short-term nurse-patient goals pertaining to relatedness were discussed. Emphasis was placed on the importance of patient involvement as soon as the nurse-patient relationship has matured to the level that the patient can trust the nurse with his goals. An example of a long-term and related short-term goals was presented.

10. The importance of the therapeutic nurse-patient relationship for a patient who has problems with relatedness was emphasized. Withdrawn patients require a consistent, patient approach with attention given to biological, psychological, and social needs. Each of these areas was discussed. Verbal and nonverbal aspects of nurse and patient behavior were considered. Issues of intervention with significant others and termination of the relationship were also presented.

11. Trust was presented as the central issue in working with a suspicious patient. Reliability and consistency are essential for the growth of trust, as is respect for the patient's need for privacy. The nursing role in terms of the patient's biological integrity was also considered. Characteristics of a trusting person were described to be used as a means of assessing the patient's progress and as a possible topic for discussion with a recovering patient.

12. Nursing intervention with the dependent patient was focused on helping the patient to express feelings and ideas, make decisions, accept pleasure, and control panic. The nurse should treat the patient on an adult-to-adult basis, although there may be an attempt by the patient to put her in a parental role. A behavior modification approach was suggested as possibly helpful with a dependent person.

13. Consistency and limit setting were primary nursing interventions suggested with manipulative patients. Channels of communication between staff members must be open, since the patient may try to capitalize on any confusion. The patient must be held responsible for his behavior. Possible nursing approaches included involvement of the patient in care planning and behavior modification.

14. Nursing interventions were suggested for patients who are unable to communicate clearly. The need to attend to both verbal and nonverbal levels of communication was discussed, as was the symbolical nature of psychotic communication. The role of the nurse in meeting the patient at his level and assisting him to feel secure enough to communicate directly was presented. Also included was the requirement that the nurse be aware of her own communications, verbal and nonverbal.

15. Accessibility of the nurse to the patient is of primary importance when the problem is one of relatedness.

16. Evaluation of nursing care was presented as a process that must involve the patient, the nurse, other staff, and significant others. The need for validation of observations was emphasized, as was the ongoing need for clinical supervision of nursing care by an experienced nurse therapist.

References

1. Aaronson, L.S.: Paranoia as a behavior of alienation, Perspect. Psychiatr. Care **15**:27, 1977.
2. American Psychiatric Association: Diagnostic and statistical manual of mental disorders, ed. 3, Washington, D.C., 1980, The Association.
3. Bartko, J.J.: Statistical basis for exploring schizophrenia, Am. J. Psychiatr. **138**:941, 1981.
4. Bateson, G.: Information and codification: a philosophical approach. In Ruesch, J., and Bateson, G.: Communication: the social matrix of psychiatry, New York, 1968, W.W. Norton & Co., Inc.
5. Bateson, G. et al.: Toward a theory of schizophrenia. In Howells, J.G., editor: Theory and practice of family psychiatry, New York, 1971, Brunner/Mazel, Inc.
6. Brown, M.M., Cornwell, J., and Weist, J.T.: Reducing the risks to the institutionalized elderly. Part I: Depersonalization, negative relocation effects and medical care deficiencies, J. Gerontol. Nurs. **7**:401, 1981.
7. Burnham, D., Gladstone, A., and Gibson, R.: Schizophrenia and the need-fear dilemma, New York, 1969, International Universities Press.
8. Cancro, R.: The genetic studies of the schizophrenia syndrome: a review of their clinical implications. In Bellak, L., editor: Disorders of the schizophrenic syndrome, New York, 1979, Basic Books, Inc., Publishers.
9. Carpenter, W.T., Jr.: The phenomenology of schizophrenia, Am. J. Pscyhiatr. **138**:948, 1981.
10. Carter, C., and Galliano, D.: Fear of loss and attachment: a major dynamic in the social isolation of the institutionalized aged, J. Gerontol. Nurs. **7**:342, 1981.
11. Field, W.E., and Ruelke, W.: Hallucinations and how to deal with them, Am. J. Nurs. **73**:638, 1973.
12. Fochtman, G.A.: Disturbances in object relations in a chronic schizophrenic patient, Perspect. Psychiatr. Care **13**:13, 1975.
13. Fromm-Reichmann, F.: On loneliness. In Bullard, D.M., editor: Psychoanalysis and psychotherapy, Chicago, 1960, University of Chicago Press.
14. Gordon, S.: Lonely in America, New York, 1976, Simon & Schuster, Inc.
15. Grosicki, J., and Harmonson, M.: Nursing action guide: hallucinations, J. Psychiatr. Nurs. **7**:134, May, 1979.
16. Hill, D.: Outpatient management of passive-dependent women, Hosp. Community Psychiatry. **21**:402, 1970.
17. Kaplan, H.I., and Sadock, B.J.: Neurophysiology of behavior. In Kaplan, H.I., Freedman, A.M., and Sadock, B.J., editors: Comprehensive textbook of psychiatry, ed. 3, vol. 1, Baltimore, 1980, Williams & Wilkins Co.
18. Leavitt, M.: The discharge crisis: the experience of families of psychiatric patients, Nurs. Res. **24**:33, 1975.
19. Lehmann, H.E.: Schizophrenia: clinical features. In Kaplan, H.I., Freedman, A.M., and Sadock, B.J., editors: Comprehensive textbook of psychiatry, ed. 3, vol. 2, Baltimore, 1980, The Williams & Wilkins Co.
20. Lehmann, H.E.: Schizophrenia: history. In Kaplan, H.I., Freedman, A.M., and Sadock, B.J., editors: Comprehensive textbook of psychiatry, ed. 3, vol. 2, Baltimore, 1980, The Williams & Wilkins Co.
21. Meltzer, H.Y.: Biochemical studies in schizophrenia. In Bellak, L., editor: Disorders of the schizophrenic syndrome, New York, 1979, Basic Books, Inc., Publishers.
22. Mullahy, P.: Psychoanalysis and interpersonal psychiatry: the contributions of Harry Stack Sullivan, New York, 1970, Science House, Inc.
23. Packard, V.: A nation of strangers, New York, 1972, The David McKay Co.
24. Rogers, C.: On becoming a person, Boston, 1961, Houghton Mifflin Co.
25. Satir, V.M.: Symptomatology: a family production. In Howells, J.G., editor: Theory and practice of family psychiatry, New York, 1971, Brunner/Mazel, Inc.
26. Schwartzman, S.T.: The hallucinating patient and nursing intervention, J. Psychiatr. Nurs. **13**:23, Nov.-Dec. 1975.
27. Searles, H.F.: Collected papers on schizophrenia and related subjects, New York, 1965, International Universities Press, Inc.
28. Shostrom, E.: Man, the manipulator, Nashville, Tenn., 1967, Abingdon Press.
29. Spitz, R.A.: The first year of life: a psychoanalytic study of normal and deviant development of object relations, New York, 1965, International Universities Press.
30. Sullivan, H.: The interpersonal theory of psychiatry, New York, 1953, W.W. Norton & Co., Inc.
31. Thomas, M.: Trust in the nurse-patient relationship. In Carlson, C., editor: Behavioral concepts and nursing intervention, Philadelphia, 1970, J.B. Lippincott Co.
32. Vaughn, C., and Leff, J.: The measurement of expressed emotion in the families of psychiatric patients, Part 2, Br. J. Soc. Clin. Psychol. **15**:157, June 1976.
33. Weiner, H.: Schizophrenia: etiology. In Kaplan, H.I., Freedman, A.M., and Sadock, B.J.: Comprehensive textbook of psychiatry, ed. 3, vol. 2, Baltimore, 1980, The Williams & Wilkins Co.
34. Wildman, L.L.: Reducing the schizophrenic patient's resistance to involvement, Perspect. Psychiatr. Care **3**:26, 1965.
35. Will, G.T.: A sociopsychiatric nursing approach to intervention in a problem of mutual withdrawal on a mental hospital ward, Psychiatry **15**(2):193, 1952.
36. Will, O.A.: Human relatedness and the schizophrenic reaction. In Stein, M.I.: Contemporary psychotherapies, New York, 1961, The Free Press.
37. World Health Organization: Report of the international pilot study of schizophrenia. Vol. 1: Results of the initial evaluation phase, Geneva, 1973, The Organization.
38. World Health Organization: Schizophrenia: an international follow-up study, New York, 1979, John Wiley & Sons, Inc.
39. Wynne, L.C.: Current concepts about schizophrenics and family relationships, J. Nerv. Ment. Dis. **169**:82, Feb. 1981.
40. Wynne, L.C., Toohey, M.L., and Doane, J.: Family studies. In Bellak, L., editor: Disorders of the schizophrenic syndrome, New York, 1979, Basic Books, Inc., Publishers.

Annotated suggested readings

Bateson, G. et al.: Toward a theory of schizophrenia. In Howells, J.G., editor: Theory and practice of family psychiatry, New York, 1971, Brunner/Mazel, Inc.

This classic paper on communicative patterns in the families of schizophrenic patients presents the "double-bind" theory.

Bellak, L., editor: Disorders of the schizophrenic syndrome, New York, 1979, Basic Books, Inc., Publishers.

This collection of papers by authorities on the study of schizophrenia is the latest in Bellak's series of books on this subject. The papers cover a broad spectrum of issues and provide the reader an opportunity to become aware of the multiple approaches that are being explored relative to this complex syndrome. Many of the papers are quite sophisticated and would probably be most meaningful to the graduate student or psychiatric nursing specialist.

Bullard, D.M.: Psychoanalysis and psychotherapy: selected papers of Frieda Fromm-Reichmann, Chicago, 1959, The University of Chicago Press.

The collected papers of Frieda Fromm-Reichmann are fascinating reading as insight is provided into the philosophy of an outstanding psychotherapist. A section on schizophrenia is included that provides application of psychoanalytical theory to therapy with schizophrenic patients.

Carser, D.L., and Doona, M.E.: Alienation: a nursing concept. J. Psychiatr. Nurs. **16**:33, Sept. 1978.

This is a thought-provoking article that presents the existential concept of alienation and relates it to application by nursing students in the classroom situation.

Carter, C., and Galliano. D.: Fear of loss and attachment: a major dynamic in the social isolation of the institutionalized aged, J. Gerontol. Nurs. **7**:342, 1981.

The authors describe group nursing interventions that were directed toward assisting elderly nursing home residents deal with fear of attachment. Social isolation was decreased by assisting the group members to recognize and express their feelings about the dangers inherent in close relationships. An excellent example of psychosocial nursing intervention at the primary prevention level directed toward improving the relatedness of a vulnerable group of people.

Cleckley, H.: The mask of sanity, ed. 5, St. Louis, 1976, The C.V. Mosby Co.

This text is a classical presentation of the characteristics of the antisocial personality. Detailed case histories are a rich source of graphic descriptive data on the behavior of these patients. The book does not focus to a great extent on treatment.

Doona, M.E., Annino, S.L., and Kelleher, M.J.D.: Professional affirmation in nursing care, J. Psychiatr. Nurs. **15**:16, 1977.

This article is written by a faculty member and two of her former students. It describes the students' experiences caring for a schizophrenic man in an inpatient setting. They describe the varied responses of students, patient, and staff through the course of the relationships. The focus is on the importance of a caring and accepting approach. This article should be very useful to beginning students who are wondering what to expect in a psychiatric setting.

Field, W.E., and Ruelke, W.: Hallucinations and how to deal with them, Am. J. Nurs. **73**:638, 1973.

The authors describe developmental phases related to auditory hallucinations and postulate nursing intervention based on this developmental process.

Fromm-Reichmann, F.: On loneliness. In Bullard, D.M., editor: Psychoanalysis and psychotherapy, Chicago, 1959, University of Chicago Press.

This is a classic presentation of loneliness as experienced by the psychotic person. It is written in a compassionate manner and includes thoughts about therapy with these patients.

Kroah, J.: Strategies for interviewing in language and thought disorders, J. Psychiatr. Nurs. **12**:3, March-April 1974.

Several disordered communication patterns are identified, and nursing approaches that are therapeutic for each identified pattern are explained. This article is particularly helpful for the neophyte.

Pyke, J.: Nutrition and the chronic schizophrenic, Can. Nurse **75**:40, Nov. 1979.

In this article, the author demonstrates the value of careful nursing assessment, leading to identification of a problem of disrupted nutritional status that appeared to be common among chronic schizophrenic patients. The author describes her investigation of the problem and recommends several nursing interventions.

Reid, L.: Approaches to the aftermath of schizophrenia, Perspect. Psychiatr. Care **17**:257, 1979.

The author presents a pragmatic approach to work with patients who are recovering from a schizophrenic episode. She advocates informing the individual about the problem, so events may be placed in the context of reality and the person may gain control of his life. A group approach is recommended.

Rickelman, B.: Brain bio-amines and schizophrenia: a summary of research findings and implications for nursing, J. Psychiatr. Nurs. **17**:28, Sept. 1979.

The author summarizes the major biological theories of schizophrenia and describes implications for nurses. An extensive biliography provides direction for the reader who wishes to explore this complex subject in greater depth.

Ruesch, J.: Disturbed communication, New York, 1972, W.W. Norton & Co., Inc.

In this work the author applies his classic work in communication theory to communication patterns associated with various psychiatric disorders. This book is helpful for conceptualizing communication problems and planning appropriate interventions.

Satir, V.: Peoplemaking, Palo Alto, Calif., 1972, Science & Behavior Books, Inc.

The focus of this book is on family development and role structure as it describes roles that facilitate or block healthy communication. How the use of blocking roles contributes to manipulative behavior is shown.

Schwartzman, S.T.: The hallucinating patient and nursing intervention, J. Psychiatr. Nurs. **13**:23, Nov.-Dec. 1975.

The author discusses auditory hallucinations in the context of the interpersonal theory of psychiatry. Case study and good discussion of nursing intervention with a hallucinating patient are included.

Searles, H.F.: Collected papers on schizophrenia and related subjects, New York, 1965, International Universities Press, Inc.

A highly respected psychoanalyst presents his views on psychotherapy with schizophrenic patients in a readable manner. The book is impressive because of the empathy with his patients that the author has obviously experienced.

Shostrom, E.L.: Man the manipulator, Nashville, Tenn., 1967, Abingdon Press.

This is a comprehensive analysis of manipulative behavior in terms of the development, manifestations, and implications of manipulation. It specifically relates theory to various interpersonal situations and describes the therapeutic approach.

Will, G.T.: A sociopsychiatric nursing approach to intervention in a problem of mutual withdrawal on a mental hospital ward, Psychiatry **15**(2):193, 1952.

This article should be read and reread by every student of psychiatric nursing. It demonstrates the use of the nursing process to problem solve and provide therapeutic nursing care for withdrawn patients.

Will, O.A.: Human relatedness and the schizophrenic reaction. In Stein, M.I., editor: Contemporary psychotherapies, New York, 1961, The Free Press.

This absorbing account of psychotherapy with schizophrenic patients is based on the interpersonal theory of psychiatry; there are excellent descriptions of Sullivan's theory applied to the etiology and course of schizophrenia.

World Health Organization: Report of the international pilot study of schizophrenia. Vol. 1: Results of the initial evaluation phase, Geneva, 1973, The Organization.

World Health Organization: Schizophrenia: an international follow-up study, New York, 1979, John Wiley & Sons, Inc.

These two volumes present the results of a longitudinal epidemiological study of schizophrenia that took place in nine countries. These reports detail the construction of the study, as well as data collected and conclusions reached. These books are highly recommended for nurses who are interested in research, education, or advanced clinical practice.

CHAPTER 12

PROBLEMS WITH
THE EXPRESSION
OF ANGER

Healthy children raised in decent conditions among loving people in a gentle and just society where freedom and equality are valued will rarely commit violent acts toward others.

Ramsay Clark, *A Few Modest Proposals to Reduce Individual Violence in America**

Learning objectives

After studying this chapter, the student will be able to:

- *define anger in relationship to anxiety resulting from a threat.*

- *describe the continuum of behavior related to the feeling of anger.*

- *compare and contrast the biological/instinctual, frustration-aggression, and social learning theories concerning the stressors related to anger.*

- *analyze biological responses to anger relative to high levels of anxiety and the fight-or-flight response.*

- *differentiate among passive, aggressive, and assertive behaviors.*

- *identify coping mechanisms relative to the experience of angry or aggressive feelings.*

- *formulate nursing diagnoses related to problems with the expression of anger, taking into consideration associated medical diagnoses.*

- *develop with the patient mutually agreed on long- and short-term goals for nursing intervention in problems with the expression of anger.*

- *examine one's own responses to anger.*

- *describe the process involved in developing assertive behavior.*

- *analyze nursing interventions for the care of the angry patient.*

- *set appropriate limits on acting-out behavior.*

- *describe safe procedures for intervention in potential or actual violent behavior.*

*Reprinted by permission from page 2 in *Violence and the Violent Individual* by J. Ray Hays, Thomm Kevin Roberts, and Kenneth S. Solway (eds.). Copyright 1981, Spectrum Publications, Inc., New York City.

403

■ *evaluate the effectiveness of nursing interventions in angry behavior.*

■ *identify suggested readings for further study.*

Anger is a feeling of resentment that occurs in response to heightened anxiety when the individual perceives a threat. It is characterized by a feeling of tension, and there is a need for the discharge of the tension. It is possible to suppress the overt expression of anger, but sooner or later, perhaps in a very different form, the tension will be released. The chronically angry person may develop a duodenal ulcer, become depressed, or explode inappropriately at a minor mishap. These are all signs that anger has not been expressed productively. Other persons may deal with anger by joining the army, kneading bread, or writing a symphony. These expressions are examples of sublimation and may be constructive for the individual. However, the basic issue is still avoided.

Direct expression of anger at the time that it occurs and toward the immediate cause is the healthiest and most satisfying way of releasing the tension. For most people this is also the most difficult response. Culturally, direct expression of anger is discouraged. Children are taught to "play nice" and to allow visitors to play with their toys, not even complaining if something is broken. Little boys who fight are chastised; little girls should never even think of fighting. Because of these attitudes, many people grow up fearing anger and viewing it as abnormal. This gives rise to the use of indirect means to express angry feelings.

Fear of expressing anger is related to fear of rejection. Parental disapproval is a powerful influence on the child's behavior. In adulthood similar disapproval is anticipated if one becomes angry at significant others. Yet it is hard not to become angry at those to whom one is close. When people are dependent or interdependent on each other, there is the expectation that needs will be anticipated and met. Sometimes there is even the irrational belief that needs will be recognized by the other without direct expression. When needs are not met, disappointment and, frequently, anger result. One then faces an inner conflict, since direct expression of anger to the other person may result in rejection, thus further reducing the possibility of gratification. On the other hand, failure to express the feeling leads to resentment and interferes with open participation in the relationship. Rothenberg[19] states that "when anger is accompanied by a clear communication, it is a sign of basic respect for a loved person."

People also become angry at life situations. If the car breaks down or the bank is closed or the taxes go up, an individual becomes angry. However, this anger seems to be much easier to express. In fact, the person may repeat the story several times, apparently becoming more emotionally aroused each time. This kind of experience can help the person express stored up anger and is a displacement of angry feelings from a threatening to a less threatening situation.

For some people, life situations become so unmanageable and overwhelming that anger builds up to the point of erupting explosively as violent behavior. It is known that poverty, unemployment, and family instability contribute to a higher incidence of family violence and violent crime.

Continuum of responses to anger

Anger may be described as on a continuum. Mild anger is an everyday part of life and is experienced as annoyance. Small annoyances may be forgotten almost immediately. For instance, most people have had the experience of undressing and discovering a small bruise, not remembering how it happened. Earlier in the day they probably bumped themselves, cried out, and promptly forgot the whole incident. Most people have no difficulty handling this level of anger.

At the next level there is interference with the accomplishment of a goal, resulting in frustration. For example, a sudden thunderstorm may cause the cancellation of a family picnic. There is temporary confusion as those affected share their feelings of angry disappointment. However, when the feelings have been expressed, verbally or nonverbally, alternatives are considered and modified goals are set. The feelings associated with the experience will be remembered but are quickly resolved.

Further along the continuum, anger is more intense when frustration occurs and acceptable alternatives cannot be found. The person who has lost a job or has been told he has a terminal illness may feel anger related to impotence. This

FIG. 12-1
Continuum of coping responses related to feelings of anger.

level of anger is more difficult to express and to resolve. Frequently the object of the anger is impervious to the person's feelings. This anger may preoccupy much of the person's attention and interfere with his ability to function productively. Concerned support from significant others, and sometimes professional counseling, may be necessary to help the person reestablish equilibrium.

The extreme experience of anger is rage or fury. Rothenberg[19] differentiates anger from violence, hostility, and revenge, which involve destructiveness. At this level the person is totally consumed by angry feelings and unable to control their expression. It is at this point that violence may occur, and there is a danger to the angry person and to others who are nearby. Rage may result from a long series of frustrating experiences that have depleted the person's coping abilities. It is also seen in psychotic states when the person is completely unable to cope with frustration. It is a primitive response and is, in fact, seen in babies and small children who have not yet developed adaptive mechanisms. The fury of a 2-year-old having a temper tantrum would be difficult to control in an adult. This extreme degree of anger is frightening. Fear of losing control and becoming violent inhibits many people from overtly expressing anger.

Novaco[16] has identified the following positive functions of anger:

1. *Energizing function.* Anger energizes behavior.

2. *Expressive function.* Open expression of anger characterizes a healthy relationship.

3. *Self-promotional function.* Anger can be used to project a positive self-concept.

4. *Defensive function.* Anger serves as an ego defense in response to elevated anxiety by externalizing the conflict.

5. *Potentiating function.* Anger gives a sense of greater control over a situation.

6. *Discriminative function.* Anger can serve as an alerting mechanism and indicate a need for coping behavior.

Awareness of the positive aspects of anger is important to the implementation of a therapeutic nurse-patient relationship. Rather than discouraging the expression of anger, the nurse may help the patient to use its positive functions constructively. Fig. 12-1 illustrates the continuum of responses to anger from constructive to destructive.

Nurses encounter anger frequently in the course of providing patient care. A disruption in health, no matter how minor it may appear, is a frustration, and frustration results in anger. In addition, the health care system is complex and may add to the patient's frustrations, leading to still more anger. It is therefore important for nurses to understand anger, to become aware of their own responses to angry feelings, and to help patients express anger in a healthy and productive way.

Unfortunately, nurses may also encounter instances in which the anger of a staff member is expressed inappropriately toward a patient. Patient abuse is a persistent problem in health care settings, particularly if staff are working under stressful conditions. Abuse may be physical, ranging from handling a patient roughly to actual physical assault. It may also be psychological, including speaking rudely, cursing, sarcasm, or ignoring a patient's needs. Whenever a nurse encounters this upsetting situation, there is a legal and ethical obligation to intervene directly if the patient is in immediate danger. If there is no immediate danger, the nurse may choose to report the incident to the appropriate supervisory nurse. Ignoring an incident of patient abuse only increases the likelihood that it will recur in the future. The principles discussed in Chapter 28 on the abusive family may also be applied to abuse that occurs in a health care setting.

Stressors

There are several theories of the nature of the process of anger. In general, they may be categorized as biological, psychological, and social. There is no definitive evidence at present that gives one theory more validity than any other. There is a strong probability that anger really results from a combination of all these factors combined with the person's unique personality structure.

Biological factors

Two major theorists, Sigmund Freud and Konrad Lorenz, have hypothesized that human aggression evolves from instinctual drives. Late in the development of his psychoanalytical theory, Freud came to believe that the person was under the influence of two basic drives. The first was the life drive, expressed through sexuality. This he called Eros. The second was the death drive, expressed through aggression. This he called Thanatos. Freud believed that life was a struggle to maintain a balance between the two drives. He hypothesized that destructive behavior such as suicide occurred when the death drive gained supremacy. Because of the strength of the drive, humans were always pressured to behave destructively, with the aim being either toward the self or toward others. This was described by Fromm as the "tragic alternative."[8:15] This particular theory of Freud's was not well received by many of his followers and was not thoroughly explored by him, since it was developed rather late in his career.[8]

Konrad Lorenz is a physician and naturalist. His theory of aggression is based on observations of animals, from fish and birds through the evolutionary ladder to humans. He believes that there is an instinctual aggressive drive that is common to all animals. Lorenz[13] acknowledges that this theory may be difficult for people to accept because of the comparison between human beings and other species. However, he maintains that human aggression derives from the same type of instinctual force as that of other species. He also states that modern man "suffers from insufficient discharge of his aggressive drive."[13:243] This inability to release aggression may result in various self-destructive behaviors, including neuroses and accidents.

An interesting and controversial aspect of the instinctive theories is that there is no allowance for the exercise of control by the individual. Essentially, they state that aggression will occur no matter what the person does. For some this idea is repugnant, since it implies that humans are simply the slaves of their drives. To others it is appealing because of the implication that the individual need not assume responsibility for his behavior. However, the hypothesis that aggression originates instinctively does not preclude the possibility of a variety of options for the discharge of aggressive feelings. The related behavior may be constructive or destructive according to the choices available to the individual.

Another biologically based theory views anger as a psychosomatic phenomenon. Stearns defines anger as a "combination of uneasiness, discomfort, tenseness, resentment (which is a response to selective stimuli) and frustration."[21:6] Anger may result from either environmental or internal stimuli and is characterized by an identifiable physiological response linked to activity of the sympathetic branch of the autonomic nervous system. Environmental stimuli have to do with the transmission of information, which, primarily through visual and/or auditory perception, provokes an angry response. Internal physiological stressors may include endocrine imbalance, such as hypothyroidism or hyperthyroidism, hypoglycemia, hunger, and fatigue,[21] as well as convulsive disorders and brain tumors.

Montague[15] describes the biological mechanisms that are believed to be associated with the experience of anger. She describes stimulus complexes that activate neural circuits, causing a tendency for the individual to behave aggressively toward environmental stimuli. The involved neurons are located in various areas of the brain and may be facilitated or inhibited by inputs from other neural systems. The limbic system plays a central role in both stimulating and inhibiting the aggressive responses. Research in this area is being pursued. This research is difficult because the affective areas tend to be buried deep in the primitive areas of the brain, and therefore much of the research so far has been performed on animals. Fromm[8] links this neural response to the "fight-or-flight" mechanism and views it as an innate method of self-preservation.

Psychological factors

One psychological approach to the evolution of aggressive behavior is the frustration-aggression theory developed by Dollard et al.[6] According to this theory, all aggression results from an experience of frustration. Frustration occurs when the person is thwarted in an attempt to achieve a desired goal, whether this is because the goal is unrealistic or an obstacle is placed between the person and the goal. The sense of frustration, and thereby the degree of aggression, is increased if the goal is highly valued or if the person has made repeated attempts to achieve it. According to Fromm,[8] this theory has been criticized recently because there is no allowance for stressors other than frustration that might lead to aggression.

Frustration may be experienced as a threat. When people are threatened, they become anxious. The emotional response to the anxiety that results from a threat may be experienced as anger. In addition to frustration, there are other threats that lead to anger. One is the threatened loss of self-esteem. In this case the stressor may be real, as in the threatened loss of a job, or imagined, as when a mother interprets her child's leaving home for college as a rejection of herself. Conflict may also be viewed as threatening and lead to an aggressive response. An important element of a threatening situation is the person's perceived lack of control. Aggression can be an attempt to overcome the threat by taking control of the situation.

Coffey[5] relates the occurrence of violence to a feeling of impotence. Several potential sources of anger have been identified by Maynard and Chitty.[14] They support the frustration-aggression theory by stating that blocked progress toward a goal may lead to anger. Another cause is the failure by a valued person to live up to one's expectations. Anger may also arise when an individual is forced to confront his shortcomings and admit his weaknesses. Finally, a threat to authority frequently leads to an angry response. A common thread in this analysis of anger is disappointment in the achievement of established expectations whether of the self or of another person.

Another psychological approach to anger and aggression is that of the behaviorists. They view aggression as a learned response that has been reinforced by facilitating goal achievement. For instance, 4-year-old Johnny wants a cookie just before dinner. When his mother refuses, Johnny has a temper tantrum. If his mother then gives him a cookie, Johnny has learned that an aggressive outburst will be rewarded. If similar situations continue to occur in his life, Johnny will use an aggressive approach to need satisfaction. It is important to note that others learn that non-aggression is rewarded. Thus the behaviorists explain the range of aggressive behaviors that exist.

As an existential theorist, Erich Fromm[8] presents a different psychological theory. He believes that behavior is based on several existential needs. These include the needs for an object of devotion, relatedness, unity and rootedness, effectiveness, and stimulation and excitation. These needs must be met. For each need there are both positive and negative behavioral means to achieve satisfaction. The need for effectiveness may be met by loving productive behavior or by sadistic destructive behavior. When the person is not able to meet his needs through positive constructive behavior, he will resort to negative destructive behavior. Fromm describes the latter person as an "existential failure, a man who has failed to become what he could be according to the possibilities of his existence." The failure is a result of social conditions, combined with the individual's reason and will.

Sociocultural factors

Social and cultural factors may also have an influence on the occurrence of angry behavior. Cultural norms help to define acceptable and unacceptable means of expressing aggressive feelings. Sanctions are applied to violators of the norms through the legal system. By this means society controls violent behavior and attempts to maintain a safe existence for its members. Unfortunately, this prohibition against violent behavior is often extended to include any form of expression of anger. This inhibits people from healthy expression of angry feelings and thereby leads to behavior indicative of suppressed anger.

Urban life tends to foster increased aggressive behavior. In part, this may be related to the theory of personal space. Crowding is prevalent in cities. When people have little privacy or when they feel that their area of personal space has been invaded, there is frequently an aggressive response. In ghetto areas, where overcrowding is common, this anger becomes a smoldering resentment, which can erupt into violence, as was demonstrated in the riots of the late 1960s. Fast[7] reports on a study by Kinzel in which personal space needs of men who were imprisoned for violent behavior were compared to those of prisoners with no history of violent behavior. It was found that the violent group required twice the personal space of the nonviolent group.

What would seem to most people to be a comfortable interpersonal difference would for these men be a provocation to a violent outburst. This tendency combined with alcohol use is particularly explosive, since usual social inhibitions are decreased as a result of drinking.

Issues related to personal space are also pertinent in a hospital setting. Nursing and medical care that involves touching is a direct invasion of intimate space. Patients may attempt to identify areas that belong to them, usually including the area immediately surrounding the bed, but sometimes extending to other areas, such as a particular chair in the day area or dining room. Intentional or accidental use of this space by another can lead to an angry outburst. Lathrop[10] has identified other characteristics of the hospital milieu that can lead to aggressive behavior, such as the following:

1. Staff disagreement concerning the treatment of a patient
2. Anger, distrust, and conflict among the staff
3. Staff inconsistency
4. A significant change in medication

She identifies the common element in these situations as the removal of a source of support for the patient. This is experienced as a threat, leading to a feeling of vulnerability. Aggression may result as the person tries to gain control of the situation. When aggressive behavior occurs in a hospital setting, it is important to analyze the characteristics of the milieu, as well as those of the patient. Intervention in staff behaviors sometimes results in positive behavioral change for patients.

Social psychologists have formulated the social learning theory to explain the development of aggressive behavior. According to Roberts, this theory was originated by Miller and Dollard and later extended by first Rotter and then Bandura and Walters.[18] According to these theorists, aggressive behavior is learned as a part of the socialization process. This is essentially a behaviorist model of personality development. Children who grow up in violent settings learn to use aggression as an acceptable means of meeting their needs. Aggressive behavior may be learned by imitation or by direct experience.[18] Imitation may be related to the family, subculture, or symbolical models. It has been noted that parents who were victims of child abuse are more likely to abuse their own children. This is an example of imitation of a familial pattern. Subcultural

patterns that lead to imitation of aggressive behavior involve the acceptance of violence as a means of achieving status. These include such diverse activities as violent crime, aggressive sports, and war. Symbolical modeling is best exemplified by the probable influence of television on the occurrence of violent behavior. There have been court cases in which the defense for a violent crime was the fact that the assailant had watched a similar act on television. It has also been observed that following a well-publicized act of violence, such as an assassination or mass murder, there is frequently a spate of similar assaults or threats of assaults. A cultural paradox in the United States is the contrast between the generally stated value that peace is good and the fascinated attention that is given to violence.

According to social learning theory, the other way of learning aggressive behavior is by direct experience.[18] This aspect of the theory draws heavily on behavioral theory: behavior that is rewarded will recur. This approach has been discussed as a psychological stressor related to aggression. Social learning theorists also accept the premise that biological components of aggressive behavior interact with the psychosocial aspects. It is most likely that overt acts of aggression occur as a result of the interaction of the person's biological, psychological, and sociocultural characteristics, and each of these factors must be considered as components of the nursing assessment.

 Data collection

Behaviors associated with the expression of anger

When a person becomes angry, the response is evident in both physiological and psychological behaviors. The physical feeling of anger is uncomfortable and, according to Stearns, results primarily from activity of the sympathetic fibers of the autonomic nervous system in response to secretion of epinephrine. In some instances there is also evidence of parasympathetic involvement. The cardiovascular response includes increased blood pressure and heart rate. It has been demonstrated that the tachycardia does not result from vagal stimulation. It is therefore believed to result from epinephrine secretion. Blood composition is also altered, with fewer lymphocytes and increased free fatty acids. Gastrointestinal behaviors reveal a combination of sympathetic and parasympathetic innervation.

Behaviors include an increase in salivation, nausea, either increased or decreased secretion of hydrochloric acid, decreased gastric peristalsis, and, sometimes, constipation. The central nervous system responds to anger with increased alertness. Electroencephalographic changes have also been noted when anger is induced in experimental situations. There is an increase in muscle tension and heightened deep tendon reflexes. Frequency of urination is usually increased. Sensory alertness is enhanced and dilatation of the pupils is generally noted.[21]

These behaviors are usually labeled the "fight-or-flight" response. When the individual perceives a threat, there are two alternative reactions available. One is to confront the threat—to stand and fight. Many animals choose this response only when cornered. Because of social learning, humans may place a value on fighting and may choose this response even if it is not essential. The alternative is flight—to escape from the threat by removing oneself from its influence. Flight may involve leaving the scene of the threat or may be accomplished by emotional withdrawal. In the flight situation the individual's emotional response would probably be fear rather than anger.

Since the person responds to a threat by preparing to flee or to fight, the physiological response in fear and in anger is similar. Essentially, the person is prepared for the activity that is about to take place. Hyperalertness helps him to analyze the situation, including assessing the extent of the threat and scanning the environment for any additional threatening circumstances. Since the anxiety level is increased, mental activity is stimulated—at first productively—but the person's responses may become fragmented and confused if anxiety reaches panic levels (Chapter 7). Blood flow is diverted from the viscera to the skeletal muscle groups and the brain, since more activity will be required of these areas. In addition, the rate of blood flow is greater to speed nutrients to the cells. The respiratory rate increases in proportion to the body's increased need for oxygen. Subjectively, the person generally feels tense and flooded by feelings of resentment and hostility. When overwhelmed by intense anger, the person may act spontaneously without conscious planning of the behavioral response.

Penningroth[17] relates the fight-or-flight response to the situation of the hospitalized psychiatric patient who is feeling threatened by loss of control of his life. He points out that the opportunities for flight are limited, putting the patient in the situation of having to fight. This sequence of events may lead to episodes of violent behavior, as illustrated in Clinical example 12-1.

CLINICAL EXAMPLE 12-1

Mr. B was a 32-year-old man with a medical diagnosis of paranoid disorder who was admitted to the locked ward of a psychiatric hospital becuase he had been arrested after his neighbors complained that he was letting the air out of their tires. He said that he did this because the neighbors laughed at him and talked about him when he was out walking his dog. He was angry about being arrested and wanted to leave the hospital but was held under commitment because he also threatened to burn down the house of the neighbor who had called the police.

Mr. B resisted cooperating with the admission procedure. He belligerently demanded to be released, threatening to call the governor and "sue everybody in the place." When he was asked to undress for a physical examination, he ran down the hall and barricaded himself in the dining room. As staff forcibly entered the room, he began to lash out. Several staff members removed him to a seclusion room where he was given intramuscular medication and isolated until he regained control of his behavior. He paced the floor and pounded on the door for 30 minutes before he began to appear calmer.

Several days later, when Mr. B was used to the staff and felt more comfortable in the hospital, he related to a nurse, "I hope I didn't hurt you the other night, but I didn't know what you wanted to do to me. A man has to protect himself, you know."

When this patient entered the hospital, he was already feeling threatened. He had perceived a loss of self-esteem relative to his neighbors and his conviction that they were talking about him. This feeling was reinforced by his arrest. His effort to take control and leave the situation was thwarted when formal commitment was effected. The precipitating event to his loss of control was the request that he remove his clothes. In effect, he was being asked to give up his last remnant of security. He then resorted to the fight-flight mechanism, first fleeing and then, when cornered, fighting. This situation could possibly have been avoided if he had been given time to adjust to his new situation and to establish a degree of control before being confronted with a new threat.

Wolpe is one of the major behavioral theorists. He has provided the impetus for the development of the theory of assertiveness as a positive behavioral expression of one's rights. The basic assumption of assertiveness theory is that every individual has a right to behave in a way that meets his needs, as long as he does not impinge on the rights of another person. The primary obligation is to oneself. However, assertiveness theorists believe that this approach to need gratification also enhances the esteem of the other. The assertive person assumes that the other person also has the right and the ability to act in his own best interest.

Assertiveness is at the midpoint of a continuum that runs from passive to aggressive behavior. The passive person consistently subordinates his own rights to his perception of the rights of others. When the passive person becomes angry, he tries to camouflage it, thereby creating increased tension in himself. In addition, if the other person becomes aware of the anger by observing nonverbal cues, he is deprived of the opportunity to confront the issue. This can increase his tension as well. This pattern of interaction can seriously impair growth in an interpersonal relationship. Clinical example 12-2 illustrates passive behavior.

CLINICAL EXAMPLE 12-2

Ms. J was a staff nurse on a busy surgical unit. She enjoyed her work and liked the patients. She also placed a high value on getting along with her co-workers. Other staff members always spoke positively of her. Ms. C, the head nurse, valued Ms. J as an employee, stating particularly, "She's not like the rest of them. She never complains."

Ms. J made it a practice never to refuse a request made by a patient or another staff member. If a patient who was assigned to another nurse asked her to explain his diet or straighten his bed, she would do so, even if she was then behind in her own work. She never asked for help from others, since she felt that her assignment was her responsibility. If a co-worker asked to change days off with her, Ms. J always agreed, even if she had plans, rationalizing that the other person probably had more important plans.

Ms. C began to sense a tenseness when she was around Ms. J. Since she could not think of any problem at work, she assumed that Ms. J must have been having a problem at home. She was concerned and asked Ms. J if she could help. To her amazement, Ms. J recited a long list of angry feelings related to the work situation. Ms. C then felt guilty when she realized that she and the other staff members had been taking advantage of Ms. J.

Although Ms. J had thought that she was acting in a healthy, mature way, she was actually negating her own needs and thereby diminishing her self-respect. Her co-workers, who superficially liked her, in reality felt uncomfortable with her because they were never allowed to reciprocate when she had been helpful to them. Ms. C's guilty response quickly changed to anger when she realized that she had been a victim of Ms. J's passivity. If Ms. J had informed Ms. C of her feelings, she would have treated her more equitably.

Chenevert[4] has listed 10 basic rights for women in the health professions. They are the rights to be treated with respect, have a reasonable workload, be paid an equitable wage, determine one's own priorities, ask for what is wanted, refuse without making excuses or feeling guilty, make mistakes and assume responsibility for them, give and receive information as a professional, act in the best interest of the patient, and to be human. Nurses, like Ms. J tend to ignore these basic rights, leading to passive, rather than direct, expression of anger.

A passive response to anger usually results in an indirect expression of the angry feelings. This was the the source of the tension that Ms. C felt in this situation. Bach and Goldberg[3] have written about the "nice" people. They believe that a lack of aggression must cover up a great potential for violence. In their view, direct expression of aggressive feelings is healthy and desirable. "Nice" people are frequently passive-aggressive. At a superficial level they are concerned, interested, and sympathetic. However, there is an underlying tone of hostility that contradicts the superficial message. For example, a therapist may tell a patient in a condescending tone of voice, "You're doing very well—much better than I expected." Although the verbal message is overtly supportive and complimentary, the tone of voice conveys the hostile message "You're such a loser, I'm amazed that you get along as well as you do." The patient is at a real disadvantage in this situation. If he passively accepts the statement, he keeps peace with the therapist but decreases his own self-esteem. If he challenges the hostile undertone, he runs the risk of bringing the therapist's anger to the surface and of being labeled "paranoid." This is an example of a double-bind situation (Chapter 11), which involves a passive-aggressive message.

Passivity is also expressed nonverbally. The person may speak softly, frequently in a childlike manner. There is little eye contact from a passive person. Body language communicates diffidence and self-denial. The person may be slouched in posture and generally holds his arms close to his body. Fidgeting also communicates passivity. Gestures are seldom used, although the head may be nodded in agreement (even when the person really disagrees).

Sarcasm is another indirect expression of anger. This usually provokes anger in the person who is the target. It is differentiated from assertive behavior because it usually infringes on the rights of the other. A sarcastic remark generally conveys the message "You are not worthy of my respect." Sarcasm may be disguised as humor. Confrontation may then be responded to with a disclaimer such as "Can't you take a joke?" Humor that derogates another person is hostile and is indulged in for the purpose of self-enhancement. It tends to backfire because the joker is revealed as insecure and needing to downgrade others to bolster his own self-esteem.

At the opposite end of the continuum from passivity is aggression. The aggressive person ignores the rights of others. He operates under the assumption that every person must fight for his own interests and he expects the same behavior from others. Life is a battle. An aggressive approach to life may lead to violence, either physical or verbal. The aggressive behavior frequently covers a basic lack of self-confidence. The person enhances his self-esteem by overpowering others and thereby proving his superiority. Clinical example 12-3 describes aggressive behavior.

CLINICAL EXAMPLE 12-3

Suzy was a 9-year-old girl brought to the child psychiatric clinic by her mother on referral from the school nurse. She was described as a "tomboy" who loved active play and hated school. She was the first girl to make the neighborhood Little League baseball team and had proved her right to be there by beating up several male team members. Suzy was sent to the clinic after the teacher caught her forcing younger children to give her their lunch money.

When Suzy came to the clinic, she presented a facade of toughness. She did not deny her behavior and explained it by saying that the "little kids don't need much to eat anyway. I let them keep some of the money." Suzy was saving money for a new baseball glove. When she was asked about school, she said angrily, "I'm not dumb. I could learn that junk, but who needs it. I just want to play ball."

Psychological testing revealed that Suzy's IQ was slightly below average. She attended school with a group of upper middle class college-bound children. Even in the fourth grade she was feeling insecure and

unable to compete. She masked her insecurity with her bullying behavior, striving for acceptance in sports, where she did have ability. The medical diagnosis was conduct disorder, undersocialized, aggressive. When Suzy's problem was explained to her parents and the school, some of the pressure for academic achievement was alleviated. Her parents spent extra time helping her with her homework. Also, she was given genuine recognition for her athletic ability, demonstrated by the gift of a new baseball glove. Suzy gradually responded to the positive input from others by developing a sense of positive regard for herself. As she did so, she no longer needed to bully other children and began to grow into some real friendships.

Aggressive adults are not unlike Suzy. They try to cover up their insecurities and vulnerabilities by acting aggressive. The behavior is self-defeating because it drives people away, thus reinforcing the low self-esteem and vulnerability to rejection.

Aggressive behavior is also communicated nonverbally. The aggressive person usually speaks loudly with great emphasis. He may invade personal space and usually maintains eye contact over a prolonged period of time so that the other person experiences it as intrusive. Gestures may be emphatic and often seem threatening (e.g., the person may shake his fist, stamp his foot, or make slashing motions with his hands). Posture is erect and often the aggressive person leans forward slightly toward the other person. The overall impression is one of power and dominance.

In contrast to the passive and aggressive nonverbal behaviors, assertive behavior conveys a sense of self-assurance but also communicates respect for the other person. The assertive individual speaks clearly and distinctly. He observes the norms of personal space appropriate to the situation. Eye contact is direct but not intrusive. Gestures are utilized to emphasize speech but are not distracting or threatening. Posture is erect and relaxed. The body language may be symmetrical with that of the other party. The overall impression is one of strength, but not threatening.

The content of assertive speech focuses on the individual's interpretation of his rights in the situation at hand. The assertive person feels free to refuse an unreasonable request. He will, however, share his rationale with the other person. He will also base the judgment about the reasonableness of the request on his own priorities. On the other hand, the assertive person does not hesitate to make a request of others, assuming that they will inform him if his request is unreasonable. If the other person is unable to refuse, the assertive individual will not feel guilty about making the request.

Assertiveness also implies communicating one's feelings directly to others. This applies to both negative and positive feelings. As a result, anger is not allowed to build up and the expression of feeling is more likely to be in proportion to the situation. If dissatisfaction is verbalized, the reason for the feeling is included. Assertive people also remember to express love to those to whom they are close. Compliments are given when deserved. Assertion also involves acceptance of positive input from others. Think about the real message in this brief interaction:

MARY: **That's a pretty dress, Jane. Is it new?**
JANE: **This old thing? I've had it for years. I couldn't find anything else to wear today.**

What did Jane really say to Mary? The implication is that Mary has poor taste to admire a dress that Jane thinks so little of. If Jane were assertive, she would thank Mary for the compliment and perhaps even agree with her that it really is a pretty dress.

Within each person lies the capacity for passive, assertive, and aggressive behavior. When one is confronted with a threat, therefore, there are options in terms of how to respond. These choices are to be passive, fearful, and to flee; to be aggressive, angry, and to fight; or to be assertive, self-confident, and to confront the situation directly. It is important that all these choices do exist because none are inherently good or bad. Rather, the situation and the characteristics of the individuals involved define the appropriate response. When confronted by a mugger on a deserted street, one may assertively explain why the mugger should change his mind. However, if flight is available, it might be a better choice, or passive submission might be safer. Similarly, if the children are being persistently annoying and getting on mother's nerves, aggressively telling them to stop may be most effective. The problem related to assertiveness is not that people are sometimes passive or aggressive but that they do not have the option of being assertive because they have not learned how. Table 12-1 summarizes the major characteristics of passive, assertive, and aggressive behaviors.

A variation on the indirect expression of angry feelings is acting-out behavior. Acting out may also convey such feelings as love, fear, or guilt, but frequently it involves anger. Acting out refers to behavior that attracts the attention of others and represents the feelings or conflicts the person is experiencing. Adolescents often use this behavior as they deal with the crises of that developmental stage, but acting out is by no means limited to teenagers. Loomis[12] points out that acting out is not a controllable behavior until the person understands the reason or learns alternative behaviors. In therapy it is frequently related to transference feelings. Clinical Example 12-4 illustrates this concept.

TABLE 12-1. Comparison of passive, assertive, and aggressive behaviors

	Passive	Assertive	Aggressive
Content of speech	Negative Self-derogatory "Can I?" "Will you?"	Positive Self-enhancing "I can" "I will"	Exaggerated Other derogatory "You always" "You never"
Tone of voice	Quiet, weak, whining	Modulated	Loud, demanding
Posture	Drooping, bowed head	Erect, relaxed	Tense, leaning forward
Personal space	Allows invasion of space by others	Maintains a comfortable distance; claims right to own space	Invades space of others
Gestures	Minimal, weak gesturing, fidgeting	Demonstrative gestures	Threatening, expansive gestures
Eye contact	Little or none	Intermittent, appropriate to relationship	Constant stare

CLINICAL EXAMPLE 12-4

Peter was a 16-year-old boy who was referred to a halfway house for adolescents because he could not get along in a foster home setting. He refused to obey rules, used drugs, and constantly argued with the foster parents. He was consistently truant from school, where he had completed the eighth grade. He had been arrested once for stealing hubcaps, but the charges were dropped. Peter's family of origin had fallen apart when his parents divorced when he was 5 years old. His father left town and had no further contact with Peter. His mother was alcoholic and lost custody of her children to the city Department of Social Services when neighbors reported her for neglect. Although she never tried to regain custody of Peter, even after she remarried, she also never agreed to his adoption. Peter had spent 11 years moving from foster home to foster home—eight in all. At first, he had tried to get along, but he soon discovered that his behavior had little effect on how he was treated. He then began to use whatever means he could to meet his own needs.

When Peter entered the halfway house, he was initially agreeable, followed the rules, and seemed to be making a good adjustment. He was particularly close to a young male counselor and spent hours talking with him about his thoughts, feelings, and past experiences. However, after about 3 weeks, several small, mysterious fires were discovered in the house. They had obviously been set. After the group of residents were confronted with the situation, another boy approached a counselor and said he had seen Peter setting a fire. When presented with the evidence, Peter acknowledged that he had been the culprit and asked when he would have to leave. He seemed disbelieving when he was told that he could remain if he assumed responsibility for his behavior. He questioned why he was being trusted. Later, when talking with his counselor, he related that he had felt a need to get away from the house because he was beginning to like it. He feared that he would be hurt if he stayed and was later rejected. At a deeper level, his counselor believed that Peter was testing to see if the counselor really cared about him as he seemed to or if he would abandon him as his parents had when he was a small child. Unconsciously, Peter had always thought that he was responsible for his parents' divorce, since he had been told regularly that he was a bad person. Peter's medical diagnosis was conduct disorder, socialized, aggressive.

Peter's acting-out behavior was complex and in part unconsciously motivated. He was particularly frightened by feelings of caring, which made him vulnerable to hurt when the relationship ended. His response to this imagined threat of loss was to take the initiative and assume control of the situation by causing his dismissal from the home. If the sequence had gone as he expected, Peter would have also reinforced his beliefs about his own worthlessness and the vindictiveness of other people. When trust and concern were conveyed to Peter, he was able to begin to reassess some of his beliefs about himself and other people. Because the staff in this facility was used to working with acting-out behavior, Peter's experience became the beginning of a time of growth in self-awareness.

Misdirected anger also contributes to the development of other emotional problems. In particular, anger that is redirected toward the self and experienced as guilt is a prominent feature of depression, as described in Chapter 9. At other times internalized anger may be expressed physiologically as a psychosomatic illness. This mechanism has been considered in depth in Chapter 7.

Coping mechanisms

Many everyday activities serve to meet the demands of the aggressive drive. The competition that is so valued in Western cultures is fueled by aggression. Accomplishment of work often requires a degree of aggressiveness for succuss. People cope with aggressive feelings by using the energy they provide for productive accomplishments.

When aggression is uncontrolled, problems result. The anger that is then felt requires the implementation of psychological coping mechanisms. Since the anger is an expression of anxiety aroused by a threat, the ego defense mechanisms described in Chapter 7 are helpful. Angry feelings are frequently displaced. For instance, the man who was treated unfairly by his boss complains to his wife about the dinner she prepared. Sublimation also helps one to cope with angry feelings. Some great works of art reflect the anger that was felt by the composer or artist at the time the work was created. Music, in particular, can also help listeners to dispel some of their anger. This probably influences the popularity of musical fads such as "punk rock," whereby young people can ventilate some of their hostility toward the system in a nondestructive way.

A less healthy means of coping with anger is projection. In this case the angry feelings are attributed to someone or something else. As an example, the person who is flooded with unconscious hostile impulses may believe that others are plotting to kill him. This particular mechanism does not facilitate healthy functioning, since the person essentially trades his anger for fear. Repression may also apply to anger. However, the repression of anger contributes to what Rubin[20] refers to as the "slush fund," and later the anger reappears as hostility, explosiveness, bigotry, manipulation, and many other distorted expressions.

Reaction formation is the mechanism that underlies passive-aggressive behavior. Although the person presents an ingratiating facade, this is a defense against anger that the person is unable to express directly. Other defense mechanisms may also be used as an unconscious response to anger. The limitation inherent in any of them is that the real motivation for the observable behavior is outside of awareness. Thus the person is not able to examine his behavior and modify it.

There are also direct, conscious responses that may help to cope with anger. One is physical activity. Sometimes angry people need a time to work off the excess physical energy associated with the biological response. They can then deal more effectively with the interpersonal ramifications of the experience. Hitting a punching bag or taking a brisk walk is preferable to punching a friend and is also healthier than trying to set the feeling aside. An activity break also allows the person to review the situation and gain perspective before assertively confronting it.

Each person develops an individualized style for coping with anger. This results from past experiences, parental modeling, and cultural expectations. The key point to consider in assessing the person's coping ability is whether this personal style facilitates the expression of the angry feelings. If they are allowed to accumulate and fester or if they are expressed explosively, the person needs help in developing new, more satisfying coping mechanisms.

 Nursing diagnosis

When formulating a nursing diagnosis relative to a patient's angry behavior, the nurse needs to consider the nature of the threat or physiological disruption to which the person is responding. This would include the circumstances discussed as stressors. In addition, the observable response to the threat should be stated. The model in Fig. 12-2 summarizes the relationship between anger, anxiety, low self-esteem, and guilt. It indicates the two possible modes of expression of the anger—externally in either constructive or aggressive behavior, or internally in either nonassertive or self-destructive behavior. This model

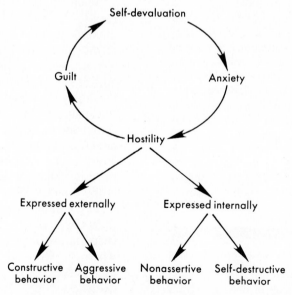

FIG. 12-2
Model representing the expression of anger.

TABLE 12-2. Comparative examples of nursing diagnoses and medical diagnoses associated with paranoid disorder

Nursing diagnoses	Medical diagnoses as described in DSM-III*
Anger related to belief that neighbors are talking about and laughing at him	**Diagnostic criteria for PARANOID DISORDER** A. Persistent persecutory delusions or delusional jealousy
Threat of violent behavior related to anger about arrest	B. Emotion and behavior appropriate to the content of the delusional system
Assaultive behavior related to panic level of anxiety resulting from fear of hospitalization	C. Duration of illness of at least 1 week
Guilt related to episode of assaultive behavior	D. None of the symptoms of criterion A of schizophrenia, such as bizarre delusions, incoherence, or marked loosening of associations
	E. No prominent hallucinations
	F. The full depressive or manic syndrome (criteria A and B of major depressive or manic episode) is either not present, developed after any psychotic symptoms, or was brief in duration relative to the duration of the psychotic symptoms
	G. Not due to an organic mental disorder

*From American Psychiatric Association: Diagnostic and statistical manual of mental disorders, third edition, Washington, D.C., APA, 1980.

TABLE 12-3. Comparative examples of nursing diagnoses and medical diagnoses associated with conduct disorder, undersocialized, aggressive

Nursing diagnoses	Medical diagnoses as described in DSM-III*
Aggressive behavior toward other children related to low self-esteem, resulting from inability to compete academically	**Diagnostic criteria for CONDUCT DISORDER, UNDERSOCIALIZED, AGGRESSIVE** A. A repetitive and persistent pattern of aggressive conduct in which the basic rights of others are violated, as manifested by either of the following:
Loneliness related to inability to make friends	1. Physical violence against persons or property (not to defend someone else or oneself), e.g., vandalism, rape, breaking and entering, fire setting, mugging, assault
Conflict with parents related to inability to meet their unrealistically high expectations	2. Thefts outside the home involving confrontation with the victim (e.g., extortion, purse snatching, armed robbery)
Achievement in sports related to natural athletic ability	B. Failure to establish a normal degree of affection, empathy, or bond with others as evidenced by *no more than one* of the following indications of social attachment:
	1. Has one or more peer-group friendships that have lasted over 6 months
	2. Extends himself or herself for others even when no immediate advantage is likely
	3. Apparently feels guilt or remorse when such a reaction is appropriate (not just when caught or in difficulty)
	4. Avoids blaming or informing on companions
	5. Shares concern for the welfare of friends or companions
	C. Duration of pattern of aggressive conduct of at least 6 months
	D. If 18 or older, does not meet the criteria for antisocial personality disorder

*From American Psychiatric Association: Diagnostic and statistical manual of mental disorders, third edition, Washington, D.C., APA, 1980.

**TABLE 12-4. Comparative examples of nursing diagnoses and medical
diagnoses associated with conduct disorder, socialized, aggressive**

Nursing diagnoses	Medical diagnoses as described in DSM-III*
Defiance of rules related to need to assume control of events influencing his life	**Diagnostic criteria for CONDUCT DISORDER, SOCIALIZED, AGGRESSIVE**
Fear of close relationships related to pain resulting from past separations	**A.** A repetitive and persistent pattern of aggressive conduct in which the basic rights of others are violated, as manifested by either of the following:
Acting out of anger related to threat resulting from staff's attempt to establish closeness	1. Physical violence against persons or property (not to defend someone else or oneself), e.g., vandalism, rape, breaking and entering, fire setting, mugging, assault
Low self-esteem related to belief that he had caused his parents' divorce and to repeated rejections by significant others	2. Thefts outside the home involving confrontation with a victim (e.g., extortion, purse snatching, armed robbery)
	B. Evidence of social attachment to others as indicated by at least two of the following behavior patterns:
	1. Has one or more peer-group friendships that have lasted over 6 months
	2. Extends himself or herself for others even when no immediate advantage is likely
	3. Apparently feels guilt or remorse when such a reaction is appropriate (not just when caught or in difficulty)
	4. Avoids blaming or informing on companions
	5. Shows concern for the welfare of friends or companions
	C. Duration of pattern of aggressive conduct of at least 6 months
	D. If 18 or older, does not meet the criteria for antisocial personality disorder

*From American Psychiatric Association: Diagnostic and statistical manual of mental disorders, third edition, Washington, D.C., APA, 1980.

may be helpful to the nurse in formulating a nursing diagnosis.

Tables 12-2 to 12-4 compare nursing diagnoses with DSM-III[2] criteria for medical diagnoses. In Table 12-2 nursing diagnoses for the assessment of Mr. B (p. 409) are compared to the medical diagnosis criteria for paranoid disorder. A comparison of nursing diagnoses for Suzy (p. 411) related to the medical diagnostic criteria for conduct disorder, undersocialized, aggressive is given in Table 12-3. Table 12-4 illustrates nursing diagnoses for Peter (p. 413) as compared to the medical diagnostic criteria for conduct disorder, socialized, aggressive.

There are multiple possible individualized nursing diagnoses related to anger. They will vary according to the source of anger, degree of anger, frequency of angry feelings, direction of anger, chosen mode of expression, and the person's physical condition. It can be challenging to recognize that a given behavior is a representation of anger and to identify the stressors involved. People often mask their anger and redirect it. Good communication among health team members can facilitate the successful accomplishment of this part of the assessment process. Fig. 12-3 illustrates the model of health-illness phenomena related to the expression of anger.

 **Planning and implementation
of nursing interventions**

Goal setting

Mutually set long- and short-term nurse-patient goals are essential to guide the intervention process. Long-term goals will be directed toward

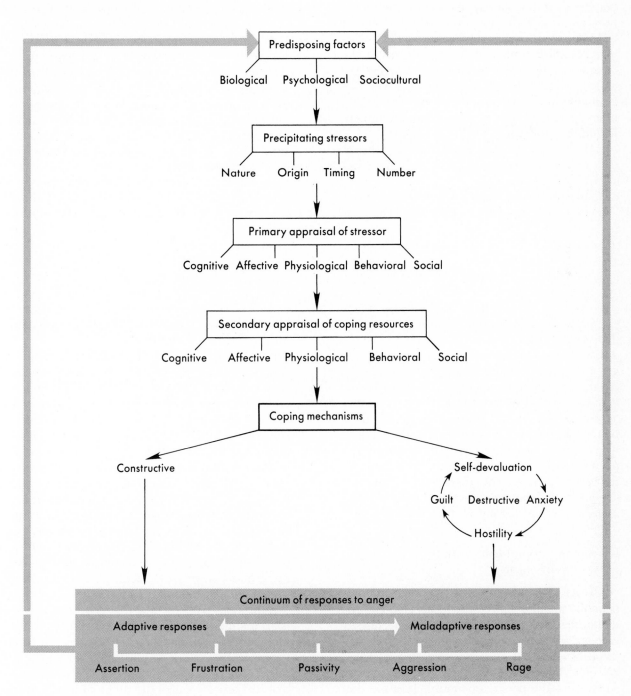

FIG. 12-3
Model of health-illness phenomena related to the expression of anger.

the constructive use of angry energy to accomplish tasks and to motivate self-growth. Short-term goals serve as guideposts along the way, helping the nurse and the patient to identify the progress of the therapeutic experience. If, for instance, the nursing diagnosis is job dissatisfaction resulting from inability to say no to the boss, a long-term goal would be "In 6 weeks the patient will assertively inform his boss when he is unable to accept a new responsibility that is offered to him." Related short-term goals might include the following:

1. In 1 week the patient will develop a list of present job responsibilities and time commitments.
2. In 2 weeks the patient will refuse a request from a salesperson whom he does not know.
3. In 3 weeks the patient will refuse a request from a neighbor.
4. In 4 weeks the patient will refuse a request from his wife.
5. In 5 weeks the patient will rehearse refusing a request from his boss that he take on more work.

This type of progression of behavioral goals gives the patient the sense of mastery and control that is sometimes the objective of aggressive behavior. It also makes a task that may at first appear overwhelming seem manageable. This is particularly important in working with a patient who becomes frustrated easily. It also meets the need for patient education, since the patient is a full participant in the therapeutic plan and should have input into devising the goal hierarchy.

Intervening in problems with the expression of anger

SELF-AWARENESS AND ASSERTIVENESS. Angry patients are frequently labeled as problem patients because of the responses of the nurses who are assigned to care for them. The attempt to provide nursing care may deteriorate into a power struggle as the nurse and the patient each strive to be the person in control. To avoid this outcome, the nurse should use the data collected about the patient to help identify the nature of his behavior and the reason for it.

If the person is experiencing anger for reasons that are primarily physiological (e.g., an endocrine imbalance, a brain lesion), the nurse may find it easier to accept outbursts of angry behavior. She can intellectually explain the reason for the patient's anger and may conclude that he "can't help it," thereby circumventing the power struggle aspect. This is particularly true if there is the expectation that medical intervention will soon bring the patient's behavior under control.

More often, the reason for the patient's behavior is hidden or not really related to the nurse. It is then harder to deal with the anger and more difficult not to take it personally, especially if it is expressed as an attack on the nurse's competency. Because it is threatening to be the recipient of anger, the nurse needs to develop an awareness of her own usual response to anxiety, threatening situations, and anger. There are several responses indicative of lack of self-awareness that are not therapeutic or productive.

One nontherapeutic response to patient anger is defensiveness. The defensive nurse interprets the patient's anger as a personal attack and immediately tries to explain her actions to prove that the perceived attack is unjustified. For example, Ms. B, a nurse, awakened Ms. R, a patient who was hospitalized for control of her diabetes mellitus. When Ms. B told the patient that she had to give her an injection of insulin, Ms. R said, "You people here don't know anything. All you do is wake me up. I'm here for a rest, you know. Some rest!" Ms. B responded with a detailed explanation of why it was important for Ms. R to have her insulin at the correct time and also offered explanations for the possible reasons for the behavior of other staff members. The more she talked, the angrier Ms. R became. Following the interaction, the nurse described the interaction to her head nurse, who pointed out that Ms. R was probably responding to multiple feelings about hospitalization. That, combined with the interruption of her plan to withdraw for a while by sleeping, led to an attack that was not really directed toward Ms. B. The nurse's response was a result of her own insecurity and discomfort with anger.

A response by the nurse that is detrimental to the patient is one of retaliation. The nurse "pulls rank" or asserts herself as the one with the authority in the health care setting. For instance, Ms. T, an elderly patient, requested a bedpan. She had already called the nurse to her bedside several times with small requests that were not really urgent. The nurse labeled her behavior as indirectly aggressive. After she gave the patient the bedpan, she went to check on another patient at the other end of the hall. Fifteen minutes later she returned to Ms. T, who had finished with the bedpan long before her return. When Ms. T mentioned this fact, the nurse responded by saying, "I do have other patients. I can't spend all my time here with you." In reality, she could have removed the bedpan before looking in on the other patient. She, too, was responding to the superficial meaning of the patient's behavior. The nurse believed that the patient was irritable and deliberately seeking attention to annoy her. Actually the patient was frightened, lonely, and angry because she knew she would be going to a nursing home instead of her own house. The nurse's retaliatory behavior only reinforced the patient's feelings.

Somewhat related to retaliation is an attitude of condescension. The nurse assumes an attitude of superiority and discounts the patient's concerns. Mr. J was in the coronary care unit after a myocardial infarction. He was a hard-driving executive who was very frustrated because his physician had forbidden any contact at all with his business. When the nurse brought his lunch, he angrily refused to eat it and referred to the food as "garbage." The nurse replied, "Now really, Mr. J, you're acting like a child. Surely Dr. A has told you that it's important for you to eat. Let's have no more of this silliness." Mr. J then sat straight up in bed and shouted at the nurse, "Get out of my room! Right now!" After the nurse left, she told a co-worker, "He certainly is obnoxious. He'll kill himself unless he controls that bad temper." This nurse's approach only increased the patient's anxiety and ultimately his anger. He was already feeling impotent and did not need to hear himself compared to a child. Furthermore, he was given the message that his anger was unjustified and should not be expressed. On the other hand, the nurse later acknowledged that Mr. J's anger could be destructive but did not recognize that suppression of his feelings could be as harmful as explosive expression of them. Had she realized this, she would have spent some time helping him to explore his feelings and acquire some sense of mastery in the situation.

Another commonly noted nontherapeutic response to the patient's anger is avoidance. In avoidance, the nurse simply refuses to recognize or to deal with the patient's feelings. For instance, Mr. M said to his nurse as she changed his dressing, "You know, I think my doctor is botching my case. That infection is no better. I think he's a real quack." The nurse continued with the procedure and after a moment said, "Did your wife visit yesterday, Mr. M? She seems like such a nice person—so concerned about you." Mr. M sighed and closed his eyes as the nurse completed the procedure. Later she said to a friend, "That Mr. M is a strange one. He hardly responds at all when you talk to him." This nurse was prevented by her own defensive system from even acknowledging Mr. M's angry statement. He felt more frustrated and resorted to withdrawal when she did not acknowledge his statement. He also extended his assessment of the physician's ability to include the nurse.

The interactions described demonstrate the need for the nurse to be aware of her own response to anger in others. Otherwise the nurse's feelings may actually interfere with her ability to provide effective patient care. The nurse who responds to anger either passively or aggressively needs to take steps to modify her approach. Assertiveness training for the nurse can help to fulfill this need. Not only will she grow in self-awareness and be better able to respond therapeutically to her patients, but she will also be more likely to experience job satisfaction.

Alberti and Emmons[1] recommend to the nurse the following process for the development of assertiveness:

1. Observe your behavior.
2. Keep a record of assertive and nonassertive behavior.
3. Select one situation for examination.
4. Review your behavior in the selected situation.
5. Observe an effective person in action in a similar situation.
6. Identify alternative responses.
7. Put yourself in the place of the effective person; imagine how you would act.
8. Practice the new approach by role playing.
9. Provide yourself with feedback; repeat step 4. Get feedback from others if available.
10. "Behavior shaping"—practice the new response until you begin to feel comfortable.
11. Practice the new approach in a real situation.
12. Repeat training if necessary or apply to other problem areas where you wish to change.
13. Take note of social reinforcement—the positive response of others to your new assertive behavior.

A nurse who undertakes a self-growth program to develop assertive behavior is also learning a process that can be helpful to patients who experience difficulty in expressing anger. A healthy approach to the expression of anger is essentially a problem-solving approach. The steps to assertiveness just described are really components of a problem-solving process. They may be compared to the steps to dealing with anger recommended by Hays[9]:

1. Acceptance of the self as a person who experiences angry feelings.
2. Exploration to find the reason for the anger.
3. Constructive direction of the energy that is generated by the anger.

Assertiveness training, in contrast, tends to deemphasize the reason for the response. This is consistent with its behavioral model origins. However, assertiveness theory provides a framework for the accomplishment of Hays' step 3.

Another model for intervention with an angry patient is described by Maynard and Chitty.[14] They recommend a seven-step approach as follows:

1. Assist the patient to identify anger by focusing on nonverbal behavior and labeling the feeling using the patient's preferred words.
2. Give permission for angry feelings by communicating that they are normal.
3. Practice the expression of anger by using nonthreatening situations, such as fantasies.
4. Identify a reality-based existing source of anger.
5. Role play a confrontation with the object of the patient's anger. Role reversal may assist the patient to understand his feelings. Provide positive feedback for successful expression of feelings.
6. Identify alternative ways to express anger. Direct confrontation is not always the most appropriate approach.
7. Confront the person who is the source of the anger. This step may not be taken, depending on the situation and the patient's preference. The nurse should be available to provide support during the confrontation.

These authors also advocate encouraging the patient to evaluate the experience and the feedback by the nurse.[14] This model includes most of the steps described in the assertiveness training approach. However, it maintains a focus on the readiness of the patient for each step of the process. The role of the nurse is to guide the patient and to provide emotional support and honest feedback.

LIMIT SETTING. At times the nurse needs to intervene with a patient who is expressing his anger in ways that infringe on the rights of others. When this happens, it is necessary to set limits on the patient's behavior. Limit setting is not a punitive response to behavior, although the patient may experience it that way. It is a nonmanipulative confrontation in which the patient is informed what behavior is acceptable, what is not acceptable, and the consequences attached to behaving unacceptably. The nurse does not assume responsibility for the patient's behavior, positive or negative. It is recognized that the patient has the right to choose his preferred mode of behavior as long as the consequences are clear as well. Limits should be clarified before the negative consequences are applied. Otherwise the consequence is punitive and the patient may feel tricked.

Once a limit has been defined, the consequences must take place if the behavior occurs. Every staff member must be aware of the plan and carry it out. If this consistency is absent, the patient is likely to manipulate staff by acting out and then pointing out areas of inconsistency in limit setting. Firm, but not hostile, enforcement of limits is preferable. If the nurse responds angrily, she is less likely to see the situation clearly. This is also an indication that a power struggle is taking place. Power struggles are usually detrimental to the treatment plan.

Loomis[12] has identified three steps in the limit-setting process:

1. State expectations to the patient in a positive way.
2. Help the patient explore the reason for and meaning of his behavior.
3. Consider with the patient alternative ways to express his feelings.

This approach avoids rejection of the patient and conveys the attitude that the patient has the right to experience angry feelings and the ability to express them appropriately. Clinical example 12-5 shows acting-out behavior and constructive limit setting.

CLINICAL EXAMPLE 12-5

Mary was a 17-year-old girl who was admitted to the hospital for suspected hyperthyroidism. She quickly become bored with the hospital routine and phoned several of her friends to visit her. When the nursing staff was making rounds at the shift change, they found several teenagers in Mary's room. There was also a strong aroma of marijuana. Since there was a hospital limit of two visitors at a time, some were asked to leave. The group was also informed that marijuana smoking was not allowed in the hospital.

After visiting hours Ms. T, a young staff nurse, sat down to talk with Mary. She initiated a discussion of Mary's restlessness and irritability, which had led to the suspicion that she had a hyperthyroid condition. Mary readily shared her frustration with being in the hospital and her anxiety about her condition. Then she said, "I suppose you guys are mad at me for the pot, but that's a dumb rule. It's healthier than cigarettes, you know." Ms. T replied that she and the other nurses were not mad, but that they did expect Mary to obey the rule, now that she knew it. She also told Mary that she was responsible for telling her friends the rule. The consequence, if the behavior occurred again, would be restriction of visitors to her parents only. The nurse then initiated a discussion of what Mary might do to help out on the unit and thereby use some of her excess energy. Mary began to look excited and shared her love for plants. She proposed that she might visit other patients and help them care for their plants and flowers.

The nurse in this example applied the problem-solving process. She planned her nursing intervention and then approached Mary in a reasonable, adult-to-adult way. Ms. T was selected by the nursing staff to work with Mary because she did not have a punitive response toward marijuana use. This facilitated her being able to help Mary look at the reasons for her behavior and to select a constructive alternative. The interaction also served as the foundation for a therapeutic nurse-patient relationship between Mary and Ms. T.

CONTROL OF VIOLENCE. Unfortunately, some patients have more difficulty controlling their feelings and using angry energy constructively. A patient who loses control of his anger becomes violent. Violence refers to behavior that is physically assaultive and risks injury to the self, others, and the environment. The nurse in the psychiatric setting must develop the ability to deal with violent behavior in a way that minimizes the danger to all concerned.

Prevention of violence is preferable if it is possible. The intense anxiety associated with violent feelings is communicated interpersonally. By empathizing and carefully observing patients' behavior, the nurse may be able to anticipate a violent outburst. Sometimes when a patient is on the verge of losing control, the atmosphere of the nursing unit becomes filled with tension. When the nurse becomes aware that tension is mounting, intervention may avoid an outburst. The nurse may isolate the disturbed patient from the rest of the patient group; may talk with the patient if he is receptive to this approach; and may give prescribed medication. Some patients respond to vigorous physical activity to express their anger, but this approach should be used with care, since it may also precipitate loss of control.

Self-protection is a concern when the nurse is working with a potentially violent patient. The nurse should never risk being hurt by failing to take adequate precautions for her own safety. Whitman[22] recommends the following precautions:

1. Never see a potentially violent person alone.
2. Call police or security staff if their help is needed.
3. Keep a comfortable distance away from the patient. Avoid intruding on his personal space.
4. Maintain a clear exit route for both the staff and patient.
5. Be prepared to move. Violent patients can strike out suddenly.
6. Be sure the patient has no weapons in his possession before approaching him.
7. If it is necessary to restrain a patient, have an adequate number of nursing staff on hand.
8. Give prescribed antianxiety or antipsychotic medication when it is needed.
9. Be supportive to the patient and intervene to increase his self-esteem.

If the patient does become violent, immediate response is essential. Penningroth[17] advises an initial assessment of the situation, followed by a plan for intervention, and then action. Enough people should be available to ensure the safety of the patient and staff. Staff members should be taught good body mechanics and methods of holding a struggling patient without causing injury. One person should direct the group action. Also, someone should talk with the patient, explaining what is happening and the reason for the intervention. Most violent patients are reassured if they see that they can be controlled and prevented from inflicting injury. Lenefsky, de Palma, and Locicero[11] recommend two to four people, depending on the situation. If the person is very disturbed, there should be one staff person assigned to restrain each limb and a fifth person to direct the activity and communicate with the patient. Roles should be assigned prior to intervention, with the person who has

TABLE 12-5. Summary of nursing interventions with a patient who has difficulty with the expression of anger

Goal: To recognize feelings of anger and, when appropriate, assertively communicate these feelings to other people

Principle	Rationale	Nursing intervention
Assertive expression of feelings	Passive behavior reinforces low self-esteem; anger builds up internally and may lead to depression; aggressive behavior also indicates insecurity and low self-esteem; the person may become isolated from others, leading to more hostility; violent behavior can result from pent-up anger; assertive behavior reinforces high self-esteem by protecting the individual's rights without violating the rights of others	Establish a trusting relationship Assist the patient to recognize and label anger Communicate that angry feelings are normal Identify usual means of coping with anger Support effective coping mechanisms Explore alternative behaviors Assist the patient to practice assertive expression Provide feedback
Promote respect for the rights of others	Adherence to reasonable limits on acting out behavior promotes socialization; expression of feelings is a reciprocal process and involves awareness of and respect for the rights of others; anger related to limit setting can be used to teach the person more effective coping behaviors	Inform the patient of acceptable limits for behavior, including rationale Clarify the patient's responsibility for his behavior Define the consequences for failure to observe rules Achieve staff agreement on definition of reasonable limits Enforce limits by implementing consequences if violations occur Explore reasons for acting out and identify alternative behaviors Give positive feedback for adherence to limits
Protection from harm to self or others	Violent behavior entails a high risk of physical injury to the patient and to others with whom he comes into contact, psychological damage may also occur as a result of guilt related to the patient's concern that he injured someone while out of control; outbreaks of violence decrease the sense of security that is important for people to feel while they are in the process of confronting their own disturbing behaviors, thoughts, and feelings	Maintain a calm, controlled, and consistent milieu Be alert to signs of tension If possible, remove an agitated patient from a stimulating situation Give antianxiety or antipsychotic medication for agitation Avoid challenges to the patient's self-esteem If restraining the patient is necessary: 1. Maintain the patient's dignity 2. Explain the procedure to the patient 3. Gather adequate trained staff to handle the situation 4. Avoid unnecessary force 5. Protect the patient and staff from injury 6. Review the situation with the patient and staff after calm has returned Discuss episodes of violent behavior with other patients who were present

the best relationship with the patient acting as communicator. It is also the responsibility of the nurse to be sure that there are staff available to stay with and support the other patients. They should be removed from the area if possible. Sometimes a "show of force" by the presence of several staff members will be enough to assist the patient to regain control and be able to talk about his feelings. The importance of a sense of confidence on the part of the staff has been emphasized.[11] They should be well-informed about the situation before taking action. All staff members in a psychiatric setting should receive training in the prevention and management of violent behavior, including an opportunity to discuss feelings and attitudes about this aspect of nursing care. It can be reassuring to a violent patient to see that his uncontrollable behavior can be controlled and that he can be prevented from causing harm. The patient who has become violent may need medication or seclusion to help him gain control. These therapeutic techniques are discussed further in Chapter 15.

The last step in nursing intervention with a violent patient is to review the incident with the patient after he has achieved control. This helps the patient alleviate any guilt he might be feeling or fear that he might have harmed someone. The nurse can, in retrospect, review what happened and talk about alternatives should the patient become anxious and angry in the future.

Dealing with anger is a challenge for both the nurse and the patient. Nursing interventions with patients who have problems with the expression of anger are summarized in Table 12-5. Anger is not inherently good or bad. Expression of anger is not always positive or negative. Effective dealing with anger implies that the person can accept his right to be angry and the reciprocal right of others to be angry. It is not therapeutic to encourage a patient to express angry feelings indiscriminately. It is important that the patient feel free to choose whether to express anger and that, when he chooses to do so, he avoid abridging the rights of others. It is through this process that anger can facilitate growth.

 Evaluation

The evaluation of the nursing care provided to the patient who has problems with the healthy expression of anger should be based on observed behavioral change. The subjective response of the patient is also a helpful input. Maynard and

Chitty[14] recommend that the following questions be asked of a patient who has had an experience of expressing anger:

- How do you feel about the experience?
- How did the other person behave in response to your anger?
- Was the confrontation well timed?
- Did the interaction take place in private?
- What would you change in the future?
- How would you change these aspects?

Evaluation should focus on the mode of expression of anger, the appropriateness of the object, the congruence between the degree of feeling expressed and the precipitating incident, and the patient's awareness of the process. If the patient does not change in the planned direction in one of these areas, the data base, goals, and nursing interventions should be reviewed and appropriate modifications made.

There should be a staff review of any episode of violent behavior. The focus of such a discussion is to dissipate any residual staff anxiety related to the incident and to objectively evaluate their performance. The situation should be analyzed to identify the precipitating stressors and the sequence of attempts to cope with the stress. Future prevention can be directed to alleviating stressors that seem to precipitate violent outbursts and to assisting the patient to develop more positive ways to deal with anger when it occurs. Feedback should be given to colleagues about the process of restraining the patient. Procedural modifications may be made as a result of this review.

If the patient is involved in learning techniques of assertiveness, the evaluation process is an integral part of the training program. Thus the patient should be involved in eliciting feedback about his behavior in selected situations. He should be encouraged to practice assertive behavior until he feels comfortable and consistently is perceived as behaving assertively. Patients in an assertiveness group may also participate in evaluating each other.

Successful problem solving in the area of assertively expressing anger becomes a self-reinforcing process. As the patient successfully asserts himself, he experiences good feelings about himself and discovers that his needs are met more frequently. The assertive nurse experiences similar feelings and becomes increasingly effective professionally.

Suggested cross-references

Therapeutic relationship skills and self-awareness of the nurse with respect to feelings are discussed in Chapter 3. The model of health-illness phenomena and the phases of the nursing process are discussed in Chapter 4. Nursing interventions to enhance self-esteem are discussed in Chapter 8. Facilitating a patient's expression of emotions and strengthening social skills are discussed in Chapter 9. Intervening with patients who have problems with interpersonal relationships is discussed in Chapters 9 and 11. Somatic therapies are discussed in Chapter 15. Nursing intervention in family abuse and violence is discussed in Chapter 28.

SUMMARY

1. Anger is a feeling of resentment that occurs in response to heightened anxiety when a person perceives a threat. Various overt and covert expressions of anger were described.

2. Anger is experienced on a continuum from mild annoyance to intense rage. Rage is destructive, but positive functions of anger were also described.

3. Biological stressors include the instinctual drives postulated by Freud and Lorenz, as well as physiollogical disruptions such as endocrine imbalance, seizure disorders, and neoplasms.

4. Psychological stressors were described, including the frustration-aggression theory of Dollard et al., the behavioral theory, and the existential theory presented by Fromm.

5. Sociocultural stressors include the imposition of social sanctions on behavior, crowding and intrusion on personal space, and role modeling by significant others and through the media. The social learning theory of anger was discussed.

6. Physiological behaviors associated with anger result primarily from secretion of epinephrine and stimulation of the sympathetic nervous system. The behaviors resulting from this constitute preparation for fight or flight.

7. Assertive behavior was differentiated from passive and aggressive behavior as a constructive use of anger. Assertiveness theorists state that the individual has the right to pursue the gratification of his own needs so long as he does not infringe on the rights of others.

8. One may choose to be assertive or not. Assertiveness training enables the person to choose freely because he has the ability to act assertively if he wishes to accept the consequences of this behavior.

9. Acting-out behavior is often an indirect expression of anger. It attracts the attention of others and is a representation of the feelings the person is experiencing.

10. The coping mechanisms of goal-directed behavior and use of ego defense mechanisms were discussed.

11. Examples of nursing diagnoses that identify the threat (stressor) and the resulting angry behavior were given and compared to the medical diagnoses of paranoid disorder and conduct disorder.

12. Long- and short-term goals for the development of healthy coping behaviors can guide the nurse and patient in their work together and provide a sense of accomplishment as progress is made.

13. The importance of self-awareness for the nurse was discussed. Nontherapeutic responses to a patient's expression of anger were identified as defensiveness, retaliation, condescension, and avoidance.

14. Assertiveness training is a problem-solving approach to dealing with anger that can help the nurse achieve self-awareness and improve her ability to cope with the angry patient. Steps to assertiveness were described.

15. Two approaches to nursing intervention with the angry patient, described by Hays and Maynard and Chitty, were introduced.

16. Limit setting is a nursing intervention that may be employed with angry, acting-out patients. The patient is assumed to be responsible for his behavior and is informed of the consequences if the limited behavior occurs.

17. Intervention with the violent patient should focus on immediate control and safety, followed by discussion to alleviate guilt and identify alternative behaviors to help prevent future episodes of violence.

18. Evaluation of the improved ability to express anger is based on objective and subjective feedback about the increased incidence of assertive behavior. The patient's increased self-esteem related to his improved communication skills tend to perpetuate assertive behavior once it has been learned.

References

1. Alberti, R.E., and Emmons, M.L.: Your perfect right, ed. 2, San Luis Obispo, Calif., 1974, Impact Publishers.
2. American Psychiatric Association: Diagnostic and statistical manual of mental disorders, ed. 3, Washington, D.C., 1980, The Association.
3. Bach, G.R., and Goldberg, H.: Creative aggression; the art of assertive living, New York, 1974, Avon Books.
4. Chenevert, M.: Special techniques in assertiveness training for women in the health professions, St. Louis, 1978, The C.V. Mosby Co.
5. Coffey, M.P.: The violent patient, J. Adv. Nurs. **1**:341, 1976.
6. Dollard, J., et al.: Frustration and aggression, New Haven, Conn., 1939, Yale University Press.
7. Fast, J.: Body language, New York, 1970, Pocket Books.
8. Fromm, E.: The anatomy of human destructiveness, New York, 1973, Holt, Rinehart & Winston, Inc.
9. Hays, E.: Anger: a clinical problem. In Burd, S., and Marshall, M., editors: Some clinical approaches to psychiatric nursing, New York, 1963, The Macmillan Co., Publishers.
10. Lathrop, V.G.: Aggression as a response, Perspect. Psychiatr. Care **16**:202, Sept.-Dec. 1978.
11. Lenefsky, B., de Palma, T., and Locicero, D.: Management of violent behavior, Perspect. Psychiatr. Care **16**:212, Sept.-Dec. 1978.
12. Loomis, M.E.: Nursing management of acting-out behavior, Perspect. Psychiatr. Care **8**:169, 1970.
13. Lorenz, K.: On aggression, New York, 1966, Harcourt, Brace & World, Inc. (Translated by M.K. Wilson.)
14. Maynard, C.K., and Chitty, K.K.: Dealing with anger: guidelines for nursing intervention, J. Psychiatr. Nurs. **17**:36, June 1979.
15. Montague, M.C.: Physiology of aggressive behavior, J. Neurosurg. Nurs. **11**:10, March 1979.
16. Novaco, R.W.: The functions and regulation of the arousal of anger, Am. J. Psychiatry **133**:1124, 1976.
17. Penningroth, P.E.: Control of violence in a mental health setting, Am. J. Nurs. **75**:606, 1975.
18. Roberts, T.K., Mock, L.A.T., and Johnstone, E.E.: Psychological aspects of the etiology of violence. In Hays, J.R., Roberts, T.K., and Solway, K.S., editors: Violence and the violent individual, Jamaica, New York, 1981, Spectrum Books.
19. Rothenberg, A.: On anger, Am. J. Psychiatry **128**:454, 1971.
20. Rubin, T.I.: The angry book, New York, 1969, Collier Books.
21. Stearns, F.R.: Anger: psychology, physiology, pathology, Springfield, Ill., 1972, Charles C Thomas, Publisher.
22. Whitman, J.: When a patient attacks: strategies for self-protection when violence looms, RN **42**:30, Sept. 1979.

Annotated suggested readings

Alberti, R.D., and Emmons, M.L.: Your perfect right, ed. 2, San Luis Obispo, Calif., 1974, Impact Publishers.

This practical, straightforward presentation of assertiveness gives clear descriptions of assertive and nonassertive behavior and suggests ways to become more assertive. Part Two is directed toward the use of assertiveness training with patients and is recommended for readers who have advanced preparation in psychiatric nursing.

Bach, G.R., and Goldberg, J.: Creative aggression: the art of assertive living, New York, 1974, Avon Books.

The authors describe the many ramifications of misdirected anger. This book is particularly helpful in identifying family and cultural stressors leading to disruptions in the ability to express anger.

Bowman, C., and Spadoni, A.J.: Assertion therapy: the nurse and the psychiatric patient in an acute, short-term psychiatric setting, J. Psychiatr. Nurs. **19**:7, June 1981.

This is an excellent presentation of assertiveness theory as applied in a short-term hospital setting. A detailed lesson plan outlines the six-session assertiveness therapy program that the authors have developed. They also discuss this therapeutic approach relative to behavioral therapy from which it was derived. This article is particularly recommended for nurses who have been trained to conduct assertiveness therapy and are planning to initiate a program.

Campbell, W., and Mawson, D.: Violence in a psychiatric unit, J. Adv. Nurs. **3**:55, Jan. 1978.

The authors discuss the occurrence of violent behavior in an unlocked, architecturally open hospital. They raise a question as to whether there are patients who are unable to tolerate a high level of freedom, based on their observation of episodes of violence in this setting.

Chenevert, M.: Special techniques in assertiveness training for women in the health professions, St. Louis, 1978, The C.V. Mosby Co.

This is a delightful book that applies the principles of assertiveness theory to the experience of women, especially nurses, in health care settings. The author urges nurses to develop assertive skills for the sake of their patients as well as themselves. She identifies many difficult situations and gives practical suggestions for constructive behavior.

DeFabio, S., and Ackerhalt, E.J.: Teaching the use of restraint through role-play, Perspect. Psychiatr. Care **16**:218, Sept.-Dec. 1978.

In this article, the authors describe a methodology that has been effective in teaching people to restrain violent patients. It contains a detailed presentation and discussion of the process that should be very helpful to in-service educators who are planning a class on this subject.

Freeberg, S.: Anger in adolescence. J. Psychosoc. Nurs. **20**:29, March 1982.

The author discusses anger in the context of normal adolescent development. Attention is also given to the many manifestations of anger when direct expression is blocked. Suggested nursing interventions are presented.

Fromm, E.: The anatomy of human destructiveness, New York, 1973, Holt, Rinehart & Winston, Inc.

This book develops an existential theory of the meaning and expression of anger and compares and contrasts the existential viewpoint with other basic theoretical frameworks.

Galassi, M.D., and Galassi, J.P.: Assert yourself: how to be your own person, New York, 1977, Human Sciences Press.
This is a workbook approach to learning assertive behavior. The presentation is very clear, and the directed practice exercises structure and enhance the learning process.

Gluck, M.: Learning a therapeutic verbal response to anger, J. Psychiatr. Nurs. **19:**9, March 1981.
This article is a description of a program developed by the author to teach nursing assistants to respond more therapeutically to angry patients. She advocates an understanding approach that focuses on the patient's stress and the means to relieve emotional tension.

Hays, J.R., Roberts, T.K., and Solway, K.S., editors: Violence and the violent individual, Jamaica, New York, 1981, Spectrum Books.
This collection of papers comprehensively views the problem of violence in the United States. Various theories are presented, and current research is examined. This book is recommended as a resource for someone who is interested in serious investigation of this subject.

Lenefsky, B., de Palma, T., and Locicero, D.: Management of violent behavior, Perspect. Psychiatr. Care **16:**212, Sept.-Dec. 1978.
This article focuses on the procedure used for restraint of a person who is threatening violent behavior. Photographs illustrate the recommended techniques. The authors emphasize safety and the importance of a team approach by the staff.

Loomis, M.E.: Nursing management of acting-out behavior, Perspect. Psychiatr. Care **8:**169, 1970.
This article presents theoretical concepts of the origins of acting-out behavior, including an excellent model of patient-staff interaction in the acting-out process. It also includes a helpful section on nursing intervention.

Lorenz, K.: On aggression, New York, 1966, Harcourt, Brace & World, Inc. (Translated by M.K. Wilson.)
This is a fascinating and readable presentation of the instinctual theory of aggressive behavior presented by a physician who is also a naturalist. This book is bound to stimulate reflection on the behavior of humankind as seen from the vantage point of the world of nature.

Maynard, C.K., and Chitty, K.K.: Dealing with anger: guidelines for nursing intervention, J. Psychiatr. Nurs. **17:**36, June 1979.

This excellent article very clearly describes nursing interventions with patients who are having problems dealing with anger. The nursing process model is used. This is a very useful resource for nurses who are inexperienced and can benefit from a well-developed conceptual framework.

Moritz, D.A.: Understanding anger, Am. J. Nurs. **78:**81, Jan. 1978.
The author describes anger as an expression of anxiety. She emphasizes the need for the nurse to analyze angry behavior in an effort to identify the cause. Nursing intervention is discussed in the context of two case examples.

Novaco, R.W.: The functions and regulations of the arousal of anger, Am. J. Psychiatry **133:**1124, 1976.
This author approaches anger from a positive standpoint and describes several useful functions. He then suggests a cognitive therapeutic approach to the patient who is having problems with anger.

Rothenberg, A.: On anger, Am. J. Psychiatry **128:**454, 1971.
This article differentiates anger and its growth-producing functions from the destructive emotions of hostility and vengefulness. It helps to clarify some of the hazy issues about defining aggression, anger, and other related terms.

Rumpler, C.H., and Seigerman, C.: Violent behavior in an intensive care unit, Perspect. Psychiatr. Care **16:**206, Sept.-Dec. 1978.
The focus of this article is on the use of a behavior modification approach to intervene in aggressive behavior in an intensive care setting. The authors point out that aggression can be a particularly difficult problem in a general hospital. A case history is used to illustrate their creative and successful approach to the problem.

Stewart, A.T.: Handling the aggressive patient, Perspect. Psychiatr. Care **16:**228, Sept.-Dec. 1978.
The author provides practical suggestions for physical restraint of a violent patient. Photographs are included that illustrate the text and clarify the suggested approaches.

Whitman, J.: When a patient attacks: strategies for self-protection when violence looms, RN **42:**30, Sept. 1979.
This article presents some very practical information and guidelines concerning intervention in violent behavior. The focus is on protection of the patient and the nurse from harm. The author emphasizes the need to be alert to subtle clues and be prepared for unexpected violent behavior. She points out that it is unpleasant to think about this problem but ignoring it will not make it go away.

Cogito, ergo sum.
I think, therefore I am.
Descartes

CHAPTER 13

IMPAIRED
COGNITION

Learning objectives

After studying this chapter, the student should be able to:

- *define cognition in terms of its component processes.*

- *identify three models of cognitive functioning.*

- *describe Jean Piaget's three stages of cognitive development.*

- *identify the major categories of data that should be collected regarding an individual's level of cognitive functioning.*

- *compare and contrast the medical diagnoses of organic mental disease vs. organic brain syndrome and delirium vs. dementia.*

- *discriminate between the characteristic behaviors of an individual who is delirious and one with dementia.*

- *describe the purposes of psychological testing and several commonly administered tests.*

- *identify coping mechanisms that are used by individuals with cognitive impairment.*

- *state individualized nursing diagnoses for patients with cognitive impairments.*

- *assess the relationship between the nursing and medical diagnoses of individual patients with cognitive impairments.*

- *analyze various nursing interventions in terms of priorities, nursing care principles, and rationale in planning the care of a patient with cognitive impairment characteristic of delirium or dementia.*

- *assess the importance of evaluation of the nursing process when working with cognitively impaired people.*

- *identify suggested readings for future study.*

The ability to think and to reason is one of the distinguishing features of the human being. It is this ability that created civilization and allowed progress from the Stone Age to the Space Age. Knowledge is now proliferating at such a rapid rate that Toffler[17] coined the phrase "future shock" to describe the almost overwhelming impact on the individual of the need to assimilate new information. We have moved from the time when power was equated with physical strength to the use of money to acquire power to an era where there is little power without information. Although strength and money play a part in the use of power, they are most successfully wielded by the best informed. It is now anticipated that individual computers will be required to assist the person in effectively processing information.

Because of the importance of the ability to think rationally, intellectual functioning is highly valued by the individual. Most people are threatened at the prospect of losing their cognitive abilities, including reasoning, memory, judgment, orientation, perception, and attention. These processes allow the individual to make sense of experience and to interact productively with the environment. Impaired cognitive functioning leaves the affected person in a state of confusion, unable to understand experience, and unable to relate current to past events. Memory is a key cognitive process because to exercise judgment, make decisions, or even orient oneself to time and place, one must remember past experiences and points of reference. Therefore memory loss is a particularly frightening experience.

Cognitive impairment is so threatening that it has been difficult for others, even professionals, to confront those who suffer from this problem. As a result, these people have frequently been labeled as crazy or senile. Institutionalization has frequently been society's solution to meeting the basic needs of the person who is unable to adequately process information. Custodial care has been provided by caretakers who have had little knowledge of the needs of their patients. Only recently has there begun to emerge significant medical and nursing research into the needs of this patient population.

Psychology is the discipline that has historically been most involved in research on cognition. Experimental psychologists have been interested in defining the process of learning and developing models that will explain learned behavior. Bachrach[3] defines learning as "a change in behavior potential resulting from reinforced practice." This is an associationist model of learning theory. When the individual experiences a *stimulus,* a number of behavioral *responses* are available to him. He is most likely to select the response that has been *reinforced* in the past. In other words, he has learned a particular response to a given stimulus or set of stimuli. If the response is not reinforced on subsequent occasions, an alternative behavior may be substituted. If the new behavior is reinforced, the potential will be for the person to continue to behave in that way. Clinical example 13-1 illustrates this process.

CLINICAL EXAMPLE 13-1

Johnny M, age 3, asked his mother for a cookie. Ms. M told Johnny that he could have a cookie after he picked up his toys. Johnny began to kick and scream. Ms. M cuddled Johnny, gave him a cookie, and picked up the toys. When she discussed this experience with her neighbor, Ms. P, the mother of four children, Johnny's mother learned that he had had a temper tantrum and that the behavior was likely to continue if she gave in to Johnny's demands. The next time Johnny demanded a cookie, Ms. M again requested that he pick up his toys first. Johnny began his temper tantrum. His mother placed him in another room and informed him again that when he picked up his toys, he could have a cookie. After a few minutes, Johnny quieted, then came out and put away his toys. His mother responded with cuddling and a cookie. Over time, the temper tantrums disappeared.

By reinforcing Johnny's tantrums with cookies and cuddling, Ms. M had, in effect, taught him that this was an effective behavior. When she stopped reinforcing Johnny's negative behavior, he learned that another behavior was more effective in meeting his needs. Gradually, with continued reinforcement, the potential for effective behavior increased. Learning theorists believe that this sequence is responsible for the development of much of human behavior and that behavior can be changed, or learning can take place, by altering the reinforcement.

This process is depicted in Fig. 13-1. Since response number 1 is not reinforced, it tends not to recur. Instead, the individual tries response number 2. It is reinforced and thus will tend to

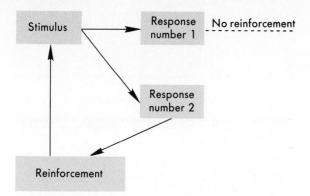

FIG. 13-1
The associationist, or behavioral, model of learning.

recur the next time the stimulus is produced. It is important to note that the reinforcement need not be a reward, although rewards are certainly powerful reinforcers. Punishment can also be a reinforcer of behavior if the alternative is lack of any response at all. Therefore, in the preceding examples, spanking Johnny would probably have been less effective than leaving him alone, since he would still be receiving his mother's attention. Also, a reinforcer need not be a material object. The cuddling may have been as effective in reinforcing Johnny's behavior as the cookie.

The associationist model of learning theory just described was developed by such theorists as Pavlov, Skinner, and Wolfe. It is also referred to as a behavioral model. Another major group of learning theorists, including Tolman and Bandura, ascribe to a cognitive model.[3] Their approach to learning is a broader one that focuses on "the acquisition of information about the environment rather than the attachment of particular responses to particular stimuli."[3] In this case, the stimulus is perceived as a *sign* that a desired resource may be available from the environment (for example, a cookie). This perception creates a *demand* that when combined with knowledge about the environment leads the individual to seek gratification. The individual's perception of the environment is referred to as a *cognitive map* that guides him in his quest to meet his need. Cognitive learning theorists would say that the change in Johnny's cookie-seeking behavior was due to a change in his perception of his mother's behavior as a part of his environment. Her changed behavior blocked the pathway that had previously led him to a cookie, so he had to find a new route.

Bachrach[3] believes that the cognitive learning theory model is closely related to the com-

puter model of cognition. The computer also relies on stored information, or *memory,* about the environment in order to make decisions. The concept of reinforcement, be it reward or punishment, has no meaning to a computer. Decisions are based on an objective evaluation of the consequences of past actions. Consequences are evaluated in terms of their effectiveness in achieving the desired result.

Further information on the behavioral model and on the modification of behavior will be found in Chapters 2 and 21.

Human cognitive development has been described by Piaget[16] and is summarized in Table 13-1. His research revealed a three-stage process of the development of thought processes. The first developmental stage is "the period of sensorimotor intelligence." This phase lasts from birth until the development of language, usually about 2 years.[16] This stage is action oriented, with the actions first directed toward the self and then gradually incorporating more space and the ability to situate the self in space. There is also the beginning of memory for objects that are out of sight, a necessary precursor for the development of language using words to describe objects that are not present. The baby who plays "peek-a-boo" is practicing this ability.

The second stage is composed of two substages, which some theorists describe as separate stages. This is the "period of preparation and organization of concrete operations: of categories, relations, and numbers." This period lasts from 2 to 12 years of age and is divided into two substages. Early in this stage, during the preoperational substage, symbolism appears in language and in play. Objects are defined in terms of function, that is, a ball is "to throw."[7] This is also the period of magical thinking, in which thoughts and words are perceived as the equivalent of action. Preoperational behavior lasts from about 2 to 5 years of age. The child then enters the substage of concrete operations. At this point, he is "capable of relatability, i.e., combinations, associations, negations and reversibility."[8] Elkind[7] states that during this period, children develop the capacity for syllogistic reasoning, which enables them to make and follow rules. They also develop the ability to quantify experience.

The third stage is "the period of formal operations."[16] This develops between the ages of 12 and 14, resulting in the ability to conceptualize

TABLE 13-1. Piaget's levels of cognitive development

Stage	Age (years)	Characteristics
Sensorimotor	Birth to 2	Action oriented
		No language
		Develops awareness of body in space
		Develops memory for missing objects
Preparation and organization of concrete operations		
Preoperational phase	2 to 5	Symbolism appears
		Objects defined by function
		Magical thinking
Concrete operations	5 to 12	Capable of relatability
		Syllogistic reasoning
		Makes and follows rules
		Quantifies experience
Formal operations	12 to 14 and older	Abstraction
		Development of ideals
		Criticism of others
		Self-criticism

at an adult level. It is only at this point that the person is "capable of abstract logic and has the ability to do manipulations in propositions, probabilities and permutations."[8] The period of formal operations enables individuals to explore idealistic concepts and to measure their own reality against their ideals.[7] This pertains to observations of significant others, such as parents, and of cultural institutions, such as government and religions. The same process is applied to the self in the form of self-criticism. This developmental process provides the foundation for continued cognitive growth as life experiences enrich and modify the individual's perception of the world.

In some individuals, cognitive processes may not develop fully or, once developed, may deteriorate. When cognitive deficiencies occur during childhood, they are generally referred to as mental retardation. The reader is referred to a textbook of pediatric nursing for a discussion of cognitive deficiencies. In this chapter, cognitive disruptions in the adult will be considered. In most cases, the individual will have developed to the level of formal operations. Although it may occur at any age, cognitive impairment is most

common in the elderly. It is highly recommended that this chapter be read in conjunction with Chapter 31, because the content of the two chapters is complementary.

Continuum of cognitive responses

Cognitive impairments include impaired memory and judgment, disorientation, misperceptions, decreased attention span, and difficulties with logical reasoning. They may occur episodically or be present continuously. Depending on the stressor, the condition may be reversible or characterized by progressive deterioration in functioning. Fig. 13-2 illustrates cognitive functioning as it occurs on the continuum of health-illness coping responses.

 Stressors

Cognitive dysfunctions are generally the result of a biological disruption in the functioning of the central nervous system (CNS). The CNS requires a continuous supply of a variety of nu-

FIG. 13-2
Continuum of health-illness coping responses relative to cognitive functioning.

trients to function. Any interference with the provision of supplies to the brain will be reflected in functional disruptions. For instance, the difficulties in cognition experienced by some elderly people result from arteriosclerotic changes in cerebral blood vessels that deprive the brain of needed oxygen, glucose, and other essential basic chemicals. Other vascular abnormalities, such as transient ischemic episodes (small strokes), cerebral hemorrhage, and multiple small infarcts in brain tissue resulting from chronic hypertension, can also result in cognitive impairments.

Wolanin[19] cites three major systemic problems that contribute to cognitive impairment: (1) hypoxia, (2) alterations in blood glucose content, and (3) toxicity. She further subdivides hypoxia into four types: anemic; histotoxic, that is, conditions that prevent cells from metabolizing oxygen; hypoxemic, that is, problems with ventilation; and ischemic.

Anemic hypoxia may be insidious in onset. Possible stressors include aspirin ingestion, resulting in occult bleeding; other occult blood loss; or deficiencies of iron, folic acid, or vitamin B_{12}. Histotoxic hypoxia may be related to such stressors as dehydration, hyperthermia, or hypothermia. A possible stressor related to hypoxemic hypoxia is chronic obstructive lung disease. Others might include asthma or an acute respiratory tract infection. Ischemic hypoxia can result from congestive heart failure, atherosclerosis, hypotension, hypertension, or increased intracranial pressure resulting from a tumor, subdural hematoma, or normal pressure hydrocephalus.[19]

Metabolic disorders frequently affect mental functioning, especially when severe or of long duration. Endocrine malfunctioning, whether it involves underproduction or overproduction of hormones, can adversely affect cognition. For example, the thyroid hormone is known to have a great influence on mental alertness. People with hypothyroidism are sluggish and retarded in their thinking. Those with severe hypothyroidism (myxedema) may develop psychotic behavior characterized by delusional thinking. People with hyperthyroidism, on the other hand, are frequently hyperalert and agitated, with acceleration of both thought and action. Other endocrine disorders that may cause cognitive disruptions include hypoglycemia, hypopituitarism, and adrenal disease. Chronic liver disease, chronic renal disease, and vitamin deficiencies are other metabolic disorders that can result in disrupted information processing. Vitamin B–complex deficiency, particularly thiamine, is believed to be the cause of the Wernicke-Korsakoff syndrome found in chronic alcoholics who have a long-standing nutritional deficiency. One of the prominent features of this syndrome is a severe deficit in cognitive functioning.

Toxic and infectious agents may also result in behavior typical of disturbed cerebral functioning. Toxins may originate either within the individual or in the external environment. An example of an internally generated toxin is the elevated blood level of urea found in a patient with renal failure. Environmental toxins would include various poisonous substances that might be ingested or animal venoms. Acute viral and bacterial infections occur in the CNS, resulting in inflammation and impaired functioning. Chronic infections also affect the brain. One such condition is the neural manifestation of tertiary syphilis, general paresis. This is seldom seen any more, since early treatment of syphilis has become more prevalent. Infections in other body systems may also have a deleterious effect on the CNS if there is an extremely elevated temperature.

Wolanin[19] emphasizes the possible significance of prescription and over-the-counter drugs as toxic stressors. Thorough assessment of drug use is particularly critical with elderly patients, because of their increased sensitivity to drugs and because of the possibility that confusion could lead to difficulty in following directions for taking drugs. Drug-drug interactions or interactions between drugs and other substances, particularly alcohol, may also lead to disruptions in cognitive functioning.

Conditions that alter the structure of brain tissue are also reflected in impaired cognitive functioning. Tumors may cause proliferation or displacement of tissue, thus altering its function. Trauma, whether accidental or surgical, will result in a change in ability to process information. The specific effect will depend on the location of the lesion.

Yet another group of stressors which may cause this type of dysfunction is that of genetic abnormalities. An example of a degenerative brain disease that is hereditary in nature is Huntington's chorea, which is inherited as an autosomal dominant trait.

Sensory underload or overload can result in cognitive dysfunction. It has been found that people who are placed in environments with minimal stimuli seem to develop internally produced stimuli in the form of hallucinations. The proliferation of intensive care units (ICUs) in general hospitals has led to an interest in sensory overload. The constant light and activity in these areas has been noted to lead to disorientation, delusional thought, and hallucinations, sometimes referred to as "ICU psychosis." However, it is difficult to differentiate how much of the cognitive impairment results from the sensory experience as opposed to other concurrent stressors, such as the introduction of multiple drugs into the system and the result of massive assaults on physical integrity.

Unfortunately, there are also several syndromes for which no specific stressor has yet been identified. One such syndrome is senile dementia or Alzheimer's disease when it occurs in individuals under age 65.[14] This problem is actually diagnosed by ruling out all possible identifiable stressors, coupled with laboratory evidence of brain degeneration. It must be noted that understanding of the biochemical processes of the brain and the response of brain and nervous tissue to stressors is still limited. As knowl-

edge grows, it is conceivable that a specific biological component will be identified in the etiology of all disorders categorized as psychiatric. The fields of psychiatry and neurology may well merge at some time as knowledge grows more sophisticated. For example, it is known that some chemical substances can create hallucinatory experiences and are popular in the drug culture for that reason. As more is learned about the mechanism of action of the hallucinogens, such as LSD and PCP, more will also be understood about processes that may take place in the brains of psychotic people.

A degree of cognitive impairment may also be found in conjunction with other disruptions in mental functioning. For instance, a delusional person may seem disoriented because he misidentifies the place he is in. People who are hyperactive related to a manic affective disturbance have short attention spans, as do depressed people. Depression may also result in memory disorders, although it is often difficult to determine whether the problem is related to memory loss or lack of motivation to try to remember or to communicate the memory. The stressors related to these disorders of cognitive functioning would be those related to the primary problem. In general, physiological causes are ruled out first, then psychosocial stressors are considered in relationship to cognitive impairment. Even when physiological factors are present, psychosocial stress may further compromise the individual's thought process. Each patient must receive a complete assessment so that nursing care can be planned in a holistic manner.

Data collection

Disruptions in cognitive functioning are most readily apparent in individuals who have a medical diagnosis of organic mental disorder (DSM-III).[1] Conditions that are not definably organic may also be referred to as "functional." The distinction between organic and functional becomes blurred, since possible organic causes are found for medical conditions formerly considered to be the result of psychosocial stressors. Lipowski[12] defines organic mental disorders as conditions caused by permanent damage to or temporary dysfunction of the brain or a combination of permanent and temporary disruptions. The problem may originate in the brain or elsewhere in the system and may be diffuse or focal. In the DSM-III,[1] a distinction is made between *organic brain syndromes,* which are not differentiated in terms of etiology, and *organic mental disorders,* in which a cause may be determined. In other words, the organic mental disorder is a defined organic brain syndrome. For example, alcohol withdrawal delirium is an organic mental disorder. Following are the six categories of organic brain syndromes[1]:

1. Delirium and dementia
2. Amnestic syndrome and organic hallucinosis
3. Organic delusional syndrome and organic affective syndrome
4. Organic personality syndrome
5. Intoxication and withdrawal
6. Atypical or mixed organic brain syndrome

The first category refers to types of widespread cognitive impairment; the second, third, and fourth categories refer to the particular functions that are affected, the fifth, to a cause of impairment, and the last, to conditions that do not meet the criteria for any of the other categories. Discussions in this chapter will focus on category 1, delirium and dementia, because these are the medical diagnostic categories that will be encountered most frequently by nurses and are not discussed elsewhere in this text. Further information on intoxication and withdrawal may be found in Chapter 14.

Behaviors associated with delirium

In the recent past, delirium was also referred to as acute, or reversible, brain syndrome and dementia as chronic, or irreversible, brain syndrome. Acute vs. chronic referred to the rapidity of the onset of the disorder and to its duration. These terms are no longer recommended because they do not discriminate between delirium and dementia. Delirium is a diffuse disruption of the cognitive state that is characterized by a clouding of awareness manifested by a limited attention span, sensory misperception, and disordered thought.[1] There are also disturbances of activity patterns and of the sleep-wakefulness cycle. Generally, there is a rapid onset and a brief course of illness. Lipowski[12] describes the disordered thought process as including disturbed attention, memory, thinking, orientation, and perception. He further notes the tendency of the degree of impairment to fluctuate throughout the day, with periods of lucidity occurring intermittently. The disturbance is generally worse at night. Delirium usually occurs in response to a specific stressor, such as infection, trauma, a toxin or drug, or alcohol intoxication.

However, the stressor may not be immediately apparent. Clinical example 13-2 will demonstrate behaviors that are typical of a patient with delirium.

CLINICAL EXAMPLE 13-2

Ms. S. was brought to the emergency room of a general hospital by her parents. She was a 22-year-old single woman who was described as having been in good health until 2 days prior to admission, when she complained of malaise and a sore throat and stayed home from work. She was employed as a typist in a small office and had a stable employment record. According to her parents, she had an active social life and there were no significant conflicts at home.

On admission, Ms. S was extremely restless and had a frightened facial expression. Her speech was garbled and incoherent. When she was approached by an unfamiliar person, she would become agitated, trying to climb out of bed and striking out aimlessly. Occasionally she would slip into a restless sleep. Her temperature on admission was 103.4° F (39.4° C) axillary, pulse was 108 per minute, and respirations were 28 per minute. Her skin was hot, dry, and flushed. Her mother said she had had only a few sips of water in the last 24 hours and had not urinated at all, although she had had several episodes of profuse diaphoresis.

Her ability to cooperate with a mental status examination was limited. She would respond to her own name by turning her head. When her mother asked her where she was, she said "home," but could not say where her home was. She would give only the month when asked for the date and said it was January, when the actual date was February 19. She also refused to give the day of the week. A neurological examination was negative for signs of increased intracranial pressure or for localizing signs of CNS disease.

The tentative medical diagnosis was that of delirium secondary to fever of unknown origin. Symptomatic treatment of the fever, including intravenous fluids, an aspirin suppository, and cool water mattress, was begun immediately while further diagnostic studies were carried out. Nurses caring for the patient noticed continued restlessness and disorientation. Her speech was still incoherent. In addition, they noticed that she was picking at the bedclothing. Suddenly she became extremely agitated, trying to get out of bed and crying out, "Bugs, get away, get bugs away." She was brushing and slapping at herself and the bed. As her mother and the nurse talked with her and held her, she gradually became calmer but periodically would continue to slap at "the bugs" and need reassurance and reorientation.

Later in the day additional laboratory results became available. A lumbar puncture was normal, as were skull x-ray films. Results of toxicological screening of blood were also negative. The electroencephalogram revealed diffuse slowing. There was an elevated white blood count and electrolyte imbalance consistent with severe dehydration. Cultures of her throat and blood were both positive for beta-hemolytic streptococci; so intravenous antibiotic therapy was begun at once while other supportive measures were continued.

As the infection gradually came under control and the fever decreased, Ms. S's mental state improved. A week later, when she was discharged from the hospital, her cognitive functioning was completely normal, with the exception of amnesia for the time during which she was delirious.

Ms. S demonstrates many characteristics that are frequently seen in patients with delirium. The behaviors are related to alterations in neurochemical and electrical responses in the brain as a result of the stressor that causes the disruption. *Disorientation* is generally present, sometimes in all three spheres of time, place, and person. Thought processes are usually disorganized. *Judgment is poor* and there is little decision-making ability. Stimuli may be misinterpreted, resulting in *illusions* or distortions of reality. An example of an illusion is the perception that a polka-dot drape is actually covered with cockroaches. Delirious patients may hallucinate. These *hallucinations* are most frequently visual and often take the form of animals, reptiles, or insects. They are real to the person and extremely frightening. Assaultive or destructive behavior on the part of the patient may be an attempt to strike back at a hallucinated image. At times, patients with delirium also exhibit a *labile affect,* changing abruptly from laughter to tearfulness and vice versa, with the affect unrelated to any environmental events. There may also be *loss of usual social behavior,* resulting in such acts as undressing, playing with food, and grabbing at others. Delirious patients tend to act on impulse.

Other behaviors may be specifically related to the causative agent of the behavioral syndrome. For example, the fever and dehydration experienced by Ms. S were a result of her systemic streptococcal infection, as was her brain syndrome. It is extremely important to differentiate behavioral manifestations, which help to identify the stressor. Treatment is usually conservative

until a specific stressor has been isolated. Although most cases of delirium are reversed, with recovery of the patient, in about 12% of the cases[12] the person dies as a result of the severity of the stressor. If adequate intervention does not take place, delirium may become dementia.

Behaviors associated with dementia

Dementia is a cognitive disruption that features a loss of intellectual abilities severe enough to interfere with usual social or occupational activities.[1] The loss of intellectual ability includes impairment of memory, judgment, and abstract thought. There are also frequently changes in personality. According to Lipowski,[12] the personality change may appear as either alteration or accentuation of the person's usual character traits. The onset of dementia is usually gradual. The course may be one of gradual deterioration or may be stable. It is also possible for the process of dementia to be reversed and for the person's intellectual functioning to improve if the underlying stressors are identified and treated.

Dementia can occur at any age but is most frequent in the elderly. It may be the result of trauma, either accidental or surgical; a chronic infection, such as tertiary syphilis; cerebrovascular disruptions, such as arteriosclerosis or chronic hypertension; or may be of indeterminate cause. "Senility" is a nonspecific term and usually applies to those who have degenerative brain disease of an unknown cause. Because of the pejorative connotation, use of the terms "senility" or "senile" is to be discouraged. Clinical example 13-3 will demonstrate behaviors associated with dementia.

CLINICAL EXAMPLE 13-3

Mr. B is a 73-year-old widower who has resided in a nursing home for 3 years. He chose to move to the nursing home after the death of his wife, although his son encouraged him to live with him and his family. Mr. B stated that he did not want to burden his family and would be happier with others of the same age. He did well for the first 18 months. He was an active participant in social groups both in the home and in his church, where he continued to attend regularly. He also visited his son once a week and enjoyed seeing his grandchildren and puttering around his son's house.

About 18 months previously Mr. B began to seem forgetful. He would ask the same question several times and on occasion would prepare for church on a

Friday or Saturday. He also became irritable and accused his son of not caring about him and abandoning him in "that place." Mr. B spent many hours taking papers from his desk and studying them. When asked what he was doing, he would say, "Attending to my business." He began to withdraw from activities, making flimsy excuses to avoid playing his favorite card game, gin rummy. When he was persuaded to play, he usually quit in frustration because he could not remember which cards had been played. At times Mr. B was quite anxious. He would periodically seem well oriented and expressed great concern about the changes he was experiencing, wondering if he was "going crazy."

Because of the concern of the nursing staff at the nursing home, Mr. B was scheduled for a complete physical examination by his family physician and a psychiatric evaluation by the geriatric psychiatric nurse consultant who came to the nursing home weekly. The physical examination revealed generally good health for a man of Mr. B's age. He suffered from a mild hearing loss and slight prostatic hypertrophy. Hypertension had been diagnosed 10 years prior to this examination but was well controlled by diuretics. Neurological examination revealed normal reflexes, normal muscle strength, a slight intention tremor, normal response to sensation, normal cranial nerves, and no disturbance of gait. An electroencephalogram was normal, as were a skull x-ray film and the results of laboratory studies of blood and urine. A brain scan and computerized axial tomography studies of the brain revealed some atrophy of the cerebral cortex.

The psychiatric examination confirmed the deficits in cognitive functioning that had been observed by the nursing home staff and by Mr. B's son. He was oriented to person and place but stated that the date was April 6, 1958. The real date was March 11, 1981. He also thought the day of the week was Friday, whereas it was actually Wednesday. He correctly identified the season of the year as spring. Mr. B was able to correctly give his birth date, the date of his son's birth, and the year he began to work at his first job. He spoke at length and with great detail about his exploits as a young man. However, he could not repeat the names of three objects after 5 minutes and could not remember what he had eaten for lunch or the last name of the man who shared his room. He became distressed when he was trying to answer these questions. His vocabulary was excellent, as was his fund of general information. However, he was unable to remember the names of the two most recent presidents. He could, however, recite the names of the eight presidents preceding them.

Mr. B's judgment was somewhat impaired. When asked what he would do if he found a stamped, addressed, sealed envelope, he said he would "read it, then mail it." His ability for abstract thinking was slightly concretized. His attention span and ability to concentrate were normal. His eye-hand coordination was disrupted, as demonstrated by his difficulty in copying simple figures. His tremor was evident both when he was drawing and when he signed his name.

He exhibited affect that was appropriate in quality and quantity to the content of the discussion. He appeared depressed when talking about his memory loss but cheerful and proud when describing his grandchildren. No abrupt mood swings were noted. The flow of speech was of a normal rate and volume. Content of speech was logical and coherent, except when Mr. B was trying to remember and describe recent events, when it became somewhat disjointed.

As a result of the data gathered in the physical and psychiatric examinations, a diagnosis was made of dementia of unknown cause.

Over the next several months, Mr. B's condition continued to deteriorate gradually. He became increasingly forgetful and began to confabulate. He was less conforming to social norms and needed reminding about hygiene and appropriate dress. He also became seductive with female residents and staff, making suggestive remarks and occasionally fondling someone. Visits to his son's home became impossible as his behavior deteriorated. His memory of the identity of family members sometimes was confused. He would misidentify his daughter-in-law as his wife and his grandson as his son. More and more, his conversation consisted of rambling reminiscences of his life in his youth. Because he is surrounded with caring people, Mr. B continues to live with dignity and respect in spite of his progressively limited ability to communicate.

The behaviors associated with dementia reflect the brain tissue alterations that are taking place. The cognitive changes are related to the actions of stressors that interfere with the functioning of the cerebral cortex. Other areas of the brain may be affected as well, which is one reason for being sure that the patient has a complete medical and neurological examination. Another reason for this is that although the condition may be irreversible, progression may be arrested by identification of the stressor and treatment of the underlying dysfunction. For instance, treatment of hypertension may prevent further occurrence of small hemorrhages, which are a possible cause of irreversible brain syndrome. Recent research has demonstrated that many cases of dementia may be reversible. It has also been found that depression in the elderly is often misinterpreted as dementia and therefore not treated appropriately. This happens so often that the condition has been labeled *pseudode-*

mentia. Depression differs from dementia in several ways.[1] A depressed person generally expresses concern about his perceived lack of cognitive ability, whereas a demented person will attempt to compensate for it and conceal it. If motivated, a depressed person is able to perform cognitive tests, and, if not, the deficits are less consistent than those found in dementia. In addition, the date of onset of depression can usually be more specifically identified than that of dementia. However, it is important to remember that the conditions can coexist, since a person who is to some extent aware of impaired cognitive ability may well experience depression.

A common behavior related to this problem is *disorientation*. Usually time orientation is affected first, then place, and, finally, person. This behavior can be distressing to the patient, who may be aware of this difficulty and embarrassed and frightened by it. This is particularly true if the person's mental acuity is fluctuating, which sometimes happens. In these instances the individual is aware, during periods of lucidity, of the confusion and disorientation experienced at other times.

Memory loss is another prominent characteristic of dementia. Immediate recall and recent memory are generally most seriously affected. Remote memory may be intact, although it too deteriorates as the condition progresses. For example, Mr. B had difficulty remembering what he had eaten for lunch but gave accurate dates for significant events earlier in his life. Most aging people dwell on the past, but people with recent memory loss have difficulty shifting to the present and at advanced stages may seem to live in the past. This was exemplified by Mr. B's misidentification of his grandson and his daughter-in-law. Another behavior related to memory loss is *confabulation*. This is the tendency of a confused person to fabricate a response to a question when he cannot remember the answer. For instance, when Mr. B was asked if he knew one of the female residents of the home, he replied, "Of course I know her. I used to play gin with her husband." Actually, the woman's husband had been dead for many years and Mr. B had never met him. This behavior should not be viewed as lying or an attempt to deceive. Rather, it is the person's way of trying to save face in an embarrassing situation. He is aware that he should know the answer to the question and gives an answer that seems reasonable, not

entirely disbelieving it himself. It is not unlike the situation in which one meets an acquaintance and cannot recollect the person's name or where they met but acts as if these facts are remembered, hoping that the other person will offer clues about his identity.

Vocabulary and general information may be less affected by dementia, at least until its very late stages. This is influenced by how recently the information was learned. Facts learned early in life may be recalled well, whereas those learned recently may be quickly forgotten, as demonstrated by Mr. B's performance in listing the last ten presidents.

These patients may have *labile affective behavior,* particularly if the limbic system has been affected by the disease process. There may also be some *deterioration in social skills*. Impulsive sexual advances toward members of the opposite sex may occur. These reflect *decreased inhibition* and *impaired judgment*. Frequently this behavior is also an attempt to establish interpersonal contact and is a way of asking for caring from others. It is also a way of reinforcing an important part of the person's identity, which is becoming less secure as mental functioning declines.

Restlessness and *agitation* are other behaviors that occur with dementia. Extreme agitation may occur at night; this is sometimes referred to as the *sundown syndrome*. It is probably due to tiredness at the end of the day combined with fewer orienting stimuli, such as planned activities, meals, and contact with people.

Disorientation results in fear and agitation. *Agitated behavior* may also occur if the person is coerced to do something he does not understand or simply does not want to do. This may reflect an effort to keep control over the person's own life, thereby maintaining self-esteem. Change is not well accepted by these patients. Efforts to change behavior patterns will probably result in increased rigidity and, if efforts persist, agitated behavior. Routine is important, particularly a routine that is congruent with the person's previous life-style. Table 13-2 summarizes the characteristics of delirium and dementia.

A term that is frequently used when referring to the person with cognitive impairment is *confusion*. Although widely accepted as nursing and medical jargon, this term has not been specifically defined. Wolanin and Phillips[20] have focused their nursing research on this topic. They define confusion as "a condition characterized by the client's disorientation to time and place, incongruous conceptual boundaries, paranormal

TABLE 13-2. **Characteristics of delirium and dementia**

	Delirium	Dementia
Onset	Usually sudden	Usually gradual
Course	Usually brief (under 1 month), with return to usual level of functioning	Usually long term and progressive; occasionally may be arrested or reversed
Age group	Any	Most common over age 65 (senile dementia); under age 65, called Alzheimer's disease
Stressors	Toxins, infection, hyperthermia, space-occupying lesion, trauma, and sensory deprivation/overload	Hypertension, hypotension, anemia, normal pressure hydrocephalus, vitamin deficiencies, toxins, slow viruses, hypoglycemia, tumors, hyperthermia/hypothermia, and brain tissue atrophy
Behaviors	Fluctuating levels of awareness, disorientation, restlessness, agitation, illusions, hallucinations, disorganized thought, impaired judgment and decision making, affective lability, loss of inhibitions, and diffuse electroencephalogram (EEG) slowing	Memory loss, impaired judgment, decreased attention span, disorientation, inappropriate social behavior, labile affect, restlessness, agitation, and resistance to change

awareness, and seemingly inappropriate verbal statements that indicate memory defects."[20:8] The term should be used with caution, however, since Wolanin and Phillips discovered a wide array of meanings when they surveyed groups of physicians and nurses.

There is dissatisfaction among many mental health professionals with the terms delirium and dementia because of the stigma of the term dementia in particular and the lack of specificity of both terms. It has been suggested that "brain failure" would be a more accurate term and would connote a similarity with other organic conditions, such as heart failure and renal failure. Although this terminology is relatively new, it seems to be gaining acceptance.

Frequently patients who have cognitive impairment are referred to a clinical psychologist for psychological testing. This referral should be made for a specific purpose, since the testing is time consuming, expensive, and tiring for the patient. Some reasons for psychological testing include identification of the stressor(s) causing the disruption, understanding of the dynamics of the problem, developing guidelines for therapeutic intervention, and obtaining a prognosis for recovery. DeCato and Wicks[6] present an ex-

cellent summary of indications for psychological referral and a description of the most common psychological tests administered to psychiatric patients. They divide the tests into three categories: intelligence, perceptual-motor, and projective tests.

Intelligence tests are used to assess the patient's general level of intellectual functioning. Those used most frequently are the *Wechsler Intelligence Scale for Children* (WISC) and the *Wechsler Adult Intelligence Scale* (WAIS). These tests must be evaluated by a skilled clinician, with consideration given to educational and sociocultural background of the patient. The result of the test is the individual's intelligence quotient (IQ), which can serve as a guideline for understanding the person's ability for intellectual performance. Some information about psychodynamics may also be obtained by analyzing the nature of the person's behavior in the testing situation.

Perceptual-motor testing is useful in determining whether an organic mental disorder is causing disturbed behavior. The *Bender-Gestalt* test requires that the patient copy a series of geometrical figures. The accuracy and facility with which the copying is done is significant in determining the presence of a biological stressor. Other factors, such as size and arrangement of the copied figures or the behavior of the patient in the testing situation, provide insight into the person's psychodynamic functioning. For example, a person who uses obsessive-compulsive behavior to cope with anxiety may try hard to make an exact copy of the stimulus figure.

Projective tests are directed specifically toward gaining information about psychodynamics. Probably the most widely known projective test is the *Rorschach* test, which consists of a standard series of inkblots. The patient is asked to respond to the inkblot, first generally and then in more detail. The response is then analyzed. Use and analysis of the Rorschach test is complex and must be done only by a qualified clinical psychologist. Another projective test that is commonly used is the *Thematic Apperception Test* (TAT). The patient is presented with a series of pictures of people engaged in nonspecific activities and asked to describe what might be happening in the situation. In both these situations the person's response is determined by his life experience as well as his current mental state. Valuable information may be gained about the person's anxiety level and the mechanisms used to cope with anxiety, which can have implications for therapy and prognosis.

There are many other psychological tests, some used for very specialized purposes. Clinical psychologists are good resource people both for explaining specific tests and for elaborating on the results of psychological testing. Frequently the psychologist is asked to determine whether or not the individual is experiencing a disruption that is organic. Further information about psychological testing may be found in Chapter 17.

Coping mechanisms

The way an individual copes emotionally with a disruption in his cognitive ability is greatly influenced by past life experience. A person who has developed an armamentarium of coping mechanisms that have been effective in the past is better able to handle the onset of a cognitive problem than is a person who already has coping problems.

The response of an individual to the onset of organic brain disease often mirrors that person's basic personality pattern. For instance, a person who has usually reacted to stress with anger directed toward other people and the environment will probably react similarly when he notices limitations in his intellectual abilities. A person who is more apt to direct anger inward and become depressed will be more likely to respond with depressive behaviors. A person who has relied on a mechanism such as intellectualization will be more threatened by loss of intellectual ability than a person who has used a mechanism such as reaction formation.

Regression is frequently used in an effort to cope with an advanced mental disorder. It may be caused in part by deterioration in mental function. It is probably also attributable to the behavioral manifestations of the problem, which result in the patient becoming more dependent on others for the fulfillment of basic needs such as nutrition and hygiene. Encouraging patients to perform self-care also supports their use of healthier coping mechanisms.

Because the basic behavioral disruption in delirium is altered awareness, which reflects the severe biological disturbance in the brain, psychological coping mechanisms are not generally used. For this reason, the nurse must protect the patient from harm and substitute for the person's own coping mechanisms by constantly reorienting him and reinforcing reality.

Early dementia is characterized by much use of the mechanism of denial. The person generally attempts to pursue his usual daily routine and makes light of memory lapses. He may be able to mobilize some environmental resources to help him cope. For instance, a businessman who is experiencing difficulty with recent memory might ask his secretary to remind him of all his appointments and provide him with a summary of the names of the people with whom he is meeting and the purpose of the meeting. As the impairment progresses, the individual may become very resistant to any limitations being placed on his independence. For instance, the family of a patient with a medical diagnosis of Alzheimer's disease might become very concerned about his ability to continue to drive a car safely. It is likely that the patient would be very reluctant to give up his driver's license and would deny that he was having any problem.

As the individual becomes more affected by decreasing cognitive ability, efforts to cope will be more obvious. The behaviors that become a concern to significant others and bring the person into contact with the health care system are frequently attempts to cope. For instance, a family member may complain that a relative has "always been irritable, but is now belligerent when he doesn't get his way." In other cases, the patient's behavior may be experienced by others as a personality change. Some behaviors that are probably attempts to cope with loss of cognitive ability include suspiciousness, hostility, jocularity, depression, seductiveness, and withdrawal. Because it is threatening to admit that a close relative has dementia, family members may also focus on the coping mechanism as the real problem, participating in the denial of the underlying cognitive impairment.

Nursing diagnosis

The nursing diagnosis of the individual with cognitive impairment must take into consideration both the possible underlying stressors and the patient behaviors that have been observed by the nurse. A comparison of nursing diagnoses and the DSM-III[1] criteria for the medical diagnosis of delirium is given in Table 13-3. Nursing and medical diagnoses for dementia are compared in Table 13-4. These tables relate to Clinical examples 13-2 and 13-3. Fig. 13-3 summarizes the model of health-illness phenomena as related to cognitive functioning.

Planning and implementation of nursing interventions

Goal setting

Goals that are related to cognitive impairment may be directed toward an improved ability to process information, if this is realistic, or toward optimal utilization of the abilities that the patient retains if the impairment is irreversible. For example, a goal for a patient who is disoriented because of drug withdrawal might be "The patient will verbalize the complete date within 3 days." In contrast, a goal for a patient who is disoriented because of chronic alcoholism and who is not in withdrawal might be "Within 1 month the patient will find his own bed every night without assistance." The latter patient may never be able to remember the exact date but may not need that information if he is to function in a protected setting. The first patient,

TABLE 13-3. Comparative examples of nursing diagnoses and medical diagnoses associated with delirium

Nursing diagnoses	Medical diagnoses as described in DSM-III*
Agitation related to fear of strangers	**Diagnostic criteria for DELIRIUM**
Visual hallucinations related to elevated temperature	**A.** Clouding of consciousness (reduced clarity of awareness of the environment), with reduced capacity to shift, focus, and sustain attention to environmental stimuli
Disorientation related to hyperthermia and unfamiliar environment	**B.** At least two of the following:

Elevated temperature related to streptococcal infection	1. Perceptual disturbance: misinterpretations, illusions, or hallucinations
	  2. Speech that is at times incoherent
	  3. Disturbance of sleep-wakefulness cycle, with insomnia or daytime drowsiness
	  4. Increased or decreased psychomotor activity

Dehydration related to minimal fluid intake and diaphoresis	**C.** Disorientation and memory impairment (if testable)
	D. Clinical features that develop over a short period of time (usually hours to days) and tend to fluctuate over the course of a day
	E. Evidence, from the history, physical examination, or laboratory tests, of a specific organic factor judged to be etiologically related to the disturbance

*From American Psychiatric Association: Diagnostic and statistical manual of mental disorders, third edition, Washington, D.C., APA, 1980.

TABLE 13-4. Comparative examples of nursing diagnoses and medical diagnoses associated with dementia

Nursing diagnoses	Medical diagnoses as described in DSM-III*
Memory loss (recent) related to cerebral cortical atrophy	**Diagnostic criteria for DEMENTIA**
Moderate level of anxiety related to periodic awareness of cognitive impairment	**A.** A loss of intellectual abilities of sufficient severity to interfere with social or occupational functioning
Withdrawal related to attempts to cope with impaired memory	**B.** Memory impairment
Irritability related to attempts to cope with impaired memory	**C.** At least one of the following: 1. Impairment of abstract thinking, as manifested by concrete interpretation of proverbs, inability to find similarities and differences between related words, difficulty in defining words and concepts, and other similar tasks 2. Impaired judgment
Disorientation related to cerebral cortical atrophy	3. Other disturbances of higher cortical function, such as aphasia (disorder of language due to brain dysfunction), apraxia (inability to carry out motor activities despite intact comprehension and motor function), agnosia (failure to recognize or identify objects despite intact sensory function), "constructional difficulty" (e.g., inability to copy three-dimensional figures, assemble blocks, or arrange sticks in specific designs)
Impaired judgment related to cerebral cortical atrophy	4. Personality change, i.e., alteration or accentuation of premorbid traits

D. State of consciousness not clouded (i.e., does not meet the criteria for delirium or intoxication, although these may be superimposed)

E. Either 1 or 2:
1. Evidence from the history, physical examination, or laboratory tests, of a specific organic factor that is judged to be etiologically related to the disturbance
2. In the absence of such evidence, an organic factor necessary for the development of the syndrome can be presumed if conditions other than organic mental disorders have been reasonably excluded and if the behavioral change represents cognitive impairment in a variety of areas

*From American Psychiatric Association: Diagnostic and statistical manual of mental disorders, third edition, Washington, D.C., APA, 1980.

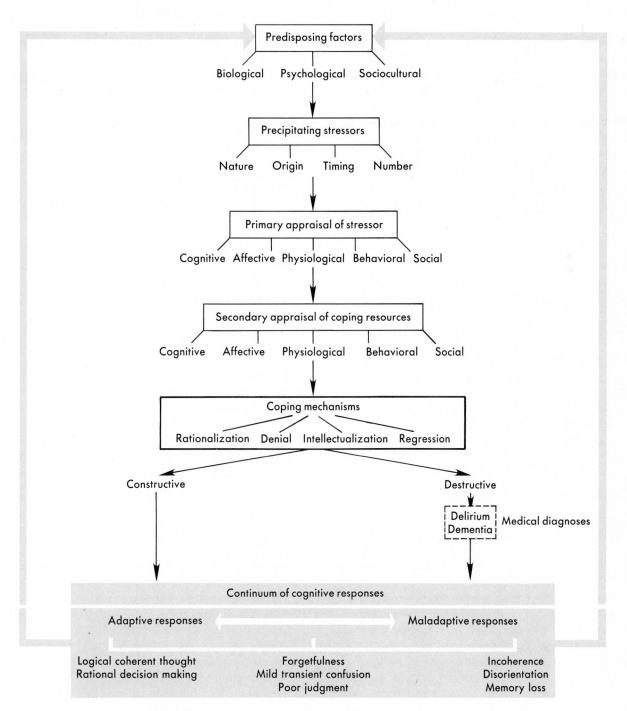

FIG. 13-3
Model of health-illness phenomena related to cognitive functioning.

however, will need that information. In addition, the nurse can use the assessment of the patient's orientation to time to assess the current status of his mental functioning. Goals should be realistic to avoid discouragement for both the nurse and the patient. If the second person had been required to learn the date, it would result in a frequent confrontation with his deteriorated cognitive skills, leading to frustration, higher anxiety, and possibly less effective coping. Realistic long-term goals may be difficult to formulate while the evaluation process is taking place. During this time the nurse may elect to focus on short-term goals directed toward maintaining the patient's basic needs.

If there is an identified stressor that is causing the patient's behavioral disruption, goals should also be developed that focus on the stressor. For instance, if a person is delirious because of a fever, a goal might state, "The patient's temperature will be maintained below 100° F (37.8° C)." When the cause of the elevated temperature is identified, appropriate goals will be written to address that problem. For example, dehydration may be a stressor contributing to an elevated temperature. A related nursing goal would then be: "The patient's fluid intake will be at least 3000 ml in each 24-hour period." As the various elements of the person's behavior are explored and documented, nursing goals must be updated and modified; new goals must be added and accomplished goals deleted.

Intervening in delirium

In providing nursing care for a patient with delirium, highest priority is given to nursing interventions that will maintain life. If the individual is too disoriented or agitated to attend to basic physiological needs, nursing care must be planned to meet these needs. Nutrition and fluid balance may be maintained by intravenous therapy. If the patient is very agitated or restless, restraint may be necessary to keep the intravenous line open. Restraints should be applied only when absolutely necessary because the patient can become more agitated and frightened when restrained. A disoriented patient should never be restrained and left alone.

Sleep deprivation may be another problem with these patients. Intervention is important because lack of sleep can add to already existing cognitive dysfunction. If the stressor that is

causing the disruption has not been identified, the physician may be reluctant to prescribe sedation for the patient, since sedative medication may confuse attempts to identify the original stressor. Nursing measures such as a back rub, a glass of warm milk, and soothing conversation may help a less agitated patient relax and fall asleep. The presence of a family member is also reassuring to the patient. Disoriented patients need to be in a lighted room. Shadows may be misinterpreted and add to the patient's fear. Also, it is less confusing to be able to use environmental objects to orient oneself to place and person.

The disoriented patient may need to be protected from hurting himself or others, particularly if he is hallucinating. The visual hallucinations of delirium are often very frightening and the patient may try to escape by running away, even to the extent of jumping out of a window. The patient's room must be safe, with security screens and a minimum of extra furniture or other objects placed where he might hurt himself. Frequently these patients require one-to-one nursing observation and repetitive verbal reorientation.

It is tempting to respond to a patient who is experiencing frightening visual hallucinations by trying to eliminate the hallucinated object. For instance, the patient might request help in brushing the bugs off the sheets. Agreeing to do this is not usually therapeutic. By participating in this activity, the nurse is nonverbally communicating to the patient that the hallucinated objects are real and can be made to go away. In reality the hallucinations will continue until the underlying stressor is eliminated. The nurse's reinforcement of the reality of the hallucination is likely to make the patient even more frightened. A more appropriate response would be to continually orient the patient to the reality situation of being sick and hospitalized. In addition, the patient can be assured that the nursing staff and physician are helping him and will keep him safe. Family members should also be helped to respond in a supportive way.

Patients who are having difficulty processing information need clear messages and instructions from other people. Choices should be kept to a minimum because the patient will not be able to think of alternatives and decide priorities. Independent decision making can be introduced into the plan of nursing care as the patient's sensorium becomes clearer. Decisions related to orientation may be especially difficult for the patient. To respond appropriately to the question "What time would you like to take your bath?" one requires knowledge of the present time and some idea of the usual routine so that one does not decide to bathe during visiting hours or at mealtime.

Simple direct statements are reassuring to the patient and have the best potential for resulting in an appropriate response. Orienting phrases such as "here at the hospital" or "now that it's June" can be woven into a conversation. A patient who is having difficulty dressing or feeding himself needs matter-of-fact, specific direction from the nurse. A very confused patient will need to be fed or dressed, again in a manner that allows him to maintain his dignity. This is another nursing function with which families can often assist. It may alleviate the family member's anxiety to be able to do something helpful for the patient and the patient may be reassured by the family's physical closeness and concern.

As the patient recovers, he may be concerned about what happened to him. The health team needs to discuss this issue and arrive at a conclusion about the disruption in functioning that occurred. This should then be explained to the patient and family. The nurse should assess the patient's understanding of the nature of his problem, the stressors which were involved, any ongoing therapy that will be required, and preventive measures that will decrease the probability of a recurrence. Teaching may have to be repeated several times before the patient copes with the feelings the illness has aroused and then grasps the information that has been conveyed. If written materials are available, they can be helpful to patients who are having residual problems processing information. The teaching should include at least one responsible family member so that the information can continue to be reinforced when the patient goes home.

If the patient is discharged from the hospital with a residual deficit in cognitive functioning, a community health nursing referral may be helpful. The community health nurse can then continue to implement the nursing care plan and can validate the patient's compliance with the treatment plan.

Davidhizar, Gunden, and Wehlage[5] have recommended the following nursing interventions for the delirious patient:

1. Regulate lights and provide a window to show diurnal variation.
2. Verbalize orienting information which includes name and purpose of persons entering the room.
3. Provide proper functioning of eyeglasses and hearing aids.
4. Avoid rough excessive handling of patient during procedures or turning.
5. Minimize forced feeding.
6. Elevate the head of the patient or allow him to partially sit up, since *visual hallucinations are increased when the patient is confined to his back.*
7. Provide for presence of familiar personal objects in the room.
8. Encourage visits from family members and friends as indicated by condition.
9. Assign the same personnel to give care.
10. Convey warmth and reassurance. Physical presence can have a calming effect.
11. Maintain firmness when dealing with the agitated, hostile patient.
12. Encourage verbal and nonverbal expression.
13. Provide for diversional activities and meaningful use of time.
14. Protect from situations where judgment and intellectual capacity would be overtaxed.
15. Schedule medications, treatments, or other procedures at times that won't interrupt nighttime sleep.
16. Limit treatments and procedures and schedule them in a predictable way in order to avoid an overwhelming situation for the patient.
17. Provide clocks and calendars.
18. Inform patient of his condition and his progress during periods of lucidity.
19. Allow patient control over aspects of his environment as he is able.
20. Recognize cultural variables that affect patient's response to stimuli.

Intervening in dementia

Nursing care of the patient with dementia is similar in some respects to that of the patient with delirium. Usually the stressors involved do not present an immediate threat to life; so highest priority is given to providing nursing care that will help the patient to maintain an optimal level of functioning. This will differ for each individual. Frequently an attitude of hopelessness evolves in those who work with chronically ill people. This can lead to stereotyping and decreased ability to see and appreciate the uniqueness of each person. It is challenging to search for this uniqueness and rewarding to find it. Individualization of nursing care is probably most important for those who will be institutionalized for a long time.

Recently gerontological nursing has been receiving more recognition as a separate specialty area within the profession. Nursing research is beginning to focus on nursing intervention with the chronically ill person and with the aging person. One finding has been that individualized attention may stimulate enhanced functioning in people who appear to have severely limited cognitive abilities. Jones[11] has described the effect of social isolation and sensory deprivation on institutionalized elderly people. In her work with one such patient she was able to stimulate renewed interest in the environment by providing consistent social interaction. Peer[15] has developed a team approach to the geriatric patient that uses a number of group activities to assist the person in maintaining an optimal level of functioning. These include kinetic therapy, which focuses on body movement; reality orientation; sensory training, using restimulation of all the senses; activities of daily living; bowel and bladder retraining; occupational therapy; poetry therapy; recreational activities; and church services. This type of approach attends to the person as a complete individual with a many-faceted personality. It is a hopeful way of providing nursing care because it communicates to the patient that there is potential for activity and growth.

Disorientation is a common problem of people with cognitive impairment. Nursing interventions should be directed toward assisting the patient to function in the environment. In an institution it is helpful to mark patient rooms with large, clearly printed signs indicating the occupant's name. This has the additional benefit of reminding forgetful people of others' names. Personal possessions can also be orienting devices. A favorite rocking chair, a handmade afghan, or a family picture give the person a sense of identity and help to identify a personal area of the institution. Everyone needs a personal space. A light in the room at night helps the person remain oriented if he awakens and helps decrease nighttime agitation. Some authorities recommend the use of small amounts of antipsychotic medications, such as phenothiazines and butyrophenones, to assist patients to rest, since barbiturate sedatives may cause paradoxical agitation in people with organic brain syndromes.[14]

Clocks with large faces assist with orientation to time. A digital clock is probably not a good idea, since the confused person may not identify it as a clock. Calendars with a separate page for each day and large writing also help with time orientation. Newspapers provide other orienting stimuli and also help to stimulate interest in current events. An institutional newspaper provides a creative outlet and focuses on patient strengths and also helps patients maintain awareness of the environment.

Reality orientation is a nursing approach that is generally helpful to patients with cognitive impairments. Orientation includes the dimensions of time, place, and person. Systematic reality orientation includes attention to each of these dimensions. Voelkel[18] compared a structural reality orientation approach to the use of a less structured group resocialization approach. She concluded that the most important factor in causing a positive behavioral change seemed to be the involvement in a caring group. Personal and physical contact was found to have a positive impact on group members. Hogstel[10] reported the results of a research project to study the effects of a reality orientation program. She also found that the most positive results were in the area of social interaction. Even if the level of confusion did not change significantly, patients who received reality orientation were noted to be happier and more involved with other people. Mulcahy and Rosa[13] used a reality orientation approach with a group of cognitively impaired patients in a general hospital. In addition to consistent orientation to person, place, and time, their nurse-patient goals included the following: awareness of the need to be hospitalized; cooperation with treatment; maintenance of self-esteem and development of self-confidence; relatedness to the environment through the use of sight, touch, and hearing; bowel and bladder continence; interpersonal interaction; accurate identification of others; and involvement in discharge planning. They developed a standardized nursing care plan and taught other nurses to use it.

Recent memory loss is another frequently encountered behavior. It may be frustrating to the patient to be constantly confronted with evidence of his failing memory. Conversational focus can be directed toward topics that the patient initiates. Most patients will feel more comfortable talking about remote memories and may derive pleasure from discussing past experiences. Misperceptions of the present situation can be dealt with gently and diplomatically. As an example, if an elderly woman who has been widowed for 10 years says that she expects her husband to come home soon, the nurse might reply, "You must have loved your husband very much. Sometimes it seems to you that he's still here." Explicitly or implicitly agreeing that her husband will "come home" is fostering false hope, perhaps leading to a disappointment. Abrupt confrontation with the reality of her husband's death is cruel and will increase her anxiety.

Previously useful coping mechanisms are often emphasized by the patient with cognitive deficit. Sometimes these attempts to cope may be hard to understand unless placed in the appropriate context. An older man who pats and pinches the nurses and makes lewd remarks may have had past success dealing with his anxiety in heterosexual situations by behaving seductively. An elderly woman who hoards food in her room may equate food with security and may be hoarding because she feels insecure. An aging person who has been suspicious of others in the past may become more suspicious as time goes on. Because of the protective nature of these behaviors, they should not be actively confronted. Rather, the nurse should try to discover the source of the person's anxiety and attempt to alleviate that, thus allowing the person to behave less defensively.

Patients may also become agitated when pushed to do something unfamiliar or unclear. Expectations should be explained simply and completely. If the patient can handle choices, they should be offered. An individual daily schedule of activities can help the person prepare for expectations and plan his day. If a patient refuses to participate in an activity, continued insistence usually leads to increased agitation. The best approach may be to wait a few minutes and then return to see if the patient will agree to the request. In the interim the nurse can examine her approach to the patient to see if she might have contributed to the problem. Perhaps the nurse seemed to the patient to be too controlling and a power struggle developed, or perhaps the nurse initiated the request abruptly, not allowing the patient a time for transition from the activity in which he had been engaged.

Bartol and Storrie[4] have developed the following guidelines for communication with the demented patient:

I. Verbal
   A. Speech construction
      1. Short words.
      2. Simple sentences (not compound or complex).
      3. No pronouns; only nouns.
      4. Begin each conversation (particularly at night) by identifying yourself and calling the person by name.
   B. Speech style
      1. Speak slowly.
      2. Say individual words clearly.
      3. If you increase your speech volume, *lower* the tone, raise the volume *only* for *deafness,* not because you do not get a response you understand.
      4. If you ask a question *wait* for a response.
      5. Ask only one question at a time.
      6. If you repeat a question, repeat it exactly.
      7. Utilize self-included humor whenever possible.
II. Nonverbal (facial motion, torso position, upper extremity gestures).
   A. General
      1. Convince yourself that your nonverbal style can be felt all the way across the room and by several people; not just the patient or staff person you are addressing.
      2. Every verbal communication is delivered by proper nonverbal gestures.
   B. Specific
      1. Stand in front (or directly in line of vision) of person.
      2. Maintain eye contact.
      3. Move slowly.
      4. If person starts or continues to walk while you are talking to him, do not try to stop him as your first move. Instead keep moving along in front of him and persevere.
      5. Use overemphasis and exaggerated facial expression to emphasize your point, particularly if vision and/or hearing is impaired.
III. General guidelines
   A. Listen actively. If you don't understand, say you don't understand and ask for a repeat of the statement. If this request precipitates a catastrophic reaction, offer your best guess. If you receive a "no," try another guess. Continue until resolution.
   B. Assume there is a capability for insight. If someone refuses to join an event he normally engages in, assume he has become sad, angry, frustrated, embarrassed, anxious about his condition. Your first job is to *check* and see if that is so—not just ask "are you okay" or some ritualistic expression.
   C. Chart all phrases and nonverbal techniques utilized that consistently "get through" for a particular person and a particular situa-

TABLE 13-5. Summary of nursing interventions in impaired cognition
Goal: Promotion of optimal cognitive functioning

Principle	Rationale	Nursing action
Conservation of energy	Physiological disruptions deplete energy; energy is used to ensure survival before supporting other functions; cognitive functioning is enhanced when adequate energy is available; patient survival and safety are always the highest priority nursing care activities	Maintain adequate nutrition Monitor fluid intake and output Monitor vital signs Provide opportunities for rest and stimulation Assist with ambulation if necessary Assist with hygiene activities if necessary Provide appropriate nursing care for identified physiological disruption Identify stressful situations to assist patient to avoid them Assess mood and intervene in identified disruptions (Chapter 9)
Conservation of structural integrity	Cognitive impairment usually involves sensory and perceptual disorders that can endanger the patient's safety	Assess sensory and perceptual functioning Provide access to eyeglasses, hearing aids, canes, walkers, etc., if needed Observe and remove safety hazards, e.g., obstacles, slippery floors, open flames, inadequate lighting Supervise medications if necessary Protect from injury during periods of agitation with one-to-one nursing care; restraints only if absolutely necessary
Conservation of personal integrity	Cognitive impairment is a threat to self-esteem; a positive nurse-patient relationship can assist the patient to express his fears, and feel secure in his environment; recognition of accomplishments also raises self-esteem	Provide reality orientation Establish trusting relationship Encourage patient to be as independent as possible Identify patient's interests and skills; provide opportunities to utilize them Give honest praise for accomplishments Use therapeutic communication techniques to assist patient to communicate his thoughts and feelings
Conservation of social integrity	Caring relationships with others promote a positive self-concept; communication by significant others can often be understood more easily than that of strangers; family and friends can provide help in knowing patient's habits and preferences; involvement of significant others in caregiving often helps them cope with the stress of patient's health problem	Initiate contact with significant others Encourage patient to interact with others; involve him in group activities Teach family and patient about the nature of the problem and the recommended health care plan Allow significant others to assist in patient care if they wish Meet with significant others regularly and provide them with an opportunity to talk Involve patient and family in discharge planning

tion. Use each others' techniques. Compare notes on successes and failures.

D. When encouraging participation in activities, regulate your exuberance on the following criteria: if you push hard enough to precipitate a catastrophic reaction you must have planned your time and energy so that you can now treat the reaction with verbal/nonverbal techniques.

E. When possible utilize an observer to watch your exchange, make suggestions, and perhaps trade off with you. If you have not really "gotten anywhere" in 5 minutes or less, you will probably do better to leave and either return in 5 minutes or have a colleague try.

F. Finally, if you say you are going to do something, *do it*. If you forget, find the person and apologize. Assuming that the person has forgotten the episode insults both your intelligence and his/hers.

G. If you need to stop a patient-patient interchange do it firmly and quickly, get them out of each others territory, wait 5 minutes then return and explain to each one why you acted as you did. Use *factual* explanations, not guilt induction.

Hirschfeld[9] recommends structuring the nursing care of the cognitively impaired older adult around Myra Levine's four principles of conservation: conservation of energy, conservation of structural integrity, conservation of personal integrity, and conservation of social integrity. Conservation of energy is related to the need to understand physiological disruptions that might deplete the person's energy supplies. Anxiety and depression are noted as other behaviors that use energy. Nursing intervention in these areas can free energy for other purposes, such as improving cognitive abilities. Conservation of structural integrity implies nursing attention to sensory and perceptual deficits that make it more difficult for the person to comprehend the environment. Patients may need to be protected from injury, and medication use may need to be supervised. Conservation of personal integrity can be accomplished through sensitivity to the person's need to maintain self-esteem. This requires awareness of one's own feelings about organic mental disorders. The encouragement of self-care and the establishment of trust are essential. Reality orientation and listening are important nursing interventions, as are the provision of privacy and respect for personal space. Conservation of social integrity focuses on the maintenance of relationships with significant others. The nurse can help to interpret behavior and encourage frequent visits. Families

need help to maintain healthy relationships with the cognitively impaired member, neither withdrawing nor fostering unnecessary dependency. These principles may be used as an organizing framework for planning the nursing care of the cognitively impaired patient (Table 13-5).

 Evaluation

Expectations of the patient who has cognitive difficulty must be realistic but not pessimistic. A brain-damaged person may never remember the correct date but may be able to find his own bedroom. However, if he is never asked to find his room, he has no opportunity to demonstrate his level of orientation. One evaluation criterion, then, is the appropriateness of the nursing goal to the individual. The nurse should assess whether the expectation might have been either too high or too low. Levels of expectation can be increased until a level is reached where the patient is clearly unable to function and then lowered to the realistic level.

Improved performance on tests of orientation to time, place, and person are concrete measures of the person's level of orientation. The frequency of social interaction is another criterion that may be used to evaluate patient progress. The ability to assist with or perform self-care may also be measured and compared over time. For the person with a progressive disorder, these evaluation measures not only provide a way of assessing the effectiveness of nursing care, but also give a picture of the rate of progression over time, thus allowing the nurse to adjust her interventions appropriately. Nurses in long-term care settings may wish to develop flow sheets identifying critical behaviors to facilitate this comparison over time. Anderson[2] developed a simple flow sheet relative to dementia for use by nurse practitioners (p. 448). A comparable flow sheet that she developed for use in evaluating delirious patients is given on p. 448.

If the disruption in behavior is reversible, it can be helpful to know the patient's usual lifestyle and level of functioning. A college professor is likely to have more highly developed cognitive skills than a laborer. A patient who is visited by numerous friends and relatives probably has different communication patterns than the person who is only visited by immediate family members. Knowledge of usual behavior serves as a

CHRONIC ORGANIC BRAIN SYNDROME FLOW SHEET*

If a majority of the following categories are marked "yes," the organic brain syndrome is probably chronic. *All or parts of these categories have changed insidiously.*

Yes	No	Behavior	Yes	No	Behavior
☐	☐	Memory impaired and immediate	☐	☐	Nocturnal restlessness
☐	☐	Difficulty in use of names and numbers	☐	☐	Disorientation to person, place, and time
☐	☐	Age greater than 70	☐	☐	Paranoia
☐	☐	Confabulation	☐	☐	Alert facade
☐	☐	Bowel or bladder incontinence	☐	☐	Decreased response to interviewer
☐	☐	Easily distracted			
☐	☐	Intellectual grasp reduced	☐	☐	Caution becomes suspiciousness
☐	☐	Rigidity of response	☐	☐	Compulsive orderliness
☐	☐	Wandering	☐	☐	Moodiness and depression
☐	☐	Confused by new places or situations	☐	☐	Poor judgment

*From Anderson, D.J.: Confusion in the elderly: a protocol to determine acute organic brain syndrome versus chronic organic brain syndrome. In Wolanin, M.O., and Phillips, L.R.F.: Confusion: prevention and care, St. Louis, 1981, The C.V. Mosby Co.

ACUTE ORGANIC BRAIN SYNDROME FLOW SHEET*

If a majority of the following categories are marked "yes," organic brain syndrome is probably acute (onset within 1 to 4 weeks). *All of these changes, or parts, occur rapidly.*

Yes	No	Behavior	Yes	No	Behavior
☐	☐	Fluctuating level of awareness	☐	☐	Delusional denial of illness
☐	☐	Recent medical, surgical, and neurological disease	☐	☐	Inappropriate sexual behavior
☐	☐	Recent change in alcohol/drug intake	☐	☐	Displacement, such as correct name and wrong address
☐	☐	Stupor progressing to delirium	☐	☐	Anxious when unable to find correct response
☐	☐	Visual hallucinations	☐	☐	Euphoria/blandness
☐	☐	Misidentification	☐	☐	Inappropriate joking
☐	☐	Great restlessness	☐	☐	Spatial inattention
☐	☐	Febrile, debilitating, or exhausting illness	☐	☐	Disorientation, but with ability to handle cognitive tasks
☐	☐	Dehydration	☐	☐	Paranoia/agitation
☐	☐	Delusional reduplication	☐	☐	Anxiety/depression
			☐	☐	Misnaming

*From Anderson, D.J.: Confusion in the elderly: a protocol to determine acute organic brain syndrome versus chronic organic brain syndrome. In Wolanin, M.O., and Phillips, L.R.F.: Confusion: prevention and care, St. Louis, 1981, The C.V. Mosby Co.

gauge against which to measure progress. Friends and family are good judges of when the patient is "back to normal." However, this should also be validated with the patient. He may have different self-expectations and may use his therapeutic experience to progress beyond his pretherapy level of functioning.

Colleagues are also helpful in evaluating the nursing care plan. They may have suggestions of alternative interventions. They may also provide the nurse with feedback about transference-countertransference issues that may be occurring outside of her awareness. For instance, a nurse who is working with an aging patient with dementia may respond to concerns about her own aging or that of her parents and have difficulty seeing the patient as a unique person. Hallucinating patients frequently arouse anxiety in the nurse, who may then be responding under the influence of her own defense mechanisms. Regular supervision can help the nurse to develop enhanced self-awareness and to assess when

a particularly anxiety-provoking situation has bothered her and why.

Suggested cross-references

Therapeutic relationship skills are discussed in Chapter 3. The health-illness model, including the phases of the nursing process and social support systems, is discussed in Chapter 4. Depression is discussed in Chapter 9. Substance abuse is discussed in Chapter 14. Psychological testing is discussed in Chapter 17. Behavior modification techniques are discussed in Chapter 21. Cognitive development of the child is discussed in Chapter 26. Gerontological psychiatric nursing is discussed in Chapter 31.

SUMMARY

1. Cognition is the ability to think and reason, including the processes of memory, judgment, orientation, perception, and attention.

2. Learning theorists have developed models of cognitive functioning, including the associationist model (Pavlov, Skinner, and Wolfe), the cognitive model (Tolman), and the computer model.

3. The developmental process of cognition was described by Piaget and is composed of three stages: the sensorimotor stage; the stage of preparation and organization of concrete operations, subdivided into the preoperational phase and the concrete operations phase; and the stage of formal operations.

4. Biological stressors, such as impaired delivery of nutrients to brain cells, metabolic disorders, exposure to toxic and infectious agents, tumors, trauma, and genetic abnormalities can cause cognitive impairment. In many instances the stressor cannot be identified.

5. Impairments in cognition are experienced by patients with the medical diagnoses of organic brain syndromes, including delirium and dementia.

6. Behaviors associated with delirium may include fluctuating levels of awareness, disorientation, disorganized thought processes, impaired judgment and decision making, illusions, visual hallucinations, affective lability, loss of inhibition, restlessness, agitation, diffuse EEG slowing, and behaviors directly attributable to the stressor.

7. Behaviors associated with dementia may include disorientation, memory loss, decreased attention span, labile affect, deteriorated social skills, impaired judg-

ment and decision making, restlessness and agitation, and resistance to change.

8. Psychological testing is an assessment tool provided on consultation by a clinical psychologist. Examples of common psychological tests were presented.

9. Coping mechanisms used by patients with impaired cognition may be exaggerations of past methods of coping with anxiety.

10. Examples of nursing diagnoses pertinent to impairments in cognition were presented and compared to the medical diagnostic criteria for delirium and dementia.

11. Nursing intervention with patients who have delirium includes life support, emotional support, and protection from impulsive behavior. Family members can provide valuable assistance.

12. Nursing intervention with patients who have dementia includes reality orientation, stimulation, encouragement of independent functioning, socialization, protection from accidental injury, maintenance of optimal biopsychosocial functioning, and encouragement of relatedness with significant others.

13. Evaluation of nursing care focuses on the appropriateness of the long- and short-term goals and the adequacy and effectiveness of the nursing interventions. Feedback can be obtained from the nurse's supervisor and colleagues, the nurse's self-assessment, the patient's significant others, and the patient. A flow sheet may be useful to record behavioral change over time.

References

1. American Psychiatric Association: Diagnostic and statistical manual of mental disorders, ed. 3, Washington, D.C., 1980, The Association.
2. Anderson, D.J.: Confusion in the elderly: a protocol to determine acute organic brain syndrome versus chronic organic brain syndrome. In Wolanin, M.O., and Phillips, L.R.F.: Confusion: prevention and care, St. Louis, 1981, The C.V. Mosby Co.
3. Bachrach, A.J.: Learning theory. In Kaplan, H.I., Freedman, A.M., and Sadock, B.J.: Comprehensive textbook of psychiatry, ed. 3, vol. 1, Baltimore, 1980, The Williams & Wilkins Co.
4. Bartol, M.A.: Nonverbal communication in patients with Alzheimer's disease, J. Gerontol. Nurs. **5:**21, July-Aug., 1979.
5. Davidhizar, R., Gunden, E., and Wehlage, D.: Recognizing and caring for the delirious patient, J. Psychiatr. Nurs. **16:**38, May 1978.
6. DeCato, C.M., and Wicks, R.J.: Psychological testing referrals: a guide for psychiatrists, psychiatric nurses, physicians in general practice and allied health personnel, J. Psychiatr. Nurs. **14:**24, June 1976.
7. Elkind, D.: Developmental structuralism of Jean Piaget. In Kaplan, H.S., Freedman, A.M., and Sadock, B.J.: Comprehensive textbook of psychiatry, ed. 3, vol. 1, Baltimore, 1980, The Williams & Wilkins Co.
8. Engelhardt, K.: Piaget: a prescriptive theory for parents, Maternal-Child Nurs. J. **3:**1, Spring 1974.
9. Hirschfeld, M.J.: The cognitively impaired older adult, Am. J. Nurs. **76:**1981, Dec. 1976.
10. Hogstel, M.O.: Use of reality orientation with aging confused patients, Nurs. Res. **28:**161, May-June 1979.
11. Jones, J.A.: Deprivation and existence or stimulation and life, J. Gerontol. Nurs. **2:**17, March-April 1976.
12. Lipowski, Z.J.: Organic mental disorders: introduction and review of syndromes. In Kaplan, H.I., Freedman, A.M., and Sadock, B.J.: Comprehensive textbook of psychiatry, ed. 3, vol. 2, Baltimore, 1980, The Williams & Wilkins Co.
13. Mulcahy, N., and Rosa, N.: Reality orientation in a general hospital, Geriatr. Nurs. **2:**264, 1981.
14. Mulder, D.W.: Organic brain syndromes associated with diseases of unknown cause. In Kaplan, H.I., Freedman, A.M., and Sadock, B.J., editors: Comprehensive textbook of psychiatry, ed. 3, vol. 2, Baltimore, 1980, The Williams & Wilkins Co.
15. Peer, S.M.: Therapeutic programs for the long-term care geriatric patient, J. Gerontol. Nurs. **2:**24, Jan.-Feb. 1976.
16. Piaget, J.: The child and reality: problems of genetic psychology, New York, 1973, Grossman Publishers.
17. Toffler, A.: Future shock, New York, 1970, Random House, Inc.
18. Voelkel, D.: A study of reality orientation and resocialization groups with the confused elderly, J. Gerontol. Nurs. **4:**13, May-June 1978.
19. Wolanin, M.O.: Physiologic aspects of confusion, J. Gerontol. Nurs. **7:**236, April 1981.
20. Wolanin, M.O., and Phillips, L.R.F.: Confusion: prevention and care, St. Louis, 1981, The C.V. Mosby Co.

Annotated suggested readings

Adams, M. et al.: Psychological responses in critical care units, Am. J. Nurs. **78:**1504, 1978.

These authors relate concepts of nursing care for confused patients to critical care areas. The article includes a good example of the use of the mental status examination.

Adams-Woodward, C.: Wernicke-Korsakoff syndrome: a case approach, J. Psychiatr. Nurs. **16:**38, April 1978.

This discussion of a cognitive impairment disorder that is related to thiamine deficiency uses a case study to illustrate the behaviors. There is also a discussion of the pathophysiological processes involved.

Bartol, M.A.: Nonverbal communication in patients with Alzheimer's disease, J. Gerontol. Nurs. **5:**21, July-Aug. 1979.

This author draws on her experience as a nurse working with a ward group of patients with Alzheimer's disease. She integrates communication theory as the rationale for nursing intervention, considering the nonverbal communication of the patient and the nurse. Descriptive case vignettes are used to clarify the theory.

Burnside, I.M.: Alzheimer's disease: an overview, J. Gerontol. Nurs. **5:**14, July-Aug. 1979.

This is a companion article to Bartol's discussion. It is a comprehensive overview of the assessment of the patient with Alzheimer's disease. Of particular interest is a glossary of terms describing behaviors associated with the disease.

Busse, E.W., and Pfeiffer, E.: Behavior and adaptation in late life, ed. 2, Boston, 1977, Little, Brown & Co.

A variety of experts in the field of gerontology have contributed to this book. The chapters on mental functioning are particularly recommended.

Butler, R.N., and Lewis, M.I.: Aging and mental health: positive psychosocial approaches, ed. 2, St. Louis, 1977, The C.V. Mosby Co.

The spectrum of problems inherent in aging is presented from a biopsychosocial framework. There is extensive information on the treatment of the aged in the community and in the institution. An excellent section on diagnostic evaluation is included.

Davidhizar, B., Gunden, E., and Wehlage, D.: Recognizing and caring for the delirious patient, J. Psychiatr. Nurs. **16:**38, May 1978.

These authors concisely present the prominent features associated with delirium. The emphasis is on nursing care in relation to the observable behaviors that are commonly seen in these patients.

DeCato, C.M., and Wicks, R.J.: Psychological testing referrals: a guide for psychiatrists, psychiatric nurses, physicians in general practice and allied health personnel, J. Psychiatr. Nurs. **14:**24, June 1976.

This article describes psychological evaluation, including descriptions of several tests and their purposes, and discusses reasons for psychological referral, when not to refer, and what to expect in a psychological testing report.

Langston, N.F.: Reality orientation and effective reinforcement, J. Gerontol. Nurs. **7:**224, April 1981.

This author identifies two aspects of reality orientation: a formal class providing specific information and 24-hour reality orientation using objects that are present in the environment. A helpful feature of the article is the comparison that is drawn between reality orientation and behavior modification.

Mulcahy, N., and Rosa, N.: Reality orientation in a general hospital, Geriatr. Nurs. **2:**264, 1981.

The authors describe a reality orientation program for confused patients that they introduced in a general hospital setting. They include an excellent example of a nursing care plan for use with a confused patient.

Trockman, G.: Caring for the confused or delirious patient, Am. J. Nurs. **78:**1495, 1978.

This article presents behaviors and nursing interventions relative to the delirious patient in a well-organized format. It should be particularly useful to the novice.

Wolanin, M.O.: Physiologic aspects of confusion, J. Gerontol. Nurs. **7:**236, April 1981.

This well-known authority in the field of geriatric nursing identifies the major physiological causes of confusion in the elderly. Nursing assessment is emphasized as a critical factor in determining the cause of confusion. Nursing interventions are described. The article is highly recommended for beginning students and nurses, including those in community settings who work with elderly individuals.

Wolanin, M.O., and Phillips, L.R.F.: Confusion: prevention and care, St. Louis, 1981, The C.V. Mosy Co.

This book is an effort to clarify and operationalize the concept of confusion. Understanding this concept is central to the provision of effective nursing care to individuals with cognitive impairment. There is an emphasis throughout the book on nursing interventions as applied to various aspects of confusion.

Sleepmonger,
deathmonger,
with capsules in my palms each night,
eight at a time from sweet pharmaceutical bottles
I make arrangements for a pint-sized journey.
I'm the queen of this condition.
I'm an expert on making the trip
and now they say I'm an addict.
Now they ask why.
Why!

Anne Sexton, The Addict*

*From "The Addict," in *Live or Die* by Anne Sexton. Copyright © 1966 by Anne Sexton. Reprinted by permission of Houghton Mifflin Company and The Sterling Lord Agency, Inc.

CHAPTER 14

SUBSTANCE
ABUSE

Learning objectives

After studying this chapter, the student should be able to:

- *define substance abuse.*

- *discuss the role of cultural attitudes in determining the definition of substance abuse.*

- *describe statistically the seriousness of the substance abuse problem.*

- *compare and contrast the major categories of abused substances.*

- *discuss the occurrence of substance abuse among members of the nursing and medical professions.*

- *analyze the problem of substance abuse as it relates to the stress response and the health-illness continuum.*

- *describe various hypotheses concerning the stressors that have been proposed as influencing the occurrence of substance abuse.*

- *compare and contrast the major categories of abused substances in terms of usual route of administration, expected behavioral responses, behaviors related to overdose, and withdrawal syndromes.*

- *formulate nursing diagnoses that incorporate the stage of substance abusing behavior, the substance abused, and the relevant stressors.*

- *assess the relationship between relevant nursing and medical diagnoses.*

- *identify realistic long- and short-term goals with substance abuse patients.*

- *analyze the biological components of intervention with the substance abuser.*

- *compare and contrast interactive approaches to nursing intervention with substance abuse patients.*

- *describe common themes in the therapy of substance abuse patients and appropriate nursing interventions.*

- *discuss social support systems that may be engaged to assist the substance abuse patient.*

- *apply principles with an appropriate rationale to planning the nursing care of substance abuse patients.*

- *identify five components of substance abuse prevention programs.*

- *list five questions that may be used to evaluate nursing intervention with the substance abuse patient.*

- *identify suggested readings for future study.*

Continuum of chemically mediated coping responses

The use of mind-altering substances is widespread in the world today. A statement such as this usually brings to mind the use of narcotics, hallucinogens, and, perhaps, alcohol. However, one should also consider prescription drugs and materials containing nicotine or caffeine. To add to the complexity of the issue, some people believe that any substance use should be defined as abuse, whereas others maintain that abuse only exists within the norms of the culture and has no objective basis. For the purposes of this discussion, substance abuse will be defined as the use of any mind-altering agent to such an extent that it interferes with the individual's biological, psychological, or sociocultural integrity.

Interference with biological integrity might be exemplified by the heavy smoker who develops emphysema, the anxious politician who becomes physically dependent on diazepam, or the alcoholic who is in delirium tremens. Psychological consequences of substance abuse could include the acute psychosis of a teenager who has been taking PCP or the inability of an office worker to feel able to function without a morning cup of coffee. Sociocultural effects are experienced by the high school student who is expelled from school following arrest for the possession of marijuana or by the young woman who prostitutes herself to make money to buy narcotics.

Volumes have been written about the various types of substance abuse and a great deal of research has been conducted. Still, definitive answers to questions about the origin and nature of these problems are yet to be found. Theories cover the gamut of conceptual models of psychology, psychiatry, sociology, and the other behavioral sciences. Some drugs, such as tobacco, alcohol, caffeine, and over-the-counter remedies are legal. Other drugs are illicit, including heroin, marijuana, cocaine, and hallucinogens. Others are legal only if obtained with a physician's prescription. The reason for these classifications is frequently unclear. Compounding the lack of clarity about the nature of substance abuse is a great deal of ambivalence present in society regarding acceptance or rejection of this behavior. This is perhaps best demonstrated by considering the issues that have arisen around the use of marijuana in the United States. There are those who believe very strongly that marijuana use is harmful to the individual and/or society and should be strictly prohibited by law. Others believe that marijuana is harmless and should be as freely available as tobacco and alcohol. Still others advocate little or no penalty for personal use of the drug but stiff penalties for its sale. Meanwhile, marijuana is widely used and in some settings, such as rock concerts, is used openly and generally ignored. However, it has been extremely difficult to obtain governmental approval for the medicinal use of marijuana, even though it has demonstrated effectiveness for problems such as the alleviation of the discomfort of people who are terminally ill with cancer and receiving chemotherapy. These various attitudes reflect the confused values that exist concerning the use of mind-altering substances.

In addition, abuse of substances is viewed differently, depending on the substance being abused, the person who is abusing it, and the setting in which abuse takes place. For instance, the upper middle class businessman who has several martinis at lunch and is therefore unable to accomplish much work in the afternoon is not necessarily thought of as a substance abuser. However, if his secretary kept a bottle of wine in her desk drawer and sipped it as she worked, she would probably be counseled to seek help for her alcoholism problem. Is there a real difference in the behavior of these two individuals? Tobacco abuse is so widely accepted in this country that there is serious debate about whether or not smokers have the right to inflict their habit on others even if it may cause them actual physical damage. Yet, a person who smoked opium would certainly be considered as deviant even if the behavior took place in private.

It is important for nurses to be aware of these cultural attitudes and to recognize their impact on the individual who abuses substances and on that person's significant others. Alcohol abuse may not be noticed because use of alcohol is generally acceptable. There is great stigma attached to alcohol abuse, thereby leading to reluctance on the part of the individual and the family to admit that there is a problem and seek help. Nurses must also take care that their own attitudes do not perpetuate the stigma and prevent them from providing help to the substance abuser. Self-awareness is especially critical when caring for these individuals. Substance abusers are very sensitive to the attitudes of others and may feel guilty because of their own basic acceptance of the culture's value system that has labeled their behavior as unacceptable. The nurse must be able to help them learn to accept themselves. This is difficult if the nurse is caught up in her own value judgments.

Substance abuse is one of this country's major public health problems. In fact, alcoholism may be the single most important health problem at the present time if one considers morbidity rather than mortality.[23] It has been estimated that 10% of adult men who drink and as many as 3% of adult women drinkers are abusers of alcohol.[7] About 7% of the adult population (over 18) of the United States, or approximately 9.3 to 10 million persons, are alcoholics.[7] Alcohol abuse among adolescents has been increasing. An estimated 3.3 million 14- to 17-year-olds are problem drinkers.[6] Alcohol abuse also affects people other than the drinker. Families of alcoholics experience increased stress and stress-related health problems as an indirect result of alcoholism. It has also been documented that alcohol is a factor in over 50% of traffic accidents, causing more than 28,000 fatalities per year.[6] Citizen pressure in several states to legislate stiffer penalties for driving under the influence of alcohol has been increasing recently.

Opiate use is much less widespread than alcohol use, but is still a serious problem. In 1978, 1.6% of high school seniors had used heroin at some time, and 9.9% had used other opiates, excluding those prescribed by a physician. This figure had decreased very slightly from that of a year earlier.[18] Opiate use is more prevalent in urban areas, among males and minority groups, although there has been a slight increase recently in use by white middle class adolescents and young adults.[9] Estimates of the total number of heroin users in the United States range from 1 to 3 million.[9] Accurate figures are difficult to determine because users can only be identified when they come to the attention of the legal or health care systems.

Opiate abuse is of great concern because it leads to severely deteriorated functioning on the part of the individual and frequently to criminal activity to raise money for purchasing drugs.

Another type of substance abuse that is of great concern is the habitual use of prescription medications, including sedatives and hypnotics, stimulants, and antianxiety agents. This problem frequently has an insidious pattern of onset. An individual may receive a prescription, like the feeling that the drug gives, and gradually take more pills at a time or take them more frequently. Next to alcohol, diazepam is probably the most frequently abused drug. Yet it is generally viewed as a relatively harmless substance and is freely prescribed for people who are anxious about problems of living. Categories of prescription drugs that are frequently abused include narcotics, barbiturates, amphetamines, benzodiazepines, meprobamate, methaqualone, and occasionally tricyclic antidepressants, particularly amitriptyline. Control of these drugs is difficult because of the many legitimate medical uses for them. There have been efforts to ban production of amphetamines based on the belief that medical uses of these drugs can be accomplished with other less dangerous medications, but so far, they remain on the market. Most of these substances have been placed under some degree of control by the Food and Drug Administration of the federal government, but the black market thrives. In addition, abuse is difficult to control because patients quickly learn that they can obtain prescriptions from several physicians and have them filled at different pharmacies, thus acquiring a large supply of drugs. Multiple addiction to prescription drugs in combination with each other and/or alcohol is becoming more prevalent.

Among the groups with the highest incidence of abuse of alcohol and of prescription drugs are physicians and nurses. The narcotic addiction rate for physicians is estimated to be between 1% and 2%. This is contrasted to the national rate for the total population of 0.3%.[9] The National Institute on Alcoholism estimates that 18% of physicians are alcoholics, compared to 10% of the general population.[15] It has been estimated that 40,000 nurses are alcoholics.[16] Known rates of substance abuse by nurses are probably artificially low. This is partially because the problem is hidden by the abuser. However, colleagues often work as enablers and fail to confront the nurse who has the problem. Whether this is due to the individual's ambivalence about substance abuse or the result of a misguided attempt to protect the addicted nurse, it is unfortunate, because it jeopardizes the well-being of the nurse and the safety of the patients for whom she is providing care. It is the absolute responsibility of any nurse to take whatever steps are necessary to intervene when a co-worker is practicing under the influence of alcohol or drugs. In recognition of the severity of this problem, in a few states, such as Maryland and Ohio, state nurses' associations have established peer-assistance groups to work with addicted nurses. These groups are comprised of volunteer nurses, many of whom are recovered addicts. They offer support and referral services to addicted nurses. This helps them to avoid loss of licensure and ultimately assists them to return to work as effective and safe practitioners. At a national level, the Division of Psychiatric and Mental Health Nursing Practice of the American Nurses' Association has also begun to study this serious problem.

Since the early 1960s, another group of substances has been abused, particularly by adolescents and young adults. These substances induce a state similar to psychosis. They include hallucinogens, the most common of which has been LSD. Another substance that is unrelated to LSD, but also leads to an altered state of awareness is PCP. Other drugs included in this psychotomimetic group are tetrahydrocannabinol (THC), which is the active ingredient of marijuana, mescaline, psilocybin, and peyote. Discussion in this chapter will be limited to LSD and PCP, since they are most likely to be encountered by the nurse. In 1978, about 14% of high school seniors had used a hallucinogen at some time, and 10% had used at least one during the last year.[18] Use of these drugs is of concern to society because of the erratic and unpredictable behavior they produce. They are not generally addictive, but are inexpensive to produce and widely available. They may also be substi-

tuted by the seller for other more expensive drugs, thus making it difficult to determine exactly what the individual has taken.

The drug that is currently most popular and the use of which has the highest status in the United States is cocaine. According to a cover story in *Time Magazine*,[5] conservative estimates of cocaine use in the United States were that 10 million people are regular users, and another 5 million have experimented with the drug. Although classified as a narcotic, cocaine is really a stimulant, more similar in effect to the amphetamines than to the opiates. Habitual use can lead to deteriorated functioning, although users claim that they perform better under the influence of cocaine. It tends to be readily available in most cities, and its use continues to rise.

Marijuana use in the United States is pervasive. Although it is still illegal, marijuana is widely available and in some settings its use is acceptable and even expected. According to a study sponsored by the National Institute on Drug Abuse (NIDA), in 1978, 59.2% of high school seniors had used marijuana or its stronger derivative, hashish, at least once. Twenty-eight percent reported that they used it at least once a week. These figures reveal an upward trend in the percentage of marijuana users in the high school population.[18] When marijuana use began to proliferate in the 1960s, the majority of users were young. However, 15 to 20 years later, many of these people still use marijuana and are now beginning to struggle with the issue of how to advise their own children on the use of drugs. One serious concern about marijuana use is that it does seem to serve as a transition to the use of more harmful drugs. Most users of marijuana do not become heroin addicts. However, it is rare for a person who has never used marijuana to use opiates, hallucinogens, or cocaine.

A serious and increasing problem related to substance abuse is the rapidly increasing occurrence of the simultaneous or sequential use of more than one substance. For instance, barbiturates and amphetamines may be used alternately to achieve relaxation and then stimulation. Cocaine use is sometimes followed by heroin to moderate the stimulant effect. Such experimentation can be dangerous, particularly if synergistic drugs, such as barbiturates and alcohol, are used. It also complicates assessment of and intervention in substance abuse, since the

FIG. 14-1
Continuum of chemically mediated coping responses.

individual may be experiencing withdrawal from several drugs at the same time.

Some relate the high prevalence of substance use and abuse to the need to blunt or escape from the anxiety created by the stresses of life. It is interesting to note that there have been efforts to find means of achieving a "natural high" as an alternative to the use of chemicals to achieve euphoria or relaxation. Advocates of meditation, yoga, and self-hypnosis claim that they are able to find peace from within themselves. There has been an upsurge of interest in Eastern religions, which frequently teach followers to achieve states of altered awareness. Others have found that they can relieve tension through physical activity. Joggers report the occurrence of a "runner's high." Neurochemical research has begun to reveal possible biological explanations for these experiences. Snyder[24] has reported on the discovery of enkephalins and endorphins. These naturally occurring peptides bind with opiate receptors in the brain and pituitary gland. They have been described as natural opiates. It is hypothesized that experiences which result in a feeling of euphoria stimulate the release of these neurochemicals. Research in this area has great promise for increasing understanding of and the potential for treatment of the addictive phenomena.

An individual may achieve a state of relaxation, euphoria, stimulation, or altered awareness by a number of means. The range of these activities is illustrated in Fig. 14-1.

Stressors

The use or abuse of substances is often viewed as a way to shield the individual from the stressful events of life. Unfortunately, this attitude can lead rapidly to a spiral in which stress occurs, the substance is used, the effects wear off, more stress occurs, more substance is used, and so on. Eventually, the use of the substance becomes an additional stressor because of interference with the person's biopsychosocial functioning.

Biological factors

Stressors related to substance abuse may be biological, psychological, or sociocultural, but are most frequently a combination. Biological stressors may include a familial tendency for substance abuse. This has been observed in the case of alcoholism. This problem tends to run in families and also tends to occur in families that have a concurrent high incidence of manic-depressive illness. About half of the children of alcoholics become alcoholics even though many are repelled by parental behavior while drinking. This is also suggestive of an inherited tendency for alcoholism. Another theory that has been proposed as a cause for alcoholism is that it is an allergic response to alcohol. This is an attempt to explain the fact that some people can control drinking behavior and others cannot. However, the only truly allergic response to alcohol that has been documented is an aversive one. A high percentage of Oriental people in particular have a physiological response to alcohol that includes flushing, tachycardia, and an intense feeling of discomfort.[11] This has been used to explain the low rate of alcoholism among people of Oriental descent.

Psychological factors

A number of psychological theories have been proposed to explain substance abuse. For in-

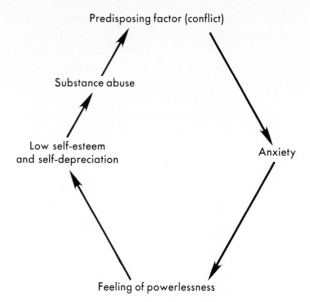

FIG. 14-2
The cycle of substance abuse. (Modified from Gold, S.R.: The CAP control theory of drug abuse. In Lettieri, D.J., Sayers, M., and Pearson, H.W., editors: Theories on drug abuse: selected contemporary perspectives, NIDA Research Monograph 30, Rockville, Md., 1980, National Institute on Drug Abuse.)

stance, it has been hypothesized that the person who comes to depend on drugs (including alcohol and tobacco)* is dependent and unable to rely on his own resources for gratification. Freudian psychoanalytical theory describes the oral-dependent personality type. This person is fixated at the oral stage of development and seeks need satisfaction through oral behaviors, including smoking or the ingestion of various substances. A related theory emphasizes the low self-esteem of the substance abuser. Gold[10] has described a cycle of behavior that is illustrated in Fig. 14-2. Substance use is reinforced because it gives the individual a sense of power regarding the area of conflict, thus reducing anxiety. Unfortunately, the substance using activity itself may create a new source of conflict and contribute to the individual's low self-esteem if guilt or fear of discovery are associated with the behavior. Eventually, the substance abuse itself perpetuates the need to continue taking the drug.

Substance abuse frequently arises during adolescence. Insecurity related to a poorly developed sense of identity may cause the young person to take drugs. In addition, adolescents are engaged in a conflict between the need to remain dependent on their parents and the need to assert their own independence. This conflict can erupt into rebellious behavior. The use or abuse of various drugs may be an expression of adolescent rebellion that is often reinforced by peer group approval.

The pleasure principle has been proposed as another explanation for substance abusing behavior. This theory suggests that organisms are motivated to seek pleasure and to avoid pain. The use of drugs induces a pleasurable state and reduces the experience of physical or psychological pain. Since the pain returns when the effect of the drug wears off, the individual is powerfully attracted to repeated drug use. This aspect of drug use is reflected in the use of the term "high" to describe the drug experience. A related factor is the described oversensitivity of substance abusers, suggesting that they might be particularly susceptible to the euphoria-inducing effects of drugs. Wurmser[27] has even described a relationship between various types of emotional pain and the type of drug that is abused. He states that narcotics and hypnotics combat rage, shame, and jealousy; stimulants alleviate depression and weakness; psychedelics ease boredom and disillusionment; and alcohol intervenes in guilt and loneliness. Some also relate the use of drugs to a mystical experience and claim that there is a drive to experience altered states of consciousness that is expressed through the use of drugs.[12] This is an existential approach to drug abuse and theorizes that drug use can lead to a spiritual experience which is achieved by most people without the use of drugs.

Family traits that predispose the individual to drug abuse have been identified. Chein[4] has described a family that is too overwhelmed to treat children as persons, lacks a male role model, has no stability, distrusts society, and has no expectations of the child. Stanton[25] reports a higher than average number of deaths in the families of drug abusers. The usual family interaction picture is that of overinvolvement of the opposite-sex parent while the same-sex parent is "punitive, distant and/or absent."[25] The following characteristics are described as distinguishing the families of drug abusers from those with other types of disrupted behavior[25]:

1. A history of multigenerational addictive

---

*The term "drug" will be used to refer to all abused substances, including alcohol, nicotine, and caffeine. Specific agents will be referred to by name or category when appropriate.

behaviors, including nonsubstance-related activities, such as gambling and television watching

2. More primitive and direct expression of conflict
3. Absence of schizophrenic behavior in parents
4. An illusion of independence of the drug abuser through peer group membership
5. Higher level of maternal symbiosis
6. The presence of death themes and untimely deaths
7. Immigrant parents, possibly resulting in cultural disparity between parents and children.

Sociocultural factors

Sociocultural stressors are also generally present when substance abuse occurs. The complexity and tension of modern life often causes individuals to seek avenues of escape. Drugs are readily available and provide a tempting respite from pressure. The legal drugs, alcohol, caffeine, nicotine, and over-the-counter drugs, are readily available and are socially approved tension-reduction agents. Advertising bombards the average person with information on the relaxing properties of a variety of drugs. Even many illicit drugs are easily obtainable by those who are familiar with the drug culture. Marijuana and cocaine are frequently available at the social gatherings of all socioeconomic classes. Miller and Cisin[19] point out that illicit drugs are not usually sought by beginning users, but are offered by others. Ausubel[2] has identified ease of access as the primary precipitating factor for drug abuse. A related predisposing factor is acceptance of drug use by the relevant sociocultural group.

Group influence and peer pressure frequently induce people to experiment with drugs. This is a particularly important factor for adolescents who are developmentally in a stage of concern about peer group acceptance. Peer influence is also reflected in the fact that fashions in drug use change as do fads in other areas. At the present, alcohol use is increasing among young people, as use of hallucinogens decreases. Cocaine is popular with older drug users as well as with the young, and its prevalence is increasing rapidly.

Failure to assimilate a value system that op-

poses drug use is also a stressor. The ambivalence of society in general about the use or abuse of various substances is perceived by the young and may be interpreted as permissiveness. Children of parents who use drugs, including alcohol and tobacco, grow up with attitudes of acceptance toward this behavior. It has been observed that members of religious groups with strong sanctions against the use of alcohol have much lower rates of alcohol use and alcoholism than members of religions that accept or encourage the use of alcohol. Cultural factors also play a role in alcohol use patterns. It has been found that Northern Europeans have higher alcoholism rates than those from Southern Europe. Of the major religious groups in the United States, Roman Catholics have the highest rate of alcoholism and Jews the lowest.

There are also sexual differences in the incidence of substance abuse. More men than women are abusers of alcohol and opiates. More women than men abuse prescription drugs such as diazepam. It must be noted, however, that the incidence of alcohol abuse by women may be higher than has been believed. Cultural attitudes toward drinking behavior differ for men and women. There is much less acceptance of female alcoholism. Therefore it is often hidden, and women tend to deny that they have a problem even longer than men do. Whereas the ability to drink large amounts is considered to be *macho* behavior for men, use of antianxiety drugs is viewed as weak and unmasculine. The latter behavior is acceptable for and even sometimes expected of women.

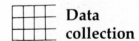 **Data collection**

Behaviors associated with alcoholism

For the purpose of this discussion, the alcoholic will be defined as any person whose drinking behavior interferes with his ability to carry out his usual daily activities and/or adversely affects his interpersonal relationships. This encompasses the person who indulges in episodic excessive drinking as well as the one who is addicted to alcohol. Excessive alcohol use can result in both physical and psychological dependency. *Physical dependence* occurs when there is a biological need in the body for the abused substance. If the substance is not supplied, physical withdrawal symptoms result. *Psychological dependence* is the craving for the subjective effect of the substance on the user. The

TABLE 14-1. Comparison of blood alcohol concentrations to behavioral manifestations of intoxication*

Blood alcohol level	Behaviors
Up to 0.1% (100 mg/100 ml)	Loud speech, decreased inhibitions, silliness
0.1% to 0.2%	Slurred speech, moodiness, unsteady gait, decreased coordination shortened attention span, impaired memory
0.2% to 0.3%	Ataxia, tremor, irritability, stupor
0.3%	Unconsciousness

*Modified from Butz, R.H.: Intoxication and withdrawal. In Estes, N.J., and Heinemann, M.E.: Alcoholism: development, consequences, and interventions, St. Louis, 1977, The C.V. Mosby Co.

onset of alcoholism is often insidious. Many heavy drinkers fantasize that they are able to control their behavior when in reality they are addicted.

Several behaviors have been identified that are warning signs of impending alcoholism. These include sneaking drinks, morning drinking, blackouts, binge drinking, arguments about drinking, missing time at work, and an alcohol-related police record. The development of tolerance, so that more and more alcohol can be consumed without causing intoxication, is also a sign that alcoholism has developed. Intoxication has been defined as a blood alcohol level of 0.1% or more. Table 14-1 compares blood alcohol levels and behaviors.

Seixas[22] has identified several other behaviors that are indicative of progressive alcoholism. One is an increased incidence of suicide in alcoholics. This may also be related to the losses that alcoholics usually experience. In other cases, people who are already depressed may begin to drink as an attempt at coping and may then become alcoholics. Since drinking usually reinforces depressed feelings, suicide may result. A second behavior is increased incidence of accidental injury to alcoholics. For example, about 50% of fatal automobile accidents are related to alcohol use.

Physically, there are a number of behaviors that are frequently related to alcoholism. Since the liver detoxifies alcohol, excessive ingestion eventually results in impaired liver functioning. Fatty liver, hepatitis, and cirrhosis of the liver are frequently complications of alcohol abuse. Other problems include esophagitis, gastritis, pancreatitis, cardiomyopathy, pulmonary function changes, myopathy, osteoporosis, various anemias, disruptions of the immune system, peripheral neuropathy, and brain damage.[22] It is obvious that hardly any organ escapes adverse effects in the alcoholic.

Psychologically, the alcoholic may be depressed, hostile, and suspicious or exhibit many other painful emotions. Specific behaviors related to these types of disruptions may be observed. It is often debatable how much of the emotional response precedes and how much follows the development of alcoholism. Alcoholics are usually reluctant to confront or even admit to their problems. They may behave very dependently toward significant others and health care givers, expecting to be shielded from stress and using any conflict to justify drinking. An alcoholic patient once explained her drinking episode by saying, "It was Christmas Eve and I knew everybody in the world was drinking, so why shouldn't I?" Another person said, "If I stub my toe, it's a good enough reason to drink." This combination of dependency and rationalization can be difficult for significant others and often contributes to the breakdown of interpersonal relationships.

Socially, alcoholics may be inhibited people. Alcohol reduces the inhibitions enough to make them able to relate more comfortably to others. However, these relationships tend to be transient and superficial. The intoxicated person may also exhibit poor judgment in his selection of companions, making himself vulnerable to mugging and other forms of victimization.

Clinical example 14-1 illustrates many of the behaviors described. This person has the medical diagnosis of alcohol dependence and alcohol withdrawal delirium.

CLINICAL EXAMPLE 14-1

Mr. H was admitted to the detoxification center of a large metropolitan hospital in acute alcohol withdrawal. He was delirious and having visual hallucinations of bugs crawling on his body. He was extremely frightened, thrashing around in bed and mumbling incoherently. Since he had a long and well-documented history of alcohol abuse, family members were contacted and confirmed that he had recently stopped drinking after a 2-week binge.

The patient had been a successful lawyer with a large practice. He specialized in corporate law and conducted much business over lunch or dinner. He also kept a well-stocked bar in his office to offer clients a drink. Without his really being aware of it, Mr. H's drinking gradually increased. After a few years he was drinking almost nonstop from lunchtime to bedtime. He then began to have a Bloody Mary with breakfast "just to get myself going."

His wife reported that he had become irritable, particularly if she questioned his drinking. On two occasions he had hit her during their arguments. She was seriously considering divorce. He had also become alienated from his children, who appeared frightened of him. Infrequently he would feel guilty about his neglect of his family and plan a special outing. Most of the time he was too drunk to carry out his plans. The family had also become less involved in activities with friends. Mrs. H and the children felt embarrassed about his behavior and so did not invite anyone to their home. On two occasions, Mr. H had tried to stop drinking. The first time he went to a private hospital, where he was detoxified and remained abstinent for about a month after discharge. He then lost an important case and decided to have "just one drink" to carry him through the crisis. Soon his drinking was again out of control. His second hospitalization was at a general hospital with an active alcoholism rehabilitation program. He was introduced to Alcoholics Anonymous and started taking disulfiram (Antabuse). This program worked until he decided that he could manage without medication. A couple of weeks later his co-workers persuaded him to "help celebrate" at an office party. This was the start of a binge that ended when he had an automobile accident on the way home from a bar. A passenger in the other car was killed and Mr. H was charged with vehicular homicide and driving under the influence of alcohol. He stopped drinking abruptly, which resulted in his current hospital admission 3 days later.

Alcohol withdrawal begins shortly after drinking has ended and lasts 5 to 7 days. It is characterized by a number of behaviors, some of which are dangerous. According to Butz,[3] the earliest and commonest behaviors are "anxiety, anorexia, insomnia, and tremor." In addition, there is hyperalertness and a feeling "often described as internal shaking." There may be a mild disorientation, which usually lasts a short time. If it persists, it may be a sign of impending delirium. Tachycardia (120 to 140 beats per minute) continues throughout withdrawal and may be used to monitor the patient's condition. Alcoholic hallucinosis is another withdrawal syndrome and is characterized by auditory hallucinations in a patient who has no other psychotic behavior. This condition generally lasts for just a few hours or days, although in rare instances, it becomes chronic.[1] These hallucinations may be distinguished from those of alcohol withdrawal delirium because they are auditory, whereas the latter are usually visual.

Delirium tremens, now called alcohol withdrawal delirium, is a very serious withdrawal syndrome also described by Butz.[3] Behaviors associated with it include "marked tremor, anxiety, insomnia, anorexia, paranoia, and disorientation." Frequently these patients have episodes of uncontrolled behavior. Delusions and visual hallucinations often occur. Other behaviors may include elevated temperature, tachycardia, tachypnea, hyperpnea, vomiting, diarrhea, and diaphoresis. Occasionally, delirium tremens may lead to death. Alcohol withdrawal delirium usually occurs on the second or third day after the last drink has been taken. It rarely occurs more than a week later. The episode is usually over within 48 to 72 hours after onset.[1]

Another serious behavioral manifestation of alcohol withdrawal is grand mal convulsions, sometimes called "rum fits." Other causes of seizure activity should be explored, including trauma and the use of other drugs. There is generally not any long-term problem related to these seizures.[3] Further information on alcohol withdrawal syndromes may be found in the suggested readings at the end of this chapter.

Alcoholics frequently are malnourished and have vitamin deficiencies. Shortage of the B vitamins contribute to the occurrence of peripheral neuropathies. Thiamine deficiency may result in the development of alcoholic amnestic syndrome,[1] also referred to as Korsakoff's disease. Individuals with this problem exhibit severe problems with memory. It frequently occurs following an episode of Wernicke's encephalopathy, which is manifested by neurological disturbances, such as confusion, ataxia, and abnormal eye movements. Wernicke's encephalopathy may be treated successfully with large doses of thiamine, but if it progresses to alcoholic amnestic syndrome, the prognosis for reversal of the memory loss is poor.[1]

Behaviors associated with drug abuse

Drug abuse refers to the use of any mind-altering substance (except alcohol, which has been considered separately) except as prescribed by a physician. Categories of drugs that are commonly abused include narcotics, stimulants, depressants, antianxiety agents, and hallucinogens.

All the drugs mentioned except the hallucinogens can be addictive. Drug addiction may involve physical dependency, psychological dependency, or both. The combination of these two factors is a powerful incentive to continue using drugs. It should also be remembered that many drugs abusers are simultaneously addicted to more than one substance.

OPIATE ABUSE. The opiates include opium, heroin, meperidine, morphine, codeine, and methadone. The first two drugs were used for medical and, in the case of opium, religious and recreational purposes in the past, but are generally no longer used. Meperidine, morphine, and codeine are frequently used analgesics that are found in any hospital medicine room. Methadone is a narcotic substance that is used as a treatment for addiction to other opiates, either to facilitate withdrawal or at a stable dose for maintenance purposes. Its usefulness lies in the fact that it does not interfere with the ability to function productively as other narcotics do. Individuals who are on a methadone maintenance regimen may work and carry on a normal life, although still addicted to narcotics. Opiates may be introduced into the body by ingestion; inhalation; smoking; or intravenous, intramuscular, or subcutaneous injection.

Narcotics addiction is a great social problem. People who are addicted to opiates generally deteriorate mentally and physically to the point that they are unable to function productively. Illegal behavior may be related to addiction as one steals or prostitutes oneself to acquire money for drugs. The obtaining and use of drugs becomes an all-consuming passion. Behaviors associated with addiction to narcotics include the development of *tolerance*. Tolerance refers to the increasing need for more and more of the drug to create the same effect. This, of course, also increases the expense of the habit. Physiological effects of narcotics include decreased response to pain, respiratory depression, nausea, constriction of pupils, drowsiness, decreased response of the hypothalamus to external input, depressed pituitary functioning, decreased secretion of digestive juices, slower peristalsis, and constipation caused by increased intestinal absorption of water.[20] Psychological responses to opiate use include most importantly a sense of euphoria, referred to as feeling "high." It is this powerful pleasurable response that causes the individual to use the drug repeatedly, ultimately leading to addiction. Other psychological effects of narcotics include apathy, detachment from reality, and impaired judgment. The phrase "nodding out" is used to describe this complex of behaviors in combination with drowsiness. Clinical example 14-2 will demonstrate the behaviors associated with opiate abuse.

CLINICAL EXAMPLE 14-2

Mr. C was a 35-year-old black man who had been jailed for auto theft. He was believed to be a member of a large ring of automobile thieves in a major metropolitan area. His previous arrest record included several episodes of armed robbery and breaking and entering. A few hours after he had been jailed, Mr. C complained of abdominal cramps and appeared very anxious. His nose and eyes were running, there were beads of perspiration on his brow, and he was rocking back and forth on his bunk. The guard called Ms. V, the correctional health nurse.

Ms. V observed Mr. C and performed a brief physical assessment. She noted that his pupils were dilated, his blood pressure was elevated, and he had "gooseflesh." In addition, there were multiple needle "tracks" on his arms. She asked him directly about drug use and he admitted that he had been addicted to heroin. He stated that his addiction began in 1967 while he was stationed with the army in Viet Nam. When he returned to the United States, he remained in the army for 18 months and was able to stop using drugs altogether. He planned to get a job and attend school after leaving the service. He related that he was disturbed by the attitude of people toward Viet Nam veterans. While he was still in the service, he was able to use peer support to cope with his feelings. However, after his discharge, he was reluctant to talk about his military experience. Others seemed disinterested, embarrassed, or hostile when he talked about it.

Mr. C had difficulty finding a civilian job. He was an artillery specialist in the army and found that it was difficult to apply this experience. He began to have nightmares and "flashbacks" of his combat experiences. Because of the anxiety associated with this, he finally returned to drugs. Without a job, he used illegal means to finance his habit and therefore repeatedly went to jail.

Ms. V discussed Mr. C's problem with the physician in the prison health department. They decided to assess Mr. C's eligibility for a methadone drug treatment program and to request consultation from a counselor at the local Viet Nam veterans counseling center. He was given the medical diagnoses of opioid dependence, opioid withdrawal, and posttraumatic stress disorder.

Withdrawal from narcotics is extremely uncomfortable, but not usually life threatening. It may be accomplished with the aid of methadone, which can be substituted for heroin or other opiates and then gradually decreased if total withdrawal is desired. When withdrawal is not mediated by the use of drugs, behaviors may include initially anxiety, yawning, diaphoresis, abdominal cramps, lacrimation, and rhinorrhea. These are followed by mydriasis, piloerection, achiness, muscular twitching, and anorexia, and later by insomnia, hypertension, elevated temperature, increased rate and depth of respirations, restlessness, nausea, vomiting, diarrhea, spontaneous ejaculation or orgasm, and blood chemistry alterations, including hemoconcentration, leukocytosis, eosinopenia, and hyperglycemia. Overdosage of narcotics can lead rapidly to coma, respiratory depression, and death. Accidental overdoses among narcotics addicts are not uncommon, particularly if the user is uncertain of the strength of the drug being used. Drugs are usually cut with inert substances before they are sold, thus resulting in the availability of varied strengths on the streets.

BARBITURATE ABUSE. The use of barbiturates results in a psychological experience that is very similar to that induced by alcohol. Barbiturate drugs include barbital, amobarbital (Amytal), phenobarbital, pentobarbital (Nembutal), secobarbital (Seconal), and butabarbital. These drugs are widely prescribed for their sedative and hypnotic properties. Like alcohol, they are basically depressants, but induce an initial response of euphoria. It is for this reason that barbiturates are popular street drugs. They do lead to both physical and psychological dependence. Behaviors that result from intake of barbiturates include euphoria followed by depression and sometimes hostility. Inhibitions are decreased and judgment may be impaired. There is a lack of coordination and slurring of speech. The person may become quite drowsy, depending on the size of the dose taken and the individual's level of tolerance. Barbiturates are generally swallowed or injected. Tolerance occurs, resulting in the use of increasing amounts to achieve the desired effect. Because of the similarities in their actions, the use of barbiturates with alcohol is dangerous and may lead to accidental overdose.

Withdrawal from barbiturates, can be dangerous and therefore is frequently conducted in the hospital. Withdrawal symptoms from barbiturates include postural hypotension accompanied by tachycardia, elevated temperature, insomnia, tremors, and agitation. If barbiturates are withdrawn abruptly, behaviors include apprehension, weakness, tremors, postural hypotension, twitching, anorexia, grand mal seizures, and psychosis.

**STIMULANT ABUSE: AMPHETAMINES AND CO-
CAINE.** Stimulant use has been increasing rapidly in recent years. The alertness and feeling of extra energy that are the results of taking these drugs have resulted in widespread use. Caffeine is the most pervasive stimulant in current use. It is found in coffee, tea, chocolate, and many soft drinks. The wide acceptance of caffeine use may make the use of other stimulants seem more acceptable. The amphetamines are prescribed medically for the treatment of obesity and, rarely, narcolepsy. They are also given to hyperactive children because of a paradoxical calming effect. As other treatments for these conditions have been found, serious questions have been raised about whether there is any legitimate medical use for amphetamines, and serious consideration has been given to placing a ban on their production. Illicit users of these drugs include truck drivers on long trips; students who are cramming for examinations; and people, such as nurses, who work night shifts.

Addiction to barbiturates and stimulants, particularly the amphetamines, frequently occurs simultaneously. Sometimes, a patient who has been using "downers" finds he needs "uppers" to give him enough energy to function. Clinical example 14-3 illustrates this pattern.

CLINICAL EXAMPLE 14-3

Ms. W was a 34-year-old woman who was moderately overweight. She had tried various diets on her own with little success. A friend told her about a "diet doctor" who had a reputation for helping his patients lose weight with minimal deprivation from eating their usual diet. Ms. W decided to see the physician and was accepted for treatment. She was given a diuretic and appetite depressant medication. The latter contained amphetamines. She began to lose weight as soon as she started the prescribed regimen and was delighted. She also liked the additional burst of energy she felt every time she took her medication. She completed projects that she had been planning to work on for months. However, her family began to complain because she was irritable and very restless. In addition, she developed insomnia and roamed about the house at night.

On the urging of her husband, she went to her family physician. She felt guilty about seeing another physician for her weight problem, so neglected to tell her regular physician about this. With the history of insomnia, irritability, and recent weight loss, her physician thought she might be depressed; so he ordered an antipressant medication and a barbiturate sedative. Ms. W soon found that she was able to sleep well with her sedative. However, she felt slightly hung over in the morning and still wanted to lose more weight, so she continued with her diet pills as well. For a while she was able to function well. Gradually, however, she found that she needed two sedatives and then she also began to use extra stimulants. Her husband questioned her drug use. Ms. W had read about drug abuse and with her husband's help identified that she had a problem. She decided to see her family physician again and this time told him the whole story. He then advised a brief hospitalization so she could be withdrawn from both drugs under medical supervision. Ms. W was very embarrassed by her addiction. While in the hospital, she needed a great deal of nursing support to integrate this experience. The medical diagnoses that were applied to Ms. W included amphetamine dependence, amphetamine withdrawal, barbiturate dependence, and barbiturate withdrawal.[1]

Ms. W's pattern is not uncommon. Aside from street use, many people slip into drug abuse without being aware of the consequences of their behavior.

The amphetamine drugs include amphetamine, methamphetamine, dextroamphetamine, and benzphetamine. The effects of amphetamine use include euphoria, hyperactivity, irritability, hyperalertness, insomnia, anorexia, weight loss, tachycardia, and hypertension. It is not generally believed that these drugs cause physical dependence, but they do cause psychological dependence and tolerance occurs. Prolonged or excessive use may result in psychotic behavior. Withdrawal of the drugs usually results in a "crash," manifested by depression and lack of energy. This discomfort provides motivation to take more drugs.

Cocaine is a stimulant drug that is also becoming a symbol of sophistication. It is fashionable to inhale (snort) cocaine through rolled up $100 bills. Those who want a more intense experience may smoke the drug after processing it chemically. This process is called "freebasing." Use of cocaine has been glamorized by the publicity given to its use by movie stars, sports figures, and other well-known people. This makes it particularly inviting to adolescents who use famous people as role models. Historically, cocaine use was advocated for a time by Sigmund Freud. He later became disenchanted with it. The drug

was also a part of the life-style of Sherlock Holmes as created by Sir Arthur Conan Doyle.

Cocaine is relatively short acting, with its effects lasting 20 to 30 minutes when it has been inhaled. The experience is very similar to that induced by the amphetamines. A cocaine high is also usually followed by a crash, leading to repeated use. The most serious long-term effect of cocaine that has been identified so far is deterioration of the mucous membrane of the nose, eventually resulting in destruction of the nasal septum. Cocaine use does not seem to result in physical dependence.

ABUSE OF HALLUCINOGENS AND PCP. One behavior that became representative of the "dropout" generation of the 1960s was the use of drugs that create experiences very similar to those which are typical of a psychotic state. These substances have been called hallucinogens, psychedelics, and psychotomimetics. LSD is representative of the hallucinogenic drugs. PCP use results in behaviors that are similar in many respects to those produced by hallucinogens. Because of the entirely different chemical structures, it is important to be able to compare and contrast these drugs.

LSD is generally swallowed. It is colorless and tasteless and is therefore often added to a drink or food, such as a sugar cube. It may also be given to a person without his being aware that he has taken a drug. Pleasurable effects of hallucinogen use include intensification of sensory experiences, with colors described as more brilliant, and sounds, smells, and tastes are heightened. Sometimes users of these drugs will report synesthesia, or a crossover of sensory experiences during which music may be seen or colors may be heard. Space and time become distorted.

The hallucinogens have not demonstrated addictive properties. They do, however, lead to self-destructive behavior because of the impairment of judgment that results from their use. LSD, peyote, mescaline, and psilocybin are commonly used hallucinogens. Vulnerable individuals who take these drugs may experience "bad trips," which may deteriorate into psychotic episodes. The patient may experience paranoid, grandiose, or somatic delusions, usually accompanied by vivid hallucinations. The hallucinatory experience may be pleasant or frightening. The patient who is psychotic is not in contact with reality and frequently misinterprets environmental events. He may be unable to attend to any of his biological needs. He may also inadvertently hurt himself either in response to hallucinations or as an attempt to escape from the frightening experience. Since there is no physical dependence, withdrawal symptoms do not occur. Usually there is a gradual dissipation of psychotic behavior, although the patient may experience "flashbacks" for several months. These brief recurrences of the hallucinogenic experience can be frightening. Patients often express the fear that they are crazy and will never be free of the aftereffects of the drug.

PCP use has become more widespread than that of LSD and related drugs. It may be ingested and is frequently smoked in a mixture with another substance, such as marijuana or parsley flakes. PCP use may precipitate an intensely psychotic experience characterized by extreme agitation. The patient may become violent or exhibit other antisocial behaviors, such as insistence on removing his clothing or the use of profanity. Physical manifestations of PCP intoxication include hypertension, hypersalivation, diaphoresis, nausea and vomiting, ataxia, dysarthria, increased deep tendon reflexes, and decreased pain response. Nystagmus frequently occurs and may be lateral, vertical, or sometimes rotary. At high doses, serious physiological consequences can occur, including seizures, coma, and death.[13] PCP use may evoke the occurrence or exacerbation of an existing and previously controlled psychosis. The unpredictability of the reaction to PCP makes it an extremely dangerous drug.

MARIJUANA USE. Marijuana will be discussed briefly because it is an illicit drug. Nurses will rarely see anyone admitted to the health care system with a primary diagnosis of marijuana use. Use of marijuana generally produces an altered state of awareness accompanied by a feeling of relaxation and mild euphoria. Inhibitions are reduced and reflexes are slowed. Prolonged use may lead to a sense of apathy and loss of motivation, sometimes referred to as the amotivational syndrome. Psychosis may occur in individuals who are already at risk. The physiological effects of marijuana use are still being investigated, but do include drying of the oral and pharyngeal mucous membranes and reddening of the eyes. Pulmonary changes similar to those associated with tobacco use have also

been found. Other long-term effects are yet to be identified.

ABUSE OF ANTIANXIETY DRUGS. Antianxiety agents, particularly the benzodiazepines, constitute a large part of legal drug abuse in the United States. Chlordiazepoxide (Librium) and diazepam (Valium) were welcomed by the medical profession and the public as the answer to the stresses of life. Because they were initially described as relatively safe drugs, the benzodiazepines were prescribed and used freely. However, it has now become apparent that these agents can be physically and psychologically addictive and that tolerance to their use does occur, resulting in the ingestion of gradually increasing amounts. Long-term abuse of benzodiazepines can be debilitating with psychological and social consequences very similar to those associated with alcohol abuse. The person who takes an antianxiety drug experiences a sense of relaxation and a feeling of confidence. As with most drugs, it is this pleasurable experience that leads to repeated use of the drug. This progression is illustrated in Clinical example 14-4.

CLINICAL EXAMPLE 14-4

Ms. T was a 28-year-old law student. She had always done well in school and had no difficulty with the theory portion of her law studies. However, she had always felt self-conscious and inadequate when she was required to speak before a group of people. She would become tremulous, her pulse and respiratory rate would increase, and her mouth would become dry. On occasion, she would lose track of her thoughts and be unable to continue speaking. This problem became a real handicap in her law classes. One of her professors gave her a failing grade for inadequate participation in class discussions. She went to her family physician and described her problem. He reassured her that could give her medication that would help her overcome her "stress response." She was given diazepam, 5 mg, one tablet to be taken every 4 hours as needed for anxiety.

Ms. T was reluctant to take drugs because she recognized the danger inherent in the use of medication. However, she knew that she would never be able to stay in law school if she did not overcome her anxiety. Before her next class, she took a pill. She quickly felt relaxed and self-confident. She described the feeling as "like I had had a martini, only nicer." When the professor asked her a question, she was able to respond and was complimented for her answer. She felt a little drowsy after class but decided that she was probably tired because she had not been sleeping well.

Initially, Ms. T only took diazepam when she anticipated that she would need to speak in class. However, she was introduced to an attractive man by a friend and he asked her out for dinner. She felt anxious before the date and decided that it would do no harm to take a pill to help her relax. She was confident and charming on the date. Gradually, she began to use the drug more frequently. She rationalized that she needed the help to get through school and would stop during summer break. One day, she discovered that she had run out of pills just before she was scheduled to participate in a classroom debate. She went to the school health service, described her anxiety about the class and received another prescription for diazepam. She began to take more than one pill at a time and took them more frequently.

As her drug intake increased, Ms. T's performance in school deteriorated. She turned in papers late and missed classes. Her speech was slurred and she was uncoordinated. Her grades slipped. A year after she began to take pills to enable her to stay in school, she flunked out.

The case of Ms. T demonstrates the seductive quality of the use of antianxiety drugs. Avoidance of anxiety is a powerful motivator of behavior. As with other drugs, as use escalates, guilt about drug taking develops, leading to anxiety that combines with the anxiety related to giving up the drug and results in increased intake. Antianxiety drugs have physiological as well as psychological effects. These may include drowsiness, hypotension, ataxia, and slurred speech. The withdrawal syndrome associated with abrupt cessation of benzodiazepines for patients who have taken the drugs for an extended period of time is similar to barbiturate withdrawal. Benzodiazepines have anticonvulsant properties, and withdrawal can lead to seizures, particularly in patients with a history of prior episodes of convulsive behavior.

Multiple drug abuse is becoming more common. The foregoing discussion reveals that many of the abused substances have similar effects. Abusers may use them interchangeably or simultaneously. Simultaneous use can lead to inadvertent overdose, since some of the substances are synergistic. It is extremely important that the exact nature of drug-abusing behaviors be identified, so that unanticipated occurrence of withdrawal symptoms can be avoided.

Table 14-2 summarizes the behaviors associated with substance abuse.

Coping mechanisms

The presence of substance abuse indicates that the person is experiencing serious difficulty coping. Healthier defense mechanisms and other adaptive behaviors are either inadequate or have not been developed. Therefore the person must resort to methods of coping that may provide temporary relief of anxiety but eventually involve even more anxiety as the person becomes aware that he is harming himself. Drug and alcohol addicts tend to resist this awareness by employing ego defense mechanisms and other behaviors that represent attempts to delude the self. Seixas[22] describes three such defensive maneuvers characteristically used by alcoholics: denial that there is a problem, projection that the drinking behavior is the result of outside experiences beyond the individual's control, and dissociation of the drinking behavior from its effects. Drug abusers also use denial. However, in contrast to alcoholics and users of prescription drugs who tend to isolate themselves from others, users of illicit drugs tend to band together into a drug culture. Although there may be little, if any, meaningful interaction while group members are high, there is the reinforcing effect of the group identity, which may be viewed as a justification for the behavior. A part of the group support is often an attitude of scorn and hostility toward "straight" people, which includes anyone who is not involved in drug abuse.

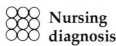

Nursing diagnosis

The nursing diagnosis of an individual who abuses substances must reflect the substance used or abused, the degree to which it is used or abused, and the possible stressors involved. Jellinek[17] has proposed the following four phases of alcoholism that may assist the nurse in determining the degree to which alcohol is being used:

Phase 1   *Prealcoholic phase.* This phase is characterized by social drinking, control over drinking behavior, and occasional alcohol use for stress reduction. At later stages of this phase there may be frequent drinking related to tension reduction.

Phase 2   *Early alcoholic phase.* This phase begins with the first blackout. There is a slow increase in alcohol tolerance and progressive preoccupation with alcohol. The person may begin to drink alone and his behavior may be embarrassing to others. Guilt feelings lead to excuses for drinking. There may be periods of total abstinence, which are used as evidence of the person's control over his drinking behavior.

Phase 3 *True alcoholic phase.* Everything revolves around alcohol. The person is avoided by significant others and resents this. It is impossible for the individual to stop after one drink.

Phase 4 *Complete alcohol dependence.* Drinking begins in the morning and continues all day. Physical dependence is present. Severe liver damage may occur. There is usually some brain damage. If drinking continues, death will occur. The person cannot stop drinking without help.

Similar phases may be identified for abuse of drugs other than alcohol. They are as follows:

Phase 1 *Experimentation.* The person takes a drug to see what it is like or to conform with peers. No further use develops from the initial experience.

Phase 2 *Early drug abuse.* A specific drug or various drugs are used with some degree of regularity for the pleasurable effects or to reduce anxiety. Drugs may be used socially.

Phase 3 *True drug addiction.* Drugs are used regularly, several times a day. Physical dependence begins if it is a characteristic of the drug. Psychological dependence is present. The life-style is drug focused. Social functioning deteriorates.

Phase 4 *Severe drug addiction.* The person does whatever is necessary to obtain drugs. Criminal behavior occurs. There is total alienation from the non–drug using culture. The physical condition deteriorates. Continued drug use will lead to death.

The case of Mr. H (p. 459) will be used as an example of appropriate nursing diagnosis for an individual who abuses alcohol. Table 14-3 compares these nursing diagnoses with medical diagnostic criteria for alcohol dependence and alcohol withdrawal delirium.[1]

The case of Ms. W (p. 462) was included to depict the abuse of amphetamines and barbiturates. Nursing diagnoses that would apply to Ms. W are compared in Table 14-4 to medical diagnostic criteria for amphetamine dependence, amphetamine withdrawal, barbiturate dependence, and barbiturate withdrawal.[1]

The case of Mr. C (p. 461) is representative of opiate abuse. The nursing diagnoses that were developed for Mr. C may be compared with the medical diagnostic criteria for opioid dependence, opioid withdrawal, and posttraumatic stress disorder (Table 14-5).

The case of Ms. T (p. 464) illustrates the abuse of antianxiety drugs. Representative nursing diagnoses for Ms. T include the following:

1. True drug addiction (phase 3) to diazepam related to the stress of law school
2. Failure at law school related to the effects of diazepam use
3. Inability to speak assertively related to low self-esteem

The medical diagnosis that would apply to Ms. T is other specified drug dependence.[1] Diagnostic criteria would be similar to those described for dependence on other substances.

In summary, the model of health-illness phenomena may be applied to substance abuse as illustrated in Fig. 14-3.

 Planning and implementation of nursing interventions

Goal setting

The establishment of nursing goals with a substance abusing patient must be done with recognition of the realities of the person's life-style and habits. The ideal long-term goal is frequently permanent total abstinence. However, the patient may be unable to face that level of commitment and is frequently very anxious at the thought of never again using the substance to which he is addicted. Recognition of this fact is reflected in the Alcoholics Anonymous (AA) approach to abstinence. AA members are advised to take 1 day, or sometimes 1 hour or 1 minute, at a time. The alcoholic is then able to take satisfaction in achieving short-term goals for sobriety. The thought of never drinking again is sometimes enough to send an alcoholic out to find a drink.

The nurse must also be aware that it is rare for an addicted person to suddenly stop substance use forever. Most addicts have to try at least once and usually several times to use the substance in a controlled way. Although some research indicates that this may be possible for some alcoholics, it is generally not a realistic goal. It should also be noted that people who tend to become addicted to one substance, such as antianxiety drugs, also have a tendency for other types of addictions. A new addiction that is substituted for the old one will only add new problems.

In general, the long-term goals for an individual who abuses substances are withdrawal
Text continued on p. 474.

TABLE 14-2. Summary of behaviors associated with substance abuse

Substance	Route (most common listed first)	Physical dependence	Psychological dependence	Expected behaviors	Behaviors related to overdose	Withdrawal syndrome	Special considerations
Alcohol	Ingestion	Yes	Yes	Euphoria, followed by depression and sometimes hostility; decreased inhibitions; impaired judgment; incoordination; slurred speech	Unconsciousness, coma, respiratory depression, death	Tremors, hallucinosis, seizure disorder, delirium tremens (alcohol withdrawal delirium)	Chronic use leads to serious disruptions in most organ systems; malnutrition and dehydration are common; vitamin deficiency may lead to Wernicke's encephalopathy and alcoholic amnestic syndrome; alcohol-dependent people are susceptible to other dependencies as well
Opiates							
Heroin	Injection Ingestion Inhalation	Yes	Yes	Euphoria, relaxation, relief from pain, lack of concern, detachment from reality, drowsiness, constricted pupils, nausea, constipation, slurred speech, impaired judgment	Unconsciousness, coma, respiratory depression, circulatory depression, respiratory arrest, cardiac arrest, death	Watery eyes, dilated pupils, anxiety, abdominal cramps, piloerection, yawning, diaphoresis, rhinorrhea, achiness, anorexia, insomnia, fever, nausea, vomiting, diarrhea	Chronic use leads to lack of concern about physical well-being, resulting in malnutrition and dehydration; criminal behavior may take place to acquire money for drugs; injection sites may become infected; multiple drug use is common
Morphine Meperidine	Injection Ingestion	Yes	Yes				
Codeine	Ingestion Injection	Yes	Yes				
Opium	Smoking Ingestion	Yes	Yes				
Methadone	Ingestion	Yes	Yes	Relieves craving for drugs without causing impaired functioning	Same	Same	

Continued.

TABLE 14-2. Summary of behaviors associated with substance abuse—cont'd

Substance	Route (most common listed first)	Physical dependence	Psychological dependence	Expected behaviors	Behaviors related to overdose	Withdrawal syndrome	Special considerations
Barbiturates	Ingestion Injection	Yes	Yes	Euphoria, followed by depression and sometimes hostility; decreased inhibitions; impaired judgment; slurred speech; incoordination; drowsiness	Respiratory depression, coma, death	Postural hypotension, tachycardia, fever, insomnia, tremors, agitation, anxiety; rapid withdrawal causes apprehension, weakness, tremors, postural hypotension, anorexia, grand mal seizures	Frequently used alternately with stimulants; combination with alcohol enhances effects and may lead to overdosage; paradoxical responses of hyperactivity may occur in children and the elderly
Amphetamines	Ingestion Injection	No	Yes	Euphoria, hyperactivity, irritability, hyperalertness, insomnia, anorexia, weight loss, tachycardia, hypertension	Restlessness, tremor, rapid respiration, confusion, assaultiveness, hallucinations, panic	Depression, fatigue	Prolonged use can result in psychotic behavior; a paradoxical depressant reaction occurs in children; frequently used alternately with depressant substances
Cocaine	Inhalation Smoking Injection	No	Yes	Euphoria, elation, agitation, hyperactivity, irritability, grandiosity, pressured speech, tachycardia, hypertension, diaphoresis, anorexia, weight loss, insomnia	Restlessness, tremor, rapid respiration, confusion, assaultiveness, hallucinations, panic	Depression, fatigue, anxiety	Psychotic behavior may occur following large doses; prolonged use by inhalation may result in destruction of the mucous membranes in the nose and deterioration of the nasal septum; use in combination with other substances is dangerous

Drug	Route			Effects	Overdose	Withdrawal	Comments
Hallucinogens (psychedelics)	Ingestion Smoking	No	No	Distorted perception, heightened sense of awareness, grandiosity, hallucinations, illusions, distortions of time and space, depersonalization, mystical experiences, dilated pupils, increased blood pressure, increased salivation	Panic, psychosis	None	A "bad trip" may result in panic, unpredictable behavior, and psychotic behaviors; "flashbacks" may occur for several months after use; self-destructive behavior may occur while under the effect of the drug
Phencyclidine (PCP)	Smoking Ingestion	No	No	Euphoria, perceptual distortion, agitation, violence, delusions, antisocial behavior, elevated blood pressure, increased salivation, diaphoresis, ataxia, increased DTRs, nystagmus, decreased pain response	Drowsiness, stupor, coma, grand mal seizures, death	None	Use may lead to psychotic behavior, irrationality, panic
Marijuana	Smoking Ingestion	No	Yes	Relaxation, mild euphoria, loss of inhibition, decreased motivation, red eyes, dry mouth	Psychosis	None	Physiological consequences of use are under investigation
Antianxiety drugs (benzodiazepines)	Ingestion Injection	Yes	Yes	Relaxation, increased self-confidence, relief of anxiety, drowsiness, ataxia, slurred speech, hypotension	Drowsiness, confusion, hypotension, coma, death	Tremors, agitation, anxiety, grand mal seizures, abdominal cramps, vomiting, diaphoresis	Dependence may occur insidiously; users may underreport the actual amount taken because of guilt about multiple prescriptions and abuse

TABLE 14-3. **Comparative examples of nursing diagnoses and medical diagnoses associated with alcohol dependence and alcohol withdrawal delirium**

Nursing diagnoses	Medical diagnoses as described in DSM-III*

True alcohol addiction (phase 3) related to the pressures of a busy law practice and family demands
 	
Delirium related to withdrawal from alcohol following a 2-week drinking binge
 	
Guilt related to his responsibility for the death of a passenger in the car with which he collided when driving while intoxicated
 	
Estrangement from wife and threatened divorce related to repeated bouts of drinking
	Diagnostic criteria for ALCOHOL DEPENDENCE
	
	A. Either a pattern of pathological alcohol use or impairment in social or occupational functioning due to alchol use:
	
	Pattern of pathological alcohol use: need for daily use of alcohol for adequate functioning; inability to cut down or stop drinking; repeated efforts to control or reduce excess drinking by "going on the wagon" (periods of temporary abstinence) or restricting drinking to certain times of the day; binges (remaining intoxicated throughout the day for at least 2 days); occasional consumption of a fifth of spirits (or its equivalent in wine or beer); amnesic periods for events occurring while intoxicated (blackouts); continuation of drinking despite a serious physical disorder that the individual knows is exacerbated by alcohol use; drinking of nonbeverage alcohol
	
	Impairment in social or occupational functioning due to alcohol use: e.g., violence while intoxicated, absence from work, loss of job, legal difficulties (e.g., arrest for intoxicated behavior, traffic accidents while intoxicated), arguments or difficulties with family or friends because of excessive alcohol use
	
	B. Either tolerance or withdrawal:
	
	    Tolerance: need for markedly increased amounts of alcohol to achieve the desired effect, or markedly diminished effect with regular use of the same amount
	
	    Withdrawal: development of alcohol withdrawal (e.g., morning "shakes" and malaise relieved by drinking) after cessation of or reduction in drinking
	
	Diagnostic criteria for ALCOHOL WITHDRAWAL DELIRIUM
	
	A. Delirium occurs within 1 week after cessation of or reduction in heavy alcohol ingestion
	
	B. Autonomic hyperactivity, e.g., tachycardia, sweating, elevated blood pressure
	
	C. Not due to any other physical or mental disorder

*From American Psychiatric Association: Diagnostic and statistical manual of mental disorders, third edition, Washington, D.C., APA, 1980.

TABLE 14-4. Comparative examples of nursing diagnoses and medical diagnoses for amphetamine dependence and withdrawal and barbiturate dependence and withdrawal

Nursing diagnoses	Medical diagnoses as described in DSM-III*

True drug addiction (phase 3) to amphetamines related to anxiety about weight gain and pleasurable response to drug taking
 	
True drug addiction (phase 3) to barbiturates related to insomnia secondary to amphetamine use
 	
Low self-esteem related to disparity between self-concept and ideal self in terms of body weight
 	
Low self-esteem related to guilt about abuse of amphetamines and barbiturates
	Diagnostic criteria for AMPHETAMINE OR SIMILARLY ACTING SYMPATHOMIMETIC DEPENDENCE
	
	Either tolerance or withdrawal:
	
	Tolerance: need for markedly increased amounts of substance to achieve the desired effect, or markedly diminished effect with regular use of the same amount
	
	Withdrawal: development of amphetamine or similarly acting sympathomimetic withdrawal after cessation of or reduction in substance use
	
	Diagnostic criteria for AMPHETAMINE OR SIMILARLY ACTING SYMPATHOMIMETIC WITHDRAWAL
	
	A. Prolonged heavy use of amphetamine or a similarly acting sympathomimetic
	
	B. After cessation of or reduction in substance use, depressed mood and at least two of the following:
	
	   1. Fatigue
	   2. Disturbed sleep
	   3. Increased dreaming
	
	C. Not due to any other physical or mental disorder, such as amphetamine or similarly acting sympathomimetic delusional disorder
	
	Diagnostic criteria for BARBITURATE OR SIMILARLY ACTING SEDATIVE OR HYPNOTIC DEPENDENCE
	
	Either tolerance or withdrawal:
	
	Tolerance: need for markedly increased amounts of the substance to achieve the desired effect, or markedly diminished effect with regular use of the same amount.
	
	Withdrawal: development of barbiturate or similarly acting sedative or hypnotic withdrawal after cessation of or reduction in substance use
	
	Diagnostic criteria for BARBITURATE OR SIMILARLY ACTING SEDATIVE OR HYPNOTIC WITHDRAWAL
	
	A. Prolonged, heavy use of barbiturate or similarly acting sedative or hypnotic, or more prolonged use of smaller doses of a benzodiazepine
	
	B. At least three of the following due to recent cessation of or reduction in substance use:
	
	   1. Nausea and vomiting
	   2. Malaise or weakness
	   3. Autonomic hyperactivity, e.g., tachycardia, sweating, elevated blood pressure
	   4. Anxiety
	   5. Depressed mood or irritability
	   6. Orthostatic hypotension
	   7. Coarse tremor of hands, tongue, and eyelids
	
	C. Not due to any other physical or mental disorder, such as barbiturate or similarly acting sedative or hypnotic withdrawal delirium

*From American Psychiatric Association: Diagnostic and statistical manual of mental disorders, third edition, Washington, D.C., APA, 1980.

TABLE 14-5. Comparative examples of nursing diagnoses and medical diagnoses associated with opioid dependence and withdrawal and posttraumatic stress disorder

Nursing diagnoses	Medical diagnoses as described in DSM-III*
Severe drug addiction (phase 4) related to the stress of involvement in combat in Viet Nam and difficulty readjusting to civilian life Anxiety, abdominal cramps, lacrimation, rhinorrhea, piloerection, diaphoresis, and dilated pupils related to withdrawal of opiates Nightmares and severe anxiety related to the stress of combat experiences in Viet Nam Lack of community support system related to alienation of significant others who were not involved in the drug culture	**Diagnostic criteria for OPIOID DEPENDENCE** Either tolerance or withdrawal: *Tolerance:* need for markedly increased amounts of opioid to achieve the desired effect, or markedly diminished effect with regular use of the same amount *Withdrawal:* development of opioid withdrawal after cessation of or reduction in substance use **Diagnostic criteria for OPIOID WITHDRAWAL** **A.** Prolonged, heavy use of an opioid (or administration of a narcotic antagonist following a briefer period of use) **B.** At least four of the following symptoms due to the recent cessation of or reduction in opioid use: 1. Lacrimation 2. Rhinorrhea 3. Pupillary dilation 4. Piloerection 5. Sweating 6. Diarrhea 7. Yawning 8. Mild hypertension 9. Tachycardia 10. Fever 11. Insomnia **C.** Not due to any other physical or mental disorder **Diagnostic criteria for POSTTRAUMATIC STRESS DISORDER** **A.** Existence of a recognizable stressor that would evoke significant symptoms of distress in almost everyone **B.** Reexperiencing of the trauma as evidenced by at least one of the following: 1. Recurrent and intrusive recollections of the event 2. Recurrent dreams of the event 3. Sudden acting or feeling as if the traumatic event were reoccurring, because of an association with an environmental or ideational stimulus **C.** Numbing of responsiveness to or reduced involvement with the external world, beginning some time after the trauma, as shown by at least one of the following: 1. Markedly diminished interest in one or more significant activities 2. Feeling of detachment or estrangement from others 3. Constricted affect **D.** At least two of the following symptoms that were not present before the trauma: 1. Hyperalertness or exaggerated startle response 2. Sleep disturbance 3. Guilt about surviving when others have not, or about behavior required for survival 4. Memory impairment or trouble concentrating 5. Avoidance of activities that arouse recollection of the traumatic event 6. Intensification of symptoms by exposure to events that symbolize or resemble the traumatic event

*From American Psychiatric Association: Diagnostic and statistical manual of mental disorders, third edition, Washington, D.C., APA, 1980.

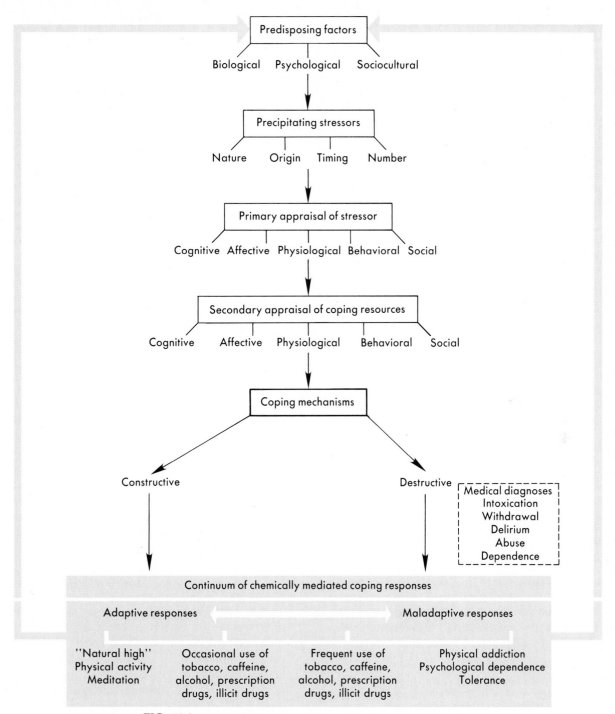

FIG. 14-3
Model of health-illness phenomena applied to substance abuse.

from the drug if dependency is present and future abstinence. It is important that the patient participate in this decision-making process and agree about the approach to abstinence that will be tried. For instance, a heroin addict who is to be referred to a methadone program must decide whether to be on a maintenance or a withdrawal regimen and must agree to abide by the rules of the program. Goals for such a patient might be as follows:

Long-term goal

The patient will refrain from using narcotics other than methadone for 1 year, at which time the goal will be renegotiated.

Short-term goals

1. The patient will attend the methadone maintenance program daily for 3 months.
2. After 3 months, if there is no evidence of drug abuse, the patient will attend the methadone maintenance program three times a week, using take-home doses of methadone on the other days.
3. The patient will attend group discussions once a week and share his experiences with the group.
4. The patient will inform his counselor if he is unable to keep a scheduled clinic appointment.

It is very important that goals for a substance abusing patient be phrased so that it is clear that the patient has responsibility for his behavior. Displacement of responsibility onto others is a frequent behavior of dependent people. Writing the goals into a contract to be signed by the patient and the nurse and providing the patient with a copy of the contract will also help reinforce the patient's responsibility for complying with the stated goals.

The nursing goals for patients who are experiencing drug withdrawal must attend to any life-threatening behaviors that are present. The highest priority will be given to stabilization of the patient's physiological status until the crisis of withdrawal is over. Emotional support will then be necessary as the person comes to terms with his behavior and begins to look to the future. The setting and constant modification of goals during this process convey to the patient the nurse's belief that there is hope for a more productive life in the future.

Intervening in substance abuse

Many theories have been described concerning the origin of substance abuse. There are also multiple theories about the effective treatment of this problem. The nurse will need to select the approach to intervention that seems most appropriate for each individual for whom she provides nursing care.

BIOLOGICAL ASPECTS OF INTERVENTION. Substance abusers frequently come into contact with the health care system because of a crisis in their physiological state. The crisis may be related to overdose, withdrawal, allergy, toxicity, or physical deterioration due to the deleterious effects of drugs, including such conditions as malnutrition, dehydration, and various infections. When an acute physical condition is present, it takes priority over the other health needs of the patient. It is particularly important with substance abuse patients to attend to the condition that they have identified as the problem. The nurse is then perceived as potentially helpful and will have added credibility when other aspects of the addictive problem are addressed.

If the person is physically dependent on a drug, withdrawal must be accomplished with medical supervision. This process is referred to as *detoxification*. Gradual weaning from the substance may be instituted, especially if the person is addicted to prescription drugs, such as barbiturates, amphetamines, or benzodiazepines. Another approach is the use of alternative drugs to block the occurrence of withdrawal symptoms. For instance, chlordiazepoxide may be given to assist with alcohol withdrawal. The dose of the substituted drug is then tapered down and eventually discontinued. The danger in this approach is that the alcoholic can become dependent on the substitute drug or may even have been taking it in addition to alcohol. A variation on this approach is used when methadone is substituted for heroin. However, the treatment program may be aimed toward gradual withdrawal from methadone or toward indefinite maintenance on a stable dose of methadone. The decision between these two alternatives is based on assessment of the likelihood of recidivism if the person becomes drug free. This treatment approach has been controversial because methadone is a narcotic. However, addiction to methadone does not cause impairment in functioning, thus allowing the person to be productive while addicted. Proponents of methadone maintenance point out the benefits of avoiding the debilitating effects of narcotic addiction.

Withdrawal symptoms may occur even when efforts are made to prevent this. Substance abusers do not always give accurate drug-use histories, although it is extremely important for the nurse to obtain as specific an assessment as possible. If the amount of substance used has been understated or if multiple abuse is undetected, withdrawal symptoms may emerge. The possibility of seizures should always be anticipated and emergency equipment at hand. Drug abuse should always be considered as a possible condition when unexpected seizure activity occurs. If drug abuse is suspected, it is prudent to be sure that the physician is apprised of the situation so blood and urine specimens can be collected for laboratory analysis.

Drug overdose is treated supportively, depending on the characteristics of the drug taken. It is, of course, important to identify the drug. In cases of narcotic overdose, narcotic antagonists, such as nalorphine may be given. After the person recovers from the acute illness, it is necessary to assess the circumstances of the overdose and particularly important to determine whether it was intentional or accidental. If the motivation is in doubt, it is best to assume that a suicide attempt has occurred until the nurse can obtain more information about the patient's mental state.

Users of LSD and PCP often have an acute toxic psychosis. The behavior may be very similar to that of the schizophrenic patient. However, there may be no history of prior abnormal behavior. Careful assessment of an acute psychotic reaction, particularly in an adolescent or young adult, should include exploration of drug use. it may be necessary to interview friends of the patient to obtain this information. An attempt should be made to identify the specific drug used, although LSD and PCP may be taken without the knowledge of the person involved.* There is an important difference in the nursing approach to users of PCP as opposed to those who have an adverse reaction to LSD. Victims of PCP-induced psychosis do not respond well to attempts at interaction. They require an environment that has minimal stimuli and is safe. Agitated PCP users may strike out in response to their fear and panic and are potentially harmful to themselves and others.[26] LSD users experiencing a "bad trip" do respond to reassurance and may be "talked down." It seems to be most helpful if support is given by a friend or by someone who has experienced LSD. However, calm empathic reassurance and reorientation by the nurse will also help decrease the patient's panic. Provision must also be made for the safety

of these individuals because they may act impulsively out of fear and harm themselves. Adequate staff should be present to control impulsive behavior of both PCP and LSD users. Vital signs should be monitored and other physiological needs met. Excretion of PCP is aided by acidifying the urine by giving the patient cranberry juice or ascorbic acid. Gastric lavage may be necessary for persistent symptoms or if an overdose has been taken.[26]

Once the initial crisis is over, biofeedback has been used as an approach to the treatment of substance abuse. The patients learn emotional control by natural, rather than chemical, means. Another long-term biological approach to substance abuse is the prescription of disulfiram (Antabuse) for alcoholics. This drug sensitizes the person to alcohol, and an aversive physiological response occurs if the person uses alcohol in any form. The response consists of a severe headache, nausea and vomiting, flushing, hypotension, tachycardia, dyspnea, diaphoresis, chest pain, palpitations, dizziness, and confusion. It can also lead to respiratory and cardiac collapse, unconsciousness, convulsions, and death. It is therefore important that the patient agree to take disulfiram only after careful instruction about the potential consequences of drinking while on the drug. This educational process should include a written list of alcohol-containing preparations to be avoided, including cough medicines, rubbing compounds, vinegars, aftershave lotions, and some mouthwashes. Drinking must be avoided for 14 days after disulfiram has been taken. This medication cannot prevent drinking by someone who is determined to drink, because that person can wait until the disulfiram has been excreted. However, it helps to prevent impulsive drinking because the person does have to wait for a period of time to be able to drink safely. This treatment is used in conjunction with other supportive therapies.

Since most of the drugs that are abused cross the placental barrier, women should be counseled about the possible effects of substance use during pregnancy. There have been incidents of congenital abnormalities in infants of mothers who have taken drugs. A fetal alcohol syndrome has been identified. In addition, use during pregnancy of drugs that cause physical dependency will result in the birth of an addicted baby who must then be withdrawn from the drug. The safest pregnancy is one in which the mother is totally drug free.

---

*To assist in assessment of drug use, a glossary of drug terminology has been included in Appendix E.

**INTERACTIVE INTERVENTIONS IN SUBSTANCE
ABUSE.** Before attempting to initiate nursing
intervention with a substance abusing patient,
the nurse must develop an awareness of her own
feelings and attitudes toward the problem. It
is recommended that a values clarification approach be used, as described in Chapter 3. Most
people have had personal contact with substance
abuse by family, friends, or colleagues. This
problem evokes many negative feelings. It is important that the nurse be able to differentiate
feelings associated with past situations from
those aroused by professional contacts with patients and their families. A supervisor, teacher,
or senior clinical nurse can be of assistance
when a nurse is having difficulty sorting out
feelings.

The multiplicity of stressors relative to substance abuse have been discussed. It is very important that nursing intervention be directed toward alleviating the stressors that apply to each
individual patient and identified in the nursing diagnosis. If the motivation for drug use has
been peer pressure, the patient will need help in
planning how to deal with the same kind of pressures in the future. This may be a particularly
difficult problem for adolescents who rely very
much on peer group approval to maintain their
self-esteem. A group support approach to treatment is helpful to these patients. They also
have a tendency to deny the potential for future
problems. Peers in a group setting can confront
the individual with the realities of social pressure. Alcoholics also need to learn how to refuse
a drink, even when urged to indulge. Role playing can be a helpful approach by the nurse, especially in a group setting. Two patients can act
out a social situation involving drinking and then
receive feedback from the group about their behavior.

Another nursing intervention that can be implemented effectively in a group setting is patient education. Substance abusers should be
well informed about the drug they have used, its
biological and psychosocial effects on the person, and community resources for future assistance. Films and other audiovisual materials
reinforce important concepts. Handouts should
be used for future reference.

Individual counseling is frequently used as an
approach with patients who are substance users.
Commonly encountered problems include denial, dependency, low self-esteem, manipulation, and anger. Concepts related to these behaviors are discussed elsewhere in this book.
However, it is necessary to address the special
application of these concepts to substance
abuse.

Denial must be dealt with because it is a
potential obstacle to recovery from chemical dependency. Most patients deny that they are unable to control their substance abusing behavior
even when drug-related problems have become
serious. For instance, an intoxicated person who
has caused an automobile accident may assert
that he "just had a few beers." A barbiturate
addict may claim that he can stop whenever he
wants to do so. The denial is partially related to
the stigma attached to drug abuse. It is difficult
to apply the term "alcoholic" or "addict" to oneself. Denial also protects the person from admitting that he is unable to control his behavior.
Self-control is a prized attribute that is central
to the self-concept of most people. Admission of
a problem is also the first step toward behavioral
change. This commitment to change is very
frightening to a substance dependent person. It
involves a decision to stop using a substance
that has become the major focus of the person's
life. Anyone who has tried to stop smoking cigarettes or diet can understand to some extent the
anxiety aroused by this decision.

It is essential that denial be overcome and that
the patient make the commitment to behavioral
change. Repeated confrontation with evidence
of substance dependence may be necessary to
evoke this response. However, this must be done
carefully so the patient is not antagonized. Repeated contacts with the health care system may
be necessary before the patient admits to the
nature of the problem.

Many therapists use behavioral contracts
when working with substance abusers. The
nurse and the patient discuss and agree on realistic behavioral objectives for the patient.
These are written down, and the document is
signed by both the nurse and the patient. Most
therapists who work with substance abuse patients insist on a provision in the contract that
the patient be drug and alcohol free when attending a therapy session. This communicates
the therapist's belief that the patient is able to
control his behavior and take positive action in
his own behalf.

Dependency is generally a personality characteristic of people who become involved in substance abusing behavior. This dependency may
also be evident in the individual's interpersonal
relationships. If the person is too dependent on

others, it may drive them away, thus increasing the need to depend on alcohol or drugs. Clinical example 14-5 illustrates this problem.

CLINICAL EXAMPLE 14-5

Mr. B was a 45-year-old man who was admitted to the medical unit of a general hospital with a diagnosis of gastritis. He complained of abdominal pain, nausea, and vomiting. He had a slightly elevated temperature of 37.5° C (100° F). When the admitting nurse who was completing the nursing assessment asked Mr. B about alcohol use, he said he had "a couple of beers" after work every day. He also reported that his wife had left him the day before admission. He said he was not sure why she left, but he was sure she would be back. Ms. B did come to the hospital to visit her husband. His primary nurse met with them together and asked Ms. B why she left. She said she was tired of putting Mr. B to bed every night after he passed out from drinking and did not want to continue to call his employer saying he was sick when he was really hung over. She had threatened to leave before, but Mr. B had always begged her to stay and she had relented. She had married him because she felt sorry for him. He had been living alone and was not taking good care of himself. She revealed that her first husband was also an alcoholic. She would agree to try again to make the marriage a success if he would agree to stop drinking and seek counseling. Mr. B said to the nurse, "I'll be good and do what she says. You tell her I'll be good."

Mr. B used alcohol to avoid responsibility for his actions and his life. He used his wife in a similar way. When she confronted him with her expectations, he responded in a childlike way and tried to place the nurse in the parental role. This avoidance of responsibility is one of the behaviors that is very difficult for the substance abuser to change. The nurse must be careful not to fall into the trap of making decisions for the patient. In Clinical example 14-5, the nurse suggested that Mr. B communicate directly with his wife about how he planned to change his behavior.

Ms. B represents another problem that is also encountered when working with a substance abusing patient. She is a woman who appears to be drawn to dependent men. She is probably a very maternal person who likes to take care of others. This increases the possibility that she will assume the role of *enabler*. The enabler perpetuates the substance abuse problem by not confronting the substance abuser and by helping to cover up the problem. When Ms. B called Mr. B's employer to say he was sick, she was being an enabler. When significant others play an enabling role, family counseling is necessary to help the family accept and support the changing behavior of the patient. Ms. B had left her husband, but he was her second alcoholic spouse, indicating that she was probably attracted to dependent men. Any increase in assertiveness by Mr. B would have further disrupted the equilibrium of their relationship.

Assertiveness training can be very helpful in assisting both the dependent substance abuser and significant others to accomplish a behavioral change. This therapeutic technique is described in detail in Chapter 11. An increase in assertiveness may also have the added advantage of a positive effect on the person's self-esteem. Although some substance abusers present a facade of self-confidence, most basically have little regard for themselves. The relaxation, euphoria, or release of inhibitions imparted by the drug helps the person overcome this sense of inferiority. Another goal of nursing care must be to find ways of bolstering the person's self-esteem. This can be very difficult because many of these people have destroyed the relationships and activities that normally build self-esteem. They may have lost jobs, friends, and family. The nurse needs to help the person identify his remaining strengths and to build on them. Strengths may be related to overcoming the substance abuse problem itself. This was so in the case of Bobby F in Clinical example 14-6.

CLINICAL EXAMPLE 14-6

Bobby was a 17-year-old who was admitted to the hospital acutely psychotic with a history of recent use of PCP. The emergency room nurse noted scarring of the veins in Bobby's arm and surmised that he was also a user of heroin. Blood and urine testing confirmed this suspicion. Bobby recovered from his psychotic episode in 24 hours but was then extremely uncomfortable due to opiate withdrawal. The decision was made to use titrated doses of methadone to assist with the withdrawal. Mr. L, a young nurse, established a close relationship with Bobby during this time. Bobby requested the nurse's help in planning for his future, but doubted that he had the strength to stay away from drugs. He was advised to take a day at a time. Mr. L took Bobby on a visit to a drug treatment program, and he agreed to try membership in one of the groups at this center. Bobby did well in the group and was very helpful to new members, describing his experiences and encouraging them to "take 1 day at a time." Bobby expressed an interest in finishing school and said he would like to become a drug counselor. The staff of the drug treatment program agreed that Bobby seemed to have an aptitude for that role and encouraged him to pursue his goal.

■■■■■■■■■■■■■■■■■■■■■■■■■■■■■■

Mr. L used his relationship with Bobby to convey his belief that the patient could succeed in giving up drugs. This message had a core of positive regard for Bobby's potential strength. The staff of the drug treatment program added to this seed of self-esteem by encouraging Bobby to help others in the program and then to aim higher at becoming a counselor himself. This process taught Bobby that there were rewards in life other than those attached to drug use. Gradually, he learned to value the interpersonal rewards more than the drug rewards while making positive use of his past difficulties. Employment in drug programs has been a positive step for many ex-addicts who frequently become excellent counselors.

Manipulative behavior is another frequent characteristic of the substance abuser. This is often focused on obtaining access to drugs or alcohol. The hospitalized person may promise to give up the abused substance to get discharged, only to start using it again as soon as he returns home. Drug abusers sometimes manipulate the health care system by getting prescriptions from more than one physician or by forging prescriptions. This behavior must be confronted when it is discovered, and the patient should be helped to understand the self-defeating nature of this behavior. Although the behavior would appear to be directed toward others, the real victim is always the patient who perpetuates his self-destructive behavior.

When substance abusers are confronted with their behavior and are pressed to assume responsibility for it, they may become angry. The root of the anger is related to the pain that is felt when the person realizes he must give up a behavior that has been central to his existence. In addition, the patient is raging over the emerging understanding of the problems he has caused for himself. Huberty and Malmquist[14] have compared the family response to the drug abuser to Kübler-Ross' stages of dying. This comparison seems particularly applicable to the anger experienced by the addict who is mourning the loss of the abused substance and the loss of life experience during the period of addiction.

The nurse must realize that the anger felt by the patient may be directed toward her but generally is not related to her behavior. The patient should be assisted to express this anger in nondestructive ways. Exercise may be helpful. Expression through art or music may also provide an outlet for rage. A danger associated with this anger is that the patient may use it as an excuse to return to using drugs or alcohol. The substance abuser needs to learn that human support can also be of help in confronting painful feelings. It is important that the person be helped to label the feelings he is experiencing. Drug users become so accustomed to avoiding feelings chemically that they have difficulty even recognizing what it is that they are feeling. Group counseling may also be helpful because individuals can see and identify feelings in others as well as themselves. Group support can help to decrease the sense of isolation that these patients often have.

Work with substance abusing patients can be frustrating. Behavioral change is very difficult for them so there is a high rate of recidivism. It may be very difficult for a nurse who has struggled to help someone overcome withdrawal symptoms and to rebuild his life to then see that person return to the health care agency readdicted. Rejection of the patient at this point is not helpful. These patients are very sensitive to rejection or criticism. They use such reactions to justify further substance abuse. They may make statements such as, "You're absolutely right. I'm not worth caring about. Nobody cares for me so why should I care for myself?" The nurse may communicate to the patient her disappointment that he did not continue to progress. However, the focus should be on beginning again, using the fact that the patient succeeded once to foster an optimistic attitude toward the future.

While the nurse is establishing a helping relationship with the patient, she should be alert to signs of other psychosocial disruptions. Some people become substance abusers because of their efforts to deal with underlying emotional problems. Alcohol and other drugs may be used in this way. Unfortunately, most of the substances which may be abused also have characteristics that tend to make problems worse, although there may be temporary relief. For instance, alcohol or barbiturates may be used to combat depression. There is an immediate sense of euphoria from these drugs. However, they are basically depressant substances and lead to later feelings of gloom. Amphetamines and cocaine bring about a "high," but there is also an inevitable "crash." People who use drugs to release inhibitions and relate more easily with others will find that they may develop a greater number of superficial relationships, but drive away the few people to whom they have been able to feel close. The nurse needs to explore these motivations for substance abuse and help the patient find other ways to alleviate his psychological pain.

SOCIAL SUPPORT SYSTEMS. Reliable support from caring people is crucial to the recovery of substance abusers. Families are often frustrated with the patient's behavior. Family counseling by a qualified health care provider is likely to be necessary to assist the family in adjusting to the patient's changing behavior. Family members may need sources of support so they can be supportive to the dependent member.

Formal family counseling is one approach to providing support to the social system. Self-help groups are another way of helping the substance abuser and his significant others. AA is the prototype for self-help groups. AA is an organization that is composed entirely of recovering alcoholics. They believe that mutual support can give the alcoholic strength to abstain. AA aims for total abstinence. The member must admit to alcoholism openly and publicly by introducing himself at meetings, saying, "My name is John and I am an alcoholic." The other members promptly respond, "Hi John!" At each meeting, one or several members share their life histories with the group. This demonstrates that individual members are more alike than different, removing a resistance to involvement that is often cited by alcoholics. AA members also commit themselves to helping each other. As a member recovers, he is eventually assigned to be a sponsor for a new member. The sponsor role entails availability and accessibility to the other member whenever he feels the need to drink. This reciprocal relationship gives the new member caring support and the sponsor improved self-esteem. AA also involves a strong religious orientation that is experienced as supportive by some alcoholics. Most cities have many AA groups. These groups often differ from each other in the characteristics of the members. There may be groups that are mostly blue collar workers, housewives, or physicians. A nurse who is referring an alcoholic patient to a group should become familiar enough with the characteristics of that specific group to know whether the patient is likely to feel comfortable with the other members. AA meetings are frequently open. It is highly recommended that every nurse arrange to attend an AA meeting to help her to understand the problem and to gain an appreciation for the work that is done by this organization.

Two other support groups have developed as extensions of AA. Alanon is a self-help group that was established to meet the needs of spouses and significant others of alcoholics. The alcoholic need not be involved in AA for the significant other to join Alanon. In fact, this organization is often very helpful to spouses of alcoholics who are actively drinking. The members support each other and offer advice on moving forward with their own lives without becoming totally absorbed in the alcoholic's problem. Alateen performs a similar function for adolescents who are involved with alcoholic family members. The message of both of these organizations is that the family member is not responsible for and cannot control the alcoholic's drinking. They can, however, still live meaningful lives of their own.

Many communities have transitional living programs, such as halfway houses, for alcoholics and drug abusers. These facilities serve as a transition between detoxification and complete return to the community. They usually have structured programs that include individual and group counseling, education about the addictive problem, AA meetings, and vocational rehabilitation. It is believed that this intensive program helps the patient readjust slowly to the community. These facilities are especially helpful for people who are alienated from their families.

There are a variety of community programs that may be available for drug abusers. Drug treatment programs generally offer individual and group counseling, family counseling, vocational counseling, and drug and health education. Some also include methadone withdrawal or maintenance for opiate addicts. These programs must have special licensure to operate and have specific federal guidelines to follow. Peer group relationships are an important aspect of most drug treatment programs. The clientele of these programs may differ, but most are directed toward "street people."

The nurse is responsible to know about the treatment programs that are available in the

TABLE 14-6. Summary of nursing interventions with the substance abusing patient

Principle	Rationale	Nursing actions
Goal—To substitute healthy coping responses for substance abusing behavior		
The nurse and patient should mutually define the problem and plan the nursing interventions	Motivation for change is related to recognition of a problem that is upsetting to the individual The patient must assume responsibility for his behavior Identification of predisposing and precipitating stressors must precede planning for more adaptive behavioral responses	Confront the patient with his substance abusing behavior and its consequences Assist the patient to identify his substance abuse problem Encourage the patient to agree to participate in a treatment program Involve the patient in describing situations that lead to substance abusing behavior Develop with the patient a written contract for behavioral change that is signed by the patient and nurse Assist the patient to identify and adopt healthier coping responses Consistently offer support and the expectation that the patient does have the strength to overcome his problem
Goal—To maintain safety and an optimum level of physical comfort		
Physical dependence must be managed in a safe environment with minimal withdrawal symptoms	Detoxification of the physically dependent person can be dangerous and is always uncomfortable The patient's physical safety must receive high priority for nursing intervention Withdrawal symptoms provide powerful motivation for continued substance abuse	Supportive physical care: vital signs, nutrition, hydration, seizure precautions Administer medication according to detoxification schedule Observe the patient carefully for withdrawal symptoms and report suspected withdrawal immediately
Goal—To engage social support systems in the patient's behalf		
Human support is to be substituted for dependence on chemicals **Peer confrontation and support is often more acceptable than that of professionals**	Substance abusers are often dependent and socially isolated people who use drugs to gain confidence in social situations Substance abusing behavior alienates significant others, thus increasing the person's isolation It is difficult to manipulate people who have participated in the same behaviors Social support systems must be readily available over time and acceptable to the patient	Identify and assess social support systems that are available to the patient Provide support to significant others Educate the patient and significant others about the substance abuse problem and available resources Refer the patient to appropriate resources and provide support until the patient is involved in the program.

community in terms of the services offered and the characteristics of the population that is generally served. Referral of a registered nurse who has been stealing narcotics to an inner city drug treatment program will not work. It is difficult to persuade a substance abuser to seek help at all. It is worthwhile to put forth the effort to find a treatment program that will meet the patient's needs as closely as possible.

Another potential resource for the substance abusing patient is the employee assistance program that may be part of an employee health service. Many businesses and industries have found that it is profitable for them to help substance abusing employees. These programs generally offer counseling and health education. The employee is usually required to participate in the program to retain his job. Nurses are often key staff members in employee assistance programs. The health care system has been rather slow in developing these programs for health care providers. Since there is such a high prevalence of substance abuse among nurses and physicians, there is a great need for programs that can focus on their problems. Nurses can be advocates for the establishment of employee assistance programs in the agencies where they work. Nursing interventions with patients who abuse substances are summarized in Table 14-6.

Prevention of substance abuse is an important public health problem. Nurses need to be aware of the need for primary prevention and incorporate this into their professional practice. Resnick[21] suggests several components for drug abuse prevention programs. The first is to work toward improvement of the social conditions that affect families. Strengthening of the family unit decreases the probability that a member will become involved in deviant behavior. The second component is to have an impact on the environment in which drug abuse takes place. There must be a focus on the schools, including their role in drug education. Legislative action may be needed. Another part of the prevention program is to strengthen the interpersonal and social skills of individuals. This leads to increased self-esteem and a positive self-concept, allowing the individual to resist peer pressure to use drugs. The fourth component is to create a strong network of interagency linkages. When different agencies work closely together, they can share resources and have a greater impact on the system. The final component is the sharing of resources between the federal and state governments.[21] This also helps to maximize the return on the investment of limited resources. Nurses can play an important part in developing and initiating policies that support the development of good substance abuse prevention programs.

 Evaluation

The evaluation of success in work with a substance abuse patient must be based on realistic expectations. Setting unreasonably high goals is discouraging to the nurse and the patient. For instance, it would be unrealistic to set a goal of total abstinence forever with a substance abuser. A more realistic goal would be to lengthen periods of abstinence with the hope that the patient would eventually achieve control over his behavior.

Estes, Smith-DiJulio, and Heinemann[8] have identified evaluation criteria for the treatment of alcoholics. These criteria apply to abusers of other drugs as well:

1. Has the patient been able to progress significantly toward achieving the stated goals?
2. Can the patient usually communicate without being defensive?
3. Is the patient able to react appropriately, managing the demands of daily life without use of a drug?
4. Is the patient actively involved in a variety of activities, using external social and activity resources?
5. Does the patient use internal resources to be consistently productive at work and involved in meaningful interpersonal relationships?

The evaluation process should take place at regular intervals during the course of the nurse-patient relationship.

Suggested cross-references

Therapeutic relationship skills are discussed in Chapter 3. The model of health-illness phenomena and the phases of the nursing process are discussed in Chapter 4. Interventions in social support systems are discussed in Chapter 5. Alterations in self-concept are discussed in Chapter 8. Assertiveness training is discussed in Chapter 13. Group therapy is discussed in Chapter 24. Working with adolescents is discussed in Chapter 27.

SUMMARY

1. Substance abuse was defined as the use of any mind-altering agent to such an extent that it interferes with the individual's biological, psychological, or sociocultural integrity.

2. The importance of cultural attitudes in determining the response to substance use or abuse was discussed.

3. Statistics were presented to demonstrate the prevalence and seriousness of the problem of substance abuse.

4. Categories of drugs that are frequently abused were described.

5. Substance abuse is a very serious problem among nurses and physicians.

6. Substance abuse was illustrated in terms of the health-illness continuum.

7. Biological, psychological, and sociocultural stressors relative to substance abuse were described. There is no agreement on the existence of a specific stressor or set of stressors that is always present when substance abuse occurs.

8. A comparison of the various categories of abused substances was done, including the usual route of administration, expected behavioral manifestations, behaviors related to overdose, and withdrawal syndromes.

9. Nursing diagnosis of the substance abusing patient was discussed relative to the stage of drug-using behavior, specific substance used, and relevant stressors.

10. Goal setting must be realistic, taking into account the need for multiple short-term goals to enable the patient to experience success.

11. The biological aspects of nursing intervention included attending to physiological needs, detoxification, drug overdose, management of acute toxic psychosis, biofeedback, methadone treatment for opiate abusers, and disulfiram treatment for alcoholics.

12. Interactive interventions include peer group discussions, role play, patient education, and individual counseling.

13. Common themes in therapy with substance abuse patients include denial, dependency, low self-esteem, manipulation, and anger.

14. Social support systems for substance abusers include families, self-help groups, transitional living programs, drug treatment programs, and employee assistance programs.

15. Five components of drug abuse prevention programs were presented.

16. Evaluation of nursing care was described in terms of five questions to be asked about the behaviors of the patient.

References

1. American Psychiatric Association: Diagnostic and statistical manual of mental disorders, ed. 3, Washington, D.C., 1980, The Association.

2. Ausubel, D.P.: An interactional approach to narcotic addiction. In Lettieri, D.J., Sayers, M., and Pearson, H.W., editors: Theories on drug abuse: selected contemporary perspectives, NIDA Research Monograph 30, Rockville, Md., 1980, National Institute on Drug Abuse.

3. Butz, R.H.: Intoxication and withdrawal. In Estes, N.J., and Heinemann, M.E., editors: Alcoholism: development, consequences, and interventions, ed. 2, St. Louis, 1982, The C.V. Mosby Co.

4. Chein, I.: Psychological, social and epidemiological factors in juvenile drug abuse. In Lettieri, D.J., Sayers, M., and Pearson, H.W., editors: Theories on drug abuse: selected contemporary perspectives, NIDA Research Monograph 30, Rockville, Md., 1980, National Institute on Drug Abuse.

5. Demarest, M.: Cocaine: middle class high, Time **118:**56, July 6, 1981.

6. Dusek, D., and Girdano, D.A.: Drugs: a factual account, Reading, Mass., 1980, Addison-Wesley Publishing Co., Inc.

7. Estes, N.J., and Heinemann, M.E.: Alcoholism: development, consequences, and interventions, ed. 2, St. Louis, 1982, The C.V. Mosby Co.

8. Estes, N.J., Smith-DiJulio, K., and Heinemann, M.E.: Nursing diagnosis of the alcoholic person, St. Louis, 1980, The C.V. Mosby Co.

9. Freedman, A.M.: Opiate dependence. In Kaplan, H.I., Freedman, A.M., and Sadock, B.J., editors: Comprehensive textbook of psychiatry, ed. 3, Baltimore, 1980, The Williams & Wilkins Co.

10. Gold, S.R.: The CAP control theory of drug abuse. In Lettieri, D.J., Sayers, M., and Pearson, H.W., editors: Theories on drug abuse: selected contemporary perspectives, NIDA Research Monograph 30, Rockville, Md., 1980, National Institute on Drug Abuse.

11. Goodwin, D.W.: The bad-habit theory of drug abuse. In Lettieri, D.J., Sayers, M., and Pearson, H.W., editors: Theories on drug abuse: selected contemporary perspectives, NIDA Research Monograph 30, Rockville, Md., 1980, National Institute on Drug Abuse.

12. Greaves, G.B.: An existential theory of drug dependence. In Lettieri, D.J., Sayers, M., and Pearson, H.W., editors: Theories on drug abuse: selected contemporary perspectives, NIDA Research Monograph 30, Rockville, Md., 1980, National Institute on Drug Abuse.

13. Grinspoon, L., and Bakalar, J.B.: Drug dependence: nonnarcotic agents. In Kaplan, H.I., Freedman, A.M., and Sadock, B.J., editors: Comprehensive textbook of

psychiatry, ed. 3, Baltimore, 1980, The Williams & Wilkins Co.

14. Huberty, D.J., and Malmquist, J.D.: Adolescent chemical dependency, Perspect. Psychiatr. Care **16:**21, Jan.-Feb. 1978.

15. Hughes, R., and Brewin, R.: The tranquilizing of America: pill popping and the American way of life, New York, 1979, Harcourt, Brace, Jovanovich, Inc.

16. Isler, C.: The alcoholic nurse: what we try to deny, R.N. **41:**48, July 1978.

17. Jellinek, E.M.: Phases of alcohol addiction, Q. J. Stud. Alcohol **13:**672, 1952.

18. Johnston, L.D., Backman, J.G., and O'Malley, P.M.: Drugs and the class of '78: behaviors, attitudes and recent national trends, Rockville, Md., 1979, National Institute on Drug Abuse.

19. Miller, J.D., and Cisin, I.H.: Highlights from the national survey on drug abuse: 1979, Rockville, Md., 1980, Department of Health and Human Services.

20. Ray, O.S.: Drugs, society, and human behavior, ed. 3, St. Louis, 1982, The C.V. Mosby Co.

21. Resnick, H.S.: It starts with people: experiences in drug abuse prevention, Rockville, Md., 1978, Department of Health, Education, and Welfare.

22. Seixas, F.A.: The course of alcoholism. In Estes, N.J.,

and Heinemann, M.E., editors: Alcoholism: development, consequences, and interventions, ed. 2, St. Louis, 1982, The C.V. Mosby Co.

23. Selzer, M.L.: Alcoholism and alcoholic psychoses. In Kaplan, H.I., Freedman, A.M., and Sadock, B.J., editors: Comprehensive textbook of psychiatry, ed. 3, Baltimore, 1980, The Williams & Wilkins Co.

24. Snyder, S.H.: Opiate receptors and internal opiates, Sci. Am. **236**(3):44, 1977.

25. Stanton, M.D.: A family theory of drug abuse. In Lettieri, D.J., Sayers, M., and Pearson, H.W., editors: Theories on drug abuse: selected contemporary perspectives, NIDA Research Monograph 30, Rockville, Md., 1980, National Institute on Drug Abuse.

26. Vourakis, C., and Bennett, G.: Angel dust: not heaven sent, Am. J. Nurs. **79:**649, 1979.

27. Wurmser, L.: Drug use as a protective system. In Lettieri, D.J., Sayers, M., and Pearson, H.W., editors: Theories on drug abuse: selected contemporary perspectives, NIDA Research Monograph 30, Rockville, Md., 1980, National Institute on Drug Abuse.

Annotated suggested readings

Betemps, E.: Management of the withdrawal syndrome of barbiturates and other central nervous system depressants, J. Psychiatr. Nurs. **17:**31, Sept. 1981.

This excellent article provides information on recognition and nursing management of withdrawal from central nervous system depressant drugs. It includes a system for judging the seriousness of impending withdrawal. The detoxification process is discussed in detail.

Brink, P.J.: Rehabilitating heroin addicts, J. Psychiatr. Nurs. **12:**14, Nov.-Dec. 1974.

This is an interesting discussion of the process of "turning on" and "turning off" to drugs. It identifies several personality styles that seem prone to drug abuse. There is a good description of the various types of rehabilitation programs.

Celentano, D.D., McQueen, D.V., and Chee, E.: Substance abuse by women: a review of the epidemiologic literature, J. Chron. Dis. **33**(6):383, 1980.

These authors reviewed the research literature pertaining to substance abuse by women. They found that very little research has been done on "substance abuse" as opposed to drug or alcohol abuse and still less explores the problem in the female population. Several areas for research are identified. This article would be very useful to the graduate student or the nurse researcher who is interested in investigating substance abuse.

Dusek, D., and Girdano, D.A.: Drugs: a factual account, Reading, Mass., 1980, Addison-Wesley Publishing Co., Inc.

This book provides a wealth of information about the use and abuse of alcohol and other drugs. It provides a good overview of the scope of the problem, including information on risk factors and epidemiological data.

Elaine, B., et al.: Helping the nurse who misuses drugs, Am. J. Nurs. **74:**1665, 1974.

This article is highly recommended reading for all nurses. The issue of drug abuse by nurses is confronted directly. The authors are four nurses who have abused drugs. They provide practical information about drugs that are frequently abused, recognition of the substance abusing nurse and confrontation. Also included are autobiographical accounts of each author's experiences with drug abuse and recovery.

Estes, N.J., and Heinemann, M.E., editors: Alcoholism: development, consequences, and interventions, ed. 2, St. Louis, 1982, The C.V. Mosby Co.

This edited volume provides an extremely comprehensive survey of current literature on alcoholism. The broad spectrum of topics make this a useful resource book. In addition, it is interesting reading.

Estes, N.J., Smith-DiJulio, K., and Heinemann, M.E.: Nursing diagnosis of the alcoholic person, St. Louis, 1980, The C.V. Mosby Co.

This book is highly recommended as a nursing reference on alcoholism. The authors are experienced in providing nursing care to alcoholic patients. They have used a nursing process framework to discuss nursing care. Of particular interest is the inclusion of interviewing guides and tools that may be used in the assessment of the alcoholic patient.

Fultz, J.M., Jr. et al.: When a narcotic addict is hospitalized, Am. J. Nurs. **80:**478, 1980.

The authors pay particular attention to the legal ramifications of treating a patient who is addicted to narcotics. Methadone maintenance and withdrawal are clearly discussed. Signs and symptoms of opiate withdrawal and opiate overdose are described.

Gareri, E.: Assertiveness training for alcoholics, J. Psychiatr. Nurs. **17:**31, Jan. 1979.

This article discusses the relationship between lack of assertiveness and alcohol abuse and describes an assertiveness training group specifically for alcoholics.

Huberty, D.J., and Malmquist, J.D.: Adolescent chemical dependency, Perspect. Psychiatr. Care **16:**21, Jan.-Feb. 1978.

This article relates the developmental tasks of adolescence to drug-abusing behavior. It includes a discussion of recovery as well. The authors compare the family process when a teenage member abuses drugs to Kübler-Ross' stages of death and dying.

Jaffe, S.: First-hand views of recovery, Am. J. Nurs. **82**:578, 1982.

The author describes her experience in treating a group of nurses who were alcoholics. She addresses issues that concern substance-abusing nurses in particular. This article is recommended as a means of sensitizing nurses to the needs of their addicted colleagues.

Jefferson, L.V., and Ensor, B.E.: Confronting a chemically impaired colleague, Am. J. Nurs. **82**:574, 1982.

This article applies concepts related to substance abuse to the addicted nurse. Case studies are used to illustrate the characteristics of drug- and alcohol-abusing nurses. The authors describe clues that should lead one to suspect the presence of substance abuse. Of particular importance is the section on intervention, including advice concerning confrontation of a nurse colleague who may be alcoholic or abusing drugs. This is highly recommended reading for all nurses.

Lettieri, D.J., Sayers, M., and Pearson, H.W., editors: Theories on drug abuse: selected contemporary perspectives, NIDA Research Monograph 30, Rockville, Md., 1980, National Institute on Drug Abuse.

This publication includes reports of a number of research studies exploring the causes of substance abuse. It is recommended for a reader who wishes to explore theories about predisposing factors and stressors in greater depth. An ability to critique research is also helpful.

McCoy, S., Rice, M.J., and McFadden, K.: PCP intoxication: psychiatric issues of nursing care, J. Psychiatr. Nurs. **19**: 17, July 1981.

This is an excellent article that provides a wealth of information relative to PCP intoxication. Patient behaviors and related nursing interventions are presented in depth and with clarity. This would be a worthwhile reference to keep close at hand in any setting providing health care services to adolescents and young adults.

Michael, M.M., and Sewall, K.S.: Use of the adolescent peer group to increase the self-care agency of adolescent alcohol abusers, Nurs. Clin. North Am. **15**:157, March 1980.

This publication provides a good example of the application of a particular conceptual model to a specific therapeutic modality. They used a reality therapy approach in a group setting with adolescent drug abusing patients. This article is especially recommended for experienced nurse therapists who are interested in exploring an innovative therapeutic approach.

Morgan, A.J., and Moreno, J.W.: Attitudes toward addiction, Am. J. Nurs. **73**:497, 1973

This article should be particularly helpful to the inexperienced nurse who needs help in analyzing her own feelings about working with addicted patients. It presents many of the realities of drug addiction that may be hard to handle emotionally.

Personatt, J.D.: Couples therapy: treatment of choice with the drug addict, J. Psychiatr. Nurs. **16**:18, Jan. 1978.

The author reviews several group treatment modalities and assesses the appropriateness of each for the drug abuser. She then describes a couples group which she co-led and states her belief that the family can provide the best support for a drug abuser who is trying to become drug free. This is a good example of an appropriate role for a clinical nurse specialist in a drug abuse program.

Pisarcik, G.: Management of phencyclidine toxicity, J. Emerg. Nurs. **4**:35, Sept.-Oct. 1978.

This article is recommended for nurses who are likely to have contact with patients experiencing toxic reactions to PCP. It includes a very clear description of the behaviors characteristic of this condition. There is also a practical discussion of nursing intervention.

Ray, O.S.: Drugs, society, and human behavior, ed. 3, St. Louis, 1982, The C.V. Mosby Co.

This book is highly recommended as a basic resource on all aspects of chemical dependency. In addition to discussion of the relevant psychosocial factors, there is also presentation of the pharmacological aspects.

Symposium on alcohol and drug abuse, Nurs. Clin. North Am. **11**:479, 1976.

This symposium includes several excellent articles pertaining to nursing care of drug- and alcohol-abusing patients. It is highly recommended as an overview of current thinking about chemical dependency.

Szasz, T.: Ceremonial chemistry, New York, 1974, Doubleday & Co., Inc.

In this provocative book, the author looks at drug use from a cultural point of view. He presents the case that drug "abuse" is culturally defined and serves the purpose of providing society with a group of scapegoats. He views the use of drugs as a type of religious observance in terms of its significance to the user. This is a thought-provoking work that forces one to reassess attitudes about drug use and abuse.

Van Gee, S.J.: Alcoholism and the family: a psychodrama approach, J. Psychiatr. Nurs. **17**:9, Aug. 1979.

This article describes the enabler role of the wives of alcoholics. Intervention into the spouse's behavior can have impact on the alcoholic. Wives frequently overcompensate, becoming dominant and making all the decisions. Psychodrama can assist her to refuse to be an enabler.

Vourakis, C., and Bennett, G.: Angel dust: not heaven sent, Am. J. Nurs. **79**:649, 1979.

This excellent article presents a thorough overview of the manifestations of PCP use and related nursing care. The authors organize the presentation of theory around a primary, secondary, and tertiary prevention model. There is also a discussion of the pharmacological characteristics of the drug.

Westermeyer, J.: A primer on chemical dependency: a clinical guide to alcohol and drug problems, Baltimore, 1976, The Williams & Wilkins Co.

This book provides a good overview of the range of chemical dependency problems. It is recommended for the person who needs a general reference on the nature of substance abuse. Clinical case studies are included to illustrated the theoretical material.

CHAPTER 15

SOMATIC
THERAPIES AND
PSYCHIATRIC
NURSING

Canst thou not minister to a mind diseas'd,
Pluck from the memory a rooted sorrow,
Raze out the written troubles of the brain,
And with some sweet oblivious antidote
Cleanse the stuff'd bosom of the perilous stuff
Which weighs upon the heart?

William Shakespeare, Macbeth, Act V

Learning objectives

After studying this chapter, the student
will be able to:

- state reasons for the use of physical restraint of patients, including mechanical restraints and seclusion.

- discuss the nursing care of a patient who is in restraints or seclusion.

- identify issues associated with psychosurgical treatment.

- describe the nursing care of a patient receiving electroconvulsive therapy, including patient education, patient care during the treatment and recovery period, and assessment of the patient's response to the treatment.

- analyze legal and ethical issues related to the use of restraint, seclusion, psychosurgery, and electroconvulsive therapy.

- compare and contrast the major groups of psychotropic medications in terms of indications for use, usual dosage, expected actions and side effects, and contraindications.

- describe nursing considerations relative to medicating special groups of psychiatric patients, including individuals who are suspicious, dependent, suicidal, and noncompliant.

- identify potentially harmful interactions between psychotropic medications and other substances.

- identify suggested readings for further study.

In the past, many somatic treatments have been used in psychiatric settings. As research into the pathophysiology of mental illness continues, it is likely that more and increasingly sophisticated somatic treatment modalities will be developed. Psychopharmacology has exploded in importance over the last 25 years and yet has far to go in identifying specific agents for specific problems, based on a well-defined mechanism of action. At the same time, treatment modalities such as restraint, which was among the earliest means of providing nursing care for psychiatric patients, are still used. Psychiatric nursing therapy, like psychiatry, is in a time of transition. Old therapies are being reassed and reconsidered. New therapies are being discovered and investigated. Nurses will be important contributors to the growth of knowledge in this area and need to scientifically study the effectiveness of the various somatic therapies.

The treatment modalities described in this chapter are presented in a way that should also provide some historical perspective regarding the progression of knowledge in this area of psychiatric care. Although several treatment forms may have been used by clinicians at a given time, generally one form was more frequently used than others. Few therapies of the past have been totally abandoned. There also seems to be a tendency for relatively unused treatments to be repopularized. Therefore some treatments that are rarely used today, such as insulin coma therapy, are presented briefly. The emphasis in all cases will be on the nursing implications applicable to the treatment described. However, since some treatments and medications are viewed as specific to certain psychiatric diagnostic categories, there will be reference to these diagnoses, and parts of the chapter will incorporate the medical model more heavily than do other portions of this book.

Use of physical restraints

Physical restraint was one of the earliest means used to try to cope with people who were unable to control their behavior. Prior to the early nineteenth century, shackles and fetters were used to control the "insane" in "asylums." Some persons spent years bound hand and foot or chained to the wall. Small wonder that families tried to keep disturbed members at home.

Modifications in these practices took place after Philippe Pinel campaigned for humane treatment of the mentally ill in France. Similar objectives were pursued in this country by Benjamin Rush and Dorothea Lynde Dix. Gradually the chains fell into disuse. However, other forms of physical restraint, including camisoles ("straitjackets"), sheet restraints, wrist and ankle restraints, sheet packs, and seclusion were commonly used until the advent of the convulsive therapies and psychopharmacotherapy. Good psychiatric nursing care was essential to humanize what could be a dehumanizing experience.

It is still necessary at times to physically restrain patients. In this era of increasing sensitivity to civil liberties and the rights of the individual, restraint should be used with great discretion. The discussion in Chapter 16 of the legal aspects of psychiatric nursing is pertinent here. When restraint is absolutely necessary as a last resort for the protection of the patient or others from harm, good nursing care is a necessity and a great challenge.

Mechanical restraints

Mechanical restraints include camisoles, wrist restraints, ankle restraints, sheet restraints, and sheet packs. Any of these measures should be applied only with a physician's order. The patient should be released from restraints as soon as any dangerous behavior has subsided or other less drastic means of restraint such as medication become effective. Nursing care of patients with restraints other than sheet packs will be discussed first. Care of patients in packs differs slightly and will be discussed separately.

Prevention of restraint is the emphasis of Rosen and DiGiacomo.[20] They recommend that informed consent for the use of restraints be obtained from the patient and family at the time of admission to the psychiatric unit. Verbal intervention and medication should be attempted before physical restraints are introduced. They have found that failure to respond to alternative approaches is generally related to one of several factors, including failure by the staff to respond soon enough, failure to explain what is planned or expected, ambivalent or hostile staff attitudes, and approaches by staff who are unfamiliar to the patient. They also describe several reasons for using physical restraint with psychiatric patients: violence directed toward the self or others; agitated behavior when medication is contraindicated, for example, a delirious patient; hyperactivity accompanied by regressed socially unacceptable behavior that alienates others; refusal to meet basic biological needs for rest and nutrition, resulting in the threat of physical collapse; the need for decreased stimuli, mutually determined by the patient and the therapist; and the patient's request if it does not represent an untherapeutic need for dependency and regression.

The patient in mechanical restraint may be confused or delirious and will probably be frightened at the limitation of movement. The nurse should not assume that the patient understands the need for restraint. Support and reassurance are essential. Restraints should be applied efficiently and with care not to injure a combative patient. Adequate personnel need to be assembled before the patient is approached and should be assigned responsibility for controlling specific body parts. Restraints should be available and in working order. Padding of cuff restraints helps to prevent skin breakdown. For the same reason, the patient should be positioned in anatomical alignment. Provision of privacy is important. If visitors are allowed, an explanation of the treatment and the reason for it before they see the patient may help them accept the situation. Physical needs must be included in the nursing care plan. Vital signs should be checked. Regular observation of circulation in the extremities is necessary. Fluids should be offered regularly and opportunities for elimination provided. Skin care is also essential. Restraints must be released at least every 2 hours to allow exercise of the extremities. Good nursing care and the communication of concern for the patient will contribute to better behavioral control. Immobilization for any reason is physically hazardous and should be avoided whenever possible.

Whaley and Ramirez[24] recommend that restraints or seclusion be terminated when a therapeutic alliance with the patient has been established and violent behavior has subsided. Release should be gradual with intervals out of restraints increased over time.

Cold, wet sheet packs may be ordered occasionally for extremely disturbed patients who are refractory to treatment with medication. In this procedure the patient is immobilized by being wrapped mummy fashion in several layers of linens. The innermost layer of sheets is soaked in ice water. The patient is in a bed with a waterproof mattress and dressed in a hospital nightgown. The sheets are wrapped so that no skin surfaces are in contact, since this could cause chafing and perhaps skin breakdown. The wet sheets are covered by layers of blankets, preferably wool. Although the pack is initially experienced as very cold, it quickly becomes warmed by the patient's body heat, which is retained in the pack. The combination of the warmth, wetness, and swaddling are very soothing and can have a calming effect on even extremely agitated patients. A patient in a pack needs constant nursing observation. Temperature, pulse, and respirations should be monitored, and the pack should be discontinued with any significant change in vital signs. The patient will perspire and fluids should be offered frequently. Soothing verbal contact may be helpful, but the environment should be quiet and conducive to rest. In general, the patient should remain in the pack for about 2 hours. Maximum calming does not usually occur in less than this time, but hazards of immobility increase as the duration of restraint increases. When the pack is removed, the skin should be thoroughly towel dried and skin care given. Privacy should, of course, be provided throughout the procedure.

Seclusion, or isolation

A patient who is restrained by the use of seclusion is confined alone in a single room. Degrees of seclusion may range from confinement in a room with a closed but unlocked door to a locked room with a mattress without linens on the floor, limited opportunity for communication, and with the patient dressed in a hospital nightgown or a heavy canvas coverall. The latter are minimally acceptable conditions for seclusion, which is to be used only when essential for the protection of the patient or others.

Seclusion is prescribed for a number of reasons. It may be used as a means of controlling the behavior of a patient who has been acting destructively and cannot be controlled by interpersonal contact, either physical or verbal. Seclusion is often helpful to patients who are hyperactive and extremely responsive to environmental stimuli. Sometimes these patients will ask to be isolated for a period of time and this should be allowed. Behavior modification protocols sometimes include seclusion as a negative reinforcer. This use of seclusion borders on punishment and should be used judiciously.

Guthiel[14] has identified three theoretical bases for the use of seclusion. The first is containment. This implies that the patient is at immediate risk for causing harm to himself or others. Seclusion protects him from this danger until his internal behavioral controls have been re-established. He is also protected from the guilt that would potentially be experienced as a result of loss of control. Another theoretical base concerns isolation. The patient is relieved of the burden of needing to relate interpersonally. There is a limitation on the amount of space available to the patient. allowing him to master a reasonable area before being confronted with the need to relate appropriately in the setting of the whole ward. The last concept is that of a decrease in sensory input. Seclusion may be calming to a person who is hyperalert and feeling bombarded by the many sensory stimuli that occur in the hospital environment.[14]

When the decision has been made to place a patient in isolation, the procedure should be carried out quickly and in a manner that demonstrates concern for the patient's dignity. The room should be prepared before the patient is approached. The plan and the reason for seclusion should be explained to the patient. A combative patient will probably not agree to be secluded; if this is the situation, it is essential to have adequate personnel present to carry out the procedure with minimal danger of injury to the patient or others. Any items of clothing or possessions that could be harmful to the person should be removed and placed in safekeeping.

Legal requirements for the care of the secluded patient vary from state to state and are minimal at best. Good nursing care should always provide for optimal fulfillment of basic human needs and concern for the dignity of the person. The nurse must assist the patient to meet biological needs by providing food and fluids, a comfortable environment, and opportunity for use of the bathroom. Frequent observation is essential, and the room must be constructed so the patient can be observed without being unnecessarily exposed to those who are not involved in his care. There should also be a means provided to allow communication with the patient. Careful records should be kept of all nursing care and observation of the isolated patient. The need for continued isolation should be assessed on a regular basis. It may be necessary for the nurse to initiate this review of the patient's condition with other health team members.

Whenever the use of seclusion has been re-quired, the nursing staff should review the events that led up to the decision to undertake this means of treatment.

Several negative effects of the injudicious use of seclusion have been identified.[14] One is the jealousy other patients might feel over the attention given to the patient who has needed seclusion. This has been termed *seclusion envy*. Another potential problem is the creation of a lasting rift between the staff and the patient who was secluded. This will occur if the patient does not understand or agree with the reason for the procedure. The use of seclusion for the wrong reasons can also lead to negative consequences. Seclusion should not be used as a punishment or as a way to relieve the staff of the care of a demanding patient. Secluded patients require frequent and intensive nursing care.

Timely nursing intervention before loss of control occurs can often avert the need for seclusion of an agitated patient. Spending time with the patient may be helpful. Sometimes the energy of agitation can be channeled into nondestructive physical activity. If a patient is angry and feels misunderstood, an effort to understand may avoid an explosion. Medication may also be useful in calming a patient if it is given in time. Allowing a patient to be alone without being forcibly isolated may also be helpful at times. Careful nursing assessment and the establishment of a trusting nurse-patient relationship are a good foundation for deciding on an effective plan of action when a patient becomes upset. Any form of physical restraint should be used as a last resort when other nursing interventions have been tried and failed.

Psychosurgery

Psychosurgery refers to the surgical interruption of selected neural pathways that involve the transmission of emotional impulses in the brain. First introduced in 1936, the early operations were referred to as lobotomies because the focus of the surgical intervention was the pathway from the thalamus to the frontal lobes of the cerebral cortex. These surgical procedures were nonspecific because of the limited knowledge at that time of brain functioning. Extensive personality change was almost inevitably a result of surgery. A nursing article from that era describes vividly the deterioration in social skills that resulted from psychosurgery and the retraining which became an integral part of the nursing care for these patients.[11] Because of the pervasive influence on the individual's ability to function adequately, the procedure was most often done as a last resort and fell into relative disuse following the introduction of new psychopharmacological agents.

Recently, however, there has been a resurgence of interest in psychosurgery as knowledge of neuroanatomy and physiology has become increasingly more sophisticated. Progress has been made in "mapping" the cortex, which has led to the possibility of the surgeon being more able to isolate and sever tracts that relate more directly to the patient's individual behavioral problem. Technology has also contributed sophisticated surgical tools, such as lasers, which cause far less generalized tissue damage. Proponents of this approach now claim that psychosurgery can be beneficial to patients who are unresponsive to other forms of therapy with minimized damage to the personality and to social functioning. Patients who benefit from various types of psychosurgery are those with chronic neurotic and chronic depressive behaviors. Contrary to the practice of the past, schizophrenic patients are not good candidates because of their basically inadequate personality structure.[10]

The nursing care of the psychosurgical patient will not be discussed in detail here, since it is more pertinent to the specialty of neurosurgical nursing. However, the nurse should be aware that the major effect of surgery is on the *emotional* component of the patient's behavior. Intelligence is not affected. Also, the patient may continue to have some preoperative symptoms, such as hallucinations, but will not have the same emotional response, thus facilitating improved functioning in activities of daily living.

The renewal of interest in this form of therapy has raised moral and ethical questions for many professionals relative to the issue of mind control. Although other somatic therapies, such as pharmacotherapy and the convulsive therapies, undoubtedly exert some degree of control over the person's thought process, psychosurgery seems to many to be more drastic because it is permanent and irreversible. Nervous tissue, once damaged, does not regenerate. These questions arise particularly when psychosurgery is suggested as a possible treatment for antisocial and violent behavior, such as murder and rape. The responsible professional nurse must form independent opinions about such issues, collecting facts and objective data. Knowledge about the functioning of the brain is in a period of rapid growth. Therefore forms of therapy such as psychosurgery will also be changing and improving. An open mind is an asset in evaluating varied approaches to the treatment of psychiatric disorders.

Electroconvulsive therapy

Electroconvulsive therapy (ECT), also referred to as electric shock therapy (EST), was first described by Cerletti and Bini in 1938 as a treatment for schizophrenia. At that time it was believed that epileptics were rarely schizophrenic and hypothesized that convulsions would cure schizophrenia. Later research did not support this hypothesis. Further experience with ECT demonstrated that it is much more effective as a treatment for affective disturbances than it is for schizophrenia. It has also been noted that epilepsy and schizophrenia do occur concurrently. ECT is now most frequently used as a treatment for severe depression.

ECT is a treatment in which a grand mal seizure is artificially induced by passing an electrical current through electrodes applied to the temples. The electrodes are generally applied bilaterally, although some therapists have used unilateral electrodes and claim that patients treated in this way experience less confusion. For the treatment to be effective, a grand mal seizure must occur. The voltage is generally adjusted to the minimum level that will produce the therapeutic effect. The number of treatments given in a series varies according to the patient's presenting problem and therapeutic response as assessed during the course of treatment. The most common range for affective disorders is from 6 to 10 treatments, whereas as many as 20 to 30 may be given for schizophrenia. ECT is most commonly given three times a week on alternate days, although it can be given daily or more than once a day. Recently some therapists have been using multiple ECT in which several convulsions are induced immediately following each other. The proponents of this approach claim greater therapeutic effectiveness with no increase in confusion or untoward responses seen in the patient. However, the American Psychiatric Association has refused to endorse this practice.[1]

Nursing intervention

Nursing intervention with a patient who is to receive ECT begins as soon as the individual and family are presented with this treatment alternative. Most people respond emotionally when told that they or a loved one needs "shock therapy." When discussing the subject with them, one should talk about "treatment" and avoid unnecessary use of the term "shock." This places the emphasis on the therapeutic value of the procedure. However, people also need an opportunity to express their feelings about ECT. Fear is usually present. Many people have heard or read about or seen movies portraying ECT. Many of these are done in a sensationalistic manner, emphasizing the frightening aspect of the experience. Also, the very idea of an electric current passing through their head causes fear in most people. The nurse must assess the patient's response and provide opportunity for communication. As the patient reveals feelings and concerns, the nurse can listen for misconceptions and clarify information about which the patient is confused. The very act of discussing ECT openly and directly communicates the attitude that it is a usual method of treatment, without undue risk. However, as with any procedure requiring general anesthesia, there is a degree of risk. Therefore the patient is asked to sign a consent form indicating that he has been fully informed about the procedure and the risks involved.

When the patient has had an opportunity to express feelings to a receptive person, teaching about the procedure of ECT should take place. Learning will be facilitated when the patient's anxiety is slightly increased but not overwhelming. Some information will probably have been given to the patient by the physician at the time informed consent was obtained. However, a thorough review by the nurse is recommended to reinforce what the patient already knows, remind him of what was forgotten, and provide an opportunity for questions. Enough time should be provided to create a relaxed atmosphere conducive to a free exchange of communication. The nurse should also be observant for nonverbal cues of the patient's response to the teaching. Asking the patient to repeat what has been explained also helps identify areas of confusion.

Much of the nursing procedure related to ECT is similar to that which is needed when a patient undergoes surgery. The patient is not given anything orally after midnight when ECT is scheduled for the morning. One exception to this may be to give prescribed sedation with a small amount of water to a patient who has dif-

ficulty sleeping. Prior to the treatment the patient is asked to remove jewelry, hairpins, eyeglasses, and hearing aids. Full dentures may be removed. Partial plates should be left in the mouth to provide even pressure on the teeth and jaw during the tonic phase of the convulsion.[4] Dress should be loose and comfortable, usually bed clothing. The bladder should be emptied. The patient awaiting ECT should also be accompanied by a trusted, understanding nurse staff member. Under no circumstances should a patient waiting for ECT see another patient during or immediately following a treatment.

In the early days of ECT no medication was given prior to the administration of the shock. Therefore the individual experienced a full-blown, and frequently violent, grand mal convulsion. Although the patient was amnesic for the convulsive episode, it was a frightening experience. Some complications, particularly fractures and dislocations, were also associated with the unmedicated procedure. Current American Psychiatric Association standards unequivocally state that ECT should be given under general anesthesia with the use of a muscle relaxant drug.[1] The patient therefore has no memory of the procedure and the convulsion occurs in an attenuated form. This change has also resulted in the involvement of an anesthesiologist as a member of the treatment team.

The following medications are commonly given prior to ECT:

1. Atropine sulfate is administered for its vagolytic effect.[4] It is frequently given subcutaneously or intramuscularly 30 minutes prior to treatment but is most effective when given intravenously with the other premedications.

2. A short-acting barbiturate such as sodium methohexital (Brevital Sodium) is administered intravenously to induce anesthesia.

3. Succinylcholine chloride (Anectine), a muscle relaxant, is administered intravenously after the anesthetic. If it is given prior to the anesthetic, the patient will feel paralyzed. The inability to breathe resulting from paralysis of the respiratory muscles can be very frightening and may be remembered after the treatment. The face and extremities are observed for muscle fasciculations, which indicate that the muscle relaxant has taken effect. Some authorities recommend isolating one extremity from the general circulation by the use of a tourniquet or blood pressure cuff before administration of the muscle relaxant. This limb can then be observed for unmodified seizure activity when the ECT is given.

These medications may be injected directly

into the vein or through the tubing of a previously started intravenous (IV) infusion. The advantage of the latter route is that the IV line is in place should complications arise during the procedure.

ECT may be given in the operating room or in an especially equipped room in the inpatient or outpatient psychiatric setting. It is a nursing responsibility to check all emergency equipment, including oxygen, suction, and cardiac resuscitation equipment prior to ECT. The ECT machine and IV equipment, if used, should also be in readiness.

The patient lies supine on a bed or cot. Usually, 100% oxygen is administered for 1 to 2 minutes while an IV infusion is being started. This hyperoxygenation prepares the patient for the period of apnea that will result from the muscle relaxant and the convulsion. The patient will also need reassurance while these preparations take place. The medications are then administered. As soon as muscle paralysis has occurred, the treatment is given. Electrodes are placed on the temples or on the nondominant side temple for unilateral ECT. A mouth gag is inserted between the teeth, and the jaw is gently supported. There is no need to restrain the limbs. The shock is administered. The fingers and toes are watched carefully for a rhythmic twitching, which is the only visible evidence that a grand mal convulsion has occurred. When the twitching has stopped, oxygen is given by bag-breathing the patient through a mask until spontaneous respiration resumes.

During the period immediately after ECT the patient requires close nursing observation in a recovery area. Emergency equipment should be readily available, although adverse reactions are rare. While unconscious, the patient should receive the same nursing care as is required by any comatose patient. A patent airway must be maintained. Occasionally, suctioning may be required to remove excessive secretions from the mouth and throat. Positioning should be on the side to prevent aspiration of secretions or in the event of vomiting. Blood pressure, pulse, and respirations should be monitored closely until the patient has fully reacted.

The patient will generally begin to respond after 10 to 15 minutes. Some drowsiness will be experienced even after the anesthesia wears off. When the patient responds to his name, the nurse should provide orientation to time, place, and situation. Most patients are confused immediately following a treatment and become frightened if they are not oriented. Since ECT is frequently given in the morning, the patient

may not remember getting out of bed and preparing for the treatment and may assume that something happened to him during the night while he was asleep. Following is an example of this type of disorientation:

One patient, who was receiving ECT in the operating room, began to talk about people "cutting on" him and suspected that one of his fingers had been removed and another sewn on in its place. This was viewed as his attempt to make sense of a situation about which he was confused. He responded well to an explanation that he did indeed go to the operating room but received a treatment other than surgery when he was there. It was further explained that the treatment was for his depression.

Orientation may need to be repeated several times following ECT. It must also be repeated every time the patient has a treatment because confusion may occur each time and for some persons becomes more severe as they have more treatments. This is particularly true for older persons, who may already have some organic brain changes associated with aging.

When vital signs are stable, the patient should be assisted to ambulate. Postural hypotension sometimes occurs, and it is wise to check the blood pressure and pulse in sitting and standing positions before allowing the patient to walk.

On occasion, a patient may become quite agitated as consciousness returns. These persons should be restrained gently to prevent injury. Forceful restraint increases the agitation by frightening the patient. The period of agitation is usually brief. However, it does tend to recur after each treatment. An injection of an antianxiety agent such as hydroxyzine hydrochloride (Vistaril) 30 minutes prior to ECT may alleviate this problem. There is no way to predict prior to the first treatment how a patient will respond during the recovery phase.

When the patient is ambulatory, he may be returned to his own bed and allowed to sleep for about an hour if he wishes. A light breakfast with others who have had ECT is often reassuring and helps orient the patient to the beginning of the day. Patients should then be included in the usual hospital routine. Resumption of normal activity soon after treatment places it in proper perspective as one part of the patient's therapy and not incapacitating.

As stated, confusion may persist to varying extents following the treatment. Nurses must be sensitive to this and provide needed orientation. There may also be some amnesia for the period of time just prior to beginning ECT, which usually subsides gradually after the course of treatment is completed. This may also be frightening to the patient who may fear that he is "losing his mind." Reassurance can be very helpful to these people. Observations about the degree of confusion the patient exhibits should also be reported to the physician, who can sometimes minimize the problem by decreasing the frequency or modifying the technique of administering the ECT.

Some physical discomfort is frequently experienced after ECT. Most patients have a headache ranging from mild to severe. An analgesic should be included in routine ECT orders. Nursing assessment of the patient should include an inquiry about headache, since the patient may be confused about who to ask for medication. There is no need to be concerned about creating a headache when there is none, since the majority of patients do develop one. Analgesia after ECT also helps relieve any muscle soreness. Occasionally, patients also complain of nausea, which is readily relieved by the administration of an antiemetic medication such as trimethobenzamide (Tigan) or prochlorperazine (Compazine).

The amount of information about the actual treatment that is shared with the patient by the nurse should be individualized, based on the patient's ability to understand, his anxiety level, and coping mechanisms. Some people become less anxious when they know and understand a great deal about an anxiety-provoking situation. Others want to know only generalities. It is the nurse's responsibility to assess this prior to initiating patient teaching.

The family should also be included in teaching. At times, when the patient is incapable of decision making, they may be asked to give informed consent for ECT. This is an extremely difficult decision to make for someone else, particularly when the treatment is frightening and surrounded by myth, as is ECT. The nurse can be helpful to the family by providing time for them to discuss their concerns and answering their questions honestly and directly. Frequently the family can be helped to be supportive to the patient, which can alleviate the patient's anxiety. Family members also need to be informed about what to expect of the patient after ECT. Confusion, particularly, may be distressing to them unless they understand that it is ex-

pected and temporary. Hospitalized patients are usually completely recovered from the treatment, dressed, and engaged in their usual activities by the time the family visits. This is reassuring to the family. Family members should never be left alone to watch a patient who is recovering from ECT. Predischarge teaching should include both the patient and the family. They need to know that some lingering confusion may exist. For this reason it is helpful to explain medication dosages and schedules to both the patient and a responsible family member. Outpatient appointments should also be communicated to both the patient and a significant other person.

If a patient is receiving ECT on an outpatient basis, it is important that the family understand the expected posttreatment behavior. Usually, these patients arrive at the treatment facility in the morning, receive ECT, and remain there until fully awake and ambulatory. They may receive a light breakfast before leaving. The patient must be accompanied by someone who can escort him home after ECT. This is necessary because of the probable presence of confusion and because there will probably be some aftereffects of the anesthesia. The accompanying person should be instructed in how to orient the patient and what to do for headache or nausea, if present. A telephone number should be provided in case any questions arise after the patient has returned home. Outpatient ECT is generally done about once a month as a maintenance treatment for a person who has recovered from a severe depression. The procedure usually goes smoothly, without complications. Outpatient ECT is less frequently given to patients who are acutely ill or who have not had this treatment previously. These patients are usually hospitalized because of the severity of their conditions.

Indications

Although ECT was originally considered as a treatment for schizophrenia, it did not prove to be particularly helpful to most schizophrenic patients. Affective disturbances, however, were frequently alleviated by treatment with ECT. Until the development of antidepressant medications and the discovery of lithium therapy, ECT was a treatment of choice for affective disorders. It is still useful for patients who cannot tolerate or fail to respond to treatment with medication. ECT may also be used as an emergency therapy for a patient who is extremely suicidal or so hyperactive that he is in danger physically. ECT is given in these cases to avoid the lag time between initiation of pharmacotherapy and the establishment of a therapeutic level of medication for the individual. For some older persons who tend to be very sensitive to side effects from medication, ECT may be a safer therapeutic modality.[16]

On occasion, ECT may be used for conditions other than affective disorders. It has been effective in the treatment of catatonic stupor or catatonic excitement. It is sometimes still given to paranoid schizophrenic patients but generally with little success. A recent survey conducted by the American Psychiatric Association revealed that most psychiatrists who use ECT recommend it for patients with diagnoses of affective disorders or schizophrenia. A few practitioners use it with other patients, including neurotics and those with organic mental disorders, and a very few use it with children and adolescents. The American Psychiatric Association strongly recommends that research be conducted to validate these less common applications of ECT. It does endorse the helpfulness of ECT for affective disorders and some schizophrenic disorders, particularly those with an affective component.[1] Although some patients may view ECT as punishment, it should certainly never be used for this purpose, nor should a patient be threatened with punishment by ECT.

Mechanism of action

The specific way in which ECT works is the subject of a great deal of research, but it has not yet been identified. It used to be believed that ECT alleviated depression because the patient viewed it as punishment. The depressed person was supposed to feel better because the self-directed anger that was at the root of the depression was expressed through the electric shock and the frightening experience of the treatment. This point of view is no longer widely accepted.

It is now more commonly believed that there is a biochemical response within the brain to the passage of the electric current in ECT. The observable behavior that indicates that this response has occurred is the convulsion. Several possible mechanisms of action have been identified. The most promising of these is that the seizure activity in the brain produces biochemical changes similar to those induced by antidepressant medications. This and other hypotheses require further research. It is also believed that

the mechanism of action which is effective with schizophrenia differs from that which occurs with depression.[1]

Complications

Complications associated with the administration of ECT are infrequent.[16] The only real contraindication to ECT is the presence of a brain tumor, which would cause dangerously increased intracranial pressure during ECT. Prior to the use of muscle relaxants, spontaneous fractures, especially of the spine, occasionally occurred. Cardiac complications, when they do occur, are more likely to be a result of the anesthesia than the ECT. In fact, some authorities believe that it is better not to anesthetize patients with cardiac problems when they receive ECT.[16] Since anesthesia is generally given and since tonic and clonic seizure activity may occur even with the use of muscle relaxants, the pre-ECT workup usually includes an EKG and x-ray films of the spine, skull, and chest. Potential problems can then be prevented.

Ethical considerations

The legitimacy of ECT as a form of treatment continues to be debated in psychiatric circles. Many professionals believe that it is a punishment rather than a treatment and that administering a shock to a person is inhumane. Others feel that it is more inhumane to allow a person to suffer the pain of a severe emotional disturbance when ECT frequently provides relief in a short time. Some are concerned that permanent brain damage could result. Others say that it should be given prophylactically to prevent recurrence of problems. It is up to each professional to reach a personal resolution of this debate. Hopefully, this will be based on objective data, including experience with patients who have been treated with and without the use of ECT. Kalayam and Steinhart[15] conducted an attitude survey of a group of patients, professionals, and members of the general public concerning their perceptions of ECT. There was general agreement by all of these groups that ECT is an appropriate treatment for certain conditions and that it does cause clinical improvement. If there is an opportunity to observe ECT being administered, the nurse should take advantage of this. Fantasy is usually much different from the reality of the treatment experience. Also, nurses who are unable to accept the use of ECT should try not to communicate negative attitudes to the patient who will have this treatment. ECT continues to be used because it has been found to be helpful to many patients.

Insulin shock therapy

Prior to the use of medication as a treatment for serious emotional disorders, insulin shock therapy was a frequently used treatment modality. Use of insulin therapy was first reported by Sakel in 1933. It is rarely used in contemporary psychiatric facilities.[21] This is primarily because equally good results can be achieved by pharmacotherapy. Insulin shock therapy required a large, specialized nursing staff who could provide intensive nursing care to a small group of patients for several hours. The usual course of therapy was 50 treatments, given at a rate of one per day 5 days a week. Both of these factors made insulin coma an expensive form of therapy. It was also dangerous. If a coma was allowed to continue too long, it became irreversible.[19]

Insulin therapy was induced by the administration of a large dose of insulin intramuscularly. The exact dose needed to cause a coma was individual and was found by starting with a low dose and increasing it over several days until coma resulted. The patient would usually begin to have hypoglycemic symptoms about an hour after the injection, progressing through a stage of disorientation and restlessness to coma after about 3 hours. The length of the coma was then gradually increased to a maximum of an hour. The coma was terminated by administration of glucose solution by nasogastric tube or intravenously or glucagon intramuscularly or intravenously. Close observation of the patient was required for the rest of the day because repeat comas sometimes occurred during the afternoon of the treatment day. Contraindications to insulin coma therapy included serious medical illness, such as cardiovascular, renal, liver, or respiratory disease, untreated hyperthyroidism, and pregnancy.[21]

Pharmacotherapy

The present time is the era of pharmacotherapy as the primary form of somatic treatment in psychiatry. Extensive use of pharmacotherapeutic agents has grown steadily since World War II. The discovery in the early 1950s of reserpine and the phenothiazines as treatment for schizophrenia provided the impetus for concentrated research in this area. Concurrently, psychiatric care was revolutionized as previously unmanageable behavior was controlled by the use of medication. Recalcitrant patients became accessible to interpersonal therapeutic approaches. Some chronically institutionalized persons were able to leave the hospital for the community. Average length of patient stay in psychiatric hospitals became shorter, and more people were treatable on an outpatient basis.

For nursing, the pharmacotherapeutic revolution has brought a wealth of new opportunities and some problems as well. In many ways psychiatric nursing care has been facilitated by the advent of medication. Fewer patients need custodial nursing care. The nurse-patient relationship can be implemented more effectively when the patient's level of anxiety has been reduced to manageable proportions with medication. In the therapeutic milieu the nurse is able to work with groups of patients to explore their adjustment to life together in the hospital and to help them develop more effective living skills. Short-term hospitalizations and gradually increasing emphasis on outpatient treatment have given an aura of hope to psychiatry.

It is also challenging and stimulating to be a participant in the tremendous growth of knowledge that is taking place in the area of neurochemistry and neurophysiology. Some of the impetus for research that is being done in these fields has originated in exploration of mechanisms of action of psychotropic medications. Through investigation of the ways in which these drugs influence neural pathways in the brain, much is being learned that may ultimately result in information about the cause of many psychiatric disorders. As more is learned, treatment becomes more precise and effective.

However, psychopharmacology has not been a panacea. It can be frustrating to work with a patient who does not respond predictably to medication, and idiosyncratic reactions do occur. Close nursing observations are always necessary when a patient is receiving psychotropic medications. Other medications should be used cautiously in combination with these drugs because numerous drug interactions can occur. Table 15-1 presents a summary of the types of interactions that can occur. In addition, some medications require dietary restrictions about which the patient must be taught. Most of these medications produce side effects, generally more

TABLE 15-1. Interactions of psychotropic drugs and other substances*

Drug	Interacting drug/class	Possible consequences
Antipsychotic agents		
Phenothiazines	Antacids, oral	Antacids may inhibit absorption of orally administered phenothiazines
Phenothiazines Aliphatic (Chlorpromazine) Piperidine (Thioridazine)	Central nervous system depressants Ethanol Barbiturates Nonbarbiturate sedative-hypnotics Antianxiety agents Antihistamines Narcotic analgesics	Additive central nervous system depression, increasing the risk of mental or physical impairment of performance
Phenothiazines Aliphatic Piperidine	Anticholinergic agents Antiulcer Antiparkinsonism	Additive atropine-like side effects Anticholinergics reduce gastric motility, resulting in enhanced intestinal metabolism of phenothiazines and reduced absorption
Phenothiazines Thioxanthenes Butyrophenones	Levodopa (Bendopa, Larodopa, Levopa)	Antiparkinsonism effects of levodopa may be antagonized by antipsychotic agents
Phenothiazines Chlorpromazine	Guanethidine (Ismelin) Amphetamine-like drugs	Chlorpromazine antagonizes antihypertensive effects of guanethidine Phenothiazines may antagonize appetite-suppressing effects of these drugs
Antianxiety agents		
Benzodiazepines	Alcohol	Potential additive central and autonomic nervous system depression
Diazepam	Barbiturates	Intravenous administration of diazepam and barbiturates for the treatment of status epilepticus and non-epileptic convulsive disorders has been reported to result in respiratory depression or hypotension
Antidepressant agents		
MAO inhibitors Isocarboxazid Phenazine	Tricyclic antidepressants	Concurrent use has resulted in severe toxicity, including excitation, fever, delirium, convulsions, and death; 10 days should elapse prior to administering tricyclics after last dose of MAO inhibitor
Tranylcypromine	Sympathomimetic amines Dextroamphetamine Ephedrine Metaraminol (Aramine) Phenylephrine Phenylpropanolamine	MAO inhibitors block metabolism of many sympathomimetic amines, resulting in marked rise in blood pressure, fever, convulsions, and death; patients should be advised to use nonprescription cough and cold preparations containing these drugs with extreme caution
	Meperidine (Demerol)	Potentiation of central and autonomic nervous system depressing effects of meperidine (respiratory depression and hypotension), restlessness, muscle twitching, fever, and death; combination is contraindicated
	Barbiturates	Potentiation of barbiturate depression
	Insulin Oral hypoglycemic agents	MAO inhibitors may potentiate the reduction in blood sugar levels when these drugs are administered to diabetic patients

*From Gerald, M.C., and O'Bannon, F.V.: Nursing pharmacology and therapeutics, © 1981, pp. 116, 130, 141, 142. Reprinted by permission of Prentice-Hall, Inc., Englewood Cliffs, N.J.

Continued.

Drug	Interacting drug/class	Possible consequences
Tranylcypromine—cont'd	Levodopa	Transitory elevation in blood pressure
	Tyramine-rich foods and beverages	MAO inhibitors prevent normal metabolism of tyramine, which accumulates and stimulates the release of norepinephrine. Adverse effects include severe headaches, hypertensive crises, heart palpitations, and possible death
	Cheeses (cheddar, Camembert, Gruyére)	
	Wines (Chianti), beer	
	Chicken liver	
	Pickled herring	
	Broad beans	
	Bananas	
	Doxapram (Dopram)	Adverse cardiovascular effects of doxapram (hypertension, arrhythmias) are potentiated
Tricyclics	MAO inhibitors	
Amitriptyline **Nortriptyline** **Doxepin**	Alcohol, other central nervous system depressants	Additive central nervous system depression, resulting in potential physical or mental impairment
Tricyclics, except doxepin	Guanethidine (Ismelin) Methyldopa (Aldomet)	Antagonism of antihypertensive effects with loss of control of blood pressure
Imipramine	Chlorpromazine (Thorazine) Haloperidol (Haldol) Anticholinergic agents	Additive atropine-like effects
Lithium	Vasopressin (endogenous)	Lithium may interfere with antidiuretic action of vasopressin, resulting in diabetes insipidus, which causes excessive urination
Lithium	Diuretics	Diuretic-induced sodium depletion enhances lithium toxicity; conversely, increased sodium intake interferes with antimanic effects of lithium
Sedative-hypnotics **Barbiturates** **Nonbarbiturates**	Alcohol, acute Analgesics, narcotic Antihistamines Antidepressants Antipsychotics	Combined use of sedative-hypnotics with other central nervous system depressants may impair mental and physical performance (e.g., motor vehicle operation) and result in lethargy, respiratory depression, coma, or death
	Antidepressants, MAO inhibitors Sulfonylurea oral hypoglycemic agents	These drugs may enhance the sedative effects of barbiturates and nonbarbiturates
Chronic barbiturates **Chloral hydrate** **Ethchlorvynol** **Glutethimide** **Meprobamate**	Anticoagulants, oral (Coumarin)	Increased rate of coumarin anticoagulant metabolism, decreasing plasma levels of coumarin and reducing its ability to prevent blood coagulation; higher dose of coumarin required; when barbiturate withdrawn and dose of coumarin not reduced, bleeding episode may occur
Barbiturates	Corticosteroids	Increased metabolism of corticosteroids when used for treatment of asthma; worsening of asthma
	Doxycycline (Vibramycin)	Increased metabolism of doxycycline, decreased plasma levels, possible reduction in antibacterial effects
	Griseofulvin (Fulvicin, Grifulvin, Grisactin)	Decreased antifungal effects of griseofulvin due to increased rate of metabolism and inhibition of absorption

distressing than dangerous. However, the nurse must be alert to the side effects that may occur and is responsible for patient teaching and for notifying the physician of any untoward reactions. The tables included in this chapter provide a summary of the most common side effects associated with the various psychopharmacological agents. Whenever a patient complains of a physical symptom while on medication, the possibility of a side effect, allergic response, drug interaction, or toxic reaction should be considered. Each person responds differently to medication, and symptoms should not be brushed aside as "just a result of the patient's anxiety." This attitude could even result in an increase of the medication that is causing the patient's problem. The nurse as the patient's advocate can investigate the problem by questioning the physician. It can also be helpful to talk with a pharmacist, who may have the most current information on pharmacological research. Elderly patients in particular may be sensitive to medications and may be prone to side effects. They need especially vigilant nursing assessment. Also, in caring for women of childbearing age, determination of pregnancy is important and use of medication should be highly selective, since the effect of some of these medications on fetal development has not yet been determined.

Problems associated with the administration of medication

Medication administration in the psychiatric setting generally progresses rather smoothly. Most patients accept medication as helpful to them, particularly if they have received thorough explanations of the reason for their treatment. However, because of the nature of the behaviors that result in psychiatric hospitalization, problems do sometimes occur related to giving medication to the patient. Some of the more common problem areas will be reviewed.

SUSPICIOUS PATIENT. Suspicious persons may believe that others are trying to control their behavior or are trying to do them harm. For either of these reasons, they may be reluctant to take medication. It is important that they have medication because it is usually being given to decrease the severe anxiety that is contributing to the patient's difficulty in trusting others.

Even though the nurse may be aware that a particular patient has been refusing medication, the initial approach to the patient should be confident and convey the expectation that the medication will be taken. A hesitant approach may arouse the patient's suspicion about the procedure. Verbalized directions should be clear and succinct, for example, "Here is your medication, Mr. Jones." If the patient hesitates, this can be followed by "Put it in your mouth and swallow it." Nonverbal communication should reinforce the verbalization. Also, to prevent confusion, the patient should be offered the same form of medication each time. For instance, if the order is for chlorpromazine, 150 mg, the nursing staff should agree to always give one 100 mg and one 50 mg tablet or three 50 mg tablets. If the liquid concentrate form of medication is used, it should be used consistently, and if it is mixed with fruit juice, it should be mixed with the same flavor each time. Attention to these details can save much time and discussion when medications are given. Another potential area of confusion for the patient occurs when the medication dosage is changed. If the patient can comprehend the information or if medication is being given in tablet form, the physician should inform the patient when a dosage change is made.

The nurse who is administering medicine to psychiatric patients should observe the patient's behavior carefully while the medicine is being taken. A suspicious patient may secrete tablets or capsules in the cheek or under the tongue, removing these as soon as the nurse looks away. If the nurse suspects this behavior, a mouth check should be initiated. This involves directing the patient to open his mouth and using a tongue depressor to look thoroughly for hidden medication. If possible, a better solution to this problem is to give the medication in liquid form. Occasionally a patient will swallow medication when it is given and then immediately go into the bathroom and induce emesis. If a patient fails to respond to medication as expected, an initial nursing action should be to observe carefully the individual's behavior following medication administration. It may be necessary to provide one-to-one observation for the patient until enough time has passed for the medicine to be absorbed.

Sometimes patients absolutely refuse to take any medication by mouth. The nurse should never try to trick the patient to take medicine by putting it in food or fluids. Discovery of this by the patient will destroy any trust that he has in the staff and give his suspicions a basis in objective reality. In addition, the patient may then also refuse to eat or drink because of the possibility that medicine is concealed, thus compounding nursing care problems and jeopardizing his nutrition and hydration. For the suspicious patient, there should be a clear separation between medication and food.

Patients who adamantly refuse oral medications may at times need to be given an injection. This requires a physician's order. The nurse should also be aware of the laws in her area concerning the patient's right to refuse treatment. Generally, only life-saving treatments may be given without the patient's permission. The patient will sometimes take medication by mouth if given the alternative of "by mouth or by needle." However, the nurse should not become embroiled in a long debate trying to persuade the patient to take oral medicine. If the patient must have the medicine and refuses it by mouth, the injection should be given quickly with as much physical restraint as is necessary for the patient's safety. The procedure should also be carried out with regard for the patient's right to dignity. Injections should be discontinued promptly as soon as the patient accepts oral medication. When they are feeling better, patients rarely object to having been medicated when they were very disturbed.

SUICIDAL PATIENT. Some of the problems encountered when giving medication to a suicidal patient are the same as those which occur with a suspicious patient, but for different reasons. Tablets or capsules given to a suicidal patient may not be swallowed so that they can be hoarded by the patient until a lethal amount has been accumulated. Seriously suicidal people should be observed with great care when medications are indicated. Mouth checks may again be required. The nurse should listen carefully for any verbal clues the patient might give such as "I know what I'm going to do. In a few more days, I'll be ready." Observation of the patient's behavior after medicine is given can also be helpful to see if he always goes to the same area or tries to be alone at that time. The person may be trying to add to a cache of drugs. Failure to swallow medicine should also be considered if the person is not responding as expected to medication.

Aside from mouth checks, the nurse may confront the patient with the observations that have been made. This should be done as an expression of concern and a desire to protect the patient from his self-destructive impulses. The nurse may also decide to conduct a search of the patient's room and possessions. The patient should be informed of the procedure and the reason for it and should be encouraged to observe while the search takes place. This procedure also has legal implications. If possible, the patient's permission should be obtained. If this is impossible, there should be clear evidence of a threat to the patient's life. Family members may also be helpful in giving permission for and helping with a search. Bear in mind that in a psychiatric unit where patients usually move about at will, a suicidal person has innumerable places to secrete medications and may be ingenious in doing so. Close observation of the suicidal person is the best way to prevent self-destructive activity.

Sometimes, suicidal patients, like suspicious patients, may refuse oral medication. This may be a more passive means of self-destruction, in which the individual invites death by doing nothing to support life. Very withdrawn suicidal patients may accept parenteral medication without resistance, although without giving explicit permission. Others may actively resist injections, in which case the legal implications mentioned in the discussion of the suspicious patient again apply. Whether the suicidal person is actively or passively pursuing self-destruction, the nurse's primary responsibility is to protect him from these impulses until self-control has been reestablished.

DEPENDENT PATIENT. Contemporary culture is drug oriented. Pills and potions are promoted as the panacea for all ills. It is not surprising that many patients expect that a magical pill will be provided that will solve all life's problems and allay all anxieties. It is hard to convince these people that pills may ease pain but rarely take it all away and that hard work is necessary to resolve psychosocial problems. A pill will not mend a broken marriage or a broken heart, however much one longs for that to happen.

Dependent people are prone to be seekers of the perfect pill. Sometimes this search can lead to overdependency on medication, even to the point of addiction. The nursing problem presented by these patients is twofold. They persistently demand medication and, at the same time, resist being engaged in exploration of their behavior. The following interaction demonstrates this dilemma.

Mr. M is a 45-year-old man who is mildly depressed, anxious, and has multiple somatic complaints. A thorough medical workup has ruled out any physiological basis for his symptoms. He is receiving diazepam (Valium), 5 mg, PO, q4h, prn for anxiety. He approaches a staff nurse, Ms. J.

MS. J: **May I help you, Mr. M?**

MR. M: **I need my Valium.**

MS. J: **Tell me how you're feeling.**

MR. M: **I feel bad. Just get me my Valium.**

MS. J: **You feel bad?**

MR. M: **Look, I need my pill now!**

MS. J: **Your Valium is ordered to help you when you're anxious. I want to try to understand how you're feeling when you ask for the pill.**

MR. M: **Well, I'm anxious and I'm getting more anxious standing here talking to you about whether I'm anxious. Now, how about my pill?**

MS. J: **Well, it has been just 4 hours since your last one. Do you think you could try to hold out for a few minutes longer? Perhaps we could talk or play ping-pong to take your mind off your anxiety.**

MR. M: **Look, the doc says I can have Valium every 4 hours. For the last hour, I've been counting the minutes. My head aches, my stomach is in knots, and look how my hands are shaking. Please get me my pill.**

MS. J: **OK. If you can't wait, I'll get it for you. I'd like to talk to you later, though, to see if we can come up with some ideas of other ways you can handle your anxiety. Pills don't get to the root of the problem, you know.**

MR. M: **Sure, sure. I'll talk to you sometime when I'm calm. I'll wait right here while you get my pill.**

In this interaction the nurse and the patient were pursuing different goals, resulting in frustration for both. The nurse's concern about Mr. M's dependence on his medication was well founded. Her timing in approaching the idea of alternative coping mechanisms was not ideal. However, she was acting responsibly in asking Mr. M to describe his feelings before giving him medication. It can be tempting with dependent patients like Mr. M to automatically give medicine every 4 hours without question to avoid a hostile confrontation. Medication that is ordered "whenever necessary" can be withheld by the nurse if there is no objective evidence of need on the part of the patient. Of course, if the nurse is dealing with a patient whom she finds to be annoying, she must also evaluate whether her feelings are influencing her decision not to give medicine.

Close communication within the health team is helpful when working with patients like Mr. M. Frequency of medication should be reviewed regularly. All team members should be united in an effort to be supportive and to encourage the patient to confront his problems and to explore other coping mechanisms.

Placebos are sometimes given to dependent patients. This is, of course, done only with a physician's order. This plan of care should be thoroughly discussed and evaluated by the health care team before it is initiated. Deception of the patient is involved and could result in loss of trust in caregivers by the patient. It is imperative that this course of action not be undertaken as a retaliation against a frustrating patient. As a professional, the nurse should explore her own feelings about the use of a placebo and make her own decision about participating in this treatment.

Patients who are dependent on medication have great potential for addiction to medication. Nursing care of the addicted patient is addressed in Chapter 14. Nurses do have a role in combating addiction by discouraging indiscriminate use of medication and by helping patients explore healthier ways of meeting their needs.

THE NONCOMPLIANT PATIENT. The other major problem related to the nursing care of patients who are taking antipsychotic medications is that of nonadherence to the treatment plan. Patients need careful explanations about the medication schedule and encouragement to take medicine regularly. Suspicious patients may not continue with medicine at home. Other patients may stop taking medicine because they feel better. Connelly[5] has reviewed the literature relative to noncompliance with a mental health care plan. This includes refusal to take prescribed medications. She identified the following 15 factors that have been implicated as contributing to noncompliance:

1. The individual's perception that his condition is not serious enough to require treatment

2. A lack of a feeling of personal susceptibility to future episodes of illness

3. The type and number of behaviors that have been included in the plan of care

4. The type of behaviors that have been proscribed

5. The amount of change required in personal habits

6. Any increase in the number or complexity of recommendations

7. The side effects of drugs

8. Fear of dependence on drugs

9. Lack of adequate knowledge

10. Lack of understanding of the importance of the treatment regimen

11. Either very high or very low levels of anxiety

12. The presence of an internal locus of control

13. Family discord

14. A negative relationship with the provider

15. Lack of continuity of care

O'Brien[18] has identified the additional factors of pressure from significant others not to take medicine, the inability to afford the drugs, and the embarrassment about taking them at work. These factors can be used by nurses as guidelines when planning care that involves compliance with a treatment regimen. Some noncompliant patients are given their antipsychotic medication by depot injection rather than orally. Fluphenazine enanthate or decanoate may be given intramuscularly every 10 days to 3 weeks depending on the patient's response. Medication is usually started orally to evaluate the patient's reaction to it before the injections are started. Nurses must do the same teaching about possible side effects and the necessity for medicine that they do with patients who take oral drugs.

Medications commonly used in psychiatry

Psychopharmacotherapy is a specialized field that is presently involved in a knowledge explosion. Research is being conducted in many areas, and information about medications seems to expand and change every day. Nurses need to be aware of important developments in this field. One way to accomplish this is by regularly reviewing professional literature, particularly periodicals. Pharmacists are good resource people and can recommend helpful research reports or can assist in evaluation of conflicting research findings. Information provided by pharmaceutical companies should be used with discrimination; it may be valid, but they rarely disseminate findings that reflect negatively on their product.

This discussion is not an attempt to provide exhaustive information on psychotropic medications. Interested readers may find such information in great detail in pharmacology texts. The focus here will be to delineate the major categories of medication commonly prescribed for psychiatric patients and the most frequently encountered nursing implications. These are all powerful drugs and may cause responses that have not been mentioned here. Any concern expressed by a patient about medication should be taken seriously and reported to the physician. The major categories of medications that will be discussed are (1) antipsychotic agents, (2) antianxiety agents, (3) antidepressants, (4) lithium carbonate, and (5) sedatives and hypnotics. Sedatives and hypnotics are frequently used in psychiatry and are common in other specialty areas as well. Stimulant drugs are prescribed occasionally, but many experts doubt that their effectiveness outweighs the potential for abuse of these medications. The potential for abuse of the last two groups of drugs is covered in Chapter 14.

ANTIPSYCHOTIC DRUGS. Medication was introduced as a treatment for psychotic behavior in the early 1950s. The earliest drugs were reserpine and chlorpromazine. Reserpine is no longer in wide use and will not be discussed in detail. Chlorpromazine was the first of many drugs of the phenothiazine group to be used in the treatment of psychosis. More recently drugs of the butyrophenone and thioxanthene derivative groups have also been introduced. The generic names, brand names, dosage ranges, dosage forms, common side effects, and complications of representative drugs from these groups are presented in Table 15-2. Since these drugs are chemically related, the side effects and complications tend to be similar and have been presented as a group. However, there is some variation of frequency of side effects within the group. Parkinsonian effects tend to occur more frequently with haloperidol, fluphenazine, thiothixene, and trifluoperazine. Sedation, anticholinergic effects, orthostatic hypotension, allergic responses, and seizures are more frequent with chlorpromazine, thioridazine, chlorprothixene, promazine, mesoridazine, triflupromazine, carphenazine, and acetophenazine.[3] Therefore, if a patient develops side effects from one medication, the physician may prescribe an equivalent dosage of another drug to make the patient more comfortable. Many of the side effects are probably related to the mechanism of action of these drugs, which is not yet completely understood. It is suspected that there is probably an interference with dopamine reception or synthesis at the neural synapse.[13] This hypothesis would also lead to the suspicion that an excess of dopamine contributes to psychotic behavior, but this is as yet unproved.

There are implications for nursing care related

TABLE 15-2. Antipsychotic medications*

Generic name	Trade name	Dosage range (mg/24 hr)	Dose form	Side effects†	Complications†
Phenothiazines				Oversedation, impaired psychomotor function, akathisia, Parkinson's syndrome, dystonia, orthostatic hypotension, anticholinergic effects, impotence, photosensitivity, weight gain, lactation, menstrual irregularity, potentiation of other drugs and alcohol	Tardive dyskinesia, seizures, cholestatic jaundice, agranulocytosis, rash, pigmentary eye change (thioridazine only), alterations in lenticular opacity (chlorpromazine only), metallic blue pigmentation of the skin (only after long-term use of chlorpromazine)
Acetophenazine	Tindal	40 to 120	Tablet		
Butaperazine	Repoise	15 to 100	Tablet		
Carphenazine	Proketazine	25 to 200	Tablet, concentrate		
Chlorpromazine	Thorazine	25 to 2000	Tablet, Spansule, concentrate, parenteral, suppository, syrup		
Fluphenazine	Prolixin, Permitil	1 to 20	Tablet, concentrate, elixir, parenteral		
Fluphenazine decanoate	Prolixin	12.5 to 50	Depot IM (given every 7 to 21 days) or SC		
Fluphenazine enanthate	Prolixin	12.5 to 50	Depot IM (given every 7 to 21 days) or SC		
Mesoridazine	Serentil	30 to 400	Tablet, concentrate, parenteral		
Perphenazine	Trilafon	12 to 64	Tablet, concentrate, syrup, Repetabs, parenteral		
Piperacetazine	Quide	40 to 160	Tablet, parenteral		
Prochlorperazine	Compazine	30 to 150	Tablet, Spansule, parenteral, concentrate, suppository		
Promazine	Sparine	150 to 800	Tablet, concentrate, parenteral, syrup		
Thioridazine	Mellaril	75 to 800	Tablet, concentrate		
Trifluoperazine	Stelazine	4 to 40	Tablet, concentrate, parenteral		
Triflupromazine	Vesprin	30 to 150	Tablet, parenteral, suspension		
Butyrophenones					
Haloperidol	Haldol	2 to 15	Tablet, concentrate, parenteral		
Thioxanthene derivatives					
Chlorprothixene	Taractan	25 to 600	Tablet, concentrate, parenteral		
Thiothixene	Navane	6 to 60	Capsule, concentrate, parenteral		

*Based on data from Cain, R.M., and Cain, N.N.: A compendium of psychiatric drugs, part I, Jan. 1975, and Veterans Administration: Drug treatment in psychiatry, Washington, D.C., 1970, The Administration.

†Applies to all drugs in table; see text.

to the side effects of antipsychotic medication. The nurse should be aware of the most common side effects and be prepared to teach the patient about them when they occur. Most side effects are uncomfortable but not dangerous. Following is a summary of those which appear most frequently and the appropriate nursing care:

1. *Oversedation.* Patients usually feel groggy when they begin to take antipsychotic medication. This side effect tends to diminish after the patient has taken the medication for a time. It can also be minimized by giving the whole daily dose of medication at bedtime, since the sedating effect does not last as long as the antipsychotic effect.[7] If a patient is very upset by the drowsiness, the nurse could suggest altering the dosage schedule to the physician. It can also be helpful to explain the side effect to the patient and offer the hope that it will decrease with time.

2. *Extrapyramidal effects.* There are four groups of extrapyramidal symptoms associated with the use of antipsychotic medications: parkinsonian equivalents, dystonias, akathisia, and tardive dyskinesia.[17] All of these symptoms are probably related to the dopamine blocking properties of the medications.

Parkinsonian symptoms are behaviors similar to those observed in persons with Parkinson's disease, such as fine tremors, pill-rolling tremor of the fingers, drooling, and the characteristic petit pas gait.

Dystonias occur suddenly and are frightening to the patient. One dystonic reaction is a sudden spasm of the muscles of the face and neck, generally pulling the jaw to one side and twisting the neck. Another consists of the eyes uncontrollably rolling back into the head. Other dystonic reactions include opisthotonos and a variety of bizarre facial and head movements combined with salivation.[7]

These conditions are generally relieved immediately by intramuscular injection of diphenhydramine hydrochloride (Benadryl), 50 mg, or benztropine mesylate (Cogentin), 2 mg. A great deal of reassurance is also necessary. Long-term preventive treatment of parkinsonism, the dystonias, and akathisia may include a change to a different antipsychotic medication or the addition of an oral antiparkinsonian drug, such as trihexyphenidyl hydrochloride (Artane), procyclidine hydrochloride (Kemadrin), or benztro-

pine mesylate. There is, however, growing concern about using these latter medications over an extended period of time because of the potential for toxic effects related to their anticholinergic activity, including confusion, dry mouth, blurred vision, or possibly bowel or bladder paralysis.[22] The trend is to use them briefly to deal with parkinsonian side effects but to then discontinue them. It has been found that dystonic reactions tend not to recur after the patient has been taking medication for a time. Any remaining parkinsonian symptoms may be less disturbing to the patient than the side effects of the drugs taken to alleviate them.

Akathisia is a feeling of restlessness that results in an inability to sit still. The patient may complain of a twitching or crawling sensation in his muscles. This is usually dealt with by substituting another antipsychotic drug.

Tardive dyskinesia is a complication of antipsychotic medication that has recently received much publicity. McAfee[17] has described the behaviors that are characteristic of tardive dyskinesia. There are athetoid or choreiform movements that are generally rhythmic and coordinated. The buccolinguomasticatory triad includes a complex of lip, tongue, jaw, and head movements, such as sucking, lip smacking, protrusion of the tongue, lateral jaw movement, and jerking of the head and neck. Early in the development of the syndrome there may be vermiform, or wormlike, movements of the tongue when it is protruded. Extension and flexion of the fingers occurs. This is called *piano-playing restlessness.* Axial hyperkinesis refers to a to-and-fro clonic motion of the spine. There may also be hemiballistic movements that are swinging motions of the arms or side-to-side swaying. It was believed that tardive dyskinesia occurred only after many years of treatment with antipsychotic drugs. However, recent research has revealed that it may begin within a matter of months, but its development may be screened by the medications. It is believed that this problem is related to a dopamine-acetylcholine imbalance in brain tissue as a result of the biochemical action of these drugs.[9] There has been some promising research conducted using cholinergic drugs as a treatment for tardive dyskinesia. Prevention and early detection of the problem can be facilitated by the use of "drug holidays," which are scheduled periods of time when the patient takes no medication. Long-term use of anticholinergic medications, such as benztropine mesylate (Cogentin) or trihexyphenidyl hydrochloride (Artane), is also discouraged be-

cause they appear to aggravate tardive dyskinesia.

Nursing interventions should focus on close
observation of patient behavior for identification
of the development of tardive dyskinesia. Prompt
reporting of observed symptoms is essential so
that intervention can begin. Patients who have
advanced tardive dyskinesia require supportive
treatment, including provision of a high-calorie
soft diet, encouragement to wear dentures if
needed, lubrication of the lips, and careful fit-
ting of shoes. Adequate rest should be promoted
because the choreiform movements are quite
tiring, but cease during sleep. These patients
need a great deal of understanding and emotional support.[17] They are aware of their bizarre
uncontrollable movements and the alienating
effect that they have on other people. The occurrence of tardive dyskinesia serves as a reminder that antipsychotic medications are powerful chemicals and that their effect on the body
is not totally understood. They should be used
only when necessary to alleviate a person's emotional pain and should be discontinued if they
are no longer needed. Wendt[23] has described
graphically the discomfort associated with being in a "chemical straitjacket."

3. *Anticholinergic effects.* The anticholinergic
effect of the antipsychotic drugs influences
functioning of the autonomic nervous system
and results in a number of side effects, for the
most part uncomfortable but not dangerous.
One effect that could be serious is orthostatic hypotension. This occurs with particular frequency
in the elderly and may require change in medication. The nurse should warn these patients
against sudden changes in position and check
sitting and standing blood pressure when medications are being introduced. Dry mucous membranes are annoying. Sucking on glycerine-
based cough drops sometimes helps the mouth
feel moist. Constipation may occur. The nurse
should chart bowel movements and offer a laxa-
tive as necessary to prevent fecal impaction.

4. *Endocrine effects.* These may include gy-
necomastia, lactation, menstrual irregularities,
and increased libido in women and impotence
in men. Patients may be concerned and embarrassed by these problems. The nurse can help
by providing explanations and reassurance.

5. *Allergic reactions.* Rashes occasionally occur with antipsychotic medications and should
be evaluated by the physician. Usually the medication is changed and the rash is treated with
topical or systemic medication. Cholestatic jaundice occurs infrequently and requires discon-

tinuation of the medication. Liver function tests
should be done periodically or if a patient shows
any evidence of jaundice.

6. *Serious blood dyscrasias.* These are rare
but serious. The nurse should be aware that
serious blood dyscrasias can occur and report
any indication of this complication.

7. *Photosensitivity.* This side effect, which is
similar to a severe sunburn, is particularly associated with chlorpromazine. Patients taking
this medication should be warned against
exposure to direct sunlight and informed about
the use of sunscreening creams. Long-term use
of chlorpromazine may also result in a metal-
lic blue discoloration of the skin, especially in
areas that are exposed to the sun.

Informed consent is now being obtained for
the use of psychotropic medication in some
places. Whether or not informed consent is obtained, nurses should assume the responsibility to educate patients about the nature of the
side effects that might be associated with their
medication and the importance of reporting
these to a health care provider promptly.

ANTIANXIETY DRUGS. As antipsychotic drugs
were being discovered in the early 1950s, so
were drugs in the antianxiety group (Table 15-
3). Meprobamate, the first, was synthesized in
1950. Chlordiazepoxide, the first of the benzodiazepines, followed in 1957. These drugs have
become a fixture in contemporary society.[8] Our
pill-oriented culture has embraced these medications as the easy answer to life's anxieties.
Widespread prescription by nonpsychiatrists has
made them readily available and acceptable to
people who would not dream of using "street
drugs." Of course, these drugs are available on
the street as well. As one patient said, "Why
should I pay to see you (her therapist) so I can
get a prescription for my Valium when I can
get them cheaper on the street anyway?" Unfortunately, many patients rely on medications to the point of refusing to engage in a therapeutic relationship.

On the other hand, antianxiety agents can be
of great benefit to people who would otherwise
be nearly immobilized by anxiety. They can
help individuals cope with crises and may reduce anxiety so that the motivated person can
become fully involved in psychotherapy. These
drugs have sedative properties and lower abuse
potential and lethality than other sedatives

TABLE 15-3. Antianxiety medications*

Generic name	Trade name	Dosage range (mg/24 hr)	Dose form	Side effects	Other considerations
Glycerol derivatives					
Meprobamate	Equanil, Miltown	1200 to 1600	Tablet, capsule, liquid	Drowsiness, ataxia, confusion, slurred speech, headache, lethargy, giddiness, dizziness, vertigo, impaired visual accommodation†	Potential for physical dependence at high doses; withdrawal syndrome similar to barbiturate withdrawal; alcohol, sedatives, and hypnotics potentiated by these drugs; hazardous activities to be avoided‡
Tybamate	Tybatran	250 to 2000	Capsule		
Benzodiazepines					
Clorazepate	Tranxene	15 to 60	Capsule	See above	See above
Chlordiazepoxide	Librium	15 to 100	Capsule, tablet, parenteral		
Diazepam	Valium	6 to 40	Tablet, parenteral		
Oxazepam	Serax	30 to 120	Capsule, tablet		
Antihistamines					
Hydroxyzine	Atarax, Vistaril	75 to 400	Tablet, syrup	Drowsiness, dry mouth	Hazardous activities to be avoided; potentiates other central nervous system depressants

*Based on data from Cain, R.M., and Cain, N.N.: A compendium of psychiatric drugs, part II, Feb. 1975, and Veterans Administration: Drug treatment in psychiatry, Washington, D.C., 1970, The Administration.

†These are usually mild and apply to both glycerol derivatives and benzodiazepines.

‡These apply to both glycerol derivatives and benzodiazepines.

and hypnotics. They are therefore useful for the treatment of patients who tend to develop drug dependency or who are suicidal. Small amounts of medicine should be given to these patients, however, since these drugs can be abused and can be lethal if taken in great enough quantities. When addiction to an antianxiety agent occurs, there is potential for serious withdrawal symptoms, including grand mal seizures. Also, the combination of antianxiety medication with alcohol can be lethal. Patients should be informed of these dangers, so they understand that these are potent drugs and not to be taken unnecessarily. One of the benzodiazepines, flurazepam (Dalmane), has marked hypnotic properties and is not classified as an antianxiety agent.

As a responsible professional person and citizen, the nurse has an important role as educator of the public in the use of medication. She can be a guide in encouraging those who need medicine to use it and in encouraging discontinuation of medication that is no longer needed. Professional people also serve as role models for the general public in the responsible use of medicine. The nurse should take care not to share medications with friends and relatives or to recommend medication. Referral to a physician is the appropriate course of action if a significant other needs help. All psychopharmacological agents are powerful medications and to be used with great discretion.

ANTIDEPRESSANT DRUGS. In the late 1950s, antidepressant medications were discovered. These agents had a specific effect on the symptoms of depression and have led to extensive research on the biochemistry of depression. There are two major groups of antidepressants: the monoamine oxidase (MAO) inhibitors and the tricyclics. Biochemically, antidepressants appear to facilitate transmission at the neural synapse. At the present time tricyclics are used more frequently than MAO inhibitors because they have proved to be safer and at least equally effective for the majority of patients. Pertinent data about the antidepressants are presented in Table 15-4. An advantage of the antidepressants is that they are not addictive. However, it should be remembered that depressed patients are frequently suicidal, and overdoses of antidepressant medications can have very serious consequences, including cardiovascular and renal dysfunction.

Nurses caring for patients who are receiving antidepressant medication need to be aware that response to the medication may not occur for up to 3 weeks after the first dose is taken.[6] The patient will need supportive nursing care and much encouragement while waiting for the medication to reach a therapeutically effective level. Especially if side effects are also present, the patient may become discouraged and request to stop taking medicine. Elderly patients are particularly vulnerable to side effects, especially postural hypotension, and may need to start on very low dosages, gradually building to a therapeutic dose. Cardiovascular side effects may also occur. Nursing care includes careful monitoring of vital signs.

Particular attention should be given to vital signs of the patient who is receiving MAO inhibitors. There is a danger of hypertensive crisis when these drugs are combined with any of a wide array of other medicines and tyramine-containing foods. Some foods that contain tyramine are aged cheeses, red wines, beer, chicken livers, pickled herring, cream, chocolate, yeast extracts, and fava beans.[3] The patient should be provided with a list of these foods and also instructed not to take *any* other medication without first checking with the physician. Any incidence of headache should be reported to the physician immediately, since hypertensive crisis can be fatal if it results in a cerebrovascular accident.

Antidepressant medicine has given new hope to patients who are depressed. Although most depressions eventually resolve themselves, these drugs can significantly decrease the duration of the disorder and facilitate the patient's return to a productive life. Generally, antidepressants can be gradually reduced and eventually discontinued if the patient tolerates the dosage reduction. These patients do not usually need to resign themselves to lifelong medication but should be taught the signs of impending depression so they can seek psychiatric help promptly in case of recurrence.

LITHIUM CARBONATE. Lithium carbonate is a naturally occurring salt that is specifically effective in controlling behaviors associated with manic-depressive disease in the manic phase or to prevent the periodic mood swings that occur with this disorder. Lithium was introduced by Cade in Australia in 1949 but not approved for use in the United States until 1970.[12] Like the antidepressants, a systemic therapeutic level

TABLE 15-4. Antidepressant medications*

Generic name	Trade name	Dosage range (mg/24 hr)	Dose form	Side effects	Other considerations
Tricyclics					
Amitriptyline	Elavil	75 to 300	Tablet, parenteral	Dry mouth, blurred vision, constipation, drowsiness (except protriptyline), jitteriness, nausea, heartburn	Caution needed with suicidal patients; hazardous activities to be avoided; potentiated by alcohol; not to be combined with MAO inhibitors
Desipramine	Norpramin, Pertofrane	75 to 300	Tablet		
Doxepin	Adapin, Sinequan	75 to 300	Capsule, concentrate		
Imipramine	Presamine, Tofranil	75 to 300	Tablet, capsule, parenteral		
Nortriptyline	Aventyl, Pamelor	50 to 100	Capsule, liquid		
Protriptyline	Vivactil	15 to 60	Tablet		
MAO inhibitors					
Isocarboxazid	Marplan	10 to 30	Tablet	Hypertensive crisis if combined with tyramine-containing foods, severe headaches, dry mouth, constipation, insomnia, overstimulation, dizziness	Not to be combined with tricyclics; inhibited by alcohol; potentiates amphetamines, barbiturates, chloral hydrate, antiparkinsonian agents, antianxiety drugs, phenothiazines, sympathomimetics
Phenelzine	Nardil	15 to 75	Tablet		
Tranylcypromine	Parnate	10 to 30	Tablet		

*Based on data from Cain, R.M., and Cain, N.N.: A compendium of psychiatric drugs, part I, Jan. 1975, and Veterans Administration: Drug treatment in psychiatry, Washington, D.C., 1970, The Administration.

of lithium must be reached before any behavioral effect occurs. Analysis of blood samples can be done to monitor the lithium level. This is usually done as the therapeutic dosage is approached and periodically for as long as the person takes the medication. Since lithium is prescribed prophylactically to prevent future episodes of manic-depressive behavior, the patient will probably take it indefinitely.

Nursing care of the patient on lithium therapy should center around health teaching. Many patients respond well to instruction about the nature of their problem. For people who have been repeatedly hospitalized for unpredictable mood swings, it can be a relief to know that medication can stabilize their moods. There is always, however, a need to adjust to the idea that medicine must be taken regularly, perhaps for the rest of one's life. The nurse can help by being available to discuss this with the patient and to reinforce the need to take medicine and to have blood levels taken. Maintenance dosages of lithium range from 600 to 1200 mg/ 24 hr, which should maintain a blood level of 0.5 to 1.5 mEq/L. A blood level about 2.0 mEq/ L is considered to be toxic.[3]

The patient should know early symptoms of lithium toxicity and understand that the physician should be notified immediately if these symptoms occur. Toxic symptoms include at early stages a feeling of sluggishness, lethargy, a fine tremor or muscle twitching, ataxia, slurred speech, anorexia, nausea, vomiting, and diarrhea. If untreated, the condition can progress to semiconsciousness and coma with hyperactive deep tendon reflexes, tremors, and fasciculations. Seizures can occur, as can serious electrolyte changes, cardiac impairment, and sometimes death.[12] The patient should also contact the physician if any conditions that influence fluid and electrolyte balance, such as vomiting, diarrhea, or excessive perspiration have occurred, since lithium is an electrolyte and the level may have been affected. For the same reason, the patient needs to consume adequate fluids and salt.

Burgess[2] has cautioned about the use of lithium during pregnancy, especially during the first trimester. It does cross the placental barrier, and the effect on the fetus is unknown. As pregnancy progresses, renal clearance of lithium increases and the dosage may need to be adjusted based on blood levels. The daily dose should be decreased by half during the last week of pregnancy and discontinued when labor begins. The prepregnancy dose may be resumed postpartum,

unless the mother breast feeds. Lithium is transmitted in human milk so should probably not be given to nursing women. The effects of lithium absorbed in utero on the newborn include cyanosis, cardiac arrhythmia, and generalized hypotonia. These disappear when the serum lithium level becomes normal.

Some side effects may also occur, especially as lithium therapy is begun. They usually disappear as the appropriate dosage level is established. Side effects include fine tremor of the hands, abdominal cramps, nausea, vomiting, diarrhea, thirst, polyuria, fatigue, and weight gain. In some cases goiter has occurred, and lithium should be used with caution if the patient has known thyroid disease.[12] The nurse can provide reassurance if the patient complains of side effects.

SEDATIVES AND HYPNOTICS. Sedative and hypnotic medications are frequently used in psychiatric settings. Emotionally disturbed people often suffer from insomnia. These medications must be used with care. They are usually addictive, and dependent people are vulnerable to developing drug dependencies. This aspect of sedative use is discussed in Chapter 14. Depressed patients generally have difficulty sleeping. They also have a high suicide potential. Overdoses of sedatives are lethal, particularly since these drugs are potentiated by many other medications and by alcohol. Accidental deaths also occur when sedatives and alcohol are combined.

The effects of sedatives and hypnotics are very similar to those of the antianxiety drugs and alcohol. There is an initial feeling of euphoria followed by relaxation and sleep. It is the euphoric feeling that is sought when these drugs are used illicitly. However, they are central nervous system depressants, which accounts for their sleep-inducing properties. Unfortunately, sedated sleep is not usually natural sleep. Many sedatives interfere with normal sleep patterns, especially the occurrence of rapid eye movement (REM) sleep. This is believed to contribute to the hangover that is often experienced following a night of sedated sleep. Over a period of time, it may also lead to irritability.

The most commonly used group of sedative and hypnotic drugs are the barbiturates.[8] They are also typical of all the limitations just described. Nonbarbiturate sedatives, such as glute-

TABLE 15-5. Sedative-hypnotic medications*

Generic name	Trade name	Dosage range (mg/24 hr)		Dose form	Side effects	Other considerations
		Sedative	Hypnotic			
Barbiturates						
Phenobarbital	Luminal	15 to 30	100 to 200	Tablet, liquid, parenteral	Residual sedation, dizziness, headache, nausea, vomiting, rash, excitement, confusion, depression, anemia, respiratory depression, circulatory depression	These drugs are addictive, causing both physical and psychological dependence; they should be used only when necessary and for a short time only; there is an additive effect with alcohol and antianxiety drugs
Amobarbital	Amytal	65 to 200	100 to 200	Tablet, capsules, parenteral		
Pentobarbital	Nembutal	30 to 40	100 to 200	Capsule, liquid, parenteral, suppository		
Secobarbital	Seconal	—	100 to 200	Capsule, liquid, parenteral, suppository		
Butabarbital	Butisol	15 to 30	50 to 100	Tablet, liquid		
Nonbarbiturates						
Glutethimide	Doriden	250 to 500	500	Tablet, capsule	Rash, nausea, hangover, blurred vision, blood dyscrasias, respiratory depression	Course following overdose is unpredictable; requires careful monitoring
Methyprylon	Nolud	50 to 100	200 to 400	Tablet, capsule	Dizziness, nausea, diarrhea, headache, rash, hangover	
Ethchlorvynol	Placidyl	—	500 to 750	Capsule	Nausea, vomiting, dizziness, blurred vision, facial numbness, hypotension, rash, hangover	
Chloral hydrate	Noctec, Kessodrate, Felsules, Aquachloral	250	500 to 2000	Capsule, liquid	Gastric irritation	
Flurazepam	Dalmane	—	15 to 30	Capsule	Dizziness, drowsiness, ataxia, oversedation, lethargy, coma, headache, gastrointestinal upset, irritability, weakness, chest pains, joint pains	

*Based on data from Davis, J.M.: Minor tranquilizers, sedatives and hypnotics. In Kaplan, H.E., Freedman, A.M. and Sadock, B.J., editors: Comprehensive textbook of psychiatry, ed. vol. 3, Baltimore, 1980, The Williams & Wilkins Co.

thimide and methyprylon, share the drawbacks of the barbiturates and are even more toxic in overdoses. Probably the safest sedative drug currently available is flurazepam (Dalmane), a benzodiazepine. This drug shares the characteristics of the antianxiety drugs of the same class. It is relatively safe and less addictive than other sedative drugs. Table 15-5 summarizes the major sedative-hypnotic drugs.

Nurses should give sedatives with discretion. They are not a substitute for good nursing care. Many other nonmedication, sleep-inducing nursing interventions should be tried. A disturbed patient may benefit more from an opportunity to talk about his problems than from taking a pill for sleep. Providing a back rub or other physical comfort measures may also be helpful. Warm milk is a traditional soporific that is often effective. Creative nursing care can be extremely beneficial to an insomnic patient.

Future directions

Somatic therapies have always had an important place in the psychiatric nurse's repertoire of skills and will undoubtedly continue to do so. The rate of the growth of knowledge at the present time makes it mandatory that nurses maintain their awareness of current practice through continuing education. Public education is also essential as more and more information is disseminated to the community at large. The consumerism movement has stimulated interest in mental health and psychiatric treatment. Because abuses have occurred in the past, professionals are being held accountable for their actions. Consumer education will be a more and more important priority for the nurse.

At the same time, nurses must examine and resolve their own feelings about the treatments that have been presented in this chapter. Many are intrusive to some extent on the person's exercise of free will and personal decision making. Some seem barbaric and unscientific because the reason for effectiveness is vaguely understood, if at all. Yet the consequences of treatment may be vastly preferable to the continuing pain and disability of a serious mental illness. Each nurse must arrive at a personal answer to the questions raised through experience with these treatment modalities. Each nurse has a contribution to make in adding to the growing store of knowledge about the biological aspects of psychiatric disorders. As knowledge grows, so will satisfaction with the treatment that is given.

Suggested cross-references

Ethical decision making is discussed in Chapter 3. Care of suicidal and noncompliant patients is discussed in Chapter 10. Nursing interventions with suspicious and dependent patients are discussed in Chapter 11. Legal issues in psychiatric care are addressed in Chapter 16.

SUMMARY

1. Physical restraint has been used for centuries and is still appropriate at times for treatment of psychiatric patients. Civil liberties must be considered when physical restraint is used.
   a. Mechanical restraints include camisoles, wrist and ankle restraints, sheet restraints, and cold wet sheet packs. The nurse should be familiar with the procedure of applying restraints. Good nursing care includes attention to the patient's biological integrity, interpersonal needs, and right to dignity.
   b. Seclusion or isolation involves the confinement of a patient alone in a room. This procedure should be used infrequently for a short time and with a specific rationale. Good nursing care includes frequent observation of the patient, provision for biological needs, and concern for the

patient's dignity and privacy. An open channel of communication with the patient must be maintained.
2. Psychosurgery refers to the surgical interruption of selected neural pathways that govern transmission of emotion between the frontal lobes of the cerebral cortex and the thalamus. Nursing care focuses on postoperative needs plus whatever retraining might be necessary for the patient to function in the usual social setting.
3. Electroconvulsive therapy is the passage of an electrical current through the brain to induce a grand mal seizure. On the average, six to ten treatments are given in a series. Nurses must be supportive to patients who are receiving this frightening treatment. Patient teaching and reassurance are helpful. Later, orientation and supervision are necessary if confu-

sion occurs. The patient may also need help meeting physiological needs.

4. Insulin shock therapy is infrequently used at the present time. A state of physiological shock is induced by injection of high doses of insulin. The patient is gradually brought to the point of coma. Intensive nursing care is required to monitor the patient's condition both during and following the treatment.

5. Pharmacotherapy is now the most frequently used of the somatic therapies. Major groups of psychopharmacological agents are somewhat specific to various kinds of behavior, although more research needs to be done in the area of specificity. Health teaching is an important nursing function that helps to ensure patient compliance with therapy. Careful observation of patient response to medication, including alertness to side effects, is also essential. Suspicious, suicidal, and dependent patients need especially skillful nursing intervention when they are receiving medications. Major psychotropic groups include the following:

a. Antipsychotic agents, including the subgroups phenothiazines, butyrophenones, and thioxanthene derivatives. Common side effects and complications include extrapyramidal symptoms, anticholinergic reactions, endocrine responses, and allergies. Potential for drug abuse and suicide with these medications is relatively low.

b. Antianxiety agents, including meprobamate, the benzodiazepines, and some antihistamines. Common side effects include drowsiness, dizziness, slurred speech, and blurred vision. There is potential for physical dependence on meprobamate and the benzodiazepines. These drugs potentiate the effect of alcohol and hypnotics

and may be lethal in high doses or in combination with other agents.

c. Antidepressants are divided into two major categories: tricyclics and monoamine oxidase (MAO) inhibitors. Tricyclics are safer and more frequently used. Side effects are generally mild, except that the elderly are sometimes sensitive to hypotensive effects. MAO inhibitors predispose the user to hypertensive crisis if foods containing tyramine are eaten. They also interact with numerous other medications and are therefore usually used only when there is no response to tricyclics. Nurses must teach the patient and family about these reactions. All medications should be used cautiously with depressed patients because of suicidal risk.

d. Lithium carbonate is used specifically to treat the manic phase of manic-depressive disease or preventively to prevent mood swings of known manic-depressive patients. The therapeutic dosage range is narrow and must be monitored by regularly assessing serum lithium levels. Patients must be taught signs of toxicity, including tremors and gastrointestinal disturbances. Health teaching also includes information about situations that might affect the electrolyte balance, such as vomiting, diarrhea, and diaphoresis. Dependency is not a problem, but adherence may be, since the patient may have to commit himself to a lifelong regimen of therapy.

e. Sedative and hypnotic drugs are used in psychiatric settings to assist insomnic patients to sleep. They should be used with caution because they are highly addictive and lethal when taken as an overdose or in combination with alcohol or antianxiety drugs. These properties are characteristic of barbiturates and most nonbarbiturate sedatives. The exception is the benzodiazepine drug flurazepam (Dalmane). It is reasonably safe and not readily addicting.

References

1. American Psychiatric Association: Task force report 14: electroconvulsive therapy, Washington, D.C., 1978, The Association.
2. Burgess, H.A.: When a patient on lithium is pregnant, Am. J. Nurs. **79:**1989, 1979.
3. Cain, R.M., and Cain, N.N.: A compendium of psychiatric drugs, parts I and II, Drug Ther. **5:**77, 105, Jan.-Feb. 1975.
4. Cohen, R.: EST and group therapy = improved care, Am. J. Nurs. **71:**1195, 1971.
5. Connelly, C.E.: Compliance: a review of the research with implications for psychiatric–mental health nursing, J. Psychiatr. Nurs. **16:**15, Oct. 1978.
6. Davis, J.M.: Antidepressant drugs. In Kaplan, H.I., Freedman, A.M., and Sadock, B.J., editors: Comprehensive textbook of psychiatry, ed. 3, vol. 3, Baltimore, 1980, The Williams & Wilkins Co.
7. Davis, J.M.: Antipsychotic drugs. In Kaplan, H.I., Freed-

man, A.M., and Sadock, B.J., editors: Comprehensive textbook of psychiatry, ed. 3, vol. 3, Baltimore, 1980, The Williams & Wilkins Co.
8. Davis, J.M.: Minor tranquilizers, sedatives and hypnotics. In Kaplan, H.I., Freedman, A.M., and Sadock, B.J., editors: Comprehensive textbook of psychiatry, ed. 3, vol. 3, Baltimore, 1980, The Williams & Wilkins Co.
9. Doller, J.C.: Tardive dyskinesia and changing concepts of antipsychotic drug use: a nursing perspective, J. Psychiatr. Nurs. **15:**23, Nov. 1977.
10. Donnelly, J.: Psychosurgery. In Kaplan, H.I., Freedman, A.M., and Sadock, B.J., editors: Comprehensive textbook of psychiatry, ed. 3, vol. 3, Baltimore, 1980, The Williams & Wilkins Co.
11. Ewald, F.R., Freeman, W., and Watts, J.W.: Psychosurgery: the nursing problem, Am. J. Nurs. **47:**210, 1947.

12. Fieve, R.R.: Lithium therapy. In Kaplan, H.I., Freedman, A.M., and Sadock, B.J., editors: Comprehensive textbook of psychiatry, ed. 3, vol. 3, Baltimore, 1980, The Williams & Wilkins Co.

13. Gerald, M.C., and O'Bannon, F.V.: Nursing pharmacology and therapeutics, Englewood Cliffs, N.J., 1981, Prentice-Hall, Inc.

14. Guthiel, T.G.: Observations on the theoretical bases for seclusion of the psychiatric inpatient, Am. J. Psychiatry **135**:325, 1978.

15. Kalayam, B., and Steinhart, M.J.: A survey of attitudes on the use of electroconvulsive therapy, Hosp. Community Psychiatry **32**:185, March 1981.

16. Kalinowsky, L.B.: Convulsive therapies. In Kaplan, H.I., Freedman, A.M., and Sadock, B.J., editors: Comprehensive textbook of psychiatry, ed. 3, vol. 3, Baltimore, 1980, The Williams & Wilkins Co.

17. McAfee, H.A.: Tardive dyskinesia, Am. J. Nurs. **78**:395, 1978.

18. O'Brien, J.: Teaching psychiatric inpatients about their medications, J. Psychiatr. Nurs. **17**:30, Oct. 1979.

19. Peasley, E.L.: The patient having coma shock treatment, Am. J. Nurs. **49**:623, 1949.

20. Rosen, H., and DiGiacomo, J.N.: The role of physical restraint in the treatment of psychiatric illness, J. Clin. Psychiatry **39**:228, March 1978.

21. Surawicz, F.G., and Ludwig, A.M.: Miscellaneous organic therapies. In Kaplan, H.I., Freedman, A.M., and Sadock, B.J., editors: Comprehensive textbook of psychiatry, ed. 3, vol. 3, Baltimore, 1980, The Williams & Wilkins Co.

22. Veterans Administration: Drug treatment in psychiatry, Washington, D.C., 1970, Veterans Administration.

23. Wendt, R.L.: "Good morning, world. I'm glad to be back!" Am. J. Nurs. **79**:949, 1979.

24. Whaley, M.S., and Ramirez, L.F.: The use of seclusion rooms and physical restraints in the treatment of psychiatric patients, J. Psychiatr. Nurs. **18**:13, Jan. 1980.

Annotated suggested readings

American Psychiatric Association Task Force: The current status of lithium therapy: report of the APA task force, Am. J. Psychiatry **132**:997, 1975.

This is a comprehensive review of issues relevant to lithium therapy, including indications for use, contraindications, biochemistry, side effects, and research needs. It is an excellent resource for those who are involved with patients receiving lithium.

American Psychiatric Association: Task force report 14: electroconvulsive therapy, Washington, D.C., 1978, The Association.

This is a comprehensive report of a task force that was formed by the APA to study the use of ECT. The report is based on an extensive survey of psychiatrists and a thorough review of the literature. It is an excellent source of current information, including recommendations for policies and procedures relative to ECT. There is also a good model for obtaining informed consent.

Backinsky, M.: Geriatric medications: how psychotropic drugs can go astray, R.N. **41**:50, Feb. 1978.

The author describes the effects of psychotropic medications on elderly patients. Changes in metabolism and biological responses alter the reactions of the elderly to drugs. This reference will be useful to nurses who work with this age group. A summary chart of drugs and adverse effects is included.

Bridges, P., and Williamson, C.: Psychosurgery today, Nurs. Times **73**:1363, 1977.

This article provides a good update on current use of psychosurgery, including indications, evaluation of candidates and preoperative and postoperative care. The authors address the ethical issues related to this procedure and offer suggestions about conducting a psychosurgery unit in an ethical manner. This is a thorough article that is of interest to nurses in neurosurgical and psychiatric settings.

Buckman, R.W.: Drug interactions and the practice of psychiatry, Curr. Concepts Psychiatry **2**:1, Jan. 1976.

This is a tabular presentation of potential drug interactions between psychopharmacological agents and other drugs. It is presented in summary form, so lacks rationale.

Cain, R.M., and Cain, N.N.: A compendium of psychiatric drugs, parts I and II, Drug Ther. **5**:77, 105, Jan.-Feb. 1975.

This is an excellent overview of the therapeutic effects, side effects, toxic effects, and other pertinent data regarding the major classifications of psychopharmacological agents. A wealth of information is compactly presented.

Cohen, R.: EST and group therapy = improved care, Am. J. Nurs. **71**:1195, 1971.

This article gives a description of the use of EST in one clinical setting, including integration of group interventions with patients who are undergoing electroconvulsive therapy. Particularly useful for the practitioner or student is the inclusion of a sample nursing procedure for EST.

Evans, F.J.: The power of a sugar pill, Psychol. Today, **7**:55, April 1974.

This article presents the arguments for and against the use of placebos. Especially worthwhile for the nurse is the description of the placebo effect that is present with many medications if the caregiver transmits a positive attitude.

Guthiel, T.G.: Observations on the theoretical bases for seclusion of the psychiatric inpatient, Am. J. Psychiatry **135**:325, 1978.

The author has identified conditions under which it is appropriate and inappropriate to seclude a patient. He conveys the belief that this can be a helpful treatment for some patients. However, he also presents drawbacks and contraindications for its use. This is a good overview of some of the debatable issues relative to seclusion.

Hitchens, E.A.: Helping psychiatric outpatients accept drug therapy, Am. J. Nurs. **77**:464, 1977.

The author addresses issues of patient compliance with drug therapy as related to antipsychotic medication. These can be applied to discharge planning with inpatients, as well as work with outpatients. The article presents nursing approaches to maximize the probability of compliance and is recommended for nurses engaged in discharge planning or outpatient therapy.

Kline, N.I., and Davis, J.M.: Psychotropic drugs, Am. J. Nurs. **73**:54, 1973.

*This comprehensive discussion of the most commonly
used psychopharmacological agents includes a wealth of
information useful to nurses at all levels of expertise,
whether used as an introduction to medication in psychiatry or as a review for the experienced nurse.*

Laitinen, L.V., and Livingston, K.E.: Surgical approaches in
psychiatry, Baltimore, 1973, University Park Press.

*This highly technical description of the various pro-
cedures being developed in the area of psychosurgery is
recommended only for the nurse who is directly involved
in care of these patients and who has extensive knowledge
of neuroanatomy, neurology, and neurosurgey.*

McAfee, H.A.: Tardive dyskinesia, Am. J. Nurs. **78:**395,
1978.

*This article presents recent data on tardive dyskinesia,
a side effect of the neuroleptic medications, and includes
possible biochemical explanations for this problem. It emphasizes nursing responsibilities in detecting incipient
tardive dyskinesia and interventions with patients and
families.*

Morgan, A.J.: Minor tranquilizers, hypnotics, and sedatives,
Am. J. Nurs. **73:**1220, 1973.

*This article focuses on criteria for the appropriate use
of these medications, with attention to the potential for
drug abuse and the nurse's responsibility in dispensing
"prn" medications. It is a good basic reference.*

Mulaik, J.S.: Nurses' questions about electroconvulsive therapy, J. Psychiatr. Nurs. **17:**15, Feb. 1979.

*This author has comprehensively and concisely de-
scribed the nursing considerations related to ECT. This
article would be an excellent resource for nurses who are
about to have their first experience with patients who are
receiving ECT. It would also be very helpful to nurses
who are planning nursing care with ECT patients.*

O'Brien, J.: Teaching psychiatric inpatients about their
medications. J. Psychiatr. Nurs. **17:**30, Oct. 1979.

*This article describes the development and implementa-
tion of medication classes for patients as a result of a
nursing staff's concern about readmissions related to noncompliance. It describes in general the teaching approaches used and specifies the areas in which nurses
can and cannot actively educate the patient.*

Pilette, P.C.: The tyranny of seclusion: a brief essay, J. Psychiatr. Nurs. **16:**19, Oct. 1978.

*This is an admittedly emotional essay opposed to the
use of seclusion. It can be a stimulus to thought, leading to discussion and, hopefully, more scientific approaches to this issue.*

Pilette, W.L.: What is an adequate trial of psychotropic medication? Perspect. Psychiatr. Care **15:**170, Oct.-Dec. 1977.

*The author reviewed the literature regarding the dos-
age range and length of time recommended for a therapeutic trial of antipsychotic and antidepressant medications. He found that there were no generally accepted
guidelines incorporating both of these factors. He strongly
recommends that research be conducted to establish reliable guidelines.*

Sclafani, M.: Medication classes for the emotionally ill, J.
Psychiatr. Nurs. **15:**13, April 1977.

*The author briefly describes a medication education
class developed for patients in a state hospital setting. Of
interest are the samples of a pretest and posttest questionnaire assessing the patient's drug knowledge and a
drug information sheet. These tools were developed for use
in this program and may be helpful to others who are planning a similar activity.*

Shader, R.I., editor: Manual of psychiatric therapeutics, Boston, 1975, Little, Brown & Co.

*This collection of papers on a multitude of topics related
to psychopharmacotherapy is a good reference for nurses
with a particular area of interest relative to the use of
medications.*

Thomas, S.P.: Uses and abuses of electric convulsive shock
therapy, J. Psychiatr. Nurs. **16:**17, Nov. 1978.

*The author has thoroughly reviewed the literature per-
taining to ECT and has presented the major controversial issues concerning this treatment. The material is
presented objectively. A good bibliography is included.*

White, J.H.: Pediatric psychopharmacology: a practical guide
to clinical application, Baltimore, 1977, The Williams &
Wilkins Co.

*This book is recommended for nurses specializing in
pediatric or child psychiatric nursing. It is a thorough
consideration of the use of psychopharmacological agents
with children. The material is illustrated with selected
case histories.*

Pinel immediately led Couthon to the section for the deranged, where the sight of the cells made a painful impression on him. Couthon asked to interrogate all the patients. From most, he received only insults and obscene apostrophes. It was useless to prolong the interview. Turning to Pinel, Couthon said: "Now, citizen, are you mad yourself to seek to unchain such beasts?" Pinel replied calmly: "Citizen, I am convinced that these madmen are so intractable only because they have been deprived of air and liberty."

Philippe Pinel, Traité Complet du Régime Sanitaire des Alienes 56 (1836)

CHAPTER 16

LEGAL ASPECTS
OF PSYCHIATRIC
CARE

Learning objectives

After studying this chapter, the student should be able to:

- state the admission, discharge, and status of civil rights as they pertain to informal, voluntary, and involuntary admission to a psychiatric hospital.

- describe the legal justification for commitment, the procedural elements of the commitment process, and the three types of resulting hospitalization.

- analyze the moral, legal, and psychiatric implications of involuntary commitment, including the issues of assessing dangerousness and freedom of choice.

- identify the common civic and personal rights retained by psychiatric patients.

- define the following terms: testamentary capacity, incompetency, confidentiality, privileged communication, and malpractice.

- evaluate the potential benefits and problems that may arise from the right to treatment, the right to refuse treatment, and the right to treatment in the least restrictive setting.

- discuss the rights, responsibilities, and potential conflict of interest attendant in the three legal roles of the nurse: as provider, employee, and citizen.

- compare and contrast the four sets of criteria commonly used in the United States to determine the criminal responsibility of a person believed to be mentally ill.

513

■ *critique the five forces currently affecting the mental health delivery system and the mechanisms and resources needed to improve the quality of mental health care in this country.*

■ *identify suggested readings for future study.*

To assess the awareness of psychiatric professionals of the legal rights of their patients, Trancredi and Clark[24] conducted a study that included psychiatrists, psychiatric residents, nurses, and social workers. The results indicated that they were generally unaware of a patient's legal rights at the time of admission and during hospitalization. Yet the relationship between psychiatry and law reflects the tension between individual rights and social needs, and the two areas have many similarities. Both psychiatry and law deal with human behavior, interrelationships between people, and responsibilities people assume based on these relationships. Both also have a role in society's desire for control of undesirable behavior. Together they mutually analyze when psychiatric treatment is therapeutic, custodial, or incarceration.

There are also discrete differences between the two disciplines. Psychiatry is concerned with the meaning of behavior and personal life satisfaction. Law addresses the outcome of behavior and has developed a system of rules and regulations to facilitate orderly social functioning. These differences are evident in terminology when it is recognized that "insane" and "legal commitment" are predominantly legal, not psychiatric, terms. Lawyers, judges, and juries determine whether a person was insane when he acted and whether a psychotic individual should be legally committed for a period of treatment.

The practice of psychiatric nursing is influenced by the law, particularly in concern for the rights of patients and the quality of care they are receiving. In the past 20 years, civil, criminal, and consumer rights have been established and expanded through judicial decision. Previously powerless and neglected groups such as the mentally ill are now using the legal system as both a forum for the expression of legitimate grievances and as a vehicle for social change. Many of the laws vary from state to state, and professionals are required to become familiar with the legal provisions of their own states because knowledge of the law enhances the freedom of both the nurse and patient.

Hospitalizing the patient

One out of every eight Americans needs some form of mental health services, and a fourth of the people receiving psychiatric care are hospitalized. Not everyone who requires psychiatric care receives it, but the population statistics of mental hospitals are still imposing. Ten of every 10,000 Americans are patients in public mental hospitals, and state hospitals provide a major portion of long-term care for those patients with chronic illness. More than 25% of all hospital beds in the country are occupied by psychiatric patients, and there are three times as many patients on record at psychiatric hospitals as there are criminals in prison.[18] The process of hospitalization can be traumatic or supportive for the individual, depending on the institution, attitude of family and friends, response of the staff, and type of admission. Three major types are used at present: informal, voluntary, and involuntary. Characteristics that distinguish them are summarized in Table 16-1.

Informal admission

This type of admission to a psychiatric hospital occurs in the same way a person is admitted to a general medical hospital, that is, without formal or written application. The individual is then free to leave at any time, as he would be in a general medical hospital. The patient is often requested to sign himself out "against medical advice," but he is not required to do so.

Voluntary admission

Under this procedure any citizen of lawful age may apply in writing (usually by use of a standard admission form) for admission to a public or private psychiatric hospital. He agrees to receive treatment and abide by the hospital rules. His reason for seeking help may be his own personal decision or may be based on the advice of family or a health professional. If a person is too ill to complete the admission process but voluntarily seeks help, a parent or legal guardian may request admission for him. In most states a child under the age of 16 may be admitted if his parents sign the required application form.

This is a preferred type of admission because it is similar to that of any medical hospitaliza-

TABLE 16-1. Distinguishing characteristics of the three types of admission to psychiatric hospitals

	Informal admission	Voluntary admission	Involuntary admission
Admission	No formal application needed	Formal application must be completed by patient	Application did not originate with patient
Discharge	Initiated by patient	Initiated by patient	Initiated by hospital or court but not by patient
Status of civil rights	Retained in full by patient	Retained in full by patient	Patient may retain none, some, or all, depending on state law

tion. It indicates that the individual acknowledges problems in living, is seeking help in coping with them, and will probably actively participate in finding solutions. The majority of patients who enter private psychiatric units of general hospitals are voluntary.

When admitted in this manner, the patient retains all his civil rights. These include such privileges as the right to vote, possess a driver's license, buy and sell property, manage personal affairs, hold office, practice a profession, and engage in a business. It is a common misconception of the public that all admissions to a mental hospital involve the loss of civil rights.

If the voluntary patient wishes to be discharged from the hospital, most states require that he give written notice to the hospital. In some states he can be released immediately; in others he can be detained from 48 hours to 15 days before being discharged. This allows the hospital staff time to confer with the patient and family members and decide if additional inpatient treatment is necessary. If it is and the patient will not withdraw his request for discharge, the family may initiate involuntary commitment proceedings and thereby change the status of the patient.

Although voluntary admission is most desirable, it is not always possible. Sometimes a patient may be acutely disturbed, suicidal, or dangerous to self or others and yet rejecting of any therapeutic intervention. In these cases involuntary commitments are then initiated.

Involuntary admission (commitment)

In the late 1940s the World Health Organization reported that almost 90% of admissions to state mental hospitals in the United States were involuntary commitments. Conversely, only little more than 10% were voluntary. The trend has definitely shifted to more voluntary admissions. In 1963, 30% were voluntary, and by 1971 nearly half of all admissions to psychiatric hospitals were initiated by the patient himself.[3] This trend is due to the greater variety of admission statuses and more stringent limitations placed on the use of involuntary commitment. This is still in striking contrast to England, however, where over 80% of the patients are admitted voluntarily.

Although involuntary commitment has come under more intense scrutiny, the United States Supreme Court continues to recognize it based on two legal theories: first, under its "police power," the state has the authority to protect the community from the dangerous acts of the mentally ill; second, under its *parens patriae* powers, the state has an interest in providing care for citizens who cannot care for themselves, such as some mentally ill persons. In the past 20 years, and particularly over the most recent ones, the police power rationale for civil commitment has been supplanting the *parens patriae* doctrine by means of statutory changes. In addition, there has been a related trend toward increasing the requirements for standards of proof and procedural due process for such commitments.

Involuntary commitment does not always imply compulsion. It means that the request for hospitalization did not originate with the patient and may signify that either it was actively opposed by him or he was indecisive and did not resist. The criteria for commitment vary among states and reflect the confusion present in the medical, social, and legal arenas of society. Most laws justify commitment of the mentally ill on three grounds: (1) dangerous to others, (2) dangerous to self, and (3) need for treatment. The important element appears to be whether the person can function in a reasonable manner in the outside world without becoming an undue burden on his family or the community. The vagueness of these criteria is reflected in the patients committed to psychiatric hospitals. Those suffering from psychoses account for less than half of all admissions, and the aged, the neurotic, and others account for the majority.[13]

State laws on commitment vary, but they attempt to protect the individual who is not mentally ill from being detained in a psychiatric hospital against his will for political, economic, family, or other nonmedical reasons. Certain procedural elements of the commitment process are common. Action is begun with a sworn petition by a relative, friend, public official, physician, or any interested citizen stating the person is mentally ill and is in need of treatment. Some states allow only specific individuals to file such a petition. An examination of the patient's mental status is then completed by one or two physicians. Some states require at least one of the physicians be a psychiatrist.

The decision as to whether the patient requires hospitalization is then made. Precisely who makes this decision determines the nature of the commitment. Medical certification means a specified number of appointed physicians make the decision. This power to certify is given to all physicians and not limited to psychiatrists. Court or judicial commitment is decided on by a judge or jury in a formal hearing. In this case the court is required to notify the patient so that he can retain legal counsel to prepare for the hearing if he desires to contest it. A jury trial is not mandatory in most states but can be requested by the patient. Most states recognize the right of the patient to have legal counsel, but only about half actually appoint a lawyer for the patient if he does not have one. Administrative commitment is determined by a special tribunal of hearing officers. The Fourteenth Amendment to the United States Constitution protects citizens against infringements on liberty without "due process of the law." Because of this, medical certification is used infrequently and primarily in emergency situations, and administrative commitment is subject to judicial review.

If the individual is determined to be in need of treatment, the final step of the commitment process then occurs and he is hospitalized. This may be for varying lengths of time, depending on the needs of the patient. Fig. 16-1 presents a diagrammatical model of the involuntary commitment process. It identifies three types of hospitalization: emergency, temporary, and indefinite.

EMERGENCY HOSPITALIZATION. Almost all states have provisions for emergency commitment for patients who are acutely ill. The goals

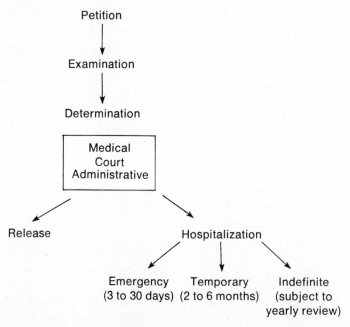

FIG. 16-1
Diagrammatical model of the involuntary commitment process.

for the commitment are short term, and it is primarily intended as a means of controlling an immediate threat to self or others. In those states lacking such a law the acutely ill individual is often taken into custody by the police and kept in jail on a disorderly conduct charge, which is a criminal charge. Such a practice is inappropriate and frequently detrimental to the mental status of the patient.

To obtain an emergency commitment, the patient's family, a physician, or someone designated by the state must file a petition that includes a supporting report by a psychiatrist. It is then reviewed by a judge or hospital official, and hospitalization is provided. Most state laws limit the time the person can be detained under emergency commitment to from 3 to 30 days. Emergency hospitalization allows for detainment in a psychiatric hospital only until proper legal steps are taken to provide for additional hospitalization.

TEMPORARY OR OBSERVATIONAL HOSPITALIZATION. This type of commitment is primarily used for the purpose of diagnosis and short-term therapy and does not require an emergency situation, as does the emergency hospitalization. Again, the commitment is for a specified period of time, but in this case it ranges from 2 to 6 months. The commitment process is similar to that just described. Some states require a court order for all temporary commitments, whereas others require one only if the person protests the hospitalization. If at the end of the stipulated period of time the patient is still not ready for discharge, a petition can be filed for an indefinite commitment.

INDEFINITE HOSPITALIZATION (FORMAL COMMITMENT). A formal commitment provides for the hospitalization of a patient for an indeterminate amount of time or until he is ready for discharge. The process is usually that of a court commitment. Patients in public or state hospitals more frequently have indefinite commitments than patients in private hospitals. Even when committed, these patients maintain their right to consult a lawyer at any time and to request a court hearing to determine if additional hospitalization is necessary. The hospital ultimately discharges the patient, however, and a court order is not necessary to do this.

Commitment dilemma

In nine states involuntary commitment assumes incompetency and is accompanied by the patient's loss of his civil rights. He is restricted in his ability to make contracts, vote, drive, obtain a professional license, serve on a jury, marry, or enter into civil litigation. In addition, the patient must suffer the stigma attached to the label "committed" in all his future activities. Because of the large number of people affected by involuntary commitment and the loss of personal rights that it entails, it becomes a matter of great legal, moral, social, and psychiatric significance. In the practice of general medicine there is no equivalent divestment of individual rights except for rare cases of mandated quarantine for carriers of some potentially epidemic diseases.

The question may be asked "How disturbed or ill does one need to be to merit commitment as insane?" A psychotic state is not a necessary or sufficient cause for commitment, as evident in the number of elderly, addicted, and neurotic patients hospitalized, as well as the many psychotic individuals who remain at liberty. Perhaps a person's dangerousness to himself or others is a more pertinent consideration. Certainly psychiatric professionals consider hospitalization in this instance as a humanitarian gesture and as a protection of the individual and society. "Dangerousness," however, is an undefined, unspecified term.

DANGEROUSNESS. It is interesting to note that people who are mentally healthy and dangerous have their freedom guarded by the courts so that after a prison sentence is served, the individual is automatically released and can no longer be retained. However, someone who is mentally ill and dangerous can be confined indefinitely. Ennis makes the following observation:

Of all the identifiably dangerous groups in society, only the mentally ill are singled out for preventive detention and . . . they are probably the least dangerous as a group. Why should society confine a person if he is dangerous and mentally ill but not if he is dangerous and sane?"[8:101]

To support his suggestion that the mentally ill are probably less dangerous than the mentally healthy, he cites a 5-year study of 5000 patients discharged from a state mental hospital in New York. The results showed that their arrest rate was one twelfth that of the general population. The idea of preventive detention does not exist in most areas of the law where the ability to predict an action does not confer the right to control the action in advance. Only illegal acts result in a prolonged loss of liberty for most citizens, except the mentally ill.

Another aspect of this dilemma also revolves around this idea of dangerousness. Extensive reviews of the literature have concluded that there are no reliable indicators of dangerousness.[22] Furthermore, even if some mentally ill individuals are potentially dangerous, it has not been proved that psychiatrists are good predictors of future violence. Frequently psychiatrists overpredict the patient's potential for dangerous acts and the extent of his illness. Oran[15] believes this is because of the medical training of the psychiatrist, which has taught him that underdiagnosis is more harmful than overdiagnosis. It is compounded by his conflicting roles as agents of both the patient and community, which require him to be therapist, warden, and judge. If he underpredicts a psychiatric illness and the patient later causes harm, the community's anger is directed at him. If he overpredicts illness, however, a patient is subjected to treatment against his will.

Szasz[23] states that whether a person is dangerous is not the real issue, but it is rather who he is and how he is dangerous. He believes society condones danger in some ways but not others. For example, drunken drivers are very dangerous and kill many more people than people with paranoid ideation. But drunken drivers are not committed, and people labeled paranoid are. In fact, some kinds of dangerous behaviors required in certain roles, such as race car driver, trapeze artist, and astronaut are admired and valued. It has been suggested that the assessment of danger involves four separate questions[6]:

1. What type of harmful act is to be considered dangerous: physical or psychological harm, harm to persons, or harm to property?
2. What degree of injury constitutes harm: verbal abuse, assault, or assault with a weapon?
3. How likely is it that the harmful act will occur? Do actuarial tables or clinical judgment give us predictive ability?
4. How frequently will the harmful act recur? Do the compulsively repeated acts of the exhibitionist make him more dangerous than a man whose only violent act was the murder of both his parents?

The answers to these questions can be very sub-

jective, which suggests that the underlying issue is one of noncomformity in ways that offend others. In this context social role becomes important.

Before the law all men are equal, but it is also true that the majority of committed patients are members of the lower classes. Scheff has observed the following:

There is a large portion of the patient population, 43 percent, whose presence in the hospital cannot readily be explained in terms of their psychiatric condition. Their presence suggests the punitive character of the societal reaction to deviance.[20:168]

The behavioral criterion of dangerousness for commitment can be said to change the function of the psychiatric hospital from a place of therapy for mental illness to a place of confinement for certain offensive behavior. It suggests that the covert function of the psychiatric hospital is that of social control. This idea is supported by the various behavioral disorders that justify commitment, including drug addiction, alcoholism, and sexual offenses. In addition, epileptics are vulnerable to commitment in almost 40% of the states despite the fact that epilepsy is not a mental illness but a controllable physical abnormality.

FREEDOM OF CHOICE. The legal and psychiatric question being raised is one of freedom of choice. Some professionals believe that at certain times the individual cannot be responsible for himself. For his own protection and the protection of society it is necessary to confine him and to make decisions for him. An example is the suicidal patient. In most states it is against the law to kill oneself. Law and psychiatry join therefore to protect the person and help him resolve his conflict. How does this compare with the cancer or cardiac patient who may reject medical advice and his identified therapeutic regimen? Should society, through law and medicine, attempt to cure him by involuntary methods? Some physicians, like Chodoff,[4] view civil commitment as basically a benevolent system that can make bona fide treatment available. He disagrees with the assumption that the mentally ill are competent to exercise free will and make decisions in their own best interest, such as decisions about whether to take medications or whether to be out in the streets instead of in a hospital. He contends that there are mentally ill people who may not be physically dangerous but nevertheless endanger their own prospects for a normal life. Chodoff believes institutions can at least protect them and in many cases help them. Thus he views the abolition of involuntary civil commitment as gravely immoral.

Other individuals, such as Szasz, oppose intervention. Szasz argues for responsibility for self and the right to choose or reject treatment. Should one's actions violate criminal law, he suggests the individual be punished for those actions through the penal system:

For some time now I have maintained that commitment—that is, the detention of persons in mental institutions against their will—is a form of imprisonment; that such deprivation of liberty is contrary to the moral principles embodied in the Declaration of Independence and the Constitution of the United States; and that it is a gross violation of contemporary concepts of fundamental human rights. The practice of "sane" men incarcerating their "insane" fellow men in "mental hospitals" can be compared to that of white men enslaving black men. In short, I consider commitment a crime against humanity[23:113]*

There is currently a trend toward due process and evidentiary procedures and standards that approach or adopt the rigor of procedures and standards used in the criminal process. These changes are reflected in the Massachusetts Mental Health Act of 1970, which recoded the statutes governing the admission, treatment, and discharge of the mentally ill and mentally retarded. The changes in the Massachusetts statute were both substantive and procedural. The most significant substantive change was the elimination of very broad and vague criteria for commitment. These vague criteria were replaced by ones which required that the likelihood of serious harm to self or others be proven prior to involuntary hospitalization. There were at least two important procedural changes made. One was the abolition of an indefinite period of involuntary hospitalization. The commitment was required to be for limited periods. The second important change was the requirement of fact evidence, rather than just expert opinions, as to whether the prospective patient met the legal criteria for commitment. The significance of these changes is indicated by the fact that nine other states (Maine, Nebraska, New Mexico, Ohio, Rhode Island, South Carolina, Tennessee, Washington, and Wisconsin) have statutorily adopted either the identical or substantially the same language as the Massachusetts standard for civil commitment.

Whether to take a stand for or against com-

mitment is an issue each nurse must resolve for herself. What should be done if the nonconformist does not wish to change his behavior? Does he maintain his freedom to choose even if his thinking appears to be irrational or divergent from the norm? Does the concept of mutuality exclude coercion? Can social interests be served by a means less restrictive than total confinement, such as outpatient therapy? Every nurse should assume the responsibility for reviewing the commitment procedures in her state and work for legislative amendments that would facilitate the necessary reforms.

The commitment dilemma therefore exposes present practices and opens areas of controversy for the future. The present mental hospital has been described as a jail, hospital, poorhouse, and home for the elderly. It protects, treats, feeds, maintains, and houses socially incompetent individuals who are often feared by society. When they are discharged from the hospital, they are frequently left without alternatives and come to the attention of law enforcement agencies or welfare offices. Local communities deny the problem by resisting the establishment of halfway houses or sheltered homes in their neighborhood. Third-party insurance seldom covers extended outpatient psychiatric care. In today's mobile and impersonal society, family and friends are often unwilling or unable to care for the newly released patient, who may end up in a dismal run-down hotel or boarding house with nothing to do but watch television and wander the streets.

These issues need to be addressed by psychiatric nurses, patients, and citizens across the country. The value of commitment, goals of hospitalization, quality of life, and rights of patients must be closely aligned and resolved through the judicial, legislative, and medical systems.

Discharge

A patient who voluntarily admits himself into the hospital can be discharged by the staff when he has received "maximum benefit" from the treatment, or he may initiate his own discharge request. Most states require that he give written notice of his desire for discharge, and some hospitals will also request he sign a form that states he is leaving "against medical advice." These forms then become part of his permanent record. He is usually released 24 to 72 hours after submitting a discharge request. In the event that

*Excerpt from *Ideology and Insanity* by Thomas Szasz. Copyright © 1970 by Thomas S. Szasz. Used by permission of Doubleday & Co., Inc.

a voluntarily admitted patient elopes from the hospital, he can be brought back only if he again voluntarily agrees. Staff frequently attempt to contact such a patient and discuss alternatives with him. If he refuses to return to the hospital, he must either be discharged or involuntary commitment procedures must be initiated.

An involuntarily admitted or committed patient has lost the right to leave the hospital when he wishes. Temporary and emergency commitments specify the maximal length of detainment. Indefinite commitments do not, although periodic reviews of the patient's status should be held, and the patient may apply for another commitment hearing to determine if additional hospitalization is necessary. If a committed patient elopes, the staff has the legal obligation to notify the police and committing courts. Frequently these patients return home or visit family or friends and can be easily located. The legal authorities then return the patient to the hospital, and additional steps are not necessary, since the original commitment is still effective.

There are three specific kinds of discharges. These include the conditional discharge, absolute discharge, and judicial discharge.

Conditional discharge

Many committed patients are assisted in the transition from the hospital into the community by specified leaves of absence or liberties. These are known as conditional discharges because certain things are expected of the patient. Most frequently he is required to attend outpatient therapy through the hospital or community mental health center. If he is progressing well, his leaves may be extended for 30 to 90 days or more. During this time the commitment order is still in effect, and, should he relapse while in the community, he can be brought back to the hospital and treatment continued.

This type of discharge planning allows for a gradual integration into the community, and many patients have benefited from it. If at the end of the conditional period the patient demonstrates a good adjustment, the hospital can issue an absolute discharge of the patient.

Absolute discharge

As the name implies, absolute discharge is the termination of the patient's relationship with the hospital. It is a final discharge, and if the patient needs to return to the hospital at some future time, new admission proceedings must be initiated. Usually the hospital is required to notify the court when a committed patient is given an absolute discharge.

This type of discharge is employed most often when substantial progress has been made by the patient and he is able to function well in the community. However, there are also instances when patients who have not improved and are unlikely to improve in the future are granted absolute discharges. In these instances arrangements are made with the families or guardians to provide satisfactory care for the patient. In addition, some laws require that other state officials be notified by the hospital.

Judicial discharge

Nearly 40 states now have laws that allow a patient or his family the right to appeal to the court for a discharge even though the hospital does not agree with the discharge request. The process and requirements for such cases vary from state to state, but they allow the patient an additional recourse for grievance if he believes hospitalization is no longer appropriate. Such legislation may be instrumental in further defining patients' rights in future years.

Patients' rights

In 1973 the American Hospital Association issued a Patient's Bill of Rights, which many general hospitals throughout the country have adopted. Psychiatric hospitals, however, continue to struggle with the issue of the basic civil rights of the individual. In recent years the civil and personal rights of the mentally ill have been supported in legislative acts throughout the country. In retrospect the new laws also reflect the restrictions and discriminations suffered by the mentally ill in the past. Some states are now allowing the committed patient to retain all his civil rights, similar to the voluntary patient, except the right to leave the hospital and to terminate treatment.

Allowing for great variation among states, patients presently have the following rights[11]:

■ Right to communicate with people outside the hospital through correspondence, telephone, and personal visits
■ Right to keep clothing and personal effects with them in the hospital
■ Right to religious freedom

- Right to be employed if possible
- Right to manage and dispose of property
- Right to execute wills
- Right to enter into contractual relationships
- Right to make purchases
- Right to education
- Right to habeas corpus
- Right to independent psychiatric examination
- Right to civil service status
- Right to retain licenses, privileges, or permits established by law, such as a driver's or professional license
- Right to sue or be sued
- Right to marry and divorce
- Right not to be subject to unnecessary mechanical restraints
- Right to periodic review of status
- Right to legal representation
- Right to privacy
- Right of informed consent
- Right to treatment
- Right to refuse treatment
- Right to treatment in the least restrictive setting

Some of these rights merit exploration in greater detail.

RIGHT TO COMMUNICATE WITH PEOPLE OUTSIDE THE HOSPITAL. This right entails the freedom of the patient to visit and hold telephone conversations in privacy and send unopened letters to anyone of his choice, including judges, lawyers, families, and staff. On occasions hospital staff have intercepted letters presumed to be threatening or abusive and disposed of them. In states where this is not illegal, such activity raises the moral question of individual freedom vs. the good of the community.

RIGHT TO KEEP PERSONAL EFFECTS. This establishes the right of the patient to bring clothing and personal items with him to the hospital, taking into consideration the amount of space available for storage of them. It does not make the hospital responsible for their safety. Valuable items should preferably be left at home. If the patient brings something of value to the hospital, the staff should place it in the hospital safe or make other appropriate provisions for its safekeeping.

RIGHT TO BE EMPLOYED IF POSSIBLE. This includes the right to work whenever possible and the right to be compensated for it, including payment for work-therapy programs within the hospital. Involuntary servitude or work without pay within institutions is on the decline because courts have held that the Thirteenth Amendment, which abolished slavery, also applies to psychiatric patients. The consequence of these decisions is that mental institutions cannot force patients to work, either by punishing them or by making privileges or discharge dependent on work. If patients choose to work, they must be assigned jobs on documented therapeutic grounds and they must be paid the minimum wage.

The Department of Labor is notifying all institutions that if they fail to pay patient workers, they are violating the law. The ultimate effect of this move is not yet known. Some professionals fear that the money to pay patients will come out of treatment funds and that the patients will fare worse in the end. Others fear that hospitals will hire regular labor and leave the patients with nothing to do. Some argue that institutions will charge patients for room and board and recover much of the money. A further fear raised is that if the Department of Labor enforces the law and if institutions comply, they may be forced to close because of lack of funds.

RIGHT TO EXECUTE WILLS. A person's competency to make a will is known as *testamentary capacity*. He can make a valid will if he (1) knows that he is making a will; (2) knows the nature and extent of his property, and (3) knows who his friends and relatives are and what the relationships mean. Each of these criteria must be met for the will to be considered valid. This means he must not be mentally confused at the time he signed his will. It does not imply that he must have the exact details of his property holdings or specific bank account figures. But he cannot attempt to give away more than he possesses. Furthermore, the law requires that he know who his relatives are but does not require him to bequeath anything to them.

The fact that a patient is committed or is diagnosed as psychotic does not immediately invalidate his will. The will is valid if it was made during a lucid period and the patient met the three criteria. The problem most debated in determining testamentary capacity is the delusional patient, particularly if the delusional thinking could alter the outcome of the will. The important question in this regard is whether the false belief or delusion caused the person to dispose of his property in a different way than he would have otherwise.

Two or three persons must witness the will

by watching the person as he signs it and each other as they sign it. It is necessary therefore that they all be together at this time. At a later time a nurse may be summoned into court to give testimony on the condition of the person at the time he drew up his will. The nurse should testify relative to the three criteria, as well as report pertinent observations, recall information as accurately as possible, and express herself concisely and objectively. Hospital charts may also be used in the court proceedings, and the nurse's notes relative to the patient's behavior and mental status may provide additional information.

RIGHT TO ENTER INTO CONTRACTUAL RELATIONSHIPS. Contracts are considered valid by the court if the person understands the circumstances involved in the contract and the natural consequences of it. Once again, a psychiatric illness does not invalidate a contract, although the nature of the contract and degree of judgment needed to understand it would be influencing factors.

Incompetency. An issue related to this right is the one of mental incompetency. Every adult is assumed to be mentally competent and possess the mental ability to carry out his affairs. To prove otherwise requires a special court hearing to declare him "incompetent." This is a legal term without a precise medical meaning. To prove that an individual is incompetent it must be shown that (1) he has a mental disorder, (2) this disorder causes a defect in judgment, and (3) this defect makes him incapable of handling his own affairs. All three elements must be present, and the exact diagnostic label is not as important in this regard. If a person is declared incompetent, a legal guardian will be appointed by the court to manage the patient's estate. This frequently is a family member, friend, or bank executive. Incompetency rulings are most often filed for persons with senile dementia, cerebral arteriosclerosis, chronic schizophrenia, and mental retardation.

The trend in legislation is to separate the concepts of incompetency and involuntary commitment, since the reasons for each are essentially different. Incompetency arises from society's desire to safeguard a person's assets from his own inability to understand and transact business. Involuntary commitments are usually initiated to protect the patient from himself (in the case of suicide), protect others from the patient (in the case of homicide), and administer treatment. However, many states still consider the two equivalent, and the policies and procedures of the hospital may impose the incompetent status on the patient.

As a result of an incompetency ruling, the person cannot vote, marry, drive, or make contracts. A release from the hospital is not necessarily an automatic restoration to competency. Rather, another court hearing is required to reverse the previous ruling and declare the individual competent and allow him to once again manage his own affairs.

RIGHT TO EDUCATION. This right is being exercised by many parents on behalf of their emotionally ill or mentally retarded children. Everyone is guaranteed this right under the constitution, although many states have not made provisions for the adequate education of all groups of citizens and are now being required to do so.

RIGHT TO HABEAS CORPUS. Habeas corpus is an important right the person retains in all states even if he has been involuntarily admitted to the hospital. It originated in English Common Law and is provided for in the Constitution of the United States. The object of the writ is the speedy release of any individual who claims he is being deprived of his liberty and detained illegally. A committed patient may file such a writ at any time on the grounds that he is sane and eligible for release. The hearing takes place in a court of law where those people who serve to restrain the patient must defend their actions. A jury is sometimes impaneled to determine the sanity of the patient. A determination is then made, and if the court finds the patient to be sane, he is discharged from the hospital.

RIGHT TO INDEPENDENT PSYCHIATRIC EXAMINATION. Under the Emergency Admission Statute the patient has the right to demand a psychiatric examination by a physician of his own choice. If this physician determines that he is not mentally ill, the patient must be released.

RIGHT TO MARRY AND DIVORCE. Since marriage is a formal contract, the same general criteria for validity apply; that is, the marriage is considered valid if the individual understands the nature of the marriage relationship and the duties and obligations it entails. The crucial element is his mental capacity at the time of the marriage, not before it or after it. In general, courts are reluctant to declare a marriage void. Many states have laws forbidding the marriage of mentally ill persons. This is based on the notion that mental illness, whether genetically or environmentally induced, often runs in families. Thus the primary objective of such laws is to prevent the procreation of children who might be mentally ill. In these cases the law is not based on any scientific evidence of the inheritability of mental illness.

In most states psychiatric illness is not in itself grounds for divorce. However, some states will grant divorces if the mentally ill spouse has been committed to a hospital for a certain number of years (usually 3 to 5). It is sometimes also necessary to specify that the spouse is "incurably insane." Many psychiatric professionals are hesitant to make such a determination.

RIGHT TO PRIVACY. The right to privacy implies the right of the individual to keep some information about himself completely secret from others. *Confidentiality* involves the disclosure of certain information to another person, but this is limited to specifically authorized individuals. It is the responsibility of every psychiatric professional to safeguard a patient's right to confidentiality in all aspects of psychiatric treatment, including even the knowledge that a person is in therapy or in a hospital. Revealing such information might damage a person's reputation or hamper his ability to obtain a job. This was most dramatically evident when Senator Eagleton was running as a vice-presidential candidate in the 1972 presidential election. Unfortunately, as with most rights, the protection of the law cannot be applied in a discriminative manner, and thus potential ethical and professional dilemmas can be created, such as the one experienced by the nurse in the following true case,[10] Clinical example 16-1.

CLINICAL EXAMPLE 16-1

On a Wednesday morning in 1981 in Springfield, Illinois, a man walked into Lauterbach's Cottage Hardware Store, grabbed an ax and began swinging. When he left, one person was dead and two others were critically injured. Ten days later, police received a call from Mr. K who was a patient in the 49-bed psychiatric unit at St. John's Hospital. Mr. K told the police that his roommate at the hospital confessed the crime. However, he didn't know his roommate's name. He asked Nurse M to identify him but she refused to do so, since she believed his name was shielded by a state law guaranteeing the privacy of mental

health records. Hospital administrators supported her decision even after she was fined $250 by a county judge for refusing to give the man's name to a grand jury. Nurse M did tell the police that the suspect was not a patient in St. John's at the time of the murder and that he resembled their composite sketch.

The issue of confidentiality is becoming increasingly important, since various agencies demand information about a patient's history, diagnosis, treatment, and prognosis and sophisticated methods for obtaining information (such as wiretapping and computer banks) have been developed. These threaten the individual's right to privacy. The clinician is free from legal responsibility if information is released with the patient's written and signed request. As a rule it is best to reveal as little information as possible and discuss with the patient what the material will be.

The concept of confidentiality builds on the element of trust necessary in a patient-therapist relationship. The patient places himself in the care of others and reveals vulnerable aspects of his personal life. In return he expects high-quality care and the safeguard of his interests. Thus the patient-therapist relationship is an intimate one and demands trust, loyalty, and the maintenance of privacy.

The phrase *privileged communication* is a legal one and applies only in court-related proceedings. It includes communications between husband and wife, attorney and client, and clergyman and church member. The right to reveal information belongs to the person who spoke, and the listener cannot disclose the information unless the speaker gives permission. This privilege exists for the protection of the patient who could sue the listener for the disclosure of privileged information. Another purpose of it is to inspire confidence in the patient to encourage making a full account of symptoms and conditions so that they may be properly cared for and treated. Privileged communication between other professionals and a patient exists only if a law specifically establishes it. Thirty-three states currently recognize privileged communication between physicians and patients; twelve do not. Five states have laws providing for privileged communication between nurses and patients, including Arkansas, New York, Oregon, Vermont, and Wisconsin.[16] In these states the nurse is exempt from giving information obtained in a professional capacity if the information was necessary to implement nursing care. All the other states do not, and a nurse would be required to reveal what the patient said to her in a court of law. In general, however, it is rare that a nurse is called into court to divulge information of this kind.

In 1975 the Federal Rules of Evidence were revised to extend physician-patient privilege only to psychotherapist-patient privilege. Acknowledging, however, that sometimes it was necessary to obtain information for the good of the public interest or to avoid fraud, the following exceptions were noted[25]:

1. Communications *not* made for purposes of diagnosis and treatment
2. Commitment and restoration proceedings
3. Issues as to wills or otherwise between parties claiming by succession from the patient
4. Actions on insurance policies
5. Required reports (venereal diseases, gunshot wounds, child abuse)
6. Communications in furtherance of the crime of fraud; mental or physical condition put in issue by the patient (personal injury cases)
7. Malpractice actions
8. Some or all criminal prosecutions, depending on the state

Most hospitals keep psychiatric records separately and provide that they are less accessible than medical records. They are viewed by the law and psychiatric profession to be more sensitive than general medical records. Psychiatrists, for the most part, retain the right to decide if they should release medical information to the patient, and in some states patients are barred from viewing them at all. A hospital chart can be summoned into court, however, and anything that is written in it can be used in a lawsuit. Privileged communication does not apply to hospital charts, and nursing notes should be written carefully in all cases. Furthermore, it is a general rule that only those persons involved in a patient's care may read his chart. This includes physicians, nurses, aides, students, and others directly involved in the treatment process.

RIGHT TO INFORMED CONSENT. Informed consent includes the disclosure by a physician of a certain amount of information to the patient about the proposed treatment and the attainment of the patient's consent, which must be competent, understanding, and voluntary. The physician must explain the special treatment, its possible complications, and its risks. The patient must be capable of giving consent and not be a minor or judged incompetent or insane by the court. Failure to obtain consent may be the basis for lawsuits of "assault and battery" or negligence.

Psychiatric outpatients usually express their consent by their willingness to come for treatment, and only unusual treatments, such as experimental drugs or ECT require specific written consent. Informally admitted and voluntary patients usually sign a paper on admission consenting to psychiatric treatment, which includes milieu therapy, chemotherapy, psychotherapy, and occupational therapy. Unusual treatments again need special permission. In the care of the involuntarily admitted patient, the commitment procedure gives the hospital the right to treat the patient.

Consent forms usually require the signature of the patient, a family member, and two persons who witnessed their signing it. Nurses are frequently called on in this regard. It then becomes a part of the patient's permanent hospital record.

RIGHT TO TREATMENT. The concept of the right to treatment is a relatively recent development. In 1960 Birnbaum, a graduate student in both medicine and law, wrote, "there does not appear to have been any significant and realistic consideration given, from a legal viewpoint, to the problem of whether or not the institutionalized mentally ill person receives adequate medical treatment so that he may regain his health, and therefore his liberty, as soon as possible."[2] This cause received its impetus with a 1966 case in the District of Columbia (*Rouse vs. Cameron*). The court held that mental patients committed by criminal courts had the right to adequate treatment. Furthermore, it said that confinement without treatment was tantamount to incarceration and thus transformed the hospital into a penitentiary. It affirmed that the purpose of involuntary hospitalization was treatment, not punishment, and if this treatment was not provided, the patient could be transferred, released, or even awarded damages for his period of confinement. The court clarified that the hospital did not need to show that the treatment would improve or cure the patient but only that there was a true attempt to do so.

This right to treatment was extended in 1972 to all mentally ill and mentally retarded persons who were involuntarily hospitalized in a case in Alabama (*Wyatt vs. Stickney*). The court stated:

> To deprive any citizen of his or her liberty upon the altruistic theory that the confinement is for humane therapeutic reasons and then fail to provide adequate treatment violates the very fundamentals of due process.[28]

It further defined criteria for adequate treatment in three areas: (1) a humane psychological and physical environment, (2) a qualified staff with a sufficient number of members to administer adequate treatment, and (3) individualized treatment plans. The keystone of the Wyatt decision is the requirement that an individualized treatment plan be formulated. Failure to provide it means the patient must be discharged unless he agrees to remain voluntarily. This case is presently being appealed to a higher court, and if this decision is upheld, it will be an important one because it goes beyond the earlier right-to-treatment case and states that judicially enforceable standards of care in mental hospitals are required. It will also have economic implications, since meeting the three criteria of a humane environment, qualified staff in sufficient numbers, and individualized treatment plans will clearly cost more money. Upholding the court's decision might very well force states to reconsider the economic resource allocation presently allotted to mental health.

A landmark court decision in this area was given in June, 1975, by the Supreme Court in the case of *Donaldson vs. O'Connor* in which a Florida State psychiatric patient was freed after 15 years of confinement. The court ruled that he was not dangerous and was not receiving treatment and therefore to continue to confine him would be in violation of his right to liberty.

The constitutional basis for the right to treatment is found in the Eighth and Fourteenth Amendments. The Eighth Amendment deals with the issue of cruel and unusual punishment and the Fourteenth deals with due process and equal protection under the law. Various right-to-treatment cases have been introduced in the state courts throughout the country, and the outcome of them will greatly affect the care of the mentally ill. This new right, however, also poses several questions. One involves the appropriateness of treatment and whether confinement itself can be considered therapeutic. A second problem raises the question of what to do with the patient who is untreatable. Should a

length of time be set after which the patient is released? Another problem is the unwilling patient. Might a person refuse treatment and then seek his release, claiming he was denied his right to adequate treatment? A more pressing question is whether the public is willing to pay the magnitude of the costs required to provide adequate treatment to the mentally ill in public institutions? In current times of high inflation and reduction in government funds, programs are often struggling for survival at existing funding levels, let alone expansion. Thus fiscal constraints may play an even greater role than judicial decisions in affecting the care of the mentally ill.

RIGHT TO REFUSE TREATMENT. The relationship between the right to treatment and the right to refuse treatment is a complex one. The right to refuse treatment includes the right to refuse involuntary hospitalization and has been called the "right to be left alone." Some people believe that therapy has the power to control a person's mind, regulate his thoughts, and change his personality, and the patient should be protected against this by the right to refuse treatment. This argument states that involuntary therapy conflicts with two basic human and legal rights. The first is freedom of thought and the second is the right to control one's own life and actions as long as they do not interfere with the rights of others. An issue related to this is the right to refuse experimentation. A minimum requirement for any experimental treatment is the written consent of the patient. But evidence exists that in certain institutions inadequate consent had been obtained and in others no attempt at all was made to obtain consent.[21]

The landmark case in establishing this right for psychiatric patients was decided in 1979 in *Rogers vs. Okin*. In this case the court went farther than in any previous case in establishing the rights of hospitalized psychiatric patients to refuse medication by reinforcing the standard that restraint may be used only in cases of emergency, such as the occurrence of, or serious threat of, extreme violence, personal injury, or attempted suicide. In writing the opinion for the court, Judge Tauro held that:

> The committed patient has a right to be wrong in his analysis of that information (regarding a particular treatment program)—as long as the consequences of such error do not pose a danger of physical harm to himself, fellow patients or hospital staff. And so, while

the state may have an obligation to make treatment available, and a legitimate interest in providing such treatment, a competent patient has a fundamental right to decide to be left alone, absent an emergency.[19]

Thus the fundamental premise of the court's decision in this case was that committed psychiatric patients were presumed competent to make decisions with respect to treatment in nonemergencies.

The questions raised by the right-to-refuse-treatment concept are many. Does the right apply to all treatment techniques, including medications, or only to those which are hazardous, intrusive, or severe, such as psychosurgery? How can staff meet the obligation to implement the right to treatment when a patient refuses to be treated? How does one differentiate between refusal, resisting treatment, and noncompliance and does each of these interpretations require a different course of action? There are no existing solutions to these complex issues, but they are of concern to nurses, who are frequently responsible for delivering prescribed treatment modalities such as medications.

At this time nurses should make their judgments on a case-by-case basis. The Task Force on Behavior Therapy has examined the issue of coerced treatment and suggested three criteria that may justify it[1]:

1. The patient must be judged to be dangerous to himself or others.
2. It must be believed by those administering treatment that it has a reasonable chance to benefit the patient and those related to him.
3. The patient must be judged to be incompetent to evaluate the necessity of the treatment.

They stress that even if these three conditions are met, the patient should not be deceived. He should be informed as to what will be done to him, the reasons for it, and its probable effects.

Future court decisions will certainly explore the many aspects of this issue. Peck indicates possible outcomes:

> The right-to-treatment movement . . . will undoubtedly do away with some of the injustices and deplorable conditions that have resulted in support for the right to refuse treatment and involuntary hospitalization. The end result might be more humane hospitals and treatment, which would lessen the impact of this movement. On the other hand, the right to treatment will probably also tend to make hospitals force their treatment, out of fear of being sued, on persons who were previously ignored. This in turn might result in an increase in cases maintaining the right to refuse treatment.[17:315]

RIGHT TO TREATMENT IN THE LEAST RESTRICTIVE SETTING. The right to treatment in the least restrictive setting is closely related to the right to adequate treatment. It refers to the goal of evaluating the specific needs of each patient and maintaining the greatest amount of personal freedom, autonomy, dignity, and integrity in determining the treatment or services he is to receive. This right applies to both community- and noncommunity-based programs. Greater consideration of this right might well limit some of the controversy surrounding the commitment dilemma and the right to refuse treatment.

The cases behind this right assert that if patients can function in some setting other than a mental hospital, the court has the responsibility of placing them in that setting. This was the ruling in the case of *Dixon vs. Weinberger* in 1973 when the judge ruled that patients in Washington, D.C., have a statutory right to confinement in the least restrictive facility.[7] Responsibility was placed on Washington, D.C., and the federal government to develop a plan to identify those who should be transferred to community-based facilities and the means for achieving this transfer, including the creation of alternative facilities if necessary. Even though the right to the least restrictive alternative tends to support patient's needs for normalization in a much more effective way than the right to treatment cases, they are complicated by the fact that new models, more facilities, and increased financial resources must be applied to the concept of aftercare, so that discharged and chronically ill patients can be supported in the community.

This right raises a number of difficult questions. Will sufficient funds be allocated to provide adequate supportive care in the community? What will happen to the remaining chronically ill patients who are not discharged into less restrictive alternatives? Will the community centers be able to provide a quality of care that is better than that provided by institutions? How can one stem the antipathy that exists in the larger community toward local placement of mentally ill patients? And most important, given the present economic constraints, will the limited resources allotted to mental health be given to community centers at the expense of large hospitals?

NURSING'S ROLE IN PATIENTS' RIGHTS. The National League for Nursing in 1977 issued a statement on the nurse's role in patients' rights.[14] Respect and concern for patients and assurance of competent care were identified as basic rights, along with patients receiving the information they need to understand their illness and make decisions about their care. The League urged nurses to direclty involve themselves in assuring the human and legal rights of patients.

Many of the patients' rights identified by the League include those previously mentioned. They also list the following rights*:

■ Right to health care that is accessible and that meets professional standards, regardless of the setting

■ Right to courteous and individualized health care that is equitable, humane, and given without discrimination as to race, color, creed, sex, national origin, source of payment, or ethical or political beliefs

■ Right to information about their diagnosis, prognosis, and treatment, including alternatives to care and risks involved

■ Right to information about the qualifications, names, and titles of personnel responsible for providing their health care

■ Right to refuse observation by those not directly involved in their care

■ Right to coordination and continuity of health care

■ Right to information on the charges for services, including the right to challenge these

■ Above all, the right to be fully informed as to all their rights in all health care settings

Perhaps the single most important factor in the implementation of the rights of patients is the attitude of psychiatric professionals. A sensitivity to patients' rights cannot be imposed by the court, the legislature, administrative agencies, or professional groups. If nurses show disdain for those rights, implement them perfunctorily, or are outwardly hostile about honoring them, patient's rights remain an empty legal concept. But if they are sensitive to the rights in all aspects of their relationships with patients, they will secure these human and legal rights.

SUMMARY. The 1978 report from the President's Commission on Mental Health[18] recommends that each state have a "Bill of Rights" for all mentally disabled people which should be incorporated in educational programs directed to patients, staff, families, and the general public. It proposes that a copy of the rights be promi-

---

*National League for Nursing: Nursing's role in patients' rights, New York, 1977, The League. Used with permission.

nently displayed in all mental health settings, be given to each patient using the services, and be explained in an easily understandable manner.

The Mental Health Systems Act of 1980 supports the recommendations of the President's Commission on Mental Health and included within the act itself is a Bill of Mental Health Rights.[12] This portion of the act is presented on pp. 528 to 530. Unfortunately, presidential commissions, mental health legislation, and litigation have primarily brought abstract victories to patients. Efforts to implement these decisions have been marked by confusing requirements, inadequate resources, and insufficient knowledge. Clearly the reforms mandated by the law will cost money, yet public willingness to pay for both more and better psychiatric care is questionable at present. The limitations on resources will continue to be a major factor, regardless of how well organized, numerous, and well intentioned are the advocates of better mental health care. Thus the protection of the rights of the mentally ill will be greatly dependent on evaluating the effectiveness of any new programs arising from executive, judicial, or legislative orders.

Legal role of the nurse

Professional nursing practice is not determined by a simplistic adherence to patients' rights. Rather, it emerges from an interplay between the rights of patients, the legal role of the nurse, and her concern for quality psychiatric care (Fig. 16-2). There are three roles that the psychiatric nurse moves in and out of in the process of completing her professional and personal responsibilities. These are the role of provider of services, employee or contractor of services, and private citizen. These roles are played simultaneously, and each role has attendant rights and responsibilities.

Nurse as provider

All psychiatric professionals have legally defined duties of care and are responsible for their own work. If these duties are violated, malpractice exists. *Malpractice* involves the failure of a professional person to give the kind of proper and competent care that is given by members of his profession in the community, resulting

TITLE V—MENTAL HEALTH RIGHTS AND ADVOCACY*

Bill of rights

Sec. 501. It is the sense of the Congress that each State should review and revise, if necessary, its laws to ensure that mental health patients receive the protection and services they require; and in making such review and revision should take into account the recommendations of the President's Commission on Mental Health and the following:

(1) A person admitted to a program or facility for the purpose of receiving mental health services should be accorded the following:

(A) The right to appropriate treatment and related services in a setting and under conditions that—

(i) are the most supportive of such person's personal liberty; and

(ii) restrict such liberty only to the extent necessary consistent with such person's treatment needs, applicable requirements of law, and applicable judicial orders.

(B) The right to an individualized, written, treatment or service plan (such plan to be developed promptly after admission of such person), the right to treatment based on such plan, the right to periodic review and reassessment of treatment and related service needs, and the right to appropriate revision of such plan, including any revision necessary to provide a description of mental health services that may be needed after such person is discharged from such program or facility.

(C) The right to ongoing participation, in a manner appropriate to such person's capabilities, in the planning of mental health services to be provided such person (including the right to participate in the development and periodic revision of the plan described in subparagraph B), and, in connection with such participation, the right to be provided with a reasonable explanation, in terms and language appropriate to such person's condition and ability to understand, of—

(i) such persons's general mental condition and, if such program or facility has provided a physical examination, such person's general physical condition;

(ii) the objectives of treatment;

(iii) the nature and significant possible adverse effects of recommended treatments;

(iv) the reasons why a particular treatment is considered appropriate;

(v) the reasons why access to certain visitors may not be appropriate; and

(vi) any appropriate and available alternative treatments, services, and types of providers of mental health services.

(D) The right not to receive a mode or course of treatment, established pursuant to the treatment plan, in the absence of such person's informed, voluntary, written consent to such mode or course of treatment, except treatment—

(i) during an emergency situation if such treatment is pursuant to or documented contemporaneously by the written order of a responsible mental health professional; or

(ii) as permitted under applicable law in the case of a person committed by a court to a treatment program or facility.

(E) The right not to participate in experimentation in the absence of such person's informed, voluntary, written consent, the right to appropriate protections in connection with such participation, including the right to a reasonable explanation of the procedure to be followed, the benefits to be expected, the relative advantages of alternative treatments, and the potential discomforts and risks, and the right and opportunity to revoke such consent.

(F) The right to freedom from restraint or seclusion, other than as a mode or course of treatment or restraint or seclusion during an emergency situation if such restraint or seclusion is pursuant to or documented contemporaneously by the written order of a responsible mental health professional.

*From Mental Health Systems Act, Report No. 96-980, Amendment to Senate Bill 1177, Sept. 23, 1980.

(G) The right to a humane treatment environment that affords reasonable protection from harm and appropriate privacy to such person with regard to personal needs.

(H) The right to confidentiality of such person's records.

(I) The right to access, upon request, to such person's mental health care records, except such person may be refused access to —

(i) information in such records provided by a third party under assurance that such information shall remain confidential; and

(ii) specific material in such records if the health professional responsible for the mental health services concerned has made a determination in writing that such access would be detrimental to such person's health, except that such material may be made available to a similarly licensed health professional selected by such person and such health professional may, in the exercise of professional judgment, provide such person with access to any or all parts of such material or otherwise disclose the information contained in such material to such person.

(J) The right, in the case of a person admitted on a residential or inpatient care basis, to converse with others privately, to have convenient and reasonable access to the telephone and mails, and to see visitors during regularly scheduled hours, except that, if a mental health professional treating such person determines that denial of access to a particular visitor is necessary for treatment purposes, such mental health professional may, for a specific, limited, and reasonable period of time, deny such access if such mental health professional has ordered such denial in writing and such order has been incorporated in the treatment plan for such person. An order denying such access should include the reasons for such denial.

(K) The right to be informed promptly at the time of admission and periodically thereafter, in language and terms appropriate to such person's condition and ability to understand, of the rights described in this section.

(L) The right to assert grievances with respect to infringement of the rights described in this section, including the right to have such grievances considered in a fair, timely, and impartial grievance procedure provided for or by the program or facility.

(M) Notwithstanding subparagraph J, the right of access to (including the opportunities and facilities for private communication with any available—

(i) rights protection service within the program or facility;

(ii) rights protection service within the state mental health system designed to be available to such person; and

(iii) qualified advocate;

for the purpose of receiving assistance to understand, exercise, and protect the rights described in this section and in other provisions of law.

(N) The right to exercise the rights described in this section without reprisal, including reprisal in the form of denial of any appropriate, available treatment.

(O) The right to referral as appropriate to other providers of mental health services upon discharge.

(2) (A) The rights described in this section should be in addition to and not in derogation of any other statutory or constitutional rights.

(B) The rights to confidentiality of and access to records as provided in subparagraphs H and I of paragraph 1 should remain applicable to records pertaining to a person after such person's discharge from a program or facility.

(3) (A) No otherwise eligible person should be denied admission to a program or facility for mental health services as a reprisal for the exercise of the rights described in this section.

(B) Nothing in this section should—

(i) obligate an individual mental health or health professional to administer treatment contrary to such professional's clinical judgment;

Continued.

TITLE V—MENTAL HEALTH RIGHTS AND ADVOCACY—cont'd

Bill of rights—cont'd

(ii) prevent any program or facility from discharging any person for whom the provision of appropriate treatment, consistent with the clinical judgment of the mental health professional primarily responsible for such person's treatment, is or has become impossible as a result of such person's refusal to consent to such treatment;

(iii) require a program or facility to admit any person who, while admitted on prior occasions to such program or facility, has repeatedly frustrated the purposes of such admissions by withholding consent to proposed teratment; or

(iv) obligate a program or facility to provide treatment services to any person who is admitted to such program or facility solely for diagnostic or evaluative purposes.

(C) In order to assist a person admitted to a program or facility in the exercise or protection of such person's rights, such person's attorney or legal representatives should have reasonable access to —

(i) such person;

(ii) the areas of the program or facility where such person has received treatment, resided, or had access; and

(iii) pursuant to the written authorization of such person, the records and information pertaining to such person's diagnosis, treatment, and related services described in paragraph 1, I.

(D) Each program and facility should post a notice listing and describing, in language and terms appropriate to the ability of the persons to whom such notice is addressed to understand, the rights described in this section of all persons admitted to such program or facility. Each such notice should conform to the format and content for such notices, and should be posted in all appropriate locations.

(4) (A) In the case of a person adjudicated by a court of competent jurisdiction as being incompetent to exercise the right to consent to treatment or experimentation described in subparagraph D or E of paragraph 1, or the right to confidentiality of or access to records described in subparagraph H or I of such paragraph, or to provide authorization as described in paragraph 3, C, iii, such right may be exercised or such authorization may be provided by the individual appointed by such court as such person's guardian or representative for the purpose of exercising such right or such authorization.

(B) In the case of a person who lacks capacity to exercise the right to consent to treatment or experimentation under subparagraph D or E of paragraph 1, or the right to confidentiality of or access to records described in subparagraph H or I of such paragraph, or to provide authorization as described in paragraph 3, C, iii, because such person has not attained an age considered sufficiently advanced under state law to permit the exercise of such right or such authorization to be legally binding, such right may be exercised or such authorization may be provided on behalf of such person by a parent or legal guardian of such person.

(C) Notwithstanding subparagraphs A and B, in the case of a person admitted to a program or facility for the purpose of receiving mental health services, no individual employed by or receiving any remuneration from such program or facility should act as such person's guardian or representative.

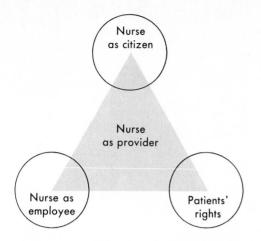

FIG. 16-2
Model of interactive influences on psychiatric nursing practice.

in harm to the patient. Most malpractice claims are filed under the law of negligent tort. A *tort* is a civil wrong for which the injured party is entitled to compensation. Because, under the law, everyone is responsible for his own torts, each nurse can be held responsible in malpractice claims. Under the law of negligent tort the plaintiff must prove the following:

1. A legal duty of care existed.
2. The nurse performed the duty negligently.
3. Damages were suffered by the plaintiff as a result.
4. The damages were substantial.

When patients are admitted to a psychiatric hospital for treatment, the problems of litigation in connection with their care are many and varied. The Bill of Rights in the Mental Health Systems Act helps to clarify the sometimes conflicting role of mental health professionals when it asserts the following[12]: a health professional is not obligated to administer treatment contrary to her clinical judgment, prevent the discharge of any person for whom appropriate treatment is or has become impossible as a result of the person's refusal to consent, admit any person who has repeatedly frustrated treatments in the past by withholding consent to the proposed treatment, or provide treatment to any person admitted solely for diagnostic or evaluative purposes. Such legislation helps to shed some light on the role of nurses and other health providers in such issues as right to treatment and right to refuse treatment.

In the past, lawsuits against nurses were relatively uncommon. However, they can occur when errors are made by the nurse in either her dependent or independent functioning. The most common causes of malpractice suits against nurses are negligence in the areas of suicide precautions and assisting in ECT. When a patient is believed to be suicidal, the psychiatrist writes an order for suicide precautions. The nurse then has the responsibility to implement that order in a way that assures the patient's safety. The exact procedure varies from hospital to hospital, but it should include close observation of him, limiting his activity to the ward only, and removing from him any objects that may possibly be used to injure himself. Another potential problem area concerns the patient receiving ECT. Proper precautions must be taken by the nurse to prepare him before the treatment and to monitor his status when he returns until he is fully conscious and alert.

Creighton[5] stresses that the nurse is responsible for reporting pertinent information about her patient to her co-workers involved in caring for him. The degree of nursing care she must use with patients must be dependent on the patient's condition, with the seriously ill demanding a higher degree of care to protect them from injury and self-destruction. Reporting information includes written as well as oral communication, and the importance of accurate records cannot be overemphasized. Many potential problems can be avoided with clear, concise nursing notes. For example, notes that record the specific suicidal precautions that were implemented with a patient clarify the nurse's functioning. The nurse should also record the occasion when she explained to a patient and his family the food precautions he needed to observe when taking his MAO inhibitor medication. Such a note would prevent a possible lawsuit should the patient violate his dietary restrictions and become ill while on a leave of absence from the hospital. Accurate reporting is an element of good nursing care and should be completed promptly and with diligence.

The exact legal responsibilities of nonphysician therapists have not yet been well defined. It would be valuable for the nurse to practice the following preventive measures to avoid possible lawsuits:

1. Implement nursing care that meets the Standards of Psychiatric–Mental Health Nursing Practice as described by the American Nurses' Association.
2. Know the laws of the state in which one practices, including the rights and duties of the nurse as well as the rights of the patients.

3. Keep accurate and concise nursing records.
4. Maintain the confidentiality of patient information.
5. Consult a lawyer should any questions arise.

Nurse as employee

The role of employee, or contractor of service, is much less known and less frequently scrutinized, but is also very important. This is the role that mandates the practitioner's rights and responsibilities in relation to one's employers, partners, consultants, and other professional colleagues. The rights and responsibilities of employees and contractors of service are not widely known by professionals. But it is here that one's economic security, professional future, and peer relationships are based.

As an employee, a nurse has the responsibility to provide adequate supervision and evaluation of those under her authority for the quality of care given, to observe her employer's rights and responsibilities to clients and other employees, to fulfill the obligations of the contracted service adequately, to adequately apprise the employer of circumstances and conditions that impair the quality of care given, and to report observations of negligent care by others when and where appropriate.

In return for fulfilling these responsibilities, a nurse can expect certain things from her employer, including the right to consideration for service, the right to provision of an adequate working environment and conditions, the right to adequate and qualified assistance where necessary, and the right to respect all of her other rights and responsibilities.

Nurse as citizen

The third role that the nurse plays is that of citizen. This role is particularly significant because all other roles, rights, responsibilities, and privileges are awarded because of the inherent rights of citizenship. Our form of democratic government grants these rights as inherent: civil rights, property rights, right to protection from harm, right to a good name, and right to due process. These rights form the foundation for the extension of other legal relationships of the nurse.

CONFLICT OF INTEREST. Unfortunately, the best interests of the patient, the nurse, and the employer do not always merge, and conflict can occur when, for example, the nurse's right to live and work without threat to personal security is violated by a patient who causes the nurse physical or emotional harm. The many dimensions of this potential conflict are illustrated in the case of a psychotic patient who has hallucinations that are adequately controlled with psychotropic medications but who refuses to take them. Intervention with this patient needs to take into consideration the following possibilities:

■ Failing to medicate the patient may be a denial of his right to treatment.
■ Failing to medicate the patient could have harmful side effects, such as the unnecessary and possibly irreversible continuation of his illness.
■ Failing to medicate the patient may lead to a psychotic episode and result in violence and injury to himself, other patients, or the staff.
■ Failing to medicate the patient may lead to a psychotic episode but no violence.
■ Medicating the patient in the absence of an emergency situation and without a clear threat of violence is in violation of his right to refuse treatment.

In this case, the staff decided not to medicate the patient. When the night nurse went to check on the patient in his room that evening the patient struck the nurse in the face, which resulted in severe bruises and the loss of some teeth. This development leads to a host of new questions.

■ Was the patient competent and legally liable for his actions?
■ What were the circumstances of the incident?
■ Was the nurse sufficiently aware of the potential hazard and, if so, was she responsible for assuming the risk?
■ Was the staffing pattern adequate to discourage, respond to, and control a potentially violent situation?
■ Was there a provision in the environment of the unit for potentially violent patients and, if so, why wasn't it used for this patient?

Obviously, there are no simple or perhaps even equitable resolutions to such dilemmas; yet they are real and ever present. It would appear that prevention needs to be the focus of concern by mental health professionals. This requires a knowledge of legislation, rights, and responsibilities with a serious appreciation of the potential conflicts that might emerge. Nurses

MARYLAND NURSES' ASSOCIATION
The Bill of Rights for Registered Nurses*

We, the Council on Human Rights of the Maryland Nurses' Association, in order to promote increased knowledge and understanding of the rights and responsibilities of all registered nurses, have developed The Bill of Rights for Registered Nurses. We propose that this Bill will aid in educating consumers and health care professionals about the rights of registered nurses, as well as their corresponding responsibilities. Therefore, we submit the Bill of Rights for Registered Nurses as a positions statement of the Maryland Nurses' Association.

The nurse has a right:	**The nurse has a responsibility:**
Individual	
to practice according to the Maryland Nurse Practice Act.	to assume personal accountability for individual nursing judgments and actions which consider the individual value systems and the uniqueness of each patient/client.
to make independent nursing judgments.	
to question any delegated medical order or any plan of care that may cause possible harm to the patient/client or others.	to implement the nursing process in providing individualized nursing care.
to refuse to carry out any delegated medical order or any plan of care that may cause possible harm to the patient/client or others.	to safeguard the patient/client and the public from incompetent, unethical, or illegal health care practices.
to pursue quality continuing education.	to refuse to perform any nursing action which will jeopardize the patient/client or the public, and the obligation to communicate the rationale to the proper authority.
to teach individuals and groups health care practices that facilitate treatment, prevent illness, and provide optimal wellness.	to avail one's self of opportunities which will broaden knowledge and refine and increase skills.
	to educate the patient/client and the public.
Employment	
to competitive hiring and promotion which is based on knowledge and experience and which is unrestricted by consideration of sex, race, age, creed, or national origin.	to maintain competence and prepare one's self adequately for promotion.
to realistic assignments that can assure the patient/client quality care that includes safety, dignity, and comfort.	to evaluate one's own work environment and to communicate and document unrealistic work loads through appropriate channels.
to negotiate salary and individual conditions of employment.	to make known individual convictions and preferences prior to hiring.
to work in a safe and adequately equipped environment.	to assess, evaluate, document, and correct unsafe conditions and to communicate such information to the appropriate authority promptly.
to work with qualified, competent nursing personnel.	to objectively document and report to appropriate authority evidence of competent, as well as incompetent performance and to evaluate, inform, counsel, and teach nursing personnel when indicated.
to periodic, fair, objective evaluations by peers.	

*From the Council on Human Rights. Approved by the Maryland Nurses' Association, Baltimore, 1980, The Association.

Continued.

MARYLAND NURSES' ASSOCIATION
The Bill of Rights for Registered Nurses—cont'd

The nurse has a right:	The nurse has a responsibility:
Employment—cont'd	
to pay increases based on demonstrated performance.	to participate in the development of reliable and valid evaluation criteria for peer review.
to due process whenever accused of unethical, incompetent, illegal, or unqualified practice or of prejudicial or inappropriate conduct.	to maintain competence, incorporate new techniques and knowledge, and continuously upgrade the quality of health care.
to be an advocate for the patient/client and the public when health care and safety may be affected by incompetent, unethical, or illegal practices.	to participate in the planning, establishment, and implementation of procedures to ensure due process.
to representation by a negotiator in labor matters.	to be alert to any instances of incompetent, unethical, or illegal practices by any member of the health care system and to take appropriate action regarding these practices.
	to select and utilize a knowledgeable and impartial negotiator.
Professional	
to receive support from the nursing profession at all levels.	to participate in activities that contribute to the ongoing development of the profession's body of knowledge.
to belong to an autonomous nursing organization.	to be an active member and to participate in the nursing organization's effort to implement and improve standards of nursing.
to have expert testimony supplied by the nursing organization for both legal and legislative issues.	to provide knowledgeable, objective, articulate expert testimony.
to full and equal representation on all decision-making bodies concerned with health care.	to provide knowledge, active, and effective collaborating with members of the health professions.
to be involved actively in the political decision-making process at all levels of the government.	to be knowledgeable, active, and effective in the legislative process by direct involvement, effective education and selection of representative legislators, lobbying, and creating citizen awareness in promoting local, state, and national efforts to meet the health needs of the public.

in one state, Maryland, have demonstrated an awareness of these issues and have developed a bill of rights for registered nurses (p. 533 and above). This document is commendable in that it serves to educate nurses and the public and also to clarify rights and responsibilities. In addition, professional nursing judgment requires a careful examination of the context of nursing care, the possible consequences of one's actions, and the feasible alternatives one might employ. Only then do rights and responsibilities take on any real meaning.

Psychiatry and criminal responsibility

The determination of criminal responsibility concerns the accused person's condition at the time of the alleged offense. It has received much public attention when used in the "insanity defense." This defense proposes that a person who has committed an act that in a usual situation would be criminal is held not guilty by reason of "insanity." This is a difficult decision to make; usually the defense attorneys and prosecutors offer many arguments pro and con and frequently psychiatrists are called on to testify. Nurses are seldom directly involved in the legislative process, but they should have an understanding of the law in this area both as citizens and psychiatric professionals.

The idea behind this type of defense is an essentially humanitarian one. The rationale for it is that a person should not be blamed if he "did not know what he was doing" or "could not help himself." With the complexity of today's society and the judicial system, however, many believe this defense is being abused, and it has created great controversy in the legal and psychiatric professions.[27] Much of this controversy has been stimulated by the attempt on President Reagan's life. The conflict among citizens, legal authorities, mental health professionals, and in the news media has been heightened by the "not guilty by reason of insanity" verdict by the John Hinckley, Jr., case in 1982. This might precipitate changes in the present law.

At the present time there are four sets of criteria used in the United States to determine the criminal responsibility of an offender who is suffering from a mental illness: the M'Naghten Rule, the Irresistible Impulse Test, the Durham Test, or "Product Rule," and the American Law Institute's Test, or the ALI Test, the most frequently used criteria.

M'Naghten Rule

This law originated with the trial of Daniel M'Naghten in London in 1832 when he was tried for the murder of Edward Drummond, the private secretary of Sir Robert Peele. M'Naghten had suffered from delusions of persecution, and on numerous occasions had complained to public authorities. Receiving no help, however, he decided to resolve the situation himself. He began watching the house of Sir Robert Peele and one evening, under the belief he was shooting Peele, shot Edward Drummond as he emerged from the house. When he came to trial, his attorney entered an appeal of "partial insanity" and M'Naghten was declared of unsound mind and was committed to an institution for the criminally insane. In deciding the case, the judges identified two rules to use in determining the

criminal responsibility of a person who pleads insanity. The first rule states that the individual at the time of the crime did not "know the nature and quality of the act." The second states that if he did know what he was doing, he did not know that what he was doing "was wrong." These two rules are simply referred to as the "nature and quality" rule and "right from wrong" test.

This case was the first major test for determining criminal responsibility, and it is still used in most states and criminal courts. It has become less popular in recent years, however, because of the narrow wording, which some people believe ignores aspects of the whole personality such as emotions and will.

Irresistible Impulse Test

About 15 states have adopted this test along with the M'Naghten Rule. It is never used in isolation. According to this test, a person may know the difference between right and wrong but finds himself impulsively driven to commit the criminal act. It is usually necessary to show a lack of premeditation and that the strength of the urge was so great that it would have been carried out regardless of the circumstances. This test is frequently used as a defense for sudden, violent behavior displayed under stress.

Durham Test, or "Product Rule"

This test is based on a 1954 decision that took place in the District of Columbia. The rule states that the accused is not criminally responsible if his act was the "product of mental disease." Thus it is sometimes called the "Product Rule," although this phrase and "mental disease" have been difficult to define. Many people object to the use of this test because it greatly expands the number and scope of individuals who may use the insanity defense. At this time it is only used in New Hampshire, Maine, and the Virgin Islands.

American Law Institute's Test

This test is similar to the combination of the M'Naghten Rule and Irresistible Impulse Test. It states that a person is not responsible for his criminal act if he lacks the capacity to "appreciate" the wrongfulness of it or to "conform" his conduct to the requirements of the law. It also excludes "an abnormality manifested only by repeated criminal or otherwise antisocial conduct." This last condition thereby excludes the psychopath who has repeated criminal conduct. This test has become popular over the years, and it is now used by all the federal circuit courts and at least ten states' courts.

Disposition of mentally ill offenders

If a person is found not guilty by reason of insanity, he is not often set free. In some states he may be committed at the discretion of the court, and in almost a third of the states he is automatically hospitalized. Some offenders are treated in special hospitals, others are sent to state mental hospitals, and still others are sent to treatment facilities provided in the penal institution. Since the insanity defense is used most often in capital offenses, it is usually desirable to make security provisions available and penal institutions lend themselves best to this.

After hospitalization and on recovery, the patient may be discharged by the court that ordered his commitment. In other states he may be discharged by the governor. Still others allow the mental institution to make that decision. The major criteria for discharge of the patient are that he is not likely to repeat his offense and that it is relatively safe to release him to the community.

Future challenges

The interface between psychiatry and the law is becoming increasingly complex. Historically, the mental health delivery system had only two components—mental health professionals and the patient. Now, however, the system has grown to include five forces, each of which must be taken into account when dealing with any mental health problem. This pentagonal relationship (Fig. 16-3) has been described by Kopolow[9] to be composed of consumers, providers of services, governmental regulators and lawmakers, the judiciary, and third-party insurers. Members of each of these groups have related, but slightly different, interests. The consumer is concerned that services be available when and where he wishes them, that they are appropriate to his needs, and that he is involved in establishing the priorities of the program. The provider has clinical and professional biases. If outside controls must exist, the provider wants

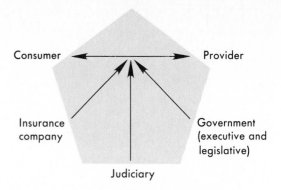

FIG. 16-3
Pentagonal relationship that characterizes the mental health delivery system. (From Kopolow, L.: Patient's rights and psychiatric practice. In Barton, W., and Sanborn, C., editors: Law and the mental health professions, New York, 1978, International Universities Press, Inc.)

them equitably applied and with one's responsibilities and liabilities clearly defined. The government wants citizens to have access to quality care at the least cost and wants the providers to be accountable for the care they provide. The courts, after years of neglect, have recently assumed the role of guardian of patients' constitutional rights and have begun to scrutinize patient care and treatment. Finally, insurance companies are concerned with either making a profit, or remaining solvent while seeking assurances that they are paying for covered services by appropriately licensed and credentialed professionals. The changing priorities and interactions of these five forces affect the quality, availability, and responsiveness of mental health services in this country.

At present there is a simultaneous urge to adequate treatment of the psychiatrically ill and protection of their constitutional rights. Both of these trends are emerging at a time of fiscal restraint. It would appear as if one's choice is between abandoning former patients to their rights in the community or warehousing them in large institutions, whether these be hospitals or jails.[26] Mental health professionals are concerned about the quantity and quality of care received by psychiatric patients. Legal reformers are indignant about the lack of rights experienced by these patients and object to a law that justifies commitment under the uncertain prediction by a single professional of some unproven and unknowable harm. Criminal court judges are angry that in the day-to-day implementation of the commitment law, the only option left to them is to prosecute the mentally ill defendant. Psychiatric hospitals are understaffed and underfunded and are attacked on all sides for their inability to "care" for and "cure" psychiatric patients. Community programs are few and poorly supported and have resulted in deinstitutionalized patients living without treatment in urban ghettos or finding their way into the criminal justice system. The public is frightened at the thought of having psychiatric patients in their neighborhoods, and concerned citizens demand that mental health programs exercise greater control over this population perceived to be dangerous.

Clearly, mechanisms are needed by which patients, mental health professionals, attorneys, and concerned citizens can work together to improve mental health care and advance the rights of all patients. The priorities of the mentally ill extend beyond protection of their legal rights to protection of their clinical needs and general welfare. No one profession or group unilaterally can fulfill all of these needs, but increased cooperation among the various mental health advocates can make this goal possible.

Mental health advocacy is evolving into one effective method for protecting and advocating the rights of all citizens to high-quality mental health care that is clinically and constitutionally appropriate. New Jersey, for example, has a Division of Mental Health Advocacy mandated by the state legislature that works to produce a better system of mental health care and delivery. It is staffed by lawyers, psychologists, psychiatric nurses, social workers, and others who work as advocates for those caught up in the psychiatric system. Other states, such as Minnesota, New York, Michigan, and California, have adopted similar programs. The purpose of mental health advocacy is to assure that both clinical and legal considerations of the patient are properly weighed, and it is increasingly being considered as part of the range of services to which patients are entitled.

It has been noted that the ratio of patients to prisoners is three to one and suggested that for every public defender there should be three mental health lawyers. Whether or not such an idea becomes a reality, it is still possible to safeguard the rights of patients by (1) periodic reviews of those involuntarily committed, (2) considering the least restrictive setting when determining treatment or services, and (3) greater use of alternatives to hospitalization, including foster home and day treatment programs. Impetus for change in this area is requiring that states reorder their priorities, yet it is occurring at a time when a number of states have been forced to cut their mental health budgets. One can only speculate on what the impact of all this activity will be in the future.

> In the Sixteenth Century the deranged were expelled, shipped off, or executed; in the Seventeenth Century the insane were locked up in jails and houses of correction; in the Eighteenth Century madmen were confined in madhouses; in the Nineteenth Century lunatics were sent to asylums; in the Twentieth Century the mentally ill are committed to hospitals; in the Twenty-first Century . . .
>
> **K. Jones,** *Lunacy, Law, and Conscience*

Suggested cross-references

Ethical decision making is discussed in Chapter 3. Issues related to the right to refuse treatment are discussed in Chapter 15.

SUMMARY

1. Informal admission to a psychiatric hospital occurs without formal or written application. The patient admitted in this way is free to leave at any time.

2. Voluntary admission requires the individual to make written application to a psychiatric hospital and agree to receive treatment and abide by hospital rules. If he wishes to be discharged, it is usually required that he give written notice to the hospital. Both the voluntary and informal types of admission are preferred by many psychiatric clinicians because the patient is an active participant in the process and retains all his civil rights while in the hospital.

3. Involuntary admission means that the request for hospitalization did not originate with the patient, and when he is committed, he loses the right to leave the hospital when he wishes. It is usually justified on the grounds of (a) dangerous to others, (b) dangerous to self, and (c) need for treatment. The procedure for commitment includes filing a petition, completing a mental status examination, and determination of the need for hospitalization, which can be a medical, court, or administrative decision. Involuntary admission in some states assumes incompetency and is accompanied by the loss of all civil rights. This is not true of most states, however. This issue of involuntary commitment raises the questions of assessing dangerousness and freedom of choice, and there are differing opinions on the moral, legal, and psychiatric implications of it.

    a. Emergency involuntary admission may be used for patients who are acutely ill, and most states limit the amount of time the person can be detained to from 3 to 30 days.

    b. Temporary or observation involuntary admission is used for the purpose of diagnosis and short-term therapy. The commitment is for a specific period of time ranging from 2 to 6 months.

    c. Indefinite involuntary admission, or formal commitment, detains a person for an indeterminate length of time or until he is ready for discharge. It usually involves a court decision.

4. Voluntarily admitted patients may either be discharged by the staff or they may initiate their own discharge requests. Most states require that they give written notice of their desire for discharge. Involuntarily admitted patients have lost the right to leave the hospital when they desire. Indefinite commitments are subject to periodic reviews.

    a. A conditional discharge is a patient's specified leave of absence from the hospital. Certain expectations are placed on him, the most common being that he attend outpatient therapy. This type of discharge assists his transition from the hospital into the community. If he demonstrates a good adjustment, he may then receive an absolute discharge.

    b. An absolute discharge is a final one and marks the patient's termination of his relationship with the hospital. New admission proceedings must be initiated if the patient wishes to return to the hospital after receiving an absolute discharge.

    c. A judicial discharge is one issued by the court. It is provided for by laws that allow a patient or his family to appeal for discharge even though the hospital may oppose this request.

5. The civil and personal rights of psychiatric patients are presently being supported in legislative acts throughout the country. The nature of these rights varies greatly from state to state. At present they include the right to communicate with others, keep clothing in the hospital, practice religious freedom, be employed, manage personal affairs, execute wills, form contracts, make purchases, be educated, file a writ of habeas corpus, obtain an independent psychiatric examination, be eligible for civil service status, retain licenses, sue, marry, divorce, be free of mechanical restraints, obtain periodic review of status, secure legal representation, maintain privacy, be informed before giving consent, receive treatment, refuse treatment, and be treated in the least restrictive setting.

    a. The person's competency to execute wills is called the testamentary capacity. To make a valid will, it is required that he (1) know he is making a will, (2) know the nature and extent of his property, and (3) know who his friends and relatives are and how he is related to them.

    b. "Incompetency" is a legal term that must be proved in a special court hearing. To determine incompetency, it must be shown that the person has a mental disorder that causes a defect in judgment, and this defect makes him incapable of handling his own affairs. As a result of this ruling he is deprived of many of his civil rights. This can be reversed only in another court hearing that declares him competent.

    c. Habeas corpus is an important right all patients retain. It provides for the speedy release of any individual who claims he is being deprived of his liberty and detained illegally. The hearing for this determination takes place in a court of law where the patient's sanity is at issue.

    d. The right to privacy implies the right to keep some information about oneself completely secret from others. "Confidentiality" involves disclosure of certain information to another specifically authorized person. "Privileged communication" applies only in court-related proceedings and must be established by law. At present, most states do not provide for privileged communication between nurses and patients.

    e. The right to informed consent requires that a physician explain the treatment to the patient, including its possible complications and risks. The patient's consent to it must imply competency, understanding, and volition. All unusual and experimental treatments require special permission.

    f. The rights to treatment, refuse treatment, and receive treatment in the least restrictive setting are recent developments that are being delineated in various court decisions. They reflect an important movement that will greatly affect hospital conditions, the care of patients, the extent of involuntary commitment, and the community.

6. The psychiatric nurse has rights and responsibilities attendant to each of three legal roles: nurse as provider, nurse as employee, and nurse as citizen.

    a. As a provider, every nurse is responsible for the quality of care she gives to patients and can be held responsible in malpractice claims. For a nurse to be proved negligent it must be shown that (1) a legal duty of care existed, (2) the nurse performed the duty negligently, (3) the patient suffered damages, and (4) the damages were substantial. Although lawsuits against psychiatric nurses are uncommon, they can occur if the nursing care is not competent or does not meet the standards of the profession.

    b. As an employee, the nurse has responsibilities to her peers, employer, and colleagues. As a citizen, her rights form the foundation for the extension of the nurse's other legal relationships. It is possible for the nurse to experience a conflict of interest among these rights and responsibilities, which can pose serious problems. A knowledge of one's obligations and an appreciation of potential conflicts are necessary preventive measures for the nurse.

7. Criminal responsibility concerns the accused person's condition at the time of the alleged crime. The "insanity defense" has received much attention in this regard. At present, three tests are commonly used in the United States to determine criminal responsibility. These are the M'Naghten Rule, the Irresistible Impulse Test, and the American Law Institute's

Test. A fourth test, the Durh Test, or "Product Rule," is seldom used.

8. Five forces currently affect the mental health delivery system—the consumer, provider, government, judiciary, and insurance companies. No one group or profession is able to fulfill the multifaceted advocacy need of the mentally ill. The future must provide for independent and collaborative approaches to advocacy so that it can become an effective mechansim for the creation of a more responsive mental health system.

References

1. Arkin, A., et al.: Behavior modification, N.Y. State J. Med. **76:**190, Feb. 1976.
2. Birnbaum, M.: The right to treatment, Am. Bar Assoc. J., p. 499, 1960.
3. Brakel, S.J., and Kock, R.S.: The mentally disabled and the law, revised ed., Chicago, 1971, University of Chicago Press.
4. Chodoff, P.: The case for involuntary hospitalization of the mentally ill, Am. J. Psychiatry **133:**496, 1976.
5. Creighton, H.: Law every nurse should know, Philadelphia, 1975, W.B. Saunders Co.
6. *Cross vs. Harris,* 418 F 2d (D.C. Cir. 1969).
7. *Dixon vs. Weinberger,* No. 74285 (C.D.D.C. Feb. 14, 1974).
8. Ennis, B.J.: Civil liberties and mental illness, Criminal Law Bull., p. 101, 1971.
9. Kopolow, L.: Patients' rights and psychiatric practice. In Barton, W., and Sanborn, C., editors: Law and the mental health professions, New York, 1978, International Universities Press, Inc.
10. Law briefs, Time, p. 44, July 6, 1981.
11. McGarry, L., and Kaplan, H.: Overview: current trends in mental law, Am. J. Psychiatry **130:**627, 1973.
12. Mental Health Systems Act, Report No. 96-980, Amendment to Senate Bill 1177, Sept. 23, 1980.
13. Merton, R.K., and Nisbet, R.A., editors: Contemporary social problems, New York, 1961, Harcourt, Brace & World.
14. National League for Nursing: Nursing's role in patient's rights, Pub. No. 11-1671, New York, 1977, The League.
15. Oran, D.: Judges and psychiatrists lock up too many people, Psychol. Today **7:**27, Aug. 1973.
16. O'Sullivan, A.: Privileged communication, Am. J. Nurs. **80:**947, 1980.
17. Peck, C.: Current legislative issues concerning the right to refuse versus the right to choose hospitalization and treatment, Psychiatry **38:**303, Nov. 1975.
18. President's Commission on Mental Health: Report to the president, vol. I, Washington, D.C., 1978.
19. *Rogers vs. Okin,* 478, Fed. Supp. 1342, 1979.
20. Scheff, T.: Being mentally ill: a sociological theory, Chicago, 1966, Aldine Publishing Co.
21. Spece, R.: Conditioning and other techniques used to 'treat'? 'rehabilitate'? 'demolish'? prisoners and mental patients, South Calif. Law Rev., p. 616, 1972.
22. Stone, A.: Mental health and law: a system in transition, Rockville, Md., 1975, National Institute of Mental Health, U.S., Department of Health, Education, and Welfare.
23. Szasz, T.: Ideology and insanity, New York, 1970, Doubleday & Co., Inc.
24. Tancredi, L., and Clark, D.: Psychiatry and the legal rights of patients, Am. J. Psychiatry **129:**328, 1972.
25. 28 USCS Appendix 476, 1975.
26. Whitmer, G.: From hospitals to jails: the fate of California's deinstitutionalized mentally ill, Am. J. Orthopsychiatry **50**(1):65, 1980.
27. Williams, R., and Robitscher, J.: Should psychiatrists get out of the courtroom? Psychol. Today, p. 85, Dec. 1977.
28. *Wyatt vs. Stickney:* 344, Fed. Supp. 373, 375, 1972.

Annotated suggested readings

After *Wyatt vs. Stickney:* Progress reports from Alabama, Hosp. Community Psychiatry **28:**351, 1977.

This issue examines the impact of the Wyatt ruling on mental health care in Alabama. It attempts to explore whether litigation is a viable and effective means of intervention into a mental health system. Articles included in the issue discuss implementing the Wyatt standards at Bruce Hospital, an administrative viewpoint, community mental health services in Alabama after Wyatt, and the outcome of patients released after Wyatt. It presents a thorough analysis, and the overall tone is generally positive.

Barton, W., and Sanborn, C., editors: Law and the mental health professions, New York, 1978, International Universities Press, Inc.

This is a compilation of papers by recognized authorities in both the legal and mental health professions. They examine the implications of recent judicial decisions that have affected psychiatric practice and suggest possible routes toward a smoother interface between law and psychiatry. Topics covered include informed consent, malpractice, confidentiality, competence, patient rights, involuntary admissions, and dangerousness.

Chodoff, P.: The case for involuntary hospitalization of the mentally ill, Am. J. Psychiatry **133**:496, 1976.

The author examines three points of view on the question of involuntary hospitalization. He believes that there is an overreliance on the dangerousness standard, and he favors a return to the use of medical criteria by psychiatrists.

Ennis, B.: Prisoners of psychiatry, New York, 1972, Harcourt, Brace, Jovanovich, Inc.

This book contains specific case histories of men and women whose lives were changed by the label "mental illness." It is written by a lawyer who represented mental patients, and it makes interesting reading on a more personal level.

Ennis, B., and Siegel, L.: The rights of mental patients, New York, 1973, Avon Books.

This guide was published in cooperation with the American Civil Liberties Union and presents a brief description of the various rights of psychiatric patients. It also suggests how these rights can be protected. The appendixes are particularly valuable in that they present the mental hygiene statutes of all the states, a bibliography, the judge's opinion in the Wyatt v Stickney *case, and the minimum standards for adequate treatment of the mentally ill as determined by the courts.*

Feileger, D.: The battle over children's rights, Psychol. Today **11**:89, July 1977.

Thirty-eight states have laws allowing parents or guardians to commit their children as voluntary patients to mental institutions. This article questions if children should have the right to be heard independently. It describes the federal court decision of Kremens v Bartley, *which decided that children are entitled to protection against abuses in the commitment process. The issue is a complex one because the child's right to liberty is pitted against the parent's authority and claim to control of the child. Resolving this conflict is difficult, and before the Bartley case no previous federal court decision had ever dealt with a similar situation.*

Golann, S., and Fremouw, W., editors: The right to treatment for mental patients, New York, 1976, Irvington Publishers, Inc.

This book is a result of the Amherst Conference on the Right to Treatment, which focused attention on the rights of institutionalized persons and the professional and political issues involved in implementing these rights.

Gonzalez, H.: The consumer movement: the implications for psychiatric care, Perspect. Psychiatr. Care, **14**:186, Oct.-Dec. 1976.

This worthwhile article briefly examines the consumer movement and its two major components: the consumer as consumer and the consumer as a provider of health care. The author then analyzes the implications of the consumer movement for health care providers in the delivery of psychiatric care. It is a thought-provoking article.

Kesey, K.: One flew over the cuckoo's nest, New York, 1962, Viking Press.

This is a popular novel that has also been adapted for the theater and movies. It describes the plight of the central character, MacMurphy, who has been committed to a state mental hospital. The story records his attempt to fight the hospital system and obtain a release. Many of the elements of institutionalization are dramatized in this powerful and enjoyable tale.

Kittrie, N.: The right to be different, Baltimore, 1971, Johns Hopkins University Press.

The author describes the conflict between the humanitarian ideals of the therapeutic state and the practical results of the administration of criminal law. He examines the problems of mental illness, commitment, and due process and the future implications of implementing a therapeutic state. Particular attention is devoted to delinquent youths, psychopaths, addicts, alcoholics, and methods of dealing with the population explosion. This book provides advanced reading in this controversial area.

Kopolow, L., and Bloom, H., editors: Mental health advocacy: an emerging force in consumers' rights, Rockville, Md., 1977, U.S. Department of Health, Education, and Welfare.

This publication seeks to stimulate interest in patient advocacy. The first part reviews major concepts in advocacy; the second part describes statewide mental health–advocacy programs. The third part describes a unique judicial decision, and the appendix includes a model state advocacy statute and an excellent bibliography.

McGarry, L., Schwitzgebel, K., Lipsitt, P., and Lelos, D.: Civil commitment and social policy, Rockville, Md., 1981, U.S. Department of Health and Human Services, National Institute of Mental Health.

This monograph is the final report from a research project that documented the impact and consequences of the new mental health law in Massachusetts on the civil commitment of the mentally ill. This is one of the few studies to actually examine the consequences of such legal changes.

Means, H.: Criminal case number 16836: *the State of Maryland vs. Sherry Windt*, The Washingtonian **38**:102, Feb. 1978.

This article describes the interplay between psychiatry and the law in a true case presentation of 16-year-old Sherry Windt, who killed her mother. The reporter has access to both legal and psychiatric records, and he presents the complex sequence of events relative to her trial and psychiatric assessment. It is a stimulating article that provokes numerous questions regarding psychiatry and the law.

Meisel, A.: Rights of the mentally ill: the gulf between theory and reality, Hosp. Community Psychiatry **26**:349, 1975.

The author briefly reviews some of the procedural and substantive rights of mental patients and discusses the difficulties of translating the rights promulgated in the courts into reality. It is a clearly written, concise article that summarizes some pertinent legal issues in psychiatry.

Murchison, I., Nichols, T., and Hanson, R.: Legal accountability in the nursing process, ed. 2, St. Louis, 1982, The C.V. Mosby Co.

The authors contend that knowledge of the law must be an integral part of all nursing theory and practice, and the theme of this reference book is the incorporation of law into the nursing process to support independent nursing action. It presents fundamental concepts all nurses should know, although issues particularly pertinent to psychiatric nursing are not specifically addressed.

Nations, W.: Nurse-lawyer is patient advocate, Am. J. Nurs. **73**:1039, 1973.

This article describes the innovative role of a nurse who has both nursing and legal qualifications as she acts as an ombudsman for psychiatric patients in a Veterans Ad-

ministration Hospital. *The functions she performs are
identified as responding to requests for help from patients and families, serving as consultant and advisor
about patient problems to administration, and helping the
director see the operation of the institution through the
eyes of the patient.*

Offir, C.W.: Civil rights and the mentally ill—revolution in
bedlam, Psychol. Today **8**:61, Oct. 1974.

*The struggles of psychiatric patients in state mental
hospitals are vividly described in this article. These patients, aided by civil libertarians, are suing physicians,
hospitals, and government officials in an attempt to win a
wide assortment of rights. The article examines the issues
of involuntary servitude, the right to treatment, preventive detention, and the right to due process in commitment procedures. It is written in an informal manner
with the purpose of informing the public rather than documenting specific judicial decisions.*

Peck, C.: Current legislative issues concerning the right to
refuse versus the right to choose hospitalization and treatment, Psychiatry **38**:303, Nov. 1975.

*This article outlines the issues and the most important
legal decisions between 1970 and 1975 with respect to involuntary civil commitment, the right to refuse treatment,
and the right to treatment. It gives examples of states
who have not reformed their laws and suggestions for improvement. The reader is provided with an understanding of the philosphical controversy and the general direction of the legislation in this area.*

Rubin, J.: Economics, mental health and the law, Lexington, Mass., 1978, D.C. Heath & Co.

*This is a most timely exploration of the economic bases
and implications of recent mental health litigation. Important issues of the book are the need to consider what
is being demanded and supplied in regard to mental health
care, at what cost is it produced, and the willingness
of people to pay for it.*

Stachyra, M.: Nurses, psychotherapy, and the law, Perspect.
Psychiatr. Care **2**:200, Sept.-Oct. 1969.

*The purpose of this article is to alert psychiatric nurses
to the legal issues involved when nurses practice psychotherapy and to urge them to support legislative reform
that would explicitly sanction qualified nurses doing psychotherapy. It compares existing nurse practice acts, psychology practice acts, and medical practice acts, and
identifies specific recommendations for amending existing
laws.*

Szasz, T.: Law, liberty, and psychiatry, New York, 1963, The
Macmillan Co., Publishers.

*This text presents a critical inquiry into the current
social and legal uses of psychiatry. The author's aim is
to show that psychiatry today in the United States is often
used to subvert traditional political guarantees of individual liberty. He describes many of the faults committed
in the name of mental illness and proposes solutions for
them. The 20 chapters cover more of the pertinent issues
that arise between law and psychiatry and this text is
considered to be a classic in its field.*

Szasz, T.: Psychiatric slavery, New York, 1977, The Macmillan Co., Publishers.

*The author supports the concepts of freedom and per-
sonal responsibility and in this text he examines the problem of involuntary mental hospitalization. He parallels it
to involuntary servitude and illustrates his thesis through
the use of the Donaldson case.*

Tancredi, L., Lieb, J., and Slaby, A.: Legal issues in psychiatric care, New York, 1975, Harper & Row, Publishers,
Inc.

*This current text is written for students in all areas of
mental health. It explores the many complex legal issues
that confront the psychiatric professional in a thorough
and concise manner and clearly understood language.
Illustrative case examples are used to provoke discussion
and apply pertinent theory. It can serve as a valuable
and ready reference for psychiatric nurses.*

Thorner, N.: Nurses violate their patients' rights, J. Psychiatr. Nurs. **14**:7, Jan. 1976.

*The author reports on a study she conducted on the
refusal of medication by patients. Her findings revealed
that medication refusals do not occur with a high frequency in the psychiatric setting, and nurses deal with
refusals by first using psychological methods. She also
reported that nurses in the study did not have an adequate knowledge of the patients' right to refuse medication and the legal responsibility in medication administration.*

Wilhelm, Y.: A look at psychiatric commitment, Perspect.
Psychiatr. Care **9**:49, April-June 1971.

*The commitment process is reviewed in this article and
the author points out the great discrepancy that exists between the theoretical and practical ways by which people
are committed to mental institutions. She cites two interesting studies—one exlores the legal screening of persons
alleged to be mentally ill and the other reviews the hearing
procedures involved in commitment, which lasted an average of 4.1 minutes. The author shares her own clinical
observations and concludes that often commitment procedures do not satisfy the minimum requirements for ethical
practice of the legal or medical professions. This is a recommended reading for concerned nurses.*

Williams, R., and Robitscher, J.: Should psychiatrists get
out of the courtroom? Psychol. Today **11**:85, Dec. 1977.

*Psychiatrists have become increasingly active in pre-
trial screenings for mental competence, courtroom debates
about sanity and responsibility, and posttrial decisions on
the probability of rehabilitation. In this article the author
debates the role of the psychiatrist in the courtroom. His
final recommendation is to make forensic psychiatrists
more responsible and to refine the theory of criminal responsibility so that judges and juries get less confusing
advice.*

PART TWO

PRACTICE OF

PSYCHIATRIC NURSING

Information is of no value for its own sake,
but only because of its personal significance.

Eric Berne

CHAPTER 17

PSYCHIATRIC EVALUATION

E. Susan Batzer

Learning objectives

*After studying this chapter, the student
should be able to:*

- *state the role of the nurse in the psychiatric evaluation of patients and the knowledge and skills needed by nurses to function in this area.*

- *identify the two basic elements of a psychiatric evaluation and the purpose of each.*

- *describe the stages of the psychiatric evaluation as they relate to the collection of data on the presenting problem, patient's history, mental status examination, formulation of a diagnostic impression, and case disposition.*

- *identify the major categories of data that should be collected by the nurse with regard to the patient's presenting problem, history, and mental status.*

- *analyze the specific aspects of the patient's behavior that should be assessed in each of the five major categories of the mental status examination.*

- *discuss additional resources the nurse can use to complete an assessment of the patient.*

- *relate the formulation of a medical diagnosis with that of a nursing diagnosis.*

- *describe the factors that need to be considered in making a decision about a case disposition.*

- *discuss future trends in the psychiatric evaluation of patients.*

- *identify suggested readings for future study.*

CLINICAL EXAMPLE 17-1

Late one night two police officers escort a young woman into the emergency room. The nurse observes her to be an attractive brunette, but her manner of dress is rather bizarre. She is wearing a bright purple satin shirt, cut-off jeans, white boots studded with rhinestones, and sunglasses. She is demanding to be released, stating that she has important business that must be taken care of immediately. The young woman approaches the nurse and states in a quiet, polite tone of voice that she is being held against her consent and that the authorities will be contacted about the matter. The police inform the nurse that the woman was picked up at the courthouse that evening after they received a phone call from the security guard. She had been walking around the state office building placing flyers on all the doors. She approached the security guard, demanding entrance to the courthouse for a scheduled private meeting with the chief judge.

This vignette, which might be typical of a person with a manic episode, might also represent other conditions, such as substance-induced organic disorder or schizophrenic disorder. What information does the nurse need to assess this woman's current mental functioning and to determine whom to ask for further assistance?

CLINICAL EXAMPLE 17-2

A 57-year-old unemployed mailman who recently stopped drinking and is an avid member of Alcoholics Anonymous is admitted to the medical unit of a general hospital for a gastrointestinal workup because of bowel complaints, which he attributes to recent minor surgery he had for a rectal abscess. The results of the x-ray examinations and laboratory tests are all within normal limits. This man is to be discharged to his home, where he lives with his 90-year-old mother, who suffered a mild stroke 6 months ago. The nurse enters his room the evening before discharge and finds that he has stabbed himself in the abdomen with a pocket knife.

Was this man's depression so well masked that no clinical symptoms were evident during his hospital stay? Were there any clues recorded in the initial interview and assessment? Was a psychiatric evaluation done along with evaluation of the gastrointestinal, genitourinary, cardiopulmonary, and other systems medically scrutinized by all on admission?

These clinical examples demonstrate the importance of a psychiatric evaluation. They have several things in common: a psychiatric problem, nurse-patient interaction, and a lack of sufficient data to effectively assess and plan a treatment program. As vital members of the health care team, nurses must assume a role in the psychiatric evaluation of patients.

Role of the nurse

At one time the task of psychiatric evaluation was ascribed to the physician, usually a psychiatrist. However, Imboden[8] points out the need for a psychiatric evaluation as part of the routine physical examination of patients. If the patient's problem is psychologically based, a psychiatric evaluation might save the patient the time and expense of costly tests and procedures. The holistic approach to the study of humans implies assessment of psychological needs and potential. Nurses who are trained in caring for the patient as a total being will include the psychiatric evaluation as part of the assessment skills they acquired in nursing school.

A psychiatric evaluation is not something totally new to be learned. It is primarily a reorganization of knowledge and skills acquired by nurses. Basic knowledge of human behavior and psychodynamics, psychopathology, and psychotherapy, combined with interviewing and assessment skills are the tools nurses need to perform a psychiatric evaluation. Like most things, it is a skill easily learned with practice. What might often impede nurses in their performance is not a lack of knowledge but an uneasiness with psychiatric problems in their patients. It is important therefore that nurses be aware of their own negative reactions or feelings toward patients with psychiatric symptoms.

As in other areas of nursing, the role assumed by the nurse will depend on the level of nursing preparation achieved and the health care setting in which the nurse is employed. The general practitioner should include the psychiatric evaluation as part of the nursing history obtained to identify the nursing diagnoses and related plan of care. Clinical example 17-3 illustrates such an assessment.

CLINICAL EXAMPLE 17-3

An attractive 21-year-old woman is admitted to the gynecological service for a dilation and curettage.

While orienting her to the unit, the nurse observes that she is chain smoking and continuously moving about the room. When asked some general questions about her illness, she begins to cry and tells the nurse about her boyfriend, who was recently killed in an automobile accident. The nurse pursues the conversation and from an assessment decides to call the psychiatric liaison nurse for assistance.

This illustration presents the roles of two nurses. The staff nurse performed an assessment of the patient, including a brief psychiatric evaluation, and then called on the liaison nurse. This nurse consultant has advanced knowledge in the area of psychiatric nursing that will enable her to determine the nature of the patient's problem and assist the staff nurse in designing a plan of care to meet the patient's psychological and physiological needs.

Nurses working in a community mental health center may have advanced knowledge in psychiatric nursing through education at the master's degree level or through experience and in-service education in the mental health field. They often perform the initial evaluation of the patients seen in the center and call on other health team members such as the psychiatrist and psychologist for consultation to confirm the psychiatric diagnosis and treatment plan. Nurses in this setting may also be involved in certain aspects of the identified plan of care, such as arranging for hospitalization or engaging the patient in a form of psychotherapy, including crisis intervention, insight-oriented therapy, or other modes of therapy.

Nurses working in a psychiatric inpatient setting can perform a variety of functions based on the philosophy of the unit where they are employed. Whether this includes primary nursing, patient advocate, or other conceptually defined roles, nurses need to assess and continuously review their patient's mental functioning. This provides for a focus on the patient's problems and a vehicle for ongoing evaluation of the patient's needs.

Interview

The basic elements of a psychiatric evaluation are the psychiatric interview and the mental status examination. For the purpose of clarity these will be addressed separately in this chapter. However, this is not to imply a clear-cut demarcation in the clinical performance of the psychiatric evaluation. The interview provides the structure for assessment of the patient. Assessment denotes systematic collection of pertinent data about the patient. A data base on which nursing judgments can be made is collected through history taking and the mental status examination. Throughout the interview valuable data are obtained by observation of and communication with the patient.

There is no best way to perform a psychiatric evaluation. The nurse's approach and line of inquiry will vary depending on the nature of the presenting problem and the individual patient being assessed. There are many formats for performing and recording the psychiatric evaluation.[1,8-10] This chapter presents one framework for organizing and systematically recording assessment data.

The purpose of the psychiatric interview is to establish rapport with the patient, gain knowledge of his characteristic patterns of living and coping behaviors and assess how his mind is working. The interview is goal-directed communication that provides an opportunity for the nurse to experience who the patient is and to understand how he has developed through the course of life events. This attempt at fully acknowledging and understanding the patient as a unique human being enables the nurse to more effectively determine the patient's needs and an appropriate plan of care. How often does the plan of care fail or the problem reappear because of a lack of concern for the patient as an individual? Consider the patient with high blood pressure who is told to relax by the nurse who does not know he has six children to feed and bills to pay and is the only working member of his family. It is not surprising to find that this man has both uncontrolled blood pressure and is depressed when he next visits the hospital. The loss of appetite and inability to sleep, characteristic of an affective disorder, have compounded the original problem of high blood pressure.

Establishment of rapport is often taken for granted or viewed as an intuitive skill. However, it is a goal to be achieved by the nurse and should be thought about and planned for as any other nursing goal. A basic factor is respect for and awareness of the feelings of security in the patient. A threat to the individual's security produces anxiety, which, in turn, influences the nature of the data obtained in the interview. The nurse conveys a sensitivity to the patient's feelings by demonstrating a genuinely warm and concerned approach. This atmosphere of acceptance facilitates the expression of feelings and concerns by the patient.

Addressing the patient by name and introducing herself by name and title is a way the nurse conveys respect to the patient. Following this identification, a definition of purpose should be established so that a framework for the interview is set. This provides an opportunity for the sharing of expectations and the allaying of anxiety of the participants, since both individuals are clear about what is to follow. The nurse as interviewer is governed by the purpose of the interview, which is distinct and specific for each situation encountered. For example, with a patient who has had a thoracotomy as part of the treatment for Hodgkin's disease and is struggling with acceptance of this chronic condition and its effects on her current life-style, the psychiatric liaison nurse will provide consultation for the purpose of advising and perhaps facilitating the securing of competent psychiatric treatment elsewhere. A second type of interview is the initial meeting in brief psychotherapy or in a continued treatment situation. The nurse's purpose here is to both establish a diagnosis and a professional acquaintance with the intent of carrying on treatment herself. A third type of interview with a different purpose would be with the parents of a child who is handicapped or has a chronic disease. Although the focus of the interview might be a discussion of an identified problem the child is having, an assessment of the particular difficulties and needs of the parents must be considered in planning for the child's treatment.

Whenever the nurse conducts an interview the environment should be one that provides for an atmosphere of privacy. Ideally, this would include a comfortable room used solely by the interviewer and the person being interviewed. More often than not, this kind of privacy only occurs in settings where there are private offices in which the patient and nurse can meet. The nurse must often overcome environmental constraints, and her creativity is called on to convey an atmosphere of privacy to the patient. This can be accomplished by turning chairs in a crowded room away from others so that distractions are at a minimum or by leaving a message with other personnel that the interview is being conducted and should be interrupted only for identified reasons.

Thus far, understanding the patient through demonstrating respect, acceptance, and concern for him as an individual has been stressed. However, setting the stage for self-disclosure is not enough. The nurse must actively participate in the process by being what Sullivan[11] refers to as a participant observer. This implies both participation with and observation of the patient in an attempt to collect relevant data on which nursing care can be based.

Skill in the art of communication is a valuable tool of the participant observer. Maintenance of eye contact and the use of open-ended questions and reflection are familiar techniques used by the nurse in promoting communication. It should be noted, however, that active participation in the interview is not synonymous with increased verbalization by the nurse. A facial expression that reflects interest and concern is just as effective as a verbal message in denoting participation with the patient.

Two skills of utmost importance in conducting a psychiatric interview are listening and observation. Here they are specifically addressed because they are perhaps the most difficult skills to acquire. Attentive listening to and observing another involves transcending oneself and this is a difficult task. Being sure that what is spoken is what is heard as the sender of the message intended, and not as the receiver of the message had either expected or hoped for, requires continuous introspection on the part of the nurse who is the receiver of valuable information about the patient.

When communicating with the patient, the nurse must listen both to what is being said and what is not being said. A patient's verbal description of his mother is that she was "kind, loving, helpful, someone he could always turn to." However, as more information is shared, the patient describes his mother as "having been out of the house a lot working and leaving him with various babysitters throughout his childhood." From these limited data the nurse might begin to wonder how the mother was able to communicate the kind, helpful, loving attitude that her son describes. Or the nurse might question if this is more a description of what the patient as a child needed and wanted but did not receive from his mother. As a result of this conflict, the defense mechanisms of denial and fantasizing may be operating to protect the patient as he tells the nurse the story of his early childhood. Much more information is needed before an assumption such as this one can be made. What is implied in this description is that the nurse strives to understand what the patient is trying to communicate. Does she know what he means by his statements? Could it mean something other than what immediately occurs to her?

Throughout the interview the nurse must also listen for the themes that develop as the patient describes himself and his current and past history. In describing his life events a 22-year-old patient pointed out that his parents taught him at an early age to please other people. It also became evident to the nurse that his parents were consulted on most of the decisions he made throughout his life, such as the friends he had, the schools he attended, what his major was in college, and where he chose to live with his wife. He expressed trouble at work in placing limits on his co-workers who constantly asked him to do favors for them and join clubs, which he was not able to refuse. One of the themes inherent in this description is the patient's inability to assert himself. It is important to focus on this, since it may be one of the predisposing stressors related to his complaint of depression.

Observation also requires a special kind of attentiveness in the nurse. It is important to observe the verbal content as well as the nonverbal communication of the patient represented in the body language he uses. Does he look older or younger than his stated age? Is there a message in his style of dress or the gestures he uses in the interview? Does his manner of communicating reflect his educational level? Is his affective response to a particular topic congruent with the content he presents? In Clinical example 17-4 there are many nonverbal cues that the nurse should note.

CLINICAL EXAMPLE 17-4

Although Mrs. S is only 31 years of age, her torn clothing that fits loosely and her slumped posture and furrowed brow give an appearance of someone much older who has weathered many storms. She continuously wrings her hands as she talks about the death of her husband 6 years ago when her children were still infants. At one point she begins to tear while talking about her inability to give her children the things she would like them to have.

These observations, along with others obtained in the mental status examination, form the data base on which nursing diagnoses and a treatment plan is made. Other observations will be addressed in more depth in the discussion of the mental status examination.

If the skills described are used by the nurse,

an open atmosphere that encourages self-disclosure by the patient will be created. A tense, hurried, and anxious approach should be avoided. The nurse's awareness of her feelings, subjectivity, and misperceptions before meeting the patient should help her to avoid communicating her anxiety to the patient. If immobilized by her own insecurity and anxiety, the nurse will prevent the open atmosphere that allows for participation in the other individual's, her patient's, experience.

A vital concern of the beginning clinician is where to begin with the patient. Simply stated, it is best to start where the patient is. Yet few patients spontaneously begin on their own; rather, they will wait for the nurse to open the interview. A brief statement of what the nurse has learned about the patient, either from observation or from a referral, is usually enough to provide him with the opportunity to tell his story in his own way. The patient with Hodgkin's disease described earlier was approached by the nurse in the following way.

MS. J: **Good afternoon, Ms. X. My name is Ms. J and I am a psychiatric nurse.**
MS. X: **(Looks up) Hello.**
MS. J: **The head nurse, Ms. K, asked me to come and talk with you today. She is concerned about you because she has noticed that you had been crying on several occasions when she entered your room.**
MS. X: **(Beginning to tear) I'm tired of talking, I'm tired of tests, I just want to be left alone.**
MS. J: **It sounds like you are feeling frustrated.**
MS. X: **(Looking directly at the nurse) What would you know? All of this, and for what? Most people with cancer end up dead, so what's the use?**

The nurse has provided the patient a chance to ventilate and begin to disclose some of her feelings about her illness and her fear of death. From this point, considering the patient's emotional status and readiness, the nurse can proceed with the psychiatric evaluation.

With the hospitalized patient an account of the presenting problem and events leading up to the hospitalization as well as historical data about the patient may have previously been obtained and recorded in the chart by other health care professionals. If so, the nurse would modify her approach and discuss particular areas not included in the original evaluation or areas believed to be important to the patient's current mental functioning. The nurse can rely on collateral sources of information such as the medical history or social history and select the focus for the interview.

Presenting problem

A clear account of the presenting problem must be obtained. This consists of a detailed chronological reconstruction of the present illness. If it is not spontaneously offered by the patient or identified elsewhere, the nurse uses her skills in obtaining this information from the patient. How is the problem perceived by the patient? Is it interpersonal, somatic, or sociological? When was the problem first noticed (onset)? How long has it lasted (duration)? Does the patient have any ideas as to the possible causes of the problem? Has it become worse (progressed) or changed in degree? If so, when did the change occur? Has the patient found any solution or obtained any type of relief?

In eliciting this information from the patient, the nurse would look for other factors related to the current problem of which the patient may not be consciously aware, such as a change in personal relationships, job, financial condition, and other circumstances surrounding the initial occurrence. In the preceding dialogue it was assumed, perhaps because of the nurse's own conflicts, that the patient's crying spells were related to her present condition—the thoracotomy for Hodgkin's disease. When specifically asked about the onset of her crying, the patient then proceeded to tell the nurse about her husband's recent loss of his job and inability to find another. Just this amount of information could change the entire assessment of this patient's needs. She may have already worked through acceptance of the chronic illness and currently be concerned with medical insurance for future treatment. Although the original statement she makes about cancer leading to death might reflect an ongoing conflict for her, without more specific inquiry by the nurse her immediate concerns could go unnoticed.

It is therefore necessary to strive for specificity. At times the nurse will need to guide the patient in an attempt to obtain an accurate account of events. Encouraging the patient to describe actual incidents and recording these in the patient's own words rather than making a general statement will be useful in achieving a correct assessment of the patient's conflicts and in the formulation of appropriate nursing diagnoses. Skill in discouraging trivia and repetitions will be needed in helping the patient to focus on the current problem.

After a clear concise statement is obtained about the presenting problem and the incidents that led to its occurrence, the patient's view of responsibility for the problem needs to be assessed. Does he see the problem as something he needs to change, something someone else is responsible for, or something that no one can control, as in the case of someone who believes the devil has entered his body and is controlling his actions?

Whom the patient views as being responsible for the problem directly relates to what changes are desired. The 22-year-old man previously described felt depressed and questioned what he could do to overcome these feelings. Although the relationship he had with his parents may have been a causative factor in his depression and a conflict he could work through in therapy, this was not his current focus. However, placing limits on expectations he had of himself and that others at work had of him was something he consciously desired to do. This allowed for a focus on an identified problem and a definition of goals. Agreement between the nurse and patient on problem identification is essential if resolution is to occur. Whether the nurse's task is to refer the patient for treatment or to personally undertake therapy with the patient, a mutually agreed on nursing diagnosis is essential.

In the initial stage of the psychiatric interview the nurse has created an open atmosphere by demonstrating a genuinely warm concerned approach to the patient and has also gathered information about his present illness. The major symptoms have been described by the patient in behavioral terms, such as a desire to be alone or frequent fighting with spouse, and in body disturbances, such as an inability to sleep, loss of weight, or palpitations of the heart. How the presenting problem is viewed by the nurse would depend on whether there were previous episodes, if the problem is an exaggeration of long-term trends, or something entirely new. To make an assumption about the characteristic patterns of living and coping behaviors of the patient, further data collection will be necessary.

History taking

A brief survey of the patient's past life in the second stage of the interview provides the nurse with a rough social sketch of the patient. Of particular significance are events in the patient's life that may contribute to a psychological disruption, which may be secondary to maladaptive coping behaviors or indicate resources and strengths to consider in treatment planning. To help the patient see the relevance of questions about the past, the nurse can summarize briefly what the patient has said of his problems and then make a transition to the past history, for example, "For me to understand you better and the events of your present situation, I will need to learn something about your past life."

There are significant variations in the methods and forms used in obtaining historical information about the patient.[8-10] However the history is obtained, information about medical and psychiatric history, family history, and a personal history are necessary. The historical information should also include a sexual history and a drug history. The latter two areas are not usually covered spontaneously because of the anxiety-laden material. Starting with a survey of the patient's past life provides for an initial discussion of areas that are perceived by the patient as less threatening. In this way the nurse guides the patient without arousing undue anxiety by progressing from topics that promote the least anxiety to those which promote the most. The interview will have a smoother progression if the nurse asks questions in a logical sequence without abrupt changes from one topic to another.

MEDICAL HISTORY. The depth of information included in the medical history will depend on the age of the patient, the problems encountered in his life, and the resources available to the nurse. If the patient is a young woman who reports being in good physical health throughout her life, the amount of detail required would be less than from the middle-aged man who states that he has always had some physical ailment since childhood. Other family members or significant others in the patient's life, such as mother or family physician, can be vital sources of data. This is true especially if the patient is uncertain about the events surrounding a particular illness or hospitalization.

Following are areas addressed in the general medical history of the patient:

1. Illnesses and operations, with a focus on when they occurred, the outcome, and the chronicity of the condition
2. Congenital, biological, chemical, or physical injury to the nervous system, specifically any head injuries sustained
3. Current medical treatments the patient is involved in or medication he is taking

When an account of these experiences is given, it is important to place emphasis on the patient's reaction to the illnesses, operations, or accidents he has had in his life.

PSYCHIATRIC HISTORY. Following the medical history, inquiry about any previous psychiatric illnesses or encounters with a psychiatrist, psychologist, or other mental health professional is made. Have there been any psychiatric problems in the past? Is the current episode similar to these or different as the patient perceives it? What were the frequency and duration of the past episodes? If the patient was involved in treatment, what kind was it and how did he feel about it?

The psychiatric history would also include related data about the patient's family. Relatives who have had psychiatric illnesses along with the prevalence of suicide in the family should be identified. The significance of this to the patient's present illness is twofold. In certain psychiatric disorders, such as the affective disorders, heredity is considered to be one of the predisposing factors.[3] The occurrence of a psychiatric illness or suicide in the patient's family may also give a perspective on how individuals in the patient's life coped with stress and whether this has influenced the patient's repertoire of coping behaviors. It is essential to point out, however, that the patient's reaction to mental illness in his family is of more significance than the isolated fact itself.

FAMILY HISTORY. Assessment of the patient's capacity to form interpersonal relationships begins with the family history. It is through the relationship the infant has with the significant adults in his life, usually the parents, that the basis of his security is formed. Sullivan[11] believes that the goal of life is interpersonal security. By assessing the patient's interpersonal relationships throughout his life, data can be obtained about his interpersonal needs and level of self-esteem. The family environment provides the first learning situation for the individual. Areas of dysfunction and support need to be determined, since the family can be considered one of the support systems available to the patient throughout his life.

Although the patient may not remember a lot about his early childhood, he has often been told of certain significant events. These may include when and where he was born, his place in the family structure, what the family circumstances were, including any financial stresses, and whether the patient's birth was planned. He may know of any problems his mother experienced during the pregnancy or labor and delivery, who besides the parents was frequently in the home, what the characteristics of discipline were, and what his parents' attitudes toward his development and life events seemed to be. The interactions the patient had with parents, siblings, and other family members during childhood with specific reference to brutality, rejection, deaths, or separations from significant others would be important factors influencing the patient's original development of his sense of self as being either "good" or "bad."

PERSONAL HISTORY. These data will give the nurse an impression of what the emotional climate was for this individual's beginning personality development from his point of view. When and how early developmental tasks were achieved, such as toilet training and entering school, leads into the personal history of the patient. A continuation of the chronological approach in pursuit of the individual's personal history incorporates important areas of life experiences. These areas include schooling, vocational pursuits, sexual experiences, and drug experimentation. These life experiences are more easily addressed if they are presented in a historical perspective of when they first occurred.

Starting school is a big event in childhood. It is also the first opportunity the individual has to compare himself to others. Socialization patterns have begun to develop. The age on entering school, type of school (private, parochial, public), grades repeated, level of academic performance, including special achievements, episodes of truancy, and disciplinary difficulties will portray the early attitudes developed about study and work. The relationships with teachers and fellow students, friendships formed, and special interests and activities, such as scouts, will portray the early social values established. If the individual developed close relationships during this time, he can usually remember the names of his closest friends and may know something about what they are doing now. Conflicts experienced during the early primary years are expressed in behaviors such as nail biting, nightmares, sleepwalking, and enuresis. Although most children exhibit some of these behaviors, the response of the parents and what the individual remembers about the behavior are important to elicit.

As the individual approaches adolescence, a time of rapid physical development and emotional turmoil, he begins the task of identification of self and the formation of intimate relationships. During this period of the individual's life, people outside the family structure become important sources for comparisons of values, attitudes, and experiences. Experimentation with drugs, including alcohol, and sex are likely to occur and should be addressed while information about this stage of development is being obtained.

On entering high school, what was the extent and type of participation in sports, parties, church, and political activities? What was the individual's experience with groups and leadership, especially during school? Was he a member of the "in group"? Did his level of academic performance change? What was his age and status on leaving school? Did he graduate or leave school to work? Did he have any special interests or hobbies? Were they solitary or group activities? When did he first drink alcohol, smoke marijuana, and experiment with other drugs, such as LSD, amphetamines, or barbiturates? What pattern was established at the time and how has it changed? Being asked questions about drug use can be intimidating to the individual. It is important to phrase the questions so that the individual feels free to answer without having a value judgment placed on him. Phrases such as "when" or "how often," rather than "do you," assume that the behavior has occurred and make it easier for the individual to answer than when he first must decide if he wants to admit to the behavior being addressed.

With the onset of puberty, sexual attitudes become important. How and from whom did the patient learn about sexual matters? With the woman, information surrounding the time of menarche is elicited. Who told her about menstruation? Her reaction to the first and subsequent periods should be ascertained. With both women and men it should be determined at what age pubic and axillary hair appeared. Did the individual experience an early or delayed onset of body development and what was the reaction to this in relation to peers? When did the man first experience an erection and orgasm and was it with or without ejaculation? When did the individual first masturbate? What were the experiences with necking, petting, and intercourse? How were these experiences viewed by family and friends? Friendship, dating, and early sexual experiences, including autosexual, homosexual and heterosexual activities are usually important issues for the adolescent. Were these experiences comfortable or pleasurable ones or associated with guilt?

The sex life of an individual can be viewed as a barometer of emotional health. It is therefore important to ascertain if there have been any changes in the individual's sexual habits. The nurse must feel comfortable discussing sexual matters with the patient to be able to talk about the patient's sexual habits in each stage of his life. This is an area that is sensitive to most people, and further information about what areas to address and how to discuss sexual material with patients can be obtained in the publication *Assessment of Sexual Function.*[7]

An individual's occupational and marriage history are included in the assessment of the period of maturity. What are his goals and ambitions, positions held, promotions, and relationships with bosses and peers? Are there any discrepancies between stated goals and the individual's efforts to achieve them? Continuing education and military experiences can be discussed as part of the occupational history of the patient when applicable.

The marriage history should include a history of dating and courtship, the circumstances of the marriage, sexual adjustment, frequency of relations, living conditions, financial difficulties experienced, and previous marriages. If there are any children in the family, what were the reactions to the pregnancies and births and are there any prominent problems in the family now? What is the patient's relationship with his parents? If they are deceased, what was the patient's reaction to the loss?

To complete the social sketch of the patient, it is essential to determine his talents, strengths, and assets to gain a total view of him as a person. Asking him to describe his daily activities can give a clue as to what the patient is trying to achieve. The richness or poverty of activities in his life-style may indicate the meaning of life for him. Church, community, and leisure time activities are often sources of emotional support for an individual that can be used especially in times of stress.

The second stage of the evaluation has simply been an attempt to understand how the patient comes to be there in relation to the prominent landmarks that have characterized his course of life up until the present. This information depicts the development of the patient's self-concept. As with any assessment that the nurse

would perform, the amount of detail required will depend on the individual patient, his presenting complaint, and the environmental constraints such as time. Hopefully, the areas just addressed will be included in some detail in each psychiatric evaluation completed by the nurse.

Clinical example 17-5 illustrates the type of data obtained in the first two stages of the psychiatric evaluation.

CLINICAL EXAMPLE 17-5

Ms. T is a 22-year-old single, white, unemployed clerical worker who comes to the mental health clinic stating that she does not socialize any more and is becoming increasingly self-conscious about going out of the house for fear of "making a fool" of herself. She is currently living with her father, three siblings, and an aunt in the aunt's home. She states she would like to "make something" of herself but is afraid that people won't accept her.

Ms. T relates the onset of her feelings to the problems that occurred at work 18 months ago. She states she felt a lot of pressure at work, felt "extremely nervous" around her boss, was denied two promotions for "trivial reasons," and began to feel inferior to other workers, which made her depressed and led to her resignation.

During the time when problems were occurring at work, several incidents happened at home that also affected how Ms. T was feeling. Her younger sister was using drugs and the police had been called to the home several times. Ms. T was concerned about the effect this had on her aunt for whom she has a great deal of affection and gratitude. Her paternal grandmother had died in February and her twin brother had married and left the home in June. Both these individuals were a source of support to Ms. T. She wishes that her siblings and father would move out of the house, leaving only herself and the aunt because "none of them are decent people anyway and they only cause trouble for my aunt."

Her medical history includes hospitalization at age 6 for a tonsillectomy. Ms. T says she enjoyed being in the hospital and remembers playing in the play area. She had no major illnesses during childhood or adolescence that she could recall. She believes that she had the usual childhood illnesses, measles and mumps.

Ms. T's psychiatric history was negative for herself and her family. She was seen by Dr. X at the Community Health Facility 6 months ago for a questionable somatoform disorder. Her father has been seen by Dr. X for 10 years for multiple physical complaints.

Ms. T was born and raised in Baltimore. She is the eldest, along with a twin brother, of five children. She has two sisters, age 21 and 19, by her father's first marriage and one sister, age 15, by his second. Ms. T states she has little recollection of her biological mother. She remembers going to the movies with her at about age 4 and has heard from other family members that she was a "nice lady." Her father was described as a "very emotional" person who gets "very upset" easily. He drank heavily when the children were young and was taken out of the house several times by the police for disorderly conduct. Ms. T and her siblings were basically raised by her paternal aunt and grandmother. Even after the father's second marriage, she and her siblings lived with the aunt and the grandmother. Her father remarried when Ms. T was 6 years old and lived with his second wife in an apartment close to her aunt's home. She states that the family would celebrate holidays together and go on picnics but that she never felt close to any of her siblings or to her father.

Ms. T started school at age 5 and achieved "above average" grades. She was a safety in grade school and a cheerleader for 3 years in high school. She graduated from high school at age 17 without any failures. Ms. T says she was a "shy kid" most of her life but had several girl friends. However, she rarely brought them home because of her father's drinking.

She had dated one boy steadily from age 18 to 20. Her sexual experience included kissing and petting. Ms. T states she wants to be a virgin when and if she marries. She learned about menstruation from girl friends and a movie at school and her first period was at age 13. She states that she has never talked with family members about sexual matters.

Ms. T feels she has cut herself off from friends during the past 2 years. Several of them still call or drop by but she never goes out with them. She spends most of her day cleaning the house, making the meals, and listening to music in her room.

The only position Ms. T held was as a clerical worker at the bank. She acquired the job after graduation and believes that she did okay until 18 months ago. She gives a vague description of her boss, stating he just "didn't like me" and was "always on my back about something."

Ms. T denies any experimentation with drugs. She used to drink wine on social occasions when dating but stopped after she broke up with her boyfriend.

Mental status examination

The historical information obtained will give the nurse a perspective on areas with which the patient may have difficulty, such as forming interpersonal relationships, consistent job performance, and other significant life experience areas. Further supportive data for assessment of both the patient's limitations and strengths will be obtained in the mental status examination, which is the third stage of the psychiatric evaluation.

The mental status examination is a way of organizing observational data about all aspects of a patient's mental functioning. While obtaining information about the presenting problem and taking a history, the nurse is informally and indirectly accumulating information about the patient's mental functioning. However, formal questioning is usually needed at the end of the interview to complete an accurate and comprehensive mental status examination. Verbatim samples of the patient's speech and thought content are useful to present a precise picture of the patient. For clarity, the mental status examination should be recorded in a certain order and organized according to certain categories, that is, general observations, sensorium and intelligence, thought processes, mood and affect, and insight. Each item will be addressed with clinical examples for clarification followed by a continuation of the case history presented earlier.

General observations

Specific aspects of the patient's behavior are included in detail in the remainder of the mental status examination. It is useful, however, to record in the beginning the general observations of the patient, especially those characteristics which appear outstanding to the interviewer.

APPEARANCE. The patient's appearance should be described in terms of consistency with his age and station in life, his manner of dress (conservative, tasteful, meticulous, inappropriate), his personal habits (clean, unkempt, disorderly), his characteristic facial expression (alert, vacant, sad, bewildered, hostile, masklike), and his state of health and general nutrition.

REACTION TO INTERVIEW. The patient's reaction to the interview, with the circumstances surrounding it taken into account, is addressed. Has he been cooperative, friendly, evasive, ingratiating, indifferent, passive, dependent, or hostile in his responses to the interviewer? If he has been observed in various situations, does he respond differently to various types of people (physicians, nurses, other patients)? Each patient will react to the situation whether he is hospitalized, referred for psychiatric evaluation by the court, or voluntarily seeking counseling.

CONSISTENCY OF BEHAVIOR. As previously discussed, throughout the interview, communication is both verbally and nonverbally expressed. Examples of the patient's verbal and nonverbal behavior are included and the consistency of both is noted. Characteristics of the patient's speech, such as speed, vocabulary, and goal directedness are observed. Any overt motor behaviors, such as finger tapping, hair twirling, hand wringing, pacing, posturing, gait, and bizarre movements are described.

RESPONSE TO PATIENT. It is important that the nurse also become aware of the response she has to each of the patients she interviews. The response can contain diagnostic information about the patient. A depressed patient may elicit a sense of sadness and hopelessness in the nurse. In contrast, the nurse might experience anger toward a patient who is angry and hostile. The principal feeling elicited should be identified and the behaviors observed that are associated with the feeling should be clearly stated, as in Clinical example 17-6.

CLINICAL EXAMPLE 17-6

The patient was interviewed in her room on the fourth day of hospitalization. She was a white woman slightly overweight, neatly dressed in jeans and a sweater and appeared younger than her 36 years of age. Although she was cooperative, her guarded responses to all questions seemed excessively self-centered. She gave the interviewer the feeling that she didn't trust anyone and was preoccupied during the interview. When asked how other people treated her, she refused to answer with an angry "I'd rather not say!"

Sensorium and intelligence

This section describes the patient's state of consciousness and his ability to accurately perceive the environment. The patient's state of consciousness, orientation, memory, intellectual function, judgment, and comprehension are assessed. Impairment in more than one area may relate to a diagnosis of an organic mental disorder.[9] Since the disorder can vary from mild transient alterations to a permanent disruption of all areas, it is important to carefully document each area.

LEVEL OF CONSCIOUSNESS. A variety of terms can be used to identify the patient's level of consciousness. Is the patient alert and awake or stuporous and sleepy? Is he easily distracted or hyperalert? Can he sustain attention to both external and internal stimuli? A clouded state of consciousness is an essential feature in delirium and is therefore essential to assessment for accurate diagnosis and treatment.

ORIENTATION. The patient is questioned regarding his orientation to time, place, person, and situation. Does the patient know who he is, where he is, who the people around him are, and the date? Does he seem to understand the rationale for the interview and his role in it? Patients with organic disruptions may give grossly inaccurate answers, especially for time relationships.[3] In contrast, the schizophrenic disorders may cause the patient to say he is someone else or somewhere else or in some way reveal his personalized orientation to the world.

MEMORY. Memory impairment is a prominent behavior observed in dementia that can range from forgetfulness to a total lack of understanding of significant persons and events in the individual's life. There are three areas to be tested under memory: immediate recall, recent memory, and remote memory. Immediate recall involves attention and concentration as well as an ability to retain material just learned. The digits-span test requires that the patient repeat digits either forward or backward within a 10-second interval. The nurse recites a series of randomly selected digits to the patient, beginning with three digits and progressing until the patient is unable to repeat the digits in proper sequence. The same procedure is then repeated, but the patient is asked to say the numbers with the order reversed. An example may need to be given so that the procedure is understood. An approximate comparison to educational level can be made: five digits forward and four digits backward equals an eighth-grade education, and seven digits forward and five digits backward indicates a twelfth-grade education. However, high anxiety may interfere with the patient's ability to concentrate and should be considered if the performance is poor.

Recent memory can be tested by asking the patient when he came to the hospital and to recall the events of the past 24 hours. A reliable informant may be needed to verify the statements made by the patient. A test of recent memory can be performed by asking the patient to remember three words (an object, a color, an address) and then having him repeat them back 15 minutes later in the interview.

The patient's ability to give a consistent account of his past history requires an intact remote memory. Available records or reliable informants are needed to verify information, such as date of birth, age, when started and finished school, date of marriage, birth dates of children, and other significant life events.

INTELLECTUAL FUNCTION. A patient's intellectual functioning is assessed in relation to his educational, occupational, and attainment levels. Testing the patient's vocabulary, counting and calculating ability, abstract ability, and fund of general knowledge provides some information about the patient's intelligence. Vocabulary can be assessed by asking for word definitions or synonyms. Counting and calculating involve doing simple arithmetic problems (9×6, $21 + 7$) and asking the patient to serially subtract 7 from 100. If he has difficulty subtracting 7 from 100, he can be asked to subtract 3 from 20 in the same manner. This task also involves the ability to concentrate and complete a task.

The ability to conceptualize and abstract can be tested by having the patient explain a series of proverbs. The patient is given an example of a proverb with its interpretation and then asked to tell what several proverbs mean to him. Following are frequently used proverbs: "When it rains, it pours," "A stitch in time saves nine," "A rolling stone gathers no moss," and "The proof of the pudding is in the eating." Most adults are able to interpret proverbs as a representation or symbolization of human behavior or events. Cultural background is a set factor that should be considered when the patient is not able to complete the task. If the patient's educational level is less than ninth grade, asking him to list similarities between a series of paired objects will assess his ability to abstract. The following series of paired objects are frequently used: bicycle, bus; apple, pear; television, newspaper. A good reply would be in terms of function, whereas an answer in terms of structure may indicate a tendency toward concrete thinking.

To determine the patient's fund of general knowledge, he can be asked to name the last five presidents, the mayor, five large cities, the capital of France, or other similar questions congruent with his educational background. With all these tests it is essential to keep in mind the patient's educational and vocational background so that he is given tasks he is able to perform. If the patient cannot read or does not work, he may not be able to state recent events or local news but could relate plots of television shows or local neighborhood information. On completion of some general tests of intelligence, if the nurse has doubts about the patient's intelligence level or suspects deterioration from a history of changes at work, home, or school, a referral for psychological testing should be considered.[5]

JUDGMENT. The patient's judgment can best be assessed from an account of past decisions and how they were reached and from the patient's responses to the interview situation. Judgment involves the ability to understand facts and draw conclusions from relationships. In discussion of recent events does he appear to exercise sound judgment? The young teenage boy referred for counseling after repeated arrests for car theft exhibits poor judgment. It is useful to determine if the judgments are deliberate, impulsive, or inappropriate. Several hypothetical situations can be presented for the patient to evaluate: What would he do if he found a stamped, addressed envelope lying on the ground? How would he find his way out of a forest in the daytime? What would he do if he entered his house and smelled gas?

COMPREHENSION. Throughout the interview the patient's ability to understand the meaning of the questions is assessed, as well as his ability to comprehend incidents in his environment, such as local, political, and personal events that affect him and his community. Does he understand his role as a patient, and, if hospitalized, does he understand the hospital routine? An organic brain syndrome could interfere with the patient's level of comprehension.[9]

The assessment data obtained in the area of sensorium and intelligence is of particular importance in determining disorders classified as organic mental disorders. The acute picture presented to the clinician is often easy to identify, whereas the more subtle changes that can occur as a result of a degenerative disease or brain lesion require attentive observation by the nurse and, as previously mentioned, carefully documented behaviors, as shown in Clinical example 17-7.

CLINICAL EXAMPLE 17-7

It was apparent that the patient was alert and awake but almost totally distracted by something within himself. Questions and directions were repeated frequently so that they were understood. He was oriented to person, place, and situation. He performed six digits forward and three digits backward and remembered two of three objects after 15 minutes. He remembered the third with help. He listed presidents to Truman and performed serial sevens with relative ease, making two mistakes. He could not identify any recent events or discuss television shows and seemed limited in his fund of general knowledge. This may relate to his social isolation since quitting school at age 16, as described by his mother.

Thought processes

FORM OF THOUGHT. Observation of thought process is made through the patient's speech. The patterns or forms of verbalization, rather than the content of speech, are assessed. What is the rate or flow of speech? Is it overly fast or retarded? Does the patient's speech proceed in a clear, logical, goal-directed manner? As he talks about topics relating to himself, the nurse should note if the patient is able to express himself in an understandable manner or if his ideas are vague, leaving her uncertain about their meaning. Is he able to move freely from one topic to another with relative ease and flexibility? Is there continuity of thought or are his associations disconnected (loose), constantly changing (flight of ideas), wide of the point (tangential), interrupted suddenly (blocked), or distorted and bizarre, as when new words are made up to express ideas symbolically (neologisms).

CONTENT OF THOUGHT. Recurring patterns of content, such as delusions, hallucinations, or illusions may be observed and reflect a disruption in perception. Misperceptions include a variety of thoughts, feelings, or fears the patient may have that interfere in some way with his reality testing.

Hallucinations refer to sensory perceptions for which there are no external stimuli. Sometimes the patient's behavior will indicate that he is hallucinating; he may adopt a listening attitude, mumble, pick at unseen objects, or stop suddenly as if he is guarding himself. Asking if he has heard noises or voices when no one was around or had any unusual experiences will provide an opportunity for the patient to describe any such experiences to the nurse. Characteristics such as the source, manner of reception, content, and time of the experience should be described.

Delusions are recurring false beliefs that are not congruent with the patient's culture or background. Again, tactful questioning will be useful in helping him to focus on delusional material. Does he misinterpret what happens to him, giving it special or false meaning? Does he feel that he has been singled out or watched? Does he experience his thoughts or actions as being controlled by an external force? Can people read his mind or does he have psychic powers? These concerns may be complicated and will be concealed by the patient and require extensive questioning.

Illusions refer to misperceptions that have an external stimulus. The hospitalized patient may believe his room is a jail cell and the staff members are security guards. A schoolteacher with an organic mental disorder may perceive her family as pupils and the bedside table as her desk.

The patient's thoughts can be focused on obsessions, compulsions, or phobias that also interrupt the normal thought process. Repetitive thoughts, impulses, or behaviors unwanted by the individual are defined as obsessions or compulsions. These can be assessed by asking the patient if there are any intrusive recurring thoughts or actions that he feels unable to control and that occupy an extensive amount of his time. Objects and/or situations irrationally feared by the patient in a persistent manner are identified as phobias. The individual can exert great energy avoiding certain situations or thinking about the feared object.

Disruptions in both the form and content of thought are seen in the schizophrenias, affective disorders, anxiety disorders, organic mental disorders, and paranoid disorders in varying degrees of intensity and varying combinations. In the following example, the nurse includes a detailed description of the patient's form and content of thought in an assessment of his thought processes:

The patient's speech was rapid and he acknowledged feeling as if his thoughts were coming too fast, "My mind is racing ahead." The rapidity of his speech compounded the difficulty understanding him as he quickly moved from one topic to another in what appeared to be an unrelated manner. He denied any visual or auditory hallucinations; however, he believed that he could talk with God if he needed a consultant on his life situation. He felt this was a special blessing given to him over other men.

Affect

Observations of the range, appropriateness, and intensity of the patient's emotional expressions (affect) in relation to the circumstances of the interview and the ideas expressed are documented. Does the patient demonstrate variability in the expression of feeling or does his affectual response appear blunted or restricted in some way? Does he report significant life events without any emotional component (flat)? Is the patient's affectual response congruent with the content of his speech? Does he report that he is being persecuted by the police and laugh? Does he rapidly shift from one affectual response to another (labile)? The patient's statements of emotion and the nurse's empathic responses to the patient may provide clues to the appropriateness of the affect or character of the prevailing mood.

Mood

The pervasive, relatively enduring, emotional state of the patient reflects his mood and can influence his perception of his life situation. Does the patient's appearance reflect his mood? Does he look "down in the dumps"? A description of the patient's appearance, as well as his verbalizations about his mood, are recorded. How would he describe his mood? Does it remain the same or change during the day or from day to day? Asking the patient to rate his mood on a scale of 0 to 10 can be useful for an immediate rating of his mood and valuable for comparison of changes that occur during treatment. When the clinical picture is highlighted by a continuous intensification or change in the patient's mood, an affective disorder is suspected.

While eliciting the patient's feelings, if the nurse perceives a potential for suicide, she should attempt to bring out the patient's thoughts about self-destruction. Information about suicidal or homicidal thoughts should be directly addressed. Has he had the desire to harm himself or someone else? Has he made any previous attempts, and, if so, what events surrounded the attempts? To make a judgment about the suicidal or homicidal risk present,

the nurse assesses the details of the plans, ability for implementation (availability of guns), patient's attitude about death, and support systems available to him as shown in the following example:

The patient responded to most of the questions asked in a flat dull manner. Although he stated he felt sad about the recent changes in his life, his lifeless posture and tone of voice did not convey any emotional response. He denied any suicidal or homicidal ideation or plans. He related having made two previous suicidal gestures in the past year by "taking pills."

Insight

The degree of insight the patient has about the nature of his problem and how it affects his feelings, thoughts, and behavior may be assessed informally as he talks about his problems. It is important to determine if he sees the problem as something brought on by external factors or from within himself. Whether he can see his treatment needs realistically would affect the treatment plan and the setting of mutual goals to meet the patient's needs. Several questions may be helpful to ascertain the patient's degree of insight. What does he think about all he has told the nurse? What does he want to do about it? What does he want others, including the nurse, to do about it? The following example illustrates a patient's level of insight:

The patient enumerated on several problems he encountered at work. He reluctantly stated that he might have to change, but really thought that his difficulties were because of his wife's drinking. He believed he could do nothing until she changed.

This third stage of the psychiatric interview completes the assessment of the patient. The mental status examination describes comprehensive data about the patient's mutual functioning in an organized manner. Clinical example 17-8 completes the clinical portrayal of Ms. T.

CLINICAL EXAMPLE 17-8

Ms. T was a stylishly dressed, neatly groomed, slender female, in apparent good physical health who appeared her stated 22 years of age. She was cooperative during the interview but had difficulty expressing herself in specific terms. Her vague responses at times left the interviewer feeling perplexed about the difficulties she was describing.

The patient was alert and awake and oriented to person, place, and situation. Immediate recall and recent memory were intact, demonstrated in her ability to recall three unrelated objects immediately and again in 15 minutes. Some of the historical information given was inconsistent with historical factors reported by her father. Although the vocabulary used by Ms. T and her knowledge of general information was congruent with her twelfth-grade education and past employment, she had difficulty completing the serial sevens but performed serial threes with relative ease. She stated she was "nervous," which may be a factor related to performance. She was able to abstract two of three proverbs presented.

Proverb	Interpretation
Don't cry over spilled milk.	"If something happens, then forget about it. Maybe things will get better."
A rolling stone gathers no moss.	"A good person gathers no enemies. If a person stays active, he won't get depressed."
People who live in glass houses shouldn't throw stones.	"The glass will break."

Her responses to hypothetical situations were appropriate; however, the manner in which she coped with difficulties at work and home showed impairment in judgment about personal issues.

Ms. T's speech was clear, coherent, and of normal rate and tone. Except for the vague tangential manner in which she discussed her concern for her aunt, her communication was goal directed. There were no apparent delusions, hallucinations, or illusions. She denied any obsessions, compulsions, or phobias.

The central theme during the interview was her fear of being irresponsible and hurting her aunt. Her sadness and concern about her behavior in relation to the aunt pervaded the interview. She appeared nervous (looking away, fidgeting) and cried whenever she talked about her aunt. She described her mood as "low" and rated it as a four. She denied any suicidal or homicidal ideation or plan previously or at the present time.

Her insight is questionable, since she questioned her need for treatment, although she agreed to return. She knew a problem existed but was unaware of the causative factors related to her behavior.

The nurse has assembled a comprehensive data base through history taking and the mental status examination. She has collected objective facts based on observation of the patient's behavior during the interview. In the final stage of the psychiatric evaluation the nurse critically examines the information she has organized in the preceeding stages and interprets these data to formulate a treatment plan based on identified patient problems and nursing diagnoses. The elements of a psychiatric evaluation are summarized at right.

ELEMENTS OF PSYCHIATRIC EVALUATION

A. Data collection
  1. Presenting problem
    a. Onset, duration, symptoms noted, and progression
    b. Solutions attempted
    c. Significant changes in the patient's life
    d. How responsibility for the problem is viewed
  2. Characteristic patterns of living and coping behaviors
    a. Medical history and current problems
    b. Psychiatric history for self and family
    c. Family history and personal history: Chronological approach with emphasis on interpersonal relationships and major areas of life experiences
  3. Mental status examination
    a. General observations: Appearance, reaction to the interview, consistency of behavior, and response to the patient
    b. Sensorium and intelligence: Level of consciousness, orientation, memory, intellectual functioning, judgment, and comprehension
    c. Thought processes: Characteristics of speech, patterns of verbalizations, manner of communication of thoughts, organization of ideas, coherence of associations, recurring patterns of thoughts, and misperceptions described
    d. Affect and mood: Range, appropriateness, and intensity of affect; behavioral manifestations and description of mood; and suicidal/homicidal ideation or plan
    e. Insight: Understanding of current situation and solutions
B. Organization and interpretation of data
  1. Problem identification: Medical and nursing diagnoses
  2. Identification of patient resources
C. Treatment plan

Additional resources

The psychiatric interview provides the structure to obtain pertinent information about the patient. Additional resources are often utilized to complete a comprehensive assessment of the patient. The medical chart is one resource the nurse can use to collect information about the patient's medical and social histories. This information is recorded in designated sections of the patient's chart by various health team members.

Significant others in the patient's life, including family, friends, a minister, or the family physician can participate in the interview and share valuable perceptions about the patient and his current situation. Family theorists, such as Bowen,[4] stress the importance of the patient's social system in both diagnosis and treatment of psychiatric problems.

The expressive therapies are essential resources for the assessment and treatment of

---

SITUATIONS WHERE TESTING IS FREQUENTLY INDICATED*

Children

1. *Presence of a learning disorder*
   Psychological testing can help delineate the probable etiology and appropriate course of treatment in learning disabilities which may involve central nervous system dysfunction, intellectual deficiency, and/or personality and emotional factors. Tests often provide clues to family and/or school influences in the situation.

2. *Emotional-social disturbances*
   Psychological testing can be useful in gaining understanding of such problems as hyperactivity; antisocial behavior; excessive withdrawal; difficulty adapting to peers, home, and/or school; and language disorders.

3. *Developmental deviations*
   Testing gives information relative to the age-appropriateness of the child's functioning in a wide variety of areas (intellectual, personal-social, perceptual-motor coordination).

Adults

1. *Mental retardation/intellectual deficiency*
   Testing can throw light on the factors interfering with an adult's use of intelligence, as well as provide an assessment of the degree of mental ability in the case of mental retardation. State laws may require an IQ score as part of the diagnosis of mental deficiency in certain situations, such as for custodial care, and support for children with learning disabilities.

2. *Psychotherapy*
   A psychological evaluation can help determine the most appropriate therapeutic mode and goals and is often useful in deciding when to terminate therapy, or understand changes that are occurring during therapy.

3. *Differential diagnosis*
   Psychological evaluations provide measures of a person's functioning ranging from perceptual-cognitive and ego level factors to personality structure, dynamics, and unconscious factors. The analysis of strength and weakness contributes to an understanding of the patterns of the whole person that can be used to derive a differential diagnosis. For adults, testing is often helpful in detecting borderline psychosis, early signs of organicity, and early signs of schizophrenia before symptoms become clearly manifest in clinically observable symptomatology.

4. *Forensic psychiatry*
   A psychological evaluation is often a helpful adjunct in cases involving mental illness or central nervous system impairments following injury. Psychological testing also has many applications in the criminal justice system.

*From DeCato, C.M., and Wicks, R.J.: J. Psychiatr. Nurs. **14:**25, June, 1976.

children. Children are often brought for psychiatric evaluation by the family or referred by the school system for behavioral disruptions. Art, dance, or play therapy can provide the means for establishing an initial relationship with the child. These therapies are especially important when the individual is unable to express his ideas verbally or does not want to talk. The family is, again, a vital resource to the clinician working with children.

Research in recent years has provided a variety of formalized questionnaires and standardized tests as adjunctive methods for assessment. Computers are now utilized for the collection and collation of data, the diagnosis of symptom clusters, and the evaluation of specific treatment modalities.[6] Rating scales can be used to gather information from the patient and significant others. Self-report questionnaires filled out by the patient give an account of the subjective distress experienced by the patient. This description can be a more accurate account of the emotional state of the patient than that inferred or elicited in the interview. Questionnaires directed to family members or friends can relate specific characteristics of the patient's social or family life. Some of the circumstances in which psychological testing may be useful are given on the facing page.

Psychological tests are of two types: those designed to evaluate intellectual and cognitive abilities and those designed to describe personality functioning. Some of these are briefly described in Table 17-1. Commonly used intelligence tests are the Wechsler Adult Intelligence Scale (WAIS) and the Wechsler Intelligence Scale for Children (WISC). Although intelligence tests are often criticized for being culturally biased, their ability to determine an individual's strengths and weaknesses within the culture provides essential therapeutic information.

Material obtained from projective tests reflects aspects of an individual's personality functioning, including reality testing ability, impulse control, major defenses, interpersonal conflicts, and self-concept. A battery of tests are usually administered to provide comprehensive information. The Rorschach Test, Thematic Apperception Test (TAT), Bender Gestalt Test, and Minnesota Multiphasic Personality Inventory (MMPI) are commonly used by the clinical psychologist for assessment.

A more detailed discussion of the types of psychological tests available and their clinical applicability can be found elsewhere.[5] It is important for the clinician to be aware of the resources available and the general information that can be obtained from standardized scales and tests. These tests may be administered by the nurse or may require the knowledge and skill of the psychologist for administration and interpretation. Collaboration with the psychologist to review the assessment data obtained and to plan treatment is a responsibility of the nurse as a member of the health team.

Special diagnostic procedures are especially important when the patient or his family describes abrupt changes in his manner of behaving or incidents of loss of consciousness for even brief periods of time. These are the electroencephalogram (EEG), CAT scan, lumbar puncture, and blood chemistry values. Electroencephalography provides a mechanism for recording any changes in the electrical activity in various areas of the brain. The test is useful in diagnosis of epilepsy, brain lesions, and other diseases of, or injury to, the brain. According to the area of the lesion in the brain, specific symptoms would be demonstrated. The symptom complex would reflect the disruption in the function of the area of the brain involved. Distortion of the senses of taste, smell, sight, or hearing could occur. The patient's ability to speak clearly or understand what is being said to him could affect his pattern of communication. Changes in his personality or mental ability could be displayed in lapses of memory, absentmindedness, or loss of initiative. All these behaviors would be ascertained in the mental status examination. However, if the symptoms are treated from a psychopathological frame of reference, a brain tumor or seizure disorder could be overlooked and the appropriate treatment denied. The EEG, CAT scan, and lumbar puncture are essential procedures for the detection of specific brain dysfunctions.

Chemical analysis of various substances in the blood can provide the clinician with diagnostic information. This is especially valuable when a drug-induced delirium is suspected. Many drugs and poisons can cause an organic mental disorder. The most commonly implicated are the opiates, barbiturates, amphetamines, and hallucinogens. The patient may display behaviors ranging from mild confusion and drowsiness to overwhelming anxiety and hallucinations. The blood level and toxic level of the particular drug involved would be important, possibly life-

TABLE 17-1. Commonly used psychological tests*

Name	General classification	Description	Special features
Bellak Children's Apperception Test	Projective technique	Drawings of animals for children	Designed specifically for children
Bender (Visual-Motor) Gestalt Test	Graphomotor technique; may be used as projective technique	Geometric designs that the patient is asked to draw or copy, with design in view	Useful for detecting psychomotor difficulties correlated with brain damage
California Personality Inventory	Objective personality test	Seventeen scales developed presumably for normal populations for use in guidance and selection	Less emphasis on mental illness than MMPI scales, such as, dominance, responsibility, socialization
Cattell 16 Personality Factor Questionnaire (16 PF)	Objective personality test	Questionnaire covering 16 personality factors derived from factor-analytical studies	Bipolar variables allow for interpretation of scores varying either above or below the norm, such as reserved vs. outgoing; trusting vs. suspicious, timid vs. venturesome
Draw-a-Person Test	Graphomotor projective technique	Patient asked to draw a person and then one of the sex opposite to the first drawing	Projects body image, how the body is conceived and perceived; sometimes useful for detecting brain damage; modifications include: draw an animal; draw a house, a tree, and a person (H-T-P); draw your family; draw the most unpleasant concept you can think of
Minnesota Multiphasic Personality Inventory (MMPI) (Forms: Individual, Group, and Shortened R)	Objective personality test	Questionnaire yielding scores for 9 clinical scales in addition to other scales	Includes scales related to test-taking attitudes; empirically constructed on basis of clinical criteria; computer interpretation services available
Rorschach Technique	Projective technique	Ten inkblots used as basis for eliciting associations	Especially revealing of personality structure; most widely used projective technique
Rosenzweig Picture Frustration Test	Projective technique	Cartoon situations, dialogue to be completed by subject	Designed specifically to assess patterns of reaction to typical stress situations; child, adolescent, and adult forms
Sentence Completion Test	Varies from direct-response questionnaire to projective technique	Incomplete sentence stems that vary as to their ambiguity	Highly flexible; may be used to tap specific conflict areas; reveals generally more conscious, overt attitudes and feelings
Symonds Picture Story Test	Projective technique	Pictures of adolescents	Designed specifically for adolescents
Thematic Apperception Test (TAT)	Projective technique	Ambiguous pictures used as stimuli for making up a story	Especially useful for revealing personality dynamics; some pictures are designed specifically for women, men, adolescent girls, and adolescent boys
Wechsler Adult Intelligence Scale (WAIS)	Intelligence test	Eleven subtests: vocabulary, comprehension, information, similarities, digit span, arithmetic, picture arrangement, picture completion, object assembly, block design, and digit symbol	Most commonly used intelligence scale that yields a measure of intelligence expressed as IQ scores; differences in subtests can also be useful clinically
Wechsler Intelligence Scale for Children (WISC)	Intelligence test	Similar to the WAIS	Standardized for children ages 5 to 15
Wechsler Preschool and Primary Scale of Intelligence (WPPSI)	Intelligence test	Similar to the WAIS and WISC	Standardized for children ages 4 to 6½
Word-Association Technique	Projective technique	Stimulus words to which patient responds with first association that comes to mind	Flexible; may be used to tap associations to different conflict areas; generally not as revealing as SCT responses

Modified from Freedman, A.M., Kaplan, H.I., and Sadock, B.J., editors: Comprehensive textbook of psychiatry, ed. 3, Baltimore, 1980, The Williams & Wilkins Co.

saving, information needed to determine a plan of care.

Symptoms of cerebral dysfunction, including mental confusion, hallucinations, and convulsions, might also occur in certain hypoglycemic states. In this instance the patient's behavior reflects a variation in the normal amount of glucose found in the blood. The etiological factors that might be involved are numerous. It is of particular importance in the organic mental disorders to differentiate these factors so that the appropriate treatment can be instituted.

At this point in the psychiatric evaluation a diagnostic impression is formulated from an integration of significant historical data, observations of the mental status examination, and results of specific tests that have been assembled. Formulating a diagnosis implies an awareness of identified problems, which can be overt, covert, existing, or potential. When an identification of the patient's problems and needs has occurred, it is important to validate these with the patient so that a plan of care can be implemented.

Diagnostic impression

Organization and interpretation of the data collected involves formulating a diagnostic impression. The presenting problem has been identified in terms of the nature of onset, duration, and course. The nurse has clarified the relationship of the patient's behavior to stressors, or the precipitating factors that resulted in his seeking help at this time. These behaviors, along with those assembled in the interview, are compared to documented norms to identify deviations. One's theoretical base may include personality development theory, behavior theory, or systems theory. Each provides a framework for comparing behaviors and identifying deviations. Personality development involves the completion of identified tasks and incorporation of certain skills at various points in an individual's life. Behavior theory encompasses the broad spectrum of human behavior and incorporates individual set factors, such as culture and nationality, in determining the function of certain behavior for an individual in terms of its usefulness. Systems theory can also be used to provide a framework for evaluating factors in the patient's environment (family, community, nation) that influence his behavior.

The patient's behavior is the critical evidence used in formulating a diagnostic impression, regardless of the theoretical framework of the observer. The difficulty that arises in psychiatric diagnosis is in part due to the lack of specificity and simple, valid criteria for the classification of human behavior. Thus psychiatric diagnosis is a complex and controversial issue.

The most recent edition of the DSM-III[2] has attempted to increase the reliability of symptomatic diagnosis through the inclusion of specific diagnostic criteria to define each diagnosis. These criteria were utilized in clinical facilities throughout the United States during the development process to identify and solve problems in the classification of disorders. The predecessors to the DSM-III, DSM-I and DSM-II, lacked sufficient detail in the classification for either clinical or research purposes.

In the DSM-III clinically significant behavioral or psychological syndromes that include symptom clusters of patient behaviors are classified as mental disorders (Chapter 2). A descriptive approach is utilized in the discussion of each disorder and in the division of each disorder into diagnostic classes. This results in the grouping together of syndromes that have common clinical features.

The DSM-III points out that the new classification categorizes disorders, not individuals, and that each disorder is not an entity unto itself. Thus the need for an individualized approach to diagnosis is warranted. The approach of the DSM-III is atheoretical in relation to etiology unless a specific pathophysiological process is known to be causative, and then it is included in the definition of the disorder.

The nurse should possess a working knowledge of the DSM-III so that effective communication can occur through the sharing of a common terminology among health team members. The nurse's knowledge can also be beneficial in helping her to ascertain other behavioral characteristics present in the patient who displays some behaviors suggestive of a particular syndrome. With certain disorders, especially the schizophrenic and affective disorders, effective treatments can be considered according to the similarity of problems exhibited within each category.

Although the DSM-III follows a medical model in its description of symptoms of illness, the identification of specific observable behaviors of the clinical syndromes makes correlation with the nursing process model possible. The nurse, knowledgeable of the clinical syndrome involved, would focus on the nursing diagnosis identified from the assessment data obtained in the evaluation. The nursing diagnosis is a statement that reflects a discrepancy between the patient's behavior and the expected behaviors for a person with similar set factors as related to the stressors involved. For example, disturbance in self-concept might be inferred from certain patient behaviors: shabby clothing, unkempt hair, preoccupation with physical concerns, refusal to participate in social activities. Specific nursing actions are then correlated with the nursing problem identified. The patient exhibiting a disturbance in self-concept might benefit from specific information on grooming and self-care.

The organization and interpretation of the assessment data depend on the purpose of the interview and the background of the interviewer. As previously discussed, the nurse is guided by the purpose of the interview in determining the assessment data to be collected. A complete psychiatric evaluation is not always warranted, as in an emergency situation, but could be conducted over several interviews with the patient. The nurse may perform the mental status examination along with clarification of the presenting problem and rely on other resources, such as the medical chart, to obtain the pertinent historical data needed in an emergency situation.

The woman described in the beginning of this chapter may not be able to give an accurate account of historical factors when seen by the nurse. However, her mental status at the time needs to be assessed to determine the degree of incapacitation present and the immediate ramifications of it, if any. She was disturbing the peace, but should she be kept in jail overnight or allowed to leave the hospital in her current state of functioning? These are examples of the type of judgment in which the nurse will be involved when assessing patients in an emergency room or crisis clinic.

The educational background and experience of the nurse will also determine the comprehensiveness of the psychiatric evaluation and interpretations made. Nurses employed in mental health facilities will have more opportunity to practice skills in psychiatric evaluation. However, it should be stressed that all nurses need to be knowledgeable about the psychiatric evaluation process and be able to identify deviations from the norm in the patients they assess. The nurse may need to call on someone more knowledgeable in the area of psychiatry, such as the clinical specialist, for assistance in identifying particular disorders and determining a plan of care. The importance is in assessing the patient as a total being, including his state of mental health. This involves a basic knowledge about psychological behaviors as well as the sociological and biological behaviors.

Case disposition

A brief summary of factors to consider in making a decision about a case disposition will be presented. The three general areas to consider are the identified problem, the limitations and strengths of the individual, and the treatment resources available. Each area will be discussed separately and followed by a continuation of the case study of Ms. T.

The problem areas identified in the psychiatric evaluation are addressed in order of priority. The symptoms described by the patient in the presenting problem should be addressed first, since they are usually those causing most discomfort to the patient at the time he seeks treatment. However, as in other areas, the patient may not always be aware of or admit to problems that are of importance. Priority is always given to those which, if not treated, will threaten the life of the individual or the life of another. An individual's suicidal or homicidal potential must be considered first and an appropriate treatment plan provided. Another factor to consider in deciding priorities is whether the behavior observed is an expression of a failure of the individual's coping mechanisms, as in a crisis, or an expression of lifelong maladaptive behavior. The limitations of the individual in coping with the identified problems, especially in self-protection, are considered. In certain instances of psychotic behavior the individual may not be aware of his inability to care for himself and therefore may need brief hospitalization. The depressed individual is also a candidate for hospitalization, and his suicidal risk must be evaluated at all times. The support system available to the patient is considered in determining what modality of treatment is used. A number of factors should be considered in determining whether the patient should be hospitalized or referred for outpatient treatment. These include the family and significant others available to the patient; his strengths, including past coping abilities; the values and beliefs he has regarding his life; and his ability to meet the demands of the situation.

The nature of the problem will indicate the treatment modality and related goals. For example, the patient who complains of an inability to form intimate relationships may benefit from both individual and group therapy. The man who complains of impotence with his spouse may be best able to work on this problem and related issues in couples therapy.

If the nurse is involved in the implementation of therapy, the problem should be defined in measurable terms so that both the nurse and the patient can evaluate if change is occurring in the therapeutic process. It is useful to ascertain what change the patient wants, since this allows for a focus on a particular issue and the definition of goals for therapy.

Whatever the nurse's goal might entail, on completion of the psychiatric evaluation she should be able to make a recommendation to the patient. This involves being knowledgeable about the community agencies available to the patient and what services they can and cannot provide.

Clinical example 17-9 illustrates how the data obtained in a psychiatric evaluation are used in a final disposition with identified problem areas and a formulated treatment plan. The techniques of interviewing, differentiating symptoms, establishing a diagnosis, and formulating a treatment plan are skills the inexperienced nurse will develop with experience and a sound theoretical base.

CLINICAL EXAMPLE 17-9

Ms. T stated she does not socialize any more, as evidenced by her leaving her job and withdrawal from family and friends. She spends her day at home cleaning, cooking, and listening to the radio alone in her room, which are solitary activities. She stated she felt inferior to her peers at work and was denied two promotions. She feels fearful about going out because she might make a fool of herself.

Ms. T's history reveals a lack of consistent nurturing in the home and an unstable family structure. The grandmother seemed to be a source of support and nurturance to Ms. T and has recently died. There was no evidence of role models for the development of intimate relationships in the home. Ms. T described herself as a "shy kid" who had few friends in childhood. She expressed feelings of hatred for most of her siblings. The aunt has provided for her, and the overwhelming concern Ms. T has about hurting the aunt may relate to fear of rejection, thereby losing the one stable relationship she believes she has left.

Ms. T presented an attractive appearance. She appeared to have difficulty relating to the interviewer, which was evidenced in her vague responses. She seemed to hide behind the sunglasses that she wore throughout the interview. She stated a concern about her decreasing ability to relate to others and a fear of attempting to do so.

The developmental tasks of the young adult include an increase in socialization and intimacy. It is a time when an individual's involvement in relationships and special interests provide for a sense of self-satisfaction. A pursuit of career goals occurs. The relationships formed and goals attained related to work or school become a source of positive feelings about oneself. In comparing the data obtained in the interview with developmental norms, a discrepancy exists. Two problem areas are evident: a decrease in socialization and a decrease in self-esteem.

The related nursing diagnoses would include (1) social isolation related to increased stress at work and home evidenced in withdrawal and (2) disturbance in self-concept related to feelings of guilt evidenced by statements of self-blame.

The treatment modality selected is long-term individual psychotherapy with the following goals. The patient will (1) establish a relationship with the therapist, (2) reestablish contact with friends, (3) resume vocational activities (school or work), and (4) experience activities within her capabilities to increase self-esteem. Conjunctive therapies considered are group and family therapy. Group therapy would provide the patient with the opportunity to develop and test socialization skills. Family therapy would focus on the interrelationship of the patient's problem with the family process. The selection of the type of therapy depends on the framework of the therapist and the availability of other modalities.

As in other areas of nursing, it is essential that the nurse become aware of the health team members working with the patient in the health care system. The treatment plan identified must be congruent with the plans of the other health care professionals working with the patient. Communication among those involved in the patient's care, such as the physician, social worker, and psychologist, should occur throughout all stages of the nursing process if a successful outcome is to be achieved.

The psychiatric evaluation is similar to the nursing process model in that it is a systematic problem-solving approach to patient care. Assessment data are obtained during the initial stages of the evaluation, and a treatment plan with identified goals is formalized in the final stage of the psychiatric evaluation. Whether the nurse is involved only in the initial contact with the patient or participates in the treatment plan identified, she has completed the stages of the nursing process. Through interaction with the patient the nurse has been involved in assessment, planning, intervention, and evaluation even though the actual time spent in the last two stages may be minimal if a referral is made.

Future trends

It is difficult to project what might occur in the future. The experience and wisdom developed in the past century have brought changes no one could have foreseen. The study of the psyche is something that has historically perplexed human beings. Various schools of thought have emerged in an attempt to understand the development of the uniqueness of the human species. Theories of personality were developed by Freud, Sullivan, Erikson, and others as they observed and recorded the behavior of their patients over extended periods of time. Objective evaluation of behavior as an expression of the inner self remains a difficult task for the practitioner. Psychiatric evaluation still takes place in the subjective experience which evolves in the relationship that develops between the individuals involved. As advancement in technology has influenced the efficiency and effectiveness of the care a patient receives in the health care field, in the future the evaluation of the subjective side of humans will become increasingly more objective.

Psychological testing is being used more by practitioners in an attempt to expand or validate their objective impressions, as described earlier in the discussion of the resources available to the practitioner. Research has produced a variety of assessment tools, such as questionnaires, that aim to elicit certain information about the patient which can be compared to standardized results. A method for computerized psychiatric evaluation has been developed.

The role of the nurse in the health care system is being redefined as nurses continue to increase their independent functions and identify their unique contribution to the health care team. Nurses with advanced knowledge and experience in psychiatry are becoming private practitioners to meet the psychosocial demands of the population. Nurses in private practice often utilize other nurses, as well as psychiatrists, as consultants to their practice.

In considering the future trends in psychiatric evaluations, the legal implications increase as the population becomes more health oriented and adept at pursuing the right to health care. Diagnosis and treatment of health problems are scrutinized by the population and by the courts. Reported cases of negligence and malpractice are on the rise. This trend makes objective evaluation essential for the future practitioner. The integration of research and clinical practice is crucial for optimum care of human psychosocial needs. Care implies prevention and maintenance in the realm of mental health, and it should complement the established goal, cure.

Suggested cross-references

DSM-III and the medical model are discussed in Chapter 2. Therapeutic relationship skills are discussed in Chapter 3. Impaired cognition is discussed in Chapter 13.

SUMMARY

1. As vital members of the health care team, nurses must assume a role in the psychiatric evaluation of patients. Basic knowledge of the concepts of psychodynamics, psychopathology, and psychotherapy combined with interviewing and assessment skills are the tools nurses need to perform a psychiatric evaluation. The role assumed by the nurse will depend on the level of nursing preparation obtained and the health care system in which the nurse is employed.

2. The basic elements of a psychiatric evaluation are the psychiatric interview and the mental status examination. The interview provides the structure for systematic collection of pertinent data about the patient through history taking and the mental status examination. The purpose of the psychiatric interview is to establish rapport with the patient, gain knowledge of his characteristic patterns of living and coping behaviors, and assess his mental functioning. Listening and observation skills are used by the nurse to create an open atmosphere that encourages self-disclosure by the patient.

3. A clear account of the presenting problem and the events that led up to the occurrence, or history of the presenting problem, is obtained in the initial stage of a psychiatric evaluation.

4. Data collection through history taking involves obtaining information about the patient's medical and psychiatric history, family history, and personal history, including a sexual and drug history. These data are collected in the second stage of the psychiatric evaluation.

5. The mental status examination organizes observational data about a patient's mental functioning in five categories: general observations, sensorium and intelligence, thought processes, mood and affect, and insight. These data represent the third stage of a psychiatric evaluation.

6. Additional resources for data collection include the medical chart, significant others in the patient's life, formalized questionnaires, and standardized tests.

7. A diagnostic impression is formulated from an integration of significant historical data, observations of the mental status examination, and the results of special tests and diagnostic procedures. The nurse critically examines the comprehensive data obtained and interprets her findings on the basis of the comparison of patient behaviors to documented norms.

Formulating a diagnostic impression entails the identification of the clinical syndrome displayed and the nursing diagnoses identified.

8. The organization and interpretation of the collected data and identification of a case disposition complete the final stage of a psychiatric evaluation. Making a case disposition involves awareness of the identified problems and related nursing diagnoses, the limitations and strengths of the individual, and the treatment resources available. Communication with other health professionals involved in a patient's care is imperative to ensure goal achievement.

9. Psychiatric evaluation is similar to the nursing process model in that it is a systematic, problem-solving approach to patient care. The assessment data obtained and their organization and interpretation depend on the purpose of the interview and background of the interviewer, the nurse.

10. Future trends in the psychiatric evaluation of patients include the development of more objective tests and measurements in computerized form. A practical consideration in obtaining skill in the psychiatric evaluation of patients is the legal implication of an undiagnosed psychiatric problem.

References

1. Alston, J.F., and Levet, J.M.: What's happening: practical application of the mental status exam, Nurs. Pract. **2**:37, July-Aug. 1977.
2. American Psychiatric Association: Diagnostic and statistical manual of mental disorders, ed. 3, Washington, D.C., 1980, The Association.
3. Balis, G.U., Wurmser, L., and McDaniel, E.: Clinical psychopathology, Woburn, Mass., 1978, Butterworth Publishers, Inc.
4. Bowen, M.: Family therapy in clinical practice, New York, 1978, Jason Aronson, Inc.
5. DeCato, C.M., and Wicks, R.J.: Psychological testing referrals: a guide for psychiatrists, psychiatric nurses, physicians in general practice, and allied health personnel, J. Psychiatr. Nurs. **14**:24, June 1976.
6. Freedman, A.M., Kaplan, H.I., and Sadock, B.J., editors: Comprehensive textbook of psychiatry, ed. 3, Baltimore, 1980, The Williams & Wilkins Co.
7. Group for the Advancement of Psychiatry: Assessment of sexual function: a guide to interviewing, New York, 1973, Mental Health Materials Center, Inc.
8. Imboden, J.B.: Practical psychiatry in medicine. Part 16. Psychiatric evaluation of the medical patient, J. Fam. Pract. **10**:4, April 1980.
9. Nyman, G.: The mental status examination. In Balis, G.U., Wurmser, L., and Grenell, R.: Psychiatric foundations of medicine, Woburn, Mass., 1978, Butterworth Publishers, Inc.
10. Snyder, J.C., and Wilson, M.F.: Elements of a psychological assessment, Am. J. Nurs. **77**:235, 1977.
11. Sullivan, H.S.: The psychiatric interview, New York, 1954, W.W. Norton & Co., Inc.

Annotated suggested readings

American Psychiatric Association: Diagnostic and statistical manual of mental disorders, ed. 3, Washington, D.C., 1981, The Association.

This book presents the most recent classifications of mental disorders with a comprehensive description of each diagnostic category.

Bowen, M.: Family therapy in clinical practice, New York, 1978, Jason Aronson, Inc.

This book presents a collection of papers by the author depicting the evolution of his family systems theory. It covers a wide range of topics useful to the clinician in the assessment, diagnosis, and treatment of family problems.

Cheah, K.C., and Beard, O.U.: Psychiatric findings in the population of a geriatric evaluation unit: implications, J. Am. Geriatr. Soc. **28**:4, April 1980.

Research findings demonstrate the importance for professionals to be aware of the needs of geriatric patients with acute illness in order to intervene in potential problem areas.

Critchley, D.L.: Mental status examination with children and adolescents: a developmental approach, Nurs. Clin. North Am. **14**:3, Sept. 1979.

The author describes the developmental framework she utilizes for organization of the mental status examination with children and adolescents. Suggestions for age-appro-

priate activities, such as play and art, are included in a discussion of the structure of the interview.

DeCato, C.M., and Wicks, R.J.: Psychological testing referrals: a guide for psychiatrists, psychiatric nurses, physicians in general practice and allied health personnel, J. Psychiatr. Nurs. **14:**24, June 1976.

This article describes the nature of psychological evaluation and gives general guidelines for making referrals for psychological testing.

Eggland, E.T.: How to take a meaningful nursing history, Nursing '77 **7:**22, July 1977.

A general overview of the nursing history and the basic interviewing techniques used in data collection are presented. Also highlighted are the family reactions to the illness of the individual.

Eisdorfer, C., and Cohen, D.: Diagnostic criteria for primary neuronal degeneration of the Alzheimer's type, J. Fam. Pract. **11:**4, Oct. 1980.

This article provides an overview of the dementing illnesses and utilizes a review of current literature to discuss diagnostic criteria for assessment of clinical features of primary degenerative dementia of Alzheimer's disease.

Folstein, M.F., and Rabins, P.V.: Psychiatric evaluation of the elderly patient, Primary Care **6:**3, Sept. 1979.

The authors present pertinent information on the evaluation and treatment of the common syndromes found in the geriatric population with emphasis on dementia and delirium. A brief description of the mini-mental assessment tool is included with reference to the common causes for the cognitive impairment detected with this tool.

Francis, G., and Munjas, B.: Manual of social psychologic assessment, New York, 1976, Appleton-Century-Crofts.

This useful text written by nurses presents a systematic method for assessing the sociological and psychological aspects of clients.

Freedman, A.M., Kaplan, H.I., and Sadock, B.J., editors: Comprehensive textbook of psychiatry, ed. 3, Baltimore, 1980, The Williams & Wilkins Co.

An in-depth discussion of the diagnosis and classification of symptoms observed in the psychiatric patient is presented in the chapters that address psychiatric evaluation. Specific guidelines are provided to the clinician in a well-organized, easily understood format for obtaining pertinent information in the psychiatric interview, taking a history, and performing the mental status examination.

Fromm-Reichmann, F.: Principles of intensive psychotherapy, Chicago, 1971, University of Chicago Press.

Chapters 1 to 6 present material helpful to the beginning practitioner in psychiatry. Problem areas the therapist may encounter in the initial sessions with patients are addressed. A process-oriented approach to the collection of assessment data is provided with clinical examples.

Group for the Advancement of Psychiatry: Assessment of sexual function: a guide to interviewing, New York, 1973, Mental Health Materials Center, Inc.

The publication gives a straightforward approach to the assessment of sexual function of the individual. Specific questions are included with the discussion of various age-groups and particular problems that might occur at the stages of development.

Hagarty, J.R.: Psychological assessment of the mentally handicapped, Nurs. Mirror **143:**59, 1977.

This brief article describes the use of the psychologist and how to ask questions and interpret data from psychological tests to formalize the best treatment plan for learning for the mentally handicapped person. Emphasis is placed on the strengths and potential of the individual.

Haley, J.: Problem solving therapy, San Francisco, 1977, Jossey-Bass, Inc., Publishers.

This book focuses on the social context of a client's presenting problem. A discussion of how to define the problem within the social system of the client and methods or strategies to change the system and modify the problem through therapy are provided.

Imboden, J.B.: Practical psychiatry in medicine. Part 16. Psychiatric evaluation of the medical patient, J. Fam. Pract. **10:**4, April 1980.

The importance of a psychiatric evaluation of the medical patient is conveyed in the discussion of the relationships between biological and psychosocial factors in illness. A general review of the broad classification of psychiatric illness, elements of a psychiatric diagnosis, factors to consider in a psychiatric interview, and the format for a psychiatric evaluation are clearly and concisely described.

James, M., and Jongeward, D.: Born to win: transactional analysis with gestalt experiments, Reading, Mass., 1978, Addison-Wesley Publishing Co., Inc.

This book is primarily concerned with transactional analysis theory. The experiments included are useful in helping the reader to understand himself and also his relationships with others. It gives a different approach that can be used in obtaining historical information about a person.

Lancaster, J.: Adult psychiatric nursing, New York, 1980, Medical Examination Publishing Co., Inc.

Chapter 6 presents an assessment tool for the psychiatric setting. The tool outlines the areas included in a psychiatric evaluation and incorporates specific questions that address each area.

McIntyre, J.S.: Mania: the common symptoms of several illnesses, Postgrad. Med. **66:**1, July 1979.

Case histories of patients coming to the emergency room with mania are utilized for discussion of the assessment data necessary for evaluation and appropriate treatment.

Nyman, G.: The mental status examination. In Balis, G.U., Wurmser, L., McDaniel, E., and Grenell, R.: Psychiatric foundations of medicine, Woburn, Mass., 1978, Butterworth Publishers, Inc.

A comprehensive discussion of the mental status examination is presented here. Case histories are included and compared as each section of the mental status examination is discussed. This is an excellent reference for a more thorough examination of the psychiatric patient.

Rapp, M.S.: Re-examination of the clinical mental status examination, Can. J. Psychiatry **24:**8, Dec. 1979.

The author questions the objectivity of the data obtained in the mental status examination, especially in the areas of insight, memory, judgment, and intelligence. He implies that individual differences in the examiner and patient could distort the judgments made. He stresses the importance of listening to the patient for the most valuable assessment of the patient's problems.

Snyder, B.D.: An efficient approach to the mental status examination, Minn. Med. **62:**12, Dec. 1979.

The author reviews the areas included in the mental status examination and techniques to utilize in the collection of information about the patient. Particular emphasis is placed on the cognitive assessment of patients.

Snyder, J.C., and Wilson, M.F.: Elements of a psychological assessment, Am. J. Nurs. **77**:235, 1977.

This article approaches the psychological evaluation of a patient from a conceptual model rather than a medical model. Ten elements are described as the essential factors the nurse should consider in an assessment of the patient.

Spitzer, R.L., Skodol, A.E., Gibbon, M., and Williams, J.B.W.: DSM-III case book, Washington, D.C., 1981, The American Psychiatric Association.

This collection of case vignettes is helpful in its descriptive correlation of clinical material to the principles of the DSM-III. The discussion following each vignette includes the rationale for the diagnosis according to the diagnostic criteria outlined in the DSM-III.

Sullivan, H.S.: The psychiatric interview, New York, 1954, W.W. Norton & Co., Inc.

In this book Sullivan describes both the patient and therapist as they interact during the psychiatric interview. He stresses the importance of the patient-therapist relationship in understanding the patient as a unique person. Assessment of the patient is incorporated throughout the book as the stages of the interview are presented.

Taylor, M.A., Abrams, R., Faber, R., and Almy, G.: Cognitive tasks in the mental status examination, J. Nerv. Ment. Dis. **168**:3, March 1980.

A neuropsychological approach to the mental status examination is presented. The article outlines cognitive tasks, dysfunctions, abnormal responses, and suggested localization of cortical dysfunction.

Thompson, T.L., and Feinberg, L.E.: Evaluation of postoperative changes in mental status, Postgrad. Med. **67**:3, March 1980.

The article discusses the common causes for changes in the mental status of postoperative patients and provides guidelines for conducting an initial evaluation.

Zeldow, P.B.: Sex differences in psychiatric evaluation and treatment: an empirical review, Arch. Gen. Psychiatry **35**: 1, Jan. 1978.

The author reviews the literature of the 1970s concerning the sex-related differences of diagnosis and treatment of psychiatric disorders. The question of bias of both male and female raters with male and female patients is discussed. A consistent finding was that both sexes hold separate standards of mental health for males and females.

"We're all mad here. I'm mad.
  You're mad."
"How do you know I'm mad?"
  said Alice.
"You must be," said the Cat, "or
  you wouldn't have come here."
Alice didn't think that proved
  it at all.

Lewis Carroll, Alice's Adventures in Wonderland

CHAPTER 18

EVOLUTION OF INPATIENT PSYCHIATRIC NURSING

Kay Sienkilewski

Learning objectives

*After studying this chapter, the student
will be able to:*

- describe the historical events that have influenced the role of the psychiatric nurse in an inpatient setting.

- discuss the advantages and disadvantages of the utilization of a primary nursing model for the delivery of psychiatric nursing care.

- compare and contrast the educational preparation and functional roles of the major mental health care disciplines.

- analyze and compare the concepts of milieu therapy as described by Cumming and Cumming and the therapeutic community as described by Jones.

- identify the role of individual, group, and family therapy programs in the inpatient setting.

- describe psychodrama in terms of major concepts and the therapeutic process.

- discuss the utilization of the various occupational and activity therapies in the inpatient setting.

- compare the characteristics of acute intensive and long-term custodial inpatient psychiatric units and discuss the nursing implications of the differences in the settings.

- identify suggested readings for further study.

The practice of inpatient psychiatric nursing is rich in history and tradition. It would be impossible to separate the evolution of "modern day" psychiatric nursing from the developmental stages of medical practices in psychiatry, mental health concepts, and the growth of nursing as a profession. Years of progress and successful attainment of knowledge and skills in the areas of psychiatric treatment and nursing care delivery systems have given rise to inpatient psychiatric nursing practice that is exciting, innovative, and challenging. No longer is the inpatient nurse the "keeper of the key." Inpatient psychiatry offers the nurse an opportunity to use the nursing process and employ a variety of skills in responding directly to the needs of the patient and significant others.

Inpatient psychiatric nurse as a caretaker

Early inpatient psychiatric nursing was characterized by custodial care, which ranged from humanistic to neglectful and cruel. In the early Middle Ages the mentally ill were admitted into general hospitals and treated with kindness. Seventh century writings reveal that treatment of the "insane," particularly those "subject to melancholy," bore close resemblance to some practices followed in the mental hospital of the late 1930s and early 1940s.[17] Frequent baths, a wholesome diet, and "suitable exhilaration" of the mind were the primary modes of treatment for the depressed patient. The more severely disturbed were also provided these forms of therapy but were restrained in their beds to prevent them from injuring themselves or others. It was in the three centuries following the Reformation that the system of "appalling neglect and revolting cruelty" developed in the treatment of the mentally ill. This lasted until the drastic reforms of the nineteenth century.

The nurse's role was primarily to oversee the care given to the patients and to ensure the smooth operation of the ward. It was not uncommon that tasks of housekeeping, dietary management, and laundry care became the responsibility of the nurse. Thus the early inpatient psychiatric nurse was more a manager of a unit than a provider of direct patient care.[7]

The reforms of the nineteenth century had great impact on inpatient psychiatric nursing. The care of patients once again became humane, and the scientific understanding of the nature, causes, and treatment of mental illness was of primary concern. As this scientific body of knowledge increased, there was great demand for advancement in psychiatric nursing to ensure that psychiatric treatment kept pace with the rapid growth in other branches of medicine and nursing.

Despite this "new era," the role of the inpatient nurse remained primarily custodial in nature. Much of the emphasis was placed on performing tasks and administering somatic therapies. However, the seed had been planted, and the future of psychiatric nursing as a viable specialty was taking root.

Inpatient psychiatric nurse as a member of the team

With the development of social psychiatry, the role of the inpatient psychiatric nurse began to change. Nurses became key figures in milieu therapy and therapeutic communities. The nurse was used as a role model for the patients and their families. There was a dramatic shift in emphasis from the importance of performing tasks to the importance of establishing interpersonal relationships. Nursing was given "almost free rein" to involve the patient in activities of daily living. Together the nurse and the patient would problem solve important issues centered around self-care and interactions with others within the community.

As early as 1949 nursing was to enter yet another "hallowed hall."[20] For the most part, individual inpatient psychotherapy had been limited to physicians. Nurses were often instructed to observe and record the patients' behavior but not to make any type of interpretation. With the advent of the health team concept, nurses were encouraged to learn more about the psychodynamics of mental illness and to engage in individual nursing therapy. It was not infrequent that a physician would supervise a "promising nurse therapist" who was providing individual therapy to a patient.

By the mid-1950s nurses were recognized as being capable of functioning as group leaders and therapists. This was a major breakthrough, since no longer was nursing limited to custodial care and unit management. Nurses were finally participating in collegial relationships with psychiatric social workers, occupational and recreational therapists, psychologists, and physicians.

In 1949 Dr. Robert H. Felix, Director of the

National Institute of Mental Health, U.S. Public Health Service, spoke of the importance of a team approach to psychiatric care. At this time "teamwork" was still in an early experimental stage, and in some institutions even the concept of the team approach was not yet accepted, let alone practiced.[18]

In these early days of the team concept the psychiatric team was defined as consisting of the psychiatrist, clinical psychologist, psychiatric social worker, and psychiatric nurse. According to Robinson,[18] professional "rivalries" were often evident, and territoriality became a block to progress. The psychiatrist continued to view himself as "the sole dispenser of psychotherapy rather than the captain of a therapeutic team." Psychiatric social workers and psychiatric nurses were often more concerned about "delineating their separate areas of professional responsibility than about cooperating for the total welfare of the patient."[18] To overcome these early stumbling blocks, advocates of the team concept in psychiatric treatment were pressed to clarify the purpose and to demonstrate the desirability of this approach.

The definition of a clinical team comprises several explicit and implicit characteristics. The purpose of the psychiatric team is to provide a forum in which the psychiatrist, psychiatric social worker, clinical psychologist, and psychiatric nurse democratically share professional knowledge and together evolve a therapeutic plan of action.[15]

There are many implications that arise from this definition of the psychiatric team. It implies that all members have an equal opportunity to share what they have learned about the patient and that these inputs will be welcomed when it is time to develop a definite goal-directed plan of action. Implicit to the concept of a clinical team approach is the need for a team leader. It is the psychiatrist who most frequently functions in this capacity. According to Mereness, it is the responsibility of the leader to "help mold into an understandable unity the specialized information which is brought to the group by other team members." A final implication is the presence of mutual respect and understanding of the contributions that each team member brings to the situation.[15]

In the early stages of the team approach most nurses were receptive to the concept and grateful for the opportunity to contribute to patient care. However, old stereotypes of the subordinate role that nurses usually played and inadequate communication skills placed nurses at a disadvantage. It became apparent that "the nurse's academic and professional background must be equivalent to that of her colleagues if she is to feel secure and be accepted as a fully participating member of the team."[15]

Nursing educators responded to the challenge and began to make needed changes in their educational systems. Curriculum changes included the addition of scientific psychiatric nursing education, with specific emphasis on psychodynamics and interpersonal theory, communication skills, and skills in understanding and working with other disciplines. Thus there began to develop a new breed of psychiatric nurses who viewed themselves as professionally and academically competent to be fully participating members of the psychiatric clinical team.

There is little doubt that the joint endeavor of a team approach promoted mutual respect among the various disciplines, and nursing was a definite benefactor of this new-found mutuality. However, what ground nursing may have gained in collegiality may have been lost in its search for autonomy. Thus the nagging doubts about nursing being a "true profession" continued to remain as many nurses adopted a compensatory role of "junior psychiatrist."

Inpatient psychiatric nursing and the nursing process

Once nurses had been accepted as a member of the health team and psychiatric nursing had developed sophistication, skills, and knowledge in the specialty of psychiatry and psychiatric treatment, there came a need for reassessment and clarification of purpose and identity. Psychiatric nursing returned to the nursing process.

If there is anything that is unique to nursing, it is the nursing process. Sundeen et al.[21] describe the nursing process as an "interactive, problem-solving process used by the nurse as a systematic and individualized way to fulfill the goal of nursing care." They distinguish problem solving, which is used by many disciplines, and the nursing process as follows:

Many disciplines incorporate aspects of the problem-solving process. The nursing process, however, is distinguished from the problem-solving process in its purpose and method. The purpose of the problem-solving process is the development of new knowledge. The purpose of the nursing process is to maximize a client's positive interactions with his environment, his level of wellness, and his degree of self-actualization. The methods also differ. With the scientific process one can problem-solve in isolation, manipulating objects and ideas without interacting with other people. The nursing process, however, is founded on the helping, interpersonal relationship; the nurse interacts with a client to analyze and meet his biopsychosocial needs.[21:5]

Today's inpatient psychiatric nurses use the nursing process to provide care to individuals, families, and groups. Through this process the nurse strives to assist the patient to establish more effective ways of handling those stresses which led to his immobilization. It is the goal of the nurse to participate with the patient in planning the nursing care. By capitalizing on the patient's strengths, the nurse may help him to establish more harmonious interpersonal relationships and function more independently. These successful accomplishments will lead to a more positive self-concept and a sense of well-being.

The manner in which inpatient psychiatric nurses implement the nursing process may vary from institution to institution or from nurse to nurse. However, there are several factors that remain constant. The collection of a data base is the initial step in the process. This is usually accomplished in an individual interview, which is conducted by the nurse within 24 to 48 hours after the patient's admission to the unit. Depending on the patient's ability to be an accurate historian, the nurse may choose to use family members or friends as sources of information. Once a data base is gathered, the nurse develops a diagnostic impression and plans the appropriate nursing actions to be implemented. The results of these nursing actions are evaluated as frequently as necessary, and changes and modifications are made when appropriate.

It is important to stress that the nursing process does not exist in a vacuum. It is essential to the patient that each discipline on the health team work toward common goals and objectives. However, within these common goals and objectives, each discipline has a variety of dependent, independent, and interdependent functions. The most familiar dependent nursing functions are those of carrying out the physician's orders. It is the responsibility of the nurse to give treatments and medications accurately and on time. The nurse must facilitate the process by which the patient is assured of receiving all the prescribed laboratory tests, psychological tests, and other appropriate consultations. Despite the fact that these are truly dependent functions, the nurse has the right and the obligation to question any physician's orders that are unclear or possibly unsafe. Interdependent functions of the inpatient psychiatric nurse may range from the mutual sharing of information with the health team to acting as cotherapist with physicians or social workers in family or group therapy, providing she has appropriate preparation for these roles.

It is those independent functions of nursing which often give rise to the greatest sense of job satisfaction for the inpatient psychiatric nurse. It is within the realm of the nurse to implement nursing action ranging from the taking of vital signs to carrying out special types of nursing observations and supervision. Together the nurse and the patient develop goals and determine the course that seems most likely to lead to the accomplishment of those goals. Along the way the nurse must decide what teaching is necessary to provide for the patient, his family, and significant others. The nurse must answer the questions of how much can be learned from the patient's milieu and what needs must be met within the patient's home environment, community, or employment situation. It is the inpatient psychiatric nurse who often provides the vital link in bridging the gap between inpatient hospitalization and successful reintegration into the community.

It is difficult, if not impossible, to accomplish these objectives without the active participation of the patient. One method of encouraging the patient's participation is the use of nursing rounds. In nursing rounds the patient is interviewed by a "nurse consultant" in front of members of the nursing staff who are working directly with him. The nurse consultant encourages the patient to discuss both those experiences in his hospitalization which are useful and those which are nonproductive. The patient is requested to say how he believes the nursing staff can best help him reach his goals. He is urged to identify his internal and external resources and to capitalize on these strengths during the period of his hospitalization as well as when he returns to the community.

Patient response to this particular format of nursing rounds has been favorable. Many patients have articulated that in nursing rounds they have experienced being treated as "intelligent adults." They believe that they are given the right, as consumers of health care, to demand to be informed participants in that care.

Clinical example 18-1 demonstrates the implementation of the nursing process on an inpatient psychiatric unit.

Primary nursing and the nursing process

CLINICAL EXAMPLE 18-1

Ms. R was a 17-year-old, single, high school student who was admitted to an inpatient psychiatric unit with the diagnosis of manic-depressive psychosis. She was admitted for uncontrollable behavior (i.e., sexual promiscuity, running away from home, hyperverbalization, extreme irritability).

The initial nursing assessment provided a data base that revealed a chaotic family system with a long history of mental illness on both sides of the family, a social and cultural environment in which drug and alcohol abuse were prevalent, and a community that, because of its low socioeconomic status, possessed limited mental health resources. However, the patient was very bright, cooperative, and motivated to benefit from her hospitalization.

The initial nursing actions were to carry out the dependent functions of administering the prescribed medications and assuring that blood levels were checked three times a week until a therapeutic level was reached. The nurse assessed that there was an immediate need to protect the patient from her impulsive uncontrollable behavior. The patient was placed under close nursing observation at all times until she was able to be in control of her own behavior.

Once the patient's mood had stabilized, she was presented in nursing rounds. During this time the patient was able to identify a great need for the nurse to teach her and her family about manic-depressive illness and the importance of continued lithium treatment. The patient and staff agreed that a home visit would reveal the pressures that the family placed on the patient to function as surrogate mother to her eight siblings. The patient also believed that it was important that her illness not be viewed in exactly the same manner as that of her sister, who was diagnosed as schizophrenic. The patient viewed her intellectual ability and the "love" that existed in her family system as her best resources. She thought that, with the assistance of the nursing staff, she and her family could develop more understanding of her illness and decrease the chaos within the family system.

After discharge the patient was treated in outpatient therapy by a nurse therapist. The family was being seen by a psychiatric social worker.

Thus today's psychiatric nursing practice is characterized by a body of knowledge that is founded in behavioral science theories, biopsychological aspects of stress, and sound effective interpersonal relationships. This body of knowledge is translated into action by way of the nursing process. The question now becomes, What modality of care delivery is best suited for the implementation of the nursing process?

This portion of the chapter will be devoted to a discussion of primary nursing as a modality of care delivery on an inpatient psychiatric unit and the experiences of inpatient psychiatric nurses who, in becoming primary nurses, "rediscovered" the nursing process.

Primary nursing is a modality of care delivery that is characterized by the assignment of one nurse to coordinate the total nursing care of a patient from the time of admission to discharge. This care delivery system provides highly individualized, comprehensive care with a degree of continuity that other nursing modalities have failed to provide. It is the assumption of 24-hour responsibility that sets the primary nurse apart from other nurses. It is the primary nurse who assesses the patient's nursing needs, develops a plan of care to be implemented around the clock, and evaluates the results of that care. Primary nurses may delegate the responsibility of implementing the care plan in their absence, but it is they who are accountable for providing the directions through written and verbal communications. Marram, Barrett, and Bevis[14] view the primary nurse as a "triple A" nurse who has "three basic characteristics: autonomy, authority, and accountability."

These three characteristics, more than any other, differentiate between a nursing practice that is professionally oriented and one that is task oriented. A primary nurse who has autonomy functions in a collaborative manner with other disciplines. Other health professionals are used by the primary nurse as resources and consultants. However, the nursing care plan is developed by the primary nurse and the patient. In a professionally oriented practice, the person who is providing direct care must have the authority to make decisions concerning that care. Primary nurses have the authority to develop and implement a total comprehensive nursing care plan on a 24-hour basis. A true test of a professional is the demonstration of a willingness to stand accountable for all his decisions and actions. The primary nurse is accountable for all decisions made and actions taken in the nursing care of her patients.

The departments of nursing of several inpatient psychiatric facilities across the United States have chosen to use primary nursing as their care delivery system. Many have reported that primary nursing has led to increased job satisfaction among the professional nursing staff and increased satisfaction among the patient population. On the surface it appears that a transition to primary nursing in an inpatient psychiatric setting could be accomplished with ease. The nature of psychiatric nursing lends itself to the establishment of one-to-one relationships. For years psychiatric nurses have been engaging in individual nurse-patient interactions. Despite this past experience, many institutions have encountered numerous difficulties in implementing primary nursing.

Two types of problems are likely to be encountered during the transitional period. First are those problems which are internal to nursing. Second are the problems which result from the impact that implementing change in one discipline has on other disciplines. Internal problems center around the redefinition of all nursing positions from the director of psychiatric nursing to the psychiatric aides and unit clerks. How to include the nonprofessional nursing staff in primary nursing remains an unsolved problem in need of further exploration. The primary nurses themselves seem to encounter the most difficulty in accepting accountability for their decision making and practice.

To successfully implement primary nursing, there must be support and acceptance of this care delivery system from both the administrative and staff levels. Unfortunately, hierarchical authority and bureaucracy continue to be predominant characteristics of the nursing culture. Hospital and nursing administrators are reluctant to provide the adequate staffing pattern and the decentralization of decision making that is imperative to the success of primary nursing.[14]

Thus nursing administrators must view themselves as facilitators of change and must be willing to delegate certain authority to make decisions about patient care to the nurses at the clinical levels. Administrators must also be committed to providing adequate staffing patterns and resource people for clinical supervision, staff development, and inservice education. Once nursing administration has made this commitment, it must realize that organizational change alone will not lead to successful implementation of primary nursing.[11] However, by lending support and leadership through active participation, nursing administration can provide an environment that fosters an enthusiasm toward viewing change as a challenge and as an opportunity for personal and professional growth.

Can all psychiatric nurses be primary nurses? This is perhaps the most difficult of the internal problems encountered in the transitional period of implementing this system. In their study on the use of psychiatric nurses, Anderson and Apostoles[1] found that all 26 nurses in their research program were able to successfully complete their rotation through the 18-month project. It was only after the completion of the program that two of the 26 nurses resigned.

A closer look at this project reveals that in this study population associate degree and baccalaureate graduates were "overrepresented," and diploma and master's degree graduates were "underrepresented." The project nurses generally agreed (75%) that "any new graduate has the basic skills to function as a primary care nurse." However, these nurses added a qualifier to this statement by making the provision that the guidance of a clinical specialist, support from the physician, and team cooperation were essential.[1]

In their study on primary nursing Coates, Falck, and Sienkilewski[2] observed that the essential ingredients to being a successful primary nurse on an inpatient psychiatric unit were innovation, motivation, and a patient-centered orientation. They further observed that, with few exceptions, those primary nurses possessing these "essential ingredients" who did not already have their baccalaureate degrees soon began working toward them.

It is obvious that not all psychiatric nurses can be primary nurses. No one care delivery system is able to satisfy the needs of all. There is some evidence that, given a supportive nursing administration, most nurses who are willing to stand accountable and are motivated to accept the challenge will experience some success as primary nurses.

The transition to primary nursing has an impact on other health care providers, and the responses to this impact may vary from humorous to serious. An initial response from the resident physician group is often to become territorial about their patients. This phase may be referred to as the "not with my patients, you don't" phase. In a similar manner, psychiatric social workers may respond to the threat of boundary encroachment by countering, "Not with my families, you don't." Occupational and recreational therapists, who are often involved in their own search for autonomy, may be heard to say, "Here we go again."

Once the initial impact is over and resolutions to many of the internal and external problems are found, the multidisciplinary team enters into the second phase of transition. This phase is frequently characterized by the beginning development of mutual sharing, respect, and trust. "Not with my patient" becomes "What can nursing offer the patient?" "Not with my family" is replaced by "Would you like to sit in on a family assessment" or "Shall we do a joint home visit?" It is at this stage that the "here we go again" truth tellers may ask, "Have we really made it this time?"

The benefactor of a collaborative approach to care is the patient. When the psychiatric team works in a collegial fashion, there is little need for energy to be wasted on protecting boundaries and territories. Thus the team's attention is focused on the needs of the patient. Clinical example 18-2 is an actual patient's account of her experience as a primary patient in an inpatient psychiatric unit.*

CLINICAL EXAMPLE 18-2

When I came here I was completely immobilized. I was afraid of everything. The fears started as small silly things that my family and I tried to laugh off. But soon the little fears became bigger and bigger, and soon I wasn't able to function as a wife, a mother, or a human being.

Do you know that I hadn't been able to do any shopping for 2 years. I hadn't been out of my house at all for the past 6 months—except to come to the hospital. I had often thought of killing myself, but I was even too afraid to do that.

I can't tell you what being here has meant to me. Everyone has been understanding and supportive. My psychiatrist saw me three times a week in therapy and helped me learn about my illness and what caused my fears. The more I understood, the less frightening things seemed.

But I give most of the credit for my recovery to my primary nurse. She was the person who helped me to function again. She made me feel less ashamed and helped me to realize that I wasn't a total, no good weakling.

Together we planned strategies of how to get me moving. We started very slowly with short trips off the ward. The next step was to go to the market to buy cake mix for the ward bake sale. The big step happened just a few weeks ago when my nurse and I went all the way downtown to Christmas shop for my family. My family and I cried together when I gave them their gifts on Christmas Day. It was the first time in 2 years that I was able to buy them anything. I'm preparing for discharge with my primary nurse. Last weekend I went home, and I was able to shop

*Excerpt from an interview I conducted for nursing rounds.

alone. I am still apprehensive, but my nurse says that this is not unusual.

I'm being discharged next week and the plans are for me to see my doctor on an outpatient basis for awhile. My primary nurse is going to make a follow-up home visit in 2 weeks to see how things are going. I really feel comfortable with this arrangement.

Are all the other wards going to start primary nursing? I think that all the patients here should have the opportunity to have a primary nurse.

The three major characteristics of the primary nursing modality (autonomy, authority, and accountability) are the same in inpatient psychiatric nursing as in any other clinical specialty. However, unique complications do arise because of the nature of the specialty of psychiatry. More than in other areas of medicine, psychiatric care providers share an almost universal ingredient. That ingredient is the therapeutic use of self. Frequently, clinical territory is shared and skills are equalized, and "gender and character style rather than strict professional discipline lines are drawn."[23] Psychiatric nurses are often asked to expand their roles to include psychotherapy and social work. If this occurs too frequently, and if primary nurses are supervised exclusively by other disciplines, the nurse can lose her identity with her own profession. At this point she can no longer be considered a primary nurse.

Thus primary nursing in psychiatric settings must be clearly defined in relation to other professionals and paraprofessionals. Primary nurses must maintain their involvement in the milieu. They must participate in experiences with patients "because they are part of patients' everyday lives."[23] The primary nurse teaches the patient how to use all his social, interpersonal, and environmental experiences within the hospital system. It is from these experiences that the patient can often learn more effective ways of dealing with those real-life stresses which can lead to the need for hospitalization.

It is this involvement in the patient's everyday life that places the primary nurse in the position of being able to provide and integrate data from many sources. It is also this involvement that best differentiates the role of the primary nurse from other psychiatric professionals.

Recent legislative changes and budgetary constraints have had great impact on mental health care and the utilization of professional personnel. As previously mentioned, psychiatric nurses are being asked to expand their roles to include such functions as psychotherapist and case manager. Nursing administrators must be responsive to these current trends and creative in their approaches in meeting these additional service demands. The consequences of a lack of responsiveness could result in a professional loss of identity for psychiatric nurses and a decrease in the quality of nursing care provided to psychiatric patients.

It is possible to combine the concepts of primary nursing and primary care in psychiatric settings. This combination provides a system in which nurses are encouraged to expand their roles and are expected and supported to continue their primary nursing activities and milieu involvement. The amalgamation of these two concepts should be tailored to meet the organizational, treatment, and fiscal policies of the institution. However, the integrity of the modalities must be maintained. Two models of a primary nursing–primary care system are given in Table 18-1.

Model A was developed for a small psychiatric department in a general hospital. The department housed one 20-bed inpatient unit and an active outpatient clinic. In this model, the nurses functioned exclusively as primary nurses on the inpatient unit. Each primary nurse spent approximately half a day in the outpatient clinic where she functioned as a psychotherapist. Thus the primary nurse's case load consisted of three or four primary nursing patients and two or three psychotherapy outpatients.

TABLE 18-1. Comparison of two models for the implementation of primary nursing

Models	Primary nurses	Outpatient therapists
Model A		
Who assigns patients?	Head nurse	Treatment team
Who provides supervision?	Clinical nurse specialist	Clinical nurse specialist
	Peer group	Psychiatrist
Specific role functions	Nursing assessments	Individual psychotherapy
	Nursing care plans	Group therapy
		Family therapy
	Direct nursing care, that is, activities of daily living, giving and monitoring medications and treatment	Coordinating activities, such as agency referrals, housing arrangements, vocational placement, monitoring medication
	Milieu involvement	
	Nursing discharge planning	
	Home visits	
	Family and patient teaching	
Model B		
Who assigns patients?	Head nurse	Psychiatrist
Who provides supervision?	Clinical nurse specialist	Psychiatrist
		Clinical nurse specialist
Specific role functions	Nursing assessments	Psychiatric history
	Nursing care plans	Mental status examination
	Direct nursing care, that is, activities of daily living, giving and monitoring medications and treatment	Social assessment and history
		Family contacts
	Milieu involvement	Medical and psychiatric coordination
		Community resource coordination
	Nursing discharge planning	Discharge planning
	Home visits	Therapist: individual, family, group
	Family and patient teaching	

In this model, the head nurse was responsible for assigning the nursing case loads. Supervision for nursing care was provided by clinical nurse specialists with graduate education in psychiatric nursing and in peer groups with other primary nurses. The assignment of outpatients was made by the treatment team responsible for planning the follow-up care of the patients on the inpatient unit. The supervision for outpatients was provided by the same clinical specialists (who were also qualified therapists) with regular consultations from assigned medical-psychiatric backups. The primary nurses had direct input into the selection process of both the inpatient and outpatient case loads.

Model B was developed for a large state psychiatric hospital. In this model the primary nurse functioned as both case manager and primary nurse on an inpatient admissions unit. As in Model A, the head nurse was responsible for assigning the primary nursing patient case load, and supervision for these patients was provided by clinical nurse specialists with graduate education.

The patients for whom the nurse functioned as case manager and therapist were assigned by the psychiatrist in charge of the treatment team. Supervision for these patients was provided by the psychiatrists and the clinical specialists. The average case load for these nurses was approximately five or six primary nursing patients and two or three case management patients. The primary nurses maintained direct input into the selection process of both case loads.

Essential to the success of both models was a comprehensive inservice educational program and qualified clinical nurse specialists. If primary nurses are to expand their roles, they must have an adequate theoretical and clinical base. Participation in an in-depth inservice program that is balanced in didactic theory and related clinical experience should be a required activity for all primary nurses who are expanding their roles. These program models should be designed, implemented, evaluated, and controlled by nursing. In this way, primary nurses are given the support they need to maintain the integrity of the nursing model and of their professional identity.

The immediate future of primary nursing in inpatient psychiatric settings will more likely be influenced by political, legislative, and financial factors rather than therapeutic objectives or philosophies. Those in the public sector have already been subjected to severe budget cuts that have seriously curtailed the numbers of professionals hired into the system. Hospitals must utilize their financial resources and personnel to provide timely patient evaluations, family involvement, relevant treatment modalities, and appropriate dispositions. The long-term future of primary nursing will depend on psychiatric nurses' ability to demonstrate that this modality of care provides quality therapeutic interventions in a cost-effective manner.

Mental health team

The mental health team concept and multidisciplinary approach to patient care has been used by some psychiatric and mental health professionals since the late 1940s. Yet today the desirability and effectiveness of this approach has not been fully accepted or implemented. In some instances it has taken state legislation to guarantee that psychiatric patients be provided with an active team treatment plan.

The early mental health teams were composed of the psychiatrist, psychologist, psychiatric social worker, and psychiatric nurse.[18] More recently other significant members have been added to this original group. These newcomers include the psychiatric assistant or technician, occupational therapist, recreational therapist, art therapist, dietitian, and auxiliary personnel. It is highly unlikely that any one system will contain all these team members. For example, in many systems the occupational therapist may serve as recreational therapist and more infrequently as art therapist.

The list of team members grows longer as new educational programs are developed to prepare new groups of mental health professionals and paraprofessionals. Many community colleges are now offering a 2-year course that leads to an associate in arts degree in "mental health technology," and there are also a number of master's level programs in mental health counseling. The question arises: Should there be more effective use of those team members which now exist before more new groups of mental health workers are created?

Although the actual functions of the various health team members vary from system to system, the educational preparation requirements remain rather consistent. The psychiatrist, clinical psychologist, psychiatric social worker, occupational therapist, art therapist, recreational therapist, and dietitian all require specialized training in their specialty areas and most require advanced degrees. Table 18-2 compares the educational requirements for the mental health disciplines at the professional entry level. The psychiatric assistant and auxiliary personnel usually receive "on-job training." Psychiatric nurses need only basic preparation at the diploma, associate in arts, or baccalaureate level. However, advanced preparation at the master's level is required for those psychiatric nurses who engage in independent practice.

Functionally, the psychiatrist is traditionally viewed as the team leader. The tasks of making a diagnosis and other medical functions are prime ingredients of this role. The degree to which the psychiatrist becomes involved in direct patient care is largely dependent on the system. In some systems the psychiatrist functions mainly in an administrative or consulting role. In other systems there may be active involvement in group and individual therapy.

An almost universally accepted role of the clinical psychologist is that of administering and interpreting psychological testing. The clinical psychologist is invaluable in assisting the health team in differentiating many of the causative factors of a patient's behavior. Like that of the psychiatrist, the system in which the psychologist functions will largely determine the extent of participation in direct patient care. However, the clinical psychologist is adequately prepared to work with patients in both group and individual psychotherapy. The psychologist is prepared at the doctoral level in clinical psychology. This person is prepared for independent practice but cannot prescribe drugs for medical or psychiatric illnesses.

The psychiatric social worker may be involved in many aspects of the patient's therapy. Traditionally the social worker is the team member who plays the key role in evaluating families to identify the environmental and social factors in the patient's illness. As with other team members, the social worker functions in accordance with the philosophy of the system. Other common and recognized roles of the social worker include individual, family, and group therapy; discharge planning; and community referrals.

The task of assessing patients for rehabilitative planning has generally been assigned to the occupational therapist. This is a complex and frequently monumental job. The occupational therapist is often the one team member who discovers untapped strengths within the patient and uses these strengths in various innovative therapeutic programs.

The art therapist is used as an adjunct in making a diagnosis and in individualized treatment situations. The art therapist works with groups or individuals, encouraging patients to make and analyze drawings, which may often be an expression of underlying problems.

With the advent of modern technology in industry, people have been provided with more and more leisure time. Inept social skills and poor use of leisure time can lead to boredom, increased anxiety, and further isolation. The recreational therapist is instrumental in teaching patients useful pastimes that can lead to reintegration into the community.

The dietitian can be a most valuable member

TABLE 18-2. Comparison of entry-level educational requirements for the mental health care disciplines

Discipline	Entry-level education (as defined by the profession)	Education beyond high school
Nursing generalist	Associate degree, diploma, baccalaureate degree	2 to 4 years
Clinical nurse specialist	Masters degree	5 or 6 years
Psychiatric social worker	Baccalaureate degree	4 years
Occupational, recreational, activities therapist	Baccalaureate degree	4 years
Art, music, dance therapist	Masters degree	5 or 6 years
Mental health associate	Associate degree	2 years
Mental health counselor	Masters degree	5 or 6 years
Clinical psychologist	Doctoral degree	8 to 10 years
Psychiatrist	Doctorate in medicine; psychiatric residency	10 to 12 years

of the health team. Good food plays a vital role in the health teaching of all patients. The dietitian should be actively and directly involved in the treatment of specific food-related illnesses, such as anorexia nervosa, pica, bulimia, and eating-control disorders.

The composition of the mental health team and the ways in which the individual members function varies from system to system. The commonality seems to be that patients benefit from a plan of care that is developed by a team of qualified health care providers who are interested in his well-being.

Design of an inpatient psychiatric unit

The design of an inpatient psychiatric unit is important to the patients, families and friends, and the members of the health care team. The design of the facility should reflect the philosophy of the department, the methods of care provided, and the types of patients to be served. It should make the statement that patients are "worthy of an attractive facility" and that the facility's environment should "correspond as much as possible" to the environment to which he will soon return.[6]

Despite changing tastes in architectural and interior design, there are several principles that seem to continue to hold true. Adequate space is of utmost importance. Patients must be provided with an environment that promotes socialization but allows room for privacy. The unit should have flexibility. Day areas and dining rooms can be designed to easily convert into group meeting rooms. Adequate storage space should be provided to prevent a cluttered unkempt look.

There would be offices provided for individual sessions, charting, and dictating functions. An adequate treatment room facility is essential to the provision of quality medical treatment for the patient. In the more modern inpatient units there is no nurses station per se. Instead there is likely to be a reception desk with work areas that are open and accessible to patients.

In addition to a day area, dining room, and lounge facilities, space should be provided for kitchen and laundry and linen area. The bedrooms should be furnished with comfortable, attractive, sturdy beds and chairs. There should be a combination of single and semiprivate rooms. Small dormitory rooms of three or four patients may be desirable in some hospital settings.

Room for occupational and recreational activities is provided either on the unit or in a separate activities wing adjacent to the inpatient wing. These activities wings may include an arts and crafts room, and music room, and areas for indoor exercise and sports such as yoga, table tennis, and basketball.

Occasionally psychiatric patients need to be secluded or isolated. Isolation rooms can be designed to maintain the privacy and dignity of the isolated patient but still allow for free flow of traffic. This is accomplished by constructing a vestibule between the door of the isolation room and a door that opens onto the main corridor. Often private bathrooms are located in these vestibules. Depending on the degree of disturbance of the isolated patient, one or both of the doors may be locked.

The use of color, furniture, plants, paintings, graphics, and decorator pieces is of great importance. The walls of the rooms are usually painted with subtle quiet hues. Colorful accents are added with graphics, paintings, and furniture. The development of new materials that withstand long-term use and maintenance, as well as meet safety requirements, has enabled architects and interior designers to create noninstitutionalized inpatient units at "reasonable" costs.

Modalities of therapy on an inpatient psychiatric unit

Many inpatient psychiatric facilities for acutely ill patients offer a variety of therapies in the treatment of psychiatric and behavioral disorders. The inpatient psychiatric nurse is involved to some extent with all therapeutic modalities. The extent of involvement depends on the nurse's relationship with the patient and the philosophy of the institution.

Milieu therapy

Milieu therapy is "a scientific manipulation of the environment aimed at producing changes in the personality of the patient."[3] The actual use of the word "milieu" to mean a scientifically planned environment came into being in the work of Bettleheim and Sylvester in the late 1930s and early 1940s.

Early research and experiments in milieu therapy almost exclusively used psychological or psychiatric theories of illness and from these theories attempted to determine the kinds of environments that would be most therapeutic. There were attempts to "prescribe" minutely detailed interpersonal environments based on the psychodynamic needs of a "carefully diagnosed" patient. This ambitious undertaking included attempts to prescribe and program staff attitudes and responses as well as patient activities.

In 1954 Stanton and Schwartz introduced the concept that the environment can be the primary treatment as well as a supporting or complementary influence to other forms of treatment. They presented the fact that the environment may frequently have components that are irrelevant to the psychodynamics of the patient but may be important to his general welfare. Later Caudell described the effect that culture, organized values, norms, and customs have on patient care. In 1958 Freeman, Cameron, and McGhie developed the relationship between ego psychology and specific characteristics of the environment. Despite all this accumulated information, until the work of Cumming and Cumming in 1962 there had been a reluctance to consider the possibility that "the milieu might itself bring about specific changes in the behavior of patients and thus specific changes in their personalities."[3]

Milieu programs may differ widely from system to system. Despite these differences there appear to be several basic assumptions that are common to all therapeutic milieu approaches to inpatient psychiatric treatment. The first assumption is that patients have strengths and conflict-free portions of their personalities. It is these strengths which are optimally used by the scientific manipulation of the institutional environment. Second, patients have abilities to constructively influence their own treatment, the treatment of others, and to some degree the organizational structure of the hospital. The third assumption is that successful treatment of seriously disturbed patients is extremely dependent on a pervasive, therapeutic staff involvement. The final assumption is that all levels of hospital personnel have the potential for exercising a therapeutic influence.[22]

There is little question that the advent of milieu therapy helped to change the course of psychiatric nursing. Before 1946, psychiatric nursing literature stressed the importance of the management of a safe and secure environment. With milieu therapy the role of the nurse in the environment began to change from custodial to therapeutic and rehabilitative. Sills recommends a "social learning model" as an appropriate guide for nurses to use for their interventions in a therapeutic milieu. This would shift the emphasis away from "caring for the patient" to teaching the patient social skills. This would complement and support the basic goals of milieu therapy. These two basic goals are limit setting and learning the basic social skills of orientation, assertion, occupation, and recreation.[22]

Cumming and Cumming[3] view the nurse as a "facilitator and a helper to the patients rather than a therapist." In a therapeutic milieu the nurse keeps the focus on action and problem solving. Discussions of interpersonal relationships are kept in the context of a "goal-directed activity." The following nurse-patient interaction may help to distinguish between a nursing intervention in a milieu therapy setting and one in a psychoanalytical setting.

PATIENT: **I can't stand the sight of you. You are always getting in my way.**
NURSE: **We are supposed to go look at the halfway house today. I wonder how your being angry with me is going to affect our plans?**

In this intervention the nurse has attempted to bring the interpersonal discussion back to the social task at hand. On a unit where the approach is more psychoanalytical, the nurse may respond in the following manner:

PATIENT: **I can't stand the sight of you. You are always getting in my way.**
NURSE: **Can we talk more about your anger? We may be able to learn what it is that is making you so unhappy with our relationship.**

This approach is an invitation to the patient to explore his feelings and the possible transference phenomena in the nurse-patient relationship.

What is the outcome of milieu therapy? Because of the lack of standard assessment tools and techniques, studies related to treatment environment and treatment outcome have been limited. However, some consistent findings have been discernible. It appears that a treatment environment which emphasizes involvement, a practical orientation, order and organization, and a reasonable degree of staff control is most successful in keeping patients out of the hospital.[22] Therefore staff and patients should work together to provide an environment that is physically safe and secure; in which expectations, norms, rules, and standards are clear and concise; and where staff and patients have the freedom to communicate openly.

Therapeutic community

According to Kraft, "The therapeutic community is a very special kind of milieu therapy in which the total social structure of the treatment unit is involved as part of the helping process.[10:543] How does this differ from the concept of milieu therapy and what are the implications of those differences? Perhaps the clearest distinction is that in the therapeutic community it is believed that all social and interpersonal interactions in the hospital are the main therapeutic tools used to bring about specific changes in the patient. As previously mentioned, in milieu therapy the emphasis is on the manipulation of the environment to bring about changes in patient behavior, with effort being invested in keeping all interpersonal discussions in the context of a goal-directed activity.[3]

It is impossible to discuss the treatment modality of therapeutic community without exploring the original concept as set forth by Maxwell Jones. According to Jones,[8] what most distinguishes a therapeutic community from other comparable treatment programs is the way in which the total resources of the staff, the patients, their relatives, and the institution are pooled for the purpose of treatment. Thus the patient must undergo a change in status. The staff must encourage his active participation in his care planning. This would be a marked contrast to the conventional passive recipient role.[9]

In the structuring of a therapeutic community, Jones suggested that the emphasis should be placed on free communication both within and between staff and patient groups. The end results of free communication were hoped to be the examination of roles, the clarification of what behavior is regarded as appropriate, some loss of apparent distinctiveness of particular roles, and attempts to modify some overall cultural attitudes and beliefs that are antitherapeutic. Thus the therapeutic community would be democratic as opposed to hierarchical; rehabilitative rather than custodial, permissive instead of limited and controlled, and, finally, communal as opposed to emphasizing the specialized therapeutic role of the physician. In the early Maxwell Jones models of a therapeutic community, the environment was essentially permissive and flexible.

Roles of the participants were purposely unspecified, the patients' activities were highly individualized, and participation was completely voluntary. The one exception was a daily community meeting that all staff had to attend and all patients were encouraged to attend. Group responsibility was emphasized, and opportunities for corrective learning experiences were deliberately provided. The primary role of the staff was to assist the patients to gain new insights and to test new behavioral patterns.

Jones believed that each treatment unit should ideally be free to operate in the manner which was best suited to its own particular style and approach. However, he offered several components that he believed were characteristic of a therapeutic community. The daily community meeting was used as a format for discussing day-to-day life on the unit. Since these gatherings were often composed of 80 or 90 patients, many of the tensions and concerns of the individual patients were "worked through" in small group therapy sessions that followed the community meeting.

Another component of the therapeutic community is patient government. The purpose of the patient government or ward council is to deal with practical unit details such as privileges and housekeeping rosters. Jones suggested that a staff member be available to the patient government and that all decisions be fed back to the community through the community meetings.

Jones viewed the staff meeting or review as essential to on-the-ward training. He saw these as taking place for at least 30 minutes following each community meeting. In this meeting the staff would examine their own responses, expectations, and prejudices. Another important characteristic of the therapeutic community is the living-learing opportunities provided to the patient within the social milieu. Thus the therapeutic community is like a "school for living" in which the patients learn to meet the demands of everyday life.

According to Jones, "Feedback is one of the fundamental concepts in therapeutic community practice."[9] It is of great importance that all decisions, disputes, progress, and accomplishments be conveyed to the community as a whole. There is very little, if anything, that is purely confidential in a therapeutic community. The staff must be sensitive in their role of demonstrating how and when to feed back information to the community.

Although there have been additions and modifications of Jones' original concept of the therapeutic community, it is still considered as a viable model. The Marlborough Hospital in London has used the Maxwell Jones model of therapeutic community and has added some creative and innovative activities. Included in their program are the typical community meetings, staff meetings, small psychotherapy groups, work groups, admission meetings, badminton groups, and pottery groups. In addition, this therapeutic community offers individual reviews, encounter groups, projective art sessions, gestalt groups, occupational therapy workshop sessions, patient meetings, and a dream group. There are three other groups that have been created for this particular community. The "Leavers Group" is designed to look at the feelings and problems related to leaving the community. It is in this group that the need for further treatment is discussed. The "Concern Group" is composed of patients who the community believes are not able to make use of their therapy. The purpose of this group is to clarify the aim and purpose of the hospital and the individual's role within it. "The Committee" is composed of five patients, one from each small psychotherapy group, and a number of staff. It functions as a feedback source to the community meetings and to the business and patients' meetings.[12]

As in milieu therapy, the nurse's role in the therapeutic community requires maturity and a willingness to have one's own behavior the subject for discussion. Holmes and Werner suggested that nursing interventions in a therapeutic community reflect three features: patients are included in almost all information-sharing processes, patients' opinions are included in decisions about other patients, and the democratic community process is considered treatment. The "social learning model" is another appropriate guide to nursing interventions in a therapeutic community as well as in milieu therapy.[22]

Nurses are involved in the various group activities within the therapeutic community. Therefore it is essential that the nurse be skilled in group behavior and dynamics. It is interesting to note that a basic assumption in Jones' concept of therapeutic community is that patients have strengths and should be active participants in their care planning. This is exactly the basic assumption of primary nursing and the nursing process.

There are many problems related to the concept of the therapeutic community. Some concerns are that patients are taught patterns of behavior that are basically inappropriate outside the hospital. Therefore they cannot generalize these newly learned skills to the community environment.[22]

Other problems include staff anxiety because of the threat of loss of professional identity, the fact that "group responsibility" can easily be distorted to mean "no responsibility," and the possibility that the individual patient may become lost in the concern for the group.[10]

If these problems can be resolved, the future of the therapeutic community will be more assured. It will be interesting and challenging to be part of that future.

Individual psychotherapy

Traditionally, individual inpatient psychotherapy is conducted by the psychiatrist, who sees the patient on the average of one to three times weekly. The purpose of individual psychotherapy is to offer the patient an opportunity to develop insights into the sources of his thoughts, feelings, perceptions, and behavior. By developing these insights, the patient is able to improve his skills in establishing and maintaining interpersonal relationships and use more effective behaviors in dealing with stress. Despite the fact that it has recently come under attack as an effective modality of treatment, most acute psychiatric facilities continue to view individual psychotherapy as a viable and desirable practice.[4]

In a multidisciplinary approach to patient care other health care providers may function as psychotherapists. In this type of setting it is possible for the nurse to function as primary nurse for a selected number of patients and as psychotherapist for others. It is important that the "expanded role" of the nurse as a psychotherapist not be confused with primary nursing. Although primary nursing is purely a modality of nursing care delivery, the expanded role of psychotherapist requires additional training in the fields of human growth and development, psychodynamics of human behavior, and the art and science of psychotherapy.

Family therapy

The focus of family therapy is to treat as the primary unit a social system, rather than an individual member who has been defined as a "patient." A variety of techniques and practices may be used in the process of family therapy. There may be any combination of pairing or grouping in each session or a series of sessions. For example, Ackerman recommends that the entire family unit be seen for therapy, but for the diagnostic phase he conducts sessions with various individuals, pairs, or triads. Wynne varies the member composition to discover which family members should be included in treatment. Bowen will see the entire family in what he calls "family group therapy" for brief periods. He views the optimum approach as starting with the husband and wife together and continuing with both for the entire period of family therapy. Bowen will often see a single family member to assist that person to achieve a higher level of differentiation.[19]

The goals of family therapy are to reduce conflict and anxiety, to make the family members more aware of each other's needs, to increase the family's ability to deal with external and internal crises, to develop more appropriate role relationships, to help individual family members to cope with destructive forces within and without the family, and to promote health and growth.

The psychiatric nurse should have special training in family systems and conjoint family therapy before attempting to function as a family therapist. The role of the therapist is to penetrate family secrets and myths, to counteract the process of scapegoating, and to pick up nonverbal communication and make it explicit. At other times the therapist may serve as a parent figure or a personal instrument for reality testing. The family therapist must be sensitive to the needs of the individual members and the family unit as a whole and respond appropriately.

A more comprehensive discussion of family therapy is presented in Chapter 25.

Group therapy

There are various types of group therapy. Traditionally the term "group therapy" is used to describe a form of psychiatric treatment in which six to eight patients attend a specified number of meetings that are conducted by a therapist. The advantages of group therapy lie in the fact that most people's problems involve their feelings and behavior toward others. In a group setting the patient is able to develop an awareness of how his thoughts, feelings, and behavior affect others. Through group feedback and support the patient will be able to change his behavior and establish more effective interpersonal relationships.

Too frequently groups are established as a "time-saving" device or because there are not enough therapists to care for individual patients. There are times when unskilled personnel are made "group leaders." This is a grave misuse of an effective therapeutic modality. Nurses who become group leaders or therapists should ensure that their group is being offered because for those patients involved it is the most appropriate form of treatment. The nurse should be skilled in group dynamics and behavior as well as have a thorough understanding of individual psychodynamics and psychopathology.

The types of group psychotherapy used on inpatient psychiatric units vary in aim, purpose, and intensity. The selection of specific groups will be determined by the philosophy of the unit, the skills of the staff, and the capacities of the patient population. Some of the more common inpatient group therapies are personality reconstruction groups, insight without reconstruction groups, problem-solving groups, remotivation and reeducation groups, and supportive groups.[13]

Recently, assertiveness training has become a popular form of group therapy. The goal of assertiveness training is to help the patient differentiate between passive, assertive, and aggressive behavior. Opportunities are provided for the patient to "practice" using assertive behavior. The result is that the patient has a choice of how he will approach a situation. The payoff is that he develops more self-confidence and is able to make his views and needs known without infringing on the rights of others.

"Specialty groups" are used on many inpatient psychiatric units. These groups are often composed of patients within a specific age range (e.g., young adult groups), patients with common problems or needs (e.g., predischarge groups), or patients of the same sex (e.g., women's sex education groups). These groups may be open-ended discussion groups or highly structured didactic groups. They may be offered on a continuing basis or be time limited. The important factors are that all groups should serve some purpose and meet some therapeutic need and the therapist should be skilled in group process and group dynamics.

The role of the psychiatric nurse in group therapy is explored in Chapter 24.

Psychodrama

Psychodrama is a modality of therapy that uses structured and directed dramatizations of a patient's emotional problems and experiences.

The purpose of these "dramas" is to provide the opportunity for the patient to develop greater awareness of his thoughts, feelings, and actions and how they impact on others. Psychodrama was devised by Dr. Jacob L. Moreno in 1914.

Moreno established psychodrama on several theoretical principles. The *action principle* simply stated is that just as life is not limited to a single verbal dimension, so psychodramatic action overcomes the linguistic restrictions placed on understanding oneself. Moreno believed that action is "the most integrative vehicle for social learning and has the most cathartic impact."[19]

The principle of the *social atom* states that each person is the center of his "structure of primary interpersonal relationships." This interpersonal network is filled with incomplete perceptions and distortions. Psychodrama allows for the recreation of the social atom and the exploration of role function in an immediate feedback system that is conducive to learning.[16]

An important goal or outcome of psychodrama is spontaneity. Moreno[16] defined spontaneity as an ability to respond to a new situation with some "degree of adequacy" and to an old situation with a "degree of novelty."

Moreno believed that the human being was not overdetermined by his past. He thought that at any moment in time the human is in "a state of great growth-potential."[16] In psychodrama, *catharsis* is used to mean a bursting through of a personal or cultural conserve. *Tele* is a word that is used to describe a two-way feeling that cements and holds a relationship together. *Surplus reality* refers to the act of going beyond reality. An example of this may be having a dead person as represented by a group member, speak.

There are several important elements of psychodrama. Although a stage is not an absolute necessity for psychodrama, it provides a flexible, multidimensional living space. The stage should be round and should have two or three steplike levels. Since psychodrama is primarily a group process, the psychodramatist's effort is to mobilize the group to work together. It is not uncommon that the response to the action on the stage is greater in the group than it is with the people on the stage. The protagonist is the star. It is he who at the moment best typifies the concern of the group. The auxiliary egos are people in the group who take roles on stage in relationship to the protagonist and his action. Psychodramatic techniques are used to help the star and the group achieve spontaneity. Two important techniques are role reversal, in which the star exchanges his role for that of a signif-

icant other, and the use of the double, which is an auxiliary ego who gets behind the protagonist and attempts to express thoughts and feelings with which the protagonist is having difficulty.

There are three phases of psychodrama. The first phase is the warm-up. During the warm-up the psychodramatist involves the group in a discussion of issues deemed important to explore for that session. Once a group concern emerges, a protagonist is supported and encouraged to come forth. The second phase is composed of the shaping and presentation of the drama. If this stage is done properly, the entire group may benefit from the action. The final phase is the postaction group sharing. In this phase the group members express what events in their own lives were touched on by the action. The psychodramatist attempts to draw from the group some identification with the protagonist.

What are the indications for psychodrama? Advocates of this modality of therapy have reported success with treating individual patients, groups of patients with marital discord, and groups of alcoholics. Psychodrama is used in milieu therapy as a form of group therapy and as a diagnostic tool in the dealing with problems within the social system of the therapeutic community.

Psychodrama seems to have a valid place among the group treatments on an inpatient psychiatric unit, as shown in Clinical example 18-3, which is account of an actual psychodrama.

CLINICAL EXAMPLE 18-3

A member of a psychodrama group came to each session with his mattress strapped on his back. He would enter a closet, close the door behind him, and remain there until the session was finished.

During one session the group decided during the warm-up phase that they wanted to deal with rejection. They believed that the group member in the closet best typified rejection. The patient was invited to be the star and to everyone's astonishment accepted.

The psychodramatic action centered around the death of the patient's father. During the drama the patient was able to express all the anger that he had kept inside. He screamed and yelled at his father (who was described as being in hell but could hear him) for abandoning his family. Finally, he was able to say good-bye without anger.

During the group sharing phase many of the group members were in tears. Many shared their own experiences of the loss of someone close to them. The patient from that time on came to the sessions without his mattress and was able to sit on the fringe of the group.

Activities therapy

Under the general classification of activities therapy may be found a number of vital programs that are used on an active inpatient psychiatric unit either as adjunctive or primary treatment modalities. Occupational therapy, recreational therapy, art therapy, plant therapy, and dance and music therapy comprise this general classification while being specialties in and of themselves.

Occupational therapy was formally established on March 15, 1917. From a modest beginning this profession has grown into a highly complex specialty with a specific body of knowledge and several conceptual frameworks of its own. Occupational therapy is defined as the art and science of directing a person's participation in selected activity to diminish or correct pathological problems and promote and maintain health.[5]

On an inpatient unit the occupational therapy program usually consists of a wide range of both individual and group experiences that are constructed to meet the social, emotional, and occupational needs of the patients. After an initial assessment, the occupational therapist helps the patient to select group and individual activities depending on the patient's skill levels. Occupational therapy programs usually offer the traditional crafts groups in which patients learn to sew, make leather projects, work in ceramics and wood, and weave. Beyond this, these programs offer assertiveness training, daily living skills groups, and current events groups. It is the occupational therapist who is most frequently involved in adjunctive treatments, such as plant therapy and pet therapy. In the absence of an educational therapist, occupational therapists will often work with psychiatric nurses in a joint endeavor to provide patients with needed tutoring or intellectual stimulation.

Recreational therapy may be offered by a certified recreational therapist or by an occupational therapist who has special training in this area. These programs are usually geared toward those activities which are more physical or gamelike in nature. The theory behind this modality of therapy incorporates the concepts that the relationship of one's physical self to the immediate environment is important to the total health of an individual. Movement or dance therapy is a specific example of how the body can be used as a medium for change. Since body and mind cannot be separated, the dance therapist works toward integrating the muscular and cognitive expressions of the patient's feelings and thoughts. On a more traditional level, organized tournaments in volleyball, basketball, table tennis, cards, dominoes, or checkers provide the patients with useful leisure-time activities and assist them to develop skills in engaging in healthy, competitive interactions. Recreational therapists may also develop programs using community resources to help patients identify socialization activities that they can become involved with after discharge from the hospital.

Art therapy is used as both a diagnostic tool and a treatment modality. The art therapist's goals are to assist the patient to express through his drawings his thoughts and emotions, to help the patient gain relief from anxiety to graphically representing conflicts and aggressive and traumatic material wihtout guilt, to provide a socially acceptable outlet for fantasy and wish fulfillment, and to assist the patient to develop more dexterity.

The general goal of pet and plant therapy is to allow the patient to express tender, loving, and nurturing feelings without great fear of rejection. Plants and pets respond well to care but make fewer demands than families and friends usually make on the care provider. Through this form of therapy patients become alerted to the needs of other living organisms and may develop a sensitivity and sense of responsibility to respond to these needs in an appropriate manner.

Thus activities therapies are used to assist patients to develop occupational and leisure-time skills that will help to provide a smoother transition back into their communities. These programs have become an important and highly respected part of active treatment facilities throughout the country.

Somatic therapies

The somatic therapies are discussed in detail in Chapter 15. However, it is important to emphasize the role of the nurse in these vital modalities of treatment.

On the modern inpatient psychiatric unit for acutely ill patients, chemotherapy and ECT are the most frequently used of all the somatic treatments. It is imperative that the inpatient psychiatric nurse develop an in-depth knowledge of these therapies. This knowledge is essential to providing quality nursing care. The two most important functions of the nurse in relationship to these somatic therapies are the observing of the patient's responses to his treatment and teaching and preparing the patient and his family.

Other forms of somatic therapies are used infrequently on an inpatient unit. Psychosurgery is used so rarely that a nurse may never encounter this particular treatment. However, recent research indicates that new and innovative technologies may lead to safe and effective procedures which may be used as a "last resort" method of treatment. Insulin shock has all but become a treatment of the past. Cold, wet sheet packs are more frequently used but are still more of historical interest, since their use is diminishing.

Long-term custodial facilities

Although the purpose of this chapter is to present what inpatient psychiatric nursing can be when it is practiced in an environment that promotes professional, innovative, creative, patient care, it must be recognized that many long-term custodial care facilities still exist. These are the institutions in which are housed patients who (1) have not responded to treatment in an acute treatment facility, (2) will not seek treatment on a voluntary basis, (3) have been committed by the courts, (4) do not have the financial resources to seek treatment elsewhere, (5) are chronically ill and cannot function in society, or (6) are homeless and forgotten.

These facilities generally share several common characteristics. There is usually a severe shortage of staff, particularly qualified registered nurses. Conditions are often crowded, and the physical environment is frequently drab and depressing. Patients are likely to be required to wear clothing provided by the institution. Their personal possessions may be kept under lock, and access to them may be limited to rigid routine schedules created for staff convenience. The design of the units is routinely stark. Beds are most likely to be lined up in dormitory fashion, with little or no provisions made for privacy. It is not uncommon for each unit to have a large sparsely furnished day area in which the patients watch television, play games, or congregate to have a cigarette whenever the smoking lamp is lit.

The quality of care provided by these long-term facilities is extremely inconsistent. Federal, state, and local legislation has made some attempts to ensure improvements and standardization. Some of the dedicated and caring staff of these institutions have made heroic efforts to develop quality programs of treatment and rehabilitation. However, lack of funding and incredible bureaucratic snags and snarls make it painfully difficult, if not impossible, to implement change in a system that is invested in maintaining a status quo.

Consequently, patients in chronic long-term custodial care facilities are more often subjected to a program of therapeutic routine than of therapeutic design. Some of the modalities of therapy most commonly offered in long-term custodial facilities are group therapy, occupational and recreational therapy, chemotherapy, and work therapy. Most of the group therapies are remotivational groups. Since long-term hospitalization often produces apathy and social isolation, detachment, and impoverishment, activities may be used to stimulate group interactions. Activities such as games, sports, artwork, and music can be used to prepare the patients for verbal interaction. Once the patients are ready to talk, the activities are gradually decreased.[13]

Work therapy is used to describe various employment situations. In some institutions patients are used as part of the work force in housekeeping, food preparation, and maintenance of the grounds. Most institutions pay the patients for this work; others offer no monetary compensation. In a few institutions patients are involved in a planned vocational rehabilitation program, including sheltered workshops, and may be employed in the community.

Chemotherapy is frequently the primary modality of treatment prescribed for patients in a long-term custodial care facility. The reasons for this are numerous. The nature of the patient's illness often dictates an aggressive, long-term drug regimen. Shortage of staff and limited psychotherapy programs greatly influence the physician's decision about the types of chemotherapy programs to implement for his patients. In many of these institutions, one of the most noticeable elements is the staff's need for control. Thus chemotherapy may be frequently used to control patient behavior that is viewed as antagonistic, rebellious, or disruptive to the system.

We have now come full circle from the early days when psychiatric nursing was custodial in nature and the nurse's role was to ensure control and the smooth operation of the unit to the present where many of these practices still exist. This is the skeleton in our closet. Nurses cannot expect that all psychiatric patients will respond to active treatment, but they can strive to provide the best possible care they are capable of giving.

In recent years, deinstitutionalization programs have been established to assist chronically hospitalized patients to move back to community settings. Case management and community support programs provide the services that are necessary to effect this change. The nursing care of the chronically mentally ill patient is discussed in greater depth in Chapters 19 and 30.

Future of inpatient psychiatric nursing

The treatment of hospitalized psychiatric patients is continually undergoing change. At present there appear to be two major directions psychiatry may follow in the future. The first direction is the familiar interpersonal, psychodynamically oriented approach. The second is the psychobiochemical orientation that has been adopted by many of the leading research and treatment facilities throughout the country.

The role of the inpatient psychiatric nurse will certainly reflect the philosophy and direction of the treatment within the institution. With the biochemical approach, the institution is likely to stress research and the medical model. This will have an impact on the nurse in terms of specific priorities, functions, and care delivery systems. Thus the need for nursing research in this area is vital. Nurses must continue to define nursing.

Even within the interpersonal, psychodynamically oriented approach, there will be need for change and the development of new knowledge and skills. The nurse must be prepared for a reevaluation of roles and functions. It is possible that the psychiatric nurse of tomorrow will be involved in primary care. The function of this psychiatric nurse practitioner will be to coordinate the care of the patient's mental health problems. There is also likely to be increasing use of day care, partial hospitalizations, and short-term hospitalizations.

The role of the mental health team in a primary care system was a topic of animated discussion at a recent American Psychiatric Association annual convention. Leaders in the mental health field view involvement in primary care as an absolute necessity, and they frequently include psychiatric nurses as a vital part of the mental health team of tomorrow.

Despite changes in the future, one may assume that nursing care will be delivered through the application of the nursing process. Individual assessment, nursing diagnosis, planning, implementation, and evaluation are the vehicles by which any mode of treatment may be delivered. Nursing will probably continue to emphasize the importance of using the patient's strengths to assist him in reaching an optimum level of functioning. Hopefully, nursing will never lose sight of the patient as an individual with the need of respect for his privacy and human dignity.

A health care provider once said with great disgust that the problem with "all this individual assessment" is that it "makes a person a snowflake." How sad that he cannot see that just as the beauty of a snowflake lies in the uniqueness of its pattern, so does the key to wellness and recovery lie in the uniqueness of the individual's strengths and desires. That is the beauty of the human spirit.

Suggested cross-references

The roles and functions of the psychiatric nurse and the mental health team are discussed in Chapter 1. The phases of the nursing process are discussed in Chapter 4. Rehabilitation of psychiatric patients is discussed in Chapter 6. Somatic therapies are discussed in Chapter 15. Deinstitutionalization of the chronically mentally ill is discussed in Chapter 24. Family therapy is discussed in Chapter 25.

SUMMARY

1. The history of inpatient psychiatric nursing practice reflects an evolutionary process from that of custodial caretaker to active member of the mental health team. The reforms of the nineteenth century were the first major influences to have an impact on the role of the psychiatric nurse.

2. The development of social psychiatry opened the door for nursing involvement in the areas of group and milieu therapy. By 1949 nurses were functioning as individual therapists, and by the mid-1950s the role of group therapist had become a recognized and accepted part of nursing practice.

3. The concept of the health team led to needed changes in the educational preparation of psychiatric nurses. This new breed of psychiatric nurses viewed themselves as professionally and academically competent to be fully participating members of the health team.

4. The implementation of the nursing process is vital to inpatient psychiatric nursing. The steps of the nursing process include the collection of a data base, development of a diagnostic impression, planning and implementation of appropriate nursing actions, and evaluation and modification of those actions.

5. There are various modalities of nursing care delivery that may be used on an inpatient psychiatric unit. Primary nursing is a care delivery system that has recently gained much support and recognition from many professional nurses throughout the country. Advocates of this modality of care delivery report that primary nursing leads to increased job satisfaction among the professional nursing staff and increased satisfaction among the patient population.

6. The mental health team concept has been with us since the late 1940s. Yet today it has not been fully accepted or implemented. The early health teams were defined as consisting of the psychiatrist, psychologist, psychiatric social worker, and psychiatric nurse. More recently this team has included the occupational therapist, recreational therapist, art therapist, dietitian, and auxiliary personnel.

7. Inpatient psychiatric units should be designed to reflect the philosophy of the department, methods of care provided, and types of patients to be served.

8. Many active psychiatric treatment facilities use concepts of milieu therapy in their inpatient programs. According to Cumming and Cumming, milieu therapy is a planned manipulation of the environment to produce changes in the personality of the patient.

9. Maxwell Jones coined the term "therapeutic community." He believed that all social and interpersonal interactions in the hospital are therapeutic tools that should be used to bring about specific changes in the patient. Jones stressed that the patient must be an active participant in his care planning.

10. The focus of family therapy is to treat a primary social system, rather than one individual who has been defined as a "patient." The goals of family therapy are to reduce conflict and anxiety, make the family more aware of each other's needs, increase the family's ability to deal with internal and external crisis, develop more appropriate role relationships, help individual family members cope with destructive forces within and without the family, and promote health and growth.

11. Individual psychotherapy continues to be the most common modality of treatment offered on active inpatient psychiatric units. The purpose of individual therapy is to offer the patient an opportunity to develop insights into the sources of his thoughts, feelings, perceptions, and behavior.

12. Many active treatment facilities offer group therapy either as a primary treatment modality or as an adjunctive treatment to individual psychotherapy. Group therapy should never be used as a "time-saving" device. Some of the more common inpatient groups are the supportive groups, remotivation groups, personality reconstruction groups, problem-solving groups, and insight groups.

13. Psychodrama was devised by Dr. Jacob L. Moreno in 1914. The purpose of psychodrama is to allow the patient to express himself in both words and action. Psychodrama is considered to be a special form of group therapy. It is frequently used in milieu therapy to deal with problems within the social system of the therapeutic community.

14. Activities therapies are used on inpatient units to assist patients to develop occupational and leisure-time skills that will help to provide a smoother transition back into the community. Occupational, recreational, art, dance, pet and plant therapies are all highly respected parts of active treatment facilities throughout the country.

15. Somatic therapies play a vital role in psychiatric treatment. Some of the common somatic therapies are chemotherapy, ECT, and psychosurgery.

16. To this day, there still exist psychiatric facilities that offer little more than custodial care. Some patients do not respond to active treatment and must be hospitalized for long-term care. Others, because of the nature of their illness, will not voluntarily admit themselves to active treatment facilities. Efforts are being made to improve the treatment provided by these long-term hospitals.

17. The future of psychiatric nursing appears bright for those willing to accept the challenge. Primary care, day care, partial hospitalizations, and community support for chronically mentally ill patients appear to be the subjects of many future-oriented discussions.

References

1. Anderson, C., and Apostoles, F.: Primary care nursing: an exploratory project in psychiatric nurse utilization. In Kneisl, C., and Wilson, H., editors: Current perspectives in psychiatric nursing: issues and trends. vol. 2, St. Louis, 1978, The C.V. Mosby Co.

2. Coates, D., Falck, A., and Sienkilewski, K.: Primary nursing: one giant step toward professionalism, 1974 (unpublished; available from K. Sienkilewski, Springfield Hospital Center, Sykesville, Md.)

3. Cumming, J., and Cumming, E.: Ego and milieu, Chicago, 1962, Atherton Press.

4. Detre, T., and Jarecki, H.: Modern psychiatric treatment, Philadelphia, 1971, J.B. Lippincott Co.

5. Engelhardt, H.T.: Defining occupational therapy: the meaning of therapy and the virtues of occupation, Am. J. Occupational Ther. 31:666, 1977.

6. Ingenious design meets budget, space constraints for hospital's community mental health center, Hospitals, 52:41, April 16, 1978.

7. Jamieson, E., and Sewall, M.: Trends in nursing history, Philadelphia, 1941, W.B. Saunders Co.

8. Jones, M.: Towards a clarification of the therapeutic community concept, Br. J. Med. Psychol. 32:200, 1959.

9. Jones, M.: Social psychiatry in practice, Harmondsworth, England, 1968, Penguin Books, Ltd.

10. Kraft, A.: The therapeutic community. In Arieti, S., editor: American handbook of psychiatry, vol. 3, New York, 1966, Basic Books, Inc., Publishers.

11. Manthey, M.: Primary nursing is alive and well in the hospital, Am. J. Nurs. 73:83, Jan. 1973.

12. Malborough Hospital: Therapeutic community, 1976, (unpublished; available from Marlborough Hospital, 38 Marlborough Place, St. John's Wood, London, England).

13. Marram, G.: The group approach in nursing practice, ed. 2, St. Louis, 1978, The C.V. Mosby Co.

14. Marram, G., Barrett, M.W., and Bevis, E.: Primary nursing: a model for individualized care, ed. 2, St. Louis, 1979, The C.V. Mosby Co.

15. Mereness, D.: Preparation of the nurse for the psychiatric team, Am. J. Nurs. 51:320, 1951.

16. Moreno, J.: Psychodrama, New York, 1959, Beacon House.

17. Pavey, A.: The story of the growth of nursing, Philadelphia, 1937, J.B. Lippincott Co.

18. Robinson, A.: Changing of the guard, Am. J. Nurs. 50:152, March 1950.

19. Saklas, C.: Psychosocial group therapies, The Practice of Medicine and Psychotherapy 10:41.

20. Santos, E., and Stanbrook E.: Nursing and modern psychiatry, Am. J. Nurs. 49:107, Feb. 1949.

21. Sundeen, S., et al.: Nurse-client interaction: implementing the nursing process, ed. 2, St. Louis, 1981, The C.V. Mosby Co.

22. Wolf, M.S.: A review of literature on milieu therapy, J. Psychiatr. Nurs. 15:7, May 1977.

23. Zander, K.: Primary nursing: development and management, Germantown, Md., 1980, Aspen Systems Corp.

Annotated suggested readings

Carser, D.L.: Primary nursing in the milieu, J. Psychiatr. Nurs. 19:35, Feb. 1978.

In this article, the author examines the interaction between primary nursing and the therapeutic milieu. She uses case examples to illustrate the impact at the individual patient level. She also discusses the effect of the introduction of primary nursing on the treatment team and recommends interventions with the staff that are helpful during the transitional period.

Cumming, J., and Cumming, E.: Ego and milieu, Chicago, 1962, Atherton Press.

This book is considered a classic. It represents one of the first major undertakings to theoretically describe the relationship between ego and milieu. Until this time no advocate of milieu therapy had risked making the direct statement that scientific manipulation of the environment could lead to changes in behavior and personality.

Engelhardt, H.T.: Defining occupational therapy: the meaning of therapy and the virtues of occupation, Am. J. Occup. Ther. 31:666, 1979.

This volume marks the sixtieth anniversary of the occupational therapy journal. Each article presents an informative historical overview as well as current conceptual frameworks. It will give the nurse an appreciation of the struggles that another discipline has encountered in its search for professional recognition and autonomy.

Hegyvary, S., guest editor: Symposium on primary nursing, Nurs. Clin. North Am. 12:185, June 1977.

This symposium on primary nursing will give the reader an overview of the joys and pains of primary nursing. It provides a theoretical and empirical base for primary nursing, discusses patient and staff perceptions, elaborates on the structural and organizational supports needed for the implementation of primary nursing, and discusses some experimental outcomes of implementing this modality of care delivery.

Jones, M.: Social psychiatry in practice, Harmondsworth, England, 1968, Penguin Books, Ltd.

This little book is packed full of information. A large section is devoted to the concept of therapeutic community, but Jones also elaborates on the concept of social psychiatry in general. The author is outspoken in his opinions about the preparation and participation of nurses and other health team members.

Kraft, A.: The therapeutic community. In Arieti, S., editor: American handbook of psychiatry, vol. 3, New York, 1966, Basic Books, Inc., Publishers.

This is a frequently quoted reference on the concept of therapeutic community. The author attempts to pull together the thoughts, ideas, and beliefs of the leading authorities in the fields of therapeutic community and milieu therapy.

Marram, G., Barrett, M.W., and Bevis, E.: Primary nursing: a model for individualized care, ed. 2, St. Louis, 1979, The C.V. Mosby Co.

*Although there is no discussion of primary nursing as it
relates to inpatient psychiatric nursing, this book should
be considered a must. It was the only text in this field for
a long time. The reader may enjoy the introductory comparison of the growth of the women's movement and the
growth of nursing as a profession.*

Mereness, D.: Preparation of the nurse for the psychiatric
team, Am. J. Nurs. **51:**320, 1951.

*Despite the era in which it was written, this article con-
tinues to be ageless. There will always be a need for
changes in educational curricula as the role of the professional nurse continues to grow and expand.*

Sundeen, S., et al.: Nurse-client interaction: implementing
the nursing process, ed. 2, St. Louis, 1981, The C.V.
Mosby Co.

*This is a consistently excellent text. The use of clinical
illustrations is of particular value both to experienced
nurses as well as beginners. While much of the literature
"talks" about the nursing process, this work puts it into
"action."*

Templin, H.: The system and the patient, Am. J. Nurs. **82:**
108, Jan. 1982.

*This thought-provoking article looks at three aspects of
psychiatric hospitals from both the patient's view and the
view from organizational theory—the hospital as a hierarchical system, mutual adaptation and modes of transaction. It demonstrates the benefits of viewing these hospitals as social systems.*

Wolf, M.S.: A review of literature on milieu therapy, J. Psychiatr. Nurs. **15:**27, May 1977.

*This article is a comprehensive overview of the develop-
ment of milieu therapy. What makes this work of particular value is the presentation of several studies on the
effectiveness of milieu therapy, the discussion of the
nurses' role, and the all-inclusive bibliography.*

I find the great thing in this world is, not so much where we stand, as in what direction we are moving.

Johann Wolfgang von Goethe

CHAPTER 19

THE PSYCHIATRIC
NURSE'S ROLE
IN COMMUNITY
MENTAL HEALTH

JEANETTE LANCASTER
I. WADE LANCASTER

Learning objectives

After studying this chapter, the student should be able to:

- describe the history of the community mental health movement in the United States and the role of the government as reflected in the Community Mental Health Center Acts of 1963 and 1975, the 1978 President's Commission on Mental Health, and the Mental Health Systems Act of 1980.

- critique the community mental health movement with regard to its goals, staff, services, effectiveness, and clientele.

- contrast a community orientation to mental health with that of an individual orientation.

- relate the role of the community mental health nurse in assessment, including the strategies of market segmentation and target marketing.

- discuss the implementation of the role of the community mental health nurse in the areas of primary, secondary, and tertiary prevention.

- analyze the relevant stressors and appropriate nursing interventions for each of the following high-risk populations: families under stress, victims of aggression, elderly people, and the discharged mentally ill.

■ assess the importance of interdisciplinary collaboration in community mental health.

■ describe three methodologies for program evaluation and issues that must be considered in their use.

■ identify suggested readings for future study.

The twentieth century has witnessed many American social institutions undergo continuous introspection, reassessment, and reorientation. The pressure for responsiveness, openness, and humaneness revolves around a deepening concern about the human condition and the rapidly changing needs of human beings. Psychiatric nursing has not been exempt from the pressures of societal change. Nurses working in psychiatric settings have been at the forefront of change. The scope of psychiatric nursing has changed dramatically, moving from its infant state of custodial care to the present community mental health orientation. Not only has the orientation changed, but also the work environment of the psychiatric nurse has expanded from the confines of mental institutions to the everchanging boundaries of the community. To better appreciate the current role of the psychiatric nurse in community mental health, it is helpful to briefly examine the historical motivators of the community mental health movement.

Historical development of community mental health nursing

Before 1840 people diagnosed as mentally ill were housed in jails and county homes. The environmental conditions barely allowed existence and certainly offered no treatment, since mental illness was considered a permanent affliction. For the affluent and more fortunate a scarce few private and public hospitals were available.

Humanitarian reforms in mental health

Humanitarian methods in psychiatry were first seen in America in the work of Benjamin Rush, who has since been called "the father of American psychiatry." Rush is considered a transitional figure in that he encouraged humane treatment while at the same time continuing to use remedies like blood letting, purga-

tives, and a torturelike device called "the tranquilizer."

An energetic New England school teacher, Dorothea Dix, carried on the pioneering work of Rush. In 1841 Miss Dix appointed herself inspector of institutions for the mentally ill and began crusading for more humane treatment. She recommended that each state assume responsibility for its mentally ill. The result of her effort was the establishment of 32 mental hospitals in the United States. During this period most mental hospitals were built in rural areas, which offered inexpensive land, the removal of troublesome people from the mainstream of society, fresh air, and a quiet atmosphere for the patients.

As the population in the United States increased, the number of state hospitals grew steadily until 1900. However, in the years following 1900 the patient population grew more rapidly than the construction of hospitals. This trend led to overcrowding and deplorable living conditions. To further complicate the situation, the hospitals operated on meager budgets and were inadequately staffed. The hopes and plans of Dorothea Dix were not realized at this time. Although Dorothea Dix's crusade was not oriented toward community mental health, it certainly had an impact on the trend toward humane treatment for the mentally ill.

The care and treatment of mentally ill individuals continued on a downhill swing until Adolf Meyer took up the banner that Dorothea Dix had once waved. Meyer was actually the first person to espouse the basic concept of community mental health. He proposed that a clinic for mental diseases be responsible for a certain segment of the population so that studies of the social situation and the factors leading to the onset of mental derangement could be pursued.

Governmental involvement in mental health

The federal government first entered the health field in 1935 with the passage of the Social Security Act. During the depression the view was held that if the community could not care for its sick, then the government should assume this responsibility. World War II had a significant impact on the community mental health movement when an estimated 875,000 draftees out of 15 million were rejected from military service on the basis of mental or neurological impairment.[48] At the conclusion of the war the federal government assumed an active role in funding endeavors for mental health. In 1946 the United States Congress enacted the National Mental Health Act, which made grants available to states to develop mental health programs outside of state hospitals.

This act, signed into law by President Harry S Truman, radically altered the care of mentally ill Americans. Shocked at the number of young men rejected from military service for reasons of mental illness, embarrassed by the inhumane custodial treatment, and tempted by the vision of a new enlightened system, citizens, professionals, and legislators banded together to support a broad-based national program. The intent behind these efforts was to apply a public health approach to the problem of mental illness.[42] Although the intent was to focus on prevention, in actuality individual psychotherapy was supported.

Under the provisions of the act, the National Institute of Mental Health (NIMH) was organized in 1949 to serve as headquarters for the new federal mental health program. Initially the function of NIMH emphasized research into the cause and treatment of mental illness. The institute also assumed responsibility for training programs and providing assistance to individual states as they attempted to develop treatment programs.

The 1940s saw the widespread development of two important types of treatment facilities: outpatient clinics and psychiatric units in general hospitals. In contrast, advances in research had little effect on state hospitals. Meanwhile, psychiatry continued its preference for providing private care to those who could afford it, with subsequent serious inequities between private and public provisions for treatment.

In 1955 Congress enacted the Mental Health Study Act, creating the Joint Commission on Mental Illness and Health, which consisted of representatives from 36 organizations and agencies selected by the NIMH. The agencies represented were largely medical and allied medical in character.[48] In the later part of 1960 the Joint Commission submitted its report to Congress. Published in 1961 as *Action for Mental Health,* the 338-page report emphasized the need for training personnel, supporting education in the field, providing early and intensive treatment for acutely disturbed patients, and carrying out re-search activities. The report further recommended that additional clinics and psychiatric units in general hospitals be established and that regional state hospitals of not more than 1000 beds be supported. The report suggested the creation of aftercare, rehabilitation programs, and mental health education.[26]

After the publication of this report, President John F. Kennedy appointed a cabinet-level committee to review the report and to make recommendations regarding federal action. This report and that of a presidential panel on mental retardation formed the basis for President Kennedy's message to Congress in 1963 on mental illness and retardation. This first presidential message on behalf of the mentally ill called for a "bold new approach to bring psychiatry back into the mainstream of medicine and community life."[44] The president further stated that a new facility to be known as a Community Mental Health Center was needed to provide a complete range of care in the community, including a strong emphasis on prevention.

COMMUNITY MENTAL HEALTH CENTERS ACT.
Eight months later, on October 31, 1963, the Eighty-eighth Congress enacted Public Law 88-164, the Mental Retardation Facilities and Community Mental Health Centers Construction Act of 1963, which authorized federal matching funds of $150 million over a 3-year period for use by the states in constructing comprehensive community mental health centers. The intent of the act was to provide comprehensive mental health services to meet the needs of all residents in a specific area. Each center was to serve a catchment area or population base ranging from 75,000 to 200,000 residents. Geographically each catchment area ranged from a circumscribed section of a large city to an area covering several counties with a sparse population. In addition to providing new and renovated buildings, each center was also to provide a program of mental health services to the community.

To qualify for federal funds, a program had to offer the five following services:[31]

1. Inpatient care for patients requiring short-term hospitalization
2. Partial hospitalization, which included day hospital care for those patients who could return to their own homes at night and night hospital care for patients who were able to work but needed some care each day
3. Outpatient treatment, which allowed pa-

tients to live at home and go to the center at regular intervals

4. Emergency care with services available around the clock
5. Consultation and education for members of the community

Full comprehensive services in the original community mental health legislation included five additional services. Centers applying for federal support were looked on favorably if they documented a plan for the following additional services:

1. Diagnostic services, including treatment recommendations whenever possible.
2. Rehabilitative services and vocational counseling
3. Precare and aftercare with screening prior to admission and follow-up evaluation in the home after discharge
4. Training for all kinds of mental health personnel
5. Research and evaluation

The original legislation provided federal funding for a center for 8 years on a decreasing percentage formula. During the 8 years, the federal proportion of the funding decreased in nonpoverty areas from 80% the first year to 25% in the seventh and eighth years. In poverty areas the federal proportion decreased from 90% in the first year to 30% in the eighth year. At the end of the eighth year the federal grants ceased, and each center was to operate on state and local funds as well as revenue collected from services.[31]

This fiscal arrangement did not work effectively because many centers were unable to secure sufficient revenue to meet operational costs. State and local funds were not consistently available and often centers were forced to terminate services, especially those which did not produce revenue, such as consultation and educational services, in an effort to increase revenue through direct treatment services. Centers in urban areas and medical centers were often able to generate funds to support their range of services through fee-for-service or research activities. In contrast, rural centers had a difficult time sustaining themselves financially.

COMMUNITY MENTAL HEALTH CENTERS AMENDMENTS OF 1975. The Community Mental Health Centers Amendments of 1975, Title III of Public Law 94-63, was enacted by the Ninety-fourth Congress on July 22, 1975. This amendment extended the flow of funds to community mental health centers and in doing so set forth specific guidelines for services.[38] Congress reiterated the original intent of the Community Mental Health Centers Act to provide construction and operation funds to centers on a declining basis with the ultimate goal of independence from federal support. Specific requirements included providing accessible comprehensive care to people living in a designated geographical area, regardless of their ability to pay or their past or current health conditions. The amendments also urged that services in a community be coordinated between centers and other agencies and be provided 24 hours a day, 7 days a week, in a humane manner to all who seek care. Centers were to be governed by a community board and have an ongoing quality assurance program, an integrated medical records system, a professional advisory board, and an identifiable administration unit to provide consultation and education services.[11]

Additionally, the 1975 amendments emphasized that the original required services should continue to be provided and also that services for children and the elderly must include diagnosis, treatment, liaison, and follow-up care.[11] Screening services were required for residents of the catchment area who were being discharged from a psychiatric hospital. Other required areas included transitional services for residents of the community as well as treatment for alcohol and drug abuse problems.

The impact of the 1975 amendments was to legally define a community mental health center program and explicitly document the list of services required. However, the amendments were severely criticized because they limited the flexibility that centers could exercise in determining services based on the needs of the catchment area. Furthermore, the complexity of the grant process and the timetable for reduction of federal funds were criticized.

REPORT OF THE PRESIDENT'S COMMISSION ON MENTAL HEALTH, 1978. Early in 1977 President Jimmy Carter organized the President's Commission on Mental Health; of the five professionals on the commission, one was a nurse. The president's general charge to the group was "to identify the mental health needs of the nation."[12] Specific attention was directed toward the extent to which the mentally ill were served, projected needs for dealing with stress, governmental support for mental illness, including research activities and agency coordination essential in a unified program to support mental health and intervene in mental illness.

After a 1-year study period the 20-member commission released its final report containing 117 recommendations. The commission's recommendations were divided into eight sections: community support systems, service delivery, financing, personnel, patients' rights, research, prevention, and public understanding.[36] The principal recommendation called for the establishment of a "new federal grant program for community mental health services to encourage the creation of necessary services where they are inadequate and increase the flexibility of communities in planning a comprehensive network of services."[36]

In general, the report spoke to the components of the original presidential charge. Specifically the commission recommended that community networks be strengthened between existing service components and that new ways of meeting the mental health needs of underserved populations be studied, including increased flexibility in defining the parameters of a catchment area. A call was made for attention to focus on high-risk populations, such as minorities and the chronically mentally ill. An advocacy program for the chronically mentally ill was advised, since an increasing number of state hospitals were being closed.

The commission gave serious attention to evaluation, suggesting that governmental agencies consolidate their evaluation efforts into a centralized, organized approach. Furthermore, a plea was made for mental health coverage in all insurance plans with flexibility in outpatient coverage, which would support an individual who chose to be maintained in the community yet needed ongoing or periodic mental health follow-up care. Recruitment and personnel use were addressed particularly in regard to high-risk populations. Training support was given high priority for personnel choosing to work with children, the elderly, and cultural minorities.

The commission recommended increased support for research according to the following target areas: incidence of mental health problems, use of research, public knowledge related to mental health, and investigation into the major mental illnesses. Preventive measures paid special attention to the mental health needs

of children. Although the report did not cover each area in the original charge, it indicated target areas for mental health intervention and suggested ways in which goal attainment could be accomplished.

The 1980 mental health legislation continued the trend toward flexibility in planning services to meet the needs of a designated community.[40] This legislation gave states greater authority over mental health grants, allowed more flexible and innovative program planning and development, and emphasized prevention and planning of treatment approaches for priority populations. In addition, it provided linkages between mental health and other types of providers to avoid duplication of services and to foster greater coordination of resources and programs offered. Furthermore, provisions were made for funding innovative projects for retraining mental health workers whose positions were eliminated by program restructuring as more states emphasized community-oriented vs. institutional care for the mentally ill population.[40]

Criticism of the community mental health movement

The enthusiasm of the 1960s for community mental health has been overshadowed by a wide range of criticism. Former enthusiasts are dissatisfied, since the original goals and mandates are unmet. Critics contend that the most obvious shortcoming of community mental health has been a tendency to move treatment into the community without concomitant changes in treatment techniques. There has been a reluctance to view the community itself—the macrosystem—as the client. Instead, the focus continues to be on the individual within the community—the microsystem.[54]

In addition, the professional staff required to operate a community mental health program are generally recruited from traditional delivery systems. The leadership for centers is provided by staff who have been trained and educated in isolation from each other, yet the approach in community mental health calls for collaboration and team functioning. Also, the use of paraprofessionals has aroused controversy. One point of view holds that these health care providers are highly effective in that they are not hindered by a medical model or disease orientation. The counterview is that paraprofessionals have an inadequate knowledge base for providing psychiatric services.

Criticisms related to community mental health have dealt not only with the lack of collaboration and the educational background of providers but also with the type of services provided, the balance between direct and indirect services, and the lack of responsiveness to the needs of the individual community. Prevention, a mandated service for community mental health, is viewed by some as an unmeasurable activity that serves to distract from more urgent treatment approaches.

Themes of dissatisfaction with community mental health also relate to the failure to provide well-thought-out and carefully planned aftercare programs for discharged patients. As state hospitals rapidly discharged patients in the late 1960s, few communities were able to plan and implement follow-up treatment services for their chronically ill discharged patients. In many communities merely the setting changed for a large number of patients; they were moved from an impersonal state hospital to an often equally impersonal group home.

Arnhoff[1] cites studies which indicate that community treatment is no more effective than hospital care for acutely psychotic patients. He maintains that deinstitutionalization places an unnecessary burden on the family as well as the community. He further emphasizes the long-range implications of discharging psychotic patients when follow-up care is lacking or inadequate. The prematurely discharged patient has increased opportunities to procreate, provides ineffective parenting, and requires public assistance because of unemployment.

The inability to develop a comprehensive community mental health system has led to the "revolving door" syndrome, whereby patients discharged from psychiatric hospitals continue to need well-planned and individually designed follow-up services that few communities are able to provide. Hence, patients decompensate on discharge because of lack of aftercare, thus necessitating reentry into the hospital. There is mounting evidence that many chronically mentally ill patients do not require continuous hospitalization but can be maintained in the community if they are provided with appropriate medication and a variety of therapeutic services, including individual, group, and/or family therapy, as well as assistance in finding and maintaining jobs, schooling, housing, and social support.[46]

A major criticism of community mental health is that limited coordination has been achieved, and services have continued to be fragmented and specialized with no one system actually offering an integrated program of services. Tarail[51] contends that each segment of the mental health system has survival as a goal. Such a priority discounts the possibility of collaboration and organization of a comprehensive system of services. All too often patients are discharged from the hospital before community programs are developed to receive them, thereby reducing their existence to run-down hotels, inadequate boarding homes, or nursing homes supported by Medicare and Medicaid. Essentially, it is contended that the only change has been who pays the bill.[32]

Further, Langsley[32] purports that the most detrimental feature of community mental health centers has been their abandonment of treating mentally ill patients in preference to focusing on counseling and crisis intervention. He says that the initial goal of treating people with major mental health disruptions has been forgotten in favor of a focus on social action programs. He also believes that the large decrease in psychiatrists has affected treatment because in many instances, they are so few in numbers in centers that they primarily sign prescriptions.

Benefits of community mental health

Although many criticisms have been leveled against community mental health, supporters have acknowledged the benefits. Community mental health centers have been correlated with increased use by new clients as well as a change in the type of clientele. More children and adolescents are receiving psychiatric treatment in community mental health centers than received treatment previously.[2] Moreover, there has been a documented diminution of sociodemographic bias toward the consumers of mental health services since the expansion of community mental health services.[53]

The acknowledged benefits of community mental heath, its criticisms and shortcomings, as well as the commission's report provide stimuli for new directions. Once again a "bold new approach" is being called for, emphasizing the community as client and using a holistic approach to the delivery of services. This approach is to be based on a thorough assessment of community needs, awareness of existing resources, and comprehensive informed planning procedure.

Community orientation to mental health

A community orientation requires an alteration in focus. A premise basic to community mental health is that all people experience stress and have problems coping but some have fewer support systems available to them and react in a dysfunctional way to stress.[37] The community approach to mental illness focuses on prevention by identifying high-risk populations and providing services before mental health is disrupted. The aim is to strike a balance between the level of stressors and the available supports. Innumerable ways exist to actuate a community approach to mental health. Intervening in poverty, crowding, discrimination, and crime serves to decrease stressors, whereas effective health care, police, social service, and educational resources increase community supports. On a personal or small-group level, crisis intervention, anticipatory guidance, consultation, and mental health education decrease stressors and provide supports.

The treatment area is the local community within which the client is experiencing his stress. It is insufficient to deal only with the client's internal dysfunction, but, rather, treatment implies attention to sociocultural background, adaptive ability, support systems, and family interaction.[54] Community mental health identifies the root of most emotional disorders as occurring within a network of interacting systems.[35] Although it is beyond the scope of this chapter to provide a detailed systems theory framework, selected principles are incorporated in a description of the human-environment relationship. A systems approach to mental health states that a person's health status results from the dynamic interaction between his internal environment and the external multienvironments in which he exists. A systems approach is used in community mental health nursing to provide a holistic view of a person as he relates to both his intrinsic and extrinsic environments. Each person's reactions to his multienvironments are never static but rather are dynamic and ever changing. One's responses comprise ongoing attempts to maintain homeostasis. The

human system, like all living systems, is an open one in continuous interaction with the environment. Each individual's personality develops out of this interaction with the subsystems comprising his daily life. For example, interactions with family, significant groups, and the school and work environment play a crucial part in psychological development and coping. Problems or stresses in an interacting system have an effect on other systems.

The complexity of adaptive efforts is accentuated by the fact that one responds to the total environmental insult. One cannot sort out selected environmental components; adaptive responses attend to the total environmental impact. Furthermore, each human system strives to achieve a steady state or homeostasis. Symptoms of emotional disturbance signal system distress and subsequent disequilibrium. In regard to prevention, community mental health assumes that relieving stress in one component of the system will affect other components. Factors such as poor housing, lack of sanitation, unemployment, crowding, and other manifestations of economic deprivation affect mental health.

Community assessment

One of the major criticisms of the community mental health movement, as mentioned earlier, was the inability of health care professionals to focus their attention on the community as the client. The challenge for a "bold new approach" to mental health still exists; whether it is found will be determined not only by a holistic approach to the delivery of services but also by the very ways in which services are planned and delivered.

To view the community as the client is to recognize a dynamic rather than a static entity. It is inevitable that change will occur within the community. Not only will the physical environment of the community change, but also there will be changes within the health care delivery system as well as changes in health needs. Consequently, one of the most important tasks of the community mental health nurse is to plan for change. Unfortunately, good planning does not just happen; it requires a continuous monitoring and assessment of the mental health needs and status of the community.[45]

Before the development of a community mental health plan it is necessary to diagnose and assess the health needs and resources of the community. A carefully planned and implemented assessment should yield data that reveal early warning signs of trouble, such as current mental health problems that are in the greatest need of attention and the extent to which problems at various stages are unattended and unprevented. An assessment should tell what is "right" as well as what is "wrong" and suggest how the community's resources ought to be allocated.

Assessment process

A community mental health nurse faced with the task of performing a comprehensive community assessment may tend to be overwhelmed by the potential scope and magnitude of the chore. This would certainly be a natural, perhaps even an expected, reaction. However, if the assessment is approached in a scientific fashion, much of the needed data can be obtained with relative ease and a minimum of effort. This is especially true for nurses who are intimately involved in the community.

Community mental health nurses possess a wealth of knowledge about their communities. Not only do they work with the families who make up the community, but they also interact with various individuals, groups, and organizations both within and outside the community. This information about the community, which all too frequently is neither reported, assembled, nor documented, together with recorded data provides the basis for a community assessment. Thus the important thing for the nurse to keep in mind is that the key to a successful meaningful assessment lies not so much in what data to gather but, more important, in where to gather the data.

A variety of strategies are available for assessing a community. Although each of these strategies certainly has its merits, a newer, more innovative approach to community assessment is needed. This new approach should include traditional assessment data as well as recognizing the importance of the consumer. It should focus on his special needs and wants rather than the perceptions of health care providers as to what the consumer ought to have. To be truly consumer oriented, nurses should acquaint themselves with the modern philosophy of marketing, which "calls for providing real utility for the consumer, based upon an identified need and desire for goods and services."[17] Identifying consumer needs is extremely important to the modern marketer; likewise, it is of equal importance to the community mental health nurse.

Consequently, the following suggestions for community assessment are based on two interrelated concepts that have been useful to marketers in their attempts to become more responsive to both present and potential consumers.

The first concept is known as *market segmentation;* the second is called *target marketing.* In marketing terminology, markets tend to be heterogeneous and need to be segmented into several smaller homogeneous groups. Once this has been accomplished, segments or target markets become the focus of specialized programs tailored to the needs of the market. Applying these concepts to the community is an acknowledgment on the part of the nurse that the community is heterogeneous and therefore requires specialized programs that cater to the specific needs of its members.

If usable market segments are to be developed, three conditions must be considered. The first condition is measurability. This is the degree to which information exists or is obtainable about particular characteristics of the consumer. Unfortunately, many useful characteristics such as values and attitudes are not easy to measure. Likewise, many mental health stressors may not be easily identified. The second condition is accessibility. Frequently, measurable differences in consumer attributes do exist, but it is not feasible to reach them. The third condition is substantiality, which refers to the degree to which segments are large enough to be worth subdividing for separate programs.

There is no unique way to divide a community into segments. However, several segmentation variables might be useful to the community mental health nurse. One approach, for instance, might be to segment the community according to demographic variables, such as age, education, income, occupation, race, religion, and sex. A note of caution is appropriate at this point to emphasize that demographic variables are only the foundation for more detailed segmentation strategies and are rarely effective by themselves. However, even such broad segments as children and adults could be tremendously helpful. It should also be noted that the needs of the segment determine the health services needed, rather than the other way around.

Additional possibilities are to segment the community by socioeconomic variables, stages in the family life cycle, or psychographic variables such as activities, values, interests, attitudes, opinions, and life-styles. The number of different ways in which a community might be meaningfully segmented is limited only by the creative abilities of the nurse. Still another possibility is to segment in terms of identified mental health problems. Since the emphasis in community mental health focuses on prevention, one way to segment a community while maintaining an orientation toward prevention is to identify populations that are "at risk" for disruption in psychological equilibrium or mental health. For example, families under stress, victims of aggression, and discharged mentally ill persons are all strong candidates for market segmentation.

After the community has been segmented into target markets requiring mental health programs, the following information should be gathered. First, a geographical area of the community should be defined, thereby limiting the target market to those individuals who reside within a certain geographically limited area. Boundaries that result may be appropriate geographically but questionable by other standards because some people may live outside one catchment area yet be closer to its health facilities than their own. Consequently, strictly enforced boundaries tend to create time and travel problems. The solution is cooperation between communities with common boundaries.

After the establishment of geographical boundaries, there is the need to determine the size of the various target markets. Obviously the larger the target market, the more important it becomes to the health of the community. Consideration should also be given to the location of a target group within the community. For example, a target group with a widely dispersed population may require an entirely different program approach compared with a target group that is clustered in a small pocket of the community.

Once the community has been assessed in terms of its problems and needs, the community mental health nurse can then turn her attention to assessing the community's resources. Information should be gathered to determine the availability of professionals who have training in the traditional mental health disciplines, such as psychiatrists, clinical psychologists, social workers, and nurses. In addition, the availability of professionals outside the traditional mental health area, such as physicians, clergy,

and schoolteachers, should be considered. Other resources such as hospitals, halfway homes, and nursing homes should be included in the assessment, as well as existing mental health facilities and service organizations. In many communities, existing services are often fragmented and clients are frequently forced to obtain services from several different agencies, none of which is aware of the work being performed by the others.

A final input to the community assessment is identifying the community's attitudes toward mental health. Specific attitudinal information should be gathered from these groups and individuals currently working with clients, such as private practitioners, public and private hospital administrators and staff, and social workers. In addition, the attitudes of special interest and power groups as well as the attitudes of the general population should be considered in the community assessment.

Stewart[50] describes a three-phase community needs assessment approach that is similar to the marketing framework used here. He defines the three steps as problem description, desire for services, and solutions needed to solve the problems. The problem area includes (1) a description of the size and nature of the problem (number of people, where they live, and what they are like), (2) a description of the community, and (3) identification of available services that help to meet the needs identified in the problem statement.

Desire refers to the attitudes held about both the problem and the services. This step also sets priorities as to the relative importance of the identified problems. A solution is arrived at based on the previous two steps. When more than one choice of solution is suggested, then the alternatives are arranged by priority.

In summary, any assessment of the community should take into account an analysis of the existing mental health programs and facilities, an audit of the resources available, an evaluation of the attitudes toward mental health, and, most important, an identification of the specific needs of the community. Any comprehensive community analysis requires a certain depth and breadth of awareness of community needs to optimize program effectiveness.

Community mental health nursing: implementing the role

Community mental health nursing is defined as a broad continuum of activities ranging from health maintenance and promotion to curative and rehabilitative functions. Community mental health nursing is differentiated from psychiatric nursing in that in the broadest sense the community rather than the individual is the client. Psychiatry refers to a medical specialty concerned with the identification and treatment of mental disorders. Mental health refers to the maintenance and enhancement of functioning, including the prevention of disorder. Similarly, psychiatric nursing seeks to provide care to individuals who evidence psychological dysfunction, whereas community mental health nursing applies a public approach to mental health by focusing on the macrosystem or community as client. Nursing attention is directed toward factors within the community that impede the maintenance of mental health. Nursing intervention at this level focuses on such factors as the effects of poor housing, crowding, and unemployment on the mental health of residents. The nurse often serves as a catalyst in bringing stress factors to the attention of concerned groups, who then work to ameliorate the situation.

A major component of the community mental health nursing role is directed toward identifying populations at risk and seeking interventions that decrease stress and reduce the incidence of mental disorder. For example, a nurse might provide counseling for a group of divorced women to support and guide them during a crisis. Although the clients are not emotionally disturbed, the family crisis makes them "at risk" for psychological dysfunction. Activities to promote and enhance mental health can be described in accordance with Caplan's levels of primary, secondary, and tertiary prevention.[8] This schema is used to identify selected high-risk populations and describe nursing interventions designed to reduce stress and promote mental health.

Primary prevention

Primary prevention of mental disorders is described as biological, social, or psychological intervention that promotes emotional well-being or reduces the incidence and prevalence of mental illness in populations. Primary prevention attempts to lower the new cases of mental disorder over a period of time. According to Caplan's model of primary prevention,[8] the rate of mental disorder in a community is related to the interaction of both long- and short-term factors influencing the adaptive capacities of its

members. Thus mental illness occurs in a community context and the resources for helping are provided in the community.

Primary prevention in mental health is an elusive concept in that it is often difficult to document its success. DeWild[14] identified two models of primary prevention in mental health. The first provides services to ". . . increase health and reduce stress for an identified population of people who are presumed at risk, under stress, or in crisis." Such groups served by this model include single parents, expectant parents, families with preschool children or older adults in the home, those with physical handicaps, and so on. Such programs are designed to support people in working out their life stresses. The second model deals with groups who are not yet mentally ill, but who do have an educational, occupational, or social problem. For example, one program of this type works with children who were unable to adjust in school. This model seeks to reduce the vulnerability to mental illness of a group of people who are at risk because of a defined social dysfunction.

Bloom[6] points out an interesting perspective on prevention when he suggests that the previous public health paradigm used in the prevention of infectious diseases is not effective in mental illness. In the classic public health paradigm, a disease is identified, its natural history of development and progression is traced, and a program of intervention is developed. In contrast, he recommends a new paradigm for mental illness that is directed toward identifying a stressful life event which has undesirable mental health consequences. This would include identifying people at risk, studying the effects of the event, and implementing and evaluating intervention programs. The basic difference is that the specific cause or manifestation of disease or disability is not important; the focus is on preventing any form of disability from identification of known stressors.

Consistent with both the models of DeWild and Bloom, activities for primary prevention include teaching mental health principles to a variety of community groups, including the PTA, church groups, and youth organizations. Conducting interactional groups in schools, day-care centers, or children's homes also provides a medium for preventive activities. Referral constitutes a preventive approach if persons undergoing stress are directed to mental health resources before mental disorder occurs. Consultation and education comprise major tools for a community mental health framework.

MENTAL HEALTH CONSULTATION. A variety of formats are available for examining mental health consultation.[9] Community mental health nurses frequently participate in client-centered, group-centered, or program-centered consultation. Client-centered consultation focuses on helping the consultee find the most effective treatment for his client. An example of this approach is seen when psychiatric nursing consultation is requested by other professionals, such as public health nurses, to assess client behavior, determine alternative intervention strategies, and select a nursing approach to alleviate client stress and assist him to function at the highest level possible. Other target groups for client-centered consultation include clergymen, teachers, probation officers, police workers, and staff in nursing homes, day-care centers, or children's institutions. In client-centered consultation the nurse may choose either to meet the client or deal only with the staff's description.

Consultation services to schools demonstrate two of Caplan's levels of intervention. In client-centered school consultation the nurse may meet regularly with teachers on an "as necessary" basis. Primary prevention intervention is directed toward helping the teacher assess and understand a child's behavior and subsequently determine alternative approaches the teacher can take to alter the child's behavior. In addition, the nurse may provide a service to the families of children whose behavior is described as requiring alteration. The nurse often makes home visits to provide parental counseling in a type of secondary prevention activity.

The group-centered consultative role occurs when the consultant meets with a group to provide guidance regarding the consultees' work encounters. For example, the community mental health nurse might meet with a group of public health nurses to discuss individuals in their case load who evidence emotional stress.

EDUCATIONAL COMPONENT OF CONSULTATION. The educational component of primary prevention can be carried out in a variety of ways. As previously mentioned, implicit in developing any program is the necessity for assessing community needs. Certain groups tend to have a high level of stress, such as new residents. The problems that accompany relocation are numerous. Initially parents know little about community resources and services, children must adjust to new schools and peers, and both children and parents must find new friends and develop support systems. Group sessions for new residents, often in conjunction with a school or church, help ease the stress of a move. The group can focus on orientation to the community by means of identification of resources, discussion of the stress related to relocation, and suggesting adaptive coping mechanisms. It can also help parents plan ways to ease their stress and alienation and provide support to their children.

Family-centered education and consultation to courts is an innovative way for providing mental health support to families whose children are delinquent or have been defined as status offenders (school truancy and runaways). Nursing intervention includes parent-education classes, group discussion sessions, and case-centered consultation. The school provides a rich arena for mental health education and consultation. One approach for prevention is for the nurse to meet regularly with small groups of students to focus on stress and problems of daily living. A structured interaction approach such as values clarification can be used. Values clarification refers to a process for helping individuals sort out, talk about, and think through their values so as to make constructive and responsible decisions. The purpose of values clarification is not to teach values but rather to provide an arena for self-examination and articulation of one's attitudes and beliefs.[43] (See Chapter 3.)

A less structured approach to preventive psychiatry in the schools occurs when the nurse organizes or leads "rap groups." These groups serve similar purposes to those of more structured activities in that the overall goal is self-awareness and increasing one's benefit to others. In one school system "rap groups" were begun by the community health nurse who was employed as a consultant for the local mental health center for the purpose of intervention with students who evidenced behavioral difficulties, withdrawn behavior, or peer pressure problems. Weekly rap sessions were held in a selected school for eight to ten students. As the program developed, the student participants raised the question of whether others might benefit just as they had from the group experience. Subsequently volunteer leaders were recruited from social service and mental health agencies to hold weekly groups for students regardless of the identified need. All groups met simultaneously so that no schedule conflicts occurred. The objectives of this program were the following:

1. To facilitate the development of communication skills for better understanding of other people
2. To increase the opportunity for an honest expression and an exchange of opinions as a means of establishing self-worth
3. To enhance decision-making abilities
4. To provide a supportive atmosphere in which students can explore a wide spectrum of situations and consider alternatives as well as consequences in making decisions
5. To give students the opportunity to examine constructive and destructive behavior and move toward accepting responsibility for it

Initially the consultant led a group. As the program expanded, the consultant continued to lead a group but also met regularly with small groups of volunteer leaders for the purpose of group-centered consultation.

Opportunities for mental health consultation abound; success is largely determined by the consultant's sensitivity to principles of consultation as well as to the unique needs of the client. Regardless of the nature of the consultation, it is essential to involve the individuals who are to be the target of the intervention in the planning. For example, if the program is to provide consultation to school teachers, they must be involved in the original planning so that the purpose, goals, and procedure can be collaboratively discussed. The label of mental health consultation may sound threatening to individuals who perceive the purpose as imposed therapy for them.[7]

It is important to remember that even though the prospective consultees have identified a problem and often have experienced a great deal of stress, they may be resistant to intervention. Regardless of the consultant's ideas, the consultees may repeatedly counter with "yes, but. . . ." In this instance the consultant moves slowly and allows the consultee to carefully apply problem-solving techniques to his situation.

From the first moment of contact the consultant listens to everyone. It is important to listen both to what is said as well as to content areas avoided. If the consultation is being provided to a group, each member generally has a differ-

ent perception of the problem and each has his own set of data relevant to the problem. Each participant must have an opportunity to express his views as the consultant carefully avoids either agreeing or disagreeing with anyone. Additional principles and intervention techniques related to the consultation process are described in detail in Chapter 23.

Program-centered consultation adheres to the same framework as client- and group-centered consultation, although a more dramatic political-bargaining process occurs in this area. There are often considerable vested interests on the part of the consultees and differences of opinion and approach within the organization seeking consultation. Group process skills are consistently at the forefront in program-centered consultation.

Although mental health consultation to institutions, organizations, and entire communities is frequently provided, there remains considerable resistance to such efforts. The explicit goal of program-centered consultation is to help solve institution-wide problems. Although there is frequently overt agreement and often eagerness to work with the consultant, there is usually some degree of resistance to any suggested change. Berlin[4] describes several types of institutional resistance to change. The first type is inertia, which is seen when the plans for change just never get activated. Frequently, the underlying cause is anxiety and fear of the new idea or plan. This type of resistance can be dealt with in at least two different ways. One approach is to implement a major educational campaign to acquaint all people who will be involved with the new proposal to its basic tenets. The second approach is to implement the change strategy on a limited basis as a pilot or demonstration project.

The second form of resistance to change is seen in ". . . devices, built over time, that encapsulate and neutralize innovations and alterations in function or structure."[4:120] An example would be the delays encountered when a new proposal has to go through multiple levels of approval bodies. Often regulations, buck passing, and failure to support the proposal dissipate momentum for change. Similarly, ideas for change are often destroyed when a committee is assigned the responsibility for working out the details.

Change efforts are often supported by administrators yet fail because inept people are assigned the responsibility of implementing the new idea. In contrast, the administration may actually disapprove of the change and rally community leaders or other consultants to support the maintenance of the status quo. Consultants have a challenging job when they become involved in program-centered consultation. Careful and astute assessment is essential both of the administration as well as the other personnel as to their overt and covert desire for change.

Secondary prevention

Secondary prevention seeks to reduce the prevalence of mental disorder by providing interventions that decrease the stressors and shorten the duration of disequilibrium. New directions in techniques for providing secondary prevention are being sought in the area of short-term interventions designed to lessen discomfort and return the individual to effective functioning. Treatment developments include a wide variety of group therapies, marital and family therapy, and intervention strategies combining psychotherapy with environmental manipulation, such as psychodrama, dance therapy, poetry, art, or activity therapy. Each type of therapy is aimed at helping the individual gain self-awareness and thereby learn new ways of responding to stressors.

Specific techniques for secondary prevention include home visits designed to help individuals cope with high levels of stress without being removed from their home setting, suicide prevention counseling, and preadmission services, which frequently include home visits. The aim of community mental health in regard to secondary prevention is to treat the acute phase as early as possible and to use inpatient psychiatric care only when essential and when outpatient care or partial hospitalization is inadequate for the patient's needs.

Tertiary prevention

Tertiary prevention refers to measures designed to reduce the level of mental disorder in a community through rehabilitation. Implicit in rehabilitation is early planning for care on discharge from the hospital, follow-up care to reduce stressors and promote coping ability and use of a wide range of supportive activities such as transitional or halfway homes, foster homes,

home visits, and partial hospitalization. A specific plan for tertiary prevention is described in the following discussion of high-risk populations, which describes a plan for discharged psychiatric patients.

High-risk populations in community mental health nursing

Just as no community mental health program can serve all the needs of a community, this single chapter cannot identify nursing interventions for all high-risk populations. Discussion centers around four major groups of high-risk population: the family under stress, victims of aggression, elderly people, and discharged mentally ill persons. Nursing intervention with the first two groups is generally primary prevention, whereas nursing approaches with discharged psychiatric patients encompass principles related to tertiary prevention. Secondary prevention overlaps all groups. Families under stress include the developing family, working mothers, and families disrupted by divorce.

Families under stress

The whole arena of family life poses opportunities for primary prevention. In a society beset with stress and rapid change, the stability and smooth functioning of the family can no longer be taken for granted. Issues such as working mothers, divorce, and single-parent families have ramifications for nursing as does the broader area of parenting.

THE DEVELOPING FAMILY. The developmental crisis of the birth of a child demands an alteration in the family system. With the introduction of a third person, the dyadic relationship is disrupted. The goal of nursing intervention in the expanding family is that of promoting growth and ability to adapt to change, thereby offsetting the disorganizing effect of change. An efficient way for the community mental health nurse to influence the crisis of parenthood is by holding parent education classes. During these classes situations are anticipated and discussion focuses on identifying potential crisis situations and dealing with them through simulated encounters such as role playing.

Even expectant parents who eagerly await the birth of a baby often have fears about their ability as a caretaker. Many parents worry about taking a baby home from the hospital because of its small size; their lack of experience with parenting activities, such as feeding, diapering, and quieting a crying infant; or their fear of being unable to cope with the constant dependency that occurs when a baby arrives.

Additional strategies for the nurse include follow-up visits to parents who attended prenatal preparatory classes. Often the first few weeks after the birth of a child are fraught with crisis. A concerned listener who has finely tuned problem-solving abilities can be a valuable mental health resource to new parents. The community mental health nurse can also serve as a consultant to public health nurses who routinely visit many new parents.

A further avenue for preventive community mental health nursing revolves around education for parenting. Although raising children is considered a serious aspect of American life, until recently little attention has been directed to the belief that effective parenting is not an innate ability. A wide range of parent education programs are available. Whether nurses subscribe to a specific set of beliefs and strategies for parenting or choose an eclectic approach, the opportunities for promoting mental health abound. Possibly one of the most beneficial results of parent education is the acknowledgment that all parents become frustrated, angry, and ambivalent toward their children. Parent education goes beyond acknowledging feelings and includes learning and practicing alternative ways of interacting with children. Community mental health nurses can also become involved in the area of parent education by offering to conduct classes for day-care centers, church groups, or school organizations. Education for mental health addresses the needs of both children and parents as family roles shift and respond to societal change.

WORKING MOTHERS. The character of American families is rapidly changing. An increasing number of women are in the labor force because of personal career choice or financial need. Within the United States, because of the increasing divorce rate, more women are becoming the primary financial support for themselves and their children. It is often difficult to juggle three roles—wife, mother, employee. Employment outside the home can engender positive, growth-producing feelings, resulting in an increased self-esteem and heightened sense of independence, as well as negative, often immobilizing feelings of guilt and anxiety about "abandoning" one's family. It is not uncommon for a working mother to assume responsibility for everything that goes askew with the family in her absence. Many women are socialized to accept the belief that a woman's place is in the home; hence, when a woman seeks employment, she thinks she is functioning in opposition to societal norms. Three defense mechanisms seem symptomatic of underlying guilt: rationalization, projection, and overcompensation. In rationalization the mother thinks up a socially approved reason for her behavior, such as "I would just play bridge or do volunteer work if I stayed at home." Projection involves blaming someone or something else for one's need to work, and overcompensation is evidenced by trying to repay the child with gifts.[30]

How can nurses help the working mother cope with her myriad of roles?[2] First, they can encourage and provide a medium in which the mother can come to grips with her conflicting feelings. The mother needs to be aware that it is the quality rather than the quantity of mother-child interactions that has the greatest impact on growth and development. Moreover, children often benefit from their mother's feelings of self-satisfaction related to job success.

The nurse can also support working mothers as they make or change child care arrangements. Few situations have as profound an effect on the working mother as disruptions in child care. Essentially, selecting the best arrangement for each family is a problem-solving strategy whereby the family examines each available alternative and selects the one that seemingly will bring more comfort.

Another problem-solving area relates to assignment of responsibility for household chores. It is estimated that it takes 105 hours a week to carry out full-time employment and meet the domestic responsibilities of the family. A variety of household management alternatives exist and the nurse can help the mother select the one that suits the needs of her family. Five guidelines have been developed for nurses working with mothers who are experiencing role conflict[30]:

1. Help the mother examine and accept her reasons for working.
2. Encourage the woman to choose a job carefully. Working mothers cannot afford the luxury of displacing accumulated hostility from the job onto the family.
3. Communicate honestly with family members to determine their response to employ-

ment. Discussion of differences cannot occur without honest expression.

4. Assist the mother in finding a suitable surrogate whose attitudes are consistent with hers.

5. Explore ways in which help can be provided by others, the family, or the housekeeper.

DIVORCE. The divorce rate in the United States has risen sharply in the past few years, provoking a crisis situation in many families and necessitating immediate intervention directed toward stress reduction. Although the increasing divorce rate is startling, attention is also directed toward the number of marriages that do not dissolve but rather maintain themselves in a constant state of disequilibrium.

Divorce, one of the most traumatic crises a family faces, confronts each member with the task of examining and often changing his role in the family system. Although divorce is often a healthy step toward reestablishing family homeostasis, stress is involved. A body of knowledge is being accumulated regarding the reactions of both spouses and children to the experience. The first year after the divorce is particularly difficult. During this time money constitutes a major source of stress as one household divides into two, each needing financial support. Women complain of feeling helpless and physically unattractive and of experiencing an acute loss of identity. On the other hand, men describe not knowing who they are, feeling as though they have no roots, structure, or predictable home life. Many divorced men buy sports cars and flashy clothes and plunge into a wide range of social activities to offset the loneliness of apartment living.[24]

Divorce therapy is gaining attention as a tool for primary prevention. The ultimate goal of divorce counseling or therapy is to help the couple disengage from their former relationship with a minimum amount of destructive and malicious behavior toward each other or their children. Divorce is dealt with as a family systems problem, which includes not only the immediate family but also the extended family. Each person in the family has an opinion about the situation and may feel that need to lay blame on someone; each is affected by the family disruption.

One framework for understanding the dynamics associated with divorce moves through the stages of grief to explain reactions to the separation and loss.[23] Regardless of how fraught a marriage is with frustration and conflict, it is never easy to terminate. Even painful relationships have meaning for the participants. Denial serves to shield the marriage partners from the reality of the separation and their subsequent loss, since it "buys" time for individuals to reconstruct coping abilities. In nursing intervention, denial is supported by the nurse's listening to the client and helping him describe his fear and dismay at his situation. Denial is transitory and is not supported when it becomes disproportionate to the actual situation.

Anger often follows denial and may be directed outwardly toward the ex-spouse or inwardly when it is manifested as depression. As the client is forced into new roles, he may feel helpless. Since helplessness causes a person to feel vulnerable, a common coping mechanism is to become angry and attempt to impose control on the situation. Just as in the stages of grief, bargaining often follows anger. One or both spouses wonder if the marriage could have been saved "if I had just. . . ." Depression typically occurs when one or both parties realize that the emotional investment they once had in a marriage no longer exists. The final stage, acceptance, is seen when the individual can move beyond regret and begin to make plans. Throughout the counseling, but particularly once acceptance begins, the primary nursing approach is problem solving, or application of the nursing process to assess, plan, and implement coping strategies.

A major issue in relation to divorce counseling is that of family roles. Traditional family roles are often disrupted as each spouse assumes responsibilities previously carried out or shared with the other partner. Men may assume responsibility for household maintenance when previously their wives handled this task. Women may be forced to support themselves and their children; for some, employment may constitute a major alteration in role.

Specific interventions are either child centered, relationship focused, or adult centered.[29] Child-centered interventions assist the parents to understand and deal with age-related responses to divorce. Children are particularly at risk for mental health disruption during a divorce in that they are often caught in the middle of bitter parental battles, and visitation rights, custody, and child support can become bargaining issues. Children from divorced families also tend to constitute a major portion of the case

TABLE 19-1. Responses to divorce and related nursing interventions*

Behavior observed	Nursing intervention
Preschool	
Regression, confusion, irritability	Provide guidance to custodial parent who serves as child's best support person
Difficulty understanding what is happening	Teach communication skills related to interpreting meaning of divorce
Repeatedly asks same questions (e.g., "Where is Daddy?" "When is Daddy coming home?")	Examine alternatives for intervening in the child's regressive behavior
Early latency	
Often immobilized by parental separation	Open discussion may be too threatening; nurse might use a "divorce monologue" to talk about how other children react to divorce
Developmentally denial does not serve these children well, yet open confrontation with reality is traumatic	Focus on helping both parents support child's need for contact
Nearly insatiable need to maintain contact with both parents	
Anger (common reaction)	"Divorce monologue" may give child permission to express anger
Later latency	
Torn in loyalty toward parents	Encourage child to express fears and worries to parents
Worries a great deal	Support child as he deals with pain and anger
Can both express their feelings verbally and channel them into organized activities	Encourage parents to be consistent and firm in approach
Superego controls may be threatened as external controls decrease because of stress	
Adolescence	
Intense feelings of pain (anger, sadness, loss, and betrayal)	Provide an opportunity for open discussion of feelings, including helping them plan ways to express feelings directly and constructively
Strong feelings of shame and embarrassment	
Concern about their own future as a marital partner	Discuss feelings of shame, embarrassment, and fear of the future
Concern about adequacy as a sexual partner in their current dating, as well as for future married life	Use communication strategies, such as role playing or psychodrama to help adolescents learn to deal with feelings
Often unrealistic concern about finances	
Shortened disengagement from and shift in perceptions of parents	Practice improved, honest, open communication
Accelerated individuation from parents	
Heightened awareness of parents as sexual objects	
Loyalty conflicts	
Strategic withdrawal as a defense against pain	

*Modified from Kelley, J., and Wallerstein, J.: Am. J. Orthopsychiatry **47:**23, 1977.

loads in psychiatric facilities with common problems being depression, aggressive outbursts, or behavioral problems at school or in social groups. Of the 7- to 16-year-olds Shanok and Lewis studied,[47] 48% of those referred to a juvenile court clinic were from broken homes, and children of divorce constituted 49% of those referred to a child guidance clinic. Similarly, Kalter[27] reported that 41% of the children receiving services at a large university department of psychiatry were from homes in which the parents were separated, divorced, or remarried. Some frequently observed age-specific responses to divorce and pertinent nursing interventions are given in Table 19-1.[29]

Relationship-centered interventions are used when knowledge of growth and development is less an issue than is the ability to cope with the stress of divorce. Many parents become immobilized with their increased responsibility and the pressing need to make decisions and deal with the daily reactions of family members to the divorce. Frequently children get caught up in the parental conflict. Nursing intervention helps the family members remain open and honest with one another and not use each other for harmful purposes.

Adult-centered counseling focuses on helping the partner who seeks counseling adapt to his new role and cope with the stresses implicit in a major life change. Even the most desperate marriage provides some security and division of labor. Women particularly need to examine their alternatives in advance of major decisions to make the most advantageous choice as they assume expanded roles, which often include financial support of self or family.

Victims of violence

In a country such as the United States, where reported crimes appear to be on the rise, attention must focus on the mental health needs of victims of violence and aggression. Nurses working in community mental health settings are in a strategic position to provide interventions to individuals who become high risks for mental illness because of an assault against them. Often nurses have early contact with victims and can make a considerable difference in the treatment outcome. To provide beneficial care to victims, nurses must understand the range of reactions victims experience and some of the

causative factors leading to physical abuse of another. Three specific types of aggression are discussed: child abuse, battered women, and family reaction to homicide. In each type of assault the client may not actively seek mental health intervention; rather, the nurse may seek out the client through referrals from police, courts, hospitals, or other agencies.

CHILD ABUSE. Child abuse is not a new phenomenon. Occurrences of abuse to children have existed as long as parents and children have lived together. Interest in the whole area of victims as target populations for mental illness is gaining impetus; therefore child abuse is increasingly documented. The increased documentation may mean either that the actual incidence of abuse is rising or that society is assuming a more responsible and accountable stance in regard to reporting and intervening in this behavior. Child abuse is defined as a "disease" that is the single largest killer of children in the United States. Approximately 1% of American children are reported to be abused or neglected each year.[22] Although all 50 states require the reporting of incidents of child abuse, it is estimated that the majority are not reported; rather, they come to the attention of the health care providers as "accidents."

Child abuse may take the form of physical injury, sexual abuse, or emotional abuse, which occurs when children are ignored, isolated, or continually shamed and demeaned. Neglect occurs when a parent is unable to or fails to provide minimal emotional and physical care to a child. Child abuse is most likely to happen after a life crisis or significant number of family changes and often occurs in the afternoon or evening. Helfer and Kempe[22] state that 90% of the nation's abusive parents can be treated if they are given considerable support over a period of time. They further postulate that 10% of abusive parents are mentally disturbed to the extent that they cannot be easily treated, and their children should be removed from the home.

The community mental health nurse assumes a vital role in detection, education, and counseling regarding child abuse. The syndrome of child abuse tends to be self-perpetuating in that abusive parents frequently were abused as children. The only role model they had for learning about parenting was negative. A fairly accurate composite portrait can be drawn of the abusive parent. He has generally been an abused or neglected child who has never received positive nurturing so that he reaches adulthood with a vast array of unmet emotional needs. His activities center around a continual search for nuturing and security, but since his needs are nearly limitless, he constantly feels thwarted and frustrated in his search. The abusive parent fantasizes that his child will meet his emotional needs; he believes that his child will enable him to feel wanted and loved. His own dependency needs prevent him from tolerating the child's dependency. He becomes angry when the child cries, whines, or is less than a pleasing companion. Abusive parents include both fathers and mothers on all socioeconomic and educational levels. The distinguishing feature of an abusive parent is his orientation toward punishment and discipline; these parents typically expect their children to perform as adults and severely punish them when they fail to meet parental expectation.[25]

The abused child is identified by his distrust for adults and his constant fear of doing something "wrong." Past experience has taught him that the slightest inadequacy can bring untold wrath and pain. Because of a paucity of positive reinforcement these children frequently have difficulty responding to praise or caring attention.

Primary prevention of child abuse refers to impeding the onset of a potentially abusive situation. Primary prevention takes the form of public education, screening to identify high-risk families, and mental health consultation to health care providers who have substantial contact with parents. Public education begins with consciousness-raising activities. The initial goal is to call attention to the problem; once sentiment is raised about battered children, workshops on abuse and its prevention, detection, and treatment can be conducted. Similarly, parent education classes constitute a form of primary prevention. Nurses who conduct parenting classes are in a strategic position to observe parental reactions to child rearing as well as provide instruction on how to practice more effective parenting behaviors.

Nurses have a variety of opportunities for screening in relation to child abuse. Studies have indicated that parental behaviors often serve as indicators of potential abuse.[25] Signs of rejection, guilt, or extreme anxiety about the coming birth of a baby can often be detected in prenatal clinics. Parental behaviors occurring immediately postpartum and requiring follow-up assessment include a verbal or nonverbal passive reaction to the child, a hostile, reject-

ing response, or extreme disappointment about the child's sex. In follow-up home visits the nurse can detect further signs of possible rejection, such as describing the baby as "it" rather than in personal terms, finding little enjoyment in the role of parent, or continually complaining about the inconvenience the baby has caused.

Parents often make disguised pleas by taking the child to the hospital when he is in fact well. In essence the parents are asking for attention to their needs. In times of acute stress, parents and children may need to be temporarily separated. Two types of facilities can be established in communities to intervene in child abuse: a crisis nursery where small children stay for a few hours or a few days, depending on the magnitude of the family stress, and a day-care center that provides not only a setting where children can learn to interact with peers and adults but also parent-counseling groups.

In both the crisis nursery and the day-care center the community mental health nurse would serve as a consultant to the staff. Consultation is a valuable medium for preventive mental health whenever the caregivers are dealing with emotionally laden issues and problems. Staff who work with abused children day after day experience tremendous stress as they constantly face the pain and suffering of young clients. The attention of the consultant is directed toward a case-centered approach when staff are frustrated in their attempts to provide care for a child or when feelings interfere with the care given. In addition, consultation may provide support and encouragement to the staff by allowing them to acknowledge their job-related feelings.

The role of the nurse has direct implications in regard to providing assistance to the parents. It is easy to view the parents as ogres and lose sight of their problems, which are evidenced in their maladaptive parenting behaviors. The nurse makes home visits, teaches parenting courses, or meets with parent groups to assist them in examining their behavior, discussing the problems that led to abuse, and considering new ways of coping. If nurses are to provide mental health services to abusive parents, they must have a way of gaining access to their population. Some parents present themselves at a community agency requesting help before the abusive behavior leads to a serious injury or death. Other abusive parents are located through emergency room or police referral.

BATTERED WIVES. A further target or high-risk population for the community mental health nurse is the "battered wife." Wife beating is not new, but public and health professional recognition of the problem is rapidly accelerating. The term "battered wife" refers to any woman who is beaten by her mate, regardless of the legality of the marital relationship. Epidemiological attention to the phenomenon of wife beating, as with other types of victimology, is inadequate. Reporting mechanisms are not effective in determining the incidence of wife battering, since the occurrence is often documented as a "domestic disturbance" with no acknowledgment of the actual problem situation. Moreover, courts classify wife beating under assault and battery, aggravated assault, or homicide if death ensues. Victims are often afraid to actually describe what happened because of shame, guilt, or an overwhelming fear of retaliation. Hence full delineation of the magnitude of the problem is impossible.

If nurses are to provide informed interventions to victims of wife beating, it is essential to recognize that this behavior cuts across all socioeconomic levels, is seemingly more widespread than reporting indexes demonstrate, and occurs and is subsequently tolerated for diverse reasons. A woman's decision to stay with or, more likely, to not take action to leave a husband who physically abuses her is often difficult to understand. The abused wife may not know why she remains, although the most prevalent reason is fear. Women fear retaliation, inability to support themselves and their children, and loneliness and alienation.

A key to providing nursing intervention lies in assessment. Because of feelings of guilt and shame women do not always seek treatment for their assault and subsequent emotional pain. The battered woman may come to the attention of the nurse for a variety of reasons. She may identify her problem as inability to sleep, problems with her children, "nerves," or depression. As with all types of victimology, the nurse may seek out the client after a referral from hospitals or police.[33]

Cues to the identification of a victim of wife beating are similar to those used in child abuse. Victims usually have evidence of physical aggression toward them, although the signs may be well-hidden by protective clothing. The skilled batterer seeks to hit the victim in less obvious places of the body, such as the back of the head, which is covered with hair, or on parts of the body that are clothed.

Intervention with the battered wife is based on a clearly delineated problem-solving approach. Assessment of the battering situation precedes nursing action. On occasion, the assessment may be executed rapidly if the client is in danger of a future attack. Any plan for action is based on the client's own decision. Nursing responsibility includes helping the client describe her situation and critically examine her alternatives, providing information as to available resources in the community and procedures for their use, and supporting the client as she makes decisions. The nurse must remember that awareness cannot be forced on the client. She must make her own decisions.

Lieberknecht[33] identifies four commonly held misconceptions regarding the syndrome of battering that must be overcome before the nurse can provide effective interventions. The first misconception holds that a woman who is beaten must have some need filled by the experience or she would leave. In reality, a myriad of reasons prevent women from leaving what may appear to be an intolerable situation. The predominant underlying reason seems to be fear. Women are typically afraid of retaliation either to themselves or their children when they are found; they often doubt their ability to be self-supporting or fear the reactions of others to their plight. Second, many people believe that the wife is beaten because of ineffectiveness as a partner; if she loved the man more or paid more attention to his needs, she would not be beaten. In essence this belief implies that "good" wives do not get beaten, whereas "naughty" or "inefficient" wives are deservedly beaten. This misconception holds the woman solely responsible for her plight when in fact she is the victim. The third commonly held misconception is that a man, as head of the household, has the right to "control" his property. This belief dehumanizes women and equates their value to that of a piece of furniture. The fourth belief contends that battering only occurs in lower income families. As with child abuse and rape, battering transcends all socioeconomic and educational boundaries. A battered woman may be any age; she may or may not have children.

The nursing plan for the battered wife is based on the premise that the woman has experienced a significant loss. She may have lost some aspect of physical functioning, security, trust in others, especially men, and hope for a happy and mutually satisfying marriage. The woman's first reaction is shock. She may view the beatings as chance occurrences and deny the serious implications of her situation. Furthermore, she may need to use denial long enough to summon defense mechanisms for coping with the onslaught of hurt that comes with full recognition of her plight.

Once she begins to acknowledge her situation, she may be overwhelmed with rage and fear. As she develops an awareness of her situation, the nurse helps her devise a plan of action. Although she may not be ready to move out of the home, she should plan her actions in the event of another attack. The nurse helps the client consider exit alternatives from the home, who to call in an emergency, where she can go it she must leave home hurriedly, and what she can do with her children in the event of an attack.

The ultimate goal of nursing intervention is to help the woman gain control of her life. She may have limited confidence in herself, thus needing support and encouragement with each decision. Her self-esteem is often low; as she takes responsibility for herself and begins to make decisions, she increasingly sees herself as worthwhile. Not only is nursing intervention directed toward problem solving and dealing with anger, but also the impact of guilt is considered. Many battered women maintain a deep-seated belief that if they had only behaved differently, life would have taken another course. It is pointed out that men who batter their wives seem no different on the surface than other men; the battering situation is often unjust and may be unprovoked. Whatever the woman's actions, they did not warrant a physical attack.

FAMILIES OF HOMICIDE VICTIMS. According to Burgess,[7] families of homicide victims experience a two-phase trauma reaction: the acute crisis and the reorganization phase. During the crisis phase the family learns of the loss, makes arrangements for the funeral, and deals with a multitude of questions. The family experiences an acute personal loss with no warning or preparatory phase. Accompanying the emptiness and sorrow at the loss is the agony about the painful and often brutal nature of the death. Often the family becomes preoccupied with the who, how, and why of the murder. The wish for revenge can be overwhelming as the family members come face-to-face with their impotence to change the situation.

Families are generally so busy attending to details and legal matters during the acute phase that nursing intervention is not introduced until the reorganization phase begins.[7] Grief is an immediate reaction and may be accompanied by unrealistic guilt. Family members often say, "If only I had done . . . this would never have happened." Nursing intervention focuses on the family's lack of responsibility for the loss. The family is encouraged to talk about the lost family member as they move through the stages of grief. With a violent death family members do not have an opportunity for denial. They are so busy making urgent arrangements that the reality of the loss continually surrounds them.

The family's first reaction may be shock, agonizing sadness, or anger. Regardless of which reaction comes first, each must be dealt with. Pent-up anger decreases the ability to cope and deal with the grief. Both anger and grief tend to have an immobilizing effect. Before decisions can be made to move the family forward, the hurt and rage must be expressed. Essentially the reorganization phase uses a problem-solving approach to determine how homeostasis can be regained. Family responsibility and roles often shift to compensate for the lost member.

Nursing intervention supports the family's attempt to look at new roles, examine alternatives, determine priorities, and implement a plan of action. The nursing intervention continues to be supportive as new roles present difficulties and alternative plans are required. The pain and hurt in family members is not abated rapidly. Nursing intervention is also directed toward helping the family cope with the cold and impersonal nature of the legal proceedings. Their loss is one that can never be replaced; family pain is acute and agonizing. In contrast, the legal system views the lost family member as an "it," merely a statistic or case needing to be solved.

Elderly people as a high-risk group

Elderly people are at high risk for mental health disruption for several reasons, including their susceptibility to the effects of rapid social and environmental change. Since the 1950s social and technological changes have occurred at an unprecedented pace. This poses problems for elderly people who are physiologically less able to adapt to rapidly changing events in their lives.

A number of barriers exist for the elderly, which interfere with their ability to meet their mental health needs. First, a far greater share of national resources are devoted to children than to the elderly. Also, elderly people who live on fixed incomes are especially susceptible to the effects of inflation. People are at high risk for lowered self-esteem during inflationary periods when their expectations for either social mobility or maintenance of at least an adequate standard of living are destroyed by the high cost of living. Elderly people are susceptible to lowered self-esteem and resignation when they have spent a lifetime of saving for retirement only to find that they are not able to make ends meet. In addition, transportation often presents a major barrier for the elderly who do not have ready access to services. Retirement also can deal a serious blow to self-esteem, since so much of contemporary society revolves around what people do for a living.

Furthermore, society holds many myths and stereotypes about the elderly that mitigate against the maintenance of feelings of worth. Language and humor are replete with examples of clichés that cast elderly people in a negative light. Phrases like the "old goat," "silly old biddy," or "dirty old man" do not reflect a positive image of the elderly. The very word elderly tends to call forth a set of images, including graying and thinning hair, a slow stooped gait, and a tendency toward forgetfulness. In a major study by the National Council on Aging[5] it was found that older people were almost as negative in their attitudes about aging as were their younger counterparts. Few people in a sample of 4000 chose the years between 60 and 80 as "the best of my life" and about one third considered this period as the least desirable time of their life.[5]

Attitude barriers on the part of both the elderly and health care providers interfere with effective service utilization. Hagebak and Hagebak[20] described psychological barriers held by both therapists and elderly clients. They found six major attitude barriers commonly held by therapists: (1) the "you can't teach an old dog new tricks" attitude, which discounts the elderly person's ability to learn, adapt, or change; (2) the "my God, I'm mortal too syndrome," which forces therapists to acknowledge their own aging process; (3) the "why bother?" attitude, which holds that since elderly people have a shortened life span it is hardly worth the effort to work with them; (4) the "I'm a child" belief, which is seen when role reversal occurs and the therapist responds to the older person as though to a parent; (5) the "patient is a child" approach, which discounts the elderly people's abilities by treating them like children; or (6) "senility is natural," which expects the elderly person to be forgetful, slow, etc. Often the elderly respond to these attitudes like a self-fulfilling prophecy and behave accordingly.

Nurses can overcome these attitude hurdles by first recognizing that the older person is a person who just happened to grow older but is not basically different from other people. The next step is introspection or conscious examination of one's feelings toward aging and death. Attitudes, beliefs, and feelings are generally clearly transmitted to others, hence, personal awareness is extremely important.

Like nurses and other health care providers, elderly people often hold attitudes that are barriers to obtaining mental health services. They often believe that "senility is natural" and expect to evidence psychological changes. Thus they view any mental health changes as inevitable and often fail to seek assistance for problems that could be treated or reversed. Elderly people often question their value by asking "who/why am I?" They believe that since they no longer work and their children are grown they have lost their value to society. A third attitude held by the elderly is one of fierce independence, or "do for yourself," whereby they hesitate to seek the assistance of others. The counterpart to this attitude is "I'm distrustful and afraid," in which the elderly fear the services provided by anyone associated with the mental health system. Last, elderly people may evidence a "doing what's expected" syndrome in which they support stereotypes or their perceptions of what others expect of them.[20] These barriers tend to arise because both nurses and clients are unfamiliar with the aging process.

Severe psychological decline is not an inevitable part of aging. Although some physiological changes do occur with aging, many others can be prevented by modification of the environment, such as overcoming attitudes that expect the elderly to respond in less than functional ways, reducing stress, and simple techniques, such as speaking clearly and audibly. As with all age groups, stress interferes with accurate perception of environmental cues as well as problem-solving ability. Stimuli that tend to set off a stress response are those which are novel, rapidly changing, or unexpected.

The most common psychiatric problem among the elderly is depression. Old age is a time of numerous losses. For many, retirement, while eagerly anticipated, reflects a loss of meaningful involvement with the larger society. Also, friends and family members begin to die, skills and abilities may diminish, and even homes and familiar possessions are lost. The effects of several drugs commonly consumed by elderly people contribute to depression; including digitalis; antihypertensives, especially reserpine; antiparkinsonism drugs; corticosteroids; antianxiety drugs; and even some antidepressants.[19]

The interaction of drugs is a particular problem for the elderly who often mix medications. Comfort[10] says that the first operation in geriatric psychiatry is the "plastic bag test," which means to collect all the medication the patient is taking. Often some were prescribed, others were purchased over the counter, and still other medication was provided by friends or family. Not only do the elderly inadvertently mix medications but many use drugs and alcohol to cope with stress, loneliness, or feelings of fear, anxiety, or loss.

The elderly are not a homogeneous group. Each one is a unique person with needs, desires, assets, and support networks. In providing mental health services it is important to remember that most elderly people do not live in institutions but rather are able to maintain their own home or live with friends or family members. Often a primary mental health goal is that of helping the family identify and use its own strengths to support and respond effectively to elderly members. Hamrick and Blazer[21] describe a program that helps family members identify and use their own strengths to help elderly relatives. They assess areas such as recent events that may have been stressful, the developmental history of both the patient and the family, impairments in the older adult, family conflicts, and support (both tangible and intangible). Once the assessment is completed, one or more of five major approaches is generally used: (1) explain the patient's impairment and capabilities to the family, (2) inform the family about community resources and how to use them, (3) evaluate respite activities of the family, (4) allow members to express and work through their feelings, and (5) provide opportunities for the family to make decisions about the care of the older adult.

To respond effectively to the mental health needs of the elderly, nurses must use an integrated approach that takes into account the multiple stressors as well as the resources available for effective coping. Older people are not normally sick or crazy and they can learn and do respond to treatment.[10] Their mental health needs are just as great as are those of younger members of society.

Deinstitutionalization: impact on long-term psychiatric patients

With the Community Mental Health Centers Act of 1963 and the 1978 report of the Joint Commission on Mental Illness and Health come mandates for providing decentralized community care for long-term psychiatric patients. During the 15 years between these two significant mental health documents there has been a dramatic decrease in the populations of state hospitals. The question arises as to whether the patients are sufficiently well to negotiate the community system or whether many have been discharged without adequate preparation and subsequent follow-up care relative to community living.

The paradoxical nature of the *Wyatt vs. Stickney* decision of 1972 affects the goal of decentralization. Essentially the U.S. Supreme Court ordered the State of Alabama to draw up within 6 months a comprehensive plan for providing relevant treatment for all patients in mental health facilities. The court order required (1) a humane psychological and physical environment, (2) qualified staff in sufficient numbers to provide adequate treatment, and (3) individualized treatment plans.[28] The significance of this court order is that funds mandated for community mental health were reallocated for inpatient care, thereby seriously altering any attempts to plan new approaches for discharged mentally ill persons. In particular this court action emphasizes the pressure community mental health experiences from legal and, especially, federal and state funding decisions. The majority of mental health programs depend largely on external funding sources, which often limit creativity and innovation.

In a further judicial decision, *O'Connor vs. Donaldson,* the Supreme Court ruled unanimously that mentally ill patients who pose no threat to society and who are able to survive outside the hospital cannot be confined against their will and without treatment.[28] A key point relates to the definition of "ability to survive"; the whole question of quality of life can be raised. The majority of long-term psychiatrically hospitalized patients pose no societal threat; many, though, are incapable of meeting the barest needs for survival. For example, for the patient who has been hospitalized for 15 years, the reality shock resulting from spontaneous hospital discharge and the immediate need for survival can be overwhelming. Merely securing a place to live, purchasing food, and arranging for household utilities is a task compounded by gross lack of familiarity with each system involved.

Another issue that must be at the forefront of planning for a community approach is that the majority of individuals who are hospitalized for an extended period are diagnosed as schizophrenic. These individuals often lack the self-concept and confidence required to demand quality services. Furthermore, lengthy hospitalization tends to prepare individuals for a subservient role that hinders the ability to meet their needs in a societal context.

One of the basic principles of community mental health ideology refers to continuity of care. If programs are to be effective, some member of the staff must maintain contact with and responsibility for each discharged patient as he moves from one system to another.[45] Although this belief is widely held, it is infrequently practiced. Few community mental health approaches provide systematic assistance in locating housing, obtaining employment, managing finances, developing a social system for interaction, and, of primary importance, teaching basic coping skills essential to functioning outside the hospital.[48] A large number of patients discharged from public mental hospitals lack problem-solving abilities to meet the goals and demands of life outside the hospital.

Rachlin[41] contends that the major reasons why deinstitutionalization has not been successful is that the needs of patients and the directions of programs have been disjointed. In many instances, deinstitutionalization has served only to decrease the population in mental hospitals. Substitute domiciles and coordinated integrated program planning for discharged patients has been lacking in both quality and quantity. Additionally, even when unique model programs

have been successfully developed, it has been a challenge to sustain enthusiasm for the goal because dealing with chronically ill patients is difficult and does not always provide visible and immediate treatment results.

Dickey et al.[15] documented the success of a deinstitutionalization program by studying 27 patients 4 years after discharge. These patients had been hospitalized for an average of 24 years. Using interviews with both patients and caretakers, data were gathered regarding the place of residence, mental status, time spent in the hospital since discharge, level of functioning, and quality of life. The authors found that rehospitalization decreased significantly once patients moved from the hospital to the community. They also found that the best predictor of success at remaining in the community was age of hospital admission. Those who entered the hospital at an early age had increased difficulty readjusting to community life. They also found that all but two preferred their present living situation to that of the hospital. Also, patients living in the community had a better average mental status score and level of functioning than patients who were currently hospitalized. This study supported the belief that organized and systematic aftercare is a prerequisite for maintaining chronically ill patients in the community.

Personnel deployment poses a serious consideration when large numbers of patients are discharged into community-care programs. The dilemma in deployment planning is whether personnel familiar with one role can focus their attention on a new concept of mental health care. Inpatient psychiatric care has been accused of rigidity, lack of interest in the individual, and limited creativity. Each of these criticisms must be reversed if community care is to enhance mental health. For a community to establish a comprehensive program for discharged patients, inpatient services must be available. It can be anticipated that some patients will experience an exacerbation of symptoms and require short-term hospitalization.

PROPOSAL FOR NURSING INTERVENTION. A comprehensive community-based program for discharged mentally ill patients encompasses community acceptance, client advocacy, teaching basic skills of everyday living, and ongoing support in the form of individual or group supervision.[52] Although a collaborative interdisciplinary approach is required to implement the community follow-up plan, the nursing component is emphasized. Although a variety of professionals could serve as coordinators of the program, the community mental health nurse is used in the following proposal. Public health nurses are described as the actual client advocates in that they possess knowledge, skill, and an entrée in regard to community care. Ideally a plan should be developed prior to the discharge of psychiatric patients; in reality, a large number of patients already reside in the community despite lack of coping skills. Therefore a community program could begin with patients already in need of supervision or start with newly discharged persons.

Prior to the onset of a continuity-of-care program for discharged patients some degree of community responsibility should be assured. Interaction should occur in advance of purchasing or leasing any property for a transition home or similar group residence. The purpose of staff and community dialogue is to discuss plans, elicit fears from residents, and assess the degree of support available in a given community. Community residents often cite fears of physical assault, bizarre behavior, or a decrease in property values. In truth, communities may profit from a group home in that housing in poor repair is often secured because of limited funds. Residents and staff frequently attack renovations with zeal and soon increase property values.

Clients must be taught basic skills of daily living before they are discharged from the hospital. Activities such as meal preparation, budgeting, doing laundry, and use of public transportation and telephones are often foreign to individuals hospitalized for many years. They may need to practice social skills, such as job seeking, shopping, and requesting services. Teaching strategies include instruction, demonstration, and practice either through simulations, such as role playing, or actual performance of an activity, such as meal planning, shopping, and food preparation. The community mental health nurse often coordinates activities designed to facilitate reentry into society. Hospital staff provide the actual teaching with coordination and supervision from the consultant.

The concept of client advocacy has long been discussed, but there has been little comprehensive use. Public health nurses are used as client advocates, since they have ready access to both clients and the mental health system. In essence, each client has a public health nurse who monitors his functioning and progress much as in hospital rounds. Each nurse is as-

signed a certain number of clients; the nursing role is to help clients interact more effectively with the multitude of community systems supportive to daily living. Not only does the nurse make home visits and coordinate client activities, but she also includes each client in a small group that meets regularly to discuss common problems.

Each group session focuses on a specific topic. Lack of structure proves threatening for many. Topics such as side effects of medication, rehabilitation plans, or problems in getting along with others are discussed.[16] The objectives of the group session include (1) helping clients function outside the institution through support and medication monitoring, (2) reinforcing strengths, and (3) assisting clients to learn more effective ways to interact with others.[34] The community mental health nurse serves as consultant and coordinator by meeting regularly with each public health nurse or group of nurses to discuss common case load difficulties. The consultant supports the other nurses just as they support the clients.

Davies[13] describes a Continuing Care Program at Western Psychiatric Institute and Clinic in Pennsylvania that implements many of the concepts noted in the model presented. In the Pennsylvania program a model approach was designed to meet the needs of chronically ill psychiatric patients. In this program each client is provided with a continuum of care that meets individual needs. Each is assessed as to physical and psychological status, sociocultural variables, and community support network. Services are offered in three categories: direct, community, and case management.

Direct services include individual, group, or family counseling based on a crisis intervention framework. Community coping skills are also assessed, and structured activities are arranged where needed to teach basic skills. Also, outreach services include home visits or telephone calls when patients cannot come to the unit. Educational opportunities teach skills, medication maintenance, and so forth. The second set of services include the community network, which provides consultation and education to the community to strengthen resources available to chronically ill patients. The third set of services refer to case management, including coordination of services and active involvement in the treatment program.

Interdisciplinary collaboration in community mental health

Interdisciplinary interaction is a basic tenet of community mental health. In the community mental health movement, professionals increasingly seem to perform tasks using strikingly similar skills. Further rapid societal change has demanded new services to meet the mental health needs of consumers. Health professionals are attempting to adapt, change, and expand skills to provide a relevant service to consumers. The subsequent "identity crisis" in what belongs uniquely to each profession has added stress to the effectiveness of service delivery.[3] Nursing is changing rapidly, as is every other health profession. Each nurse should have a clear concept of nursing's unique role and contribution to the team. To interpret one's role and maintain accountability, one must know what is implicit in the role as well as where one's area of responsibility ends.

Interprofessional teamwork is subject to the same rules of group process as any other organized group. Considerable time and energy must be expended to facilitate team communication so as to define and delegate responsibilities and thus avoid infringing on each other's sense of territoriality. A major team goal is to determine comfortable and mutually satisfactory modes of interaction and relationship negotiation. Teamwork is a problem-solving approach both to providing services and determining ways in which members can work together. It is essential that the team be clear about the purposes, goals, and individual member responsibilities and that a mechanism be established for renegotiation of roles. Just stating the goals of the team in no way ensures consensus. Dialogue is continuous in an interdisciplinary team, with modification of goals and strategies integral to functioning.

Interprofessional teams typically go through a series of interactional stages: (1) early enthusiasm and lively interest in each other's contributions, (2) insecurity and sense of role threat combined with guarding of one's territory, and (3) role negotiation and effective functioning or abandonment of the team concept. Teams in community mental health are described as more democratic than those in other settings. Also, the leader is likely to be elected rather than designated by job title. Decisions regarding the tasks of team members are made on the basis of competence, interest, availability, and match between client or family needs and provider ability and preference.

Evaluation in community mental health

Community mental health is a new concept in a field that is defined by lack of agreement about values, modes of treatment, and standards of practice. Evaluation, although exceedingly difficult because of the intangible nature of community mental health services, is essential as a system for quality control and a catalyst for accountability. Program evaluation must answer questions both as to the quantity and quality of services.

Quality assessment methodologies

In general, three quality assessment methodologies—structure, process, and outcome—used either singly or in combination, comprise the foundation of current health care standards' procedures. In the structural approach to quality assessment, standards and criteria are designed to determine the impact of organizational patterns on the delivery of quality health care services. Two basic assumptions underlie the use of a structural approach: it is possible to assess what is "good" by identifying staff, physical, and organizational structure, and care is improved as staff qualifications are upgraded, physical facilities are improved, and sounder fiscal and administration procedures are applied.[39] Structural standards are widely used in assessment because they provide a means to assess quantifiable data. This method is traditionally undertaken by the government, since it is the easiest to apply.

In the process approach to assessing quality care the activities of health professionals are evaluated in terms of what is determined to be "good care." The assumption underlying process assessment is that health care providers can agree on what constitutes quality care. Process standards are of two types: "normative," which are derived from the formulations of recognized leaders, and "empirical," which are based on actual patterns of care. Both approaches entail observation and experimentation and change over time. This approach is largely used by the providers to pinpoint problem areas.

The outcome approach assesses care on the basis of the result of treatment. These standards measure survival, recovery, and the patient's satisfaction with his treatment. Outcome measures can be used by both government and the providers and are considered by many to be the most useful forms of evaluation, albeit the most difficult to obtain.

National standards

The National Standards for Community Mental Health Centers developed by the NIMH describe three major areas for evaluation. Attention is focused on administration and direction of the center, which includes organizational patterns, staffing, facilities, use review, and provision for requested information. The second category of evaluation calls attention to accessibility and specifically focuses on community orientation, visibility, prevention, including consultation and education, and coordination and collaboration with other agencies. The third area relates to specific service activities and includes the five major modes of treatment: inpatient, outpatient, partial hospitalization, emergency care, consultation and education, and individualized treatment plans, a range of treatment modalities, and continuity of care. As a public agency NIMH evaluates programs to ensure that grant recipients are using their funds according to stipulated guidelines. The governmental monitoring process is carried out through site visits, applications for future support, and an annual inventory completed by each center.[18]

Issues in evaluation

Within each community mental health program a decision must be reached as to the mode of evaluation. The major decision includes selecting between a structural approach, which relies largely on enumeration, and an outcome methodology, which is more difficult to complete but may be more useful in terms of program change to provide more relevant services to consumers. Although quantity of services, that is, the number of individuals who partake of any service, is far easier to measure than quality, relevant evaluation demands attention to effectiveness of services delivered. Client outcomes after treatment constitute a major criterion for evaluation. Outcome is measured against predetermined goals often stated in the form of behavioral objectives. A current disadvantage to this method of evaluation is that little outcome or follow-up data are collected in community mental health programs. Evaluation is one segment of a total monitoring package that focuses on how services affect the clients who receive them.[49] Follow-up examination is a component of evaluation that examines long-range effects of treatment approaches.

An outcome evaluation program begins with stated goals determined at the onset of treatment. Essentially the client and the nurse decide what they expect to accomplish in the treatment relationship. Many call this delineation of goals a contract. The items on the contract are stated in behavioral terms, such as "the patient will return to work with less than a 10% absentee rate due to 'nervousness.'" The major problem in outcome evaluation relates to determining the measurements to be assessed. What kinds of information or change constitute effective treatment? Outcome measures should be simple, concrete, readily observable or measurable, and open to minimal interpretation based on opinion. Both client self-reports and nurse observation comprise a component of evaluation. Although indicators, such as number of hours expended in services, number of patients seen, and scope of services offered constitute data for evaluation, these measures are no longer sufficient. Outcome and service effectiveness measures must be included despite the difficulty in establishing such criteria.

Suggested cross-references

Evolutionary perspectives of psychiatric nursing are discussed in Chapter 1. Evaluation of the nursing process is discussed in Chapter 4. Defining mental health, high-risk populations, and primary prevention activities are discussed in Chapter 5. Tertiary prevention and rehabilitation activities are discussed in Chapter 6. Violent behavior is discussed in Chapter 12. Legal aspects of psychiatric care are discussed in Chapter 16. Liaison psychiatric nursing and consultation are discussed in Chapter 23. Family abuse is discussed in Chapter 28. Psychogeriatrics is discussed in Chapter 31.

SUMMARY

1. A brief overview of the history of mental health care in the United States was presented, including the work of Benjamin Rush, Dorothea Dix, and Adolf Meyer. A summary was provided of governmental involvement in the mental health field leading up to the legislation enabling the development of community mental health centers.

2. The five essential services described in the 1963 legislation—inpatient, partial hospitalization, outpatient, emergency care, and consultation and education services—were described as were the additional services of diagnosis, rehabilitation, precare and aftercare, training and research, and evaluation. Modifications of the law included in the 1975 amendments, the 1978 report of the President's Commission on Mental Health, and the 1980 legislation were also described.

3. Several criticisms and benefits of community mental health programs were compared.

4. A brief presentation of systems theory and a holistic view of human beings was included to provide a philosophical foundation for understanding community mental health.

5. The nurse's role in community assessment was addressed. It was emphasized that attention must be given to the needs of the consumer as well as those of the community. Therefore concepts of market segmentation and target marketing were presented as they are applicable to community and consumer assessment.

6. The role of the community mental health nurse in implementation is directed toward the community rather than the individual. This role was further elaborated on according to Caplan's formulations of primary, secondary, and tertiary prevention. Consultation and education are major tools used by the nurse in community mental health.

7. Four high-risk populations were identified and discussed in terms of the applicable level of prevention and appropriate nursing interventions. They were the family under stress, victims of aggression, the elderly, and discharged, mentally ill persons. Families under stress included those with new babies, those with a working mother, and those undergoing divorce. The victims of aggression included abused children, battered wives, and families of homicide victims. Issues were presented relative to the needs of elderly people as well as the deinstitutionalization of psychiatric patients, and a model for nursing intervention was described.

8. The concept of the mental health team was described as it pertains to the role of the community mental health nurse.

9. Evaluation is an extremely important facet of community mental health and was presented in terms of both quantity and quality of services. Methods of evaluation are applied to structure, process, or outcome of services.

References

1. Arnhoff, F.N.: Social consequences of policy toward mental illness, Science **188:**1277, 1975.
2. Babigian, H.: The impact of community mental health centers on the utilization of services, Arch. Gen. Psychiatry **34:**385, 1977.
3. Bandler, B.: Interprofessional collaboration in training in mental health, Am. J. Orthopsychiatry **43:**97, Jan. 1973.
4. Berlin, I.N.: Resistance to mental health consultation directed at change in public institutions, Community Ment. Health J. **15**(2):119, 1979.
5. Beverly, E.V.: The beginning of wisdom about aging, Geriatrics **30**(7):117, 1975.
6. Bloom, B.L.: Prevention of mental disorders: recent advances in theory and practice, Community Ment. Health J. **15**(3):179, 1979.
7. Burgess, A.W.: Family reaction to homicide, Am. J. Orthopsychiatry **45:**391, 1975.
8. Caplan, G.: Principles of preventive psychiatry, New York, 1964, Basic Books, Inc., Publishers.
9. Cherniss, C.: Creating new consultation programs in community mental health centers: analysis of a case study, Community Ment. Health J. **13:**133, Summer 1977.
10. Comfort, A.: Geriatric psychiatry: mental symptoms in old age, Ala. J. Med. Sci. **18**(2):177, 1981.
11. Community Mental Health Services Support Branch: A citizens guide to the community mental health centers amendments of 1975, Washington, D.C., 1977, U.S. Government Printing Office.
12. Council of Advanced Practitioners in Psychiatric and Mental Health Nursing: Pacesetter **2:**2, Spring 1977.
13. Davies, M.A.: Continuing care unit: a model of services for chronic psychiatric patients, J. Psychiatr. Nurs. **19**(2):42, 1981.
14. DeWild, D.W.: Toward a clarification of primary prevention, Community Ment. Health J. **16:**306, 1981.
15. Dickey, B., et al.: A follow-up of deinstitutionalized chronic patients four years after discharge, Hosp. Community Psychiatry **32:**326, 1981.
16. Donlon, P., and Rada, R.: Issues in developing quality aftercare clinics for the chronic mentally ill, Community Ment. Health J. **12:**29, Spring 1976.
17. Echeveste, D., and Schlacter, J.: Marketing a strategic framework for health care, Nurs. Outlook **22:**377, 1974.
18. Feldman, S., and Windle, C.: The NIMH approach to

evaluating the community mental health centers program, Health Services Report **88:**174, Feb. 1973.

19. Filner, B., and Williams, R.F.: Health promotion for the elderly: reducing functional dependency. In Healthy people: the surgeon general's report on health promotion and disease prevention, Washington, D.C., 1979, U.S. Department of Health, Education, and Welfare.

20. Hagebak, J.E., and Hagebak, B.R.: Serving the mental health needs of the elderly: the case for removing barriers and improving service integration, Community Ment. Health J. **16:**263, 1980.

21. Hamrick, K., and Blazer, D.: Older adults and their families in a community mental health center: strategies for intervention, Hosp. Community Psychiatry **31:**332, 1980.

22. Helfer, R.E., and Kempe, C.H.: Child abuse and neglect—the family and the community, Cambridge, Mass., 1976, Ballinger Publishing Co.

23. Herman, S.: Divorce: a grief process, Perspect. Psychiatr. Care **12:**108, May 1974.

24. Hetherington, M., Cox, M., and Cox, R.: Divorced fathers, Psychol. Today **10:**42, April 1977.

25. Hopkins, J.: The nurse and the abused child, Nurs. Clin. North Am. **5:**589, 1970.

26. Joint Commission on Mental Illness and Health: Action for mental health, New York, 1961, Basic Books, Inc., Publishers.

27. Kalter, N.: Children of divorce in an outpatient psychiatric population, Am. J. Orthopsychiatry **47**(1):40, 1977.

28. Kaplan, H.A.: Institutions and community mental health: the paradox in *Wyatt v. Stickney,* Community Ment. Health J. **9:**34, Spring 1973.

29. Kelley, J., and Wallerstein, J.: Brief interventions with children in divorcing families, Am. J. Orthopsychiatry **47:**23, 1977.

30. Lancaster, J.: Coping mechanisms of working mothers, Am. J. Nurs. **75:**1322, 1975.

31. Landsberg, G., and Hammer, R.: Possible programmatic consequences of Community Mental Health Center funding arrangements: illustrations based on inpatient utilization data, Community Ment. Health J. **13:**63, Spring 1977.

32. Langsley, D.G.: The community mental health center: does it treat patients? Hosp. Community Psychiatry **31:**815, 1980.

33. Lieberknecht, K.: Helping the battered wife, Am. J. Nurs. **78:**654, 1978.

34. Lindberg, H., and Braach, C.H.: Community health nursing in the changing mental health scene, J. Nurs. Admin. **3:**41, Nov. 1973.

35. Marmor, J.: The relationship between systems theory and community psychiatry, Hosp. Community Psychiatry **26:**807, 1975.

36. MH-MR Report: A Morris Associates report from Washington, D.C. **15:**1, May 5, 1978.

37. Murray, J.: Failure of the community mental health movement, Am. J. Nurs. **75:**2034, 1975.

38. National Council of Community Mental Health Centers: Renewal of CMHC Act: amendments to PL 94-63, Washington, D.C., 1977.

39. National Institute of Mental Health: National standards for community mental health centers: report to Congress, Rockville, Md., 1977, The Institute.

40. Nation's health. Mental health bill signed into law, Washington, D.C., Am. Public Health Assoc. **10**(11):1, 1980.

41. Rachlin, S.: When schizophrenia comes marching home, Psychiatric Q. **50**(3):202, 1978.

42. Ramshorn, M.T.: The major thrust in American psychiatry: past, present, and future, Perspect. Psychiatr. Care **9**(4):144, 1971.

43. Raths, L., Harmin, M., and Simon, S.: Values and teaching, Columbus, Ohio, 1966, Charles E. Merrill Books, Inc.

44. Rubins, J.: The community mental health movement in the United States circa 1970, Am. J. Psychoanal. **31:**68, Jan. 1971.

45. Ruybal, S.: Community health planning, Fam. Commun. Health **1:**9, Spring 1978.

46. Schulberg, H., Becker, A., and McGrath, M.: Planning the phasedown of mental hospitals, Community Ment. Health J. **12:**3, Spring 1976.

47. Shanok, S.S., and Lewis, D.D.: Juvenile court versus child guidance referral: psychological and parental factors, Am. J. Psychiatry **134:**1130, 1977.

48. Snow, D., and Newton, P.: Task, social structure, and social process in the community mental health center movement, Am. J. Psychol. **31:**582, 1976.

49. Speer, D., and Tapp, J.: Evaluation of mental health service effectiveness: a start up model for established programs, Am. J. Orthopsychiatry **46:**217, 1976.

50. Stewart, E.: The nature of needs assessment in community mental health, Community Ment. Health J. **15:**287, 1979.

51. Tarail, M.: Current and future issues in community mental health, Psychiatric Q. **52**(1):27, 1980.

52. Test, M.A., and Stein, L.: Practical guidelines for the community treatment of markedly impaired patients, Community Ment. Health J. **12:**72, Spring 1976.

53. Tischler, G.L., Henisz, J., Myers, J., and Garrison, V.: Catchmenting and the use of mental health services, Arch. Gen. Psychiatry **27:**389, 1972.

54. Zusman, J., and Lamb, J.R.: In defense of community mental health, Am. J. Psychiatry **134:**887, 1977.

Annotated suggested readings

Baizerman, M., and Hall, W.: Consultation as a political process, Community Ment. Health J. **13:**142, Spring 1977.

The authors view consultation as a political-bargaining process in which actors seek to maximize, at minimal cost, expertise, organizational position, and organizational reputation. The consultant functions as an agent of his employer. From the perspective of consultation as a political-bargaining process, three social norms are

evidenced: influencing, manipulating, and negotiating. These are accepted ways to control differences, reach a settlement, or exchange expertise. The possibility exists that bargaining and influencing can provide gain to the participants, and participation in the bargaining system is "open" on some issues and "closed" on others.

Barnhill, L.R.: Basic interventions for violence in families, Hosp. Community Psychiatry **31:**547, 1980.

The author describes five basic stages for intervening in violent family situations. These include crisis management of the ongoing threat of violence, initial assessment and contract making, a complete evaluation, brief treatment, and longer term treatment. In the majority of instances these stages occur sequentially, although clients discontinue treatment when symptoms are in remission, which means that few actually stay involved from crisis management through long-term care.

Bassuk, E., and Gerson, S.: Deinstitutionalization and mental health services, Sci. Am. **238**:46, Feb. 1978.

This article discusses the many problems related to deinstitutionalization and the care of discharged psychiatric patients in the community. Major issues addressed include deficiencies in follow-up care, lack of community facilities, inadequacy of insurance coverage for mental health treatment, and role conflicts among the psychiatric disciplines.

Braff, J., and Lefkowitz, M.M.: Community mental health treatment: what works for whom? Psychiatric Q. **51**(2): 119, 1979.

A review of literature was completed to determine what type of patient functions best in what type of community setting. The findings were classified into four substantive areas, including recidivism, symptoms, social functioning, and employment. The authors failed to document from their review what type of patient functions best in what kind of community setting. They identified patient characteristics that seem to be related to the need for rehospitalization.

Feldman, S.: Promises, promises or community mental health services and training: ships that pass in the night, Community Ment. Health J. **14**(2):83, 1978.

The community mental heath system is described as one of oversell in which what was advertised and indeed promised simply was not delivered. Legislation, objectives, and unrealistic expectations account for part of this problem. Also, the problem of "overpromise" of services is compounded by the discrepancy between the services scheduled to be provided and the education and preparation of the providers. What is taught in schools for health care providers is not consistent with the skills required to provide the services promised by the community mental health movement. Feldman proposes new curricula for mental health practitioners that would reflect the needs of the population being served in contrast to continuing to emphasize traditional mental health approaches.

Forstenzer, H.M.: Planning and evaluation of community mental health programs, Psychiatric Q. **52**(1):38, 1980.

In recent years an abundance of federal reports and legislation have emphasized and in some cases mandated the need for more effective planning for community mental health services. Planners must translate this momentum on systematic planning into action in the form of programs that effectively meet the needs of the populations being served. In the past programs have been revamped without the benefit of research to support the direction being taken. The following are baseline data that must be known before planning starts: where we are, where we are going, and what changes are needed to get there. Those who undertake planning efforts need to know about the regulations under which they operate, the nature of the community, the number and type of clients needing care, and what priorities exist.

Hendrix, M., LaGodna, G., and Bohen, C.: The battered wife, Am. J. Nurs. **78**:651, 1978.

An overview of wife battering is presented in this article, which effectively directs the reader's attention to the magnitude and ramifications of the problem. Also, strategies for nursing intervention are described, which center around a problem-solving approach.

Johnson, C.L.: The American family during inflationary times, Psychiatric Opinion **16**(9):13, 1979.

The author discusses the psychological effects of inflation that are insidious and produce less dramatic changes than sudden economic upsets. Instead of a sudden change, in inflationary times people witness a steady decrease in buying power and a consequent gradual change in life-style. These economic changes also affect other areas. In fiscally tight times, families try to increase their buying power, for example, by more women entering the job market. Economic change causes family stress that is often manifested in interpersonal conflict. Lowered feelings of self-worth are seen, and the elderly are especially vulnerable.

Lamb, H.R.: What did we really expect from deinstitutionalization? Hosp. Community Psychiatry **32**(2):105, 1981.

The author asks the question of "what went wrong with deinstitutionalization?" He posits the belief that severely disabled psychiatric patients have remained a marginal population with few continuity of care programs actually helping them to effectively assimilate back into the community. He contends that the goal of making it possible for these patients to live with dignity in a comfortable low-energy but satisfying life-style is a great step toward achieving the initial goals of deinstitutionalization.

Lyon, G., and Hitchens, E.: Ways of intervening with the psychotic individual in the community, Am. J. Nurs. **79**: 490, 1979.

This article addresses an important problem—how to help the psychotic individual in a community setting. It is practical, realistic, and uses clinical examples to reinforce major points.

President's Commission on Mental Health: Report to the president, vol. 1, Washington, D.C., 1978.

This is a government report of a 1-year study commissioned by President Carter to review the mental health needs in the United States. It is strongly recommended that psychiatric nurses be familiar with the content of this report, although its actual impact on legislation and funding has been diminished with the Reagan administration.

Register, D.: Community mental health for whose community, Am. J. Public Health **64**:886, 1974.

Eight conceptual models of community are presented with brief outlines of the implications of each model. Characteristics of community mental health centers that are described include target populations, staff, awareness of community needs, and the effect of center programs on the community.

Scharer, K.: Nursing therapy with abusive and neglectful families, J. Psychiatr. Nurs. **17**(9):12, 1979.

Three major elements are described as components of the battered child syndrome: the parents must have the potential for abuse that is acquired during their childhood; the second factor is the child, since many abused children are special in some way, such as having a feeding problem as an infant or being mentally retarded, and a crisis often precipitates the abuse. The dynamics in neglect are less well defined and are often seen in aspects of mothering, such as feeding, bathing, and holding the *infant. The author recommends the mother-surrogate subrole as being a viable way to teach mothers basic mothering skills.*

Schecter, D.E.: Women in the labor force: some mental health implications, Psychiatric Opinion **16**(9):17, 1979.

Out of economic necessity an increasing number of women have entered the job market. The majority of these women continue to juggle two or three roles as they try to function as wives, mothers, and working women. The American social structure is still set up as though women are at home taking care of families. Specifically, child care facilities have not kept pace with the demand for quality surrogate environments.

Schulberg, H., Becker, A., and McGrath, M.: Planning the phasedown of mental hospitals, Community Ment. Health J. **12**:3, Spring 1976.

A basic concept in community mental health is continuity of care. How will continuity be maintained as large state hospitals are reduced in size or closed? How will patients and staff be deployed and what follow-up services are imperative?

Severin, N., and Becker, R.: Nurses as psychiatric consultants in a general hospital emergency room, Community Ment. Health J. **10**:261, 1974.

The authors describe a project to study the effectiveness of psychiatric nurses in the emergency room of a general hospital. The program objective was to involve nurses in the initial assessment of candidates for emergency psychiatric services. The nurses successfully managed 66% of the psychiatric referrals and required only telephone consultation in the majority of the remaining cases.

Skinner, P.: Marketing community health services, League Exchange No. 121, Publication No. 21-1757, New York, 1979, The League.

Since community health services are often confronted with limited funds and resources, the use of marketing is employed to attract patients, health care providers, and to promote the merits of beneficial health care services. The components of the marketing process are identified and a marketing plan is developed. The plan assesses both the internal and external environments, as well as identifies in advance potential obstacles to implementation. The application of marketing concepts to home health care agencies is clearly and concisely made.

CHAPTER 20

CRISIS
THERAPY

Sandra E. Benter

Our moulting season, like that of the fowls,
must be a crisis in our lives.

Henry David Thoreau

Learning objectives

After studying this chapter, the student
should be able to:

- *describe the history of crisis theory, specifying the contributions of Lindemann and Caplan.*

- *define crisis and explain its potential for disorganization or personal growth.*

- *relate Caplan's four phases of a crisis and impinging "balancing factors."*

- *discuss the etiology of the three types of crises: maturational, situational, or adventitious.*

- *analyze the goal, scope, and phases of crisis intervention.*

- *describe four levels of crisis intervention and eight therapeutic techniques.*

- *compare and contrast the nursing process and crisis intervention methodology.*

- *evaluate the various modalities of crisis intervention and the settings in which they may be employed.*

- *discuss future trends in crisis therapy.*

- *identify suggested readings for future study.*

Historical perspective

Historically, crisis theory is an outgrowth of psychoanalytical theory. Analytical theory proposes that there are unconscious links to behavior and that dynamic formulations can be made to explain the causes of behavior. The causes are found in one's early experiences of infancy and childhood and affect one throughout his life span. There are many areas of conflict within the individual, and for those conflicts to be resolved constructively, they must be geared toward adaptation to the environment. For example, to be socially acceptable, one's aggressive impulses can be channeled into competitive business practices rather than the physical harm of a rival.

Those who studied and practiced preventive psychiatry used psychoanalytical concepts to develop crisis theory. They explored the feasibility of intervening briefly during stressful periods to resolve the problem in an adaptive or positive way. They observed a specific sequence of phases that individuals experienced when faced with stressful situations and studied the outcomes of the crises. Crisis intervention techniques were then determined for the purpose of facilitating favorable outcomes.

Eric Lindemann,[20] in 1944, studied 101 patients in crisis. He included psychoneurotic patients who lost a relative during the course of treatment, relatives of patients who died in the hospital, bereaved disaster victims (Coconut Grove fire) and their relatives, and relatives of members of the armed forces. Lindemann observed the course of normal grief and the symptomatology of morbid grief reactions. Those bereaved individuals undergoing normal grief showed signs of somatic distress, preoccupation with the image of the deceased, hostile reactions, guilt, changes in patterns of activity, and sometimes the taking on of characteristics of the deceased. Those individuals undergoing morbid grief reactions demonstrated either delayed or distorted reactions. Distorted reactions included overactivity without a sense of loss, the acquisition of symptoms belonging to the last illness of the deceased, the development of a medical disease, an alteration in relationships to friends and relatives, the development of furious hostility against specific persons, and the development of a clinical agitated depression.

Lindemann saw the role of mental health workers to be that of helping the patient extricate himself from his ties to the deceased and find new patterns of rewarding interaction. He believed the concept of intervention during bereavement could be applied to intervention during other stressful situations such as marriage and the birth of a child. Thus the prevention of psychiatric disorders could be accomplished. He envisioned this accomplishment as taking place in the community and being patterned after a public health model so that many people could be reached. Lindemann, along with Gerald Caplan, actually set up a community mental health clinic in Massachussets where crisis intervention was practiced.

In 1964 Caplan formally introduced concepts of community mental health practice. In addressing himself to primary, secondary, and tertiary preventive aspects of practice, he clearly defined crisis theory and described crisis intervention as a formal therapy in itself.[4] He viewed primary prevention as the social and interpersonal actions that ensure the provision of basic supplies to a community to help it deal constructively with its crises. The prevention of mental disorder is the aim. Social action deals with efforts to work with political and social policies to help people cope with crises, whereas interpersonal action deals with helping individuals with their specific stresses.

Secondary prevention aims to decrease the number of existing cases through early diagnosis and effective treatment. Early referral, screening programs, and improvement in diagnostic tools are all examples of secondary prevention. This type of prevention is the more traditional treatment-oriented method of approaching mental illness. Caplan emphasizes that attention must be paid to effective use of mental health workers and knowledge so that the numbers treated successfully will be large enough to make a difference in community rates.

Tertiary prevention aims to reduce the rate of defective functioning caused by one's lowered capacity to contribute to the community after the mental disorder has ceased. Rehabilitation programs therefore focus on tertiary prevention. Secondary prevention includes primary prevention, and tertiary prevention includes both primary and secondary. Crisis therapy is a primary prevention concept and is seen as one of the most effective ways of preventing mental disorder.

In 1963 President Kennedy issued a message on mental illness and mental retardation. After the message, communities began to take on further the responsibility of caring for their own mental health needs. Although many clinicians believed that long-term psychoanalytical psychotherapy was still the preferred treatment, it was impractical in that it was expensive, required a lengthy time commitment, and generally did not meet the needs of all socioeconomic strata. It was believed that a method of treatment that was brief, direct, and here-and-now–oriented was necessary. Crisis therapy therefore became more widely used.

Definition of crisis

A crisis is an internal disturbance that results from a stressful event or a perceived threat to self. The individual's usual repertoire of coping mechanisms becomes ineffective in dealing with the threat, and the individual experiences a rise in anxiety. The threat, or precipitating event, can usually be identified. It may have occurred weeks or days ago, and its significance may or may not be linked (in the individual's eyes) to the crisis state. Precipitating events are perceived losses, threats of losses, or challenges.[4] Losses may include the death of a spouse, divorce, or loss of a job. Threats of losses may include illness of a family member or an increase in arguments with a spouse. Challenges may include a change in responsibilities at work or a change to a different line of work. Additional threats or stresses are identified in the Social Readjustment Rating Scale (Chapter 4).

In response to the threat or precipitating event the individual's level of anxiety rises and Caplan's[4] four phases of a crisis emerge. In the first phase the anxiety stimulates one's usual methods of coping into action. If these do not bring relief and there is inadequate situational support, the individual progresses to the second phase in which he becomes even more anxious as a result of the failure of his coping mechanisms. In the third phase the individual tries out new coping mechanisms or redefines the threat so that old ones can work. Resolution of the problem therefore can occur in this phase. If resolution does not occur, however, the individual goes on to the fourth phase in which the continuation of severe or panic levels of anxiety may lead to psychological disorganization. The phases of a crisis parallel the process of

*Balancing factor

FIG. 20-1
Effect of balancing factors in a stressful event. (From Aguilera, D.C., and Messick, J.M.: Crisis intervention: theory and methodology, ed. 4, St. Louis, 1982, The C.V. Mosby Co.)

the development of anxiety, as described in Chapter 7, and both these concepts are closely related. However, by definition, crises are self-limiting. A period of approximately 6 weeks is considered to be the span needed for resolution, whether it be a positive solution or a state of disorganization.

In describing the phases of a crisis, some important balancing factors need to be considered.[1] These balancing factors are one's perception of the event, situational supports, and coping mechanisms. Successful resolution of the crisis is more likely if the individual's perception of the event is realistic rather than distorted, if there are situational supports available to the individual so that others can help him solve the problem, and if the individual has coping mechanisms available to him that alleviate anxiety. These balancing factors are represented in the paradigm developed by Aguilera and Messick (Fig. 20-1). *(numerous amound)*

Symptoms of individuals in crisis are myriad. They can include helplessness, anxiety, confusion, depression, anger, withdrawal, psychosomatic symptoms, inefficiency, and hopelessness. Suicidal and homicidal thoughts may be present. Feelings of alienation from others occur frequently. Sometimes the formation of these symptoms can cause further hardships. For example, inefficiency at work may lead to the loss of a job, financial problems, and ultimately lowered self-esteem.[17] Crises can also be complicated by old internal conflicts. These previous conflicts can be reactivated by the present conflict and make the crisis resolution more difficult to attain.

An important aspect of crisis theory is that the 4 to 6 weeks of conflict are a time of increased vulnerability and can produce increased growth. Crises occur in the lives of all individuals. It is what one does with the crises that will determine whether growth or disorganization results. Growth comes from experiencing and learning in new situations. Individuals in crisis feel uncomfortable and often reach out for help. They are in turmoil and are ready to accept influence from others until they feel psychological equilibrium has returned. The fact that crises can stimulate personal growth is an important one for the nurse to consider when working with patients in crisis situations.

Types of crises

Crisis can be divided into three types: maturational, situational, and adventitious. Sometimes more than one type of crisis can occur at the same time. Thus an individual undergoing a maturational crisis can simultaneously have a situational stress that adds to his anxiety. For example, an adolescent who is having difficulty adjusting to his change of role and body image can, at the same time, experience the death of a parent.

Maturational crises

Developmental psychology describes a succession of steps one must take in the continuous task of growing toward maturity. As an individual passes from one stage to another, he goes through transitional periods during which his psychological equilibrium is upset. These periods are developmental, or maturational, crises.

Erik Erikson[10,11] described eight stages of development from infancy to old age and the relationship of each stage to the ones before and after. Each stage presents a central problem or task that must be resolved by the individual for him to move on to the next developmental stage. Within his theory Erikson emphasizes that development is a continuum in which each stage has a part, and the tasks of each stage must be completed for the individual to grow further and move toward maturity. As the personality of the individual matures, he learns to cope with the stresses of life. Erikson points out that this mastery of tasks leads to successful solutions of maturational crises.

Havighurst[14] also identified specific developmental tasks for each major developmental period from infancy through death. Table 20-1 compares Erikson's and Havighurst's developmental stages and tasks. Together they present a comprehensive view of human development and its crises.

Maturational crises are periods requiring role changes. For example, when one grows from early childhood to middle childhood, he is expected to become socially involved with people outside the family rather than limiting his involvement to the family alone. When one advances from adolescence to adulthood, he is expected to be financially responsible for himself rather than being dependent on his parents. Both social and biological pressures to change can precipitate a crisis. The nature and extent of the maturational crisis can be influenced by the adequacy of role models, interpersonal resources, and the ease of others in accepting the new role.[34] Adequate role models provide the individual with an understanding of how to act in the new role. Interpersonal resources allow the individual the flexibility to try out many new

TABLE 20-1. Comparison of Erikson's and Havighurst's developmental stages and tasks*

Developmental stage	Erikson	Havighurst
Infancy	*Trust vs. mistrust* 1. Oral needs of primary importance 2. Adequate mothering necessary to meet infant's needs 3. Acquisition of hope	1. Learning to walk 2. Learning to take solid foods 3. Learning to talk 4. Learning to control elimination of body wastes 5. Learning sex differences and sexual modesty 6. Achieving physiological stability 7. Forming simple concepts of social and physical reality 8. Learning to relate oneself emotionally to parents, siblings, and other people 9. Learning to distinguish right and wrong and developing a conscience
Toddler years	*Autonomy vs. shame* 1. Anal needs of primary importance 2. Father emerges as important figure 3. Acquisition of will	
Early childhood	*Initiative vs. guilt* 1. Genital needs of primary importance 2. Family relationships contribute to early sense of responsibility and conscience 3. Acquisition of purpose	
Middle childhood	*Industry vs. inferiority* 1. Active period of socialization for child as he moves from family into society 2. Acquisition of competence	1. Learning physical skills necessary for ordinary games 2. Building wholesome attitudes toward oneself as a growing organism 3. Learning to get along with age mates 4. Learning an appropriate sex role 5. Developing fundamental skills in reading, writing, and calculating 6. Developing concepts necessary for everyday living 7. Developing conscience, morality, and scale of values 8. Developing attitudes toward social groups and institutions
Adolescence	*Identity vs. identity diffusion* 1. Search for self in which peers play important part 2. Psychosocial moratorium is provided by society 3. Acquisition of fidelity	1. Accepting one's physique and accepting a masculine or feminine role 2. New relations with age mates of both sexes 3. Emotional independence of parents and other adults 4. Achieving assurance of economic independence 5. Selecting and preparing for an occupation 6. Developing intellectual skills and concepts necessary for civic competence 7. Desiring and achieving socially responsible behavior 8. Preparing for marriage and family life 9. Building conscious values in harmony with adequate scientific world picture
Adulthood	*Intimacy vs. isolation* 1. Characterized by increasing importance of human closeness and sexual fulfillment 2. Acquisition of love	1. Selecting a mate 2. Learning to live with marriage partner 3. Starting family 4. Rearing children 5. Managing home 6. Getting started in occupation 7. Taking on civic responsibility 8. Finding congenial social group

*From Sundeen, S.J., et al.: Nurse-client interaction: implementing the nursing process, ed. 2, St. Louis, 1981, The C.V. Mosby Co.

TABLE 20-1. **Comparison of Erikson's and Havighurst's developmental stages and tasks—cont'd**

Developmental stage	Erikson	Havighurst
Middle age	*Generativity vs. self-absorption* 1. Characterized by productivity, creativity, parental responsibility, and concern for new generation 2. Acquisition of care	1. Achieving adult civic and social responsibility 2. Establishing and maintaining economic standard of living 3. Assisting teenage children to become responsible and happy adults 4. Developing adult leisure-time activities 5. Relating oneself to one's spouse as a person 6. Accepting and adjusting to physiological changes of middle age 7. Adjusting to aging parents
Old age	*Integrity vs. despair* 1. Characterized by a unifying philosophy of life and a more profound love for mankind 2. Acquisition of wisdom	1. Adjusting to decreasing physical strength and health 2. Adjusting to retirement and reduced income 3. Adjusting to death of spouse 4. Establishing explicit affiliation with age group 5. Meeting social and civic obligations 6. Establishing satisfactory physical living arrangements

interpersonal behaviors in his attempt to achieve role changes. The use of others in accepting the new role determines the strength or resistances one comes up against in making role changes. The greater the resistance of others, the more stress the individual faces in making the changes.

Transitional periods during adolescence, parenthood, marriage, midlife, and retirement are key times for maturational crises to occur. Some of the conflicts related to parenthood are evident in Clinical example 20-1.

CLINICAL EXAMPLE 20-1

Ms. J was a 19-year-old black, single, unemployed woman who came to the mental health clinic a month after the birth of her first child. Ms. J complained of feelings of depression. Her symptoms included difficulty falling asleep, early morning awakening, crying spells, a poor appetite, difficulty in caring for the baby because of fatigue and apathy, and thoughts of wanting to hurt the baby. The patient lived with her parents and siblings and had never lived on her own. She had always been dependent on her mother to take care of her and relieve her stresses. Her mother, however, worked and the patient was totally responsible for her daughter's care each day. Also, Ms. J's mother was angry that she had had a child and usually refused to care for the baby. The patient's boyfriend, who was the baby's father, had promised to

marry her, but he had recently decided he was too young to handle the responsibility of a wife and child. In summary, a young woman who had unmet dependency needs of her own was now in a position of parenthood and had to meet the dependency needs of an infant. This precipitated a crisis state for her.

Some of the conflicts related to retirement are presented in Clinical example 20-2.

CLINICAL EXAMPLE 20-2

Mr. R was a 67-year-old white, married pharmacist who came to the mental health clinic complaining of anxiety, depression, and insomnia. His symptoms had begun 2 weeks previously and had steadily increased in intensity since that time. Two weeks ago the patient's wife had become insistent that they begin to make concrete plans to move to a retirement community in Florida. The patient described his wife as a strong willful woman who was also outgoing and charming and made friends easily. He considered himself a quiet nervous person who was comfortable only with old friends and his two sons and their families. Mr. R, although of retirement age, had continued to work as a pharmacist, doing relief work for a drugstore chain when the regular pharmacists were absent. In moving to Florida, the patient would lose his pharmacist's license, which was valid only for his present state of residence. He expressed difficulty in making the transition from a working person to a retired person. He had fears of becoming direction-less and useless. He was anxious about leaving his sons and his friends. The possibility of both complete retirement and moving to another state precipitated his present distress.

Situational crises

Situational crises occur when a specific external event upsets an individual's psychological equilibrium or the equilibrium of a group of individuals such as members of a family. Examples of situational crises include the loss of a job, the loss of a loved one, an unwanted pregnancy, the onset or exacerbation of a medical illness, divorce, and school failure or other school problems. The loss of a job can result in financial stress, feelings of inadequacy as a breadwinner, and marital conflict caused by a spouse's anger over the lost job. The loss of a loved one results in bereavement and can also cause financial stress, change of roles of family members, and loss of emotional support. The onset or exacerbation of a medical illness causes fear of the loss of a loved one. Again, financial stress and change of roles of family members often occur. Divorce is similar to the stress of the loss of a loved one, and there is, in addition, the stress of dealing with the ex-spouse. An unwanted pregnancy is a stress in that it requires decisions to be made about whether to complete the pregnancy or to abort it, and whether to keep the baby or place it in adoption. If the baby is to be kept, changes in life-style will be required. School failure or other school problems stress the individual and can lead to serious feelings of inadequacy. Parents often blame themselves or each other, and total family disequilibrium can become manifest.

Some of the stresses related to the exacerbation or onset of a medical illness can be seen in the situational crisis presented in Clinical example 20-3.

CLINICAL EXAMPLE 20-3

Mrs. H is a 55-year-old white married woman whose husband was hospitalized for mitral stenosis. Heart surgery was scheduled for the following week. Mr. H appeared appropriately concerned, but the nursing staff noticed that the patient's wife was becoming increasingly anxious. She spent each day running from her husband's bedside to the nurses' station demanding constant attention. She moved and spoke rapidly and continuously, and at times her thoughts seemed confused. Mrs. H stated that once in the past she had had a "nervous breakdown" and she hoped the stress of her husband's surgery would not result in another one.

Adventitious crises

Adventitious crises are accidental, uncommon, and unexpected crises. Multiple losses with gross environmental changes result. For example, local or mass disasters, such as fires, earthquakes, or floods, which disrupt entire communities, are adventitous crises. Recent mass tragedies, which have become all too common, are also examples of adventitious crises and include group kidnappings (the taking of hostages), nuclear accidents, group killings in communities, and floods complicated by the deposit of industrial waste material along with water.

Unlike maturational and situational crises, adventitious crises do not occur in the lives of everyone. When they do occur, however, they challenge every coping mechanism because of the severity of the stress state they impose. During adventitious crises mental health workers must reach larger numbers of people in crisis states. The multiple losses and gross environmental changes that result from adventitious crises can be seen in the following situation described in a Department of Health, Education, and Welfare publication:

In West Virginia a river filled with coal sludge overflowed when a dam broke, and an entire community was damaged. There were many deaths and injuries, loss of homes and possessions, disruption or loss of employment, sudden relocation, and extreme demands on physical endurance. The solidarity of this isolated rural community was grossly disturbed. The residents suffered a high incidence of mental illness as a result.[7,5]

Disaster-precipitated emotional problems often surface weeks or even months after the disaster. The symptoms usually occur in roughly five phases, which are described in Table 20-2.[12] If the reconstruction phase does not begin within 6 months of the onset of the disaster, the likelihood of lasting psychological problems is greatly increased. The severe psychological stress resulting from adventitious crises can be further illustrated by the findings of Terr who studied 23 child kidnap victims:

TABLE 20-2. Five phases of human disaster response*

Phase	Response
Impact phase	Includes the event itself and is characterized by shock, panic, or extreme fear; the person's judgment and assessment of reality factors are very poor, and self-destructive behavior may be seen
Heroic phase	A cooperative spirit exists between friends, neighbors, and emergency teams; constructive activity at this time can help to overcome feelings of anxiety and depression but overactivity can lead to "burnout"
Honeymoon phase	Begins to appear 1 week to several months after the disaster; the need to help others is sustained, and the money, resources, and support received from various agencies causes life to begin again in the community; psychological and behavioral problems may be overlooked
Disillusionment phase	Lasts from about 2 months to 1 year; a time of disappointment, resentment, frustration, and anger; victims often begin to compare their neighbors' plights with their own and may start to resent, envy, or show hostility toward others
Reconstruction and reorganization phase	Individuals recognize that they must come to grips with their own problems; they begin to rebuild their homes, businesses, and lives in a constructive fashion; this period may last for years after the disaster

*Data from Frederick, C., and Garrison, J.: Behav. Today **12:**32, Aug. 1981.

In the town of Chowchilla, California, a school bus containing 26 children and a bus driver was stopped by three masked men and taken over at gunpoint. The captured children were driven around in boarded over vans for 11 hours and were then transferred to a buried truck trailer. After 16 additional hours, two of the oldest boys dug them out. The children suffered from initial misperceptions, fears of further trauma, and hallucinations. Later they experienced posttraumatic play reenactment, personality change, repeated dreams, fears of being kidnapped again, and a fear of common mundane experiences.[33:14]

Crisis intervention

Aguilera and Messick state:

Crisis intervention can offer the immediate help that a person in crisis needs in order to reestablish equilibrium. This is an inexpensive, short-term therapy that focuses on solving the immediate problem.[1:1]

Crisis intervention is usually limited to a time period of 6 weeks. The goal of crisis intervention is for the patient to return to his previous precrisis level of functioning. Often the patient advances to a level of functioning that is higher than the precrisis level because he has learned new ways of problem solving. There are four phases of crisis intervention that are similar to those of the nursing process. They are assessment, planning, implementation, and evaluation.

Assessment

The first step of crisis intervention is assessment. During this phase data regarding the nature of the crisis and its effect on the patient must be collected. It is from these data that a plan for intervention will be developed. It should be kept in mind that during this phase the nurse begins to establish a positive working relationship with the patient. A number of specific areas should be assessed by the nurse. These are the balancing factors that are important in the development and resolution of a crisis:

1. Identifying the precipitating event
2. Identifying the patient's previous strengths and coping mechanisms
3. Identifying the nature and strength of the patient's support systems

To help identify the precipitating event, the nurse should explore three areas during her assessment. These areas are the patient's needs and the events that threaten those needs, the point at which symptoms appear, and the themes or memories that are verbalized by the patient. Four kinds of needs that have been identified are related to self-esteem, sexual role mastery, dependency, and biological function.[22,30] Self-esteem is achieved when the individual attains successful social role experience. Sexual role mastery is achieved when the individual attains vocational, heterosexual, and parental role successes. Dependency is achieved when a satisfying interdependent relationship with others is attained. Biological function is achieved when an individual is in a position of safety in which the continuation of his life is not threatened.

The nurse identifies which needs are not being met. She does this by questioning the patient about how he feels about himself, what areas of his life he considers to be successful, what kinds of relationships he has with others, and how safe and secure he feels in life. She looks for obstacles that might interfere with meeting the patient's needs. What recent experiences have been upsetting? What areas of life have had changes? The patient's perception of the precipitating event is of primary importance, because what may appear to the nurse as a trivial experience may have great meaning to the patient. An overweight adolescent girl may have recently been the only girl in the class not invited to a social event. This may have threatened her self-esteem. A man with two unsuccessful marriages may have just been told by a girl friend that she wants to end their relationship. This may have threatened his need for sexual role mastery. An emotionally isolated, friendless woman may have had car trouble and been unable to find someone to give her a ride to work. This may have threatened her dependency needs. A chronically ill man who has had a recent exacerbation of his illness may have had his need for biological function threatened.

The point at which coping patterns become ineffective and symptoms appear is often after the stressful incident. When did the patient begin to feel anxious? When did his sleep disturbance begin? At what point in time did his suicidal thoughts start? If symptoms began last Tuesday, ask what took place in the patient's life on Tuesday or Monday. As the patient connects life events with the breakdown in coping mechanisms, an understanding of the precipitating event can materialize.

Themes and surfacing memories the patient verbalizes give further clues to the precipitating event. Present issues of concern are symbolically connected to past issues of concern. For example, a female patient who talks about the death of her father, which occurred 3 years ago, may, on questioning, reveal a recent loss of a relationship with a male. A patient who talks about feelings of inadequacy he had as a child because of poor school performance may, on questioning, reveal a recent experience in which his feelings of adequacy on his job were threatened. Since most crises involve losses or threats of losses, the theme of losses is a common one expressed. In her assessment the nurse therefore looks for a recent occurrence that may be connected to an underlying theme.

After the precipitating event is identified, the nurse assesses the patient's strengths and previous coping mechanisms. How has the patient handled other crises in his life? To whom has he turned? How did he relieve anxieties? Did the patient talk problems out with a relative? Did he leave his environment for a period of time to think things out from another perspective? Did he participate in sports to relieve tension? Did he find relief in crying? Besides exploring previous coping mechanisms, the nurse should also note the absence of other possible successful mechanisms.

After previous coping mechanisms are assessed, the patient's living situation, with emphasis on supports in the environment, needs to be assessed. Information is sought concerning present and potential sources of support. Does the patient live alone or with family or friends? With whom is he close? Who does he think understands him and offers him strength? Is there a clergyman or church friend he thinks is supportive to him? Assessing the patient's support system is important in determining who should come for the crisis therapy sessions. It may be determined that certain family members should come with the patient so that the family members' support can be strengthened. It may be determined that since the patient has few supports in his life, he should be involved in a crisis therapy group so that the support of other group members can be elicited. Assessing the patient's support system is also vital in determining whether an inpatient hospitalization would be more appropriate than outpatient crisis therapy. If there is a high degree of suicidal and

DIAGNOSTIC CRITERIA FOR POSTTRAUMATIC STRESS DISORDER*

A. Existence of a recognizable stressor that would evoke significant symptoms of distress in almost everyone.
B. Reexperiencing of the trauma as evidenced by at least one of the following:
  1. Recurrent and intrusive recollections of the event
  2. Recurrent dreams of the event
  3. Sudden acting or feeling as if the traumatic event were occurring, because of an association with an environmental or ideational stimulus
C. Numbing of responsiveness to or reduced involvement with the external world, beginning some time after the trauma, as shown by at least one of the following:
  1. Markedly diminished interest in one or more significant activities
  2. Feeling of detachment or estrangement from others
  3. Constricted affect
D. At least two of the following symptoms that were not present before the trauma:
  1. Hyperalertness or exaggerated startle response
  2. Sleep disturbance
  3. Guilt about surviving when others have not, or about behavior required for survival
  4. Memory impairment or trouble concentrating
  5. Avoidance of activities that arouse recollection of the traumatic event
  6. Intensification of symptoms by exposure to events that symbolize or resemble the traumatic event

*From American Psychiatric Association: Diagnostic and statistical manual of mental disorders, third edition, Washington, D.C., APA, 1980.

homicidal risk along with a weak outside support system, hospitalization may be a safer and more effective treatment.

The final step in the assessment phase of crisis intervention is the formulation of a nursing diagnosis. These diagnoses may be related to any aspect of the patient's life and can reflect the nursing problems described in Chapters 7 to 14. Relevant medical diagnoses may similarly pertain to a variety of psychiatric disorders. One

type of anxiety disorder, however, is particularly applicable to crisis intervention therapy. This is the posttraumatic stress disorder. Its essential feature is the development of characteristic symptoms following a psychologically traumatic event that is generally outside the range of such usual human experiences as simple bereavement, chronic illness, business losses, or marital conflict. The trauma may be rape, assault, military combat, natural disasters, car accidents, fires, airplane crashes, torture, kidnapping, or bombing. The diagnostic criteria for this disorder are presented at left.

Planning

The second step of crisis intervention is planning the intervention. During this phase the previously collected data are analyzed and specific interventions are proposed. Dynamics underlying the present crisis are formulated from the information regarding the precipitating event. Alternative solutions to the problem are explored, and steps for achieving the solutions are designated. The nurse decides which environmental supports to engage or strengthen and how to do this. She also decides which of the patient's coping mechanisms to develop and which ones to strengthen.

Intervention

The third step of crisis intervention is implementing the intervention itself. The intervention can take place on many levels with the use of a variety of techniques. Shields[26] has described four specific levels of crisis intervention, which represent a hierarchy from the most superficial to the most in-depth:
  1. Environmental manipulation
  2. General support
  3. Generic approach
  4. Individual approach
Each step includes the lower levels of intervention. The order of the steps also represents the degree of knowledge and skill needed by the nurse for application.

Environmental manipulation includes those interventions which directly change the patient's physical or interpersonal situation for the purpose of providing situational support or removing stress. For example, a patient who is having difficulty coping with her six children may temporarily send several of the children to their grandmother's house. In this situation some stress is alleviated. Similarly, a patient having difficulty on his job may take a week of sick leave so he can be removed temporarily from that stress. A patient who lives alone may move in with his closest sibling for several days. In this situation some support is provided. Likewise, involving the patient in family or group crisis therapy provides environmental manipulation for the purpose of providing support.

General support includes those interventions which provide the patient with the feeling that the nurse is on his side and will be a helping person. The nurse's demonstration of the therapeutic elements of warmth, acceptance, empathy, and caring in addition to her offering reassurance results in this type of support.

The *generic approach* is a type of crisis intervention that is analogous to the public health model. It is designed to reach high-risk individuals and individuals of great numbers in as short a time as possible. It applies a specific method to all those individuals faced with a similar type of crisis. The course of the particular type of crisis is previously studied and mapped out. The intervention is then set up to ensure that the course of the crisis results in an adaptive resolution.

As described earlier in this chapter, grief is an example of a type of crisis with a known pattern that can be influenced toward a positive outcome. Lindemann's[20] study described the pattern of grief. He believed that helping the patient extricate himself from his ties to the deceased and find new patterns of rewarding interaction would influence the patient toward a positive or adaptive resolution of his grief. Applying this specific intervention to individuals experiencing grief, especially when a high-risk group is evident (e.g., families of local disaster victims) is an example of providing a generic approach. Use of the generic approach does not require the nurse to have a thorough understanding of the unique psychodynamics of the patient.[16]

The *individual approach* is a type of crisis intervention that is analogous to the model of diagnosis and treatment of a specific problem in a specific patient. The nurse needs to have a thorough understanding of the patient's psychodynamics that led to the present crisis and

must consequently use the intervention geared to aid the particular patient to achieve an adaptive resolution to his crisis. This type of crisis intervention can be effective with all types of crisis. It is of particular benefit in crises that are combined situational and maturational crises. The individual approach is also beneficial when symptoms include strong components of homicidal and suicidal risk. The individual approach should be applied to those crises for which a known course cannot be mapped. It also should be applied to those crises which have not responded to a trial of the generic approach. It is often helpful to consult with others when deciding which approach to use for a specific patient.

The nurse's implementation of these levels of intervention is aided by the use of some techniques of crisis intervention that are active, focal, and explorative in nature. Since the focus of crisis intervention is on the present crisis, the intervention must be now oriented to achieve the goal of quick resolution. Furthermore, the nurse must be active in guiding the crisis intervention through its various steps. A more passive approach is inappropriate for this type of psychotherapy because of the time limitations of the crisis situation. In her care the nurse is creative and flexible, trying whatever, within reason, may work. Some techniques she might use include abreaction, clarification, suggestion, manipulation, reinforcement of behavior, support of defenses, raising self-esteem, and exploration of solutions.[15,25] The technique of interpretation is not emphasized in crisis intervention because a conscious solution to an immediate problem is the goal of crisis intervention. Interpretation deals with making unconscious elements of behavior conscious and is therefore not compatible with the goal. A brief description of these techniques will now be presented.

Abreaction is the ventilation of feelings that takes place as the patient verbally recounts emotionally charged areas. Awareness of affect is experienced and tension reduction results. Usually abreaction is encouraged in crisis intervention. The nurse facilitates abreaction by asking the patient how he feels about his situation, recent events, and significant people involved in his crisis. She asks open-ended questions and reflects the patient's words back to him so that he will further ventilate his feelings. The nurse does not discourage crying or angry outbursts but rather sees them as a positive release of feelings. Only when feelings seem out of control, such as in extreme rage or despondency, should the nurse discourage abreaction and help the patient concentrate on thinking rather than feeling. For example, if a patient angrily talks of wanting to kill a specific person, it is better to help him focus on thinking through the consequences of carrying out the act rather than encouraging free expression of the angry feelings.

Clarification is used when the nurse encourages the patient to express more clearly the relationship between certain events in his life, or the nurse herself may point out possible relationships. For example, helping a patient see that it was after he was passed over for a promotion that he began feeling too sick to go to work is clarification. Clarification enables the patient to gain a better intellectual understanding of his feelings and how they led to the development of a crisis. In crisis intervention the clarification of unconscious processes is minimal.

Suggestion is the process of influencing an individual so that he accepts an idea or belief. In crisis intervention the nurse influences the patient to see her as a confident, calm, hopeful, empathic leader who can help. By believing the nurse can help, the patient himself feels optimistic and in turn will feel less anxious. He also may want to please the nurse by fulfilling her expectations of getting better.

Manipulation is a technique in which the nurse uses the patient's emotions, wishes, or values to his benefit in the therapeutic process. Like suggestion, manipulation is a way of influencing the patient. For example, the nurse may want to point out to the patient who prides himself on his independence that he is capable of as well as responsible for much of the work of solving his problem.

Reinforcement of behavior occurs when useful adaptive behavior of the patient is reinforced by the nurse. She strengthens positive responses made by the patient by agreeing with or complimenting those responses. For example, when a patient who has passively received berating from his boss states that he asserted himself in an interaction with his boss, the nurse can tell him she is pleased with his assertiveness.

Support of defenses occurs when the nurse encourages the use of defenses that result in adaptive gratification and discourages those which result in maladaptive gratification. Defense mechanisms are indirect behaviors used to cope with stressful situations. The purpose of defense mechanisms is to maintain self-

esteem and ego integrity. When defenses deny, falsify, or distort reality to the point that the individual cannot deal effectively with reality, they are maladaptive. The nurse should encourage the patient to use defenses that result in adaptive gratification and discourage those which result in maladaptive gratification. For example, when a patient denies the fact that her husband wants to break up their marriage despite the fact that he has told her and demonstrated to her what he wishes, the nurse can point out to her that she is not facing facts and dealing realistically with the problem. This is an example of discouraging the use of the defense mechanism of denial. If a patient who is furious with an authority figure writes a letter to the authority's supervisor rather than assaulting the authority, the nurse should encourage his adaptive use of the defense mechanism of sublimation.

In crisis intervention, defenses are not attacked but rather are more gently encouraged or discouraged. When defenses are attacked, the patient cannot maintain his self-esteem and ego integrity. There is not enough time in crisis intervention to help replace the attacked defenses with new healthier defenses. Returning the patient to his previous level of functioning is the goal of crisis intervention, not the restructuring of defenses.

Raising self-esteem is a particularly important technique. The patient in a crisis feels helpless and may be overwhelmed with feelings of inadequacy. The fact that he has found it necessary to seek outside help for his problem may further increase his feelings of inadequacy. The nurse should help the patient regain his feelings of self-worth. She does this by communicating her confidence that the patient can participate actively in finding solutions to his problems. The nurse also communicates to the patient that he is a worthwhile person by listening to him, accepting his feelings, and relating to him with respect.

Exploration of solutions is essential because crisis intervention is geared toward solving the immediate crisis. The nurse and patient actively explore solutions to the crisis. Alternative solutions that the patient could not conceive of originally may become apparent as he talks to the nurse and his anxiety decreases. For example, a patient who has lost his job and has not been successful in finding a new one may become aware of the fact that he knows many people in his field of work whom he could contact to get information regarding the job market and possible openings.

In addition to using these techniques, Morley, Messick, and Aguilera[23] listed attitudes that are essential for the crisis worker to have. She should see her work as the treatment of choice with persons in crisis rather than as a second-best treatment. Assessment of the present problem should be viewed as necessary for treatment, but complete diagnostic assessment should be viewed as unnecessary. The goal and time limitations of crisis intervention should be kept in mind constantly, and unrelated material should not be explored. An active directive role must be taken, and flexibility of approach is mandatory.

Evaluation

The fourth step of crisis intervention is evaluation. During this phase the nurse and patient evaluate whether the intervention resulted in the desired effect, a positive resolution of the crisis. Has the patient returned to his precrisis level of functioning? Have the patient's original needs, which were threatened by the precipitating or stressful event, been met? Have the patient's symptoms, which demonstrated ineffective use of coping mechanisms, subsided? Have the patient's useful coping mechanisms begun to function again? Does the patient have a strong support system to rely on now? The nurse reviews with the patient changes that have occurred and gives the credit for these changes to the patient so that he can see his own effectiveness. The nurse discusses with the patient how that which was learned from the experience of crisis intervention may help in coping with future crises. As in any evaluation process, if goals have not been met, the patient and nurse can go back to the first step, assessment, and continue through the four phases again. At the end of the evaluation process, if the nurse and patient believe referral for another type of professional help would be useful, the referral is made.

Clinical case analysis

The phases of crisis intervention just described can be seen in Clinical example 20-4.

CLINICAL EXAMPLE 20-4

ASSESSMENT

Mr. A is a 29-year-old, medium-built, casually dressed black man who was referred to the crisis clinic by another agency. The patient came to the clinic alone. The nurse working with Mr. A collected the following data.

The patient worked in a large steel-making company. The company was laying off many workers and reassigning others. One month ago Mr. A was temporarily assigned to an area where he had had difficulty 2 years ago. The foreman, the patient believed, was now harrassing him as he had previously. Two weeks ago the patient got angry at the foreman and had thoughts of wanting to kill him. Instead of taking violent action, Mr. A became dizzy, and his head ached. He requested medical attention but was refused. He then "passed out" and was taken by ambulance to the dispensary.

Since that time Mr. A had a comprehensive physical examination and was found to be in excellent health. His physician prescribed diazepam (Valium) on an as-needed basis, but this was only slightly helpful. The patient returned to work for 2 days this week but felt "sick" again. The agency to which Mr. A registered a complaint against his foreman was the agency that referred him to the clinic.

Mr. A complained of being depressed, nervous, and tense. He was not sleeping well, was irritable with his wife and children, and was preoccupied with angry feelings toward his foreman. He had paranoid feelings about his foreman harassing him. Mr. A denied suicidal thoughts while admitting to homicidal thoughts. He felt the homicidal thoughts were under control. At one point during the initial interview the patient was tearful despite strong attempts at control. He demonstrated adequate comprehension, above-average intelligence, a good capacity for introspection, an adequate memory, an affect more of anxiety than depression, and paranoid ideation in regard to the foreman at work. His thought processes were organized, and there was no evidence of a perceptual disorder. Ego boundary disturbance was evident in the patient's paranoid thoughts. It seemed that the foreman was, in fact, a difficult man to get along with. However, the description of personal harassment seemed distorted. There were no depressive symptoms.

Mr. A was raised by his parents. His father was "boss" and beat him and his siblings often. His mother was quiet and always agreed with his father. Mr. A's parents were Jehovah's Witnesses, and he was Baptist. The patient had a younger brother, a younger sister, and an older sister. The patient and his brother had always been close. The two of them had stopped their father's beatings by ganging up on him and "psyching him out." As a child Mr. A hung around with a "tough crowd" and fought frequently. He stated he believed that he can physically overpower others, but tries to keep out of trouble by talking to people rather than fighting and by working hard.

Mr. A had never before sought aid from a mental health facility. His physical health, as stated, was excellent. He was taking no medication at the time of his first interview. Mr. A had a tenth-grade education and had always achieved above-average grades. His work record up until this time was good. His interests included bowling and other sports. He also periodically took courses at a local community college for his own personal growth rather than in preparation for a degree.

Mr. A had been married for 9 years. His wife was 2 years younger than he. They had three daughters ages 9 and 7 and 9 months. Mr. A stated that his relationships with his wife and daughters were satisfactory. Both his wife and his brother were strong supports at this time.

PLANNING

Mr. A was in a situational crisis, an internal disturbance that resulted from a perceived threat. The threat or precipitating stress in this case was the transfer to a new boss. The patient's need for sexual role mastery was not being met, since he was not attaining vocational role success. Soon after the transfer Mr. A's usual means of coping became ineffective and he experienced increased anxiety. Symptoms that appeared included attacks of dizziness, headache, passing out, and paranoid thinking. There was no suicidal intent, but feelings toward the foreman contained some homicidal ideation. The patient demonstrated enough control over his impulses that hospitalization was believed to be unnecessary. Memories and themes in the patient's verbalizations emphasized his feelings of being harassed. He had had difficulty with his new boss before. Difficulty with his boss was speculated to be a repetition of an earlier conflict, that is, the patient's feelings toward his father, another harassing boss.

Mr. A's usual means of coping were talking calmy with the threatening party and working hard on his job, in school, and in leisure activities. These coping mechanisms failed to work for him at this time but had been successful in the past. Other strengths the patient exhibited were a good work record under the other foreman and only mild impairment in spheres of his life outside work. He had no arrest record and showed the ability of not acting impulsively but rather of thinking through his actions. Mr. A showed strong motivation for working on his problem. He was reaching out for help, and the beginning of a therapeutic relationship was developing.

Environmental supports seemed strong. The patient's wife and brother were supportive, but the patient saw his problem as not involving them. It was therefore decided that the patient would be seen alone for the sessions. The patient felt no supports at work.

The overall goal of treatment would be for the patient to return to at least his precrisis level of functioning. If possible, he could reach a level above, having learned new methods of problem solving. A crisis intervention approach was decided on that considered the patient's needs and desires, the presenting problem, and the limitations of the clinic. The patient demonstrated a good potential for problem solving and the nurse made a contract with him for crisis intervention on a weekly basis.

Possible solutions were mutually explored:

1. It was believed that the patient should remain away from work temporarily so that his rage would not be likely to explode.

2. The patient's intellectual understanding of the crisis would be sought. By understanding what had happened to cause his anxiety, the patient would be able to see more clearly ways of solving the problem. Intellectual understanding rather than affective understanding is sought because of the time limitations and goals of crisis intervention. Affective understanding involves long-term treatment with much emphasis on unconscious processes.

3. Old constructive ways of handling anger would be reinforced. These included submitting a formal complaint at work and ventilating his feelings both to the nurse during the sessions and to his family and friends at other appropriate times.

4. New ways of coping would be taught. These included seeking support at work and following several official avenues of protest.

5. Because of the strength of the patient's feelings toward his boss, it was possible that new ways of handling anger would not suffice and that a transfer to another department might be a better solution.

INTERVENTION

The level of intervention used by the nurse was the individual approach, which is the most sophisticated approach and includes the generic approach, general support, and environmental manipulation. The individual approach was chosen because the patient's crisis was not one for which a known course could be mapped. Also, since there was a homicidal component to the patient's symptoms, it was believed to be the safest approach. With a clear understanding of psychodynamics, the nurse geared the intervention to aid the patient to achieve an adaptive resolution to his crisis.

Environmental manipulation was achieved by having the patient remain home from work temporarily. Letters were written by the nurse to his employer explaining his absence in general terms. The patient was encouraged to talk to his wife about his difficulties so that she could understand his anxiety and be emotionally supportive.

General support was given by the nurse, who provided an atmosphere of reassurance, nonjudgmental caring, warmth, empathy, and optimism. The patient was encouraged to talk freely about the problem without having his feelings judged as good or bad. The nurse offered reassurance that the problem was one that could be solved and that the patient would be feeling better. The nurse let the patient know that she understood his feelings and would help him overcome his crisis.

The generic approach was used to decrease the patient's anxiety and guide him through the various steps of problem solving common to all crises. Levels of anxiety were assessed and means of reducing anxiety or helping the patient tolerate moderate anxiety were employed. The patient was encouraged to use his anxiety consciously and constructively to solve his problem and develop new coping mechanisms.

The individual approach was used in assessing the specific problems of Mr. A and treating those specific problems. An understanding of the patient's individual psychodynamics was sought and dealt with by the nurse and patient. The patient was reexperiencing harassment from a male authority figure as he had experienced with his father during his youth. Because of the repetition of harassing experiences, Mr. A perceived his treatment by his boss in a personal and paranoid way. In other words, he was strongly sensitive to unfair treatment and overreacted as a result of early repetitive childhood experiences. His emotional response was to strike out physically, as his father had struck out at him. Intellectually, Mr. A knew this would be a disastrous action, and his conflict was solved by becoming sick and passing out so that he could not assault his boss. Mr. A's intense anger was recognized and a high priority was placed on channeling the anger in a positive direction.

The first two interviews were used for data gathering and establishing a positive therapeutic relationship. Through the use of *abreaction* the patient ventilated angry feelings but did not concentrate on wanting to kill his boss. The nurse used *clarification* to help the patient begin to attain an intellectual understanding of the precipitating event and its effect on him. *Suggestion* was used by influencing the patient to see the nurse as one who can help. The nurse told the patient the problem could be worked out by the two of them and that he would soon be feeling better. The patient decided to contact several people at work to obtain information about transferring to another department or being laid off. The patient and nurse therefore were *exploring solutions*. The nurse *reinforced* the patient's use of problem solving by telling him his ideas about alternative solutions were good ones well worth his looking into. Throughout these and other sessions the nurse *raised his self-esteem* by communicating her confidence that he could participate actively in finding solutions to his problems. She also listened to and accepted his feelings and treated him with respect. By contacting others at work in his pursuits, the patient found some supportive individuals at work.

During the third session the patient described an incident in which he became furious at a worker at an automobile repair shop. The repairs on the patient's car were never right, and the patient kept returning the car there. The patient shoved the worker but limited his physical assault to that. He then felt nervous and jittery. The patient had previously expressed pride in his ability to control his angry feelings and not physically strike out at others. *Manipulation* was used by telling the patient he showed control in stopping the assault before it had become a full-blown fight and it seemed apparent he could continue to exhibit this ability. During this session, also, the patient spoke of old angry feelings toward his father. Some of this ventilation was allowed, but soon thereafter the focus was guided back to the present crisis.

In the fourth session the patient reported no episode of uncontrollable anger. He still put much emphasis, however, on being harassed by others. The nurse questioned the fact that others were out to intentionally harass the patient. Mr. A's defenses were not attacked, but his gross use of projection was discouraged. In the fifth session the patient reported that a car tried to run him off the road. At a red traffic light the patient spoke calmly to the driver and the driver apologized. The nurse *reinforced this behavior* and *supported his use of sublimation as a defense*. Discussion of termination of the therapy was begun.

In the sixth session the patient told of his plans to return to work the following week. He would be going to a different department even though it seemed he would soon be laid off. He also talked about a course he had begun at a community college. He showed no evidence of anxiety or paranoia. Termination of the therapeutic relationship was further discussed. Only a few of the techniques of crisis intervention are described here. It should be kept in mind that the techniques, in actuality, are repetitively used in all sessions to be effective.

EVALUATION

The interventions resulted in the desired effect, an adaptive resolution of the crisis. The changes that occurred were discussed with the patient. The patient's need for sexual role mastery was being met. He was returning to work in a department in which he felt comfortable and successful. His symptoms of anxiety, paranoia, dizziness, headaches, passing out, and homicidal thoughts had ended. He no longer felt harassed. His original coping mechanisms were again effective. He was talking calmly to people he was having difficulty with, and he was again working hard in a goal-oriented way (i.e., a college course). He had learned new methods of coping, which included talking about his feelings to significant others, following administrative or official avenues of protest, and seeking support. The patient and nurse discussed how Mr. A could use the methods of problem solving he had learned from the experience to help cope with future problems. The goal, return to the precrisis level of functioning, had been attained.

It was also recommended to the patient that he engage in long-term psychotherapy so that he could deal with the old angers that interfered with his present life. The patient refused the recommendation at this time and stated he would contact the clinic if he changed his mind.

A comparison of the nursing process and crisis intervention methodology

Nursing practice has been clearly systematized into a specific approach. This approach is comprised of (1) data collection, (2) nursing diagnosis, (3) planning of nursing action, (4) implementation of the plan, and (5) evaluation. The steps are used concurrently and recurrently, since they are part of a process.[2] There are loops following each step so that, when necessary, a previous step can be retraced and adjustments made. Sometimes several steps are engaged in at the same time. The nursing process is dynamic rather than concrete so that changes can be made when steps do not lead to the desired goal.

It is evident that crisis intervention methodology is similar to nursing process methodology. The crisis intervention approach is comprised of (1) assessment, (2) planning intervention, (3) implementation of the plan, and (4) evaluation. Crisis intervention is also a process and the steps are used concurrently and recurrently. For example, the suicidal potential of the patient is reevaluated and reassessed during each session, and appropriate changes in planning and implementation are made. Because of the nature of crisis intervention there are specific time limitations; so the recurrent and concurrent aspects of the process are not always clearly evident.

Settings for crisis therapy

Nurses are in the position to render crisis therapy frequently by virtue of the various settings in which they practice. The observant nurse will identify individuals in crisis and plan necessary action. Medical hospitalizations are stressful for patients and their families and are often precipitating causes of crises. The patient who becomes excessively demanding or withdrawn or the wife who becomes known as a "pest" to the nursing staff are possible candidates for crisis therapy. The loss of a limb, the limitations imposed on one's activities, and the changes in body image because of surgical intervention can

all be viewed as losses or threats that may precipitate situational crisis. Simply the stress of being dependent on nurses for care can precipitate a crisis for the hospitalized patient. Strain and Grossman[28] identified the following categories of psychological stress in hospitalized patients:

1. Threat to narcissistic integrity
2. Fear of strangers
3. Separation anxiety
4. Fear of loss of love and approval
5. Fear of loss of control of developmentally achieved functions
6. Fear of loss or injury to body parts
7. Reactivation of feelings of guilt and shame and fear of retaliation

In addition, nurses who work in obstetric, pediatric, geriatric, or adolescent settings can readily observe patients or family members undergoing maturational crises. The anxious new mother, the acting-out adolescent, and the newly retired depressed patient are all possible candidates for crisis therapy. If physical illness is an added stress during maturational turning points, the patient is at an even greater risk.

Emergency room settings are flooded with crisis cases. People who attempt suicide, psychosomatic patients, and families of accident victims are all possible candidates for crisis therapy. If the nurse herself is not in a position to work with the patient on an ongoing basis, a referral for crisis therapy can be made. Community health nurses, having the advantage of observing patients in their own environments, can often spot and intervene in family crises. The child who refuses to go to school, the man who refuses to learn how to give himself the insulin injection, and the family with a member dying at home are, again, possible candidates for crisis therapy. Community health nurses are in a position to evaluate high-risk families for their need of crisis therapy. Families with new babies, ill members, recent deaths, and a history of difficulty coping are all possible high-risk families.

The family concept of crisis defines the crisis as a family problem, regardless of who is the identified patient.[5] The identified patient is the individual who is exhibiting symptoms. Since the crisis is seen as a family problem, responsibility for the patient's symptoms is placed on the family. It is assumed that a sequence of events occurring within the family led up to the decompensation of a member. The family is viewed as a system so that each member affects and is affected by each other member. For example, when a child refuses to go to school, it is believed not only that the child fears school and wishes to remain with mother but also that the mother is afraid to be alone and wants the child home with her. The crisis is a family one, not the child's crisis. It is also assumed that role problems cause disequilibrium in families, and new role assignments may be helpful. For example, if a mother appears to be the leader of the family and the father is discounted as ineffective, the nurse can assign certain tasks to the father, such as deciding on proper bedtimes for the children, so that the father will assume some leadership. At other times, tasks are given to the entire family so that emphasis is removed from the symptoms and conflicts. The family is given the responsibility of meeting each member's needs and of changing so that the present problem can be solved.[18]

Some practitioners initiate crisis intervention programs for families with specific problems. For example, programs have been implemented for families of servicemen missing in action,[32] families going through perinatal bereavement,[24] and families with children in the intensive care nursery.[8] One innovative program was established to help patients with chronic renal failure and their families adjust to the unique demands of home dialysis.[19]

Nurses in community mental health centers or departments of psychiatry, of course, see many patients in crisis. Patients and families have varied major complaints: depression, anxiety, marital conflict, suicidal thoughts, illicit drug taking, and psychotic symptoms. Crisis therapy modalities available in mental health centers include individual, family, and crisis groups.

Crisis groups function along the same sequential phases of resolution that individual intervention follows.[29] The nurse and group help the patient to attempt to solve his problem. Thereafter the group reinforces the patient's new problem-solving behavior. The nurse's role in the group is active, focal, and present oriented. The group follows the nurse's example and uses similar therapeutic techniques. The group acts as a support system for the patient and is therefore of particular benefit to socially isolated individuals. Often the way the patient functions in the group will highlight the faulty coping that is respon-

sible for his present problem. For example, it may become apparent from a patient's interaction with group members that he does not appear to listen to anything said by others but continues verbalizing as though nothing were said. This same patient may be in a crisis because his girl friend left him because she thought he did not care about her thoughts and feelings. The nurse can comment on the faulty coping seen in the group and encourage group discussion about it.

Crisis groups can be open ended or time limited and can be geared toward a homogeneous or heterogeneous population. Donovan, Bennett, and McElroy[9] describe a limited crisis group in a health maintenance organization. They speculate that the group's success is attributable to cohesiveness of the group culture, the supportive and accepting attitude of the group, and the group's expectation that the patients will work out their problems. Chen[6] describes a successful open-ended crisis group in a community mental health center. She observes that process interventions can be creatively used to enhance the group interaction while maintaining the crisis-oriented focus. In her group, Chen uses an individual interpersonal focus and a mass group focus to help patients resolve their present crises. Homogeneous crisis groups have been initiated for groups with specific problems. For example, groups have been implemented for men accompanying women seeking abortion[13] and families in the waiting room for intensive care patients.[3]

There is a trend for psychiatric hospitalizations to be short term. Nurses practicing on these units can use crisis therapy in working with the patient and his family so that the patient can return to the community as soon as possible. This can also prevent rehospitalization. The hospitalization itself may be viewed as an environmental manipulation and thus as part of the crisis intervention.

Crisis intervention is sometimes practiced by way of the telephone rather than in face-to-face contacts. Nurses working for hot lines or nurses who become involved in answering emergency telephone calls may find themselves practicing crisis intervention without the use of visual cues. Referrals for face-to-face contact should be made, but often, because of the patient's unwillingness or inability to cooperate, the telephone remains the only contact. Listening skills must therefore be emphasized in the nurse's role. Most emergency telephone services have extensive training programs to teach this specialized type of crisis intervention. Manuals are written for the crisis worker and include content such as suicide potential rating scales, community resources, drug information, guidelines for helping the caller discuss his concerns, and advice on understanding the limitations of one's role.[21]

As part of the community, nurses are called on when adventitious crises strike the community. Floods, earthquakes, airplane crashes, fires, nuclear accidents, and other natural and unnatural disasters precipitate large numbers of crises. Frederick and Garrison[12] have described a "service model" in which mental health workers in the immediate postdisaster period should go to places where victims are likely to congregate, such as morgues, hospitals, and shelters. Later, if Federal Disaster Assistance Centers are established, mental health workers may assist in the centers. Rather than waiting for people to publicly identify themselves as persons who are unable to cope with stress, it is suggested that the mental health workers work with the Red Cross, talk to people waiting in lines to apply for assistance, go door-to-door, or, at a relocation site, ask people how they are managing their affairs and explore their experiences to stress.

Nurses providing crisis therapy during large disasters would use the public health or generic approach so that as many individuals as possible can receive help in a short amount of time. Tragedies such as group kidnappings and group killings in communities may affect fewer people and may at times require the individual approach. The nurse may choose to work with families or groups rather than individuals during adventitious crises so that individuals can gain support from others in their family or community who are undergoing stresses similar to theirs.

A good example of mental health professionals helping victims of an adventitious crisis occurred in Kansas City, Missouri, in the days and weeks following the crash of the overhead walkways at the Hyatt Hotel in July 1981. Eight mental health centers in the Kansas City metropolitan area joined to help care for the emotional sufferings of the individuals involved.

The centers formed an unofficial coalition and prepared a joint press release describing the many aspects of the grieving process and publicizing the services that they would offer to the survivors of those killed at the hotel—the injured, the observers, and the rescue workers. The services were of three kinds. First, all the centers offered phone counseling and support groups free of charge. Second, special services were planned, such as a grief workshop that was attended by about 200 people who had been at the crash scene. Other related seminars were also held. Third, the centers and media worked together to let the general public know about other resources and services as these became available and to reassure people that their strong reactions to the tragedy were normal.

Finally, crisis therapy is a major technique of preventive psychiatry. Maladaptive behavior can be prevented by identifying a crisis and intervening immediately. Crisis can actually be avoided by determining factors that can lead to a crisis and taking action to curtail the process. When the nurse sees a potentially stressful situation, she should watch the involved individual's level of anxiety. She should give time to talk and listen to those under stress so that anxiety levels can be lessened before they reach severe or crisis proportions. For example, an elderly patient with a known psychiatric illness was being seen in supportive long-term psychotherapy with his wife. The wife telephoned the nurse who was working with them to state that her husband had died 2 weeks ago and they therefore would not be coming back to the clinic. The nurse believed that the patient's death was most definitely a stress for his wife and that there was a potential for a crisis. The nurse asked the patient's wife to come into the clinic one more time so that they could evaluate how she was getting along. The wife was seen and the nurse encouraged her to talk about her husband's death and her future plans. The nurse assessed that the wife was going through the grieving process in a normal adaptive way and that as long as the wife continued talking about her feelings to family and friends, a crisis would be avoided. It is also a preventive measure to intervene when a psychiatrically impaired individual undergoes a crisis so that further debilitation can be stopped. As Aguilera and Messick point out:

All three levels of prevention are inherent and are practical in crisis intervention. It is possible that this may be a major reason why the concepts and techniques of this method of treatment have been so widely accepted.[1:140]

Nurses practice in primary, secondary, and tertiary prevention settings and can contribute greatly to prevention by case finding and treatment.

Future trends

Crisis therapy is becoming more and more popular as the treatment of choice for primary, secondary, and tertiary preventive care of psychiatric problems. It is considered both practical and effective by mental health workers and patients. Since it is a short-term therapy, it is inexpensive in terms of time and money for patients and caregivers. In our mobile and fast-moving society crisis therapy is also practical because it requires a short-term commitment from the patient and caregiver. Many people can be reached in a limited period of time.

Persons other than mental health professionals are being educated to adequately do certain levels of crisis intervention. Neighborhood workers, police, clergy, bartenders, and lawyers are but a few of the many people who come in frequent contact with the target population. These non–mental health professionals who deal with people in crisis are being taught by professionals, including nurses, how to identify individuals in crisis, how to intervene on a generic level, and how to refer individuals needing professional treatment to mental health personnel.

There are some authors who believe that there is not one systematic model of crisis therapy, but many. Conceptualization of crisis work is vague rather than detailed and refined. More research is needed so that crisis theory can be better defined operationally.[27] The choice of crisis intervention modality for specific patients seems at times to be arbitrary and dependent on the practitioner's or agency's orientation rather than based on theory. Further research is needed to identify which crisis intervention modality—individual, group, or family—is most effective under which circumstances. At present the family modality is selected when the crisis directly involves other family members and when strengthening family support is essential for the individual. At times, when family members are uncooperative and refuse to become involved in the treatment, an individual or group approach is selected. For those individuals in crisis who are isolated and have little family or friend support, a group is beneficial because the other group members form a support system. The individual approach is selected when the crisis does not seem to directly involve the family or when the patient believes he can best handle the crisis on his own. A patient whose crisis stems from his asserting his independence from his family may also want to be seen individually.

Nurses are more frequently being placed in the role of primary therapist and therefore are becoming more involved in the direct practice of crisis therapy. This trend seems to be continuing and will grow as certification procedures for nurses further develop. Nurses are also involved in indirect services in the field of crisis therapy. The theory and practice of crisis intervention is taught by nurses to other nurses in various settings and also to non–mental health professionals and paraprofessionals. Nurses are frequently in the role of consultant and advise others in their work with individuals in crisis. Additional nursing research is needed in the area of crisis therapy. What level of education and skill is needed to perform the different levels of crisis intervention? Which nursing interventions are most effective for whom? Follow-up studies are also needed so that the long-term effects of crisis therapy can be evaluated.

Suggested cross-references

Therapeutic relationship skills are discussed in Chapter 3. The phases of the nursing process are discussed in Chapter 4. Interventions in primary prevention are discussed in Chapter 5.

SUMMARY

1. The theory and practice of crisis therapy developed as an outgrowth of analytical and preventive psychiatry. Eric Lindemann and Gerald Caplan were two of the first pioneers to define and practice crisis therapy.

2. A crisis is an internal disturbance that results from a perceived threat. An individual's usual repertoire of coping mechanisms becomes ineffective in solving problems and the individual experiences a rise in anxiety. Crises are a time of increased vulnerability and can stimulate personal growth.

3. Crises can be maturational, situational, or adventitious in etiology. Maturational crises develop from stress during transitional periods of the maturing process when psychological equilibrium is upset. Situational crises occur when a specific external event upsets one's psychological equilibrium. Adventitious crisis are accidental, uncommon, and unexpected crises with multiple losses and gross environmental changes.

4. Crisis intervention is a brief, here-and-now–oriented, active mode of psychotherapy with the goal of reestablishing psychological equilibrium. On completion of the process of crisis intervention, the patient is returned to at least his precrisis level of functioning.

5. The methodology of crisis intervention includes the steps of assessment, planning intervention, intervention, and evaluation. Data are collected and analyzed, a plan of intervention is made and implemented, and results are evaluated. If goals have not been met, the patient and nurse can go back to the first step and continue through the four phases again.

6. In completing an assessment, the nurse attempts to identify the precipitating event, the patient's previous strengths and coping mechanisms, and the nature and strength of the patient's support systems. She further assesses the patient's needs and the events that threaten those needs, the point at which symptoms appear, and the themes or memories that are verbalized by the patient.

7. Levels of crisis intervention are environmental manipulation, general support, generic approach, and individual approach. Environmental manipulation includes those interventions which directly change the patient's physical or interpersonal situation for the purpose of providing situational support or removing stress. General support includes those interventions which provide the patient with the feeling that the nurse is on his side and will be a helping person. The generic approach includes those interventions which guide patients through a particular known course of a crisis so that an adaptive solution to the crisis will be the outcome. The individual approach includes those interventions which aid a particular patient to achieve an adaptive resolution to this crisis and requires a clear understanding of the patient's specific psychodynamics.

8. Techniques of crisis intervention include abreaction, clarification, suggestion, manipulation, reinforcement of behavior, support of defenses, raising self-esteem, and exploration of solutions. Abreaction is the ventilation of feelings that takes place as the patient verbally recounts emotionally charged areas. Clarification involves helping the patient see more clearly the relationship between certain events in his life. Suggestion is the process of influencing an individual so that he accepts an idea or belief, particularly the belief that the nurse can help and that he will be feeling better. Manipulation is the use of the patient's emotions, wishes, or values to his benefit in the therapeutic process. Reinforcement of behavior involves giving the patient positive responses to adaptive behavior. Support of defenses is the encouragement of the use of defenses that result in adaptive gratification and the discouragement of those which result in maladaptive gratification. Raising self-esteem involves helping the patient regain feelings of self-worth. Exploration of solutions is the examining of alternative modes of action geared toward solving the immediate problem.

9. Crisis intervention methodology is similar to nursing process methodology. In both processes the steps are used concurrently and recurrently. However, because of the strict time limitations in crisis intervention, conceptually each step is considered separately and time permits the completion of one sequence only.

10. Nurses are in the position to use crisis intervention techniques frequently by virtue of the various settings in which they practice. Settings include all areas of general hospitals, communities, mental health centers, psychiatric hospitals or units, emergency telephone services, and disaster areas. Modalities of crisis intervention used include the individual, family, and group approaches. By practicing crisis therapy in various settings, nurses are involved in primary, secondary, and tertiary prevention of psychiatric disorders.

11. Trends in crisis therapy seem to demonstrate continued use and sophistication of techniques. Nurses are involved with crisis therapy in both their direct and indirect services. Roles are growing for nurses as primary caregivers, teachers, consultants, and researchers. Further nursing research is needed so that theory can be better defined operationally. The use of specific techniques and modalities of crisis therapy need study.

References

1. Aguilera, D.C., and Messick, J.M.: Crisis intervention: theory and methodology, ed. 4, St. Louis, 1982, The C.V. Mosby Co.

2. American Nurses' Association: Standards of nursing practice, Kansas City, Mo., 1973, The Association.

3. Bloom, N.D., and Lynch, J.G.: Group work in a hospital setting, Health Soc. Work **4:**48, Aug. 1979.

4. Caplan, G.: Principles of preventive psychiatry, New York, 1964, Basic Books, Inc.

5. Chandler, H.H.: Family crisis intervention: point and counterpoint in the psychosocial revolution, J. Natl. Med. Assoc. **64:**211, May 1972.

6. Chen, M.E.: Applying Yalom's principles to crisis work . . . some intriguing results, J. Psychiatr. Nurs. **16:**15, June 1978.

7. Crisis intervention programs for disaster victims in smaller communities, Washington, D.C., 1979, Department of Health, Education, and Welfare Pub. No. (A.D.M.) 79-675, U.S. Government Printing Office.

8. Dillard, R.G., Auerbach, K.G., and Showalter, A.H.: A parents' program in the intensive care nursery: its relationship to maternal attitudes and expectations, Soc. Work Health Care **5:**245, Spring 1980.

9. Donovan, J.M., Bennett, M.J., and McElroy, C.M.: The crisis group—an outcome study, Am. J. Psychiatry **13:**906, 1979.

10. Erikson, E.H.: Childhood and society, New York, 1963, W.W. Norton & Co., Inc., Publishers.

11. Erikson, E.H.: Identity, youth and crisis, New York, 1968, W.W. Norton & Co., Inc., Publishers.

12. Frederick, C., and Garrison, J.: Disaster and mental health: an overview, Behav. Today **12:**32, Aug. 1981.

13. Gordon, R.H.: Efficacy of a group crisis—counseling program for men who accompany women seeking abortions, Am. J. Community Psychol. **6:**239, June 1978.

14. Havighurst, R.J.: Human development and education, New York, 1953, Longman, Inc.

15. Imboden, J.B., and Urbaitis, J.C.: Practical psychiatry in medicine, New York, 1978, Appleton-Century-Crofts.

16. Jacobson, G., Strickler, M., and Morley, W.E.: Generic and individual approaches to crisis intervention, Am. J. Public Health **58:**339, 1968.

17. King, J.M.: The initial interview: basis for assessment in crisis intervention, Perspect. Psychiatr. Care **9:**247, Nov.-Dec. 1971.

18. Langsley, D.G., and Kaplan, D.M.: The treatment of families in crisis, New York, 1968, Grune & Stratton, Inc.

19. Levenberg, S.B., Jenkins, C., and Wendorf, D.J.: Studies in family-oriented crisis intervention with hemodialysis patients, Int. J. Psychiatry Med. **9**(1):83, 1978-1979.

20. Lindemann, E.: Symptomatology and management of acute grief, Am. J. Psychiatry **101:**141, 1944.

21. Mills, P.: Crisis intervention resource manual, Vermillion, S.D., 1973, Educational Research and Service Center.

22. Mitchell, C.E.: Identifying the hazard: the key to crisis intervention, Am. J. Nurs. **77:**1194, 1977.

23. Morley, W.E., Messick, J.M., and Aguilera, D.C.: Crisis paradigms of intervention, J. Psychiatr. Nurs. **5:**537, 1967.

24. Quirk, T.R., O'Donohue, S., and Middleton, J.: The perinatal bereavement crisis, J. Nurse Midwife. **24:**13, Sept.-Oct. 1979.

25. Rusk, T.N.: Opportunity and technique in crisis psychiatry, Compr. Psychiatry **12:**249, May 1971.

26. Shields, L.: Crisis intervention: implications for the nurse, J. Psychiatr. Nurs. **13:**37, Sept.-Oct. 1975.

27. Smith, L.L.: Crisis intervention theory and practice, Community Men. Health Rev. **2:**5, 1977.

28. Strain, J.J., and Grossman, S.: Psychological care of the mentally ill, New York, 1975, Appleton-Century-Crofts.

29. Strickler, M., and Allgeyer, J.: The crisis group: a new application of crisis theory, Social Work **12:**28, 1967.

30. Strickler, M., and LaSor, B.: Concepts of loss in crisis intervention, Ment. Hygiene **54:**302, 1970.

31. Sundeen, S.J., et al.: Nurse-client interaction: implementing the nursing process, ed. 2, St. Louis, 1981, The C.V. Mosby Co.

32. Teichman, Y., Spiegel, Y., and Teichman, M.: Crisis intervention with families of servicemen missing in action, Am. J. Community Psychol. **6:**315, 1978.

33. Terr, L.C.: Psychic trauma in children: observations following the Chowchilla schoolbus kidnapping, Am. J. Psychiatry **138:**14, Jan. 1981.

34. Williams, F.: Intervention in maturational crises, Perspect. Psychiatr. Care **9:**240, Nov.-Dec. 1971.

Annotated suggested readings

Aguilera, D.C., and Messick, J.M.: Crisis intervention: Theory and methodology, ed. 4, St. Louis, 1982, The C.V. Mosby Co.

This book presents crisis theory and method in a detailed, comprehensive, and thorough manner. Content includes historical development, psychotherapeutic techniques, group therapy concepts, socioeconomic factors affecting intervention, the problem-solving approach, situational and maturational crises, and levels of prevention and trends as they relate to crisis intervention. Paradigms are included to facilitate understanding.

Burnside, I.M.: Crisis intervention with geriatric hospitalized patients, J. Psychiatr. Nurs. **8:**17, March-April 1970.

The author describes her work with elderly hospitalized patients. She presents a guide for crisis intervention with this type of patient, emphasizing the need for grief work.

Caplan, G.: Principles of preventive psychiatry, New York, 1964, Basic Books, Inc.

A classic in psychiatry, this book places a historical perspective on the development of crisis intervention from preventive psychiatry. A public health model is used to explain the approaches of primary, secondary, and tertiary prevention of mental disorders.

Chen, M.E.: Applying Yalom's principles to crisis work: some intriguing results, J. Psychiatr. Nurs. **16:**15, June, 1978.

Written for the serious group therapist, this article

translates some conventional group therapy principles into a crisis group theoretical framework. The literature on crisis groups is reviewed, followed by a description of an open-ended crisis group that uses Yalom's process–focused interventions. Theory is clearly defined and illustrated with clinical examples.

Crisis intervention programs for disaster victims in smaller communities, Washington, D.C., 1979, Department of Health, Education, and Welfare Pub. No. (A.D.M.) 79-675, U.S. Government Printing Office.

Although written for persons interested in the planning and delivery of disaster-related crisis intervention services, this monograph provides a wealth of information on the entire field of disasters and the use of crisis intervention to assist in disaster victims.

Getz, W., et al.: Fundamentals of crisis counseling, Lexington, Mass., 1974, Lexington Books, D.C. Heath & Co.

This general text about crisis intervention includes historical development, definitions, goals, techniques, interviewing stages, telephone crisis, and crisis with minority groups. It is useful in that it includes many clinical examples and verbatim notes.

Hall, J., and Weaver, B.: Nursing of families in crisis, Philadelphia, 1974, J.B. Lippincott Co.

This is a compilation of articles written by nurses dealing with families in crisis. The text attempts to increase the reader's understanding of crisis theory as it applies to nursing situations and provide examples of strategies and tactics that may be useful in helping families resolve crises. A variety of nursing practice settings are presented.

Harrison, D.: Nurses and disasters, J. Psychosoc. Nurs. 19(2): 34, 1981.

This brief paper reviews some of the acute psychiatric problems that can result from disaster experiences. Effective use of nurses in these emergencies is also described.

Hitchcock, J.M.: Crisis intervention, the pebble in the pool, Am. J. Nurs. 73:1388, 1973.

In this article the author stresses her belief that all nurses can implement crisis intervention. She believes that extensive theoretical and experiential backgrounds are not necessary and maps out the steps to be taken.

Jacobson, G., Strickler, M., and Morley, W.E.: Generic and individual approaches to crisis intervention, Am. J. Public Health 58:339, 1968.

The authors describe the nature of crisis and present two possible approaches in crisis intervention, the general and individual approaches. Circumstances under which each approach is selected are identified, and clinical examples of each method are presented.

Klingbeil, G.A., and Alvandi, O.M.: Concepts of transactional analysis and anxiety with persons in crises, J. Psychiatr. Nurs. 13:5, Nov.-Dec. 1975.

For a different slant this article compares crisis intervention, transactional analysis, and operational concepts of anxiety and learning.

Lancaster, J., and Berkovsky, D.: An ecological framework for crisis intervention, J. Psychiatr. Nurs. 16:17, March 1978.

This article was written for the nurse educator. The authors describe how to help baccalaureate nursing students use an ecological framework for crisis intervention with children placed in an institution for dependent and neglected children. Both theory and clinical examples are presented, making this article a useful one for students too.

Lindemann, E.: Symptomatology and management of acute grief, Am. J. Psychiatry 101:141, 1944.

This article describes an early study of the grieving process. Stages of grief are identified and normal and morbid grief reactions are differentiated. The use of crisis intervention to guide grief toward a favorable outcome is explored.

Maloney, E.M.: The subjective and objective definition of crisis, Perspect. Psychiatr. Care 9:257, Nov.-Dec. 1971.

The author of this philosophical article questions the definition and stereotyping of crisis intervention.

Messick, J.M.: Crisis intervention concepts: implications for nursing practice, J. Psychiatr. Nurs. 10:3, Sept.-Oct. 1972.

This article discusses the implications crisis intervention has for nurses in all clinical areas. Stress is placed on the need for nurses to recognize potential crises. Techniques for this recognition are described.

Mitchell, C.E.: Identifying the hazard: the key to crisis intervention, Am. J. Nurs. 77:1194, 1977.

This article concentrates on identifying the precipitating or stressful event from which a crisis develops. The author tells in detail what clues to look for and how to use the clues to intervene effectively.

Narayan, S.M., and Joslin, D.J.: Crisis theory and intervention: a critique of the medical model and proposal of a holistic nursing model, Adv. Nurs. Sci. 2:27, July 1980.

This author provides an alternative to the disease prevention orientation of crisis intervention, in describing a holistic model that emphasizes the alteration of health potential as one strives for a high level of wellness. The medical and holistic nursing models of crisis are compared both theoretically and in implications for intervention.

National Institute of Mental Health: Crisis intervention programs for disaster victims in smaller communities, Rockville, Md., 1979, U.S. Department of Health, Education, and Welfare.

This government monograph provides both theoretical and practical knowledge that can help in the planning and implementing of disaster-related mental health programs which are efficiently and effectively organized. Although primarily focused on the rural area, its recommendations have a wider interest and applicability as crisis intervention programs for various disaster victims.

National Institute of Mental Health: Training manual for human service workers in major disasters, Rockville, Md., 1978, U.S. Department of Health, Education, and Welfare.

This highly recommended manual uses crisis intervention theory and is a training instrument to help people cope after a disaster strikes. Its excellent coverage includes phases of a disaster, key concepts, community relationships, selection and education of human service workers, special risk groups, self-awareness sessions, and identification of available resources.

Parad, H., editor: Crisis intervention: selected readings, New York, 1965, Family Service Association of America.

This compilation of readings presents a range of theoretical formulations of crisis theory, and shows the way crisis intervention is used in practice. It applies crisis theory to various practice settings and a number of commonly encountered stressful situations affecting the individual, group, and family. This is a highly recommended reading.

Rogers, C.G.: The use of alienation in crisis work, Psychiatr. Nurs. 8:7, Nov.-Dec. 1970.

This article describes alienation as an estrangement resulting from the loss of previous ties and relationships. The part that alienation plays in maturational crises is focused on.

Strickler, M., and Allgeyer, J.: The crisis group: a new application of crisis theory, Soc. Work **12:**28, 1967.

This article describes a study in which individuals in crisis were treated in group therapy. The authors claim most patients made progress in the crisis group modality and explain theoretically how the progress occurred. A clinical example is given to further illustrate the concepts.

Wallace, M.A., and Morley, W.E.: Teaching crisis intervention, Am. J. Nurs. **70:**1484, 1970.

Written for the nurse educator, this article describes problems that evolve in clinical supervision of graduate nursing students learning to practice crisis intervention. Both initial and advanced problem patterns are identified and solutions are described.

Yano, B., Alexander, L., and Kuwanoe, C.: Crisis intervention: a guide for nurses, J. Rehabil. **4:**162, 1976.

This article describes intrapsychic, family, and cultural aspects of crisis intervention that need to be dealt with in practice. A case study is presented to demonstrate the described pattern of crisis intervention.

CHAPTER 21

BEHAVIOR
MODIFICATION

Helen R. Peddicord

*But humanism stands for the whole person,
the whole individual striving to become as
conscious and responsible as possible about
everything in the universe. But now you sit
there quite calmly and as a humanist you say
that due to the complexity of scientific
achievement the human being must never expect
to be whole, he must always be frightened.*

Doris Lessing, *The Golden Notebook**

Learning objectives

*After studying this chapter, the student
will be able to:*

- *define behavior in specific terms.*

- *define behavior modification.*

- *analyze the application of operant conditioning
principles to behavior modification.*

- *describe behavior modification techniques, including positive and negative reinforcement and positive and negative punishment.*

- *compare and contrast fixed interval, variable interval, fixed rate, and variable rate reinforcement
schedules.*

- *discuss the ethical issues relative to the practice of
behavior modification.*

- *identify suggested readings for further study.*

*New York, 1973, Bantam Books. Copyright © 1962 by
Doris Lessing.

The principles described in this chapter are primarily the product of the field of psychology, particularly of B.F. Skinner's work. In 1953, *Science and Human Behavior*[12] by B.F. Skinner was published. This work presented the findings of animal behavior experiments and discussed their application to human behavior in an attempt to move toward a science of human behavior. Subsequent studies during the 1950s that applied the principles to profoundly retarded and psychotic institutionalized persons indicated their effectiveness. By 1958 the *Journal of the Experimental Analysis of Behavior* was published. This journal, although largely concerned with laboratory experiments with animals, printed some articles of applied behavior therapy with humans. In 1965 this journal published the results of the first experiment with the token economy.[1] The authors, Ayllon and Azrin, had developed and evaluated an environment that consistently and systematically reinforced patients diagnosed as psychotic for adaptive behavior. The motivating environment and operant conditioning principles they described were effectively applied later to populations such as the mentally ill, mentally retarded, juvenile delinquents, preschoolers, and slow learners.[2]

The late 1960s saw applied research in operant conditioning expand into the areas of education, classroom management, parenting, community work, and self-control. During the 1970s operant conditioning principles have been used by most of the helping professionals, including nurses, physicians, social workers, teachers, and psychologists. The impact of this work can be viewed from the perspective of published bibliographies. The 1967 bibliography by Barnard listed 866 references in behavior modification.[4] Britt's bibliography,[5] covering 1924 through 1975, lists 6780 publications. Assuming that Barnard's bibliography was correct, there have been well over 5000 publications in behavior modification since 1967. These numbers give some indication of the many studies being done in the area. During the 1970s textbooks on behavior modification have appeared in the professions of medicine, social work, nursing, education, psychiatry, and rehabilitative medicine.

Behavior modification involves the application of the findings of operant conditioning principles and procedures to human affairs. Operant conditioning, according to Reynolds, "refers to a process in which the frequency of occurrence of a bit of behavior is modified by consequences of the behavior."[11:1] Careful reading of this definition may lead one to assume it is an overly simplistic approach to the obvious complexities of human behavior; however, its empirical application breaks the complexities down to a manageable level and clarifies the multiple events that affect behavior.

The terms "behavior modification" and "behavior therapy" have some distinct meanings but are often used interchangeably. Martin and Pear[9] compare where and by whom each term tends to be used. "Behavior therapy" is the term favored by psychologists and psychiatrists who treat clients in traditional clinical settings. It is also associated with an experimental foundation that is based primarily on human studies in clinical settings. "Behavior modification" is the term favored for treatment carried out in schools, homes, and other natural settings outside the traditional psychiatric setting. The subjects of its experimental research are animals and humans.

Within this chapter the term "behavior modification" will be used. It is an effective treatment modality for alleviating many human problems, among which are psychiatric disorders. Although behavior modification has not yet been proved to be the treatment of choice for strictly intrapsychic conflict, it can help to alter those behaviors which result from and exacerbate such conflict. A strictly behaviorally oriented therapist, for example, is not likely to treat a client who is experiencing a significant loss. These clients would benefit more from evocative or insight psychotherapy. A primary role of behavior modification within current treatment modalities is its emphasis on the effect of the environment on human behavior. As such, it provides an alternate way of diagnosing and treating problems.

The role of behavior modification in psychiatric nursing has been inadequately explored in nursing publications. In 1959 Ayllon and Michael[3] published an article entitled "The Psychiatric Nurse as a Behavioral Engineer" in a psychology journal. Perhaps if this had been published in a nursing journal, more inroads into this area would have been made by psychiatric nurses. The behavioral principles described in this chapter can be applied in many areas, ranging from private practice to staff nursing in psychiatric hospitals. Clark[6] explains how she combines behavioral and psychodynamic techniques in her private practice. Lee[8] describes effective teaching of behavioral techniques to psychiatric aides at a state hospital, which resulted in increased interaction between the aides and patients. It may be that the current dearth of published nursing studies in behavior modification is, as Hauser[7] suggests, due to nurses' resistance, ignorance, or both.

This chapter merely introduces behavior modification principles, and it is not written with the expectation that the reader will be able to design, implement, and evaluate a behavioral treatment program without supervision. Appropriate application of behavioral techniques can be made in any setting in which psychiatric nurses work. The frequency with which psychiatric nurses do so depends on their experiences of success or failure when they use behavioral techniques, their exposure to a skilled and helpful behavior modifier, and their familiarity with behavioral literature.

Defining behavior

Behavior is any observable, recordable, and measurable act, movement, or response of the individual. It refers to everything a person does. It is observable, if only to the person performing the behavior. Although affect, cognition, and sensation, as well as imagery, are subject to behavioral treatment, the treatment is dependent on self-observation. This chapter focuses only on behaviors that are observed by others and subject to quantitative measurement.

Before a behavior can be measured, it must be defined or accurately described. One can, in defining behavior, break it into microscopic or macroscopic elements. For example, the fire setting done by a child can be defined microscopically as gathering flammable objects, striking the match, lighting the objects, fanning the lit objects, and watching the resultant blaze or macroscopically as lighting a fire that blazes. This shows that there are several different and accurate definitions of what at first glance appears to be a simply defined behavior. Behavior definition can be a difficult task. One starts by describing what is seen and/or heard and then clarifies this until pertinent observers can agree as to whether the behavior occurs.

Consider defining the behavior of fighting. It can be described as disagreement, accompanied by raised voices, exchanging epithets, and a physical struggle of reciprocal blows and kicks. In the process of clarifying this description, questions such as the following arise: Is it fighting if there is no yelling? Is it fighting if each person hits the other only once? Is it fighting if there is a physical struggle (similar to wrestling) with no hitting or kicking? As these questions are answered, a definition that is both clear and pertinent to the purpose of the definition unfolds. If one is establishing rules and consequences for aggressive adolescents, it may be decided that there is a consequence imposed simply for one student hitting and/or kicking another student, since this is likely to prevent a fight such as that which was first described. If one is developing a treatment plan for a child who is said to "fight all the time" in a classroom, the clinician, teacher, and child together may arrive at a different definition. They may decide that the significant behavior is pulling classmates' hair or pushing them out of their seats.

These definitions exemplify that a behavior is what is observed—not conclusions, inferences, or interpretations drawn from observation. Hyperactivity is not a behavior but a conclusion about a multiplicity of behaviors. One cannot measure hyperactivity; one can measure the number of times a child looks away from an assignment within a specified amount of time, how many times he interrupts a conversation in a given time period, the number of toys he displaces, the pages of classwork completed, and the length of time he remains in one body posture. The behavioral treatment would not be directed toward hyperactivity but toward those specified behaviors which interfere with the child's success in the school, home, or community.

Other examples of conclusions instead of behaviors are psychiatric diagnoses and descriptions, such as uncooperative, aggressive, compliant, depressed, hostile, and withdrawn. When one thinks of a person to whom any of these adjectives or labels are attributed, one can readily describe behaviors associated with the adjective, but from person to person the behavioral components of the adjectives will vary. There is little chance that the conjured behavioral composite will be the same for more than one person. A clear definition of a behavior decreases the interpretative variability from person to person. A clear behavior definition is a statement of what the person does, is accessible to measurement, and is not subject to interpretation.

TABLE 21-1. Operant conditioning procedures

Maintain or increase behavior	Decrease behavior
Positive reinforcement: Addition of an environmental event as a consequence of operant, increasing probability of operant's recurrence Operant → Consequence → Operant ↑	*Positive punishment:* Presentation of aversive stimulus following operant, decreasing probability of operant's recurrence Operant → Aversive event → Operant ↓
Negative reinforcement: Removal of part of an aversive stimulus as a consequent of operant, increasing probability of operant's recurrence Aversive stimulus → Operant → Removal of aversive stimulus → Operant ↑	*Negative punishment:* Removal of something following operant, decreasing probability of operant's recurrence *Response cost:* Negative punishment in which a reinforcer is lost or withdrawn following an operant Operant → Reinforcer withdrawn → Operant ↓ *Time-out from reinforcement:* Negative punishment in which no reinforcement is available following an operant Operant → No reinforcement available → Operant ↓
	Extinction: Withholding reinforcement following an operant that was previously reinforced Operant → No reinforcement → Operant ↓

Once a behavior is reliably described, one concludes that in the person's future that behavior will increase, decrease, or remain the same. Those procedures which increase, maintain, or decrease behaviors are given in Table 21-1. Each of these operant conditioning procedures will now be briefly described.

Increasing or maintaining behavior

A behavior may increase in frequency, complexity, or duration. In the acquisition of walking skills, for example, a step occurs more often; the complexity of the step increases (forward, backward, sideways, turning, becoming longer); and the amount of time walking increases. One can observe an increase in at least these three ways in the acquisition of most skills.

Operant behavior is that behavior which is maintained, increased, or decreased according to the environmental events that follow it. For clarity, the word "operant" instead of "behavior" will be used throughout the remainder of this chapter. *When the environmental events following an operant increase the probability that the operant will recur, the process is reinforcement.* Reinforcement increases the probability that the operant will occur again. Positive and nega-

tive reinforcement both increase the chances of an operant occurring again.

The addition of an environmental event (consequence) contingent on the operant is *positive reinforcement.* An example of positive reinforcement is the response of a smile to a greeting. The operant, greeting, is followed by a smile from the person addressed. The chances that the greeting will happen in the future are increased by the smile given in response. The smile is an addition (positive in the mathematical sense) of an environmental event.

$$\text{Operant} \rightarrow \begin{matrix}\text{Positive}\\\text{reinforcer}\end{matrix} \rightarrow \begin{matrix}\text{Probability of}\\\text{operant recurrent} \uparrow\end{matrix}$$

$$\text{Greeting} \rightarrow \text{Smile} \rightarrow \text{Greeting in future} \uparrow$$

There are occasions when the intent of the person responding to an operant is to *decrease* the frequency of the operant, but the operant actually increases in frequency or remains the same. A parent may yell at a young child whenever he climbs on the table; the process in operation is positive reinforcement if he continues to climb on the table or does so more often in the future.

$$\begin{matrix}\text{Child}\\\text{on table}\end{matrix} \rightarrow \begin{matrix}\text{Parent}\\\text{yells}\end{matrix} \rightarrow \begin{matrix}\text{Child}\\\text{on table} \uparrow\end{matrix} = \begin{matrix}\text{Positive}\\\text{reinforcement}\end{matrix}$$

It is important to understand in this example that the process is defined as positive reinforcement because the child climbs on the table more often. If the child decreased his climbing on the table as a result of his mother's yelling, the process would not be positive reinforcement. Any of a number of factors may possibly explain why the mother's correction did not result in a decrease in table climbing. The relevant point is that the intent of the person providing a consequence does not determine what process is in operation. The effect of the consequence on the future occurrence of the behavior determines the process.

When the reinforcer is the removal of an aversive stimulus contingent on the operant, the procedure is *negative reinforcement.* An example of negative reinforcement is putting on sunglasses in glaring sunlight. The sunlight is an aversive stimulus; the placing of the sunglasses over the eyes is the operant; the removal of, or escape from, the sunlight's glare is the negative reinforcer. It is a reinforcer because the glare's removal *increases* the probability that the person will, in future exposure to the glaring sunlight, make use of sunglasses. A reinforcer increases the probability that an operant will recur. It is negative when what was reinforcing was the removal, or *subtraction,* of something from the environment. Negative, here, is to be understood in the mathematical sense.

Aversive stimulus →	Operant →
Glare of sun →	Use of sunglasses in bright sun →

Escape from aversive stimulus →	Probability of operant recurring ↑
Escape from sun's glare →	Probable use of sunglasses in future ↑

The example just given is one of *escaping* the glare of the sun. Putting on the sunglasses prior to going out into the sun would be an example of *avoiding* the sun.

Negative reinforcement is the procedure by which one learns to escape or avoid unpleasant situations. This is evident in the following examples.

EXAMPLE 1

A mother is reprimanding a young child; the child goes to his mother and kisses her, and her reprimand stops.

Reprimand → Kiss →	Reprimand stops →	Chance of child kissing mother when again reprimanded ↑

EXAMPLE 2

Nurse A tell Nurse B she wants to discuss the conflicts in their work relationship. Nurse B becomes too busy to talk, thus avoiding the discussion. As a result, Nurse B is likely in the future to be busy whenever she sees Nurse A.

Sees Nurse A →	Busyness →	Discussion avoided →	Busyness whenever sees Nurse A ↑

EXAMPLE 3

An adolescent's parents are displeased with their son's misbehavior in school. The adolescent runs away, thereby escaping the direct experience of his parents' displeasure. In the future he may well run away again.

Parental displeasure →	Run away →	Escape from displeasure →	Running away when parents displeased ↑

Negative reinforcement may also maintain some work habits. Employees in a work situation arrive on time for work to avoid a supervisor's reprimand or loss of wages.

Decreasing behavior

Negative reinforcement is not to be confused with punishment. *Punishment decreases the probability that the operant will recur.* Negative and positive, in the mathematical sense, describe punishing procedures. *Positive punishment* as Reynolds describes it, is "the presentation of an aversive stimulus following and dependent upon the occurrence of an operant."[11:111] In other words, an operant occurs and is immediately followed by an environmental event that is aversive to the person, and this results in a decrease in occurrence of the operant. A person wearing sunglasses on a bright sunny day removes them. Removing the glasses is the operant. Immediately the glaring light hurts the person's eyes; this is the aversive event. Subsequently the person removes the sunglasses less often in glaring sunlight. This is an example of positive punishment.

Operant →	Aversive stimulus →	Operant ↓
Sunglasses off →	Glare in eyes →	Sunglasses off ↓

The procedure is also occurring when the parent yells at a child immediately after he climbs on a table. If the child climbs on the table less often, then the procedure in operation serves as punishment, the operant being climbing on the table and the aversive stimulus being the yelling.

Child on table → Parent yells → Child on table ↓

As pointed out in the explanation of positive reinforcement, the process at work is not necessarily the one intended by the person who is responding to another's operant. One might praise a noncompliant adolescent for a particular operant whenever it occurs, but the operant may occur less and less often. The process then is not positive reinforcement but positive punishment.

Negative punishment, according to Mikulas, is "a contingent event whose offset or decrease results in a decrease in the behavior it is contingent upon. This generally consists of taking away something that is reinforcing from a person when he misbehaves."[10:97] The major forms of negative punishment are response cost and time-out.

Response cost is the loss of a previously available reinforcer following an operant. After hitting her young brother, the child is deprived of her allowance. An adolescent may lose the opportunity to use the family car after coming home beyond her curfew. A consumer pays the bank a fee after overdrawing his checking account.

Operant	→	Reinforcer withdrawn	→	Operant ↓
Child hits	→	Loses allowance	→	Hitting ↓
Late coming in	→	Loss of car privileges	→	Late coming in ↓
Overdraw account	→	Loss of money	→	Overdrawing ↓

Time-out (or time-out from reinforcement), according to Mikulas, is "the punishment procedure in which the punishment is a period of time during which reinforcement is not available."[10:99]

A young child throws toys at the wall. His mother places him on a chair in the corner. When he plays again, he is less likely to throw toys at the wall.

Operant	→	Loss of all environmental reinforcement	→	Operant ↓
Throwing toys	→	No reinforcement while in chair	→	Throwing toys ↓

Extinction is the final behavior-decreasing procedure to be discussed. Extinction is the withholding or removal of a reinforcer that was previously maintaining or increasing an operant. A fairly typical example of extinction involves temper tantrums.

A child has a temper tantrum. The mother tells the child to stop, and, because she is concerned that he will injure himself, hovers about the child. She then decides to no longer pay attention to future tantrums. When the next tantrum occurs, she completely ignores it. The previous reinforcer, mother's attention, is no longer presented. It is predictable that the tantrum will become louder and more intense, then gradually taper off. As the mother continues to ignore all tantrum behaviors, they will gradually decrease. The mother is employing the extinction process.

Operant	→	Previous reinforcer withheld	→	Operant ↓
Tantrum	→	Mother's attention withheld	→	Tantrum ↓

Extinction does not usually result in an immediate decrease in the operant. After an initial increase in rate, intensity, or duration, the operant gradually decreases.

An example, taken from group therapy, of several procedures in action follows. In human interactions there is an opulent interplay of operants, reinforcers, punishers, and aversive stimuli. When one observes a given behavior, it may be an operant of the person observed, a reinforcer to an operant of a second person, and an aversive stimulus to a third person. This example, for simplicity's sake, does not relate the content of the group's interaction. It deals only with a narrow aspect of the process to exemplify four operant procedures: positive reinforcement, negative reinforcement, positive punishment, and extinction.

Abraham, usually silent in the group, speaks. Zelda laughs while Abraham is speaking. Abraham is then silent, and Zelda speaks. While she does so, all group members look at her. Zelda verbalizes more frequently than the other group members. Each time she speaks, at least the majority of group members look at her. Later, Abraham speaks again; again Zelda laughs, and again Abraham stops speaking. He does not speak again in this session.

At least three operant procedures are in action. Zelda's laughter when Abraham speaks and Zelda's speaking are both reinforced; the former is negatively reinforced, the latter positively reinforced. The operant, laughter, is followed by Abraham's cessation of speech. Abraham's speaking is an aversive stimulus to Zelda, who removes it by the operant laughter. Zelda's laughter removes the aversive stimulus of Abraham's speaking, and her laughing when he speaks will increase. This is *negative reinforce-*

ment. Zelda's operant of speaking is *positively reinforced*. The reinforcer is the eye contact of the other members. The frequency of her speaking increases. Abraham's operant of speaking decreases in frequency. Zelda's laughter is an aversive stimulus or punisher to his verbalizing. His speaking is punished by her laughter. This is *positive punishment*.

It is imperative to note that these processes are defined by what happens. The processes are not defined before they occur. The eye contact of others (added event—positive) is defined as a *positive reinforcer* to Zelda's speaking because this is what happens when she speaks and her speaking is maintained or increased in frequency. Zelda's laughter (added event—positive) when Abraham speaks is defined as a *punisher* to Abraham's operant of speaking because this happens when he speaks and his speaking decreases in frequency (punishment). Abraham's silence (removed or terminated event—negative) following Zelda's operant laughter is a *negative reinforcer* to the laughter because what happens is an increase in the probability that Zelda will laugh when the aversive stimulus (Abraham's speaking) recurs, and the laughter will remove the aversive stimulus.

In the next group session Zelda monopolizes the group during the first 10 minutes. All group members are looking at her at least occasionally during these 10 minutes. Gradually, one person stares out the window, another gazes at a picture, two others look at one another, and the last looks from one member to another but not at Zelda. As this starts to happen, Zelda's speech rate initially increases, then gradually decreases; finally, she pauses, then is silent.

This is *extinction*. The eye contact that had been reinforcing Zelda's verbalization is withheld, and her talking eventually ceases.

As mentioned earlier, this example indicates a narrow aspect of the behaviors in question for the sake of simplicity. There are, obviously, multiple reinforcers and punishers relative to any operant. In an analysis of an operant, one begins with what is most obviously presumed to be a reinforcer. If the operant is maladaptive and is to be altered, one starts treatment with what is seen as the reinforcer that is maintaining the maladaptive operant, removes the reinforcer for that operant, and provides reinforcement for an operant that is incompatible with the maladaptive one. Schedules of reinforcements have not yet been discussed, but will be considered in the following discussion of applications of behavior modification.

Applications of behavior modification

Increasing behavior

The simplest form of behavioral treatment is rearranging the environmental reinforcers. Sometimes this is not simple. A pediatric nurse consults with the psychiatric liaison nurse about an 8-year-old girl, Carole, whose treatment requires bed rest. The child is constantly out of bed playing despite the following interventions: the need for bed rest has been explained to the child and parents, parents have been cooperative, the child life worker has provided abundant activities for the child in bed, and there are other children in the room requiring bed rest who provide companionship. Carole's noncompliance with the bed rest requirement is now imitated by the other children, and they too are frequently out of bed. All involved adults are now scolding Carole.

Initially, one must define bed rest. Does it mean simply remaining on the bed? If so, is jumping on the bed within limits? In this situation bed rest means remaining in the bed and includes only those activities which can be done in a sitting or supine position. The second step is obtaining information about what happens when Carole is found out of bed (the undesirable operant) and when she is found in bed (the desirable operant). Staff will be able to describe these events, although it may be difficult to remember a time when Carole was found in bed. The third step is designing a data collection system and obtaining a baseline, that is, the frequency at which a behavior occurs prior to intervention. During waking hours Carole will be checked every 30 minutes and it will be noted whether she is or is not in bed.

After a half day of baseline data collection, it is observed that Carole was in bed only twice and that this was at mealtime. The staff reports that this is worse than usual. Each time Carole was observed out of bed, staff scolded her. This suggests that the scolding may be reinforcing the behavior, since the staff reports that she now seems to be out of bed more often, is being checked more often, and is therefore scolded more often. A current baseline is established.

The fourth step is to establish the desirable goal of intervention. Although it might be assumed that the goal is that she remain in bed

100% of the time, it is always desirable to state the intervention goal or terminal behavior clearly. The intervention goal should also include the time period during which it is to be accomplished. The intervention goal in this situation might well be "Carole will remain in bed 100% of the time within a week of treatment."

Now intervention can begin. Staff is instructed to continue checking every 30 minutes but to say nothing, maintain a blank expression, and simply place Carole in bed if she is not already there. A second staff person is to enter the room before Carole can get out of bed, to congratulate her about being in bed, and present the designated reinforcer. If two staff persons cannot be involved, then both roles can be accomplished by one person, who reenters the room immediately after placing the child in bed.

Data collection and constant evaluation should continue throughout the week, although once Carole is remaining in bed more often, she may be checked less often. All staff and family must be informed of the treatment to increase cooperation and prevent the inadvertent positive reinforcement that scolding provided to this child's being out of bed. In this situation the environmental reinforcer, staff attention, was rearranged. Staff no longer gave Carole attention for being out of bed. The attention is given for being in bed.

Let us take the same initial situation. Perhaps the initial data indicate that it is not staff attention but the gleeful laughter of her roommates that is reinforcing Carole's getting out of bed. This may be noted by Carole's increase in remaining in bed when a particularly lively roommate is not present or Carole's looking at her giggling roommates even when being corrected. One cannot suppress the children's spontaneous laughter, but one could devise a way for Carole to engage their laughter even while in bed, for example by providing a drawing pad large enough for the others to see on which she draws funny faces. One could also solicit the aid of the children by explaining the situation, but this is not likely to help unless one provides a group reinforcement contingent on Carole being in bed a certain number of times a day. The group reinforcement could be a staff person playing a game with all of them, an extra snack, parents staying some time past the end of visiting hours, or being the last group to be awakened in the morning.

The group in the room, including Carole, could easily be told that they will receive a specific reinforcer, such as one mentioned, if Carole is in bed at least half the times that she is checked. They can also be told that it is difficult for Carole to stay in bed when they laugh each time she gets up. In this way the group is involved in rearranging the reinforcement they provide Carole. The only way in which it will be known whether the reinforcer has been correctly identified or effectively altered is by the results: does Carole stay in bed more often?

Social attention is probably the most pervasive and readily available reinforcer for human beings. There are times, however, when primary reinforcers, such as food or activity, will be the reinforcers of choice. It may be that a client is not observant of or responsive to social attention. It may also be that the history of the client and the potentially reinforcing person may be so fraught with mutual anger and rejection that the quality of the attention that would be given could not be reinforcing. In these situations a primary reinforcer, such as food, or a material reinforcer, such as money, would be more immediately effective. At other times social reinforcers may be so multiply endowed that a primary reinforcer may be necessary to gain an immediate response from the client.

The first situation, that of nonobservance or nonresponse to social attention, is seen in a client who has been institutionalized for a number of years and gives no indication that he is aware of others. A piece of sugarless chewing gum contingently delivered for eye contact will be more effective than social attention. A goal of treatment for such a client is the development of social attention as a reinforcer. This is done by pairing the primary reinforcer, chewing gum, with social attention, then occasionally reinforcing with only social attention, and finally reinforcing with social attention and infrequently with a primary reinforcer.

The second situation, mutual anger and rejection, can be seen between an adolescent with a long history of behavior problems and his parents, whose many interventions have failed. In other words, the parents have received little reinforcement for parenting from the child, and the child has received little reinforcement for being their child. Reinforcers of choice may be money, privileges, or activities.

Multiply endowed reinforcers are constantly occurring, as, for example, in a young child who has many persons laughing at his misdeeds. The child will probably not be aware of a change in the quality of attention of one person if many are laughing, but he will notice if he receives a favorite treat when he behaves in a different way.

In each of the situations just described, primary reinforcers should be accompanied by social reinforcers so that the social reinforcers alone will, eventually, effectively maintain appropriate behaviors as the primary reinforcers are gradually attenuated.

REINFORCEMENT SCHEDULES. Another consideration is the timing of the data collection and the schedule of reinforcement. In the example of the child prescribed bed rest, the data were collected and the reinforcement was delivered (if Carole was in bed) every 30 minutes. Reinforcement can be delivered according to a time schedule, as in this example, or according to a performance schedule. The time schedule is called

interval schedule reinforcement; the performance schedule is called *ratio schedule reinforcement* (see below). Each type can be delivered on a fixed or variable schedule. An interval schedule refers to reinforcement being presented for the first designated behavior after a given period of time. If it is a fixed interval (FI) schedule, the time period is stable (e.g., every 5 minutes or, as in the example of Carole, 30 minutes). If a variable interval (VI) schedule is used, an average time lapse is designated (e.g., 30 minutes), as well as a minimum and maximum interval.

Behavior performance varies according to the reinforcement schedule (see below). On an FI schedule the operant increases just prior to the

---

SIMPLE REINFORCEMENT SCHEDULES

TYPE OF SCHEDULE

Time or interval: Time lapse between behaviors before reinforcement
  Fixed interval: Specific lapse of time required for reinforcement (e.g., every 5 minutes, every month, every hour, paychecks)
  Variable interval: Various amounts of time elapse between possible reinforcement (e.g., 1 minute, 32 minutes, 3 hours, 5 minutes)

Performance or ratio: Number of times an operant is performed between reinforcement
  Fixed ratio: Same number of responses required for each reinforcement (e.g., for every fifth performance of operant, piecework in factory)
  Variable ratio: Various numbers of responses required for each reinforcement (e.g., after 3, 10, 11, 19, 29, 33, 35 performances of operant; slot machines)

CHARACTERISTICS OF SCHEDULE
Fixed interval (FI)

High rate of performance before interval ends; low rate after reinforcement, the rate gradually accelerating until interval ends
Response to extinction: Responding ceases abruptly, recurs at a high rate, ceases, and recurs, with pauses increasing until rate is zero; relatively susceptible to extinction

Variable interval (VI)

Stable high rate of performance, rate lower than VR schedule
Response to extinction: Steadily decreasing rate until response is zero; of all simple schedules, most susceptible to extinction

Fixed ratio (FR)

Quickly developed high rate of performance; rate stable, especially if ratio is small
Response to extinction: Alternating pauses and high performance rate, the pause increasing until ratio is zero; relatively resistant to extinction

Variable ratio (VR)

High rate of performance, developing less quickly than FR; high rate stable even if average ratio is relatively high, except when average ratio is increased too quickly
Response to extinction: Responses continue at high sustained rate with alternating pauses until pauses lengthen and rate gradually reaches zero; of the simple schedules, most resistant to extinction

end of the interval and then, after reinforcement, decreases. One could predict that is Carole is checked and reinforced every 30 minutes, she will get out of bed soon after being checked and given staff attention, then get into bed shortly before she thinks she will be checked again. If a VI schedule is employed, behavior is more consistent. If Carole cannot predict when she will be reinforced, she is more likely to remain in bed.

A fixed ratio (FR) schedule refers to reinforcement being provided after an operant is performed a designated number of times. A variable ratio (VR) schedule refers to reinforcement being provided for the performance of an operant a predetermined average number of times, with the minimum and maximum number of times also established.

FR and VR schedules result in higher rates of responding and greater resistance to extinction than either FI or VI schedules. If this fact is overlooked in clinical practice, one can expect treatment effectiveness to be short lived. Consider a child in residential treatment whose major problem is hitting peers in response to being teased. The child is taught an alternative response to being teased and is heavily praised every hour if he has engaged in the alternative response. This treatment is effective and the child is discharged. Suddenly the child is receiving no praise for his relatively new skill, and he quickly resorts to his old immediate feedback system of hitting.

The reinforcement schedule, while the child was in treatment, could easily have been altered to a variable interval; the average length of the interval gradually increased until the reinforcement was being received at a rate closely approximating that in the natural environment. The child would thereafter have a greater chance at permanently incorporating his new skill.

The choice of reinforcement schedules during clinical intervention depends on the severity of the presenting problem, the intended duration of the operant to be learned, the age of the client, the number of available persons, and many other factors. If the presenting problem behavior is life-threatening, one preferably designs an FR schedule with a very small ratio, graduates slowly to a VR schedule with a small average ratio, and then slowly increases the average of VR re-

inforcement. For example, a child with poor judgment runs away from a residential treatment center several times a day. While away, he engages in such behaviors as fire setting, theft, and running into heavy traffic. The initial FR schedule might reinforce him every time he walked by, instead of running out of, an exit door. The schedule is altered to every second time he walks by an exit door, then every third, then gradually a VR schedule is introduced.

The intended duration of the operant influences the choice of schedule. In Carole's case there is a time limit on her bed rest requirement; a small-interval FI schedule is likely to result in Carole rapidly learning to be in bed as the interval end approaches, although after reinforcement she is likely to get out of bed. The advantage is that Carole is receiving reinforcement for appropriate behavior. As the reinforcement becomes more important to her, a VI schedule is introduced, assuring her remaining in bed more constantly. The VI schedule is appropriate, since one need not be concerned with the operant of staying in bed as necessary for an extensive time period. Operants reinforced on a VI schedule cease quickly when reinforcement is withheld (extinction). Also, busy staff in a hospital setting seem more likely to provide reinforcement on the VI schedules.

On the other hand, if the treatment goal is a child's acquisition of appropriate classroom behavior, the ratio schedules seem more desirable. These are operants that will prove helpful to the child for many years. The reinforcement schedule should be one that will result in the operant's resistance to extinction, as well as its maintenance by the reinforcers that will occur in the natural environment.

The age of the child seems to affect the rapidity with which the fixed schedules can be increased in ratio and interval length and with which they can be changed to variable schedules. A 2-year-old learns operants so rapidly that the new behavior may be maintained simply by reinforcers as they occur in the natural environment in a few days. By the time a child is 4 years old, it seems to take longer. By adolescence, the reinforcement history is so long and complex that months of intervention may be necessary before reinforcers in the natural environment can maintain newly learned operants.

The number of persons available to implement reinforcement schedules and the number of persons in treatment affect the schedule chosen.

In general, ratio schedules require more persons because behaviors must be counted. Token economies in psychiatric hospitals and residential treatment centers usually are designed on FI and VI schedules. The number of staff needed to provide reinforcers on an FR or VR schedule to 20 to 50 clients would be exorbitant. Although the general reinforcement design of token economies is interval schedules, some provision is usually made for ratio schedules.

Decreasing behavior

Punishment and extinction are the operant procedures used to decrease behaviors. Most behaviorists do not recommend punishment except in situations in which the behavior is physically dangerous. There is no question about the effectiveness of punishment, there is question about the concomitant effects of punishment, and there are ethical considerations that do not make punishment a desirable treatment. A behaviorist is not likely to recommend hitting a child, except in situations in which his behavior must be immediately altered for his safety. If a young child, for example, runs into a busy street or picks up a sharp knife, the parent wants the child to immediately alter this behavior.

Extinction, withholding what was previously reinforcing an operant, is recommended while positive reinforcement is provided for an incompatible behavior. For example, a patient may, in verbal interactions, express a great number of nonsequential and nonsense remarks that make conversation impossible. The psychiatric nurse may note that typically when this happens the staff person comments on this to the patient and talks to him about the irrelevant material. She observes that this may well be reinforcing the nonsense talk and instructs all staff to ignore such statements, bring the conversation back to the topic at hand, and give the patient attention for attending to the topic. Extinction is being used for the irrelevant material, and positive reinforcement for relevant conversation. Whenever extinction is used, one should be careful to assure that reinforcement is given for a behavior that is incompatible with the one being treated by extinction.

Clinical case analysis

Clinical example 21-1 describes behavioral treatment initiated and carried out by a nurse.

CLINICAL EXAMPLE 21-1

Joe, a 7-year-old child, was in serious jeopardy of being removed from his home because of his playing with matches and setting fires. It was agreed that treatment would be limited to 5 days from 9:30 AM to 12 PM and from 1 to 3 PM while the child continued to live at home. The boy had within the 2 years preceding treatment set three fires that caused damage, the last fire precipitating the referral. The mother and family were frightened but were not rejecting of the child.

Prior consultation and experience with a satiation procedure treatment suggested that intensive use of the procedure might be more effective than daily 1-hour sessions. The satiation procedure for fire setting involved the client lighting and blowing out matches one by one in a well-ventilated room in the presence of the therapist. The therapist supervised the activity, maintaining a minimum of verbal interaction, neither reinforcing nor punishing the child as he lit the matches. Records were kept of the endeavor.

On the first treatment day Joe lit matches during two sessions for a total of 4 hours. Over a thousand matches were lit and blown out during this time. The child's initial response to being allowed to light matches was surprise and some confusion. It was explained that it was all right for him to light the matches only in this particular room. His rate of lighting matches remained relatively constant. The mean number lit during intervals of 5 minutes was 34, the range from 22 to 45, the mode 34, and the median 33.

Observation of Joe outside the satiation sessions revealed how much he enjoyed being praised and hugged, as well as his affinity for all social contact. Joe initiated interpersonal interactions frequently, laughed and talked while playing with peers, and often sought physical affection from staff. These observations supplied data useful in Joe's subsequent treatment sessions.

On the second day Joe lit matches for only 55 minutes; the mean rate for a 5-minute interval dropped to 21, the range being 15 to 27, the mode 20, and the median 22. During this session Joe tried avoidance maneuvers, wanting to practice throwing matches away, and stating at least five times, "I don't want to strike more." Each time he made the statement he was told quietly, "Keep doing it." Finally, he stated firmly, "I ain't gonna strike no more" and walked away from the matches.

This was greeted with a hug and praise from the nurse and a discussion with him about alternative treatment. Joe then identified, in response to questions, several areas in his home where he found matches. A book of matches was placed on the window, and Joe then rehearsed, both physically and verbally, finding the matches in a specific place at home. Initially he was not instructed what to do with the book of matches. After picking it up, he opened the book and the therapist immediately yelled, "No!" Joe replaced the matches, went through the rehearsal a second time, and the same sequence occurred. At the third rehearsal he was instructed to say aloud, "I'm not going to open up the matches" when he approached them. When he did so, he did not pick up the matches and was given a hug. Joe looked elated. His pleasure with himself increased as the rehearsals went on for over an hour and covered in his own imagery every place in his house where he could find matches.

Throughout the rehearsals several changes relating to his self-cueing and the reinforcers were gradually and progressively introduced. By the session's close, the self-cueing was inaudible and the reinforcing hug was being imagined each time he picked up and replaced a book of matches. Joe's facial expressions were so spontaneous and revealing that they left no doubt about his repeating the cue to himself and fantasizing the hugs.

These alterations were developed to increase the likelihood of Joe's continuing the behavior when not in the therapist's presence. The change from not picking up the book of matches to picking it up and replacing it was introduced to break the behavior chain of picking up matches, pulling out a match, and lighting it. It seemed important for Joe to realize that he could see and pick up matches without lighting them. Although not of major concern in comparison to fire setting, consideration was given to the possibility of the child developing a phobia of matches. A phobic response seemed more likely if he learned not to touch a book of matches. Being able to hold the matches and replace them made matches simply another object in his environment over which he had control.

On the following day, when Joe entered the room, the equipment for the satiation procedure was still in the room. Since Joe spent a few minutes looking at it, it was suggested to him that he again light the matches. Because the environmental conditions were vastly different from the previous day's rehearsal and because Joe's expression indicated a curiosity about lighting the matches, it was appropriate to continue the satiation.

The satiation session was 55 minutes long, 158 matches were lit. The 5-minute mean was 15, the range 0 to 25, the mode 20, and the median 15. During the last 10 minutes no matches were lit. There was also a qualitative difference in this session. After the first 5 minutes, during which Joe lit 25 matches, he was increasingly bored and disinterested.

The rehearsals were then started and Joe was again lively, spontaneous, and happy in his endeavor. The rehearsals were broadened to include areas outside his home where he might find matches. Joe and the therapist then went throughout the building, where he found and replaced many books of matches after the activity was explained to the occupant of each office. The social contacts, needless to say, were reinforcing to Joe, and he was lavished with encouragement and praise (perhaps too much) for his efforts.

During these rehearsals Joe was instructed to imagine his mother giving him a hug when he replaced the matches. Since it was his mother who would be giving him real hugs in the future, it would be easier over time for him to fantasize a hug from her. His image of the therapist would dim as the actual contact became a progressively distant memory.

On the final treatment day Joe showed no interest in the satiation equipment. Some time was spent on the rehearsals, but the major portion of the day Joe devoted to good-byes and playing with peers. The mother, who could not attend any of the sessions, was informed of the treatment and instructed to give Joe affection and praise periodically for not playing with matches. Phone contact with her was continued for 3 weeks. Follow-up contacts over a period of 2 years indicate that Joe has neither played with matches nor set fires since treatment.

The procedures used in this treatment were behavioral and included punishment, satiation behavior rehearsal, overt differential reinforcement, and covert positive reinforcement. The punishment was the "no" yelled at Joe as he opened the book of matches when the behavior rehearsal started. This punishment was almost immediately effective, having to be used only twice.

Satiation is what we experience when overdoing a good thing. We may frequent a favorite restaurant so often that we are tired of it or overindulge in a food until we do not want to see it again. This is satiation. There are theorists who assert that the effects of satiation are temporary. Satiation was certain to inhibit Joe's current interests in matches. The possibility that satiation's effects are temporary necessitated the development of the behavior rehearsal. In the behavior rehearsal Joe practiced an alternative response to matches, which could be reinforced. The practice response was incompatible with lighting a match; the reinforcement of this response was gradually altered from overt to covert so that it would not be dependent on others. The covert reinforcement was important also because Joe had played with matches and set the fires when he was alone. Future interest in match play and fire lighting would probably occur when Joe was alone. Having covert reinforcement in his repertoire would probably help him resist the enticement of returning to his former play with matches.

Ethical issues

Behavior modification intervention has raised many ethical issues. They are indeed issues that any therapeutic endeavor should raise, but the straight-forward assertion of behavior modifiers that they can change behavior has made them and their techniques the focal point of ethical considerations. In addition, behavior modification techniques can be applied to the environment and result in behavior change. Even as antithetical a treatment as psychoanalysis is described as successful or not by behavior change or the lack thereof. All psychiatric treatments that come to mind have at least a component of behavior change as their goal. Therefore it is not behavior change per se that has resulted in behavior modification being questioned on ethical grounds. It is that the behavior change can be effected by alterations of environmental responses to the behavior. The evocative psychotherapies seem to do so by working directly with the client, not the environment. Therefore it seems that the evocative psychotherapies alter nothing for a client without his direct cooperation and knowledge. The possibility of using behavioral techniques without such involvement necessitates special consideration.

The techniques that have been presented in this chapter are indeed effective, not always, not everywhere, but they are effective. The most basic issues related to them at present are the following: Does one human being have the right to control another? Who decides what the goals of treatment are? There are other issues also, such as obtaining client consent, guaranteeing basic human rights, weighing potential risks and benefits of treatment, evaluating treatment, and accountability for treatment.

The two major issues of control and goals of treatment will be explored. Control is a strong word—one that arouses fear in most people when they think they are being controlled by others. It arouses anger when people in power are seen to be abusing their power by controlling others. There is in this word a connotation of totality—a totality that allows no escape. It is this totality which worries people when they

think there may be a behavioral technology that can control everyone. The strong public reaction to behavior modification indicates that most people do not believe that one human being has the right to control another. Whether the behavioral technology available at present can indeed allow control, even benign control, is not as central an issue as what individuals and society as a whole can do to protect themselves from being subjected to control and to what degree control should be allowed. In a society it seems to be expected that certain human behaviors be controlled. Some of these behaviors are murder, theft, assault, and property destruction. Laws are established to ensure compliance, and a judicial system is responsible for punishing the violators of the laws. Basically these laws state that a person may not abuse others or their property.

When one gets beyond these behaviors, the issues become less clear. What about emotional abuse: the way in which one slowly or quickly pecks away at another through ridicule, sarcasm, disapproval, or bitterness. Should this be controlled? Would a society in which people are encouraged, supported, openly disagreed with, and congratulated be preferred? Many people would prefer such a society, but few would want such behaviors legislated or designed into the judicial system and controlled by a behavioral engineer. This is not desired even if it were possible because that would involve adding to the power of the government and behavioral engineer, and history documents how easily power is abused.

The fact that most behavior therapists have as their goal of treatment specific and limited behavioral change does not alter the fear that behavioral technology could, in the wrong hands, be abused. Such is the case in every scientific advance. Does this mean that it should not be used at all? Hardly. It means that one must use knowledge carefully and disseminate information about the technology as widely as possible so that use and abuse of the knowledge can be readily recognized. This is particularly helpful, since all people are affected by the reinforcers and punishments in the environment. As behavioral technology becomes more widely understood, this fear of control by others should decrease, because familiarity with it and its ensuing application increases each person's control of himself. It is also more evident that behavioral techniques indicate how one is influenced, not controlled, by the environment, and influence allows for a wide range of choices.

The issue related to the specification of goals can be a complex one. Ideally the goals of treatment are the client's goals. In reality a client's goals may be at odds with those of the therapist and the first test of the therapist may then be to establish goals with which both the client and therapist can agree. An extreme example of conflicting goals could be seen in a parent asking that a behavioral therapist help design a program, the goal of which is silent sitting in a chair 4 hours a day by a 4-year-old child. No competent therapist could agree to such a goal. The therapist in such a situation may spend a great deal of time helping the parent establish more reasonable goals. The goal of the therapist during this time is the development of such reasonable parental goals. However, is this use of time unethical because it is clearly not the parent's goal? An immediate response is that this question is nonsensical; however, it points out that glibly recommending client input into goals is not as simple as it may appear. The client who is actively hallucinating or contentedly mas-

turbating for hours on end may want nothing more than to remain in such a state. It is most unlikely that a therapist could share this same goal.

With these and other issues in mind it is possible to offer general guidelines for the ethical use of behavioral modification:

1. Treatment is to be preceded by informed consent; specification of procedure, goals, and measures to be taken; and client input.
2. Once begun, treatment should include an ongoing assessment of process.
3. Before and during treatment the therapist should recognize that the treatment should be relevant to the client's adjustment to his natural environment.

Although these guidelines are not complete answers, they may help to prevent potential abuses of therapy and contribute to client growth, and these are worthwhile pursuits for all therapy modalities used by psychiatric nurses.

Suggested cross-references

Ethical decision making is discussed in Chapter 3. Child psychiatric nursing is discussed in Chapter 26.

SUMMARY

1. Behavior modification is the application of operant conditioning principles and procedures to human affairs. Operant conditioning is modification of the frequency of occurrence of a bit of behavior by the consequences of that behavior. Behavior modification is an effective treatment modality for alleviating many human problems, and it can be used by psychiatric nurses in many areas of their practice.

2. Behavior refers to everything a person does and is observable. Behavior may be defined in specific or general terms. Specific measurable definition facilitates behavior modification.

3. Behavior modification techniques may be applied to increase or decrease the occurrence of behavior. Positive reinforcement and negative reinforcement both maintain and increase behavior. Positive punishment, negative punishment, and extinction de-

crease behavior. Negative punishment includes response costs and time-out from reinforcement.

4. Reinforcement schedules may be based on fixed or variable intervals or fixed or variable ratios of reinforcement. Advantages and disadvantages of each were discussed. FR and VR schedules result in higher rates of responding and greater resistance to extinction than either FI or VI schedules.

5. An example was given of the use of behavior modification techniques by a nurse in therapy with a fire-setting child.

6. The techniques of behavior modification have raised many ethical issues. The two major issues of control and goals of treatment were explored. General guidelines for the ethical use of behavior modification were presented.

References

1. Ayllon, T., and Azrin, N.: The measurement and reinforcement of behavior of psychotics, J. Exp. Anal. Behav. **8:**35, 1965.
2. Ayllon, T., and Azrin, N.: The token economy, New York, 1968, Appleton-Century-Crofts.
3. Ayllon, T., and Michael, J.: The psychiatric nurse as a behavioral engineer, J. Exp. Anal. Behav. **2:**323, 1959.
4. Barnard, J., and Orlando, R.: Behavior modification: a bibliography, Nashville, Tenn., 1967, J.F.K. Center for Research on Education and Human Development.
5. Britt, M.: Bibliography of behavior modification, 1924-1975, 1975, privately printed by Dr. Britt, 3000 Erwen Rd., Durham, N.C. 27705.
6. Clark, C.: Combining therapeutic approaches, J. Psychiatr. Nurs. **15:**18, 1977.
7. Hauser, M.: Nurses and behavior modification resistance, ignorance or both, J. Psychiatr. Nurs. **16:**17, 1978.
8. Lee, D.: An adjunct to training psychiatric aides in behavioral modification techniques, J. Psychiatr. Nurs. **7:** 169, July-Aug. 1969.
9. Martin, G., and Pear, J.: Behavior modification: what it is and how to do it, Englewood Cliffs, N.J., 1978, Prentice-Hall, Inc.
10. Mikulas, W.L.: Behavior modification, New York, 1978, Harper & Row, Publishers.
11. Reynolds, G.S.: A primer of operant conditioning, Glenview, Ill., 1968, Scott, Foresman & Co.
12. Skinner, B.F.: Science and human behavior, New York, 1953, The Free Press.

Annotated suggested readings

Arkin, A.M., et al.: Behavior modification: present status in psychiatry, N.Y. State J. Med. **76:**190, Feb. 1976.

This article provides a comprehensive overview of the many issues related to behavior modification. The reader is introduced to the types of behavior modification approaches. Of particular significance is the discussion of ethical issues related to this therapeutic modality, particularly when aversive techniques are used.

Becker, W.C.: Parents are teachers: a child management program, Champaign, Ill., 1971, Research Press Co.

This book contains clear programmed instruction of behavioral techniques for use by parents.

Behavior Modification, Beverly Hills, Calif., Sage Publication.

This interdisciplinary journal is published four times a year and prints research and clinical papers on applied behavior modification in a broad scope of settings.

Behavior Research and Therapy, Great Britain, Pergamon Press, Ltd.

This bimonthly, international, interdisciplinary journal publishes articles relating to the application of learning theory, broadly defined, to maladaptive behaviors.

Berni, R., and Fordyce, W.E.: Behavior modification and the nursing process, ed. 2, St. Louis, 1977, The C.V. Mosby Co.

Particularly recommended is the chapter on ethical issues. The book is appropriate for all levels of nursing students.

Carruth, B.F.: Modifying behavior through social learning, Am. J. Nurs. **76:**1804, 1976.

The author describes the application of behavior modification techniques to the care of psychiatric patients by graduate students. The students worked with mentally ill children and then chronically mentally ill adults and reported positive responses to both situations. An important side effect of the experience was that the students had an opportunity to influence staff in both settings.

Davison, G.C., and Stuart, R.B.: Behavior therapy and civil liberties, Am. Psychol. **30:**755, 1975.

This discussion of the use of behavior modification approaches to therapy as it relates to the rights of the pa-

tient is highly recommended. The authors are clearly in favor of behavior modification, but take an objective approach to describing potential abuses and the mechanisms that are required to protect civil liberties. There is a detailed delineation of protections related to the acquisition of informed consent.

Forsland, C.K., and Erickson, E.A.: A behavioral approach to physical rehabilitation: a case study, J. Psychiatr. Nurs. **16:**48, May 1978.

The applicability of behavior modification approaches in nonpsychiatric health care settings is demonstrated in this article. A case study is used to illustrate the implementation of a behavioral therapy program with a patient on a rehabilitation unit. The importance of discharge planning and follow-up is also emphasized.

Hauser, M.J.: Nurses and behavior modification: resistance, ignorance or both, J. Psychiatr. Nurs. **16:**17, Aug. 1978.

This is a thought-provoking article in which the author questions the failure of nurses to incorporate social learning theory and behavioral techniques into their practice. She raises a number of questions that merit further investigation.

Hauser, M.J.: Cognition commands change, J. Psychiatr. Nurs. **19:**19, Feb. 1981.

The author discusses cognitive models of behavioral change as they relate to work with disturbed children. The models presented include cognitive restructuring as exemplified by rational-emotive therapy, self-instruction, and problem solving. She also advocates teaching the treatment approach to parents. Cognitive restructuring and self-instruction are rather sophisticated methodologies that should only be implemented by nurses with advanced training in child psychiatric nursing.

Hersen, M., Eisler, R.M., and Miller, P.M.: Progress in behavior modification, vol. 2, New York, 1976, Academic Press, Inc.

An excellent review and analysis of published behavioral treatment by nurses is found in LeBow's chapter, Applications of Behavior Modification in Nursing Practice. Although not a nurse, the author clearly grasps the various levels of nursing practice and delineates practice models that nurses have used in behavioral models.

Journal of Applied Behavior Analysis, Lawrence, Kan., Society for the Experimental Analysis of Behavior, Inc.

This quarterly journal reports primarily experimental research.

Journal of Behavior Therapy and Experimental Psychiatry, Great Britain, Pergamon Press, Ltd.

This quarterly journal publishes papers indicated by its title as well as some that are intended to assist nonbehaviorally educated clinicians.

Lazarus, A.A.: Multimodel behavior therapy: treating the "basic id." In Franks, M., and Wilson, G.T., editors: Annual review of behavior therapy theory and practice, New York, 1974, Brunner/Mazel, Inc.

This work is appropriate for graduate students. It assumes basic knowledge of behavioral principles and their application.

Mash, E.J., Harndy, L.C., and Hamerlynch, L.A.: Behavior modification approaches to parenting, New York, 1976, Brunner/Mazel, Inc.

This book describes the broad spectrum of behavioral treatment for parents and families. It is useful for practicing clinicians.

McMorrow, M.J., Cullinan, D., and Epstein, M.H.: The use of the Premack principle to motivate patient activity attendance, Perspect. Psychiatr. Care **16:**14, Jan.-Feb. 1978.

This article includes a description of a project based on the Premack principle followed by a critique of the project. The Premack principle states that a high-probability behavior can be used to reinforce the occurrence of a low-probability behavior. The article raises several questions about the study based on the author's interpersonal approach to psychotherapy.

Mikulas, W.L.: Behavior modification, New York, 1976, Harper & Row, Publishers.

An overview of the whole field of behavior treatment is provided. This book is recommended to both undergraduate and graduate students.

Patterson, G.R.: Families: applications of social learning to family life, Champaign, Ill., 1975, Research Press Co.

This undergraduate level book presents skills families need to interact more productively.

Peterson, K.A., and Erickson, E.A.: Use of reinforcement principles to reinstate self-care activities in a deaf and blind psychiatric patient, J. Psychiatr. Nurs. **15:**15, June 1977.

This is a good illustration of the application of behavior modification principles to the care of one patient who presented a particularly challenging constellation of nursing care problems. There is a detailed discussion of nuring intervention and patient response.

Reynolds, G.S.: A primer of operant condition, Glenview, Ill., 1968, Scott, Foresman & Co.

This excellent, basic, and brief text presents findings of behavioral laboratory experiments.

Shapiro, A.K.: The behavior therapies: breakthrough or latest fad, Am. J. Psychiatry **133:**154, Feb. 1976.

The author delineates some of the potential problems associated with jumping on the bandwagon of a new therapeutic approach. He recognizes the potential benefits of behavioral therapy, but cautions that further research is needed to define better the situations in which it is applicable.

Skinner, B.F.: Science and human behavior, New York, 1953, The Free Press.

This is a basic reading in the area of behavior therapy. It is a "classic" in the field.

Steckel, S.B.: Contracting with patient-selected reinforcers, Am. J. Nurs. **80:**1597, 1980.

This article has value for nurses who are working in a variety of settings. The author describes her extensive experience with the use of performance contracts with patients who select their own reinforcements. A sample of a recommended contract is included.

Stolz, S.B., Wienckowski, L.A., and Brown, B.S.: Behavior modification: a perspective on critical issues, Am. Psychol. **30:**1027, 1975.

This paper is an extremely thorough discussion of the scope of behavior therapy and of the many associated legal and ethical issues. It is highly recommended for its completeness and for the objective approach to what can be a highly emotional issue.

Tharp, R.J., and Wetzel, R.J.: Behavior modification in the natural environment, New York, 1969, Academic Press, Inc.

This is a helpful breakdown of the many complexities of behavioral treatment. It is recommended for graduate students.

Watson, D.L., and Tharp, R.G.: Self-directed behavior, Belmont, Calif., 1972, Wadsworth Publishing Co.

This book is recommended for clinicians treating adolescents and adults.

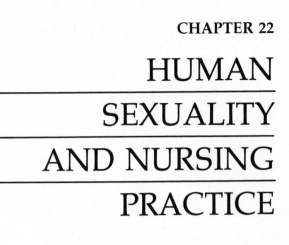

CHAPTER 22

HUMAN
SEXUALITY
AND NURSING
PRACTICE

SUSAN POORMAN

I locked myself away from you
Too long,
Tossing aside my feelings
For you.
Looking for a way out, an excuse
Not to touch you;
Because I want to,
Inciting a riot within me.

To reach out for you
Is difficult,
But less difficult
Than turning away.
Leslie Bertel

Learning objectives

After studying this chapter, the student should be able to:

- state why nurses need knowledge of human sexuality, the kind of knowledge needed, and problems encountered in obtaining it.

- describe sexuality and the difficulty in labeling sexual behavior as normal, abnormal, or problematic.

- relate the changes in sexuality that may occur throughout one's life because of illness, injury, and aging.

- contrast the following modes of sexual expression: homosexuality, transsexualism, and transvestism.

- define each of the following sexual dysfunctions: premature ejaculation, ejaculatory incompetence, impotence, female orgasmic dysfunction, and vaginismus.

- identify the two major responsibilities of the nurse in the assessment phase of the sexual counseling process.

- analyze the four phases of the nurse's growth in developing self-awareness of human sexuality.

- relate the roles of the nurse and patient in the planning phase of sexual counseling.

661

■ *describe the indications for and components of the three levels of nursing intervention in sexual counseling.*

■ *critique some commonly held myths regarding human sexuality.*

■ *state the factors that need to be assessed when evaluating the effectiveness of the sexual counseling process.*

■ *identify suggested readings for future study.*

As nursing moves toward a holistic approach to patient care, nurses are often called on to intervene in situations regarding patients' sexuality. As a profession, nursing has historically fallen short of its responsibility to counsel individuals in this area. Nurses have a wide variety of reactions to patients' concerns regarding sexuality. For example, some nurses claim that "nurses are not sex therapists and therefore do not understand sexual issues." Other nurses ignore or deny sexual issues that patients raise and "pass the buck" to physicians, social workers, or other health professionals. Nurses tell patients to ask their physician about sexuality questions, but physicians may not necessarily be more open or prepared to address these issues. Nurses may feel embarrassed when a man talks about his fear of impotence during chemotherapy. Or they may be repelled or shocked by patients who "come out" and disclose their gay identity. More than a few nurses may be hesitant to talk with a woman after her mastectomy who is worried that her husband will no longer find her sexually appealing.

Sexuality cannot be separated from the condition of being human; therefore it is imperative that nurses develop skill and confidence in addressing sexual issues with their patients if holistic health care is to be provided. Education regarding sexuality will provide professional nurses with the theoretical knowledge necessary for clinical application in nursing practice.

Implementing the nursing role

Since nurses confront difficult issues on a daily basis with patients, such as death, family problems, and life-death crises, the question can be raised as to why nurses are unable to intervene appropriately in patient situations regarding sexuality. Several factors contribute to nurses' difficulty in providing sexual counseling or health teaching:

1. Nurses often do not obtain adequate theoretical knowledge in their nursing education. Sexuality is addressed basically in terms of the anatomical and physiological functions of the male and female bodies. Nurses often do not address their feelings and thoughts about sexual issues, and in many cases nurses do not think of themselves as sexual beings. It seems that to view oneself as a professional, many nurses behave as if they believe themselves to be asexual beings. Nurses tend to deny the fact that they are human beings with needs and feelings that include sexual desires.

2. Many nursing educators are improperly prepared to address the issue of sexuality with students because of deficiencies in their own education. The effect of inadequate preparation is ignorance, which breeds ignorance and results in inadequate assessment and intervention with patients regarding issues of human sexuality.

3. Nurses often believe that physicians are more knowledgeable regarding sexuality; therefore nurses refer any sexual concern raised by patients to the physician. Several important issues arise for consideration from this assumption. First, physicians often have no more sexual education and knowledge than nurses. Second, nurses spend more time with patients on a daily basis, and therefore many patients are more comfortable talking about sexual issues with the nurse than with their physician. Most important, nurses fail to treat the "whole person" if they fail to include sexuality as a component of nursing care.[14]

Not all nurses will become experts in the area of sexuality; however, if nurses are aware of basic principles of human behavior, they will have a better understanding of a patient's sexual needs and problems. Nurses come in contact with sexual issues on a daily basis, regardless of their field of nursing practice. If nurses are comfortable with sexual issues, they will convey that comfort to the patient, which in turn gives the patient permission to discuss sexual issues with the nurse. The nurse-patient relationship is an intimate relationship in many ways. Nurses care for patients who are often experiencing painful and changing events in their lives. Thus it is appropriate that the nurse-patient relationship allow for open honest discussion of sexuality.

In answering the question "What do nurses need to know about sexuality?" several factors need to be considered. First, nurses need to know themselves, to be aware of their own feelings and values regarding sexuality. If nurses are not aware of their feelings, they cannot adequately or competently help patients meet their needs. For example, nurses may become distressed when they find patients masturbating. Many people have been raised to feel that there is something innately wrong with masturbating, even though they know intellectually that masturbation is a normal healthy expression of sexual behavior. Thus a nurse who is distressed by a patient who is masturbating will have difficulty in talking with the patient about his or her sexual needs.

Second, nurses need to understand that everyone's feelings and values regarding sexuality are not going to match their own feelings and values. Anytime the topic of sex or any issue that vaguely hints at a sexual connotation comes up, nurses frequently feel threatened and tend to lose objectivity. This may occur because of a difference of values between the nurse, patient, or norms of society. For example, the nurse who is staunchly opposed to abortion may have a difficult time caring for a patient who has just received an abortion. Nurses may ignore patients with different beliefs and values or may become passively or even actively hostile toward them. Nurses have been known to dehumanize patients with value systems that differ from their own or detach themselves from their care and then feel guilty for doing so. In such cases a vicious cycle results in which the nurse and patient both lose. When nurses have different beliefs and values from their patients, a common response is to misunderstand, feel scared and confused, and judge others' values as wrong. Although nursing textbooks tell nurses to be nonjudgmental, the ideal attitude is much easier to instruct than implement. It is critically important, if sensitive competent nursing care is to be provided to patients, that nurses get in touch with what it is they feel and believe about sexuality and about themselves as sexual beings.

Nurses also need to develop basic skills in helping patients approach their sexual concerns. Although all nurses will not become sex therapists, all nurses can become educated and enlightened about the sexual health of patients and can use practical sound counseling methods with patients. Specifically, nurses can (1) learn interviewing skills for sexual assessment and history taking, (2) develop confidence in their ability to approach or allow patients to approach sexual issues, and (3) effectively counsel or refer patients for appropriate counseling regarding sexual issues.

Most nursing textbooks address sexuality from the viewpoint of the medical model, that is, the content includes primarily charts of the anatomy and physiology of male and female reproductive organs and graphs of hormonal levels in the adult male and female bodies. Anatomical and physiological information is of vital importance in understanding human sexuality; however, such information is available and best described in anatomy and physiology nursing texts.[9,23] This chapter will depart from the traditional approach by integrating concepts of sexual counseling in a nursing process model.

Sexuality defined and described

Sexuality is broadly defined as a desire for contact, warmth, tenderness, or love.[1] It incorporates far more than genital sex. Sexuality includes looking and talking, poetry and long walks, hand holding, kissing, self-pleasuring, and the production of mutual orgasms through various means.[8] Sexuality includes one's total sense of self. Kirkendall and Rubin[13] believe people must concern themselves with sexual feelings and behaviors throughout the life cycle. Sexuality is an integral part of every human being and is lived every day of one's life. It is evident in the way one looks, believes, behaves, and relates to other human beings. Accepting a broad concept of sexuality allows the nurse to explore ways in which people are sexual beings, and understand more fully one's own feelings, beliefs, and actions related to human sexuality.

It is difficult, if not impossible, to define "normal" sexual behavior without making value judgments. One's parents, relatives, friends, and society are all likely to have different views on normal sexuality. Goldstein[6] defines normal sexual behavior as any sexual act between adults that is consensual, lacks force, and is performed in private, away from unwilling observers.

If one accepts Goldstein's definition of normal behavior, then homosexuality, the act of obtaining sexual pleasure from a member of the same sex, would be considered normal because the behavior meets the requirements of consent, adult, lacking force, and privacy. Conversely, pedophilia, the act of obtaining sexual pleasure by molesting a child, would not meet Goldstein's requirements of normal sexual behavior, since the action is not performed by consenting adults.

Experts in the area of sexuality and sexual behavior do not agree on what types of sexual behavior are problematic. For years, many people believed that any deviation from sexual relations between married partners for procreative purposes was problematic. Today, more people are beginning to view sexual behavior with a wider range of attitudes and values.

One view of problematic sexual behavior is reflected in the classification of psychosexual disorders identified in DSM-III.[2] These disorders are divided into four major groups: gender identity disorders, paraphilias, psychosexual dysfunctions, and other sexual disorders. The *gender identity disorders* are characterized by an incongruence between one's anatomical sex and

---

PARAPHILIAS

exhibitionism Repetitive acts of exposing the genitals to an unsuspecting stranger for the purpose of achieving sexual excitement, with no attempt at further sexual activity with the stranger.

fetishism The use of nonliving objects (fetishes), such as articles of clothing, as a repeatedly preferred or exclusive method of achieving sexual excitement.

pedophilia The act or fantasy of engaging in sexual activity with prepubertal children as a repeated preferred or exclusive method of achieving sexual excitement.

sexual masochism Sexual excitement produced in an individual by his or her own suffering, such as through humiliation, bondage, or beatings.

sexual sadism The infliction of physical or psychological suffering on another person to achieve sexual excitement.

transvestism Recurrent and persistent cross-dressing by a heterosexual male for the purpose of sexual excitement.

voyeurism Repetitive looking at unsuspecting people, usually strangers, who are either naked, in the act of disrobing, or engaging in sexual activity.

zoophilia The use of animals as a repeatedly preferred or exclusive method of achieving sexual excitement.

---

gender identity. The individual is uncomfortable with his or her own sex and behaves in a way usually associated with the opposite sex. Transsexualism is classified as such as disorder. *Paraphilias* are characterized by the need for unusual or bizarre imagery or acts to obtain sexual excitement, which may interfere with one's capacity for reciprocal affectionate sexual activity. These sexual deviations as described in DSM-III are identified and defined at left. *Psychosexual dysfunctions* are characterized by inhibitions in sexual desire or the psychophysiological changes that characterize the sexual response cycle. Finally, *other psychosexual disorders* include egodystonic homosexuality, which is characterized by weak heterosexual arousal and sustained homosexual arousal that is undesired and distressing to the individual.

Issues concerning sexuality are often emotionally charged, subjective, and not well understood. As a result, atypical behavior is frequently labeled problematic.

As professionals, nurses need to ask themselves for whom is the presenting sexual concern a problem? Obviously, sexual behavior that infringes on the rights of others is problematic; for example, rape and child sexual abuse. For other sexual behaviors, the nurse may not be able to easily determine if the behavior is a problem for the patient or others. Sometimes when health professionals decide a patient is displaying abnormal or problematic sexual behavior, it is so labeled because it is a problem for the professional and not the patient.

CLINICAL EXAMPLE 22-1

Ms. H is a staff nurse on an oncology unit. She has been taking care of Mr. J for the past 3 weeks. Mr. J has been diagnosed as having lung cancer in the terminal phase. Although Mr. J is experiencing discomfort, he is alert and well oriented. One day Ms. H finds him tearful and depressed. With encouragement he tells her that he misses his wife and wants to go home to see her. Ms. H tries to reassure Mr. J that he sees his wife two times each day at visiting hours. Mr. J becomes increasingly frustrated and blurts out, "You don't understand! I love my wife and I want to go home to my own bed with her. I want to be able to make love to my wife and hold her again before I die. I can't do that here!" Ms. H became embarrassed and left the room. Because of her own discomfort, she requested a different assignment for the remainder of the week. When questioned about the request for a change in assignment by the head nurse, Ms. H told the head nurse that she and Mr. J have a personality conflict and she feels unable to care for him. Later, in a staff meeting, she stated to the other nurses that Mr. J was really becoming a problem. "The man's on his death bed and all he can do is think about sex. Can you believe in his condition he wants to be discharged so that he can go home and have sex with his wife? He wanted me to help him talk with his doctor about getting discharged. He's just another dirty old man. All that work to discharge him and we'd have to readmit him in a few days."

Ms. H's behavior indicates her discomfort with planning nursing care to meet Mr. J's sexual needs. First, the nurse was unable to discuss his sexual needs with him. Second, she refused to act as the patient's advocate by helping him discuss his sexual needs with the physician. Third, the nurse presented her own judgmental values and beliefs when discussing Mr. J's problem with her co-workers.

In Clinical example 22-1 the nurse's own feelings of inadequacy interfered with her ability to allow the patient to fulfill a very important need. By labeling the patient's behavior as a problem, the nurse was exposing her own conflicting sexual values but she had not stopped to examine the feeling and values reflected in her behavior. She stated that she was upset because of the trouble the nursing staff would have in discharging and readmitting Mr. J. That is, the nurse focused on the inconvenience to the nursing staff rather than on the patient's needs as a human being. The result was to stereotype and deprecate the patient as a "problem patient" and to deny him an essential aspect of his therapeutic care.

Changes in sexuality

Feelings about oneself as a sexual being change throughout the life cycle. Sexual identity cannot be separated from one's self-concept or body image. Therefore when changes occur in one's body or emotions, they will effect a change in one's sexuality as well.

Illness and injury

Physical and emotional illness may cause alterations in a person's sexual feelings and behaviors. Nurses usually provide care to patients who experience alterations in sexual feelings and behaviors and need to discuss and therapeutically intervene in a patient's response to changes in sexual functioning. A person experiencing rheumatoid arthritis may experience body disfiguration and a change in body image because of

swollen areas around joints. The same patient may experience decreased sexual interest because of fear of joint and muscle pain during intercourse. Patients who suffer from depressive episodes often experience a decrease in libido as a symptom. People who have had a myocardial infarction in the past may have a decreased sexual interest because of fear of a heart attack from becoming sexually aroused. Psychotic patients may experience hallucinations and delusions in which they become sexually preoccupied.

Some medications contribute to sexual dysfunction, failure to reach orgasm in women, and impotence or failure to ejaculate in men. Nurses are responsible for being knowledgeable about the medications they administer and to educate patients regarding possible side effects, informing them to notify the physician when side effects occur. For example, a patient may not be aware that his medication can be the cause of his impotence, yet he may be extremely embarrassed and hesitant to talk with the physician or nurse about the problem.

Patients who become disfigured because of injury or surgery may also experience alterations in sexuality. Sudden injury leaves patients with little or no time to prepare for the loss. People who experience spinal cord injuries may lose sexual functioning because of full or partial paralysis. Such patients may need assistance and counseling to make changes in behaviors to meet their sexual needs.

Some sexual problems that arise from injury or surgery are organic in origin; others are psychological. The most common types of surgical procedures that present the potential for post-surgical difficulty with sexuality include the following[19]:

1. Loss of an external body part, such as with a mastectomy or penectomy
2. Loss of internal organs, such as with a prostatectomy or hysterectomy
3. Loss of body function, such as surgery that would result in impotence
4. Relocation of a body orifice, such as a colostomy or ileostomy

Changes in sexuality, regardless of the precipitating factor, may mean changes in sexual patterns and behaviors. The role of the professional nurse includes aiding patients with changes because of illness or injury to understand their feelings and explore their options and then facilitating a healthy adjustment. Clinical example 22-2 illustrates a nurse helping a married couple adjust to a change in sexual behavior resulting from an incapacitating physical illness.

CLINICAL EXAMPLE 22-2

Ms. C, 24 years old, is newly admitted to the hospital with a diagnosis of leukemia. Ms. C was a newlywed, having been married only 7 months. Approximately 3 weeks ago she was diagnosed with leukemia and was being rehospitalized for additional blood tests and chemotherapy. Ms. J was the nurse assigned to Ms. C's case. While Ms. J gathered assessment data from Ms. C, she inquired about sexual problems.

NURSE: **Since you learned about your condition, have you had any changes in your usual sexual activity?**

MS. C: **Yes.**

NURSE: **Are any of the changes presenting a problem for you?**

MS. C: **This is so embarrassing, I shouldn't be concerned about such a trivial thing when I have my leukemia to worry about.**

NURSE: **It is perfectly normal to be worried about your sexual life. If you would like to talk about it, I have some time.**

MS. C: **(timidly) It's OK?**

The nurse smiles and nods, encouraging Ms. C to talk.

MS. C: **My husband has been very different with me ever since we found out I was sick. He treats me like a china doll—it's like he's afraid if he touches me, I'll break. My doctor told me to continue with regular activity but to rest if I got tired. My husband doesn't seem to understand.**

NURSE: **Have you talked with your husband about this?**

MS. C: **I feel guilty for even being upset about this. I'd be too embarrassed to talk to him about this.**

NURSE: **Then your husband doesn't know that his behavior is a problem for you?**

MS. C: **I don't think so—if he does know, then he probably doesn't care (starts to cry). I didn't mean that about my husband. I know he cares about me. I guess I'm just so frustrated because I don't know what to do.**

NURSE: **Maybe it would be helpful if all three of us talked together.**

MS. C: **I don't know, I'd have to ask my husband.**

NURSE: **Well, it's up to you and your husband. I just want you to know that I will be available to talk with both of you either separately or together while you are here. Why don't you think it over and I'll check back with you about it.**

The nurse did not push the patient into any particular way of approaching her problem, but helped her explore her options. Later that week, Ms. C asked the nurse to meet with her and her husband. Ms. J reserved a quiet interview room on the unit to ensure privacy and arranged an appointment time when Mr. C was able to come in. On the day of the meeting before Ms. J had a chance to introduce herself, Mr. C blurted out the following:

MR. C: **I know why we are all here—my wife told you we have a sex problem. I can't believe she would talk to a stranger about such a private problem!**

NURSE: **It is embarrassing to talk about such a personal issue with someone you don't know. I can understand that you could feel uncomfortable talking about your sexual relationship with a stranger.**

MR. C: **You said it! I feel like a weirdo having to be counseled about sex.**

NURSE: **Let me start then by clarifying why we're here. What we'll be talking about is you and your wife's feelings and hopefully get a better understanding of how to deal with the changes in your lives since your wife's illness. You both probably have a lot of concerns and fears. I'd like to help you with them. Where shall we start?**

In this clinical situation the nurse decreased the focus on sex to allay the couple's anxiety. Ms. J then asked Ms. C to tell her husband what was bothering her. She helped them talk with each other and try to find possible solutions. For example, since Mr. C feared that his wife might be too weak or tired to engage in sex, the couple decided that Ms. C would take a more active role in initiating sex by telling her husband when she felt physically able to participate. The nurse facilitated open communication between the couple and acted as a sexual health educator by teaching the couple about the realities of Ms. C's condition. It was important for the nurse to help the couple work together to find their own solution to their problem.

Aging process

Although many researchers have documented decreases in sexual activity with aging, sexual activity remains an important part of expressing oneself throughout the life cycle. The aging process causes some changes in sexual anatomy and responsiveness for both men and women. Physiological changes in the woman are related to depleting estrogen supplies (after menopause) and include atrophy of the vaginal mucosa with decreased vaginal lubrication, actual shrinkage in size and loss of elasticity in the vaginal canal, especially in sexually inactive women, and a decrease in actual breast size.[14] In a study of 34 women from the ages of 51 to 78, Masters and Johnson[16] noted a number of alterations in sexual response patterns as compared to premenopausal women: (1) a vasocongestive increase in breast size usually seen during sexual excitement was decreased or nonexistent, (2) generalized myotonia was decreased, (3) the vasocongestive response in the breasts was decreased, (4) there is less expansion of the vagina during sexual stimulation, and (5) vaginal lubrication decreased and required a longer time to develop. The researchers also noted that some aging women experience painful uterine contractions during orgasm.

Physiological changes in the male include a gradual decrease in circulating levels of testosterone from approximately age 60 on. However, decreased testosterone levels in men are usually not as pronounced as the estrogen deficiency in postmenopausal women. Spermatogenesis does decrease with age; however, men often remain fertile until death. Aging alters the sexual response pattern of the male in that (1) longer time and more direct genital stimulation is required to achieve erection, (2) there is a decrease in the firmness of the erection, (3) a less intense ejaculation is experienced, and (4) the time interval after ejaculation when the male is physiologically unable to ejaculate again also tends to lengthen.[14]

In Western culture the myth of the older adult as an asexual being still prevails. Westerners tend to regard the older adult as one who has no interest in sexual feelings or behavior. Many personality theorists have participated in and encouraged the myth of the older adult as an asexual or childlike being. Psychoanalytical theory describes the sexuality of the aging person as a regression to oral and anal levels of gratification. Since many theories about development have had their roots in psychoanalytical theory, it is not surprising that the stereotypical myth of sexless old age is perpetuated.

Not only have people been taught that older adults have little interest in sex, but also that it is normal for the older person to have no interest in sex. Therefore when health professionals encounter older individuals who do indicate an interest in sex or who are sexually active, the professional often judges the older adult as perverted or "oversexed." Older adults themselves are not exempt from society's false beliefs about sexuality and aging. Many older adults deny sexual attractions and feelings because they also have been socialized to believe that sexual behavior in older people is abnormal or perverted. Older adults are influenced by cultural values of Western society that currently prize youth and vitality and often look with disgust at an elderly person doing anything other than sitting in a rocking chair.

Sexual capability can be maintained throughout a person's life. There are, however, several reasons for decreased sexual activity among older adults. Kolodny et al.[14] identified five categories of altered sexuality related to the aging process: general sexual disinterest, sexual boredom, impaired physical sexuality, cultural inhibition, and attrition by disuse. General sexual disinterest included people who, with advancing years, viewed sex as an unnecessary indulgence. Sexual boredom occurred in couples who realized that boredom may be a factor in the sexual relationship but failed to experiment with changing sexual habits developed over the years. Boredom may be associated with decreased self-esteem, cultural inhibitions, or changes in the health status of the aging individual.

An extremely important variable affecting altered sexuality because of aging is attrition by disuse: "use it or lose it." Prolonged abstinence from sexual activity caused more physiological problems in the older adult. For example, the older female who abstains from sexual activity will have a greater degree of shrinkage in the size of her vagina than a female of the same age who is sexually active. The older male who abstains from sexual activity may experience difficulty having erections when attempting to return to sexual activity. In general, the effects of disuse or lack of sexual activity magnify physical problems of sexuality in the older adult.[14] Most researchers at present agree with the original Kinsey studies, which indicated that persons who enjoy an active sex life as young adults will probably continue their usual pattern in older adulthood with some modifications, rather than experiencing a sudden decrease or cessation of sexual activity and interest in older adulthood.[12]

Differences in sexuality

There are numerous different modes of sexual expression. For the purposes of this chapter, three modes of sexual expression frequently encountered by nurses are discussed: homosexuality, transsexuality, and transvestism.

Homosexuality

Marmor[15] defined the homosexual person as "one who is motivated in adult life by a definite preferential erotic attraction to members of the same sex and who usually (but not necessarily) engaged in overt sexual relations with them."

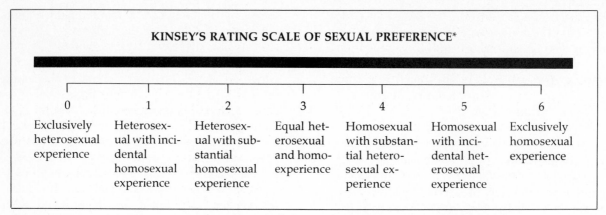

*Reprinted with permission from The Kinsey Institute for Research in Sex, Gender & Reproduction, Inc., Bloomington, Ind.

Marmor's definition excludes transitory incidental homosexual activity in adolescence and in primarily heterosexual persons. Individuals who believe in or participate in sexual practices that differ from society's norm are often termed sexual minorities. Homosexuals are the largest sexual minority. The incidence of homosexuality in the United States today has been conservatively estimated at 10% to 15% of the population.[3] Contrary to beliefs held by many individuals in our society, homosexuals are not odd or unusual, nor are they easily recognizable as homosexuals. The majority of homosexuals are everyday people who get up every morning, work, play, love, and lead normal healthy lives.

Alfred Kinsey was the first to scientifically study the incidence of homosexuality in 1948. Kinsey[12] used a seven-point rating scale in which individuals could be classified in terms of their sexual preference. This scale is presented above. Kinsey found the heterosexual vs. homosexual dichotomy meaningless. His studies indicated that a substantial percentage of men and women had experienced both heterosexual and homosexual activity. The Kinsey study indicated that 13.95% of males and 4.25% of females of the total population have had more than incidental homosexual experiences. However, many researchers today believe the incidence of homosexuality is significantly higher than the incidence reported by Kinsey.[11]

For many years the medical profession, including psychiatry, has searched for causes of homosexuality. The message in looking for the cause of a condition is that if one can find the cause then one can find a treatment or cure. Many theories have been formulated as to the cause of homosexuality; however, no cause has ever been established. Today less emphasis is being placed on curing the homosexual than on learning about homosexuality and viewing it as a sexual preference rather than a disease.

If current estimates of the incidence of homosexuality are accurate, nurses come into contact with homosexuals on a daily basis. Despite this high incidence of homosexuality, nurses generally know very little about homosexuality and almost always assume that all patients are heterosexual. Clinical example 22-3 illustrates a situation in which the nurse failed to recognize the patient's sexual preference and plan for holistic nursing care.

CLINICAL EXAMPLE 22-3

Ms. T is a 51-year-old woman who was admitted to the intensive care unit after a severe myocardial infarction. Ms. T requested that her female friend be allowed to visit her. Ms. M, the nurse taking care of Ms. T, explained to her that the intensive care unit has restricted visiting hours for immediate family only, no friends. Ms. T did not argue the regulations regarding visiting hours, but failed to recover. She began to exhibit signs of depression, loss of appetite, restlessness, irritability, and feelings of sadness.

Ms. M took excellent physical care of Ms. T and was truly puzzled at her lack of improvement. She discussed the patient with her head nurse in a case conference. The head nurse suggested that Ms. M talk with Ms. T about what was bothering her. At the head nurse's suggestion, Ms. M encouraged her patient to talk with her. Ms. T told the nurse that she really wanted her friend to visit and confided to her that she was a homosexual and that she and her friend had maintained a lover/intimate/spouse relationship for the past 25 years. Because there are no telephones in the intensive care unit, Ms. T had not been able to talk with her friend. After talking with her patient the nurse recognized her neglect in caring for her and made arrangements for Ms. T's friend to visit her on a daily basis while she was hospitalized.

Transsexualism

The word transsexual simply implies going from one sex to another. A more specific definition specifies a transsexual to be a person who is anatomically a male or female but who expresses, with strong conviction, that he or she has the mind of the opposite sex, lives as a member of the opposite sex part time or full time, and seeks to change his or her original sex legally and through hormonal and surgical sex reassignment.[20] Many times the transsexual client will describe himself as "feeling trapped in the wrong body." Transsexuals genuinely feel they belong to the other sex. Many transsexuals experience intense emotional turmoil because of the stigma from society. There are no accurate estimates of the incidence of transsexualism. However, postoperative transsexuals in the United States now number in the thousands.[20]

Several theories on the causes of transsexualism focus on organic factors, such as genes and hormone levels, whereas other theories focus on psychological factors. Many professionals today believe that transsexualism may be the result of a complex interaction of factors and are unable to identify one specific cause of transsexuality.

Transsexuality is very different from homosexuality in that homosexuals are comfortable with their anatomical identity and do not want to change their sex. Many transsexuals are heterosexual and express some distaste for homosexual activity. Transsexuals are essentially heterosexual, not homosexual, but are commonly mistaken by others or themselves as being homosexual.

CLINICAL EXAMPLE 22-4

Mr. L is a 21-year-old biological male who was admitted to the psychiatric unit for evaluation after a serious suicide attempt. Mr. L was interviewed by Mr. W, the charge nurse on the unit. Mr. L told the nurse that he tried to kill himself because he has been "sexually mixed up for years" and is tired of feeling like a freak of nature. He said that his friends make fun of him and tell him he is a homosexual, but that he does feel sexually attracted to other men and does not see himself as a homosexual. "I guess I don't feel like a man, I feel like a woman inside a man's body, and as a woman I am attracted to men."

In Clinical example 22-4, the transsexual's attraction to others of the same sex is understood in the context of his inner identification with the opposite sex. The transsexual does not want a sexual relationship with the same-sex person, but wishes to have his or her own genitals changed to that of the opposite sex. Thus the attraction is heterosexual.[11]

Transvestism

Transvestism is defined as cross-dressing or dressing in the clothes of the opposite sex. Clinically defined, "transvestism is a condition in which a male has a sexual obsession for or addiction to women's clothes, such that he periodically experiences intolerable psychic stress if he does not dress up."[20] Most often the transvestite that seeks treatment is a male; very little is known about female transvestism. No reliable statistics concerning the incidence of transvestism are available; however, many professionals believe the condition is more common than generally assumed.

Transvestites tend to be married men who report heterosexual behavior, and, although they occasionally or frequently dress in female garb, they do not wish hormonal or surgical sex change, as does the transsexual. Many transvestites try to find willing partners and often their activities of cross-dressing do not prevent sexual relationships with others.[11]

Sexual dysfunctions

Before the work of William Masters and Virginia Johnson, patients who experienced problems in the area of sexuality were generally referred to a psychiatrist for psychotherapy or psychoanalysis. Health professionals assumed that anyone who had a problem with sexuality was emotionally disturbed. Problems with sexual dysfunction are usually not psychiatric problems, but the result of sociocultural deprivation and ignorance of sexual physiology.[16]

Premature ejaculation

Premature ejaculation is the inability of a male to delay ejaculation long enough for the female partner to have an orgasm 50% of the time.[16] If the female partner is nonorgasmic for reasons other than the rapidity of the male's ejaculatory process, the definition does not apply. Premature ejaculation is the most common sexual dysfunction, with estimates indicating that millions of men suffer from this problem. Often the sexual histories of premature ejaculators have many similarities: (1) the first sexual experience is with a prostitute, in which case premature ejaculation was usually encouraged or (2) the first sexual experiences with girls in the peer group usually occurred in a hotel or the backseat of a car. In hurried or pressured sexual situations, often ridden with fears of being caught and anxieties about pregnancy, premature ejaculation was also encouraged by the situation itself or the partner. For many men, hurried or pressured sexual experiences developed into chronic patterns of premature ejaculation that were later carried into marriage relationships.

A major problem with premature ejaculation is that the condition does not allow for much sexual pleasure or for climax by the female partner. Until recently, sexual satisfaction of the female partner was often viewed with little concern. Today, however, because of a decrease in societal taboos about seeking sexual counseling, many husbands and wives are seeking treatment for premature ejaculation to achieve mutual sexual pleasure for both partners.

Ejaculatory incompetence

Ejaculatory incompetence, or retarded ejaculation, is a condition in which the reverse characteristics of premature ejaculation exist. According to Helen Singer Kaplan,[10] retarded ejaculation is defined as an involuntary inhibition of the male orgasmic reflex. A person experiencing retarded ejaculation is able to have satisfactory erections, but, even with ample stimulation, has difficulty ejaculating. Men experiencing severe cases of retarded ejaculation have never been able to ejaculate; however, severe cases are very rare and also difficult to treat. In milder conditions, the man cannot ejaculate in the woman's vagina or can only ejaculate when masturbating alone. The main factors contributing to retarded ejaculation include active

dislike for a female partner, fear of castration, religious restrictions, and performance anxieties. Ejaculatory incompetence is a high-risk condition in that it can lead to secondary impotence over a period of time.

Impotence

Primary impotence is defined as the inability to achieve and/or maintain an erection sufficient to accomplish coital connection. Secondary impotence is defined as an individual male rate of failure at coital connections in 25% of the person's opportunities.[16] No single cause of primary impotence has been identified. Several factors in personality development have been identified as recurring regularly in these patients: a seductive mother, the religious belief that sex is sinful, homosexuality, and traumatic initial failure. Frequent antecedents causing secondary impotence include premature ejaculation, excessive alcohol use, overbearing parents, religious restrictions, and long or serious physical illness.

Female orgasmic dysfunction

Primary orgasmic dysfunction can be diagnosed in women who do not attain orgasm during their entire life span. More specifically, female orgasmic dysfunction exists when every possible physical approach to sexual stimulation initiated by the patient or her partner has been unsuccessful in producing an orgasm.[16] Situational orgasmic dysfunctions include the following[16]:

1. *Coital orgasmic inadequacy.* A woman who is only capable of having an orgasm with partner manipulation, oral-genital stimulation, or masturbation.
2. *Masturbatory orgasmic dysfunction.* A woman who can be orgasmic during intercourse but with no other kind of stimulation.
3. *Random orgasmic inadequacy.* A woman who has had an orgasm at least once in either the coital orgasmic inadequacy or masturbatory orgasmic dysfunction category but is dysfunctional when referred for treatment because of changes in attitudes toward a partner, a homosexual orientation, a decrease in sexual desire, or some other accompanying complication.

Common etiological factors seen in women with primary orgasmic disorders include religious prohibitions, being raised in a protective environment that excluded acknowledgment of sexual feelings or behavior, the inability to identify with one's partner, and marriage with an inadequate man. Etiological factors observed in women with situational orgasmic disorders include the woman's attitude toward her partner, a history of homosexuality, and disinterest in sex.[16]

Vaginismus

Vaginismus is defined as a female sexual dysfunction in which intercourse is not possible because attempts at vaginal penetration evoke an involuntary spastic contraction of the vaginal entrance.[10] The condition can only be diagnosed by pelvic examination because diagnosis requires that the actual contraction of the lower third of the vagina be observed. Vaginismus is a rare sexual disorder. The condition is often seen in women who are phobic about intercourse.[10] Two prominent factors often coexist in women with vaginismus. First, many of these women are married to impotent men, but it is not known whether the husband's or wife's sexual dysfunction occurred first. Second, the family background reflects the attitude that sex was considered dirty or sinful.[16]

Assessment

Some people who experience stress in the area of their sexuality may be reluctant to accept their need for help in this area. Others seek help indirectly in that a diffuse symptom often masks an underlying sexual problem. The nurse is often the health professional who first comes in contact with these patients. The nursing process will assist her in working with patients as they develop a collaborative relationship and assess problems, assign priorities to needs, and mutually arrive at a plan of intervention.

The first phase of the nursing process, the assessment phase, includes two clearly defined responsibilities in the sexual counseling of patients: (1) the development of self-awareness in relation to sexuality and (2) the assessment of the patient. The most critical element in being able to competently counsel patients about sexuality is for the nurse to be aware of her own feelings and values. The nurse's level of self-awareness has a direct impact on her ability to intervene effectively with patients. In developing self-awareness, nurses may progress through four phases of a predictable growth experience: cognitive dissonance, anxiety, anger, and action. In assessing a patient, the nurse assesses the individual's situation and presenting problem.

Self-awareness of the nurse

The first step in developing self-awareness preparatory to sexual counseling is for the nurse to clarify values in response to her own sexuality. Foley and Davies[5] identified patterns of growth experiences developed around the nursing care of rape victims. Their model is applicable in the sexual counseling of patients as well and has been adapted accordingly. The first phase of the growth experience in developing sexual self-awareness is characterized by *cognitive dissonance*. This is defined as a state that exists when two opposing beliefs exist simultaneously.[24]

For example, nurses grow up learning what society, family, and friends believe about sexual issues. If a nurse is raised in an environment which teaches her that nice girls do not talk about sex, the nurse will carry that belief into nursing practice. When the nurse encounters a patient who wants to discuss an issue of sexual concern with her, she may experience the following two opposing reactions simultaneously:

1. As a professional, I should be able to discuss any problem, including sexual problems, with my patient.
2. Nice girls do not discuss sex.

Experiencing both of these conflicting thoughts at the same time makes the nurse uncomfortable. This feeling of discomfort eventually forces the nurse to examine her feelings and values about discussing the sexual problems of patients as part of her nursing care. The nurse will resolve the cognitive dissonance in one of two ways: (1) denying her professional responsibilities to the patient and continuing to ascribe to personal beliefs, such as nice girls do not talk about sex, or (2) examining her values and feelings about sexuality, including the fact that sexuality is an integral part of the human condition which seeks expression.

If the nurse continues to believe the myth that nice girls do not talk about sex, she may make excuses for unprofessional behavior by projecting blame onto the patient for introducing sexual topics or rationalizing that she cannot be expected to be knowledgeable about sexuality, since she is "just a nurse, and can't know everything." Rationalization encourages such behaviors as avoidance of or denial of a patient's sexual concerns. Rationalization and blaming the patient also allow the nurse to ignore her discomfort in viewing herself as a sexual human being. However, ignoring or denying one's discomfort does not allow one to move toward understanding personal feelings and values about sexuality.

Nurses need to examine what they believe about sexual issues and why they hold those beliefs. It is impossible to deny that environment and family background influence one's beliefs. In regard to sexual issues the professional nurse needs to ask: "Do I believe this because I am knowledgeable in this area and have researched the facts, or do I believe this because my parents or peers believe it?" Only when the nurse can say that the available information has been examined and an informed choice on values has been made, will the nurse have truly examined personal values and clarified them.

If one's cognitive dissonance leads to a self-examination of values, a second phase of growth occurs. In the second phase *anxiety,* shock, and fear are experienced. Anxiety is a state of "apprehension cued off by a threat to some value which the individual holds essential to his existence as a personality."[18] Fear is a subjective feeling state arising from life and limb being in danger due to a specific stimulus that is external to the person.[24] Shock is a severe "disturbance in the equilibrium or permanence of something characterized by feelings of surprise, terror, horror, or disgust."[24] In the second phase, the nurse realizes that uncertainty, insecurity, questions, and problems regarding sexuality are experienced by everyone. Often the nurse experiences anxiety because of the realization that everyone is capable of a variety of sexual feelings and behaviors and that anyone can experience a sexual dysfunction or question one's sexual identity. The nurse who is experiencing anxiety may exhibit behaviors that are ineffective in discussing sexual issues with a patient, such as talking too much (nor allowing patients to verbalize their feelings), failing to listen (failing to pick up on patient cues or messages), and diagnosing and analyzing (becoming preoccupied with facts rather than eliciting feelings from the patient).

Because anxiety is an uncomfortable feeling, the nurse strives to eliminate the discomfort. The process of learning facts about sexuality and facing the ignorance of society or one's colleagues brings the nurse to a third phase of the growth experience. *Anger* characterizes phase three of the growth experience and generally arises after anxiety and shock subside. Anger is directed at oneself, one's patients, and society. The nurse begins to recognize that issues associated with sex or sexuality are highly volatile and emotionally charged. Rape, abortion, birth control, the equal rights amendment, child abuse, pornography, and religious issues all have an obvious or subtle connection with sexuality and give rise to vehement debates. Similarly, attempts to formulate legislation relating to sexual matters is often ineffective because these issues are emotion laden. The realization of society's emotionality and irrationality in relation to issues having a sexual element often breeds anger and contempt in the nurse. For example, a nurse may become angry at what she perceives to be the ignorance, bigotry, or unprofessional attitude of a colleague or friend who judges homosexuals to be perverted deviants.

During this phase of anger nurses may begin to get on a "soapbox" and lecture others about the need for sex education to rid society of ignorance about sex and sexual issues. The nurse may develop an impatient hostile attitude toward a patient or co-worker who is not educated in the area of sexuality. For instance, a nurse may critically judge a patient who becomes pregnant because of ignorance about simple birth control methods. Furthermore the nurse is often angry with society for perpetuating ignorance about sexuality and may not understand when others do not share her enthusiasm for wanting to change society's beliefs. The nurse may also be angry with herself for her own ignorance and feel guilty and embarrassed for her lack of sexual knowledge. It is essential that the nurse be able to admit her negative feelings and lack of knowledge without fear of disapproval from colleagues or friends. Openness to one's feelings and limitations within a trusting relationship is a key step in beginning to be able to seek out and ask for information basic to understanding human sexuality.

The final step in the growth experience is the action phase. In this phase the nurse experiences a decrease in anger and an increased ability to understand that blaming herself or society for ignorance and prejudice does not aid in self-understanding and helping patients with sexual concerns. During the action phase nurses often wonder, "Why didn't anyone ever teach me what I really needed to know about sexuality?" "Why aren't people educated properly?" "Where should sex education start?" "How can I gain more knowledge for myself and others?"

Several behaviors characterize the final *action* phase of the growth experience: data inquiry, choosing values, and prizing values. Data inquiry is demonstrated when the nurse obtains information about sexuality and sexual issues so that, properly informed, values about sexuality can be freely chosen. After choosing a value position, the final behavior is one of prizing the valued position. Prizing consists of an awareness and cherishing of one's feelings and values and being willing to share them publicly. Although prizing values is considered the final step in a positive growth experience, prizing does not mean that what one values now will not change. Values are never static, but evolve and shift as a person changes, grows, and acquires new life experiences. Thus a person who once ascribed to pro-life values may later become understanding and empathetic toward women who seek an abortion. Clinical example 22-5 illustrates a nurse who prizes values enough to share them publicly.

CLINICAL EXAMPLE 22-5

Ms. G works as a staff nurse at an outpatient psychiatric clinic. One day at an interdisciplinary team meeting, Ms. G presented a new case to the treatment team for review. Her case was a 29-year-old female patient who came to the clinic because she thought she was transsexual. Ms. G began to explain the patient's history to the treatment team when one of the team members interrupted, stating "If this isn't the sickest thing I've ever heard of. . . . I hope you don't expect us to treat this woman or should I say man!" The other members of the treatment team began to snicker and continued to make jokes about the transsexual patient.

After the team meeting, Ms. G felt very confused. She usually respected her co-workers' clinical judgment and considered them to be good clinicians. But her new patient was obviously experiencing problems with her sexuality and was really serious about wanting treatment for sexual reassignment. Ms. G was also anxious because of her lack of facts and knowledge about transsexuality. She decided to do some research that evening at the library.

The next day at the office, one of the other nurse clinicians teased Ms. G about the new "half and half" patient. Another co-worker cautioned Ms. G not to see this patient in the back treatment room alone because "you never know about those perverts, they might grab you." Ms. G became irritable with her co-workers and called them ignorant bigots. Despite the problems with her co-workers she continued to research the nature of transsexualism to help her patient.

Finally, she found a psychologist in the city who worked with transsexual patients and made an appointment to talk about transsexuality.

Ms. G explained the reaction of her co-workers to the psychologist, her own difficulties in understanding transsexuality and in finding an appropriate referral for the patient. "This isn't the first time this has happened at our clinic," Ms. G told the psychologist. "Anytime we get a patient with sexual problems everybody makes jokes and nothing is ever really done for them."

After the consultation appointment, the psychologist offered to do an inservice program on sexuality for the staff. Ms. G returned to the clinic, fearful that the staff would refuse the inservice program and laugh at her for suggesting the program.

The next day Ms. G told the staff at the team meeting of the psychologist's offer to talk with them about providing care to patients expressing sexual preferences that differ from their own. One of the team members responded by laughing, "We don't need anyone to teach us about sex—I think we know everything we need to know." Everyone laughed and agreed. Ms. G, although anxious, spoke up stating, "If we all know so much, why all this nervous laughter? Look, I know it's hard to talk about sex and sexual issues but we have got to admit that we do not do a very good job addressing some of the sexual issues or problems that patients present us with here. And many patients do. We just can't go on laughing and making judgments about people—Let's face it, that doesn't help anyone."

After Ms. G spoke up there was a long silence in the room until another nurse spoke up. "You know, I think Ms. G is right. There are lots of times I just don't know what to say or do for people who come in here with sexual concerns. What could it hurt to have an inservice?" After some discussion, the staff agreed to let Ms. G call the psychologist and set up the inservice program.

Clinical example 22-5 illustrates the phases of growth health professionals experience while increasing self-awareness in the area of sexuality. These phases are represented in Fig. 22-1. Ms. G experienced cognitive dissonance when the staff called the transsexual patient sick, and she was faced with conflicting feelings. She agreed with the staff because she respected them as expert clinicians, but she also believed the patient was not sick, weird, or perverted and had a very real problem that needed professional help. Ms. G experienced anxiety when she realized that she did not know anything about transsexuality. Her anxiety also stemmed from being faced with the

FIG. 22-1

Phases of the nurse's growth in developing self-awareness of human sexuality.

reality that people express their sexuality in different ways, some of which were very different from anything she had been exposed to before. Ms. G experienced anger at herself and the staff for ignorance and judgmental attitudes and lashed out at the staff by calling them bigots. Her anger finally motivated her into action. She decided to explore her feelings, educate herself through reading and talking with a knowledgeable professional, and finally spoke up in a conflictual staff meeting to facilitate a needed staff inservice program on sexuality.

Assessment of the patient

Any basic health history needs to include questions regarding sexual history. Nurses are often involved in history gathering and assess-

ments of patients. Because of the possible anxiety and embarrassment associated with sexual issues, nurses react in a variety of ways when obtaining this assessment data. One common reaction is for nurses to ignore the sexual questions or to look at the floor and stutter while asking interview questions. Another common reaction is for the nurse to blurt out rapidly, "You don't have any sex problems, do you?" or "How's your sex life?" Patients usually respond to these statements with embarrassment and feel that these questions are intrusive. Each of these interview questions, when asked by the nurse, gives the patient a clear message that it is not appropriate to talk about sex. When the nurse is uncomfortable, the patient will be uncomfortable, often to the point that no sexual concerns will be discussed with the nurse. Comfort in discussing

SEXUAL HEALTH ASSESSMENT FORM*

1. When you were a child, how were your questions about sex answered? Where did your sexual information come from? (Appropriate for adolescents.)
   When you were a teenager, how were your questions about sex answered? (Appropriate for adults.)
2. How did you first find out about sexual intercourse (how babies are made)? (Appropriate for adolescents and young adults.)
3. How would you describe your current sexual activity?
4. What, if anything, would you change about your current sexual activity?
5. At this time in your life, how important is a sexual relationship to you?
6. Do you have any concerns about birth control?
7. Do you have any health problems that, in your opinion, affect your sexual health or happiness?
8. Are you taking any medicines that, in your opinion, affect your sexual health or happiness?
9. Is there anything about these questions that you would like clarified or explained?

*From Sexuality: a nursing perspective by F.H. Mims and M. Swenson. Copyright © 1980, McGraw-Hill Book Company. Used with the permission of McGraw-Hill Book Company.

sexual issues is the first requirement for the nurse who wishes to successfully assess a patient's sexuality. A nurse who is comfortable in discussing sexuality conveys the message that it is normal to talk about sexual health as a part of a health assessment interview. If nurses are able to remove the attitude that "sex is dirty and should not be discussed" by presenting a calm and professional manner, questions about patients' sexual health can be asked in a factual manner, and the patient is allowed the freedom to discuss sexual matters without guilt or embarrassment.

The second requirement for a nurse to successfully assess a patient's sexuality is effective interviewing skills. Many nurses who demonstrate excellent interviewing skills become uncomfortable asking questions about sex. How-

ever, concepts of effective interviewing are the same for sexual issues as for any presenting problem. For example, open-ended questions are often most helpful to initiate a discussion on sexuality. The question must be at the patient's level of understanding, because each person is a unique individual. The amount of time and depth needed to complete an interview will vary with each patient and problem. Often one or two questions may be sufficient to assess a person's sexual health. Other times, when patients have specific sexual problems, a detailed and specific assessment needs to be done. A sexual health assessment form that may be used by the nurse is given at left.

Another important factor to convey in assessing a patient's sexual health is to inform the person that information gathered during the interview is strictly confidential and that the patient's medical chart cannot be given out without the patient's written permission. Assurance of confidentiality is important in the care of all people. Many sexual minority patients are especially sensitive about confidentiality, since they often fear losing their jobs or family rejection if their sexual minority status was accidentally discovered by employers or relatives.

Planning

After obtaining assessment data regarding the sexual problem, which often includes a complete physical examination, the nurse implements the planning stage of the nursing process. It is at this point that the nurse and patient review the assessment data, define problems, and work together to establish goals that the patient wants to achieve. It is important that the nurse does not identify goals that she wants the patient to achieve, but rather helps the patient identify his own goals and develop a realistic plan to achieve these goals.

The planning phase could simply involve reviewing assessment data with the patient, exploring options, and making referral sources known and available. The nurse's level of expertise determines the amount and degree of planning done with a patient. The planning phase could also include developing a plan of sexual health teaching for the patient or for the patient and spouse conjointly. From the assessment data, the nurse and patient can discuss together what needs to be known about a specific sexual

TABLE 22-1. Myths and facts on human sexuality

Myth	Result of myth	Fact
Most individuals who suffer from sexual dysfunctions (e.g., impotence, frigidity) are deeply psychologically disturbed	Individuals who experience sexual dysfunctions are embarrassed and ashamed, often try to hide their problem, and do not seek professional help	According to Masters and Johnson, "sociocultural deprivation and ignorance constitute the etiologic background for most sexual dysfunctions, not psychiatric illness"[15]
Excessive masturbation is harmful	Individuals often feel guilty or ashamed about masturbating; some individuals deny themselves this experience because of uncomfortable feelings society perpetuates	No physical harms have been reported; no medical definition for excessive masturbation exists; masturbation seems to be a self-limiting practice; when sexually satiated, the individual will then lose interest in being sexually aroused[10]
Women can be excessively amorous (nymphomania)	Women are ashamed (and guilt ridden) of sexual desires and fantasies; in marital relationship responsibility for initiating sex is always on husband, which can cause feelings of resentment from both partners	According to Masters and Johnson classic nymphomania is statistically nonexistent; nymphomania in our culture does not refer to objectively measured states of female excitation, but rather to what males perceive as excessive[16]
Sex during menstruation is unclean and harmful	Women often view their bodies as unclean and even unfit or inferior during menstruation; women use menstruation as an excuse to avoid intercourse rather than simply saying no without a "good reason"	Medically menstrual flow is in no way harmful or dirty; if women desire, there is no reason to abstain from intercourse during menstrual flow[16]
Oral and anal intercourse are perverted and dangerous	Many individuals refrain from these behaviors or indulge in them only to feel ashamed and guilty afterward	According to Masters and Johnson, "nothing could be further from the truth"; they suggest certain precautions when performing anal intercourse, such as avoiding contamination of vaginal tract and wearing a condom to prevent bacteria from entering penile passage[16]
Teenagers are sexually promiscuous because they all learn sex education in school	Parents who believe this myth fight against comprehensive sex education programs in public education; many parents believe their children have sex education in school, when in fact, the majority do not	Recent estimates indicate that only 10% of today's youth receive comprehensive sex education;[7] existing sex education programs vary greatly in content and quality
Most homosexuals molest children	Known homosexuals are often fired from teaching jobs, and many parents will not allow their children to spend any time with anyone who is homosexual; children learn from an early age that homosexuals are "bad people," that they should stay away from them	Of all reported cases of molestations, 90% are heterosexual, adult male with minor female[21]

TABLE 22-1. Myths and facts on human sexuality—cont'd

Myth	Result of myth	Fact
Homosexuals are sick and cannot control their sexual behavior	Homosexuals are denied jobs and are sometimes jailed for their homosexuality; homosexual parents often have their children taken away by courts	According to Bell and Weinberg, who studied 979 homosexual men and women in a study conducted by the Institute for Sex Research in 1978: (1) most homosexuals' social and psychological adjustment is indistinguishable from the heterosexual majority and (2) objectionable sexual advances are far more likely to be made by a heterosexual (usually male to female) than a homosexual[2]
All homosexuals are alike: men, limp wristed, speak with lisp; women, unattractive, masculine, "butch," short hair, deep voice	Society considers any individual who does not conform to the correct "macho male" and "fluffy female" stereotypes to be homosexual	Bell and Weinberg's study indicates that relatively few homosexual men and women conform to hideous stereotypes[2]
Advancing age means end of sex	Many older adults become victims of this myth not because their bodies have lost the ability to perform, but because *they* believe that they have lost the ability to perform	Sexually men and women can function effectively into their 80's if they understand the physiological changes that occur with aging and do not let these changes frighten them[16]

issue and plan approaches that will give the patient the needed information.

Intervention

Primary intervention

Primary intervention strives to promote health and prevent problems from occurring through specific methods, such as teaching and preplanning. Before being able to engage in either sex education or counseling, however, the nurse must examine her own values and beliefs about patients who practice sexual behavior that may be different. This can be facilitated by exploring the myths commonly held by society regarding human sexuality.[17] Table 22-1 presents a list of some of these sexual myths, the result of believing the myth, and the corresponding facts.

Education is the most frequent method of primary prevention for sexual problems and issues. The controversial question of where sex education belongs stimulates much debate among different educational and religious groups throughout the country.[21] Some groups believe that sex education should be censored in public schools and that sexuality should never be publicly discussed. However, if a professional nurse believes in the principles of primary prevention, sex education is a vitally important component of a comprehensive education in today's society.[22]

According to Hacker,[8] sex education needs to be incorporated into education from kindergarten throughout one's entire educational career. When individuals are not properly educated in the area of human sexuality, they are denied the opportunity to explore their own values and beliefs about sexuality and to know themselves as sexual beings. Lack of knowledge breeds ignorance that can adversely affect the sexual counseling of patients. When individuals are not aware of facts about sexuality and do not understand their own feelings, important decisions are made on limited information that they may later regret. Sex education can help people know themselves better when the curriculum allows for expression of thoughts, feelings, and examination of behavior, while learning factual information.

Basic concepts that must underlie effective sex education include the following: (1) we are sexual from birth and sexuality is an inseparable part of our identity and (2) all sexual thoughts and feelings are considered normal, but it is our behavior that needs to be monitored in terms of its appropriateness. The key principle in effective sex education is teaching individuals when and where to act on feelings, as well as when and where not to act on them. Finally, sexuality needs to be viewed as more than genital sex. It encompasses one's total sense of self.[8]

Nurses have a professional responsibility to become educated in the field of human sexuality so that holistic health care becomes a reality. The educational process can be accomplished in nursing curricula and continuing education programs. However, some nurses elect additional education and clinical practice in the field of human sexuality. These nurses may become sex educators in schools and the community in such facilities as outpatient clinics and planned parenthood agencies. Nurses prepared at the master and doctoral levels may choose to become sex therapists through postgraduate work in the field of human sexuality and through extensive clinical supervision from qualified sex therapists.

Secondary intervention

Secondary intervention involves early detection of a problem that already exists, and interventions are directed toward avoiding maladaptive behavior. Counseling of sexual minorities and sexual dysfunctions are discussed in this section within a brief therapy (6 to 12 weeks) framework. The counseling of transsexual patients is described in the discussion on tertiary intervention.

COUNSELING THE HOMOSEXUAL. Many people accept their homosexuality without being concerned about it, whereas others have difficulties and seek professional help. The first step in counseling a homosexual patient is the counselor's acceptance of him or her. Most patients are extremely perceptive of their therapist's values and attitudes toward them. The counselor who believes she is hiding her prejudices from the patient is only fooling herself. Because the nurse has grown up in a society that believes homosexuals are sick and perverted, it is difficult to examine myths and search for facts. The patient has grown up in the same society and, although experiencing homosexual feelings or behaviors, still goes through the same growth experience about homosexuality as anyone else.

Often an important step in counseling the homosexual individual is to aid him or her in exploring values and beliefs about homosexual people. It is possible that the person has internalized some of society's prejudices about homosexuals, such as, "homosexuals are sick, evil people who should not be allowed to live homosexual life-styles." Therefore "because I am homosexual, I am sick and should not act on my sexual feelings because they are evil and bad." Common responses evidenced by patients who attempt to cope with society's prejudices include denial, confusion, and sexual promiscuity, which is especially prominent among those who are trying to prove to themselves that they are not gay.

It is helpful to have patients discuss and specifically list beliefs they hold about homosexuality and for the therapist and patient to review and discuss each one. A review of beliefs about homosexuality may not be sufficient because, although the nurse and patient work to dispel the myths, society consistently and very powerfully reinforces them. Having the individual read appropriate materials about homosexuality will also be helpful in discriminating myths from facts. Throughout this review process the patient will be extremely sensitive to the therapist and will test the therapist's acceptance or rejection.

CLINICAL EXAMPLE 22-6

Ms. A, a 25-year-old single female, came to the mental health clinic with the complaint of a "sexual problem." Her history revealed that she had been sexually inactive for the past 5 years. At the age of 20, Ms. A had a brief sexual encounter with a man she had been dating for 2 years. She ended the relationship shortly afterward because she had no interest in maintaining a sexual relationship with the man. Recently, she became involved in a relationship with a woman that was very satisfying to her. She felt she had to end the relationship because she would not tolerate thinking of herself as a homosexual. During one of the initial counseling sessions Ms. A told the nurse that she must end the relationship before "it" happens again.

NURSE: **What are you afraid will happen?**
MS. A: **I'm afraid I'll feel attracted to her again.**
NURSE: **What about that frightens you?**
MS. A: **(becoming upset) That will mean I'm homosexual!**
NURSE: **What does being homosexual mean for you?**
MS. A: **It means I'm sick. It's a sin, I couldn't go to church anymore.**
NURSE: **Are all homosexuals sick?**
MS. A: **Yes.**

NURSE: **What makes you think that?**

MS. A: **Everybody knows that homosexuals hang out in sleazy bars and don't work and are on welfare. They all have emotional problems, need therapy, and eventually wind up in mental institutions.**

NURSE: **Do you know any homosexual people?**

MS. A: **Well, not exactly. . . .**

NURSE: **What have you read about homosexuality?**

MS. A: **Nothing.**

NURSE: **Then it looks to me like you are basing all of your conclusions on hearsay and not real knowledge. I think that you and I need to explore your beliefs in more detail, then you can do some reading to find out the facts.**

In clinical example 22-6, the nurse and Ms. A developed a plan commonly used in sexual counseling to explore the issue of homosexuality over the next several sessions. Two goals that were identified by the patient and the nurse included the following:

1. Understand the facts vs. myths about homosexuals and their life-styles.
2. Understand the patient's feelings about herself in regard to her sexual identity.

Some of the actions taken to implement the plan included:

1. Ms. A listed all her beliefs about homosexuality and homosexuals.
2. The nurse encouraged Ms. A to explore the literature on homosexuality and suggested readings to help dispel the myths.
3. The nurse then discussed these with Ms. A and suggested that Ms. A attend a social gathering for gay people to test out her new-found knowledge. (The nurse suggested the social gathering because many people struggling with a homosexual identity are frightened to test out situations that would dispel the myths.)

COUNSELING THE TRANSVESTITE. Counseling the transvestite patient is primarily a supportive intervention. Many transvestites never need or seek therapy. For transvestites who do seek help, the therapist must help the person to find socially and personally acceptable ways of sexual expression. Many transvestites seek willing and cooperative partners, which alleviates problems for them. Often with transvestite patients counseling revolves around a partner or family member understanding and accepting the patient.

COUNSELING PATIENTS WITH SEXUAL DYSFUNCTIONS. Although patients with sexual dysfunctions are treated from many different treatment modalities, two brief treatment models of sex therapy commonly implemented are discussed here: the Masters and Johnson and the Helen Singer Kaplan models.

Masters and Johnson model. Masters and Johnson began pioneering research in the area of sexuality in the 1950s. Their book, *Human Sexual Inadequacy*,[16] describes their research in specific detail and their counseling methods for sexual dysfunctions. Masters' and Johnson's treatment for sexual dysfunctions includes short-term education with step-by-step instructions regarding the physical aspects of sexual activity and supportive psychotherapy. The researchers believe that attitudes and ignorance are responsible for most sexual dysfunctions, contrary to the belief by the general populace that sexual dysfunctions indicate a severe psychiatric illness.

Masters' and Johnson's therapeutic approach to patients begins by obtaining a detailed sexual and background history. They recommend a male-female therapeutic team, a dual therapist approach. On day one of the treatment program, therapists meet with the couple to review and clarify their histories taken the previous day. Meeting with the couple is called a round table discussion. After this discussion, the couple is instructed to carry out the sensate focus exercise. This exercise requires each partner to instruct the other in specific ways of caressing for the purpose of sensual pleasure without involving the breasts or genitals. The activity is done first by one partner and then the other partner. The next day the exercise is repeated, including breasts and genital areas, but without performing coitus. The purpose of the exercise is to alleviate performance anxiety and to enhance warm comfortable feelings between partners. The exercises are done in comfortable private surroundings with both partners in the nude. After the sensate focus exercises are completed, the attention of therapy is directed to the presenting sexual dysfunction. Some of the specific behavioral approaches used by Masters and Johnson are briefly described in Table 22-2. The Masters and Johnson model emphasizes education, communication, and cooperation between partners in their treatment plan.

Helen Singer Kaplan model. Kaplan's method[10] of treating sexual dysfunctions integrates psychodynamic behavioral principles into conjoint therapeutic sessions. Kaplan combines specific behavioral tasks with psychodynamic insights, dyadic approaches, dream interpretations, and

TABLE 22-2. Summary of two models of treatment techniques for sexual dysfunctions*

Sexual dysfunction	Masters and Johnson	Helen Singer Kaplan
Premature ejaculation	*Squeeze technique.* As soon as full erection is achieved, woman's thumb is placed on frenulum, located on ventral surface of penis, and first and second fingers on dorsal surface of penis immediately adjacent to one another on either side of coronal ridge; pressure is applied by woman squeezing thumb and first two fingers together for 3 or 4 seconds; pressure makes man lose urge to ejaculate; procedure is repeated so couple can enjoy 15 to 20 minutes of continuous sex play without ejaculation	*Stop-start technique.* Woman masturbates man until he feels urge to ejaculate; he then tells woman to stop; after ejaculation urge abates, he will then tell woman to begin stimulating him again and when he feels the urge to ejaculate, instructs her to stop; this is repeated four times, with final time allowing ejaculation; it is important with this technique for man to focus sharply on his erotic sensations and not allow himself to be distracted; this exercise is repeated with petroleum jelly several times and then with penis inserted in vagina with man controlling woman's hip movements
Ejaculatory incompetence, retarded ejaculation	Woman stimulates man demandingly, specifically asking him for verbal direction in stimulative techniques that are pleasurable; by doing this, woman forces ejaculation manually; hopefully when this occurs, man will identify this pleasure with her rather than regard her as threat or contaminated sexual object; after establishing competence in ejaculatory function with masturbation techniques, next step is intravaginal ejaculation; after manual stimulation of penis by woman she inserts penis into vagina (female superior position) and begins pelvic thrusting; if man does not ejaculate, shortly after thrusting, woman returns to manual stimulation	Two principles of treatment: 1. Progressive in vivo desensitization to intravaginal ejaculation; treatment goal is to gradually shape ejaculatory response toward ejaculation on coitus; specific behavioral prescriptions will vary with each individual case but will be structured with the above stated goal in mind, e.g., man who can only ejaculate if woman has left house and he is alone might have behavior prescription to masturbate behind locked doors in his bedroom with her downstairs; if successful, next step is to being her close, e.g., next room, until couple reaches goal 2. Stimulation and distraction. Person is physically stimulated intensely, while at the same time mentally distracted; mental absorption in erotic fantasy while genital stimulation is being experienced is an ideal method of releasing orgasm reflex
Impotence	Couple instructed not to have intercourse; progression from nongenital caressing and pleasuring exercises to genital pleasuring exercises; each member of couple instructs the other in specifics of their own pleasure; when intercourse is attempted, woman assumes superior position and inserts male's penis into her vagina; couple is continuously reassured in nonpressure, no hurry environment; at no time in this treatment is couple instructed to have intercourse	Client and partner are gradually led through the following sequence of events: 1. Erotic pleasures without erection 2. Erection without orgasm 3. Extravaginal orgasm 4. Intromission without orgasm 5. Coitus

*Modified from: Kaplan, H.S.: The illustrated manual of sex therapy, New York, 1975, The New York Times Book Co.; and Masters, W.H., and Johnson, V.E.: Human sexual inadequacy, Boston, 1970, Little, Brown & Co.

TABLE 22-2. **Summary of two models of treatment techniques for sexual
dysfunctions—cont'd**

Sexual dysfunction	Masters and Johnson	Helen Singer Kaplan
Female orgasmic dysfunction	After sensate focus and lowering hostile environment between couple, controlled genital play is initiated with woman showing man what her actual preferences are; gradually penis is inserted (female superior position) without thrusting; gentle movements are made by woman and finally penile insertion with male thrusting	First step is orgasm alone by digital stimulation plus distraction by fantasy (sometimes vibrator is suggested here); this gradually moves to orgasm with partner, either by masturbation or by man stimulating woman's clitoris; when this is successful couple moves to orgasm with intercourse; if orgasm with intercourse does not occur, bridge maneuver is employed; *bridge maneuver:* either partner manually stimulates clitoris while penis is contained in vagina up to point of, but not actually to, orgasm and then let coital thrusting trigger orgasmic reflex
Vaginismus	First vaginal constriction is shown to both partners during physical examination; then dilators in graduated sizes are employed in privacy of couple's bedroom; gradually size of dilation is increased until woman can tolerate man's penis	Couple is instructed to observe vaginal entrance with mirror and woman gradually inserts finger into vaginal canal, then inserts two fingers; after woman can tolerate insertion of two full fingers, man is included; he repeats procedure, gradually couple moves to penile insertion without thrusting and finally penile insertion with thrusting

gestalt and transactional techniques. Kaplan differs from Masters and Johnson in that she believes the single therapist is as effective as cotherapists of opposite sexes. According to her, the primary objective of sex therapy is symptomatic relief, which can be achieved by treating the patient without a partner in some cases.

Kaplan's treatment process begins with an extensive evaluation that includes marital, psychiatric, sexual, medical, and family history from both partners. If profound intrapsychic or interpersonal difficulties are found, the couple may be referred to appropriate individual or conjoint therapy and are not accepted for sex therapy at that time. According to Kaplan, sex therapy is usually contraindicated in couples who are severely disturbed.

Like Masters and Johnson, Kaplan employs the sensate focus exercises and variations of the exercises, such as showering together, to begin sex therapy or further evaluate a client's suitability for sex therapy. The therapy process itself consists of erotic tasks, performed at home, plus weekly or semiweekly meetings with the therapist. At the therapy sessions, clients and the therapist explore feelings experienced during the erotic exercises. The Kaplan method prescribes a unique series of home or private exercises for the couple and the dysfunction that take into account the motivations and dynamics of the relationship. The integration of experiential and dynamic modes is a major feature of Kaplan's approach. The role of the therapist includes education, clarification, and support.

• • •

Table 22-2 describes a number of commonly used behavioral techniques specific to sexual dysfunctions. The techniques in no way indicate the total comprehensive treatment for sexual dysfunctions, but give a baseline description of exercises that are implemented in sex therapy. Both Kaplan and Masters and Johnson emphasize communication between partners and the exploring of the relationship and emotional concerns during therapy. The reader is referred to original works of these sex therapists for more specific information.

Tertiary intervention

The tertiary level of intervention attempts to promote maximum functioning for patients with problems of a chronic nature and requires longer term intervention methods. Although specific and time-limited counseling methods have been described earlier in this chapter, longer term care is sometimes required for people who do not respond to brief treatment methods. This may include individual, couple, or group psychotherapy that is insight oriented and supplements the previously described treatment techniques. For example, a patient who, after 12 therapy sessions, could not accept her homosexual identity resorted to heavy alcohol abuse and needed longer term psychotherapy for approximately 3 years. Another couple who could not resolve their impotent sexual dysfunction in brief sex therapy needed longer term counseling. Patients with chronic physical problems who experience increasing deterioration of physical ability may need ongoing counseling regarding maintaining some type of sexual activity, for example, using pillows to cushion brittle bones and help minimize pain.

In tertiary intervention, the role of the nurse is to help the individual explore options, which in certain cases can be somewhat limited. The nurse helps the patient adjust to disabilities and realities that cannot be changed while reaching the maximum comfort and pleasure the person is capable of attaining.

Treatment of the person who is a transsexual has been the topic of heated debate in recent years. The debate ranges from recommending long-term psychotherapy to surgical reassignment. Recently standards of care were developed by the Harry Benjamin International Gender Dysphoria Association.[4] These standards set guidelines for individuals who are to receive hormonal therapy, psychotherapy (including qualifications of therapists), and surgical reassignment. The standards help professionals who treat transsexual patients give quality care.

Briefly, treatment advocated by the Harry Benjamin International Gender Dysphoria Association includes thorough assessment of the patient by a trained professional, hormonal therapy, and finally surgical reassignment (not all transsexuals choose surgical reassignment). Phases of treatment include the following steps:

1. The person must demonstrate a sense of discomfort with self and the wish to live in the genetically opposite sex role.
2. The person must be known to a professional therapist (who is an expert in the field of sexuality) for a period of 3 to 6

months and demonstrate a sense of discomfort with self and the desire to live in the genetically opposite sex role.

If the person meets these criteria, the therapists then endorses him or her for hormonal therapy. A male changing to a female receives estrogen; a female changing to a male receives testosterone. Before starting hormonal therapy, the patient receives a complete physical examination with specific blood work (serum glutamic pyruvic transaminase levels in females changing to males and serum glutamic pyruvic transaminase, bilirubin, triglyceride, and fasting glucose levels in males changing to females). If the person desires surgical reassignment (a penectomy, castration, or vaginaplasty for a male changing to a female; a hysterectomy, vaginectomy, or phalloplasty for a female changing to a male), they must be known to the professional therapist for at least 6 months. The individual must have been successful in living in the genetically opposite sex role for at least 1 year and up to 2 years. Before the transsexual receives the surgical alteration, the original therapist's endorsement must be agreed on by a second therapist who has evaluated the person.

It is imperative that professionals who provide care for transsexual patients be educated in the field of human sexuality. The assessment phase of the treatment process is especially important. The patient and therapist must be certain that implementing the treatment plan is the best approach because the surgery is not reversible.

Evaluation

In the evaluation phase of the nursing process model, the nurse works with the patient to evaluate the effectiveness of the sexual counseling or treatment used. Factors to consider in evaluating the process of treatment include the following:

1. *Sense of well-being.* How does the person feel about himself or herself as a person? Have his or her feelings about self improved during the treatment?
2. *Functioning ability.* If the individual was dysfunctional, is functional ability restored? Somewhat improved? What about the person's ability to function within primary relations at work? with friends?
3. *Satisfaction with treatment.* Does the patient feel that treatment was helpful? Were his or her goals adequately met?

Evaluation of any form of sexual therapy or treatment should be an ongoing process in which the nurse and the patient work together in evaluating goals, problems, and alternatives. Clinical example 22-7 illustrates the evaluation process in a nurse-patient situation.

CLINICAL EXAMPLE 22-7

Mr. and Mrs. S sought sex therapy because they had been experiencing sexual difficulties since their marriage 2 years ago. Mr. S had been suffering from premature ejaculation and Mrs. S claimed that she had lost any interest in a sexual relationship with her husband and refused to discuss the problem of premature ejaculation with him.

The couple was seen by a nurse clinician who was an experienced sex therapist. At the onset of the therapy both the couple and therapist established the following goals:

1. Improve communication between the couple
2. Discuss the premature ejaculation problem and explore options of improving the sexual relationship that would prove satisfying to both partners

During the therapy, the nurse worked with the couple to openly discuss important issues with each other and improve the patterns of communication. Behavioral sex therapy techniques were employed for Mr. S's problem with premature ejaculation. After 10 weekly sessions the couple and the therapist evaluated the course of treatment together. The following factors for evaluating treatment effectiveness were explored:

1. *Sense of well-being.* Both Mr. and Mrs. S felt better about themselves as individuals and their relationship. They were better able to discuss and solve issues of concern. They felt a renewed affection for each other and a desire to problem solve rather than ignore problematic issues.
2. *Functioning ability.* With the use of behavioral sex therapy techniques, Mr. S's premature ejaculation problem had significantly decreased and both members began to enjoy a satisfying sexual relationship.
3. *Satisfaction with treatment.* Both Mr. and Mrs. S felt that the goals of treatment had been accomplished and that there was a general improvement in the quality of their relationship.

After the evaluation, the couple, with the therapist's agreement, decided to terminate therapy, since the presenting problem was resolved and the goals of treatment were accomplished. By maintaining a facilitative position, the nurse helped the couple make their own choices in problem solving, and the responsibility for their choices remained solely with the couple. Thus their autonomy and sense of self were affirmed by the nurse and the goals of high-level wellness and holistic health care were promoted.

Suggested cross-references

Therapeutic relationship skills and self-awareness of the nurse are discussed in Chapter 3. The phases of the nursing process are described in Chapter 4.

SUMMARY

1. The need for knowledge of human sexuality in nursing was discussed. Information important for implementing the nursing role was identified and included self-awareness, values clarification, and effective counseling and communication skills.

2. Sexuality was broadly defined as a desire for contact, warmth, tenderness, and love. Criteria for normal sexual behavior were identified as sexual behavior between adults that is consensual, lacks force, and is performed in private. Difficulties in labeling behavior as normal, abnormal, or problematic were discussed.

3. What people believe about themselves as sexual beings changes throughout their lifetimes. Physical and emotional illness, injury, surgery, and the aging process were identified and discussed as specific changes that may affect sexuality.

4. Different modes of sexual expression were identified and defined: homosexuality, transsexualism, and transvestism. Sexual dysfunctions were also identified and defined: premature ejaculation, ejaculatory incompetence, impotence, female orgasmic dysfunction, and vaginismus.

5. Concepts of sexual counseling were presented in a nursing process model. The assessment phase of the nursing process includes two major responsibilities for the nurse: (1) self-awareness in relation to sexuality and (2) assessment of the patient according to situation and presenting problem. Phases of a positive growth experience in working with patients who have sexual concerns were identified and discussed as cognitive dissonance, anxiety, anger, and action. Patient assessment was described in terms of interviewing and history taking.

6. The planning phase of the nursing process requires active involvement on the part of the patient. The nurse must be careful not to develop a plan

and establish goals that she feels the patient should follow, but to help individuals identify their own goals and develop a plan to work toward achieving them.

7. Intervention with patients would depend on the person's situation and specific individualized needs. Intervention was discussed on three levels:

a. Primary, which includes sex education and preventive counseling

b. Secondary, which includes the brief treatment of sexual dysfunctions

c. Tertiary, which includes longer term counseling for sexual problems

The Masters and Johnson and Kaplan models of treatment were described.

8. In the evaluation process, the nurse and patient need to consider the following factors in assessing the effectiveness of the nursing care: the patient's sense of well-being, functioning ability, and satisfaction with treatment.

References

1. Aletkey, P.J.: Sexuality of the nursing home resident, Top. Clin. Nurs. **1:**60, 1980.
2. American Psychiatric Association: Diagnostic and statistical manual of mental disorders, ed. 3, Washington, D.C., 1980, The Association.
3. Bell, A.P., and Weinberg, M.S.: Homosexualities: a study of diversity among men and women, New York, 1978, Simon & Schuster, Inc.
4. Berger, et al.: Standard of care, 1981, The Harry Benjamin International Gender Dysphoria Association, Inc.
5. Foley, T., and Davies, M.: Rape: nursing care of victims, St. Louis, 1982, The C.V. Mosby Co.
6. Goldstein, B.: Human sexuality, New York, 1976, McGraw-Hill, Inc.
7. Graves, H., and Thompson, E.: Anxiety: a mental health vital sign. In Longo, C., and Williams, R., editors: Clinical practice in psychosocial nursing: assessment and intervention, New York, 1978, Appleton-Century-Crofts.
8. Hacker, S.S.: It isn't sex education unless. . . . J. Sch. Health **5:**209, April 1981.
9. Hole, J.W.: Human anatomy and physiology, Dubuque, Iowa, 1978, Wm. C. Brown Co., Publishers.
10. Kaplan, H.S.: The illustrated manual of sex therapy, New York, 1975, The New York Times Book Co.
11. Kelly, G.F.: Sexuality: the human perspective, New York, 1980, Barron's Educational Series, Inc.
12. Kinsey, A.C., Pomeroy, W.B., and Martin, E.C.: Sexual behavior in the human female, Philadelphia, 1953, W.B. Saunders Co.
13. Kirkendall, L.A., and Rubin, I.: Sexuality and the life cycle. In Barbour, J.R., editor: Human sexuality 79/80, Guilford, Conn., 1979, The Dushkin Publishing Group, Inc.
14. Kolodny, R.C., et al.: Textbook of human sexuality for nurses, Boston, 1979, Little, Brown & Co.
15. Marmor, J., editor: Homosexual behavior: a modern reappraisal, New York, 1980, Basic Books, Inc., Publishers.
16. Masters, W.H., and Johnson, V.E.: Human sexual inadequacy, Boston, 1970, Little, Brown & Co.
17. Masters, W.H., and Johnson, V.E.: Ten sex myths exploded. In Barbour, J.R., editor: Human sexuality 79/80, Guilford, Conn., 1979, The Dushkin Publishing Group, Inc.
18. May, R.: The meanings of anxiety, New York, 1950, Ronald Press.
19. Mims, F.H., and Swenson, M.: Sexuality: a nursing perspective, New York, 1980, McGraw-Hill, Inc.
20. Money, J., and Wiedeking, C.: Gender identity role: normal differentiation and its transpositions. In Wolman, B.B., and Money, J., editors: Handbook of human sexuality, Englewood Cliffs, N.J., 1980, Prentice-Hall, Inc.
21. Scales, P.: Barriers to sex education, J. Sch. Health **50**(6):337, 1980.
22. U.S. Dept. of Health, Education, and Welfare, National Center on Child Abuse and Neglect: Child abuse and neglect: the problem and its management, Pub. no. (OHD) 75-30073, U.S. Government Printing Office.
23. Vander, A.J., Sherman, J.H., and Luciano, D.S.: Human physiology, New York, 1975, McGraw-Hill, Inc.
24. Webster's new collegiate dictionary, Springfield, Mass., 1977, G. & C. Merriam Co.

Annotated suggested readings

Adams, G.: Recognizing the range of human sexual needs and behavior, Am. J. Maternal Child Nurs. **1:**166, May-June 1976.

This article is a thorough presentation of what human sexuality is all about. It gives simple yet useful information and principles for the nurse to use in her professional interaction with clients.

Adams, G.: The sexual history as an integral part of the patient history, Am. J. Maternal Child Nurs. **1:**170, May-June 1976.

The author convincingly and thoroughly presents the importance of the sexual history in the patient's total health history. The article gives the what, why, and how of sexual history taking. It is a highly recommended reading for all nurses.

Anderson, M.L.: Talking about sex—with less anxiety, J. Psychiatr. Nurs. **18:**10, June 1980.

This article helps the professional nurse examine the anxiety that is often involved in discussing client's sexual concerns with them. Anxiety is discussed from both the clients' and the nurse's perspective. First, the client's anxiety, what causes it, and how the nurse can help to decrease anxiety are examined; second, the author examines the anxiety of the nurse, causes for it, and what can be done to reduce it.

Barbach, L.L.: For yourself: the fulfillment of female sexuality, New York, 1975, Doubleday & Co., Inc.

This book is about a sex therapist's experiences with preorgasmic women. The author outlines steps and exercises for women to complete in order to increase sexual fulfillment. Unlike many sex therapists, Dr. Barbach worked only with women, rather than couples.

Bell, A.P., and Weinberg, M.J.: Homosexualities: a study of diversity among men and women, New York, 1978, Simon & Schuster, Inc.

This official publication of the Institute for Sex Research reports on a survey of 1456 homosexual and heterosexual men and women living in the San Francisco area. The study examines the variety of homosexual life-styles and demonstrates that homosexuality encompasses much more than people's sexual activities.

Bell, A., Weinberg, M., and Hammersmith, S.: Sexual preference, Bloomington, Ind., 1981, Indiana University Press.

This book asks why some people become homosexuals, while others become heterosexuals. It retires many cherished ideas and suggests that sexual identity is impervious to the influence of parents and psychotherapy. Controversial and important reading.

Carlson, B., and Wheeler, K.A.: Group counseling for preorgasmic women, Top. Clin. Nurs. 1:4, Jan. 1980.

This article outlines a method of group counseling for women having problems achieving orgasm. It includes specific group content, suggested reading materials, and a sample homework assignment given to group members.

Clark, D.: Loving someone gay, New York, 1978, Signet Books.

This book examines the myth and mysteries surrounding "gay" (homosexual) people. It includes an excellent chapter for professional counselors who work with gay clients.

Hacker, S.S.: It isn't sex education unless. . . . J. Sch. Health 51(4):207, 1980.

This article discusses appropriate content for sex education classes. It includes the principles of sex education and the sexual concepts that underlie an effective sex education curriculum.

Kaplan, H.S.: The new sex therapy, New York, 1974, Brunner/Mazel, Inc.

This book describes Kaplan's method of brief treatment for sexual dysfunctions. It clarifies basic underlying concepts by relating technical material to the theory of psychopathology.

Kaplan, H.S.: Disorders of sexual desires and other new concepts and techniques in sex therapy, New York, 1979, Brunner/Mazel, Inc.

This book addresses the dysfunction of inhibition of sexual desire, which occurs when one or both members of a couple have no desire for sex or find sex distasteful. Kaplan presents cases throughout the book of couples with this disorder and explains her treatment approach.

Kaplan, R., Meeks, L., and Segal, J.: Getting in touch: a design for graduate and undergraduate human sexuality courses, Health Values: Achieving High Level Wellness 1:155, July-Aug. 1977.

This article presents a human sexuality course for undergraduate students using graduate students as facilitators in small group discussions. Two examples of strategies are described: "Working with words" and "Life styles—is it really your choice?"

Kelly, G.F.: Sexuality: the human perspective, Woodbury, N.Y., 1980, Barron's Educational Series, Inc.

This is a comprehensive book on the subject of human sexuality. It includes excellent chapters on sexual response, reproduction and birth control, and gender identity. It is well written and informative, with excellent bibliographies accompanying each chapter.

Loovis, D.: Straight answers about homosexuality for straight readers, New York, 1977, Barnes & Noble Books.

This book specifically explores fears and concerns that "nongay" people have about the "gay" world. It provides honest answers and clears up common misconceptions. The author also explores theories of the origin of homosexuality.

LoPiccolo, J., and LoPiccolo, L., editors: Handbook of sex therapy, New York, 1978, Plenum Publishing Corp.

This edited handbook on sex therapy presents a unified, integrated approach to a broad range of therapies for rapid treatment of sexual dysfunction.

Masters, W.H., and Johnson, V.E.: Human sexual response, Boston, 1966, Little, Brown & Co.

This book is Masters' and Johnson's first effort to explore the physiology of sexual response. It discusses the anatomy and physiology of the male and female sex organs. The authors describe their research findings regarding sexual response and orgasm.

Masters, W.H., and Johnson, V.E.: Human sexual inadequacies, Boston, 1970, Little, Brown & Co.

This book identifies and describes sexual dysfunctions and specific treatment methods for those dysfunctions. Masters' and Johnson's dual therapy treatment approach is explained and case samples are included.

Mims, F.H.: Sexuality in the nursing curriculum, Nurse Educator 15:20, April 1977.

This article identifies levels of treatment in relation to levels of clinician competency. It can be used as a guide for planning and developing human sexuality courses and clinical experiences for various types of nursing education programs.

Mims, F.H., and Swenson, M.: Sexuality: a nursing perspective, New York, 1980, McGraw-Hill, Inc.

This text presents a nursing perspective for clinical issues in the area of sexuality. It includes thorough chapters on psychosexual development and sexuality in health disruptions such as spinal cord injuries, surgical interventions, postcoronary problems and sexually transmitted diseases. It also addresses the issue of sexual history taking and sexual health teaching.

Nass, G., Libby, R., and Fisher, M.: Sexual choices: an introduction to human sexuality, Belmont, Calif., 1981, Wadsworth, Inc.

This book presents a political analysis of sexuality in American culture. It has a wide scope and makes for very informative reading.

Satterfield, S., and Stayton, R.: Understanding sexual function and dysfunction, Top. Clin. Nurs. 1:4, 1980.

This article discusses the similarities and differences of sexual dysfunction in the male and female. The article helps the reader to understand the cause of sexual dysfunction, disorders of response, and treatment options open to the clinician specializing in sex therapy.

Silbert, D.: Human sexuality growth groups, J. Psychiatr. Nurs. 19(2):31, 1981.

This article is a condensation and overview of a program developed by the author for undergraduate nursing students. It focused on sexual self-awareness and sexual values clarification as a way of broadening acceptance and understanding of individual differences.

Thomas, S.: Bisexuality: a sexual orientation of great diversity, J. Psychiatr. Nurs. **18**(4):19, 1980.

Here is an excellent review of contemporary theorizing and research on bisexuality. It includes definition, prevalence, etiology, personal characteristics, viability as a way of life and implications for the future. This should be required reading for all nurses.

Wolman, B.B., and Money, J., editors: Handbook of human sexuality, Englewood Cliffs, N.J., 1980, Prentice-Hall, Inc.

This handbook is a comprehensive overview of important issues in sexuality. It includes an exceptional chapter on gender identity disorders. Each chapter contains recent research data and review of current literature.

*The greatest good we can do for others
is not just share our riches with them
but to reveal their riches to themselves.*

Anonymous

CHAPTER 23

LIAISON NURSING: A MODEL FOR NURSING PRACTICE

FRANCES G. LEHMANN

Learning objectives

*After studying this chapter, the student
should be able to:*

- *state the scope, functions, and role characteristics of liaison nursing practice.*

- *identify the three categories of problems encountered by the liaison nurse.*

- *describe the orientation phase of the liaison process, including setting, communication, confidentiality, and elements of a contract.*

- *discuss the four stages of the liaison process as they occur in the working phase.*

- *relate the major activities of the nurse during the termination phase of the liaison process.*

- *discuss future trends and challenges for liaison nursing practice.*

- *identify suggested readings for future study.*

Historically there are many major and minor forces that have helped shape the role, need, and use of liaison nursing. Liaison nursing is a model for nursing practice that has developed from the consultative process, and within psychiatric nursing it is considered a subspecialty.[13] It was generated out of need: the psychosocial needs of the client in a general hospital setting and the ethical needs of nursing to deliver professional health care to the holistic client in the most practical and economical method available. The liaison nurse has a high degree of expertise in psychiatric nursing and a special ability to integrate these skills with knowledge in medical-surgical nursing to provide comprehensive nursing service.

A model of liaison nursing

There are various models of liaison nursing. Blake[2] perceives the nurse consultant providing indirect client services as a collaborative agent of change through an education process. Robinson's model[14] has the liaison nurse serving two basic functions: giving direct patient care and assisting the nursing staff in making their own care more therapeutic. The model used in this chapter is an adaptation from Caplan's model of consultation. Caplan's definition is "a process of interaction between two professional persons—the consultant who is a specialist, and the consultee."[3] In his model the focus of interaction is the consultee's difficulty with a work-related problem in which the consultant has specialized competency. In this chapter the term "liaison nursing" is used to describe a particular professional process between two systems in which one of the systems (the user) has a current work-related problem and voluntarily requests help from an outside system (the provider), who is perceived to have a specialized competency in a defined area. Stated more simply, someone has a problem and believes an outside expert can help solve that problem.

There are several ways of practicing liaison nursing. Some nurses are independent private practitioners who are employed for a specific assignment by the consultee organization on a fee-for-services basis. Other clinicians are staff members of an identified liaison department within a general hospital setting who provide direct care to individual "problem" clients in a crisis or brief therapy model on a referral basis.[1,9] The approach in this chapter is explicitly an indirect service process in which an outside liaison consultant, on a limited-time basis, facilitates a separate organization's ability to develop and enhance its own staff's knowledge and skill to provide more effective and efficient direct service. This approach provides an opportunity for a liaison nurse to work effectively in a relatively short time and have a widespread effect on large numbers of consultees who are in direct contact with many clients. This approach also provides optimal benefit from the specialist's knowledge while facilitating the consultee's own professional abilities. The liaison nurse has the opportunity to deal indirectly with a larger number of "clients" than might be possible in a direct service method.

The present status of liaison nursing becomes more meaningful when viewed from the broader historical perspective of psychiatric nursing. A major influence on the evolution of psychiatric nursing was federal legislation (Public Law 88-164, the Community Mental Health Centers Act) passed in 1963, which created the authority for establishment of a comprehensive mental health delivery system in the United States to meet the psychiatric needs of all socioeconomic classes of Americans. This major mental health movement created a lack of qualified people to staff the centers. To help alleviate this deficit, several nonmedical professional disciplines, such as psychology, sociology, social service, and nursing, designed and implemented educational and training programs to prepare mental health workers. The significance of the legislation on nursing education can be measured by the number of schools of nursing that took advantage of federal training grant money and by the number of psychiatric/community mental health nurses prepared at the graduate level in the last decade. Psychiatric nurse practitioners, using specialized education, have taken their place alongside other mental health specialists in the health care delivery system.

Along with the increased demand for professionally and competently prepared psychiatric nurses to serve as established program staff members, another force within the comprehensive mental health center movement created a visibility factor affecting this same human resources pool. Mental health consultation is provided by all mental health centers as well as many other health facilities. This basic service has resulted in mental health nurse specialists having regular contact with other human service agencies and institutions. Through this broad base of contact, many disciplines have had access to and have recognized the unique viewpoint of nursing in treating individuals in relation to one another and to their environment.

The thrust toward holistic health care is relatively new, becoming popular within the last 25 years. In nursing, however, total patient care is documented as far back as Florence Nightingale's time. In contemporary times, nurses continue to minister to human beings in a holistic manner. Nursing activities are concerned with those factors which influence both the client and his environment. Traditionally interventions have focused on the client's mental, psychosocial, and spiritual needs as well as physical needs, regardless of the setting in which the nursing service is used. Nursing has long been a proponent of its members being skilled in providing service to a client in his own environment, as evidenced by community health nurses going into the home, occupational nurses being available in work places, and school nurses being regular staff members of educational institutions.

A larger number of psychiatric clinical nurse specialists are now available for both direct and indirect mental health services and their visibility and proved value are becoming widespread. Thus the evolving role of the psychiatric nurse from the traditional position of physical caretaker of patients in mental institutions into a collegial leadership position as consulting nurse seems appropriate. The psychiatric nurse's ability to provide on-the-scene direct consultation service in various professional settings is a natural unfolding of another chapter in the history of nursing.

Types of problems

The psychiatric clinical nurse specialist can function in many professional roles, applying the knowledge and theory of mental health concepts. These roles may resemble each other but have different goals, outcomes, strategies, and methods. The role of liaison nurse offers an exciting method of working closely with other members of a health team in promoting effective problem management. As previously defined, the model of liaison nursing used here is that of an expert providing problem-centered consultation service in a coordinate relationship, with problem resolution being the mutually shared goal of both partners.[6]

The identified problem can focus on one client

(*case problem*), a series of related problems (*program problem*), or a particular administrative problem (*organization problem*). In practice, there is generally an overlapping of these artificial categories. If, however, the liaison nurse has an awareness of the general nature of the identified problem and the level of the target system with which she is interacting, it helps in working through the entire liaison process from contract setting to outcome evaluation.

The case category relates to assisting the user to become more effective in direct service to the client. The liaison nurse's primary focus is on ways to increase the user's skill and knowledge in giving service to a particular client. The spotlight is on the client and alternative ways of providing direct service to that client. The program category relates to helping the user define or meet particular professional goals. The liaison's primary focus is on ways to improve the user's professional functioning in an identified area of practice in dealing with more than one client. The organization category relates to developing new programs or improving existing ones that affect the basic structure or function of the organization. The liaison's primary focus is on the administrative system and an effective course of action that involves organizational change to produce a desired outcome.

Clinical example 23-1 illustrates each category.

CLINICAL EXAMPLE 23-1

Case problem. Mr. C, a 68-year-old widower who had been living in a retirement home for about 6 months, began withdrawing from all social activities. Formerly he had been active and an initiator of planned outings for other members of the home community and generally appeared to be adjusting to the move after the death of his wife some 9 months previously. The staff of the home had vast experience in helping other clients work through similar life situations, but they believed that all the interventions implemented on Mr. C's behalf had minimum effect. The director of activities therapy and the director of nursing services requested a case consultation with Mrs. L, a clinical nurse specialist working as an independent practitioner. Mrs. L entered the user system at middle-management level and was asked to focus on Mr. C by working with the nursing staff to help it develop a more effective nursing care plan.

Program problem. The teaching staff in a private preschool facility went to the director of the program and requested more help. Mrs. B, the director of the program and a capable administrator, believed the present staffing pattern was adequate but also recognized that the faculty as a whole was experiencing more and more frustration in providing high-quality care for the youngsters enrolled in the program. She requested Mr. G, a clinical nurse specialist working in a community mental health center, to consult with the faculty regarding the problem.

Organization problem. A community hospital had received official permission to open an inpatient psychiatric unit. This challenge included the cooperation of many disciplines, many health care delivery systems, and many community and civic organizations. The director of nursing requested the administrator to include a mental health nurse consultant on the ad hoc planning committee. He contracted with a psychiatric/community mental health nurse to serve as liaison nurse for the duration of the project. She became a full-time employee of the hospital and administratively reported directly to the director of nursing service; no employees were responsible to her.

Role characteristics

Problem solving is a function of any nurse, regardless of educational preparation or defined role. There are several essential qualities of the liaison relationship, however, that contribute to the specialized problem-solving activity of liaison nursing. It is also important to differentiate commonly blurred activities, such as supervision and education, from liaison nursing. The liaison nurse should have a way of distinguishing these various activities to define her own role, responsibilities, performance, and outcome.[10,15]

An essential difference between the liaison role and supervisor role is the authority base and administrative responsibility for outcome.[16] The liaison nurse should have a coordinate professional relationship with the user. This means she should have no administrative authority or coercive power over the user. Implicit in this aspect is the factor that the liaison nurse is not responsible for implementing recommended changes, just as the user is free to accept or reject any or all parts of the recommendation.

The organizational aspect of a liaison nurse position should be that of a staff rather than a line position. This differs from a supervisory role, in which authority is explicit to hierarchy rank. By definition, the liaison nurse is outside the user system. This means she is outside the regular chain of command within the user organization. This aspect also provides the liaison nurse with the necessary freedom to work with people at any level within any needed time frame rather than in a full-time line position that fills a slot within the organizational structure.

The power of the liaison nurse rests in her own authority of ideas based on an acknowledged specialized area of expertise. The user explicitly and voluntarily asks for help. The liaison nurse respects the user as a professional partner in problem-solving activities. While dealing with the current problem, the liaison nurse works in such a manner as to add to the user's knowledge base and thereby enables the user to deal more effectively with similar situations in the future. In this way the liaison nurse facilitates the user's potential and relates in a coordinate way by asking for and using his input.

The liaison process emphasizes that the provider and user deal with aspects of the problem that are unclear and confusing to the user rather than with the issue of people who are inadequate or incompetent. The liaison nurse should project the attitude that the user is an active, interdependent partner and ultimately responsible for implementing the proposed interventions. The liaison nurse can be perceived as contributing to the user's professional development and not as an evaluator of the quality of work or job performance. This becomes especially critical in case and program-focused problems.

Although the liaison nurse may provide new information and knowledge to the user, this aspect of the liaison process differs from an educational activity in that the stated goal is not to impart a specific body of knowledge to the user. The liaison process is an activity in which the liaison nurse provides support and guidance while helping the user to enlarge and deepen his own understanding of the issues. He can then, hopefully, develop more effective ways of handling the current problem and future similar situations. How the liaison nurse guides the consultee to creatively challenge and resolve the identified problem within his own resources can be the exciting synergistic application of her own talents to produce change and growth for all concerned.

Conceptual model for liaison nursing

The liaison nurse should have a conceptual model and a theoretical framework for practice. It is this combination of style and method (structure and function) that will help the liaison

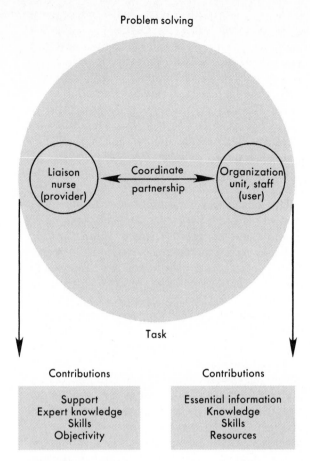

Problem solving

Task

Liaison nurse (provider)

Coordinate partnership

Organization unit, staff (user)

Contributions

Support
Expert knowledge
Skills
Objectivity

Contributions

Essential information
Knowledge
Skills
Resources

FIG. 23-1
Conceptual role model used by the liaison nurse.

nurse provide maximum return for her efforts and time and make the work exciting and rewarding. The conceptual model used in this chapter is a role model of a coordinate, nonhierarchical relationship between an outside expert and a participating human services system. This model sets the tone of the interactive relationship. Within this model, both provider and user bring distinct contributions to the problem-solving tasks, as depicted in Fig. 23-1.

Theoretical framework for liaison nursing

It is the liaison nurse's professional responsibility to use sound principles, apply concepts to the information available, and provide practical and easy-to-understand interventions founded on carefully thought out theory.[5] The practitioner therefore needs to develop a framework under which she functions in her role. The liaison nurse demonstrates a firm foundation of knowledge, organizes theory from a variety of disciplines, and uses this unique combination to formulate her own model for nursing. The

theory base should include knowledge of systems theory, change theory, staff management, organizational behavior, problem-solving theory, growth and development, cultural and ethnic norms, stress and stress reduction theory, and crisis theory, as well as environmental, interpersonal, and intrapersonal psychiatric dynamics. In one situation organizational theory may become the primary focus, another time interpersonal relationships may be the frame of reference, and yet another situation will deal directly with an intrapersonal problem.

The theoretical framework serves as a flexible reference for the nurse as she adapts to the various expected and unexpected components of any liaison situation. The particular method and approaches chosen come about through her own sense of purpose and professional identity. Within a defined framework she can shift the focus and scope of the problem to meet the needs of the users on the basis of their organizational structure, institutional policies, and perceptions of the liaison nurse's role. This framework becomes a road map and a practical frame of reference for the liaison process. It is the liaison nurse's way of organizing a wide range of skills and in-depth knowledge. It is a way of visualizing her thinking. It reflects her beliefs about the nursing profession and influences her own practice.

Liaison process

Although liaison nursing is a specialized type of nursing, the steps of the process can be compared to the traditional nursing process. Both are orderly, mutual, problem-solving activities; both relate to at least two people interacting in such a manner as to effect change; both processes hold the partners responsible for participation. The nursing process involves four steps: assessment, planning, implementation, and evaluation. These four steps comprise the actual liaison process, with an orientation and termination phase marking the beginning and conclusion of the formal liaison activity. As with any "process," liaison nursing is an ongoing activity with any component step interrelated with all other steps.

Orientation phase

As defined earlier, liaison nursing is a specialized professional activity in which the provider, as an outside expert, joins the user in problem solving in a nonhierarchical relationship. The nature of the relationship requires that certain issues in addition to the task at hand be attended to so that both systems will find it mutually satisfying and beneficial.

It is important for the liaison nurse to make face-to-face contact with key members of the staff and the appropriate authority personnel in the system as soon as possible to make her purpose and presence known. This contact also serves as a way to gather data about the organizational structure and the communication network operating there. It is also important for the liaison nurse to have an idea of the nature and scope of services provided by the organization, the philosophy, and any operating policies relevant to the target unit within the organization.

Any role is defined in relation to the social system of which it is a functioning part. The entire liaison process is affected by the type of setting and the individual and collective professional background of the personnel involved in the relationship. Settings could include health care settings, such as acute care general hospitals, ambulatory care facilities, and nursing homes; non–health care settings would be industries, schools, churches, self-help groups, and human services agencies, such as welfare departments, judicial systems, penal systems, and child care services. Each type of setting will have its own unique philosophy, organizational structure, established protocol, and vague and specific expectations of how the liaison nurse will function in that particular setting. The liaison nurse's knowledge of and experience with organization theory will benefit her intrapersonally and interpersonally as she functions within any setting.

The effectiveness of the liaison process is influenced by the user's concept of the liaison nurse's role. It is important for both sides to clarify the nature and scope of the liaison's role. This avoids two common causes of failure of a liaison process: the staff has unrealistic expectations or they distort the purpose for which the consultation was requested. The liaison nurse should also evaluate the accuracy of the user's perception of the present liaison nurse on the basis of past experience with other personnel in a similar role.

The liaison nurse will have the opportunity to work with intraprofessional (fellow nurses), interprofessional (other disciplines), and nonprofessional (technical) personnel. Needless to say, the liaison nurse will have to maintain the strength of her own identity as well as an awareness of the identities of others. The liaison nurse should interact with other people under the assumption that the other person has a sense of accountability, responsibility, and competency in his own area of work. This respect for the other person transcends educational background or professional experiences.

The liaison nurse's ability to communicate effectively with many levels of personnel is a skill that makes the process much smoother. The communication process depends on the liaison nurse, setting, and user of services. Developing communication channels involves identifying key formal and informal networks. It is important for the success of the liaison process that both sides have a working arrangement for obtaining and disseminating messages.

Basic conceptual differences will become apparent as people work together in the task of problem solving. Establishing a common language in which both partners are comfortable and feel productive will minimize differences. It is helpful for the liaison nurse to use words that are familiar to other people. Using words that others use will help prevent the nurse from talking on an inappropriate level or skirting the subject. Using abstract approaches or focusing on what seem to the user to be impractical or irrelevant issues will not promote their self-confidence. The liaison nurse's method of communicating with staff should not be by advice giving or using declarative sentences. It is preferable to use questions that guide the user to alternative ways of viewing the problem. Helping the consultee to reduce the complexities to relevant facts promotes clarity and mutual understanding of the situation.

It is important for the user to recognize that liaison discussions are confidential. This means that the liaison nurse guards against being a "switchboard" or carrier for messages that should be delivered directly within the organization. A liaison nurse should also make sure she does not take sides in differences of opinion among staff members. Promoting the attitude that any information gathered will not be used to purposely harm any person or the reputation of the organization is important. The focus of any interaction should be work difficulties and not the private personal needs of staff members. If personal issues are hindering a staff member's performance and interventions are indicated, this recommendation is not transmitted within the official liaison process. The liaison nurse restrains from gathering personal information that could turn the liaison session into a therapy session. Instead, she can tactfully encourage the troubled staff member to seek out an impartial skilled listener.

CONTRACT. The need to delineate expectations on both sides is obvious. The informal liaison process is the ongoing way in which both user and provider continually work out, modify, and change ground rules of the relationship. The formal liaison process is guided and evaluated by a written agreement between the liaison nurse and the user. This agreement is simply called "a contract." The contract represents an exchange between the partners of the terms of specific services to be rendered and the parameters of the complementary activity.[8] If the request for services comes through informal channels (via telephone or face-to-face contact), the liaison nurse needs to verify that permission at the appropriate level of authority is given for the liaison activity. The purpose behind requesting a letter of contract therefore is to prevent misunderstandings between the parties.

To avoid possible misrepresentation or ambiguity, a letter or memorandum from an authority person in the user organization should be directed to the liaison nurse. This document can describe the various aspects of the user's expectations. It eventually serves as a tool for outcome evaluation.

The contract is not so much a legal document as an agreement between professionals of two systems. It can be kept simple. It should be dated and signed by both user and provider. The main points to cover include the following:
1. A brief description of the problem situation
2. Expected goals
3. Estimated time to be used on the project
4. Means of compensation for the time
5. The key department and personnel involved, including the contact person

The liaison nurse can also use the contract to understand more fully the informal relationship. By expanding and examining the statement of problem in point 1, she can decide if it is a case, problem, or program consultation process. She can gather more background information as to what action has been taken so far to resolve the problem and what personnel have been involved in the activity to date. The stated goals in point 2 may end up as part of the original problem. Viewing both the expected goals and stated problem in context will show how the user perceives the entire situation.

Through points 3 and 4 the liaison nurse can learn about the organization's perception of both quality and quantity regarding time. It should also be established which possible dates or times are available for optimal productivity. Point 4 includes such considerations as whether the organization sees the compensation in terms of an hourly rate vs. a job rate. If the consultant is in-house, it should be clear to which department the time is to be charged. Point 5 includes the communication network to be used, the names of staff and their jobs, a list of people who are available for discussion, the scope of confidentiality expected, the kinds of information appropriate for discussion with whom, and who the authority source is for permission.

Work phase

After the orientation phase in which the initial contact and contract are completed, the actual liaison process begins. Fig. 23-2 is a representation of the process model, which depicts the four steps of assessment, planning, implementation, and evaluation. This same model is used on case, program, and organization problems. A more detailed discussion of the various steps fol-

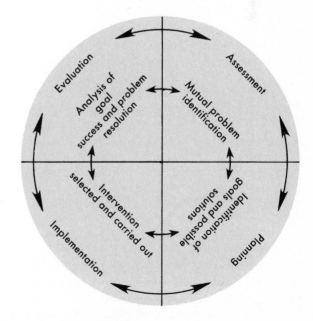

FIG. 23-2
Stages of the liaison process.

lows. The model is then applied to an actual case problem.

ASSESSMENT. This step actually begins when the contract is formulated. It continues with the two participating systems accumulating and classifying all data, clarifying the information available, and assessing it in a conceptual manner. The liaison nurse can ask questions in such a way as to stimulate the staff's thinking and communicate the message that they are capable. One technique that can guide the discussion to a deeper level is the liaison nurse asking herself, aloud, questions about the complexities of the situation. By speculating aloud, she promotes new understanding among the staff. She also demonstrates a willingness to risk and act as a role model for the problem-solving process. Beginning sentences with "I wonder if . . ." facilitates a feeling of joint endeavor. During this stage the liaison nurse should assess the strengths and weaknesses of the user, identify the real and potential barriers to action, determine what impediments have kept the user from resolving the problem, and assess the general problem-solving ability of the partners.

This step ends when an identified problem is agreed on by the two systems. The activity in this stage is most critical to the rest of the liaison process and may be repeated a number of times until the focus of the identified problem is narrow enough to manage and realistic enough to be resolved by the user organization. A concise conclusion derived from the assessment stage makes the rest of the process easier.

PLANNING. This step starts with the liaison nurse reframing the problem in such a way that the user can view the situation objectively and, it is hoped, without feeling threatened. The liaison nurse does this by using theoretical concepts that promote learning and can be generalized to similar situations. She listens to and values the staff's ideas. She may modify them by adding depth and breadth to the proposed intervention or by suggesting unusual but theoretically sound ways to implement them. Any suggested intervention should be both feasible and practical within the setting and in line with the functioning skills and capabilities of those who are responsible for their implementation. This avoids upsetting the existing lines of communication and authority. The suggestions should also be sensitive to the rights and well-being of all those affected by the potential change. The planning should reflect what presently exists and not what ought to be. It is ethically improper for the proposed interventions to be based on an idealist level of problem management.

This step ends when possible solutions to the problem are arrived at through the coordinated efforts of the liaison nurse and the user. Goals should be stated based on the outcome desired. These goals provide a framework for interpreting, planning, and evaluating ongoing activities.[11]

IMPLEMENTATION. This step begins with selection of the interventions to be tried. This decision rests with the users. In fact, this stage may actually take place after the liaison nurse has left the physical environment and the actual liaison process is terminated. This stage includes testing out any alternative suggestions that came out of the planning step. The step ends when the implemented interventions have been in effect long enough to assess observable change.

EVALUATION. This step begins with ascertaining to what extent the interventions met their stated goals. If the liaison nurse does not plan to be involved with the actual evaluation stage of the process, it is important that she help the user devise specific ways to measure the expected outcome or the interventions; therefore, in a psychological sense, the liaison nurse is involved in the complete process. The evidence used to evaluate should include obvious data, although implied data are used on occasion. The evaluation focuses on the effects of the planned interventions and not on the staff who implemented the plan. This is an important difference in that the total situation is examined, not how individual people are functioning. Another aspect of evaluation is that information may be generated that indicates gaps of knowledge or lack of skill on the part of the staff. These needs may be met through an educational approach to the problem.

This step ends when the user determines whether the defined problem has been resolved, to what degree of success the solution worked, and what additional problems, if any, were uncovered during the process.

Termination phase

Termination involves both physical and psychological closure. Wrapping up the work phase of the liaison process is important. Certain tasks such as report writing and leave taking are necessary. Much of the actual work involved in this phase depends on the liaison nurse's basic personality, the setting, and the formal contract. If the liaison nurse is a staff member of the user organization, her visibility will continue. If she has a one-time relationship, leave taking will be more formal.

LIAISON REPORT. Communication is not only a theoretical framework used in liaison nursing but a practical aspect of the experience. Throughout the interaction, progress may have been discussed, but, at the completion of the consultation activity, a formal written report is indicated. In this way all members of the organization who have been engaged in the process will have access to information relevant to the planned or implemented interventions. The report should be directed to the organization rather than to an individual staff member.

The format of the report will vary with the type of consultation, the setting, the level of organization involved, and the issues under focus. The following areas should be included:

1. The purpose, dates, and activities during the process
2. A statement of the identified problem
3. An assessment of the situation
4. Alternative plans for problem resolution
5. Specific interventions
6. Suggestions on how to evaluate the interventions

This formal report can be brief but explicit as to what the liaison nurse believed happened in the total process. The report should be consistent with the theoretical framework on which she bases her practice.

CONTINUED GROWTH AND DEVELOPMENT. The contract and summary report serve as tools for the liaison nurse to use in evaluating her own performance in the process and for making revisions in using the process on the next occasion. The liaison nurse is constantly changing and growing in her own professional development as a consultant. Self-evaluation is a necessary part of the nursing process. Areas that need evaluation are goal setting, problem solving, and communication skills (interpersonal and written), as well as theory application.

Performance evaluation is easier if criterion-referenced measurements are used. This is preferable over norm-referenced evaluation, since comparing oneself to others in the field is almost impossible. As with any profession, liaison nursing skills need constant nourishment. Atten-

dance at professional meetings and conferences allows the liaison nurse to keep in contact with other professionals and helps her assess her own growth and development. Reading professional literature and theoretical and clinical textbooks is a way of increasing one's theory base and scope of knowledge.

Clinical case analysis

The liaison process as described can be illustrated by Clinical example 23-2.

CLINICAL EXAMPLE 23-2

Assessment. Mrs. L responds to a telephone call from Mrs. K, director of nursing of the retirement home.[4,7] Mrs. L, Mrs. K, and Mrs. P, director of activities, meet. After informal conversation regarding the case problem, a contract letter is drawn up by Mrs. K: "Whereas our home has a resident whose lack of participation in planned activities keeps him isolated from other residents, we would appreciate your help in developing a treatment plan that provides opportunity for Mr. C to increase his involvement in group activity. As mutually agreed, this project should entail approximately 3 hours of joint effort. Our standard pay rate for nurse consultants is $20 per hour with no employee fringe benefits. Please feel free to talk with any staff or residents at their discretion. Mrs. P or I will arrange our time to meet your schedule." Both Mrs. K and Mrs. L sign the contract and an appointment is set for the next day with Mrs. K and Mrs. P.

The next day Mrs. L meets with Mrs. K and Mrs. P in the latter's office. A report is given regarding Mr. C's current status. Mr. C's physician administered a tricyclic antidepressant the previous week. No therapeutic effects had been noted. Mrs. L encourages both Mrs. K and Mrs. P to recount past interventions that were tried. Mrs. L uses nonthreatening questions to ascertain how both staff members see Mr. C in relation to his environment, life stage, grief phase, and physical and mental capacities. By speculating aloud to herself, she brings out different aspects of the same information in such a way as to increase the complexities and broaden the focus of the stated problem. By elaborating on certain points, she increases the staff's knowledge base. She is able to assess the collaborative relationship between nursing and activity therapy. She reflects her thoughts to the other two professionals in such a way that all three professionals engage in data gathering, investigating, and organizing the various information.

Mrs. K arranges for Mrs. L to talk with Mr. C during one of the structured activities held in the recreation room. During this time Mrs. L also talks informally with other residents and staff members in the same social setting. On returning to Mrs. K's office, Mrs. L encourages the staff to ask meaningful questions to increase their own knowledge regarding the total situation. After about 45 minutes of dialogue the three participants arrive at a concise conclusion. Mr. C is experiencing an anniversary grief reaction to his wife's death.[17] The mutually agreed on restated problem becomes, "Mr. C uses social isolation as a coping behavior as he works through the grief process." The problem statement describes an action of the client and reflects the hypothesis on which the treatment plan will be based. This identification of the problem makes it easier for the staff to focus objectively on the client and not be threatened by feelings of guilt or inefficiency in not meeting his social needs.

Planning. The grief process is the theoretical concept Mrs. L uses to help the staff reframe Mr. C's situation. The emphasis is shifted from engaging Mr. C in more activity to evaluating his behavior in terms of the stages of grief as outlined by Kübler-Ross.[12] The goal of problem resolution is to facilitate Mr. C's grief work. Although the aim is to provide individualized care for Mr. C, the staff benefits from learning about theoretical aspects of grief that can be generalized to other clients. The liaison nurse uses leading questions such as "Do you suppose Mr. C was in a state of denial when he first came here? That might explain how he got so busily involved in so many activities." Mrs. L provides information for discussing the various stages of grief and draws out examples of behaviors or attitudes that help assess which stages Mr. C has worked through. By increasing the staff's understanding of a specific need or reason for a particular behavior, approaches can be planned to help Mr. C relate to the emotional reactions manifested by his behavior.

At one point the discussion focuses on alternative housing for Mr. C. It is suggested he might live temporarily with his daughter. On closer evaluation it is ascertained that the daughter is unable to provide for her father at this time, since she recently changed jobs, moved to another city, and is living in an efficiency apartment until she decides if she likes the job and location. This alternative is discarded, since any recommendation should be sensitive to the rights of others. The treatment plan is written specific to actions of the patient with the underlying assumption that present behaviors are meaningful in helping him work through the loss of his wife, his home, his daughter, and his life-style. The liaison nurse uses the conference to have the staff look at Mr. C's behaviors as goal directed and to generate interventions that facilitate his emotional release. Mrs. K and Mrs. P mutually agree to reduce Mr. C's expected involvement in activities and to provide a psychologically appropriate environment for the various stages of grief.

Several strategies were discussed and it was agreed that Mr. C should be included in the planning stage of his treatment program. Mr. C's participation in the planning and implementing stages recognizes his strengths and allows him to remain self-reliant.

Implementation. Without describing specific interventions used in this case, a few guidelines are offered regarding this phase of liaison nursing. Short-term objectives can be used as selected steps toward reaching a long-range goal.[11] In Mr. C's case "facilitating client's grief work" is one step toward helping him adjust to his life stage and life-style. The interventions should focus on specific, expected actions of the client and not nursing care provided by staff. The interventions should be written in short concise statements (e.g., "introduce Mr. C to Mr. O, who has successfully completed grieving for his wife"). Expected measurable outcomes are established and a time frame is placed on each suggested intervention. Mrs. L negotiates with the directors to be available as a resource for 2 months as the planned interventions are tried and the results are measured.

Evaluation. Mrs. K receives a report from staff members in an ongoing manner regarding Mr. C's progress. A few minor revisions were made in the original plan. According to the evaluation of both Mrs. K and Mrs. P, the client profited, the interdepartment staff became more cohesive because of the cooperative effort at problem solving, and the staff's increased knowledge would benefit all residents of the home.

Mrs. L spent a total of 2 hours at the actual consultation site. The liaison project ended when she sent a summary letter to the retirement home at the end of the 2 months. The established relationship continued from time to time with other projects.

Following are a few of the liaison techniques used in the previous clinical example:

1. Keep the focus on the client's situation and away from the staff's handling of the situation so that the users recognize their work performance is not under investigation.

2. Avoid personal issues. If a staff member talks about personal or private material, gently and purposefully direct the discussion back on focus by asking a client-related question.

3. As information is reviewed, raise questions to discover additional details and enrich the staff's awareness.

4. Use inquiry in such a way as to show the staff's wealth of valuable information.

5. Avoid asking for information that the staff would perceive as testing its knowledge base.

6. Allow the staff to know when you are confused. Being open to your own confusion allows the staff to recognize that clarifying is one of the steps in problem solving and when the pieces are

put together, the patterns and meanings become clear.

7. Whenever possible, interview the referred client and the staff members who provide direct service to that client.

A forward look

Psychiatric liaison nursing will continue to evolve and be influenced by movements within the general practice of nursing as well as forces within the comprehensive health care delivery system. As nurses improve their professional image and internalized self-concept through education and quality performance, a separate and equal identity with other health disciplines can be achieved. National health insurance is a controversial issue, and whatever its fate, the process of looking at health care as a right promotes reevaluation of the health care industry. Consumer demands and involvement in their own care will dictate how nurses will function. The nation as a whole is becoming more mental health conscious. The social stigma of a person having an emotional problem vs. a physical illness is diminishing. With technological advances in all areas, this is the age of specialization and consultation in an effective method of providing expert knowledge or skill in a defined area.

The current educational preparation of all nursing students includes psychiatric principles. Nurse practitioners in all settings are aware of the total welfare of the client and feel increasingly comfortable in requesting consultation to provide total care. The educational preparation of psychiatric clinical nurse specialists emphasizes indirect service. The interest and use of nurse clinicians with master's degrees is being shifted to facilitate the skills of other health providers in dealing directly with clients.

There are three major dimensions in which liaison nurses can influence their own professional future. These and the tasks involved in each follow.

Accountability
1. Develop instruments for self-evaluation, since most clinicians work independently and can learn from retrospective audit.

2. Document liaison services in an official manner to validate and justify needs as well as to promote referrals.
3. Establish educational and experimental criteria for professional certification.

Accessibility
1. Participate in as many interprofessional activities as possible to provide role identity, visibility, and leadership.
2. Initiate liaison services to outreach agencies and rural and smaller outlying hospitals, even at the sacrifice of time or money, to promote improved and newly developed client care practices.
3. Utilize effective and creative marketing strategies to promote the consultation services. Competition for the declining health care dollar is a realistic component to consider in a cost-effective health care delivery system.

Application
1. Identify and practice within a sound theoretical framework.
2. Devise and implement research projects that test out established theory or validate/reject hypothetical concepts.
3. Use creative and flexible ways to effect change.
4. Be well prepared by keeping up with new developments through formal or continuing education.

Suggested cross-references

Therapeutic relationship skills are discussed in Chapter 3. The phases of the nursing process are discussed in Chapter 4. Strategies for promoting health care are described in Chapter 5.

SUMMARY

1. Liaison nursing is a model for nursing practice that has developed from the consultative process. The liaison nurse has a high degree of expertise in psychiatric nursing and an ability to integrate these skills with knowledge in medical-surgical nursing to provide expanded services. Liaison nursing is an interpersonal, coordinate, problem-solving consultation process between professionals who influence or participate in providing human services.

2. Three categories of problems are encountered by the liaison nurse:

a. Case problem, which focuses on the problem of one particular client

b. Program problem, which focuses on a series of problems related to the user's professional functioning

c. Organization problem, which focuses on developing new programs or improving existing ones within the organization.

In practice, frequently these categories overlap.

3. The liaison nurse has no administrative authority within the problem-centered organization. She is not responsible for implementing recommended changes, and the user is free to accept or reject any or all parts of the recommendation. The provider-user relationship is voluntary and time limited. The goal of the liaison nurse is to assist the staff to advance in professional efficiency and increase their ability to handle similar problems in the future. The liaison nurse should have a conceptual model and a theoretical framework for practice.

4. The liaison process is based on the nursing process and consists of four steps or stages: assessment, planning, implementation, and evaluation. It is characterized by an orientation phase, working phase, and termination phase.

5. A written agreement or contract should be obtained during the orientation phase. It should include a description of the problem situation, expected goals, estimated time for the project, amount of compensation, and key personnel involved.

6. The work phase consists of the four following stages: assessment, planning, implementation, and evaluation. The liaison nurse's assessment involves the accumulating and classifying of data, clarifying the available information, and assessing it in a conceptual manner. When this is completed, both the nurse and the user should have reached an agreement on an identified problem. In the planning stage, interventions are proposed to solve the problem and goals are identified based on the desired outcome. Implementation begins when the user decides which interventions are to be tried and alternative suggestions are tested out. This phase may take place after the liaison nurse has left the organizational setting. During the evaluation stage the user determines to what extent the interventions have met their stated goals. The liaison nurse may be directly or indirectly involved in this phase of the process.

7. Termination involves both physical and psychological closure. Tasks during this phase include report writing and leave taking. Self-evaluation by the liaison nurse is another important activity at this time because she is responsible for continued growth in her professional abilities.

8. Liaison nursing, as a subspecialty of psychiatric nursing, is evolving parallel to nursing in general. Three dimensions in which liaison nurses can influence their own professional future include accountability, accessibility, and application.

References

1. Barton, D., and Kelso, M.T.: The nurse as a psychiatric consultation team member, Psychiatry Med. **2:**108, 1971.
2. Blake, P.: The clinical specialist as nurse consultant, J. Nurs. Admin. **10:**33, 1977.
3. Caplan, G.: The theory and practice of mental health consultation, New York, 1970, Basic Books, Inc., Publishers.
4. Dawson, D., and English, C.: Psychiatric consultation and teaching in a home for the aged, Hosp. Community Psychiatry **26:**509, 1975.
5. DeLoughery, G.W., Gebbie, K.M., and Neuman, B.M.: Consultation and community organization in community mental health nursing, Baltimore, 1971, The Williams & Wilkins Co.
6. DeLoughery, G.W., Neuman, B.M., and Gebbie, K.M.: Change in problem-solving ability among nurses receiving mental health consultation: a pilot study, Commun. Nurs. Res. **3:**41, 1970.
7. Freedberg, L.E., and Altman, C.S.: Psychiatric consultation in a nursing home: a two-year experience, Gerontologist **15**(2):125, 1975.
8. Gebbie, K.M.: Consultation contracts: their development and evaluation, Am. J. Psychiatr. Health **12:**60, 1970.
9. Issachuroff, A., et al.: Psychiatric nurses as consultants in a general hospital, Hosp. Community Psychiatry **21:**361, 1970.
10. Kolson, G.: Mental health nursing consultation: a study of expectations, J. Psychiatr. Nurs. **14**(9):24, 1976.
11. Krall, M.L.: Guidelines for writing mental health treatment plans, Am. J. Nurs. **76**(2):236, 1976.

12. Kübler-Ross, E.: On death and dying, New York, 1969, The Macmillan Publishing Co.
13. Nelson, J.K., and Schilke, D.A.: The evolution of psychiatric liaison nursing, Perspect. Psychiatr. Care **14**(2):60, 1976.
14. Robinson, L.: Liaison nursing: psychological approach to patient care, Philadelphia, 1974, F.A. Davis Co.
15. Smith, M.C.: Perceptions of head nurses, clinical nurse specialists, nursing educators, and nursing office personnel regarding performance of selected nursing activities, Nurs. Res. **23**:505, 1974.
16. Stetler, C., and Downs, C.: The supervisor/consultant: a difficult role, J. Nurs. Admin. **4**(4):50, 1974.
17. Weiss, R.: Loneliness: the experience of emotional and social isolation, Cambridge, 1973, M.I.T. Press.

Annotated suggested readings

Burch, J.W., and Meredith, J.L.: Help with problem patients: nurses as the core of a psychiatric team, Am. J. Nurs. **74:** 2037, 1974.

This article deals with the importance of a liaison nurse helping the nursing staff ventilate their feelings about their work and their relationships with medical staff, nursing staff, and family. The psychiatric nurse consultation role developed in this article focuses on both direct and indirect services.

Caplan, G.: The theory and practice of mental health consultation, New York, 1970, Basic Books, Inc., Publishers.

This book is the acknowledged prototype for both consultation theory and practice. Many of the principles Caplan discusses are applicable to liaison nursing as a consultation process. It is an excellent resource book for a practitioner or student of liaison nursing.

DeLoughery, G.W., Gebbie, K.M., and Neuman, B.M.: Consultation and community organization in community mental health nursing, Baltimore, 1971, The Williams & Wilkins Co.

This book was written by acknowledged leaders in nursing education, primarily for nurse practitioners in community mental health. It is worthwhile reading to help understand the consultative process. The authors address both one-to-one and group consultation. They also raise some pertinent questions regarding the future of this specialty.

Garant, P.: The psychiatric liaison nurse: an interpretation of the role, Superv. Nurse **8**(4):75, 1977.

This article discusses in depth the role of the liaison nurse as an agent of change. The degree of acceptance of the consultant depends on how the role is perceived and interpreted by both the consultee and consultant. The author outlines some of the hurdles and responsibilities of the role.

Geist, R.A.: Consultation on a pediatric surgical ward, Am. J. Orthopsychiatry **47**:432, 1977.

This article is written by a physician and discusses the liaison psychiatry role; however, the function of a liaison nurse can be enhanced by incorporating some of the notions presented in the article. It is also an appropriate article for general staff nurses to read to understand and use liaison staff members.

Lancaster, I.W., and Lancaster, J.: Models and model building in nursing, Adv. Nurs. Sci. **3**(3):31, 1981.

This article focuses on the concept of models and the model building process. The article serves as an introduction to the relationship between model building and the role that models play in marketing the nurse practitioner's services as a consultant.

Mannino, F.V., and Shore, M.F.: The effects of consultation: a review of empirical studies, Am. J. Community Psychol. **3**(1):1, 1975.

This article does not address itself to nurse consultants but to the issue of consultation as a process. The article provides an overview on outcome evaluation. It also provides some thoughts for reflection by nurses in this subspecialty and discusses how research might be the missing link between direct service and recognition of consultation benefits.

Marcus, J.: Nursing consultation: a clinical specialty, J. Psychiatr. Nurs. **14**(11):29, 1976.

The author discusses the characteristics and qualities needed by the consultant. Various ways in which a nurse consultant can function are also discussed. This is an excellent article for those interested in entering the subspecialty.

Nuckolls, K.B.: The consultation process: a reciprocal relationship, Am. J. Maternal Child Nurs. **2**(1):11, 1977.

This article reports on a model of liaison nursing similar to the coordinate role proposed in this chapter. Both partners build on the strengths of each other in a synergistic approach to better client care. The article illustrates that this is an era of specialization in nursing.

Robinson, L.: Liaison nursing: psychological approach to patient care, Philadelphia, 1974, F.A. Davis Co.

This is an excellent book in which the liaison nurse process is described in detail with clinical examples and the theoretical framework the author uses in the process. Robinson, a pioneer in the practice and education of liaison nursing, founded the first graduate program in liaison nursing and uses her clinical and teaching experiences to provide the reader with an understanding of liaison nursing as a subspecialty of psychiatric nursing. This is a required text for any person interested in this field.

Robinson, L.: Psychological aspects of the care of hospitalized patients, ed. 3, Philadelphia, 1976, F.A. Davis Co.

This book serves as a resource for any nurse working in a general hospital setting. Typical psychological problems encountered among the client population are used as clinical examples to help the nurse understand how to better intervene. A comprehensive bibliography provides additional resources.

Severin, N.K., and Becker, R.E.: Nurses as psychiatric consultants in a general hospital emergency room, Community Ment. Health J. **10**:261, 1974.

The nursing role studied in this article is that of a psychiatric nurse employed as consultant to general physicians in a general hospital emergency department. This expanded nurse's role within the psychiatric team is discussed in depth, including a description of how resistance from the emergency nursing personnel was reduced.

Stevens, B.J.: First line patient care management, Wakefield, Mass., 1976, Contemporary Publishing, Inc.

This is a primer for all nurses who supervise delivery of client care. The first-line managerial responsibility fo-

cuses on middle-management nursing. At this authority level the initiation of liaison services often occurs. This paperback book helps the liaison nurse understand some of the organization and role problems on this level in nursing.

Wise, T.N.: The utilization of a nurse consultant in teaching liaison psychiatry, South. J. Med. Ed. **49:**1067, 1974.

This article describes how nurses are used as colleagues on a consultation team. The message is explicit that nurses can offer a unique contribution in a multidiscipline learning experience. The article validates that physicians can learn from nurses.

Zahourek, R., and Morrison, K.: Help with problem patients: mental health nurses as consultants to staff nurses, Am. J. Nurs. **74:**2034, 1974.

This article discusses the planning and implementing of a nurse-to-nurse consultation service in a general hospital. Examples of consultation cases are presented that give precise ways of handling "problem patients."

Zahourek, R., and Tower, M.: Therapeutic abortion. The psychiatric nurse as therapist, liaison, and consultant, Perspect. Psychiatr. Care **9:**640, 1971.

This article differentiates among the various functions of a qualified psychiatric nurse in one medical setting. Although the client problem discussed is abortion, the application of clinical skills makes for worthwhile reading.

Self and world are correlated, and so are individualization and participation. . . . Participation means: being a part of something from which one is, at the same time, separated.

Paul Tillich, *The Courage To Be*

CHAPTER 24

SMALL GROUPS AND THEIR THERAPEUTIC FORCES

KATHRYN G. GARDNER

Learning objectives

After studying this chapter, the student should be able to:

- define the group as a type of social system.

- compare and contrast the various types of groups, including identification of the nurse's role with each.

- identify and describe the two basic functions of groups.

- analyze group process in terms of the dynamic dimensions of communication, roles, norms, cohesion, and power.

- identify the four stages of group development.

- discuss the therapeutic aspects of group experiences.

- compare and contrast informal, therapeutic, and psychotherapeutic groups, describing indications for each and differentiating leadership roles.

- describe a variety of group psychotherapy models and theoretical frameworks.

- discuss the phases of development of a psychotherapy group, including therapist responsibilities and commonly encountered group behaviors.

- identify the need for nursing research relative to the therapeutic use of groups.

- identify suggested readings for further study.

701

Groups play a powerful role in forming society's organizational structure, influencing social behaviors of individuals, and shaping individual identities. In the last few decades the potential and actual therapeutic force of groups has been increasingly recognized. At least since 1947 when Lewin[18] observed that individuals under certain conditions are influenced more easily in group rather than individual settings, groups have been more formally studied by many disciplines. From studies on groups some phenomena of groups have become clear. These phenomena have to do with the processes that occur in groups, the structure and common dimensions of small groups, and the therapeutic aspects of groups.

Historically, nursing has been relatively slow in realizing the implications of working with groups and studying groups. This slowness is partially because of the traditional model of acute care nursing, the emphasis on the one-to-one nurse-patient relationship, insufficient knowledge about groups, and, until recently, the lack of sufficient numbers of nurses educated and experienced in group work. However, in the last two decades several things have occurred that have fostered nurses' interest in group work. The concept of the therapeutic community, the community mental health movement, the emergence of self-help groups and therapeutic groups, and the growing acceptance of group psychotherapy as a desirable treatment modality have kindled nurses' interest in groups. Additional factors that have enhanced group work in nursing have been the changing health care delivery patterns, the emphasis on preventive psychiatry, the increased amount of research in training and therapy groups, and health professionals' increased accountability to consumers and their representatives. From 1960 to the present time nursing literature has increasingly described nursing interventions within small groups. By the 1970s, groups and therapeutic intervention in groups began to be a part of both the undergraduate and graduate curricula in nursing. In the 1980s nurses have begun to study the groups they lead.

In addition to the importance of groups in clinical work, the knowledge of the group process is critical in team practice, community work, supervision, and management. The nurse often uses knowledge of groups in working with her colleagues and as a team member, team leader, and administrator. With the increased complexity of the health care system, it has become a necessity for nurses to be able to effectively participate in groups as a guest, member, and leader.

Groups as a potential therapeutic tool

To be consistently effective in therapeutic group work, one must have an understanding of some of the frequent and complex processes that occur in small groups and a knowledge of various approaches that use these processes to increase the therapeutic potential of the group for its members. This chapter will focus on these processes and approaches only as they relate to small groups. The study of processes and therapeutic techniques of large groups, such as ward or community meetings, is beyond the scope of this chapter.

Definition of group

The average size of a small group is six to twelve members. A basic definition of a group is that it is a collection of individuals who have a relationship with one another, are interdependent, and may share some common norms.[8] Thus the term "group" often refers to the interaction or relationship between three or more people. A group may be perceived as a separate entity or social system. As a separate system, it has its own structure and dimensions or properties. In other words, a group is not just a gathering together of three or more persons, but rather it is a separate entity that emerges only after the persons involved start interrelating with each other. As such, it is distinguishable from other groups within the environment and it has characteristics that differ from the sum total of all its parts.

Common dimensions in a group

Group functions

All groups have two basic needs or functions: the need to work on or complete a task or goal (there may be more than one), and the need to satisfy some psychosocial or emotional need or needs of its members. The latter function is sometimes called the group maintenance function.[26] If these two basic needs are not met, the group's effectiveness will decrease and the group may dissolve. The task or goal is usually one that connects the group to its external environment. The task of the group may or may not be well defined. The task of a group can be further divided into a primary task, which is necessary for the group's survival or existence, and secondary, or ancillary, tasks, consisting of those tasks which may enhance the group but are not basic to its survival.[23] An example of a primary task for a group of mothers might be to gain further mothering skills; a secondary task might be to improve the mother's social network. The psychosocial aspect of the group may either impede or enhance the group's accomplishment of its task.

Group structure

Group structure refers to the underlying order of the group. It describes the boundaries, communication and decision-making processes, and authority relationships in the group. The structure of the group offers it stability and helps to regulate behavioral and interactional patterns in the group. Structure describes the arrangement of the group similar to the arrangement of steps to a dance. Some of the major aspects of group structure, which will be discussed later, are communication, roles, and power.

Communication

The examination of communication patterns within the group is a common method used to study how a group approaches its task and psychosocial functions. Both verbal and nonverbal aspects of the group's communication can be observed: (1) individual member communications, (2) spatial and seating arrangements, (3) common themes expressed by the group, (4) how frequently and to whom members communicate, (5) how members are listened to in the group, and (6) what problem-solving processes occur in the group. Through studying these aspects, an observer can note interpersonal conflict in the group, the roles assumed by some of the members, the level of competition in the group, and the degree to which the members understand and are working on the task. An effective group leader will observe the group's communication, facilitate the group in clarifying and accomplishing its tasks, and assist the group in meeting some of the psychosocial needs of its members.

Role

In studying groups, it is important to observe what roles members assume in the group. Role is the position members assume in the group. Each role has certain expected behaviors and responsibilities. Persons may experience a conflict when there is a discrepancy between the role they seek or assume and the role ascribed to them by the group. In addition to roles that members bring to the group, such as nurse or parent, there are group roles. For example, a member may assume and be given the role of the group historian. In this role the member may be encouraged by other members to reminisce important events in the group. The role a member of a group assumes can be determined by observing the communication and behavioral patterns of that member while in the group. Following are factors that influence role selection: personality structure of the individual, the group size, the group's tasks and their significance to a member, the interaction in the group, and the individual's position in the group. Benne and Sheats[4] catalogued three major kinds of roles individuals can play in groups: (1) group building or maintenance roles—concerned with the group processes and functions, (2) group task roles—concerned with completing the group's task, and (3) individual roles—not related to the group's tasks or maintenance and may be self-centered and distracting for the group. A person in a maintenance role would, for example, be an individual who acts as a harmonizer and peace maker. An example of a person in a task role would be an individual who clarifies and seeks new information. The importance of group maintenance and task roles has been observed by Bales and Slater,[3] whose studies demonstrate that there is some evidence that groups encourage members to specialize in one of these two role functions.

Lewin's analysis[18] of groups describes a role pertinent to all groups, the gatekeeper. The function of this role is to provide entry into the group. Health professionals often need to determine who occupies this role when they are trying to influence families and informal groups or other social support systems in the community. One way to determine the person who occupies this role is to ask the group with whom they prefer the outsider to talk. The person who occupies this role tries to maintain and strengthen the group in its interactions with the external world.

Power

All groups have a power structure or hierarchy. Power is the member's ability to influence the group and its other members. The power structure in the group is usually resolved in its initial stages. Power implies a reciprocal relationship. To be successful all members in a power structure must have their needs met. To determine the power various members have, it is helpful to assess which member(s) receive the most attention, which members are listened to most, and which members make decisions.

Norms

Norms are standards of behavior that are adhered to by the group. They are statements of the perceived expectations of how the group will react in the future based on the past and present experiences of the group. It is important to understand the norms of a group because they influence the quality of communication and interaction within the group. The observance of norms results in conforming. If a member does not follow the norms, he may be considered a deviant by the other group members. Groups differ in how much deviancy they will allow. Norms may be expressed or communicated overtly or covertly. Overt expression of norms may be written or clearly stated. For example, members may clearly state to a new member that smoking is not allowed in the group. Covert expression of norms may be implied through the behaviors of members in the group. Norms are created to facilitate accomplishment of the group's goal(s) or tasks, control interpersonal conflict, interpret social reality, and foster group interdependence. An example of the importance of group norms is the influence of norms on health practices. For example, a family group may not eat meat and may bathe once a week.

Cohesion

Cohesiveness is the esprit de corps of the group. It is related to the attraction to and the satisfaction derived from the group by each member. Cohesiveness is a basic fiber of any group because it is directly related to the life span and success of the group. It is the force that acts on members to remain in the group.[8] Since cohesion is such an important dimension, some group leader interventions are aimed toward promoting cohesiveness. The method to foster cohesion is application of communication theory, such as encouraging members to talk directly with each other, discussing the group in "we" terms, and encouraging all members to be in similar spatial arrangements, for example, not permitting some members to move their chairs away from the group. A leader can also foster cohesion by pointing out similarities among group members, assisting members in listening to each other, and encouraging cooperation among the members.

The group leader is continually concerned with the level of cohesiveness in the group. There are various ways to measure cohesiveness in a group. Group leaders might observe to what degree members express interest in each other and to what degree members recognize each other for their individuality. Another way to measure cohesion is to determine the degree of member identity with the group as a whole and the expression of members' desire to remain in the group.[8]

Many factors contribute to the level of cohesiveness in a group. Some of these are the agreement of members on group goals, interpersonal attractiveness between the members, degree to which the group satisfies individual needs, similarities among members, and satisfaction of members with the style of leadership. For a more detailed discussion on cohesiveness the reader is referred to *Group Dynamics: Research and Theory* by Cartwright and Zander.[8]

Group development

Another important factor that will influence a leader's behavior and determine the evaluation of the group's effectiveness is the developmental stage of the group. Groups, like individuals, have an innate capacity for growth and development. Likewise, they have an ability to regress and to resist working effectively. Many authors and researchers have studied phases or developments in groups. Small groups are recognized as having various definable stages of group development. Bennis and Sheppard[5] studied phases of group development in sensitivity groups and theorized that central concepts of group development are dependent and interdependent issues. They relied heavily on Freudian theory and viewed the issues of power, authority, and intimacy to be important to the group's life. Martin and Hill[22] studied the various phases of psychotherapy groups. They described six phases of group development, ranging from the individual's unshared behaviors in a derived structure to the individual's use of a group as an effective and creative problem-solving agent. Schutz[30]

TABLE 24-1. Developmental phases in small groups*

Phases	Definition	Task activity	Interpersonal activity
Forming	Group members concerned with orientation	To identify task and boundaries regarding it	Relationships tested; interpersonal boundaries identified; dependent relationship with leaders, other group members, or preexisting standards established
Storming	Group memers resistive to task and group influence	To respond emotionally to task	Intragroup conflict
Norming	Resistance to group overcome by members	To express intimate personal opinions around task	New roles adopted; new standards evolved in group feelings; cohesiveness developed
Performing	Creative problem solving done; solutions emerge	To direct group energy toward completion of task	Interpersonal structure of group becomes tool to achieve its task; roles become flexible and functional

*Modified from Tuckman, B.: Developmental sequence in small groups, Psychol. Bull. **68:**384, 1967.

stated that every group developed according to three sequential interpersonal states: inclusion, or being "in or out"; control, or being "top or bottom"; and affection, or being "near or far." Each stage is characterized by members expressing various aspects of the same interpersonal issue or conflict. Tuckman[33] in discussing the development of the group, believed that any group is concerned with the completion of the task. He referred to the group structure as being the interpersonal relationships among the members and task activity as being the interactions directly related to the task. Tuckman summarized the various phases of group development as forming, storming, norming, and performing. These phases have been confirmed as occurring in at least one research study that observed groups in a classroom setting.[28] Table 24-1 summarizes Tuckman's categories and model.

Tuckman does not mention the termination phase. In a reclassification of Tuckman's theory of development, Lacoursiere (as cited by Dolgoff[13]) proposed that a mourning phase be added and combined in the norming stage with the performing and storming phases. Termination occurs when the group dissolves because the task is accomplished. It may also occur when interpersonal issues prevent the group from accomplishing its task.

Group development does not occur in distinct phases. Phases may overlap each other, and a group may regress to a previous phase. For example, group regression can occur with the addition of a new member. Phases of group development can be thought of as a path that a group takes to form and accomplish its objectives. The leader's task is to understand and assist the group as it goes along its growth path. Examples of specific leadership behaviors will be noted later in the discussion of the leader's responsibility in therapy groups.

Therapeutic aspects of groups

Groups have the potential of being positive (constructive) or negative (destructive) forces. The history of civilization abounds with examples of both types of groups. Persons interested in behavioral sciences have begun to isolate some of the factors that occur in groups which influence their members. Nurses and other health providers need to understand how a group can exert influences on its members so that they may consciously use these forces to enhance or modify the effects on individuals in the group.

Dr. Irvin Yalom,[35] a group therapist, has clearly described some of the positive forces that occur in group therapy. Yalom listed 11 curative factors that may occur in every type of therapy group. These factors are found in Table 24-2. Yalom's curative factors do not occur in isolation from each other. Although these factors may be

TABLE 24-2. Yalom's curative factors*

Factor	Definition
Imparting information	Receiving didactic information and advice
Instillation of hope	Increasing hopefulness of group members
Universality	Realization that others experience same thoughts, feelings, and problems
Altruism	Experience of sharing part of oneself to help another
Corrective reenactment of primary family group	Ability of members to alter learning experience previously obtained in their families
Development of social interaction techniques	Opportunity to increase one's awareness of social interactions and develop social skills
Imitative behaviors	Opportunities to increase skills by imitating behaviors of others in group
Interpersonal learning	Ability to engage in group in wider range of interpersonal exchanges, thereby increasing each member's understanding of responsibility and complexity of interpersonal relationships and decreasing members' interpersonal distortions
Existential factors	Ability of group to help members deal with meaning of their own existence
Catharsis	Opportunity to express feelings previously unexpressed
Group cohesion	Attraction of member for group and other members

*Modified from Yalom, I.: The theory and practice of group psychotherapy, ed. 2, New York, 1972, Basic Books, Inc.

more pertinent to therapy groups, they are important factors to consider in all groups, especially those which have health-related goals for their members. In the last several years researchers have begun to study various groups for their curative factors. Because of the limited number of studies, no conclusions can be made at this point. However, several studies indicate that cohesiveness, catharsis, and interpersonal learning are rated by group therapy practitioners as the most important curative factors in their groups.[20]

In a study by Lieberman, Yalom, and Miles[19] on encounter groups, cognitive learning appeared to be the most important factor in differentiating those who learned from those who did not learn from the encounter group experience. Cognitive learning is the derivation of information or insight that is useful to oneself. Cognitive learning is a frequent activity that is used by many nurses working with groups. Examples of this are groups that have the learning about a condition or disease as a primary task. In this same study on encounter groups, four major leadership dimensions were identified: caring, emotional stimulation, meaning attribution, and executive functioning. Caring included warmth,

affection, acceptance, encouragement, and communication of positive regard. Emotional stimulation was when the leader challenged and encouraged the revelation of feelings and personal values. Meaning attribution involved increasing cognitive dimensions, and executive functioning included limit setting and managing activities. In this study, the leaders who were rated most effective were high on caring and meaning attribution and moderate in emotional stimulation and executive functioning. Although, as of yet, these leadership dimensions have not been adequately studied in further encounter groups or other types of groups to be conclusive, they do offer a group leader a different way to think about leadership skills.

Groups commonly encountered in nursing practice

Many groups have therapeutic value for their members. Through belonging to a group, an individual's needs may be gratified and growth may be facilitated. Except for psychotherapy groups, most groups have not identified their primary task as the alleviation of emotional stress.

However, the prevention and alleviation of emotional stress often becomes a secondary task of groups that have as one of their goals, or concerns, the promotion of health and adaptation of their members. The therapeutic impact of groups may occur spontaneously from an already formed group or when individuals form a special group because of their vulnerability, stress, and reactions to illness. These groups are in various phases of group development, have different primary tasks, and may or may not have designated leaders. Five common types of groups that either potentially or actually have therapeutic value for their members are the family group, informal group, sensitivity training group, therapeutic group, and psychotherapy group. An understanding of these five types of groups is essential to the practice of psychiatric nursing. Knowledge of individual behaviors in these groups can be used in any of the five components of the nursing process: data collection, nursing diagnosis, planning, implementation, and evaluation.

Family

The family is a specific kind of group, often called the primary group. A primary group fosters warm, intimate and personal relationships among its members.[26] Members of a primary group can exert great influence on each other. Often stress in one member of a primary group will cause stress in other members. Thus illness in one member of a family group is felt in some way by all members.[29] When a member of a family is ill, nurses' use of the nursing process can assist families to optimize their therapeutic impact. Nurses can assess the amount of stress the individuals are experiencing, and, through a constructive use of themselves, they can intervene to decrease the stress. A common method of intervention employed by nurses is to use the curative factor of imparting information. A nurse will give information to a family regarding a patient's condition or treatment. Nurses have begun to research the relationship between family-oriented nursing interventions and the patient's rate of improvement and adaptation. For example, Eisenberg[14] studied the effects of nursing interventions with husbands who had wives undergoing mastectomies. This study compared the wives' perceptions of their adaptation to two different nursing approaches used with their husbands.

In another study[9] nurses were able to increase the recovery rate of patients after heart surgery by training their families how to do reality orientation and be reassuring to the family member immediately after surgery. This nursing intervention increased the families' therapeutic potential by decreasing the patients' postsurgical complications.

Informal groups

Informal groups are perhaps the most frequent type of group the nurse encounters. Although significant to nursing practice as a whole, they are especially significant to the practice of psychiatric nursing in a therapeutic environment or community. In a psychiatric ward setting the nurse's participation in informal groups can influence the therapeutic effectiveness of the environment. Likewise, observations of patient's participation in informal groups enhance the nursing assessment and nursing evaluation of the patient and the progress he has made.[16]

Another setting in which informal groups play an important role is the waiting room.[17] Depending on the nature of these groups, they may be more or less helpful and may align themselves with or oppose the health care staff. These groups usually form because the members share a common problem, need to communicate and share information, and need to be helped as well as to help. Each informal group will develop its own properties and culture and each has the potential of becoming a supportive group for its members.

Informal groups are groups that do not have a formalized structure and task and are often more spontaneous in nature than formal groups. Examples of these groups are various patient and staff groups that spontaneously form on a unit. Informal groups often consist of persons who are in some way interdependent and interrelated to each other. In organizations the presence of informal groups often supplements or counteracts the deficiencies of the formal group. Informal groups often improve and expedite information and communication processes. These groups may exert considerable influence among their memberships as well as on groups who interface with the informal group. For example, an informal group of patients may supplement or decrease the effectiveness of therapeutic interventions with a patient.

Because of the importance of the informal

group, psychiatric nurses should consider nursing interventions with informal groups as essential. These groups provide a setting in which assessment of the patient's interpersonal communication and social skills can be done. The nurse, by participating in these groups, can use them to make effective and powerful therapeutic interventions. As participants, nurses should be aware of the group process, aware of their role as well as that of others in the group, and ready to capitalize on some of Yalom's curative factors.

Nurses can deliver many nursing services in an informal group setting, such as patient teaching and emotional support. Nurses may enter initially or join an already formed group, and in each case their behavior will partially determine the group's therapeutic outcome. In joining informal groups, nurses must be prepared to be rejected at times by the members. The goals, roles, and norms of a group may not be enhanced by permitting a new member to join. When rejection occurs, the nurse would do well to consider the group's primary task and how she might facilitate or perhaps inhibit accomplishment of this task.

As time progresses, it has become more apparent that nursing intervention in informal groups is a skill necessary for the practice of psychiatric nursing and is increasingly useful in other areas of nursing practice. It is an area that warrants more critical study by the nursing profession. In the acute and community health care setting, informal groups of patients and families may influence the patient's compliance, self-esteem, satisfaction and health outcome. Working with informal groups is a daily challenge. It requires that the nurse be astute in determining the tasks and roles of the various members, make quick assessments, and communicate clearly and honestly. In some respects all informal groups represent unharnessed energy of human beings who want to care for each other.

Sensitivity training groups

Although nurses without specialized preparation should not lead sensitivity training groups, nurses often participate in these groups as a means to increase their understanding and effectiveness in group work. These groups are usually small, comprise eight to twelve members, and vary considerably in duration. The purposes of these groups are to increase self-aware-

ness, increase an understanding of group processes, and/or increase an awareness of the effects of one's behavior in groups. These groups usually focus on present individual and group behaviors. Most sensitivity training groups will advocate a specific theoretical framework. These theoretical frameworks may range from being individual to being group oriented, and the interventions and techniques used by the leader may vary greatly. Some of these theoretical frameworks are that of the National Training Laboratory (NTL), which has the widest range of goals and leadership flexibility; the Tavistock model, which is mainly concerned with understanding the process of a group as a whole and the member's relationship to the leader; gestalt, which emphasizes awareness of the total person; and Esalen, which emphasizes the individual and interpersonal relations in the group. It is important before participating in a training group to know the leaders' qualifications and the theoretical model that will be used. Participation in training groups is viewed by most group therapists as a valuable learning experience.

Therapeutic groups

Therapeutic groups are groups that have a broad goal of preventing emotional turmoil or disturbances. They are different from traditional psychotherapy groups in that emotional stress is secondary to physical diseases, other external stress, or crisis. The primary purpose of the therapeutic group is prevention, not treatment of emotional disorders. Education is usually a secondary goal in these groups. In contrast, the primary purpose of psychotherapy is to treat emotional disorders.[21]

In the last decade nurses have become more involved in therapeutic group work and have begun to write about their effectiveness in these groups. Nurses have led therapeutic groups for parents whose children have a disease,[7,15] for patients who are coping with a disease or stress,[2,6,10] and for patients' spouses.[11] Because of the emphasis on prevention, these groups seem especially relevant to nurses in all health care settings, especially the community. For example, these groups are useful with schoolchildren who are coping with a problem such as obesity, parents who want to improve their parenting skills, the elderly to decrease social isolation, and families of the elderly in discussing coping with an aged parent.

More recently nurses have written about groups in medical settings. According to the group's goals, they may be preparatory or adaptive groups. The preparatory group provides information in anticipation of the event, such as a preoperative surgical group. The adaptive group helps its members face an event, such as diagnosis. DeMocker[12] describes the following major helpful factors in nurse group care:

1. Providing information
2. Providing emotional catharsis
3. Sharing members' perceptions
4. Sharing feelings of fear, loneliness, and frustration
5. Improving interpersonal communication
6. Being in a helper role
7. Learning and rehearsing new skills
8. Providing role models
9. Helping to confront reality

All of these factors can be readily incorporated into Yalom's curative factors, but some of Yalom's factors are deleted in this list.

Most of the writing about these groups has been descriptive. There needs to be more systematical investigation of selection of members, leadership strategies, therapeutic interventions, and adequate measurement of therapeutic outcomes in these groups. Most of the nurse authors write enthusiastically about their perceptions of the therapeutic benefit of these groups, and there is little, if any, mention of negative aspects. The involvement of nurses in therapeutic groups seems to parallel or reflect the consumers' and nurses' increased attention to psychosocial factors in healing and health. Nurses, as demonstrated in the literature, have increasingly viewed leading or co-leading therapeutic groups as a part of their nursing practice, responsibility, and right.

The self-help group is another type of group that is often viewed as therapeutic to its members. The responsibilities of these groups lie within the membership. Professional persons, in their professional practice, are not directly involved with these groups. The extent of professional involvement is usually to refer members to a specific group or to act as a resource to the groups. Examples of self-help groups are Recovery Incorporated, Make Today Count, Alcoholics Anonymous, Weight Watchers, and colostomy groups. Self-help groups are usually formed around a specific problem or stress. Goals of these groups may include education about specific coping or adaptive techniques, suppression of harmful impulses that are related to a specific problem, and socialization. Some of these groups may be highly structured and have overt rules and norms. These groups often help and support

their members with other social systems in their environment. They also instill hope in their members by giving new members successful role models.

In addition to these groups nurses have often led small groups for patients on inpatient psychiatric units. These groups often have the following goals: (1) resolving interpersonal issues that arise from living on inpatient units, (2) helping patients increase their problem-solving ability, (3) providing information, (4) helping patients gain or regain social interaction skills, (5) preventing maladaptive regression from occurring, and (6) helping patients to integrate back into their natural communities. These groups can often be a reflection of the larger treatment milieu. The group leader(s) must be aware of individual patient goals and approaches and significant events in the milieu. Because of the complexity of leading these groups, group leaders should always have adequate preparation for group leadership and have supervision or consultation available to them. Usually these groups will require the leaders to be more flexible in their activity structure and involvement than in other types of groups.

Psychotherapy groups

Group psychotherapy is the treatment of emotional stress and disorder through the means of a group method and group process. As treatment, the group psychotherapeutic processes are systematical, planned, goal oriented, and based on theoretical formulations. The therapist, on the basis of her theoretical framework, uses her knowledge of group process to enhance the therapeutic effectiveness of the group.

Group therapy differs from individual therapy in several major ways. The most obvious difference is that the group itself is used as a treatment tool. Group therapy is effective in treating disturbances in interpersonal relations. A disadvantage of group therapy is that individuals may feel more frightened. In contrast to individual therapy, group members may feel more vulnerable and a higher sense of risk. Self-disclosure is usually viewed as being more difficult in a group setting. Compared to individual therapy, group therapy may not deal as effectively with in-depth material. Group therapy often allows for a corrective emotional experience that will facilitate a change in behavior. The therapist in group therapy is not as powerful as in individual therapy. Transference—the displacement of thoughts, wishes, and feelings from a significant person to another person—is more diluted in group therapy than in individual therapy. Group therapy allows for more reality testing than individual therapy. Some advantages of group therapy are that it allows for consensual validation, increases experiences in risk taking, and gives experiences of feeling mutually supported. An important element in all group therapy is that members feel a sense of belonging and thus feelings of isolation are decreased. Individuals learn that they may act as therapeutic agents for each other. At this point there is no clear evidence establishing either the individual or group treatment modality as being more effective or superior. Both treatment modalities can be viewed as complementing each other. Recently there has been work on outcome studies involving specific patient populations, problems, and/or target complaints. In Parloff and Dies'[27] review of group therapy research literature, they reported that studies on schizophrenics, addicts, and offenders do not clearly endorse group therapy as the most effective independent treatment modality. However, many studies on group therapy have methodological problems and do not adequately describe the specific approaches and techniques used in treatment groups.[27] Thus before one draws conclusions about the effectiveness of group therapy, more specific research studies with better descriptions of the independent variables and designs are needed.

Group therapists are from all the disciplines that practice psychotherapy—psychiatry, psychology, social work, and nursing. Within these four disciplines, nursing has been the last to practice group therapy. Within the last decade there has been wide acceptance that nurses prepared with a master's degree in psychiatric—mental health nursing are able to practice effective group psychotherapy. The American Nurses' Association Statement on Psychiatric and Mental Health Nursing Practice emphasizes that nurse therapists can use groups as a "primary treatment modality."[1] The development of group therapist skills requires specific and extensive preparation, usually including graduate study and several supervised clinical groups by qualified and experienced group therapists. A trained group therapist usually has a knowledge of dynamics of human behavior and psycho-

pathology, has taken courses in group process and group therapy, participated in a sensitivity or encounter group, observed therapy groups, and conducted several supervised psychotherapy groups.

From the mid-1960s until the present time, some nurse authors have stated that nurses, regardless of formal education, who have the appropriate experience, knowledge, and personality are capable of doing group psychotherapy.[31] This position of the importance of experience, maturity, and knowledge over arbitrary educational criteria finds some support from authors in other health disciplines. Most nurse authors, however, suggest that nurses with less than a master's degree preparation should not do insight-oriented psychotherapy. As evidenced by the literature from 1965 until the present, nurses who are not clinically prepared at the master's degree level have functioned as group therapists for supportive therapy groups. At present there is no agreement as to what are the qualifications necessary to lead these supportive therapy groups. Nevertheless, this confusion should not be understood to mean that supportive groups are less complex or easier to lead than other therapy groups, but may indicate that these groups require a different kind of leadership skill.

Types of group psychotherapy

As already implied, a wide range of treatment techniques are used in group psychotherapy. With the current emphasis on community psychiatry, models and techniques of group psychotherapy have expanded to accommodate more diverse populations. Group psychotherapy has become more acceptable and, in some situations, the preferred treatment. The various models of group psychotherapy can be best studied by considering them to be on a continuum, ranging from supportive to psychoanalytical group psychotherapy. Marram[21] described the various groups on this continuum to be support, reeducation and remotivation, problem solving, insight without reconstruction, and personality reconstruction.

The first four groups described by Marram rely heavily on theoretical frameworks of ego psychology, learning theory, social psychology, and communication therapy. All these groups are concerned with increasing the members' adaptation, self-esteem, and state of emotional well-being. The goals of support groups are aimed at reinforcing the group members' healthier defensive operations. The focus of these groups is on what the members are experiencing presently in their lives and in the group. The interactions in the group are mainly at the conscious level. The therapist is usually active and keeps anxiety engendered by the group at a minimum level. The remotivation and reeducation groups also may use behavior theory. Usually goals of these groups are to increase communication and interaction among members and to learn more socially appropriate and adaptive behaviors. These groups are frequently used for withdrawn, socially isolated, and institutionalized patients. Remotivation, or social skills, groups commonly use activities such as having coffee, going on a shopping trip, or doing an art project as a vehicle to motivate members' interaction with each other. In reeducation groups the therapist may act as a teacher. In these groups the therapist assists the patients to learn more adaptive and socially desirable behaviors. An example of a reeducation group is a group in which members learn social behaviors such as dining out.

Problem-solving groups focus on resolving specific problems that a patient may be experiencing. These groups assist the patient in better understanding the problem, suggest possible solutions, and evaluate the results of implementing a solution. These groups may be designed to focus either on one specific problem, such as admission or discharge, or on broader problems, such as those encountered while living in the hospital. The problem-solving technique is the main technique used by the therapist in these groups.

Insight-without-reconstruction groups emphasize interpersonal communication and psychodynamic theoretical frameworks. Group interventions are mainly focused at the conscious and preconscious levels. The group goals are aimed at alleviating emotional stress and effecting change by increasing an individual's cognitive and emotional understanding of his problems. Alternative ways of solving problems and behaving are explored. The interpersonal behaviors that occur among group members are studied and used to enhance the individuals' knowledge about themselves.[21]

Personality reconstruction groups actively use psychoanalytical theory and emphasize understanding unconscious materials. When appropriate, interpersonal concerns among members are worked through. These groups emphasize understanding the impact of former relationships on the present interpersonal concerns and con-

flicts. Dream analysis and free association may be used. Whereas some analysts emphasize the individual in the group, other therapists and analysts also work with the group process. The goals of these groups are for individuals to understand their personality and defensive structure and to modify behavioral patterns and defensive mechanisms.[21]

Theoretical frameworks of group psychotherapy

In leading a psychotherapy group, the therapist should act from a theoretical framework. The theoretical framework that is chosen serves as a guide to assess the group, determine the therapist's behaviors and interventions in the group, and evaluate the effectiveness of the therapeutic techniques employed. The theoretical frameworks of group therapy are mainly derived from various theories in psychiatry, such as psychoanalytical, interpersonal, and behavioral theory, and from social psychology. Differences in theoretical frameworks may range from emphasizing the individual in the group to emphasizing the group as a whole.

To enable the reader to grasp the various types of group psychotherapy theories that can be used, a few theories will be discussed briefly. However, to obtain a working knowledge of group psychotherapy theory, the reader must do further reading.

One theoretical framework that nurse therapists have found useful is Whitaker and Lieberman's Focal Conflict Model.[34] This model is based on the assumption that the therapist's primary interventions are at the group, rather than the individual, level. This theory is based on the principle that therapy groups will develop unconscious conflicts that have meaning to all members. The conflict arises from the group experiencing simultaneously a wish (a disturbing motive) and a fear (a reactive motive). When confronted with such a conflict, the group seeks resolution that may alleviate the fear and/or, at the same time, gratify the wish. The therapist's task is to help the group to understand the conflict and to arrive at a successful solution. Successful solutions will be shared by all members of the group, will reduce reactive fears, and may also partially satisfy the wish.

An example of how this model may be used can be shown through the issue of a therapist's vacation. The disturbing motive or wish is to express anger at the therapist for taking a vacation; the fear or reactive motive is fear of retaliation if anger is expressed. For example, the group may fear the therapist will not return to the group after the vacation. A possible partially successful group solution to the conflict would be for all members to be silent about the therapist's vacation and instead discuss their own past vacations. A successful solution would be for the group to openly discuss their fears and anger regarding the therapist's vacation. The therapist could facilitate the group in arriving at this solution by giving the members permission to express their anger and fears and by demonstrating acceptance when the members discuss these fears.

A communication model is another theoretical framework commonly used by nurses working in groups.[21] This model uses principles of communication theory and therapeutic communication. This model assumes that dysfunctional or ineffective communication in groups may lead to members' dissatisfaction, inadequate feedback, decrease in group cohesion, and further pathological problems. In using this model, the leader's interventions are aimed at facilitating efficient communication of group members. Through successful communication, individual members' problems and the group problems can be identified and solved, and successful feedback channels can be established.

Through the use of communication theory the leader can illustrate that (1) it is impossible for members not to communicate, (2) members must take responsibility for what they communicate, (3) communication is a phenomenon with many levels, such as verbal and nonverbal and overt and covert informational levels, (4) to be effective, a message must be understood by other members of the group, and (5) members can use communication theory to help each other communicate more effectively. An example of the application of communication theory is a therapy group that has the primary goal of helping members improve their social interactional and interpersonal skills. Communication theory is used in helping members to realize how they nonverbally communicate and in assisting them to practice different ways to communicate. One member of the group may learn that because she is always looking down, other members think she is disinterested in them. The group

also learns to acknowledge a member's nonverbal communication (shaking); their concern can motivate her to describe what her shaking means (she feels anxious about being with new people). The leader in this group, when appropriate, briefly explains some principles of communication and illustrates how these principles can be used in the group. The leader uses her interventions to model effective communication and utilizes Yalom's curative factor of imparting information. She also assists in the group in deciding when it is advantageous to analyze a specific message or communication sequence.

The interpersonal theory of interactional group theory is derived from Sullivan and the interpersonal school of psychiatry. In this theory therapists work on both the individual and group level. Group members learn by examining their transactions and feelings among themselves and between themselves and the therapist. Through this process members' disturbed perceptions are corrected and socially effective behaviors are learned. Feelings of anxiety and loneliness are focused on especially. The therapist presents herself as a humanist who is an expert in human relations.[32]

An example of the use of this theory is a women's therapy group in which the primary goal was for the members to improve their interpersonal relationships. When an interpersonal conflict occurred in the group, the leader used this situation to encourage members to discuss their feelings that were aroused by the conflict, to learn what in the conflict made the member or members involved feel anxious or emotionally distressed, and to determine the behaviors the members used to avoid or decrease the anxiety during the expression of the conflict. Through this learning, it was expected that members would be able to correct their previous maladaptive ways of relating and learn more adaptive behaviors.

Psychodrama, which was introduced by Moreno,[24] is another form of group therapy that also requires specialized training. In this model, members are encouraged to act out immediate pressing or past life situations. Members in the group are structured and given temporary assigned roles, such as the audience, stage, protagonist (the patient selected to be the major subject for the specific enactment), auxiliary egos (the therapeutic actors to whom the protagonist is responding or reacting), director, and producer. Psychodrama is a therapeutic intervention based on spontaneity, reality testing, catharsis, and role reversal. Psychodrama allows members to act out specific situations, conflicts, or problems. One example of a situation enacted is a disagreement between a group member and his landlord regarding dissatisfaction with repairs that were made. The patient (protagonist) could play himself, and another member (auxiliary ego) would play the landlord. The group leader would direct the scene. As the script is acted out, the patient would gain further understanding of himself and his behavior during the disagreement. This understanding would also increase when other members (the audience) give feedback to the patient. At another time the roles of the patient and the landlord might be reversed. The role reversal would facilitate the patient's understanding the landlord's predicament and how the patient might communicate more effectively.

In addition to these group theories, there are many other theories that can be employed in group therapy. Specific theories, such as transactional analysis, behavior therapy, and gestalt therapy have gained acceptance in group work. These theories use specific techniques, games, and rules. References about these theories can be found in the annotated suggested readings.

As stated before, many other theories can be used by the group therapist. Some group therapists use an eclectic theoretical approach and technique with groups. What is most important is that the therapist be well versed in the theories and techniques that she uses in group work and that they are chosen appropriately.

Responsibilities of leaders in group psychotherapy

Nurse therapists or leaders in therapy groups must be concerned about many factors regarding the group. Some of these factors are the manner in which the group is working toward achieving its goal or goals; the relationship of the individual members to the group; the anxiety level of individual members; the anxiety level in the group as a whole; the amount of cohesiveness in the group; the process, including communication and behaviors that occur in the group; the boundary maintenance of the group; and the leader's reaction to the group. Thus the group leader must be able to study the group and interact in the group at the same time. The leader is constantly monitoring the group and is, whenever necessary, ready to help the group toward achieving its goals.

To aid in understanding some of the many responsibilities of group therapists, the task of a group therapist will be described fully in the following discussion of the developmental sequence of a therapy group. From this discussion, the reader should not conclude that all therapy groups and all therapists function in the same way. Some groups, by decision or default, do not progress through these developmental stages, and the leaders' techniques and styles vary according to their personalities, beliefs, and their goals for their group. The principles outlined for leadership behavior will be generalized and may usually be used for therapeutic and psychotherapy groups.

Pregroup phase

The first task is to determine if the group will have one therapist or co-therapists or co-leaders. Co-leadership exists when there are two or more designated leaders for the same group. Co-leadership provides an opportunity for peer feedback and growth. Co-leadership facilitates members' work by increasing the possible assessments and areas to be covered in their analysis of the group, and, in some cases, allows for the reenactment of the primary group. If co-therapy is chosen, the nature of the co-therapy relationship must be identified. For example, co-therapists may choose to be equal partners, focus on different areas, or have a junior-senior relationship. Throughout the working relationship, conflicts between the co-therapists must be quickly resolved or usually they will be mirrored or reflected in the group. Co-leaders need to be aware of why they want to work with each other, allow for flexibility, be able to give and receive both positive and negative feedback, and plan sufficient time to become comfortable with each other and their respective leadership styles.

The most important factor to consider in starting a group is its goal or goals. The purpose of the group will greatly influence many of the leadership behaviors in the life of the group. There may be more than one group goal, and, if so, the primary goal should be clearly identified. To guarantee the success of the group, the goals of the group must be clearly understood by all persons involved, including the members and the agencies that sponsor the group. An essential task of the leader in the life of the group is to clarify and assist the group in achieving its purpose.

Once the purpose is established, the leader

GROUP PROPOSAL GUIDELINE

1. List the group goal(s).
   a. Primary goal
   b. Secondary goal
2. List group leader(s) and their related expertise.
3. List theoretical framework(s) utilized by the leader(s) to meet the group goals.
4. List criteria for membership.
5. Describe the referral and screening process.
6. Describe the structure of the group.
   a. Meeting place _____
   b. Meeting time _____
   c. Length of each meeting _____
   d. Number of members _____
   e. Length of group _____
   f. Expected member behaviors _____
   g. Expected leader(s) behaviors _____
7. Describe the evaluation process for members and the group.
8. Describe resources needed for the group, such as coffee, a movie projector, or audiovideo equipment.
9. If pertinent, describe the expected cost and financial benefits incurred from the group.

must be certain that administrative permission is given to have the group. A written group proposal is one effective way to discuss the group with the administration. A guide of what to include in a group proposal is shown above. To avoid possible future problems, the therapist should determine if there are any administrative limitations imposed on her in leading the group. For example, an agency may not want a group to meet beyond its physical facilities or may prefer that the therapist not use certain techniques in the group. Also, any financial cost factors to the agency should be clearly identified.

The leader is also responsible for obtaining the physical space for the group. In choosing a room, the leader should identify the room requirements in relationship to the purpose of the group. For example, in a therapeutic group that has didactic teaching, educational resources such as a blackboard or movie projector or screen may be needed. Likewise, in a psychotherapy group, space may be needed for comfortable chairs to be placed in a circle without a table. In a group that plans to use human relations exercises, a more spacious room will probably be needed. In all cases the room in which the group meets should be comfortable, private, and free from intrusive noises and interruptions. The room selected should remain consistent throughout the duration of the group.

The next step usually undertaken by the group therapist is to select patients or members for the group. The therapist develops selection criteria based on purposes of the group, solicits referrals to the group, and, ordinarily, interviews members to determine their appropriateness for the group. In obtaining individuals to be screened for the group, the therapist and/or the agencies must provide information to selected persons or groups about the group. All information given should clearly identify the purpose of the group, some broad criteria of membership eligibility, and the time, place, and duration of the group. The therapists' names and the appropriate professional credentials should be stated also.

The selection of patients or members of the group is one of the most important tasks of the therapist, because the composition of the group will greatly influence its outcome. In selecting members of the group, the leader should determine which variables will foster group cohesion and therapeutic problem solving. Generally, selection criteria should be based on both heterogeneous and homogeneous patient or member variables. Homogeneous variables will increase attractiveness to the group. Examples of possible homogeneous variables are individual adaptation styles, age, and education levels. Yalom[35] advocates that the therapist use cohesiveness as a primary guide for selection of patients for therapy groups and that heterogeneous factors be chosen from demographic variation. Selection criteria to be considered by the therapist include problem areas, motivation, age, sex, cultural factors, educational level, socioeconomic level, ability to communicate, intelligence, and coping and defensive styles.

If possible, the therapist should choose whether the membership of the group will be closed or open before she screens members for the group. A group is closed if no new members are added once the group is started. In an open group, members leave and new members are added throughout the duration of the group. Open-ended groups may maintain the same purpose, with both members and leaders changing. They usually continue indefinitely and have no termination date for the group as a whole.

The screening interview's primary purpose is for the therapist and patient to determine the appropriateness of the potential member to the group. Many secondary purposes are simultaneously accomplished during the screening interview:

1. To begin to develop a relationship between the therapist and the member
2. To determine the motivation of the possible member
3. To determine if the candidate's goal or goals are in agreement with the group goals
4. To educate the candidate about the nature of the group
5. To determine the kind of group experience the individual has had
6. If appropriate, to begin to review the group contract

In addition to or replacing the screening interview, some clinicians use a group intake. A group intake is when several new members meet in a group for one to three sessions to learn about the group psychotherapy process and identify some possible treatment goals. This approach is less costly and has the same objectives as the screening interview.

As soon as possible a decision should be made about group membership. If a person is not selected for a group, other possible treatment should be made available to him, and he should be told the reasons for not being selected. If it is appropriate, the referring person should also be given these reasons.

Initial phase

The initial phase is comprised of those meetings in a new group in which the group's members begin to "settle down" to work. This phase is characterized by anxiety regarding inclusion, the setting of norms, and the casting of various roles. Curative factors such as catharsis and universality begin to operate in this phase but become more influential in other phases. This phase has been subdivided into three stages by Yalom[35]: the orientation, conflict, and cohesive stages. The stages correspond to Tuckman's first three stages of group development.

ORIENTATION STAGE. During the first stage of this phase the therapist is more directive and active than in other stages. Two tasks of the therapist in this stage are to orient the group to its primary task and to assist the group in arriving at a group contract. Some common factors that therapists may include in the group con-

tract are goals of the group, confidentiality, meeting times, honesty, structure of the group, and communication rules (e.g., only one person may talk at a time). Since an important part of this phase is norm setting, the therapist should actively see that the norms set by the group will facilitate the group's achieving its primary and secondary tasks. Another task of the therapist in this stage is to foster attractiveness or cohesion among the members. In fulfilling this task, the therapist encourages interaction among members and maintains the group at a working level of anxiety. For example, the therapist could state that the group is "our" group and can suggest how group members help each other. One method would encourage members to state their expectations of what they hope to learn from the group. The therapist would then reinforce the expectations that are realistic for the group to accomplish and give examples of how the group might meet these expectations.

During the first stage the members are evaluating each other, the group, and the therapist. In this evaluation process they are deciding if they are going to be in or out of the group and are determining what their level of participation in the group will be. Some common conscious or unconscious fears or concerns of members during this stage are the fear of being rejected, fear of self-disclosure, and fear of not being seen as an individual. Social amenities are important, and the members are searching and attempting to develop their social roles. The roles members assume during this stage are often renegotiated during other stages. The group, at this time, is a dependent one and frequently members will test out their dependency needs and wishes on the leader. Members look to the leader for structure, approval, and acceptance, and they may try to please the leader with reward-seeking behaviors. The leader, in not gratifying all the dependency wishes of the members and by encouraging members to interact more with one another, supports group members in becoming more interdependent on each other and less dependent on the leader. The dependency issue between the leader and the members may lead the group into conflict and thus into the second stage.

CONFLICT STAGE. This stage of the group corresponds to Tuckman's storming stage of group development. Issues related to control, power, and authority become of prime importance.

Members are concerned about the "pecking order" or determination of who is "top or bottom" in regard to issues related to control and decision making.[30] The dependency conflict may be openly or covertly expressed, with members being polarized between independent and dependent issues. Bennis and Sheppard[5] describe this stage as being a struggle between the counterdependent and dependent members, with the counterdependent members waiting to assume the leader's role. An example of this phase would be a group that was divided over the issue of whether they could telephone each other. Some members wanted the leader to give them the correct answer, whereas others thought that the leader's statements were irrelevant and not helpful. During this phase the counterdependent members might sit in the leader's chair and let the leader know her directions have been unsuccessful or unheard. The dependent members could ask the leader for more directions. Other members who are neutral (neither dependent nor counterdependent) eventually may assist the group in resolving this conflict.

Subgroups usually form within the group and hostility is expressed. Often the hostility is directed toward the leader, but it may also be expressed toward other members. The therapist's tasks are to allow for the expression of both negative and positive feelings, to help the group to understand the underlying conflict, and to prevent and/or examine nonproductive behaviors such as scapegoating. This phase is usually the most difficult for the new therapist, because some members in the group may lead the therapist to believe she has failed the group by not living up to its unrealistic expectations. Yalom[35] described some reasons that commonly lead certain members to express resentment toward the leader: the member's awareness of the therapist's limitations, the therapist not fulfilling a "traditional leader" role, and awareness that the therapist will not give each member a favorite standing.

The therapist must be careful not to avoid or suppress the group member's anxiety and, at times, should encourage the group to express its hostility. If hostility toward the therapist is expressed indirectly, such as anger toward other authority figures (staff members, teachers, parents), the therapist should assist the group in expressing its anger more directly. A useful technique is for the therapist to give the group permission to discuss its anger, which she may do by expressing the possibility to the group that it may be disappointed or angry at the leader.

By the end of this stage the therapist may be dethroned and her omnipotent role with its magical solutions may be discarded. Slowly the therapist becomes humanized. Members learn that responsibilities for the group are shared and are not only invested in the leader. Members may also learn that expressions of anger and disappointment do not destroy the leader and may assist the group to more accurately assess its resources and limitations. The resources of the group can then be used to facilitate the group in achieving its primary and secondary tasks. Members of the group may realize that conflicts need not be avoided and, instead, through discussion, may serve to increase the group's maturity and usefulness.

COHESIVE STAGE. Tuckman's norming phase is closely related to this stage. Group members, after resolving the conflicts in the second stage, feel a strong attractiveness toward one another and a high attachment to the group. Expressions of positive feelings toward one another and toward the group are frequently verbalized and expressions of negative feelings are usually suppressed.

Members of the group feel free to give self-disclosing information and share more intimate concerns with one another. However, the group's problem-solving ability is restricted in that negative feedback and communication is usually avoided in order not to decrease the high group morale. The therapist's task is to facilitate the group in further exploring the members' disclosures in relationship to the primary task of the group. The therapist while not hindering the basic cohesiveness of the group, should encourage the group to eventually use its problem-solving ability. Through this behavior, the therapist role models how a group member can have individual concerns and values and still be a productive member of the group. In other words, the therapist demonstrates that differing and opposite opinions may not destroy the group identity.

At the resolution of this stage, members may learn that self-discoveries and differences should not be feared. They also learn that similarities and differences between the group members may help the group to achieve its tasks. At the end of this stage, task achievement is begun to be seen by the group as a reality. The group loses its false sense of happiness and hope and gains an ability to work together creatively around its primary and secondary tasks.

Working phase of the group

The working phase of a group can be compared with Tuckman's performing stage of group development. During this stage the group becomes a team. It directs its energy mainly toward completion of its tasks. Although they are hard at work, this phase is an enjoyable one for both the leader and members. Responsibility for the group is more equally shared, anxiety is usually decreased and is tolerated better than in the previous phases, and the group is more stable and realistic.

In a psychotherapy group, members begin seriously to work through their concerns related to their therapeutic goals, which were identified during the pregroup and initial phases. They begin to do a more in-depth exploration of the various goals related to the tasks of their group. For example, in a psychotherapeutic group for mothers with chronically ill children, the members may discuss their various reactions to the children, their ambivalent feelings, some of their thoughts regarding the reason for their feelings, and various alternative ways to cope with their present daily realities.

The major role of the leader is to facilitate the group's completing its task or tasks. This is accomplished by maximizing the group's effective use of its curative properties. Because the group members are fully participating in the work of the group, the therapist's activity level decreases in this phase. The leader now acts more like a consultant to the group. The leader helps to keep the group on its proper course and, if possible, tries to decrease the impact of any factors that may regress or retard the group.

Because this phase is mainly characterized as the group's creative problem-solving and resolution phase, there are few, if any, specific guidelines for the leader. The leader's interventions are mainly based on her theoretical frameworks, experiences, personality, intuition, and needs of the group and its members. In addition to monitoring the group's maintenance function through fostering group cohesion, maintaining its boundaries, and encouraging the group to work on the group tasks, the leader's interventions may be directed toward helping the group solve specific problems. Because these problems are unique to the group, many of them are not universally predictable. Some of the more common problems have been identified by Yalom[35]:

the formation of subgroups, the management of conflict, and determination of the optimal level of self-disclosure.

Subgroups that conflict with the goals of the group and are not acknowledged by the group are restrictive to its work. Other members of the group may feel excluded, and loyalties will be divided between the subgroup and the group as a whole. For example, in a women's group, two of the members become close friends. They keep secrets from the group and engage in many private conversations during the group session. Other members feel excluded from this dyad and ineffective in working with them. To decrease the negative impact of a subgroup, the consequences and reactions of the subgroup should be openly discussed by the group.

Conflict is unavoidable and can be used to foster group and individual growth. However, at some time the expressions of conflict need to be controlled so that their intensity does not exceed the group's tolerance. Examples of conflict are competition among members for the leader's attention and a disagreement between two members of a group. Some ways a leader may manage conflicts are acknowledgment that the conflict does exist, expression of the value that conflicts are natural occurrences and can be growth producing, encouragement of members to discuss the reasons behind the conflict, and thorough discussion by members giving feedback to each other. The tolerance for successful conflict resolution is related to the amount of group cohesiveness, trust, and acceptance felt by the members.

The amount of self-disclosure is usually related to the amount of acceptance and trust the discloser feels. Self-disclosure is always a risk-taking activity. If a person gives pertinent or private information too quickly, he will feel vulnerable and perhaps untrusted. Likewise, during the working phase if a person discloses too little, he may be ineffective in forming interpersonal relationships; thus his growth potential in the group may be decreased.

Resistance, or the forestalling of the therapeutic process, is one form of behavior that can be expected in therapy groups. Resistance to working on the therapeutic goal can occur at both an individual and group level. For both the individual and group, it is one matter to agree on the therapeutic goals and another to work on obtaining the actual therapeutic outcomes. Resistance by individual members may take many forms, such as avoiding discussion of a conflict area, frequent or prolonged silences, attempting to become an assistant therapist, absence of members, pairing between two members, and prolonged expression of hostility. Resistance by the group or a majority of group members also takes on many forms, some of which are similar to the previously mentioned ones. Other examples of group resistance include shared silence among the members, unusual amounts of dependency toward the leader, an unusual amount of hostility in the group, scapegoating, subgroup formations, and the wish for magical solutions to resolve the group conflict. Resistance can be perceived as occurring because of individuals' or group's increased anxiety, which is experienced around conflict or change. The management of resistance depends on the type of psychotherapy group, the group contract, and the therapist's theoretical framework. Some ways resistance can be decreased by the therapist are to make observations regarding the group process and/or individual behaviors, offer interpretations, counteract the resistant behavior, and demonstrate more adaptive behavioral patterns.

By the end of the second phase, members have learned that they, at least partially, have achieved their goals and hopefully have a sense of their own productiveness and accomplishments. The need for the group or their involvement in the group has become less apparent. The group or members of the group must begin to deal more actively with its final task—that of separation.

Termination phase

The work of termination begins during the first phase of every group. However, as the group or members of the group approach termination, certain processes are more likely to occur. The termination phase is not always discussed as a definite phase in the literature on groups. However, it is discussed as a separate phase here because of the significance that termination may have for the members.

There are two types of termination: termination of the group as a whole and termination of individual members of a group. A closed group usually terminates as an entire group; in an open group, members (and perhaps the therapist) terminate separately. Members and groups may terminate prematurely, unsuccessfully, and successfully.

Termination is a highly individualized process. Individuals and groups will terminate in ways that are unique to themselves. Since termination is inevitably a painful process, it often is denied. Termination may often cause the group to experience increased anxiety, regression, and/or a feeling of accomplishment. To permit members to avoid this subject would be the same as preventing individuals from having a possible successful growth experience. Useful or common behaviors used by therapists are to encourage an evaluation of the group or its terminating members, reminisce about important events that occurred in the history of the group, and encourage members to give feedback to each other. An evaluation usually is restricted to the achievement or lack of achievement of the group's or the individual's goals. The therapist must be careful not to collude with members in denying termination; rather, the leader must encourage termination to be fully discussed. Termination may lead to the discussion of many related topics such as other separations, death, aging, and the use and passage of time. Members, if terminated successfully, may eventually feel a sense of resolution about the group experience and may use their experiences obtained in the group in many of their other encounters in life.

Evaluation of the group

Evaluation of the group and the progress of individual members in the group is an ongoing process that begins in the selection interview of possible group members. Most clinicians use record-keeping mechanisms as a way to remember the critical events in the group. These records can later be used to evaluate the group from a descriptive point of view. To make record keeping easy it is usually helpful to have a "group notebook." In this notebook leaders can write pertinent data on individual members, such as their group goals, their telephone number(s), their addresses, the screening note, any individual comments, and a termination summary note. In another section of the group notebook, the leaders can describe each group meeting. One suggested format on how to quickly record each group meeting is given on the facing page.

In addition to these measures, it is sometimes helpful to determine each individual member's goal attainment. This can be done using subjec-

```
┌─────────────────────────────────────┐
│                                     │
│      GROUP SESSION NOTE OUTLINE     │
│                                     │
│   ███████████████████████████       │
│                                     │
│   Date _____ Group meeting No. __│
│   1. Membership:                    │
│      a. List members attending (state if new │
│         member).                    │
│      b. List members who were late. │
│      c. List absent members.        │
│   2. List individual members' pertinent issues │
│      or behaviors discussed in the group. │
│   3. List group themes.             │
│   4. Identify important group process issues │
│      (such as developmental stage, roles, │
│      norms).                        │
│   5. Identify any critical leadership strategy │
│      used.                          │
│   6. List proposed future leadership strate- │
│      gies.                          │
│   7. Predict member and group responses for │
│      the next session.              │
│                                     │
└─────────────────────────────────────┘
```

tive ratings by the group leaders, or obtaining an individual member's perceptions on how they are meeting their goals. A slightly more objective evaluation is to write the members' goals down and ask them to rate their goal achievement on a Likert scale. The evaluation of members' goal achievement should always be done at termination, and, depending on the nature and length of the group, it may be done on a regular interview basis.

In addition to the descriptive evaluation, the clinician may decide to administer a before and after group paper and pencil test(s). The test(s) selected should be congruent with the expected changes in the group. For example, an anxiety scale could be administered to members attending a group whose major goal is to reduce anxiety. If this type of evaluation is used, it is critical that the clinician use the most appropriate scale available and that the agency and the patients' permissions are obtained. It is paramount that all parties involved know the intent of using such test(s).

Future role of nurses in group work

In the last decade nurses have increasingly become aware of the therapeutic potential of groups and have begun to incorporate group work in their practice. Yet, if literature is an accurate reflection of the past, nurses have not yet fully incorporated group work in their practice. As observed by Nakagawa,[25] in the early 1970s nurses began to agree that nurses with advanced preparation did group therapy. Nurses mainly focused on the neglected or chronically mentally ill patient in the early 1970s. Examples of patient populations in which nurses practice as group therapists are geriatric patients, chronically schizophrenic patients, and chronically hospitalized patients. However, by the late 1970s nurses began to write about their group work with different populations, including crisis groups, groups for the acutely ill patient, and family groups. As reflected in the literature, nurses, like other health professionals, have recently placed more expectations on themselves in describing and evaluating their clinical work in groups.

Psychiatric nurses have been slow to view themselves as group psychotherapists. As compared to their role as individual and family therapists, their ability to work in insight-oriented group psychotherapy has only begun to be adequately illustrated in the literature. As nurses and other professionals increase their understanding of the usefulness and effectiveness of group work, they become more accurate in documenting their skills and techniques and in evaluating the treatment outcome. Only then can concepts that are systematically applicable to nursing practice in groups be taught and studied.

It is expected that pressures for nurses to work with more groups will come from within and without the nursing profession. The increasing cost of health care, the amount of stress in our society, the awareness of the benefits of primary prevention, and the increased awareness of the effectiveness of groups are all bound to increase nurses' incentives to work with groups of patients or clients. As a critical mass of nurses gain more experience in group work, they are also bound to influence the profession internally. Within the next decade it is hoped and expected that nurses will describe their work with groups in a wider population and will scientifically document these skills and the resulting client or patient outcome behaviors.

Exclusive of psychotherapy, there are several exciting areas of group work for nurses. The first area is in their work with informal groups. Nurses in acute health care settings have first-hand knowledge of patients' daily experiences and can easily interact with those patients in informal settings. Nurses have not yet fully realized the possibilities for nursing assessments and interventions in informal groups. Once nursing intervention in informal groups is understood, these interventions will need to be studied in relationship to outcome. The second area in which nurses should expand their group practice is with therapeutic groups. Nurses may make a special contribution in therapeutic groups that focus on coping with illness and on situational or developmental crises. These groups especially seem to use the expertise of nurses. A third area in which nurses can utilize their group skills is within their work group. Working with other nurses, as well as other professionals, often requires that the nurses be comfortable in group situations and can utilize the group process to assist the group in accomplishing its task. Without knowledge of group process issues, the nurse may be more likely to avoid identifying some helpful or destructive group behaviors. How nurses behave in groups of health team members is a question that warrants further study.

In the 1970s nurses had just begun to use group skills in their practice. It is expected that work with groups will expand nurses' effectiveness in at least the cognitive, psychological, and sociological aspects of their practice. Working with groups, similar to working in a one-to-one nurse-patient relationship, will become an essential part of the science and art of nursing practice.

Suggested cross-references

Working with groups in promoting mental health is discussed in Chapter 5.

SUMMARY

1. Groups are a specific social system that can be defined and studied. A group consists of individuals who are interrelated and interdependent and who may share common purposes and norms.

2. All groups have two functions: a task and a maintenance function.

3. Some common dimensions that are often used to evaluate a group's progress are communication processes, membership roles, norms, power structure, cohesion, and stages of group development.

4. There are identifiable curative or therapeutic factors that may occur in groups.

5. Nurses can use informal groups to enhance their assessments and to provide a therapeutic experience for the group's members.

6. The leading of therapeutic groups, which prevents or decreases emotional disturbances or stress, should be viewed as being in the realm of nursing practice.

7. Group psychotherapy is a useful and beneficial treatment modality for alleviating emotional disturbances.

8. There is a wide range of models of group psychotherapy from supportive therapy to personality reconstruction.

9. Specific theoretical frameworks should be used by group therapists. Theoretical models can be used to assist therapists to assess the group, intervene in the group, and evaluate the effectiveness of their interventions.

10. A group psychotherapist has specific responsibilities in leading the group. Some of these responsibilities may be studied in relationship to the phases of group development.

   a. During the pregroup phase, therapists determine the purpose of the group, arrange for a place for the group to meet, determine criteria for membership, and select group members.

   b. In the orientation stage, therapists facilitate the group's arriving at a group contract, orient the group to its task, and promote group cohesion.

   c. In the conflict stage, therapists may encourage members to express their disillusionment and hostility and maintain the group's activity within a working level.

   d. During the cohesive stage, therapists assist the group to improve its problem-solving ability by helping the group to use negative feedback and disagreement.

   e. In the working stage, therapists facilitate the group's accomplishing its tasks by acting as a resource person to the group, assisting the group in handling problems such as subgroup formation, and managing conflict and resistance.

   f. In the termination stage, therapists assist the members in evaluating what they have learned and in separating from each other.

11. Nurses need to do more clinical research in their work with groups; specifically, their intervention techniques need to be documented more scientifically and related to outcome.

References

1. American Nurses' Association: Statement on psychiatric and mental health nursing practice, Kansas City, Mo., 1976, The Association.
2. Armacost, B., Turner, E., Martin, M. et al.: A group of "problem" patients and a staff of nurses at the other end of their tether, Am. J. Nurs. **74:**289, 1974.
3. Bales, R., and Slater, P.: Role differentiation in small decision-making groups. In Parsons, T., and Bales, R.F.: Family socialization and interactional process, Glencoe, Ill., 1955, Free Press.
4. Benne, K.D., and Sheats, P.: Functional roles and group members, J. Soc. Issues **4**(2):41, 1948.
5. Bennis, W., and Sheppard, H.: A theory of group development, Hum. Rel. **9:**415, 1956.
6. Bilodeau, C.B., and Kackett, R.P.: Issues raised in a group setting by patients recovering from myocardial infarction, Am. J. Psychiatry **128:**73, July 1971.
7. Burke, C.: Working with parents of children with hemophilia, Nurs. Clin. North Am. **7:**787, 1972.
8. Cartwright, D., and Zander, A., editors: Group dynamic research and theory, ed. 3, New York, 1968, Harper & Row, Publishers, Inc.
9. Chatham, M.A.: The effect of family involvement on patients' manifestations of postcardiotomy psychosis, Heart Lung **71:**995, 1978.
10. Cohen, R.: ECT + group therapy = improved care, Am. J. Nurs. **7:**1195, 1971.
11. D'Afflitti, J.G., and Swanson, D.: Group sessions for the wives of home-hemodialysis patients, Am. J. Nurs. **75:**633, 1975.
12. DeMocker, J., and Zimpfer, D.G.: Group approaches to psychosocial intervention in medical care: a synthesis, Int. J. Group Psychother. **31:**247, 1981.
13. Dolgoff, T.: Small groups and organizations: time, task and sentient boundaries, Gen. Systems **20:**135, 1975.
14. Eisenberg, A.: The effects of working with husbands on adjustment of mastectomy patients, master's thesis, University of Rochester School of Nursing, Rochester, N.Y., 1976.
15. Ferguson, B.: A parents group, J. Psychiatr. Nurs. **17:**24, 1979.
16. Gardner, K.: Patient groups in a therapeutic community, Am. J. Nurs. **71:**528, 1971.
17. Gardner, M.E.: Notes from a waiting room, Am. J. Nurs. **80:**86, Jan. 1980.
18. Lewin, K.: Group decision and social change. In Newcomb, T.M., and Hartley, B.L., editors: Readings in social psychology, New York, 1947, Holt, Rinehart & Winston, Inc.
19. Lieberman, M.A., Yalom, I., and Miles, M.: Encounter groups: first facts, New York, 1972, Basic Books, Inc.
20. Long, L.D., and Cope, C.S.: Curative factors in a male felony offender group, Small Group Behavior, **2:**889, 1980.
21. Marram, G.: The group approach in nursing practice, ed. 2, St. Louis, 1978, The C.V. Mosby Co.
22. Martin, E., and Hill, W.: Towards a theory of group development: six phases of therapy group development, Int. J. Group Psychother. **7:**20, 1957.
23. Miller, E.J., and Rice, A.K.: Selections from systems of organization. In Colman, A., and Bexton, W.: Group relations reader, Sausalito, Calif., 1975, GREX Publishing.
24. Moreno, J.L.: Psychodrama and group psychotherapy, Sociometry **9:**249, 1941.
25. Nakagawa, H.: The state of the art of psychiatric nursing: the theory and practice of group work, presented at the State of the Art in Psychiatric Nursing Conference, Rutgers—The State University, New Brunswick, N.J., April 8-9, 1974.
26. Olmsted, M.: The small group, New York, 1959, Random House, Inc.
27. Parloff, M., and Dies, R.: Group therapy outcome research, 1966-1975, Int. J. Group Psychother. **23:**281, 1977.
28. Runkel, P., Lawrence, M., Oldfield, S., Rider, M., and Clark, C.: Stages of group development: an empirical test of Tuckman's hypothesis, J. Appl. Behav. Sci. **7:**180, 1971.
29. Satir, V.: Conjoint family therapy, rev. ed., Palo Alto, Calif., 1967, Science & Behavior Books.
30. Schutz, W.: Interpersonal underworld, Harvard Bus. Rev. **36:**123, July-Aug. 1958.
31. Smith, A.: A manual for the training of psychiatric nursing personnel in group psychotherapy, Perspect. Psychiatr. Care **8**(3):106, 1970.
32. Spotnitz, H.: Comparisons of different types of group psychotherapy. In Kaplan, H., and Sadock, B., editors: Comprehensive group psychotherapy, Baltimore, 1971, The Williams & Wilkins Co.
33. Tuckman, B.: Developmental sequence in small groups, Psychol. Bull. **63:**384, 1965.
34. Whitaker, D., and Lieberman, M.: Psychotherapy through the group process, Chicago, 1964, Aldine Publishing Co.
35. Yalom, I.: The theory and practice of group psychotherapy, ed. 2, New York, 1975, Basic Books, Inc.

Annotated suggested readings

Group dynamics

Bennis, W., and Shepherd, H.: A theory of group development, Hum. Rel. **9:**415, 1956.

This book reveals an often quoted and useful theory of group development. The theory is derived from the authors' observations of sensitivity groups; the theory is based on psychoanalytical theory. Some readers may find this article a little difficult to read.

Bion, W.R.: Experiences in groups, New York, 1959, Basic Books, Inc.

This book describes the basic premises in the Tavistock theory of groups. It is a somewhat difficult but very rewarding book to read.

Cartwright, D., and Zander, A., editors: Group dynamic research and theory, ed. 3, New York, 1968, Harper & Row, Publishers, Inc.

This book is an excellent summary and classic collection of research studies on group dynamics. The theoretical presentation and its clinical implications are especially useful to the clinician.

Colman, A., and Bexton, W.: EOS group relations reader, Sausalito, Calif., 1975, GREX Publishing.

This text is intended for the advanced student and has an excellent collection of papers representing the group relations model. It contains articles that discuss Tavistock theory and its application to clinical, educational, or organizational and architectural problems.

Luft, J.: Group processes: an introduction to group dynamics, ed. 2, Palo Alto, Calif., 1970, National Press Books.

This is a quick-reading introductory book to the study of groups. It is especially useful in applying communication theories to the group or small group.

Mills, T.: The sociology of small groups, Englewood Cliffs, N.J., 1967, Prentice-Hall, Inc.

This is a useful text on small groups for students who previously have had some introduction to this literature. The author describes groups within a sociological framework and shows the reader how to systematically observe a group.

Olmsted, M.: The small group, New York, 1959, Random House, Inc.

This is a good classic introductory book for the study of small groups. It summarizes many theories of small groups that were derived from sociology and psychology.

Shaw, M.: Group dynamics: the psychology of small group behavior, New York, 1971, McGraw-Hill Book Co.

This book examines small group process in relationship to processes of social interactions. It reviews many relevant theories and research studies in the group dynamics area.

Tuckman, B.: Developmental sequence in small groups, Psychol. Bull. **63:**384, 1965.

This is an excellent article that summarizes many theories of group development. It may be necessary to read the article several times to obtain the full benefit of the author's work.

Group therapies

Adrian, S.: A systematic approach to selecting group participants, J. Psychiatr. Nurs. **18**(2):37, 1980.

This article explores how to assess candidates for group participation by utilizing inclusion and exclusion criteria offered by the literature. An assessment format is presented and illustrated by clinical examples.

Armstrong, S.W., and Rouslin, S.: Group psychotherapy in nursing practice, New York, 1963, The Macmillan Co., Publishers.

This is one of the first books written to introduce group therapy to nurses. The authors forcibly state the importance of group work to psychiatric nursing practice. It was designed to be an introductory textbook on group psychotherapy. A person who is interested in the historical development of group work in psychiatric nursing would find this book to be a rich resource.

Aronson, M.: Resistance in individual and group psychotherapy, Am. J. Psychother. **21:**86, 1967.

The author defines resistance and describes some of its manifestations in individual and group therapy.

Authier, J. et al.: Group interventional techniques: a practice guide for psychiatric team members, J. Psychiatr. Nurs. **14**(7):19, 1976.

This article is a basic practical guide on how to intervene in groups. It was written for staff members employed in psychiatric units.

Baier, M.: Group therapy with parolees in a community mental health center, J. Psychosoc. Nurs. **20:**26, Feb. 1982.

This is a good example of a creative use of group intervention by a nurse. The author describes a short-term group that she established for recently paroled offenders. She characterizes the group as a modified self-help group.

Balgopal, P.: Variations in sensitivity training groups, Perspect. Psychiatr. Care **11**(2):80, 1973.

This article reviews various theoretical orientations of training groups in relationship to group goals, leadership roles, group composition, location and duration of group, and group process and content.

Berne, E.: Group treatment, New York, 1966, Grove Press, Inc.

This book is divided into two sections. The first gives a broad and practical guide for group treatment and the second describes transactional analysis and its application.

Borriello, J.: Leadership in the therapist-centered group as a whole psychotherapy approach, Int. J. Group Psychother. **26:**149, 1976.

This is an excellent article for the advanced student. The article describes a model of leadership that is based on practice and incorporates the therapist-centered group as a whole approach. Bion's and Ezriel's theories of group dynamics are briefly described and compared.

Burton, A., editor: Encounter: the theory and practice of encounter groups, San Francisco, 1969, Jossey-Bass, Inc.

This collection of chapters discusses various methods, approaches, and theories of encounter groups.

Dinnauer, L., Miller, M., and Frankforter, M.: Implementation strategies for an inpatient women's support group, J. Psychosoc. Nur. **19**(8):13, 1981.

This article describes how three nurses implemented an inpatient women's group, including group objectives, supervision, organizational endorsement, educational materials, and evaluation.

Fidler, J.: The relationship of group psychotherapy to therapeutic group approaches, Int. J. Group Psychother. **20:**473, 1970.

This is a thoughtful description and discussion of the differences between psychotherapeutic and therapeutic groups for patients. Group psychotherapy is differentiated from other therapeutics in the psychotherapist's diagnosis, plan, and treatments.

Fochtman, G.: Therapeutic factors of the informal group, Am. J. Nurs. **76:**238, 1976.

This short article illustrates, with clinical examples, how nurses can therapeutically intervene in informal patient groups.

Gardner, K.: Patient groups in a therapeutic community, Am. J. Nurs. **71:**528, 1971.

This is an article describing various types of informal groups in the therapeutic milieu of an inpatient setting.

Getty, C., and Shannon, H.: Nurses as co-therapists in a family setting, Perspect. Psychiatr. Care **5:**36, Jan.-Feb. 1967.

The authors describe factors that are inherent in an egalitarian model of a co-therapy relationship. Examples are used to illustrate this model.

Goldberg, C., and Goldberg, M.D.: The human circle: an existential approach to the new group therapist, Chicago, 1973, Nelson-Hall Co.

This book describes an existential analytical approach to group therapy as well as some specific group techniques. Some of the issues the authors discuss are nonverbal communication, confrontation, the therapist-patient relationship, problem solving, leadership, and group processes.

Goldberg, C., and Stanitis, M.A.: The enhancement of self-esteem through the communication process in group therapy, J. Psychiatr. Nurs. **16**(12):5, 1977.

The authors describe their interventions used in a therapy group. Communication theory is used to explain the formation of self-esteem and the leader's therapeutic techniques. This article is easy to read and is a good example of how a group therapist can apply specific theory to assess, lead, and evaluate a group.

Hager, R.: Evaluation of group psychotherapy—a question of values, J. Psychiatr. Nurs. **16**(12):26, 1978.

The focus of this paper is on the evaluation that takes place during the course of group psychotherapy rather than afterwards. The role of evaluator and criteria for evaluation are discussed.

Kadis, A. et al.: Practicum of group psychotherapy, ed. 2, New York, 1974, Harper & Row, Publishers, Inc.

This basic book on group psychotherapy is based on psychodynamic principles. The authors briefly describe basic and complex aspects of group therapy in a lucid manner. Theoretical discussion is limited, and there is an emphasis on the practical aspect of group therapy.

Kanter, S.: The therapist's leadership in psychoanalytically oriented group psychotherapy, Int. J. Group Psychother. **26**:139, 1976.

This is an excellent discussion for the advanced student of the therapist's leadership functions in a psychoanalytically oriented group psychotherapy. Leadership functions are discussed according to three phases of the group: initial, working, and termination.

Kaplan, H., and Sadock, B., editors: Comprehensive group psychotherapy, Baltimore, 1971, The Williams & Wilkins Co.

This book should be on the "must" reading list of any group therapist. It covers a wide range of issues and techniques related to group therapy. It also discusses the theories and hypotheses on which these techniques are based. The text is organized into four major parts: basic principles of group psychotherapy, specialized group therapy techniques, psychotherapy with groups in special categories, and training and research.

Krumboltz, J., and Potter, B.: Behavioral techniques for developing trust, cohesion and goal accomplishment, Ed. Technol. **13**:26, 1973.

This article describes leadership behaviors that facilitate group members' developing trust and cohesion and accomplishing their goals. An excellent article for any beginner in group work.

Latner, J.: The Gestalt therapy book, New York, 1972, The Julian Press, Inc.

The author describes the theory and application of gestalt therapy. This readable book is a good introduction to gestalt therapy. The author briefly discusses the various settings, including workshops and groups, in which gestalt therapy has been used.

Lieberman, M., Yalom, I., and Miles, M.: Encounter groups: first facts, New York, 1972, Basic Books, Inc.

This is a comprehensive study of leadership behaviors, the individual's relationship to the group, and group conditions and properties of training groups.

Loomis, M.: Group process for nurses, St. Louis, 1979, The C.V. Mosby Co.

A basic book on small group dynamics that is written to assist a nurse leading or participating in a group.

Loomis, M., and Dodenhoff, J.: Working with informal patient groups, Am. J. Nurs. **70**:1939, 1970.

A theoretical framework using group dynamics is described to aid in the understanding of informal groups and their formation.

Marram, G.: The group approach in nursing practice, ed. 2, St. Louis, 1978, The C.V. Mosby Co.

This is an excellent review of group work for nurses. Included in this book are discussions on types of group therapy, theoretical concepts of groups, and many illustrations of the application of group work to nursing practice.

Mullan, H., and Rosenbaum, M.: Group psychotherapy: theory and practice, New York, 1962, The Free Press.

A practical approach to group psychotherapy is discussed in a group psychoanalytical psychotherapy framework. The authors discuss practical details in regard to administration, organization, and therapeutic technique.

Msyzka, M.A., and Josefiak, D.: Development of the co-therapy relationship, J. Psychiatr. Nurs. **11**:27, May-June 1973.

Two co-therapists discuss the correlations between their cotherapy communication system and the group communication system. The development of the co-therapy relationship is described.

Nakagawa, H.: The state of the art of psychiatric nursing: the theory and practice of group work, presented at the State of the Art in Psychiatric Nursing Conference, Rutgers—The State University, New Brunswick, N.J., April 8-9, 1974.

This manuscript consists of a summary of the literature on groups in nursing until 1973.

Rogers, C.: On encounter groups, New York, 1970, Harper & Row, Publishers, Inc.

Carl Rogers' perceptions, beliefs, and techniques in encounter groups are discussed in this book.

Sager, C., and Kaplan, H.: Progress in group and family therapy, New York, 1972, Brunner/Mazel, Inc.

This book is equally divided between articles on group therapy, family therapy, and specific patient populations. The group therapy sections review psychoanalytical group theory approaches and some newer specific techniques and approaches in group therapy, such as the use of television and assertive groups.

Sampson, M., and Marthas, M.: Group process for the health professional, New York, 1977, John Wiley & Sons, Inc.

This is an introductory textbook that is aimed at acquainting the reader with major theories of group process. An excellent book for undergraduates who are beginning to use study groups and want to learn how to work effectively in them.

Scheidlinger, S., editor: Psychoanalytic group dynamics: basic readings, New York, 1980, International University Press.

This book contains a collection of articles on group dynamics that aids in understanding group behavior. All of the articles share an underlying assumption of psychoanalytic thought.

Slavson, S.R.: The fields of group psychotherapy, New York, 1956, International University Press, Inc.

This is a classic book on group psychotherapy that discusses specific therapy groups and specific settings.

Slimner, L.: Use of the nursing process to facilitate group therapy, J. Psychiatr. Nurs. **16**(2):42, 1978.

The author describes and illustrates three group theoretical models: the focal conflict model, the communication model, and the group dynamics model. Examples of these models are given to demonstrate how they can be used as group assessment guides.

Swanson, M.: A check list for group leaders, Perspect. Psychiatr. Care **7**(3):120, 1969.

This is a basic guide written to aid the nurse to self-assess her work in groups.

Werner, J.: Relating group therapy to nursing practice, Perspect. Psychiatr. Care **8**(6):248, 1970.

This article summarizes focal conflict theory and some principles of group dynamics and gives case illustrations on how to apply the selected principles and theory to nursing clinical practice.

Whitaker, D., and Lieberman, M.: Psychotherapy through the group process, Chicago, 1964, Aldine Publishing Co.

This book is easy to read and describes a specific theoretical model (the focal conflict model) for group therapy. Case examples are used throughout the book to illustrate the theory.

White, E.M., and Kahn, E.M.: Use and modifications in group psychotherapy with chronic schizophrenic outpatients, J. Psychosoc. Nurs. **20**:14, Feb. 1982.

The authors have analyzed their experiences as leaders of psychotherapy groups with chronic schizophrenic patients. They are advocates for the helpfulness of group approaches to these patients. Specific suggestions are made for the modification of group intervention techniques to meet the needs of chronic schizophrenic patients. This article should be very helpful to nurses who work in outpatient settings serving deinstitutionalized populations.

Williams, R.: A contract for co-therapists in group psychotherapy, J. Psychiatr. Nurs. **14**:11, June 1976.

This article discusses ten basic points that should be a part of a contract for co-therapists who are working with groups.

Witt, J.: Transference and countertransference in group therapy settings, J. Psychosoc. Nurs. **20**:31, Feb. 1982.

This article provides a good overview of the application of psychoanalytical concepts of transference and countertransference to group interaction. The illustrative clinical example should be of particular interest to beginning group leaders.

Yalom, I.: The theory and practice of group psychotherapy, ed. 2, New York, 1975, Basic Books, Inc.

This is an excellent book on group therapy that is extremely useful for both the new and experienced therapist. The author cites relevant research and uses many clinical examples to illustrate his ideas.

FAMILY THERAPY

Patricia E. Helm

We are truly heirs of all the ages;
but as honest men it behooves us
to learn the extent of our inheritance. . . .

John Tyndall, "Matter and Force" in vol. 2,
Prayer as a Form of Physical Energy

Learning objectives

After studying this chapter, the student
should be able to:

- state the focus of family therapy and the indications for it.

- identify the role of both the generalist and specialist in relation to family therapy.

- analyze the family systems model, structural model, and strategic, or brief, model of family therapy with regard to the following elements: theoretical basis, goal of therapy, and dynamics of treatment.

- within the context of a family systems model of therapy describe the relevance of differentiation of self, triangles, nuclear family emotional system, multigenerational transmission process, family projection process, sibling position, and emotional cutoff.

- within the context of a structural model of therapy describe the relevance of subsystems, subsystem boundaries, and restructuring operations.

- assess the importance of communication theory to the development of strategic, or brief, family therapy.

- identify suggested readings for future study.

In the 1950s, if a nurse therapist acknowledged that she was seeing anyone in the family other than the patient, she risked censure by the entire psychoanalytical community. She could be accused of breach of confidence and of failure to protect the boundaries of the therapeutic alliance between the nurse and patient from contamination. Today, 30 years later, the "growing edge" of family therapy encompasses many well-known persons in the field, numerous conferences and workshops, a panoply of books and videotapes, and a number of training programs in family therapy.[1]

Family therapy seeks to view the gestalt, the context in which an emotional problem is generated and played out between family members. Rather than viewing one member as sick or one relationship as pathological (such as the much-researched "schizophrenogenic mother" and symbiosed child), the family therapist focuses on the symmetrical process between family members that perpetuates and enables the "sick" behavior of one identified member. All family members are equally involved. For example, the school-phobic boy's overclose relationship to his mother can be seen as her solution to the problem of her husband's emotional withdrawal from her into his business for 16 hours of the day. The boy's attention-demanding behavior saves both spouses from confronting their conflicts with each other and the problem of their intimacy within the marriage. Seen in this context, there is no one member of the family who is to blame, no one victim to bolster with supportive therapy, but rather a skewed family process that has become fixed and requires rebalancing.

Viewing symptoms within this context requires a theoretical reorientation. To view family therapy as a modality of treatment is obsolescent; rather, it is a different way to conceptualize human relationship problems. It broadens the isolating, individual point of view to include the context in which relationship events take place.

This chapter will provide a summary of three of the major, current theoretical approaches to family therapy and delineate some of the main techniques that have evolved from these theories. The best guides to the history of family therapy, highlighting the work of the "first generation" personalities, are works of Chris Beels and Andy Ferber[4] and Phil Guerin.[20] The goal of the chapter is to develop an informed interest in the field and facilitate the pursuit of further reading and perhaps training in family therapy. For those nurses who do not work in psychiatry but who work with patients' families in some capacity, this chapter will provide some theories to help organize the wealth of information and stimuli that impinge on any observer of a family in stress.

Role of the nurse in family therapy

Nurse therapists have evolved with psychiatry. "Insanity" moved out of the hands of priests who would exorcise it, out of prisons that would contain it, and into the hands of physicians who would cure it. When "insanity" was conceived of as "mental illness," it was brought under the rubric of medicine. As medicine became more psychologically sophisticated, the intimate connection between the soma and the psyche was established. Psychiatry has gained a position of grudging legitimacy in the medical field. The development of psychosomatic medicine and psychiatric liaison services in medical hospitals attests to the increasing recognition that the emotional and psychological needs of patients must be met to maximize physical healing.

As medicine became more complex, the number of available physicians proved inadequate to perform multiple treatment procedures. Under these circumstances nurses were asked to assume more and more responsibility for total patient care. Observing emotional stress in patients and patients' families has always been an integral part of this care. Nurses responded intuitively to stress in their patients long before intrapsychic and interpersonal theories of psychiatry were conceived. Public health nurses observed the emotional stress of illness and social deprivation in patients and families in community settings. Inasmuch as one goal of psychotherapy is to reduce acute stress in a patient, family therapy is a natural evolution of the traditional role of the nurse.

Contact with patients' families is an inevitable part of patient care. For many years nurses have been making intuitive observations about functional and dysfunctional families and intervening with families without formal training in family therapy. A well-functioning family is a flexible one that can shift roles, levels of responsibility, and patterns of interaction as it passes through periods of varying stressful life changes. A well-functioning family may, under acute or prolonged stress, produce a symptomatic member, but this family rebalances in such a way that function of all members is restored and symptoms fade. A functional family has the following characteristics[18,26]:

1. It maintains a homeostatic balance and flexibility and adapts to change as it passes through transitional stages of family life and periods of stress.

2. Emotional problems are viewed as partially a function of each person, rather than residing entirely in one family member.

3. Emotional contact is maintained across generations and between family members without blurring necessary levels of authority.

4. Overcloseness or fusion is avoided, and distance is not used to solve problems.

5. Each twosome is expected to resolve the problems between them. Bringing a third person in to settle disputes or to take sides is discouraged.

6. Differences between family members are encouraged to promote personal growth and creativity.

7. Children are expected to assume age-appropriate responsibility and to enjoy age-appropriate privileges negotiated with their parents.

8. The preservation of a positive emotional climate is more highly valued than doing what "should" be done or what is "right."

9. Within each spouse there is a balance of affective expression, careful rational thought, relationship focus, care taking, and object orientation, and each spouse can selectively function in the respective models and roles.

Dysfunctional families lack one or more of these characteristics. All nurses, regardless of their area of expertise or practice setting, encounter dysfunctional families in which problems may be overt or covert and member satisfaction is low. Some of the more common dysfunctional family patterns nurses may observe include the following: the overprotective mother and the distant father (distant at work, in alcohol, or absent from the home) with a timid, whiney child or a destructive acting-out teenager; the overfunctioning "superwife" or "superhusband" and the underfunctioning passive, dependent, and compliant spouse; the spouse who maintains "peace at any price" and who whitewashes difficulties in the marriage but who suddenly feels wronged and self-righteous when the mate is discovered to be in legal difficulty or to be having an affair; the child who evidences poor peer relationships at school while attempting to parent younger siblings to compensate for ineffective and emotionally overwhelmed parents;

and the overclose three generations of grandparent, parent, and grandchild in which lines of authority and generational identity are ill-defined and the child is acting out because of a lack of effective limit setting by an agreed-on parental figure.

The decision as to when family therapy is appropriate or especially indicated over individual or group therapy is a controversial issue. Partially this decision is dictated by resources; many settings do not have anyone trained in family therapy. Even if the resources are available, the therapist's bias will have an influence. Some family therapists believe family therapy is the treatment of choice for any presenting problem or symptom. They make no distinction because they conceptualize all emotional problems within the family framework. Other family therapists recommend certain guidelines in determining which problems should be treated in family therapy. They may suggest that family therapy is indicated in the following situations[*]:

1. The presenting problem appears in system terms, such as marital conflicts, severe sibling conflicts, or cross-generational conflicts (parents vs. offspring; parents vs. grandparents).

2. Various types of difficulty and conflict arise between the identified patient and other family members.

3. The family is experiencing a transitional stage of the family life cycle, such as beginning a family, marriage, birth of the first child, entrance of children into adolescence, the first child leaving home, retirement, or the death of one spouse.

4. Individual therapy with one family member results in symptoms developing in another family member.

5. There is no improvement with adequate individual therapy. Enlarging the conceptual field to include the family in therapy may produce therapeutic movement.

6. The individual in treatment seems unable to use an intrapsychic or interpretive mode of individual therapy but primarily uses therapy sessions to talk about or complain about another family member.

In the majority of cases clinical training programs in family therapy are open to nurse specialists with graduate degrees. Workshops in

---

[*]I am indebted to Behnaz Jalali, M.D., for her ideas on this subject.

family therapy are offered across the United States. They vary in duration, theoretical model used, and in the level of clinical sophistication required of participants. The nurse therapist doing family therapy should have some formal graduate training or on-the-job education through didactic and clinical seminars. She should seek out and obtain individual or group supervision for her clinical work in treating families to refine her clinical skills and deepen her theoretical understanding of family systems.

Family therapy is being done in inpatient and outpatient settings. In the home it is used by crisis intervention teams, and it is being used with groups of families of chronically ill patients in aftercare clinics at state psychiatric hospitals. It is also being done by mental health professionals who volunteer their time to private or non-profit associations, such as the Cancer Foundation, to work with families stricken with a specific disease. Some intensive care units, such as kidney dialysis and coronary care units, are using therapists to do family therapy when a severe psychological disturbance is recognized in the patient or family as a result of the acute medical illness.

Because family therapy is practiced in a wide variety of settings and involves families at all levels of functioning, the generalist nurse, without a graduate degree, will be exposed to it in many areas of her practice. Understanding theoretical models of family therapy will benefit this nurse in many ways. She may apply certain principles of these models in her work with families of medically hospitalized patients to promote their functioning and support their methods of coping with stress and illness. Just as the functioning of the family as a whole is affected by the illness of one of its members, so too the family's method of coping with a member's illness can affect the outcome of the illness, either positively or negatively. Knowledge of family therapy theories will help her make more acute observations, more readily identify problems within family systems and assist her in selecting effective nursing interventions and evaluating the accuracy of her assessment by the interactional or functional change evident in the family. It may also assist her in initiating appropriate referrals.

The theoretical views of family therapy presented in this chapter—family systems therapy, structural family therapy, and problem-solving, strategic, or brief family therapy—are three distinct and, at times, conflicting views. They represent three major approaches in family therapy that have clearly articulated theoretical frameworks developed from clinical research with families. The opinion about which treatment approach is most effective with a family is primarily a function of the nurse therapist's theoretical orientation. There are no well-defined criteria or conclusive research in this area.

Family systems therapy

Family systems therapy was developed by Bowen[8] in the 1950s. The therapy has continued to evolve and refine as more people trained in systems theory have studied increasingly larger numbers of families and developed more training and research programs. A premise of this therapy is that a family is a homeostatic system, and a change in functioning of one family member results in a compensatory change in the functioning of other family members.[8] It could be likened to a centerless web in which, when one strand moves, the tensions in the entire web readjust. Systems therapy explains emotional dysfunction in human relationships, specifically in the family system. Symptoms in any member of the family, whether social (e.g., child abuse, delinquency), physical (e.g., alcoholism, chronic illness), emotional (e.g., depression, schizophrenia), or conflictual (e.g., marital conflict), are viewed as evidence of dysfunction in the family relationship process. Although the family is only one of the multitude of emotional systems in which an individual is involved, it is probably the most intense and influential one. Extrafamilial relationships rarely carry the voltage or toxicity of the family emotional system. This is not to say that one's family system totally determines one's behavior and function but rather that family systems foster or inhibit function. The individual's responsibility for his actions is never lost.

The purpose of any theory is to understand, predict, and thereby gain some control of the phenomena being studied. Understanding, as applied to family systems therapy, does not entail uncovering intrapsychic motivations but rather identifying the functional facts of a relationship—what happened, when, where, how, and who was involved. These observable facts are more important than the reasons why the problematical behavior occurred. A systems therapist gathers from family members descriptions of behavior rather than feeling states. The absence of conventional psychodynamic jargon in family systems writing reflects a conscious attempt by Bowen and early systems researchers to remove the cause-and-effect medical model or "why thinking." Systems therapy coined a new working language using simple descriptive words.

Bowen[6-8,10,11] has described in detail the team research he conducted in the early 1950s on schizophrenic families in a live-in hospital setting. From this live-in research evolved a new theory of family psychotherapy. This theory, which is based on clinical observations of the research families' behavior, proved applicable to relationship patterns in more functional family systems also. Bowen proposed the following:

> . . . Schizophrenia and all other forms of mental illness belong to a continuum, the difference being one of *degree* of impairment rather than a qualitative difference between schizophrenia and the neuroses.[8:391]

He believed that "patterns originally thought to be typical of schizophrenia are present in all families some of the time and in some families most of the time."[11:61]

A cornerstone of systems therapy developed from a central pattern observed in research families, which was their failure to distinguish between the intellectual process of thinking and the more subjective process of feeling. It was as if the thinking processes were so flooded with feeling that they were unable to separate intellectual opinion and belief from affective content. Routinely a person would say, "I feel that . . . ." when "I think/believe that . . . ." would have been more accurate. The families' efforts were toward fostering feelings of togetherness and agreement in relation to others, avoiding statements of opinion or belief that would establish one member as different or separate from the family "party line." A key goal of systems therapy therefore is to clarify and distinguish thinking and feeling processes in family members. Bowen's belief in the importance of distinguishing between feeling and thought is reflected in his use of the term "emotional illness or dysfunction" rather than "mental illness." He views emotional illness as a phenomenon deeper than a disorder of the mind and the thinking process; it is rather a disturbance in the basic life processes of a person.[8] The observation of this fusion between thinking and feeling led to the concept of the "undifferentiated family ego mass" (what Virginia Satir refers to as "people salad") and the conclusion that people with the greatest fusion between feeling and thinking function the most poorly and inherit a high percentage of life's social, psychiatric, and medical problems.[11]

Family systems theory consists of seven interlocking concepts. There are three concepts that apply to overall characteristics of family systems: differentiation of self, triangles, and the nuclear family emotional system. The remaining four concepts, the multigenerational transmission process, the family projection process, sibling position, and the emotional cutoff, are elaborations of the central family characteristics.

All these concepts refer to family processes that inhibit or promote individual family members' rising out of the emotional "we-ness," or fusion, that binds us all to our families. Bowen believes forces toward fusion are as instinctual in a person as opposing forces toward differentiation, and a member's movement toward either increased emotional closeness or distance is reflexive and predictable. The higher the level of differentiation in a person, the higher the level of functioning. Differentiating the self from the "we-ness" is therefore the goal of treatment. Guerin, on the other hand, sees the goal of family systems therapy as attainment of emotional freedom in the context of the family system. He is less militantly opposed to "we-ness" in the system than Bowen. In restating the goal of treatment in this way, he "leaves room for the ability either to be fused into a period of relationship refuge or to clearly draw one's boundaries and hold a functional position against the weight of the system."[20:19]

Differentiation of self

The concept of differentiation of self is Bowen's attempt to measure all human functioning on a continuum from the greatest emotional fusion of self boundaries, such as the folie à deux phenomenon, to the highest degree of differentiation or autonomy. A concise description of the differentiated person is the person who is less anxious than the family system and who is able to bring up toxic issues in a nonassaulting way without anxiety. In Bowen's earlier work he refers to the "undifferentiated family ego mass" or the "conglomerate emotional oneness" that exists in varying degrees of intensity in families. The intensity of emotional closeness in a family can be such that members know each other's thoughts, feelings, and fantasies.

There is a cyclical quality to this closeness. As the emotional intensity or fusion between two individuals increases and the self of one is incorporated into the other self, the relationship is perceived to be uncomfortably close. This is usually followed by distance-creating behavior in which there is hostile rejection of the overcloseness and the two individuals actively repel each other.[9] Relationships can cycle through these phases, since anxiety in the relationship ebbs and flows at frequent intervals. Relationships can also become fixed at an angry, repelling standoff. In people who operate at this lower reactive end of the continuum, their intellect and emotions are so fused that they are dominated by the automatic emotional system. These people are less adaptable, less flexible, more emotionally dependent on those about them, and easily stressed into dysfunction. People at the upper end of the continuum maintain a degree of separation between thought and emotion. In periods of stress they can retain a relative amount of intellectual functioning and are more flexible, adaptable, and more independent of the reactive emotionality around them.[11]

The concept of differentiation eliminates the notion of normalcy, even in its poorly defined state. It has no direct connection to presence or absence of symptoms, although Bowen believes people at the lower end of the scale tend to inherit more of life's problems. People at the upper end of the continuum, if they are stressed into dysfunction, tend to recoup rapidly.

Triangles

The concept of triangles is the key to understanding the systems approach to emotional function, and many techniques evolve from this concept. The idea of triangles is certainly not a new one. Freud's theory of the oedipal complex describes a sexual triangle. Bowen has called the triangle the basic "building block of an emotional system." A triangle is a predictable emotional process that takes place in any significant relationship when there is difficulty in the relationship. The three corners of a triangle can be composed of three people; two people and a group, such as a religious affiliation or Al-Anon; two people and an issue, such as drinking or success; or two people and an object, such as the house or drugs.[17] Obviously the possible list of groups, issues, or objects is endless; it requires only that they have an emotional significance equal to that of a person.

All people seek closeness in emotional systems. Emotional closeness but separateness is difficult for two people to maintain; the tendency is to fuse, to lose self, or parts of self, in the other. There is a natural urge to seek completeness of self by accumulating parts of other. The old adage "opposites attract" reflects this assumption. The balance is precarious between two people trying to maintain a comfortable distance so that there is sufficient emotional closeness without fusion. The inevitable result is emotional distancing, and the system is then ripe for the formation of a triangle. For example, the husband wants more expression of affection and closeness from an emotionally constricted wife. The more he pursues her, the more she withdraws, most commonly into preoccupation with her child. The husband starts working longer hours. Husband and wife then start arguing circularly: "You care more about making a new account than you do about your wife and children!" "You expect to have nice things and then blame me for working extra hours!" The key to the function of triangles is stabilizing and maintaining the status quo while at the same time avoiding tension, conflict, or talking about sensitive emotional areas. The two people can then focus on the new issue (or person or object) and avoid discussing the painful issues between them. Feelings are thus drained off, focus is taken off self and one's own part in the problem, and change in self is avoided.

The reciprocal function of a triangle and the idea of equal responsibility can be a difficult concept to convey to a couple when the distancing mechanism used by one spouse is as emotionally charged as an extramarital affair. If the wife distances from the painful issues in the relationship, by "triangling" an affair, it is difficult for the husband to relinquish his self-righteous position of the "wronged husband" and see his behavior of working 14 to 16 hours a day as serving the same distancing function in the relationship. The specific nature of the distancing mechanism has meaningful content (whether it is overwork, extramarital affairs, homosexuality, psychotic symptoms, religious preoccupation, suicide gesture, depression, or psychoanalysis), but all serve the same function as a triangular relationship within the family.[15]

The concept of a family scapegoat originally served to broaden the individual pathological view to include the part the family played in the symptomatic behavior. The tendency, however, is to view the scapegoat as the helpless victim of a persecuting family. With this bias a nurse therapist would see two parents who are unable to settle their differences and wish to avoid their

FIG. 25-1
A commonly occurring family triangle.

marital discord by focusing on the "victim child." This leads to blaming the parents. From a systems view, with the concept of triangles, this process operates with all three twosomes that make up the triangle. A diagram of this triangle is presented in Fig. 25-1. Father and mother avoid conflict by focusing on the son, mother and son avoid dealing with their overcloseness by having a common enemy in the father. Father and son avoid awareness of their emotional distance by relating through the mother as go-between. Recognizing how this emotional dysfunction process is promoted by each family member invalidates the label of victim and victimizer. Fogarty stresses, "All members of a triangle participate equally in perpetuating the triangle and no triangle can persist without the active cooperation of all its members."[17:13]

It is not a problem to be in a triangle; in fact, it is impossible to stay out of all triangles. Triangles form and re-form rapidly and are the daily reflexive way most people handle conflict or tension. Problems will arise if a triangle becomes fixed when it involves significant relationships of deep friendship, blood ties, or marriage. Triangles are not static but form and re-form around toxic, emotion-laden issues, such as money, sex, child rearing, religion, alcohol, and education. A person's position in a triangle alters depending on the issue. A mother and father may be distant on the highly charged issue of how to spend their money but may be close and in accord about the loaded issue of their adolescent daughter's sexual activity. Judgments about these issues are most often based on emotion rather than careful thought.

To determine what a person's operating principles are, that is, the governing laws of his conduct, they must be inferred from what the person does in regard to an emotion-laden issue rather than what he says. Operating principles may thus vary from intrinsically valuable ones based on conscious conviction to more immature, reactive, impulsive principles. Immature principles are other focused rather than self-focused and lead to a loss of freedom of self-determination. Any behavior that is predictable (as in behavior operated by a triangle) is not free. The loss of freedom impairs self-functioning, perpetuates problems, causes a deterioration in family functioning, and promotes symptom development.[15]

Other-focused, triangle-promoting operating principles are reflected in such ways as declaring feelings "right" or "wrong"; using plural pronouns "we" or "us" rather than "I"; accusing the other person of "you made me mad/do it"; stepping in to settle, side taking, or blaming in two other people's conflict; telling or holding secrets; telling the other person what to do; and assuming responsibility for the other person's feelings, for example, "I want to make her happy" or "I couldn't tell him because it would hurt him." These statements may commonly be interpreted as thoughtful or being very responsible. In fact, avoiding one's own feelings by focusing on the other person is fundamentally irresponsible. From taking responsibility for another's feelings it is a small leap to taking charge of the other person's behavior. Everyone tends to fall into this pattern, especially in a marriage or parent-child relationship. When a person becomes anxious, it is more comfortable to project the problem outside the self onto the other person and then work to change the other. The implicit assumption here is "I can't help my behavior, but he is behaving that way deliberately."[21]

In more dysfunctional, closed family systems, interaction between family members becomes determined by fixed interactional patterns, as observed in schizophrenic families, for example. These fixed triangles are an effort to maintain a homeostatic balance and to avoid stress. When an additional stress occurs outside or within the family, such as a job change or the birth of a new member, symptoms may arise in a dysfunctional attempt to reduce stress and restore balance. This is evident in Clinical example 25-1.

CLINICAL EXAMPLE 25-1

Mr. and Mrs. D, whose family consisted of six children, had a seventh unplanned child. The family was financially strained, and Mr. and Mrs. D had a conflictual and distant relationship. When the last child was born, a middle sibling, 13-year-old Andy, developed symptoms and became school phobic. The school insisted the child receive treatment. Late in the treatment the mother finally revealed that one of the reasons for the family's financial strain was the husband's work phobia and his occasional gambling sprees. The wife had covered for him for years, calling his boss to make excuses and taking part-time work herself. Until the birth of the last child, the family was able to maintain a precarious, minimally functional balance. The additional stress, however, produced symptoms sufficiently noticeable to cause an outside agency, the school, to become involved in an attempt to restore functioning in the family.

A major focus of treatment is to get key figures in key triangles to identify their emotional "triggers." This involves having the person identify the verbal or behavioral cues of the other person to which he reflexively reacts with a predictable behavior, maintaining his position in and perpetuating the dysfunctional triangle. When the person pinpoints what cues activate his triggers, he can take control of his part in the process. Once one person takes control and changes his part in a triangle, the whole system changes. An example of this was a mother who was overclose to her 16-year-old daughter, who had become school phobic and stayed home from school for a year before the family sought treatment. The father would come home from work, see the daughter had missed school another day, and angrily attack her with "shape-up speeches." The mother, who bitterly complained about the daughter being home all day doing nothing, would then become protective of the daughter and launch an attack on father: "How can you say those things to her; you know how upset she gets." Once the mother was able to get a "handle" on her emotional trigger and stop feeling sorry for her daughter (the mother had always been terrified of her "drill sergeant" father), she was able to control her protective reflex, step back, and permit the father to become more effective with his daughter.

The nurse must not only identify key triangles in a family and identify operating principles of family members pertaining to specific issues, but also she must be tuned into her own vulnerability to her emotional triggers. She must assume that the family will attempt to triangle her into the family's emotional system to reestablish equilibrium. The nurse's job is to maintain sufficient emotional distance to watch the process unfolding between family members while at the same time maintaining emotional contact with each family member.[12] Bowen[35] has enumerated many of the reactions a therapist might have which would indicate that the therapist is part of a triangle: feeling sorry for or pitying the other, feeling angry at the system or member, being overly positive about the system, or seeing someone doing something horrendous and feeling one has to correct it. The nurse knows she is part of a triangle in the family process when she finds herself without questions or responses in the session. The idea is to avoid becoming part of a triangle, thus diffusing the emotional process, and to limit the action to the two family members. Once the therapist steps in to take sides, progress stops and status quo is reestablished.[36] If side taking is used by the therapist, it should be a planned strategy in which she maintains the freedom to realign with specific family members.

Systems therapists do not believe they can change family members; change is possible only when it is generated within the self. Just as family members are coached on taking responsibility for and control of self within the family system rather than trying to change the other, the family therapist's responsibility is to stay relevant to the emotional flow of the family without becoming part of a triangle in the system. One way for the nurse to get herself out of an emotional process she reacts to in the session is to elicit the members' responses. For example, if she finds herself getting irritated at a critical intrusive husband, she can turn to the wife and ask, "What happens to your insides when your husband interrupts with criticism?" This feeds the process back into the system, keeping it between the spouses.

One of the areas of controversy in the field of family therapy is the importance of the therapist's working on her own family of origin (referred to as TOF, therapist's own family). Systems therapists contend that it is a major aspect of training as a family therapist. "Working on" means the nurse differentiates herself in her own family of origin. She identifies the issues in her family that she is reactive to and with whom she is part of a triangle around these issues. She then works to get out of the triangle by gaining control of her reflexive distancing and fusing in her family in order to have the freedom of emotional closeness and of some emotional distance with each family member (without using geographical distance to create emotional space). Unless a therapist is conscious of the triangles she is a part of in her own family, she will be vulnerable to the same roles and behaviors in the families she is treating.

Nuclear family emotional system

The nuclear family emotional system refers to patterns of interaction between family members and the degree to which these patterns promote emotional fusion.[16] These patterns of interaction, called operating principles, are the ways the person behaves in most significant relationships. All marriage relationships reflect a balance, or complementarity, of operating principles and reciprocal function.[21] There is the spouse who is reasonable, object oriented, and emotionally distant married to the affectively expressive, relationship oriented, emotional pursuer. These differences in operating principles provide the attraction and the balancing stability to the marriage relationship. One spouse is the subject overfunctioner, the other the emotional overfunctioner. Difficulty arises with time when dependence on attributes of the spouse reduces functional attributes in the self. Self borrows on the functioning of the spouse, and self boundaries are blurred. This is referred to as ego fusion. When these reciprocal functions become fixed positions of overfunction-underfunction, emotional dysfunction and symptoms occur, such as chronic depression or physical illness. In such a relationship, to view one spouse as strong and independent and the other as weak and dependent fails to recognize the overfunctioner's dependence on the underfunctioning of the other spouse. The underfunctioner must be one-down for the other to appear one-up.

Emotional fusion operates in all marriages to a lesser or greater extent. When the relationship is unstressed, the reciprocal function works smoothly. When stress occurs, each spouse becomes more like oneself. The distancer seeks space and objects (the job, art, alcohol); the pursuer seeks togetherness and expression of personal feelings. Both are efforts to avoid personal anxiety. The pursuer takes the distancer's withdrawal as personal rejection and reactively withdraws. No longer feeling crowded, the distancer then moves in emotionally, only to be met with "Where were you when I needed you; get lost." The distancer then pulls back, baffled and angry at the rejection, and, in time, a fixed emotional distance sets in.[21] These are the bitter standoff relationships nurses see in their practice just before the couple decides on a divorce. These relationships are ripe for triangulation with an affair or with an unsuspecting therapist.

People pick spouses who have equivalent levels of differentiation of self.[8] The greater the undifferentiation, the greater the tendency toward fusion and potential problems. If there is a high degree of ego fusion and intensity in the nuclear family, this intensity can be diffused and attenuated through active contact with the family of origin. In periods of stress, contact with the extended family or family of origin can stabilize the nuclear family. Promoting such contact can be an effective therapeutic strategy.

Bowen[9] has identified two patterns in the nuclear family emotional system, which he labels the explosive family and the cohesive family. Family units of a cohesive family are geographically close, in frequent contact and communication. The person who geographically separates from his family of origin because of the fusion or intensity of attachment there may marry a spouse from a cohesive family. The person's unresolved attachments to his own family of origin lie dormant until ritualized contact (at a wedding or funeral) stirs them up. In a nuclear family in which both spouses are detached from their families of origin the spouses tend to be more dependent on each other, and the process between them is more intense. These are the explosive families.

Bowen[8] postulates three mechanisms by which spouses maintain sufficient emotional distance from each other to handle the anxiety associated with fusion. All three mechanisms may be used by the couple, or tension may be focused in one area. If tension is great enough, it will spill over into other social systems such as mental health centers or school counselors. The three mechanisms used are (1) marital conflict, (2) dysfunction in one spouse, and (3) projection of the problem onto one or more children.

Conflictual marriages are built on a perpetual struggle between spouses to get "their fair share" (of needs met, of freedom, of love, of attention, or of control) and neither spouse is willing to compromise. A high percentage of the self is wrapped up in the "happiness" of the other, and functioning of the self is enmeshed in the function of the other. Because of the amount of investment in the other, whether positive ("Anything to make her happy") or negative ("I sacrificed the best years of my life helping him be a success; I'll never let him go now"), these relationships tend to be stable, predictably cycling through periods of intense closeness, distance-creating conflict, making up, then renewed closeness. Although it is commonly believed that this amount of conflict would harm the children of such marriages, Bowen[8] postulates that the children are, in fact, protected from overinvolvement because tension is focused between parents.

Intervention in conflictual marriages usually involves working with the most motivated spouse at first. If both spouses are seen together, frequently the uproar between them is too great to tolerate in the session. They are so reactive to each other that limit setting such as laying ground rules of no interruptions and one person talking at a time or strategies such as a "listening chair" or turning one spouse's chair to the wall to listen are ineffective. In such situations spouses must be seen separately initially. The approach is to get the focus on the self and to decrease the amount of blaming and attack and efforts to change the other. The nurse strives to focus on what part the spouse plays in the situation and gain some control of one's own reactive triggers. Once the blaming is reduced, the spouse can then reevaluate his or her own set of beliefs and values without the need to attack the other. Such reevaluation entails going back to one's family of origin in phone or letter contacts or planned visits, gaining a broader view of the source of the nuclear family conflict, and working to establish more personal relationships with one's family of origin. Bowen calls this process coaching. Usually before this point is reached in the treatment, the absent, less-motivated spouse has sought to join the sessions because of the changes that have occurred.

Significant changes in the marriage system occur when one spouse withdraws emotional overinvestment in the other and focuses on self. The spouse making changes must be warned of predictable efforts by the other to reestablish status quo by an escalation of anger-provoking behavior, threats to leave, etc. If the spouse making changes can maintain a self-focused position through the resistance, both partners may become active in the treatment. While temporarily working with one spouse, the nurse must guard against becoming part of a triangle in the system by emotionally siding with the spouse initially in treatment or by becoming the only support for the spouse in treatment. This can be especially difficult for the nurse when the unexpressed plan of the unmotivated spouse is to deposit the husband or wife in treatment and then obtain a divorce, expecting the nurse to "take care of" the spouse. Whitaker and Miller[42] explore this issue in depth.

The second mechanism used by spouses to maintain emotional distance is the dysfunction of one spouse. As mentioned earlier, one spouse may be emotionally, socially, or physically disabled to varying degrees. The degree to which the one underfunctions is the degree to which the other overfunctions. This ensures that emotional equilibrium is maintained, since both partners are locked into a mutually dependent relationship. Interventions with such a relationship are similar to those used with the conflictual marriage. Bowen suggests working with the overfunctioning spouse first, getting this spouse to tone down and pull back. Since nature abhors a vacuum, the underfunctioning spouse then moves in to take up the slack.

A striking example of pulling the overfunctioning spouse back with a resulting shift in the emotional and functional balance is evident in Clinical example 25-2.

CLINICAL EXAMPLE 25-2

Mr. and Mrs. S are a couple who sought treatment because the husband was missing so many days at work. The couple would get into huge battles about the husband not feeling like working and the wife feeling outraged at the financial stress he was creating. It became apparent that Mrs. S treated Mr. S like one of their adolescent boys. She overfunctioned to the point of cleaning up after her husband's destructive temper tantrums. Over a period of time, with considerable coaching, she was able to pull back in several areas, refusing to wake the husband or clean up after him, leaving it up to him to pay the bills, and generally holding back her critical nagging. The first sign of progress was at the husband's next temper tantrum (he did delicate electrical work and had a low frustration tolerance). He carefully selected which objects he would throw or smash in his workroom, not throwing a box of small nuts and bolts, for example. He cleaned up his own workroom and began going to work regularly. As the husband's functioning improved, the wife became significantly depressed and began addressing unresolved issues in her family of origin. This couple demonstrated the reciprocity in the mechanism of underfunctioning and overfunctioning in a marriage.

The third distancing mechanism used by spouses to control the intensity of fusion between them is the projection of the problem to one or more of the children. Prior to development of a theory of family pathology, the parents of a symptomatic child would be excluded from therapy, further reinforcing the dysfunction in the family by focusing on the child as "the problem." Child-focused families tend to be particularly entrenched in viewing the problem as exclusive to the symptomatic child, or else they deny the existence of a problem entirely. When the school or probation officer recommends treatment, they passively comply but participate reluctantly. When a couple centers on their children, it is easier to avoid marital confrontations because there is always something to worry, criticize, or complain about with the children. These families exhibit strong dependency on the children's symptoms, and they tenaciously resist exploring larger issues in therapy.[2]

How one child gets singled out as the focus of parental concern is a complex process that may have its roots in several previous generations. Key triangles tend to repeat themselves over generations; so the parent's natural tendency is to put one child in the parent's old position in the triangle. Nodal events are the normative events that occur in every family life but which generate anxiety because change ensues. These include such events as birth, death, sickness, marriage, job changes, school changes, divorce, and family relocation. Carter[13]

suggests that the amount of stress generated around a nodal event is contingent on the amount of change resultant. If a significant developmental stage of the child (e.g., in utero, birth, entering school for the first time, adolescence) coincides approximately with the occurrence of a nodal event, this child is vulnerable to the focus of family stress and impairment. The first born and the last born are also particularly vulnerable to the position of family focus.

Intervention with such families cannot be a frontal assault with logic or the family will be lost to treatment. The primary goal is to remove the focus from the child and place the conflict between the parents where it belongs. This is accomplished by placing the dysfunctions of the child within the context of the family system by taking a family history and drawing a family genogram. Drawing a three-generation family genogram is a structured method of gathering information and graphically symbolizing a large amount of factual and emotional relationship data in the initial interview.[22] A sample genogram is presented in Fig. 25-2. Drawing a family genogram in full view of the family on large

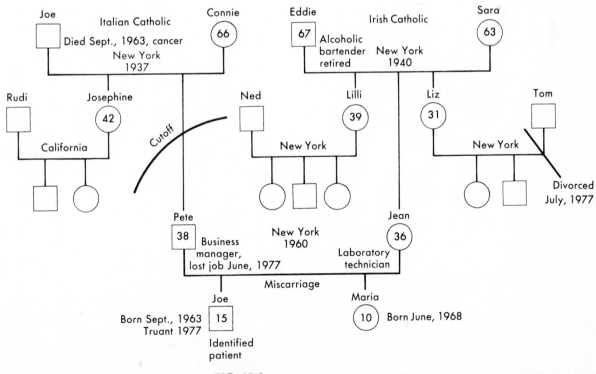

FIG. 25-2
A hypothetical family genogram.

easel paper or a blackboard broadens the family's focus and stimulates their thinking of the extended family system. The therapist's questions and comments are geared toward change of self rather than changing the child.

Strategies used to defocus the identified child as the problem include identifying or defining the behavior of other family members as problematical to spread the problem and anxiety around. Another strategy is to move the problem up one generation by asking how grandparents might handle the problem or opening discussion on conflict about disciplining the children between grandparents. With some families the nurse can coach the overinvolved parent, for example, the mother, to pull back from the focused child and send a note to her own mother telling her one thing about herself that she does not want her to know. This reveals the three-generational aspect of the presenting problem. Guerin recommends working with the sibling subset at times, separately from the parents, to promote a more positive support system among sibs. Frequently sibs mimic their parents' negative behavior toward the focused child or resent the excessive attention he gets from parents and are aggressive toward him.

Families with an acting-out child and two parents in the ineffective helpless position (or one parents set up as the "heavy" and the other as "the nice guy" saboteur) need a direct approach initially. An effective way to point out how the adults are relinquishing their authority to a young child is to use an extreme example: "If your child had third-degree burns, could you get her to take the horribly painful treatments?" or "If your child had heart disease, could you limit her activities?" Following are four guidelines for parents locked in a triangle with the acting-out "problem child":

1. The person who sets the rule must be present to enforce it.

2. With two parents in the home, divide the areas of responsibility (e.g., allowance, bedtime, nights out) so that when a dispute comes up, it is clear with whom the child must negotiate.

3. Yelling is ineffective and preempts thinking. Parents need to control their reactive buttons.

4. Calmly decide the consequences of repeated disobedient behavior and inform the child of them. When the behavior occurs, without yelling, carry out the consequence even if the par-

ent's personal plans must be changed to do so.*

As soon as the child focus is sufficiently reduced, the child is removed from the sessions. The therapist then forms the third corner of the triangle, actively relating to both spouses without taking sides and thereby keeping conflict between the spouses.

Multigenerational transmission process

The roots of the family emotional system extend back through generations. When there is emotional dysfunction, it can be scattered throughout the family tree.[19] Drawing a three-generation family genogram frequently reveals certain relationship patterns that might otherwise seem to be isolated phenomena peculiar to one nuclear family. For example, suicide of younger brothers, divorce among female siblings, or alcoholism might appear to be a pattern across a family system when four or five generations are mapped out on a genogram. A difference between family systems therapy and other forms of family therapy is the underlying assumption that a symptom in one family member in one generation has its origin several generations before, although families seeking treatment usually present symptoms as a nuclear family problem.

Family projection process

The concept of the family projection process refers to the way anxiety about specific issues is transmitted through the generations. These are the issues that are emotionally powerful, such as money, sex, child rearing, religion, work or school achievement, alcohol, politics, illness and death, and around which a rigid "party line" develops. Family members polarize around these issues, taking the family position or the direct opposite. Neither position allows freedom or flexibility of thought. Positions are reactive and fixed. Coaching a person to work on the family of origin involves helping him identify his predictable position in family triangles around specific loaded issues. By thinking about the issues he normally reacts to emotionally, he can plan strategies that will get him unhooked from his triangled position.

The family projection process also refers to the process that labels and assigns characteristics to certain members of the family. Whether the labels are overpositive ("Mary Sunshine," "The Genius") or overnegative ("the crazy one,"

---

*I am indebted to Betty Carter for her ideas on this issue.

"dummy,"), they are equally unrealistic and confining. After years of family labeling or pronouncements, the labeled person will come to volunteer for the label and deserve it.

Sibling position

The concept of personality profiles based on sibling position is borrowed by family systems theorists from Walter Toman, a Viennese psychiatrist. Toman's basic thesis[37] is that important personality characteristics are determined by the sex of one's siblings and one's birth order. For example, the younger brother of two older sisters will present a profile quite different from the older brother of a brother. Using the 10 personality profiles Toman developed, one can fairly accurately predict marital discord or harmony on issues of rank or sex. A younger brother of brothers would have more difficulty relating to his spouse than a younger brother of sisters would have. If this younger brother of brothers married a younger sister of sisters, they would both have discomfort with the opposite sex. In addition, they would be struggling for juniority rights (who's going to take care of whom). Recognizing a possible source of conflict to be sibling rank and sex can help a couple live with their differences.

Emotional cutoff

The emotional cutoff is a way some families deal with intense unresolved attachment between children and parents. The cutoff can be in the form of emotional isolation, although members still live geographically close, or in the form of physical distance from the family of origin.[11] The cutoff creates the illusion of having achieved separation from one's parents. The more intense the emotional cutoff, the more likely it is the person will recreate the same problem in his own marriage. The strongest argument for a person to reconnect emotionally with his cutoff family is to prevent the same process from occuring with his own children. Such patterns tend to repeat over the generations.

Modes of therapy

Several modes of therapy have been mentioned thus far, including therapy with both spouses or both parents present and therapy with one spouse or parent in preparation for the other spouse joining. Another mode of family therapy is therapy with one family member. This is most frequently used with the young adult who is single and self-supporting. This method involves learning about the functioning of family systems and triangles, keeping an active emotional relationship with important members of the family by planned phone calls, letters, and visits, and developing an ability to control emotional reactiveness to avoid becoming part of an emotional triangle during visits with the family.[8] The goal here, as with other modes of family therapy, is to achieve more self-differentiation from the family of origin, as well as to develop a person-to-person relationship with important family members. This therapy is referred to as coaching. Once the person is knowledgeable about triangles and methods of detriangling within his own family, coaching sessions can be held monthly or as needed to supervise ongoing self-differentiation efforts.

The last mode of therapy is multiple family therapy (MFT) developed in its present form in the late 1960s. MFT is to be distinguished from multiple family group therapy. The latter uses role playing and psychodrama and promotes interfamily group process to achieve the goal of changing family interaction and increasing its sensitivity to the family environment.[34] MFT, from a family systems framework, is different. Sessions are structured so as to ensure against emotional exchange between families, which, Bowen believes, encourages a fusion of other families into a large undifferentiated ego mass.[34] The idea behind MFT was to conserve teaching time of families, provide contact with a greater volume of families, and allow the opportunity for families to learn from the efforts and experiences of other families. While other families observe, the nurse therapist works with each family the same as she would if she were working alone with that family. She asks numerous de-detailed questions about the family's problem, defocuses feelings, and addresses one spouse while the other spouse listens. Then she turns to the silent spouse, asking for thoughts or reactions to what the other spouse has said. The family members observing can talk to the therapist about another family but cannot directly talk to the other family.

Structural family therapy

Structural family therapy is a body of theory and techniques based on a view of the individual within his social context. The assumption is that behavior is a consequence of the organization of the family and the interactional patterns between family members. With this view, changing the family organization and the feedback processes between members changes the context in which a person functions, which thereby changes the person's inner processes and behavior. The therapist temporarily becomes part of the context. This approach is most clearly conceptualized by Menuchin[26] and those associated with the Philadelphia Child Guidance Clinic.

The implicit question of a structural family therapist is "In what way is this family structure maintaining this dysfunctional symptom?" Family structure is the invisible set of functional demands that organizes the way in which family members interact. A family is a system that operates through transactional patterns. Repeated transactions establish patterns of how, when, and to whom to relate, and these patterns determine whether the system is functional or dysfunctional.

Components of structural family therapy

The first component of this family model is the family as a social system in transformation. The family system must maintain its continuity so family members can grow while at the same time it must adapt to stresses both internal and external to the system. With this view, what traditional therapists would label pathological might be seen as the normal anxiety that characterizes a transitional stage in accommodation to new circumstances. This is described in Clinical example 25-3 by Menuchin.[26]

CLINICAL EXAMPLE 25-3

An elderly widow decided to move from her apartment where she had lived for 25 years because she came home one day and found it had been robbed. Soon after a moving company moved her, she sought treatment from a psychiatrist. She complained that the people who moved her were trying to control her and had purposely lost and misplaced precious possessions. They were leaving sinister messages for each other on her furniture, and when she went outside, people followed her and signaled to each other. The psychiatrist diagnosed her as psychotic with paranoid delusions and prescribed tranquilizers. When this did not help, she sought a second psychiatric who recommended hospitalization. The third therapist she sought out was a context-related therapist. He under-

stood her symptoms as an ecological crisis precipitated by feeling forced to move into an unfamiliar environment. He explained to her that she had lost her shell—the familiarity of objects in her apartment, the neighborhood, the neighbors. As any crustacean who has lost its shell, she felt vulnerable and was experiencing reality differently than before. He instructed her to go home, unpack, and place her familiar objects, books, and pictures in the new apartment. He told her to do her daily chores in a routinized way, go to the same shops and checkout counters, and for 2 weeks make no effort to meet neighbors. She was to visit old friends and family but not discuss her recent experiences. If anyone asked, she was to explain that those had just been the problems of an illogical fearful old woman.

The interventions of a structural family therapist are toward changing the relationship between a person and the familiar context in which he functions, thereby changing his subjective experience and enabling new, more functional behavior to emerge. In this case the therapist's interventions protected the woman from the unfamiliar and frightening environment until she could "grow a new shell." He blocked the environmental feedback that was serving to confirm her paranoid fears as friends and family withdrew to secretly discuss her frightening behavior. As her experience of her environment changed, her symptoms disappeared.

The second component of Menuchin's model[26] of a viable functional family is that the family undergoes predictable stages of development over time that require adaptive restructuring. Each stage has appropriate developmental tasks that must be accomplished for the family to pass on to the next stage. One stage is the courtship period when the young person is shifting from juvenile to membership in the adult community, establishing status in relation to others, and selecting a mate. This is one of the major times when professional help is sought.[23] The stage at which a new family unit is formed by marriage is preceded by negotiation of the spouses' relationship with respective families of origin. In addition, the families of origin must adjust to partial separation of one member, inclusion of a new member, and accommodation to a new spouse subsystem in the family system functioning. Unless families of origin undergo this transformation, the new family unit may never succeed. Equally unsuccessful are couples who cut themselves off from extended families.

During the marriage stage, multiple and complex rules and transactional patterns must be established between partners. Some ways of relating are reinforced and others are shed in the process of mutual accommodation as a new family system is formed. When a child is born, the functioning of the spouse unit must be modified to include parenting functions. It must shift from an intimate unit of two to a system of three. Frequently the new child becomes the repository of or the excuse for new and unresolved old conflicts between spouses. Many old battles are fought in the arena of child rearing because the couple cannot separate parenting functions from spouse functions.

In the middle years of marriage a major task is the weaning of parents from children. For families in which spouses established communication through the children and the children are leaving (or struggling to leave) home, this is a particularly stressful time. This can be a period of enrichment for spouses if (typically) the husband is enjoying a degree of career success and the wife is freer now to pursue career plans or interests she set aside earlier to rear children. Finally, a family member enters the stage of retirement and old age. This can be a period of relative harmony or it can be problematical as spouses are thrown together 24 hours a day. In time, one of the partners dies, and adult children then face the crisis of caring for an aging parent. The family cycle continues to unfold, and as the family is transformed over time, it must adapt and restructure itself to continue functioning. It is when a family adheres inappropriately to previous structural schemas that stress builds and symptoms develop.

A third component of Menuchin's model of viable functioning family relates to the structure of the family. The major elements of structure are power and influence, sets of relationships, and boundaries (individual, sexual, generational).[32] Structure can become dysfunctional in any or each of these areas. As in any organization, the family system must have a power hierarchy with different levels of authority to function efficiently. There must also be a complementarity of functions, a team effort among family members. Over the years mutual expectations of particular family members evolve. These expectations may be openly negotiated but more often are implicit, with patterns of behavior developing around small daily events.

The family system differentiates and carries out its functions through subsystems. Subsystems can be made up of individuals or dyads and can be formed by generation, sex, interest, or function.[26] Each person belongs to a mul-

tiplicity of subsystems with different levels of power and in which differentiated skills are learned. The boundaries of a subsystem are the rules defining who participates in subsystem functions and how. Each subsystem has specific functions and interpersonal developmental tasks to be accomplished. Subsystem boundaries must be free of intrusion if functions are to be performed and interpersonal skills developed. For example, patterns of mutual accommodation as well as healthy competition cannot develop among siblings if parents or grandparents perpetually interfere. A central principle of structural family therapy is that subsystem boundaries must be clear for proper family functioning. They must be defined well enough to prevent intrusion or interference but must also permit emotional contact among members.

Menuchin[26] describes families with extreme boundary problems as either enmeshed or disengaged. Enmeshed boundaries are weak and fluid; personal space and subsystem boundaries rapidly change and impact on all subsystems. This diffuseness of boundaries inhibits the development of autonomy and competence. Perceptions of self and others are poorly differentiated.[27] A child in such a family might be so sensitized to conflict between parents that he is unable to perform in school. The parents in such a family can become upset because the child refuses his vegetables at dinnertime. Such families flood with anxiety at times of stress and have poor adaptive capacities to change.

Disengaged families have rigid boundaries. Communication between subsystems is poor; supportive or protective contact is minimal. Members of such systems may function autonomously but have a skewed sense of independence and lack feelings of loyalty and belonging and the capacity for interdependence. Stierlin[33] hypothesizes that the product of a disengaged family is the sociopath. Because of the rigidity of subsystem boundaries, members may fail to respond adequately or entirely when one member is stressed. In such a family a child's reading disorder might go unnoticed or a husband's suicidal behavior be disregarded.

The nurse often functions as a boundary maker. She may clarify diffuse boundaries by blocking interruptions or encouraging the shutting of bedroom doors. She may open overly rigid boundaries by recommending that a distant parent and child spend time together or calling attention to the expression of a nuance of feeling by a family member that would otherwise go unnoticed by other members. The nurse's assessment of family subsystems and boundary functioning provides a rapid diagnostic picture of the family and indicates the direction and goals of therapeutic interventions.

As mentioned earlier, each subsystem has specific functions and interpersonal developmental tasks to be accomplished. The spouse subsystem must develop patterns of mutual support for each person's functioning in many areas. Couples must develop a complementary routine that enables decisions to be made and arguments to be settled without domination or relinquishing of self by either spouse. Ideally, they will bring out the best in each other, with each promoting personal growth and creativity in their spouse.

What commonly occurs in most marriages, to a greater or lesser degree, is that spouses engage in an "other-improvement program." They bring into the marriage certain expectations of their spouse and work very hard to get the spouse to meet them. Interpretations in this area should be balanced and directed to both spouses and the part each plays in perpetuating the destructive process should be pointed out. A mutual interpretation would be to say to the wife, "In your efforts to make contact with your husband, you are driving him away" and to the husband, "Your strong silent style is alluring and elicits nagging." Balanced interpretations such as this emphasize the complementarity of the system, join the positive and negative in each spouse, and eliminate judgmental implications of motivation.

The parental subsystem must perform the tasks of socializing the children without sacrificing the function of mutual support and accommodation between the spouses. Children must have access to each parent but be excluded from spouse functions. Menuchin speaks with a clear voice to parents regrading the importance of parental authority in an era that tends to promote "pure democracy" between parents and children. He validates the difficulty parenting entails, noting that few do it to their own satisfaction. Parenting processes are different depending on the age of the child. Part of promoting differentiation in the family is making the differentiation in ages clear. Adolescents have certain responsibilities and certain

privileges that 12-year-old siblings do not. Children must learn to negotiate with their parents to learn to navigate in a world of unequal power relationships.

The sibling subsystem is where children first learn about peer relationships. They learn how to make friends, compete, negotiate, cooperate, and gain recognition of their skills. Knowledge of growth and development of children is valuable for the nurse who must, at times, translate age-appropriate skills, needs, and values to baffled parents. The nurse should support the child's right to autonomy while at the same time supporting the parents' authority.

Goals of the initial interview

A vital component to structural family therapy is the process of joining the family.[25,26] The nurse temporarily becomes part of the family system by adapting her behavior to the rules and manner of the particular family. She can do this either purposefully or unconsciously. The aim is to accommodate herself to the family to gain experiential entrance into the family system. Unless she does this at the outset, restructuring and change is impossible. Following are methods of joining:

1. Mirroring or mimicking—matching the family's mood, pace, communication patterns, or kinesthetic cues (e.g., becoming jovial or somber, communication becoming terse or punctuated with long pauses, becoming fidgety)

2. Respecting families' values and hierarchies (e.g., if one spouse is the central switchboard, addressing all communication through that spouse first)

3. Keying in culturally when possible or finding elements of kindship (e.g., "I have an adolescent boy too")

4. Searching for strength—observing for the minutest positive detail about individual family members that the nurse can highlight and thereby confirm the individual's sense of self and make contact with him (e.g., appreciating a clever phrase or a preteen's poised manner)

5. Supporting family subsystems (e.g., giving smaller children toys to play with while talking to older ones or having parents sit together as they discuss their difficulty with the children)

6. Tracking—asking for elaboration with concrete details and examples of specific content in the family's discussion, which serves to confirm individuals who are speaking as well as to explore family structure (e.g., tracking a mother's mentioning that she and her son are close by

asking what time of the day and in which part of the home they are closest, thus learning that the mother and son sleep together while father sleeps in another room)

Another task of the nurse during the initial formation of the therapeutic system is the struggle to assume leadership in the session. The nurse therapist must accommodate sufficiently to the family to enter the system while at the same time maintaining the leadership position. She must join while still retaining the freedom to confront and challenge. She can assume leadership by presenting herself as an expert, gaining the family's confidence and instilling hope. She establishes the rules of the system, such as who attends the session, that no one talks for another, and that no one interrupts. She controls the flow of communication and directs who is to speak to whom.

At the beginning of the session she must contact each member. At that point, she will be presented with the public mask. She must not spend more than 15 to 20 minutes with an individual before moving to contact the next member of she will get sucked into the system. Very soon she must ask two people to interact directly to enact a problem they have been describing. The public mask then falls away and the nurse can make direct observation of dysfunctional interactions. Rather than going from content issue to content issue or participating in a litany of the past, the nurse therapist can introduce the conflict inherent in small events. She can be immediately involved in a conflictual situation by highlighting a nonevent and creating an affective event.

Menuchin is a master of this technique of transforming minute simple nonevents and ballooning them for therapeutic intervention. For example, in a demonstration videotape, within the first 5 minutes of the session Menuchin transformed the nonevent of a father "helping" the identified patient, the adolescent son, adjust his video microphone wire into a therapeutic intervention around the family's infantalization of the son. Menuchin maintains that the amount of knowledge needed about the family to diagnose and begin restructuring dysfunctional interactions is available quickly.[31] Structural family therapy does not explore or interpret the past. It is active and immediate.

Diagnosis in family therapy is based on the nurse's accommodation and joining the family and observing and experiencing the pulls of the family on her behavior as well as observing her impact on the family. The interactional diagnosis is not fixed in time but alters as the family accommodates to or resists the therapist's restructuring interventions. It also varies depending on which family subsystem is active in the therapeutic situation at any one time. In this way diagnosis and therapy are inseparable.

Restructuring

The aim of restructuring interventions is to transform the dysfunctional transactional patterns that maintain symptomatic behavior. The nurse is concerned not only about symptom removal but also about changing the organization of the family so the symtpom does not get passed on. However, if an area of organization such as the parents' relationship does not contribute to the symptom Menuchin does not enter there. He feels constrained by the family's presenting symptom.

Menuchin identifies seven categories of restructuring operations: enacting family transactional patterns, marking boundaries, escalating stress, assigning tasks, using symptoms, manipulating mood, and supporting, educating, or guiding.

Enacting transactional patterns, as described earlier, involves family members actively discussing an event that they might otherwise be describing to the nurse.[26] Instead, the nurse instructs specific members to discuss the matter between themselves. In this way she disengages from the interaction to observe and watch for nonverbal confirmation or contradiction of the content, patterned sequences, interruptions, distractions, alliances, and coalitions. Thus the nurse can see the family in action and make direct observations of how they naturally resolve conflicts, support each other, or diffuse stress. The nurse may find it difficult to stay outside these transactions, permitting the family to drag her back into direct discussion. Going behind a one-way mirror after giving the family clear directions is a way to avoid this temptation. Manipulating space by rearranging seating or position can be an effective way of encouraging or intensifying dialogue. The seating pattern a family assumes when it first walks into a session provides clues to alliances, coalitions, centrality, and isolation. The nurse's manipulation of seating and space can be a diagnostic probe to see how flexible the family is to such change, as well as a graphic indication to the family of a therapeutic goal. For instance, seating the spatially isolated father next to his son where the mother was seated and placing her next to the nurse suggests the goal of more direct involvement between father and son, with the mother outside that relationship.

The *marking of both individual and subsystem boundaries* in a family promotes clarity in the enmeshed families and reduces rigidity in disengaged families. Simple rules such as that family members speak *to* each other and not *about* each other, no one speaks for another, no one may interrupt, and no one acts as another's memory bank promote individual autonomy. Subsystem boundaries are encouraged by the nurse's inclusion or exclusion of various subsystems attending a session. She would ask children to leave or not attend a session in discussing spouses' sex life. The assignment of tasks such as instructing the father and daughter to go out for a pizza once a week without the mother or younger siblings also promotes subsystem boundaries. Having the sibling subsystem interact in a session, with the mother behind a one-way mirror, gives the children the opportunity to find alternate ways to resolve conflicts normally interrupted by mother's interventions. At the same time, this gives mother the opportunity to identify more positive interaction among the children when before she could only reflexively react to their anger, rebelliousness, and selfishness by intruding on their boundaries. Rigid triads involving cross-generational interactions can be especially resistant to boundary marking.

Escalating stress in a family forces members to develop alternative, more functional, ways of resolving stress. In families seeking treatment, dysfunctional patterns have developed around the symptomatic member. Operations that escalate stress can include blocking the usual transactional patterns and emphasizing differences the family was glossing over. Asking for the customarily silent spouse's opinion following the dominant spouse's statements or asking a member to describe a disqualifying facial expression serves to highlight unspoken family disagreements. Developing implicit conflict involves making covert conflict overt.

Families develop methods for diffusing conflict rapidly, such as the noisy teasing or shoving between two young brothers that occurred before the parents' conflict could surface openly. Blocking the sibling conflict forced the parents to contact directly. Polarizing extant conflict in a family provides the nurse with an opening into the system. A husband and wife were presenting to the nurse a picture of equal helplessness in the face of their adolescent son's delinquent activities. Asking the husband if he had ever tried telling his wife she was "messing up" with the son polarized the positions of the overprotective mother and the "reasonable" distant father. The nurse can produce stress by temporarily joining one member or subsystem in alliance or coalition. This operation must be carefully planned and requires the nurse's ability to disengage or else she will be sucked into the system. She can do this serially to help members take differentiated positions or can form a coalition, usually with a spouse, when the system rigidly resists open conflict. Joining a husband's attack on the wife makes the conflict too intense for the wife to diffuse stress onto the son. She is forced to address the conflict between herself and the husband.

The *assigning of tasks*, either in or outside the session, structures the setting for alternative interactions and behavior to occur between family members. In designing tasks the nurse must have a clear idea of the family's structure and dysfunctional patterns and have specific interactional goals to be accomplished through the task. Tasks can be such simple directions in a session as asking a husband and wife to sit next to each other as they discuss an issue. In a family in which the wife carries all discipline functions with the children, excluding the father, the father is assigned the job. The mother is instructed to handle only emergencies; otherwise, the father is to be informed of infractions he does not directly observe himself. The wife may not interfere with her husband's disciplinary tactics. She is to take note of the results of the discipline on the children's behavior. This can shift the skewed balance of parental authority so both parents become active and effective.

In assigning tasks it is good to give all critically involved members a portion of the task to complete. It reduces the likelihood of one member sabotaging the new behavior of another if each has a focus on himself. It also makes it easier to relinquish a fixed behavior if another behavior is assigned to replace it. Whether the task is completed or not, the family and nurse have new information about family patterns and progress.

Symptoms can be used in restructuring operations in various ways.[26] Symptoms may be focused on, as in a family Menuchin describes in which the daughter was a fire setter. The focus remained on the daughter, but the mother was instructed to spend time daily teaching the daughter how to light matches safely. This promoted a closer mother-daughter relationship, which was previously obstructed, while retaining a helpful focus on the symptom. Symptoms can be exaggerated to increase their intensity and mobilize family resources, such as by telling a severely depressed middle-aged husband to sit Shiva (Jewish tradition of 7 days' mourning) for the part of himself that is dead. A symptom can be relabeled, as in the case of a mother who continually nagged critically at the son. Redefining her nagging as concern opened the way for more positive caring interactions. Moving to a new symptom entails shifting the family's focus and intensity onto another family member temporarily. In the family in which the husband was failing to go to work and the wife alternately protected him and threatened to leave him, identifying her behavior as seriously depressed reduce her intense focus on the husband. A symptom's effect can also be changed, thereby altering interactions around it. An example would be in the family with the fire setter when the mother was encouraged to interact with the daughter in a competent, educating fashion.

Manipulating the family's mood is another restructuring operation. An exaggerated initiation of the predominant family affect might mobilize counteraffect in the family, thereby initiating a wider range of expression. The nurse can also model a more appropriate affect for the family, for example, reacting with strong indignation to a young boy's criticism of his mother. This promotes respect and clarifies the boundaries of a passive enmeshed parental subsystem.[26]

Support, education, and guidance can be a restructuring operation. They can take the form of modeling, assigning tasks, or sharing of concrete information. Menuchin repeatedly points out to families how they program each other in the circular process of a family system.

The goal of structural family therapy is not a change in behavior but a change in the organization of the whole family, allowing individual members a new experience in the family.[26] Using a model of an effectively functioning family, the therapist joins the family in a therapeutic system with the intent of restructuring it in a defined way. The restructuring either facilitates the maintenance of functional subsystems or helps to form new subsystems that will promote healing and growth.

Strategic, problem-solving, or brief family therapy

Communication theory has undergone evolutionary changes since the well-known double-bind theory was first proposed by a group of researchers in Palo Alto, California, in 1956.[3] These changes have revolutionary implications for the practice of psychotherapy. Out of communication theory has developed strategic short-term, or problem-solving, family therapy.

The original communication theorists included Gregory Bateson, John Weakland, and Jay Haley, with Don Jackson and William Fry consulting. The focus of their early study was the nature of observable face-to-face communication, verbal and nonverbal, among members of a family or other ongoing social group, and its significance for the shaping of actual behavior.[41] The clearest explication of early communications theory is in *Pragmatics of Human Communication* by Watzlawick, Beaven, and Jackson.[39] Communication theorists contend that *all* behavior, not only verbal productions, is communication, and since there is no such thing as nonbehavior, it is impossible not to communicate.[38] The theorists recognized that most communication does not consist of simple declarative messages but rather a multiplicity of levels of communication between sender and receiver. The verbal and nonverbal levels of a message necessarily modify and qualify each other. That is, the significance of any message depends on how it is reinforced, confirmed, contradicted, or specially framed by other simultaneous, preceding, or following messages. These (along with the setting and the relationship between sender and receiver) constitute the context that must be considered in interpreting any message.[41]

Another basic tenet of communication theory is that communication is an ongoing process. Originally, for purposes of analysis, communication was broken down into discrete units of "stimulus" and "response" in a linear structure reflecting cause-and-effect thinking. It later became apparent that this was both inaccurate and inappropriate. There is no beginning point or end point in the stimulus-response-reinforcement pattern of human interaction (referred to later as a positive feedback loop). Obviously, in most relationships, the behavior of each participant is predicated on the behavior of the other. In families, complex, highly patterned, repetitive interactions become established.

With the communications model, when a two-person (or more) system is dysfunctional in its communication, there is potential for a pathological condition. Studying communication patterns in schizophrenic families, the researchers identified several forms of "pathological communication." Disqualification in communication includes self-contradictions, inconsistencies, subject switches, tangentializations, incomplete sentences, misunderstandings, obscure mannerisms of speech, and literal interpretations of metaphor and vice versa.[39] An example of disqualification is a question an older brother used to baffle his younger sister: "Do you walk to school or carry your lunch?" Disconfirmation in communication involves ignoring or invalidating essential elements of a significant other's view of himself, telling the person you do not feel the way you feel, need what you need, or experience what you experience.[32] Incongruent communication is delivering two conflicting messages simultaneously, whereby if the receiver responds to either message, he will be charged with badness or madness. This is the basis of the double-bind or paradoxical injunction. An example is the command "Be spontaneous!" or, from Greenberg's collection of maternal communications, "Give your son Marvin two sport shirts as a present. The first time he wears one of them, look at him sadly and say in your Basic Tone of Voice: 'The other one you didn't like?'"[38:111] Finally, symptoms are means of communication; the symptomatic person is convinced the symptoms are out of his control, while the symptoms can serve as a controlling mechanism in the family. Psychosomatic symptoms come under this description.

The treatment goals of family therapy, based on the early communicational view of behavior, were to correct pathological patterns of communication and to promote functional communication between family members in which members express themselves clearly and directly and ask for and receive feedback. Thus behavioral change would occur in the family as a result of direct, clear, unambiguous communication.[32] From their research of schizophrenic families, the Palo Alto group expanded their research and practice to other kinds of clinical

problems, recognizing that the manifestations of schizophrenia included much that was characteristic of other clinical problems. From their observations of here-and-now communication in families, it was a short conceptual leap to the formulation of strategic family therapy.

In 1966 Fisch proposed the establishment of the Brief Therapy Center of the Mental Research Institute in Palo Alto, California. He was joined by Watzlawick and Weakland, all previously involved in the communication research under Jackson at the Mental Research Institute. They shared an attitude toward treatment concerning the function (the "what") rather than the meaning (the "why"), of behavior and they were looking for tools to shorten treatment and facilitate change. Initially, the therapeutic interventions that seemed to do this appeared gimmicky, but they gradually evolved a conceptual framework to explain these successful interventions. Their focus was on how symptoms or human problems arise and how they are resolved, especially through paradoxical intervention.[38] Simultaneously with their work on the West Coast, Haley[24] developed the problem-focused family therapy approach through his association with Menuchin, Erikson, and Montalvo on the East Coast. What sets strategic family therapy apart from structural and systems therapy is its primary goal, which is the removal of the presenting symptom through directives or tasks in conjunction with the use of paradox.

Whether one speaks of problems or symptoms, they are not an entity in their own right. A problem is only a problem when it is labeled as such by those involved. A problem is behavior between two or more people that one or more persons do not like and which persists despite efforts to change.[19] Strategic therapists make a distinction between difficulties and problems. Difficulties are either undesirable states of affairs that can be removed by a logical solution or undesirable, common life problems that must simply be lived with.[40] Problems commonly stem from small difficulties that escalate and are maintained by mishandling of attempts to solve them. Mishandling most frequently occurs around adaptation to ordinary life events and ranges from (1) ignoring or denying difficulties on which action should be taken to (2) attempting to resolve an ordinary life difficulty that is unnecessary (e.g., a husband who would not talk to his wife before breakfast) or impossible (e.g., the generation gap) to resolve to (3) a wide area of difficulties where action is needed but the wrong kind is taken.[41]

Strategic family therapists are not concerned

with the history of the problem or the motivation behind it. They are not interested in characteristics of people (passive, hostile, hysterical) and they place no importance on insight. Little distinction is made between acute and chronic problems. Chronic problems are simply ones that have been mishandled longer. The presenting problem behavior and the problem-maintaining behavior is the primary focus of treatment.

Communication theorists borrowed from cybernetics when they identified a positive feedback loop in human interaction. This is the vicious cycle that develops from efforts by family members or the identified patient himself to stop or "help" undesirable behavior. For example, the rebellious teenager, when faced with parental discipline, will become increasingly rebellious. As the discipline becomes harsher, the boy's behavior escalates further. Thus "the action which is meant to alleviate the behavior of the other party, in actual fact, aggravates it."[14:610] From this view, the cause and the nature of a problem are essentially the same process. People try to change behavior in the most logical way possible. Common sense suggests prevention or avoidance of undesirable behavior by means of the reciprocal or opposite behavior. If this does not work, they try harder with the same behavior. The resolution of problems therefore requires a change of the problem-maintaining behaviors so as to interrupt the vicious positive feedback cycles.[41]

Interdiction in the system can be either at the point of the identified patient, the nonidentified patient, or both, depending on who is the "customer," that is, the person most uncomfortable or most concerned with the problem and thus most willing to change. Effective intervention can be made through any member of the system to break the positive feedback loop. This is illustrated in Clinical example 25-4.

CLINICAL EXAMPLE 25-4

A colonel is being militarily strict with his son, and the boy is becoming increasingly defiant. The therapist tells the father his son is "going to the dogs." The therapist then suggests that the father hold back on his discipline to get a baseline measurement of just how bad the boy's behavior will get. As pressure on the boy is reduced, his behavior improves.

Another example is a woman who suffered from urinary frequency. She was isolated both at home, feeling unable to leave the house to socialize, and at work because she had her machine set by the bathroom door where there were no co-workers. She worked from 12 to 8 PM. The therapist instructed her to urinate as many times as she felt she had

to each morning before going to work but to use the toilet only three times; after that she was to urinate sitting in the tub. She was to make no effort to change her pattern at work. The next week the woman reported she had been in agony the first morning but was unable to urinate sitting in the tub. She then figured that if she could limit herself at home, she could do so at work, and had no further urinary frequency.[5]

These examples demonstrate the use of reversal or symptom prescription, which carry the message "do not change" or "more of it," both of which stop the family or patient from trying to stop. The task of persuading people to change the very behavior that common sense tells them should help often requires treatment strategies which appear "weird," illogical, or paradoxical.

Since the focus of treatment is symptomatic, the nurse's first task is to obtain a clear statement from the patient of the presenting complaint in specific concrete terms. As Haley states, "Problems . . . should be something one can count, observe, measure, or in some way know one is influencing."[24:40] After the nurse obtains a detailed description of the problem and determines what about the behavior makes it a problem, she then gathers an account of what solutions the family has tried. This tells her which remedies to avoid and indicates the problem-maintaining behavior. Next the nurse asks what the family's or patient's minimal goal of treatment would be—what smallest identifiable change would signify progress or some success. General goals such as "improved communication" are not acceptable, nor are feeling changes such as "to feel happier" or negative goals such as "to stop certain behavior." Rather, the nurse seeks positive statement-of-action goals that delineate what people would be doing to reflect an attitude or feeling change. According to the cybernetic view, if a small but significant change can be made in what appeared to be a hopeless situation, a so-called ripple effect may occur. That is, "once a patient is mobilized and regains confidence in his ability to solve problems, he sometimes finds that he can tackle other difficulties."[30:47]

As soon as possible, the therapist attempts to grasp the patient's "language" and the ideas and values that appear central to him. "Tuning into" the family's view and then extending that view is the critical step that precedes the therapist's concisely formulated strategic intervention. This step is known as reframing. To reframe means to change the conceptual or emotional setting or viewpoint in relation to which a situation is experienced and, by using language that is congenial to the family's world view, place it in another frame that fits the "facts" of the same concrete situation equally well and thereby changes its entire meaning.[19,38] An example of reframing includes using the component of hostility when it is present in a woman's frigidity and reframing the problem as one produced by her overprotecting the male. Since, assuming there is a hostile component and protecting the husband is the last thing she would want to do, the new frame to the problem uses the hostility as an incentive to release her inhibited sexual feelings. When Tom Sawyer reframed whitewashing the picket fence as an artistic entertaining enterprise rather than a dreary chore, he utilized his derisive friends' competitiveness to vie for the opportunity to whitewash. Reframing brings about an attitudinal change and a change in emphasis of the facts of a situation. This thereby changes the meaning of the situation to permit new behavior while the concrete facts remain unchanged.

A team of Italian family therapists, lead by the psychoanalyst Mara Selvini Palazoli has gained increasing recognition in the United States for its successful short-term therapy with anorectic families[28] and most recently with schizophrenic families.[29] The team functions with two co-therapists working directly with the family while their two colleagues observe and support them behind a one-way mirror. Interventions, designed by the whole team, address each family member's cyclical behavior that perpetuates the problem. At the heart of their therapy is the use of paradoxical injunctions. Interventions are designed to produce resistance in the family, which in turn brings about the desired change in behavior.

Strategic therapists place no importance on the therapist having therapy. This is seen more as residue from earlier psychoanalytical thought. The nurse can be trained in this theoretical framework and learn the skills consistent with this approach without understanding her own involvement with her family. Structural therapists share this view.[24]

Strategic therapists are attacked for the "manipulative, insincere" nature of their approach. They emphatically acknowledge that this is the case. Communication research made clear that it is not possible not to communicate. An extension of that is that it is not possible not to influence. A nondirective, dynamically oriented therapist influences the patient's communication in hundreds of subtle ways, including body movement, intonation, and leading responses. If the therapist does this out of conscious awareness, she is said to be not manipulating. The "insight" school and the nondirective school of therapy influence patients outside of the patient's awareness throughout the process of therapy. Strategic therapists do so openly. The patient's "awareness" of the manipulation itself is irrelevant as long as the directive or strategy is given and followed. The difference between the two schools of psychotherapy is a conceptual one rather than an ethical one. The "insight" school believes that change in people comes about through the therapeutic relationship with a change in their understanding of themselves. The strategic school persuades a person to change "spontaneously" by arranging a situation so that the person initiates the change in behavior.[24]

The strategic therapy model views the therapist as an active and deliberate change agent who is expected to formulate a strategy that will bring about the change the patient is paying money to achieve. The responsibility for success or failure therefore rests on the nurse, although the nurse never takes the credit for change in the patient's eyes. In this therapy the point at which termination takes place is clear. According to Fisch and co-workers:

> If a therapist accepts the patient's complaint as a reason for starting therapy with him, he should, by the same logic, accept his statement of satisfactory improvement as a reason (and time) for terminating treatment.[14:599]

Conclusion

The theoretical models of family therapy presented in this chapter are diverse and at times conflicting. There are, however, threads of similarity in the characteristics of a well-functioning family identified by the various theoretical views. These common characteristics suggest directions any nurse might take when intervening with families to promote health or prevent illness. Reducing the intensity of anxiety and stress in a family reduces the likelihood of secondary stress symptoms, such as divorce, exacerbation of disease, death or accidental injury of a family member, or conflictual interpersonal relationships. In the high-stress setting of the general hospital, anxiety in a family escalates when their questions, feelings, and fears are not openly expressed to medical staff or when medical staff fail to listen attentively or answer directly. Family and staff mutually attempt not to "upset" the other person by bringing up emotion-laden subjects, such as terminal illness, death, or disfigurement. In an atmosphere of mutual avoidance of taboo subjects a closed communication system develops between medical staff and family. The nurse who can handle her own anxiety about the issues of acute and chronic illness and death can listen and respond empathically but nonreactively to patients and families, share factual information clearly, and thus promote open communication systems. Opening closed communication system reduces the intensity of a family's emotional reaction to illness and death.

Nurses working in obstetrics and pediatrics are in contact with families at the outset of a normative crisis in family life, that is, at the addition of another member into a homeostatic family system. The expectation of families at this time (except when the pregnancy is an unwanted one) is that the event will be joyful and satisfying. Mothers especially, when confronted with feelings of helplessness or inadequacy, severe anxiety or panic, and, perhaps, occasional almost homicidal rage at the spouse or infant, are frightened and believe something is wrong with them. They fail to perceive their reactions as predictable reactions in a crisis situation. As nurses educate families to the concept of normative life crises, the family's anxiety diminishes. They are less likely to view their emotional reactions as problems and more likely to see them as normal responses to transitional family stress.

For the nurse therapist working with couples or families in treatment, the sense of bewilderment and information overload, which is characteristic of the therapist in a family treatment situation, is what makes this work the most exciting as well as the most difficult. To stay afloat in this sea of data, it is important for the nurse to develop a thorough understanding of one conceptual framework for herself. She can then use treatment strategies and techniques from various models that are congruent with the theoretical framework she has developed. Her choice of strategy would depend on her assessment of the specific family and the level at which she decided to intervene.

The essence of family therapy is conceptualizing the nature of human relationship problems or behavioral disorders within the natural context in which they arise within the family. The family, as a system, seeks to maintain a dynamic equilibrium. Change in any one part of the system shifts the balance, resulting in alterations throughout the system. By recognizing this and using it as leverage for therapeutic change, family therapy aims to be effective.

Suggested cross-references

Assessment of families is discussed in Chapter 4. Vulnerable families are discussed in Chapters 5 and 19. Working with families of psychiatric patients is discussed in Chapter 6.

SUMMARY

1. Family therapy is not a modality of treatment but rather a way of conceptualizing human relationship problems. It focuses on the context in which an emotional problem is generated. The process between family members that supports and perpetuates symptoms is considered to be the focus of treatment rather than the individual family member who manifests the family's problems.

2. Characteristics of the well-functioning family, common dysfunctional family patterns, and indications for family therapy were described. The role of

both the generalist and specialist nurse in family therapy was identified.

3. Bowen's family systems therapy was the first theoretical model discussed. It moved away from the medical model and a psychopathological point of view to conceptualize all family systems on a continuum ranging from total dysfunction to high levels of functioning. A cornerstone in systems theory is separating the thinking and feeling processes of family members. The goal of systems therapy is for individual family members to differentiate themselves from the family emotional "we-ness" system.

4. Seven central interlocking concepts of systems theory were discussed:

 a. *Differentiation* reflects sufficient separation between intellect and emotions so that one is not dominated by the reactive anxiety of the family's emotional system.

 b. A *triangle* is a predictable emotional process that takes place in any significant relationship when there is difficulty in the relationship. The nurse must identify key triangles in her own family and work to detriangle herself to be more effective with her families in therapy.

 c. The *nuclear family emotional system* refers to patterns of interaction between family members and the degree to which these patterns promote emotional fusion. Three mechanisms used to reduce the level of fusion between spouses were discussed.

 d. The *multigenerational transmission process* is the assumption that relationship patterns and symptoms in a family have their origin several generations before. A four- or five-generation genogram reveals such patterns.

 e. The *family projection process* is the projection of spouses' problems onto one or more children to avoid the intense emotional fusion between the spouses.

 f. One's *sibling position,* that is, birth order and sex, is a determining factor in a person's personality profile.

 g. The *emotional cutoff* is a dysfunctional way in which some family members deal with intense family conflict by using either emotional isolation or geographical distance.

Various modes of therapy from a family system framework were described.

5. Structural family therapy, as conceptualized by Menuchin, was the second theoretical model discussed. Structural therapy assumes that behavior and the family's level of function are a consequence of the organization of the family and the interactional patterns between family members.

 a. According to the structural view, a family is a social system in transformation.

 b. The family goes through predictable developmental stages over time, requiring adaptive restructuring of the family.

 c. The major elements of a family structure that enable the viable functioning of the family were identified as (1) a power hierarchy with different levels of authority, (2) differentiated subsystems that have different functions and levels of power,

and (3) subsystem boundaries that are sufficiently well defined to prevent intrusion but sufficiently permeable to permit emotional contact between members. Families with extremely diffuse or extremely rigid boundaries are called enmeshed or disengaged families, respectively.

6. Tasks of the nurse according to this structural model include defining boundaries and supporting the functions of family subsystems. Goals of the initial interview include joining the family, assuming leadership in the session, and instructing family members to interact and thereby enact the family conflict. Family interactional diagnoses alter as the family reacts to interventions. Restructuring interventions serve to transform dysfunctional transactional patterns that maintain symptomatic behavior. Restructuring includes enacting transactional patterns, marking boundaries, escalating stress, assigning tasks, using symptoms, manipulating the family mood, and support, education, and guidance of the family.

7. Strategic, or brief, family therapy was the third theoretical model discussed. This model evolved on the West Coast from the earlier work of the communication theorists. Important principles of communication theory include the following:

 a. All behavior is communication; therefore it is impossible not to communicate.

 b. The meaning of a message includes the content and the context in which it was sent.

 c. Communication is an ongoing process of stimulus-response-reinforcement. Communication theorists studied the interactional patterns in schizophrenic families and identified pathological communication patterns. Correcting these patterns became the goal of treatment.

8. Strategic therapists are concerned with the removal of problematical behavioral patterns or symptoms. They assume problems arise from small difficulties and are maintained by mishandled attempts to resolve them. The focus of treatment according to this model is to intervene in the problem-perpetuating, positive feedback loop in human interaction and break the vicious cycle. Effective therapeutic intervention frequently involves the use of paradox and reverse psychology. The goals of strategic therapy include obtaining a clear statement from the client of the presenting complaint in specific concrete terms and reframing the problem, which thereby changes the meaning of the situation and thus permits new behavior to occur.

9. Knowledge of theoretical models of family therapy can assist the nurse when intervening in health promotion and illness prevention with families in a variety of settings. The nurse therapist should use one conceptual framework in her work with families and integrate various treatment strategies and techniques as appropriate.

References

1. Ackerman, N.: The growing edge of family therapy. In Sager, C., and Kaplan, H., editors: Progress in group and family therapy, New York, 1972, Brunner/Mazel, Inc.
2. Barragan, M.: The child-centered family. In Guerin, P., editor: Family therapy theory and practice, New York, 1976, Gardner Press, Inc.
3. Bateson, G., Jackson, D., Haley, J., and Weakland, J.: Toward a theory of schizophrenia, Behav. Sci. 1:251, 1956.
4. Beels, C., and Ferber, A.: Family therapy: a view, Fam. Process 8:280, 1969.
5. Berensen, D.: An interview with Richard Fisch, The Family 3(1):24, 1976.
6. Bowen, M.: Intrafamily dynamics in emotional illness. In D'Agostino, A., editor: Family, church, and community, New York, 1961, P.J. Kennedy & Sons.
7. Bowen, M.: Family psychotherapy with schizophrenia in the hospital and in private practice. In Bosormenyi-Nagy, I., and Framo, J., editors: Intensive family therapy, New York, 1965, Harper & Row, Publishers, Inc.
8. Bowen, M.: Family therapy and family group therapy. In Kaplan, H., and Sadock, B., editors: Comprehensive group psychotherapy, Baltimore, 1971, The Williams & Wilkins Co.
9. Bowen, M.: Multigenerational transmission process. In Haley, J., editor: Changing families, New York, 1971, Grune & Stratton, Inc.
10. Bowen, M.: The use of family therapy in clinical practice. In Haley, J., editor: Changing families. New York, 1971, Grune & Stratton, Inc.
11. Bowen, M.: Theory in the practice of psychotherapy. In Guerin, P., editor: Family therapy theory and practice, New York, 1976, Gardner Press, Inc.
12. Cain, A.: The role of the therapist in family systems therapy, The Family 3(2):65, 1976.
13. Carter, B.: In a family therapy workshop, Bridgeport, Conn., 1976.
14. Fisch, R., Watzlawick, P., Weakland, S., and Bodin, A.: On unbecoming family therapists. In Ferber, A., Mendelson, M., and Napier, A., editors: The book of family therapy, New York, 1972, Science House, Inc.
15. Fogarty, T.: Family structure in terms of triangles. In Bradt, J., and Moynihan, C., editors: Systems therapy, Washington, D.C., 1971, The Groome Child Guidance Center.
16. Fogarty, T.: The family emotional self system. A day with a family workshop, New Rochelle, N.Y., CFL sampler, Jan. 4, 1975.
17. Fogarty, T.: Triangles, The Family 2:165, Spring-Summer 1975.
18. Fogarty, T.: System concepts and dimensions of self. In Guerin, P., editor: Family therapy theory and practice, New York, 1976, Gardner Press, Inc.
19. Goolishian, H.: Problem focused family therapy, Orthopsychiatry Workshop, New York, April 1977.
20. Guerin, P.: System, system, who's got the system, The Family 3(1):13, 1976.
21. Guerin, P.: Theoretical aspects and clinical relevance of the multigenerational model of family therapy. In Guerin, P., editor: Family theory and practice, New York, 1976, Gardner Press, Inc.
22. Guerin, P., and Pendagast, E.: Evaluation of family system and genogram. In Guerin, P., editor: Family therapy theory and practice, New York, 1976, Gardner Press, Inc.
23. Haley, J.: Uncommon therapy, the psychiatric techniques of Multon H. Erickson, M.D., New York, 1973, W.W. Norton & Co.
24. Haley, J.: Problem solving therapy, San Francisco, 1976, Jossey-Bass, Inc.
25. Klugman, J.: Owning and disowning: the structural dimension, Fam. Process 16:353, 1977.
26. Menuchin, S.: Families and family therapy, Cambridge, Mass., 1974, Harvard University Press.
27. Menuchin, S. et al.: A conceptual model of psychosomatic illness in children, Arch. Gen. Psychiatry 32:1031, 1975.
28. Palazoli, M.: Self-starvation, New York, 1978, Jason Aronson, Inc.
29. Palazoli, M., Cecchin, G., Prata, G., and Boscolo, L.: Paradox and counterparadox, New York, 1979, Jason Aronson, Inc.
30. Rabkin, R.: Strategic psychotherapy, New York, 1977, Basic Books, Inc.
31. Ritterman, M.: Paradigmatic classification of family therapy theories, Fam. Process 16:29, March 1977.
32. Steidl, J., and Wexler, J.: What's a clinician to do with so many approaches to family therapy? The Family 4(2):59, 1977.
33. Stierlin, H.: The dynamics of owning and disowning: psychoanalytic and family perspectives, Fam. Process 15:277, 1976.
34. Strelnick, A.H.: Multiple family group therapy: a review of the literature, Fam. Process 16:307, 1977.
35. Terkelsen, K.: Bowen on triangles—March, 1974, workshop. I, The Family 1(2):45, 1974.
36. Terkelsen, K.: Bowen on triangles—March, 1974, workshop. II, The Family 2:1, 1974.
37. Toman, W.: Family constellation, New York, 1961, Springer Publishing Co.
38. Watzlawick, P.: Some basic issues in interaction research. In Framo, J., editor: Family interaction, New York, 1972, Springer Publishing Co.
39. Watzlawick, P., Beaven, J., and Jackson, D.: Pragmatics of human communication, New York, 1967, W.W. Norton & Co.
40. Watzlawick, P., Weakland, J., and Fisch, R.: Change, principles of problem formation and problem resolution, New York, 1974, W.W. Norton & Co.
41. Weakland, J.: Communication theory and clinical change. In Guerin, P., editor: Family therapy theory and practice, New York, 1976, Gardner Press, Inc.
42. Whitaker, C., and Miller, M.: A re-evaluation of psychiatric help when divorce impends. In Sager, C.J., and Kaplan, H.S.: editors: Progress in group and family therapy, New York, 1972, Brunner/Mazel, Inc.

Annotated suggested readings

Anonymous: Toward the differentiation of a self in one's own family. In Framo, J., editor: Family interaction: a dialogue between family therapists and family researchers, New York, 1972, Springer Publishing Co.

Originally published anonymously, this work by Bowen describes his efforts to differentiate himself from his family of origin. He effectively demonstrates the application of family systems theory with his own family. It is a classic in systems theory.

Bowen, M.: Family therapy and family group therapy. In Kaplan, H., and Sadock, B., editors: Comprehensive group psychotherapy, Baltimore, 1971, The Williams & Wilkins Co.

In this article, Bowen presents the theoretical framework of family systems theory. The evolution of Bowen's technique from his theory is clear from his discussion and case examples.

Bowen, M.: Family therapy in clinical practice, New York, 1978, Jason Aronson, Inc.

The development of Bowen's thinking is collected in one volume containing all his previously published articles plus several original ones. Most of the earlier articles in this volume have become "classics." This is an important text for any student who wishes to understand systems theory in depth.

Bradt, J., and Moynihan, C.: Systems therapy, Washington, D.C., 1971, Groome Child Guidance Center.

This is a collection of outstanding papers presented at the Georgetown Family Symposia from 1966 to 1971. It includes theoretical papers, research, and descriptions of clinical application and technique from a family systems framework. It is a good text for the beginning family therapist.

Cain, A.: The role of the therapist in family systems therapy, The Family 3(2):65, 1976.

A nurse therapist describes the process of systems therapy, and the pitfalls involved in working with a family in treatment.

Carter, E., and McGoldrick, M.: The family life cycle, a framework for family therapy, New York, 1980, Gardner Press, Inc.

This volume contains a series of original contributions from well-known practitioners in the family therapy field. The chapters systematically cover the developmental stages of the family life cycle and commonly encountered family problems that disrupt the life cycle, including chronic illness and death, divorce and remarriage, and poverty. The concept of the family life cycle is a clinically useful and important one to nurse family therapists, as well as nurses outside of psychiatry who work closely with their patients' families. This is a valuable text for beginning and advanced students alike.

Ferber, A., Mendelsohn, M., and Napier, A.: The book of family therapy, New York, 1972, Science House, Inc.

In conversational tones many well-known persons in the family therapy field discuss personal and theoretical views of their own work. This is a recommended book for a beginner in the field.

Fogarty, T.: Triangles, The Family 2:11, Spring-Summer 1975.

This article thoroughly examines the family systems concept of triangles. It is an important article for the advanced student.

Guerin, P., editor: Family therapy and practice, New York, 1976, Gardner Press, Inc.

This book contains a series of original contributions from the most distinguished leaders in the family therapy field. It is an excellent reference text for the beginning and advanced student. Theory and technique from several frameworks are presented in a clear organized fashion.

Haley, J., editor: Changing families, New York, 1971, Grune & Stratton, Inc.

This is a well-selected collection of articles by well-known authors in the field covering a spectrum of theoretical approaches to family therapy. Many of the articles contained in this volume have become "classics."

Haley, J.: Uncommon therapy, the psychiatric techniques of Milton H. Erickson, M.D., New York, 1973, W.W. Norton & Co.

Milton Erickson is a highly regarded pioneer and leader in the family therapy field. In this volume Haley has carefully edited and explicated hours of recorded cases Dr. Erickson has treated. The use of paradoxical intention is demonstrated in multiple examples.

Haley, J.: Problem solving therapy, San Francisco, 1976, Jossey-Bass, Inc.

In this book the author presents the problem-focused, strategic approach to family therapy in a clear, organized manner. Theory and technique are richly supported with case example. This is an important text for beginners and advanced students alike.

Haley, J.: Leaving home: the therapy of disturbed young people, New York, 1980, McGraw-Hill, Inc.

This practical, down-to-earth book focuses on the problems and solutions surrounding the transition of leaving home, when young people become self-supporting and independent of their families. It suggests and explicates a model of therapy to be used with families who are stuck in this crucial transition piont. Case histories and interview excerpts illustrate the methods of therapy.

Jones, S.: Family therapy, a comparison of approaches, Englewood Cliffs, N.J., 1980, Prentice-Hall, Inc.

As the title implies, this book comprehensively reviews and compares different theoretical models of family therapy currently in practice, including Bowenian, structural, strategic, behavioral, psychoanalytical theories. It is a valuable resource for beginning students in the field.

Klugman, J.: "Enmeshment and fusion," Fam. Process 15:321, 1976.

This concise article examines and contrasts the differences between two seemingly synonymous concepts from the structural and systems framework respectively.

Lederer, W., and Jackson, D.: The mirages of marriage, New York, 1968, W.W. Norton & Co.

This book is intended for families and therapists alike. It explodes false myths and assumptions about the marriage relationship and offers some no-nonsense suggestions for solving readily recognized marital problems from a communication theory framework.

Madanes, C.: Strategic family therapy, San Francisco, 1981, Jossey-Bass, Inc., Publishers.

This is a recent book by a leader in strategic family therapy. The focus is on destructive unequal power structures in symptomatic families. She describes both straightforward interventions and paradoxical interventions with commonly encountered family, marital, and parent-child problems. The wide range of case studies included demonstrate her theoretical framework and strategies for intervention. This is a valuable book for the beginning and advanced student alike.

Menuchin, S.: Families and family therapy, Cambridge, Mass., 1974, Harvard University Press.

This volume contains a clear exposition of structural family therapy. Numerous case examples are well integrated into theoretical discussion. This book is an important text for beginning and advanced students.

Menuchin, S. et al.: A conceptual model of psychosomatic illness in children, Arch. Gen. Psychiatry **32:**1, Aug. 1975.

This article compares the medical model of psychosomatic illness to a systems, multiple feedback model within the family structure. It describes the necessary conditions in a family for the development of severe psychosomatic illness in children and the family therapy strategies used to treat it.

Menuchin, S., and Fishman, H.C.: Family therapy techniques, Cambridge, Mass., 1981, Harvard University Press.

This highly practical book provides clear definitive coverage of the techniques and skills utilized in structural family therapy. Techniques are described, and then excerpts of parts of sessions are included to illustrate and amplify theoretical descriptions. This is Menuchin's latest book, and the logical theoretical sequel to Families and Family Therapy.

Menuchin, S., Rosman, B., and Baker, L.: Psychosomatic families, anorexia nervosa in context, Cambridge, Mass., 1978, Harvard University Press.

In this book by Menuchin and his associates he describes his successful treatment and research with the families of anorexics. Over half the book consists of clinical interviews and case examples.

Palazoli, M. et al.: Paradox and counterparadox, New York, 1978, Jason Aronson, Inc.

This book reports the early results of clinical research of the Milan Center for Family Studies with acute schizophrenic families. The unique short-term therapy approach of Palazoli and her team is described. Their use of paradoxical interventions to change the paralyzing circular patterns of disturbed communication in schizophrenic families is explained and elucidated by clinical examples. This book is recommended for the advanced student.

Rabkin, R.: Strategic psychotherapy, New York, 1977, Basic Books, Inc.

This book offers a thorough discussion of strategic therapy. It discusses in depth the use of reverse psychology, which employs the patient's resistance and paradox.

Smoyak, S.: Family therapy. In Psychiatric nursing 1946 to 1974: a report on the state of the art, New York, 1975, American Journal of Nursing Co.

Through an extensive review of the literature, the author identifies the evolving role of the nurse in family therapy. Because of its thoroughness and historical review, it is an excellent resource for nursing's involvement with families.

Toman, W.: Family constellation, New York, 1961, Springer Publishing Co., Inc.

This book describes personality profiles based on a person's sibling position, considering birth order and sex. This book is a classic and should be read by all students of family therapy.

Watzlawick, P., Beaven, J., and Jackson, D.: Pragmatics of human communication, New York, 1967, W.W. Norton & Co.

This book describes the effects of human communication, with special attention to behaior disorders. The authors define general communication theory, present basic characteristics of human communication, and offer examples of pathological communication. This is a basic text for understanding the origins of strategic, or brief, family therapy.

Watzlawick, P., Weakland, J., and Fisch, R.: Change, principles of problem formation and problem resolution, New York, 1974, W.W. Norton & Co.

The authors' efforts to understand their effective but seemingly irrational treatment strategies stimulated the development of a theory of change, which evolved into strategic family therapy. This book offers a clear explication of the use of paradox in treatment. It is the logical theoretical sequel to Haley's Uncommon Therapy *for the advanced student.*

Youth's love
Embracingly integrates
Successfully frustrates
And holds together,
Often unwittingly
All that hate, fear, and selfishness
Attempt to disintegrate.

R. Buckminster Fuller, And It Came to Pass —Not To Stay

CHAPTER 26

CHILD PSYCHIATRIC NURSING

Rita L. Rubin

Learning objectives

After studying this chapter, the student should be able to:

- describe the four major influences on the development of child psychiatry.

- state the levels, scope, and settings of child psychiatric nursing practice.

- discuss the elements of the latency period of child development, including Piaget's cognitive processes, the functions of the ego, and the role of Mahler's individuation theory.

- identify the major categories of data that should be collected by the nurse with regard to the child's health status.

- compare and contrast the characteristics of the following diagnostic labels: autistic-presymbiotic, symbiotic-psychotic, and borderline.

- discuss common areas of conflict for children with ego deficits and the nursing diagnoses appropriate to them.

- analyze the indications for and implications of the various therapeutic modalities that can be included in the plan of care.

- describe the phases, techniques, and components of nursing intervention with disturbed children.

- assess the importance of evaluation of the nursing process when working with children.

- identify suggested readings for future study.

Historical antecedents

The field of child psychiatry had its beginnings in the early 1900s. It developed from four major bodies of knowledge: psychoanalysis, education, psychology, and an outgrowth of information from work with delinquent youth. Sigmund Freud's major influence on child mental health was his recognition of the role of early childhood experiences in the mental health of the adult. He also treated a phobic child, Little Hans, by coaching his father in the technique of analysis.[13] Child psychoanalysis owes its development and practice to two analysts, Melanie Klein, who initially worked in Berlin in the 1920s and 1930s, and Anna Freud, who worked simultaneously in Vienna. Klein is considered to have utilized play in the same way an analyst would use adult free association. Thus the term *play therapy* became the key to treating mentally disturbed children.[15] Anna Freud utilized the medium of play as well, but differed from Klein somewhat in her approach. Anna Freud's major emphasis was the development of a positive transference with her child patient. Play with toys was a technique of communicating and relating to the child in a way he could understand.[9] Both child analysts were uprooted by World War II and resumed their work later in the United States and England.

The field of education promoted the idea that children needed a combination of nurturing and learning experiences to become responsible adults. As early as the mid-1800s, students of educational science recognized that children progressed through developmental stages and learned spontaneously by doing. Contributors at the turn of the twentieth century included Sully,[26] who recognized the importance of play in children's communication, and the normative studies of Binet,[3] Catell,[6] and Gisell,[14] who developed the concept of intelligence and set the groundwork for the developmental theory of Erikson.[11]

The educational psychologists, Dewey and James, furthered the study of the range of normal and also asked questions about how the child learns. Their work was instrumental in bridging knowledge from education to psychology for application in the teaching and testing of children. Influential in the field of psychology were Pavlov, Watson, and Skinner, who established the behaviorist school.[30] Their descriptions of stimulus-response (S-R) learning have been applied not only to the education of children, but also to modifying troublesome behaviors of children. In addition, Jean Piaget, a Swiss psychologist, has provided child psychiatry with a developmental theory of cognitive growth.[10]

The contribution stemming from concern about juvenile delinquents and orphans came in response to the great influx of immigrants and the Industrial Revolution, both of which occurred in the early 1900s. During this time, almshouses and foster homes were established to keep children off the streets. In 1909, Healy[16] studied the problem of delinquency in Chicago and concluded that aberrant behavior was produced by multicausal factors, not the least of which was the role of the family. Another important name associated with the treatment of delinquency is Aichhorn, who treated delinquent youths in Vienna in the 1920s, using psychoanalytical principles.[15]

A final major influence on the field of child psychiatry was the child guidance movement that began around 1930. The psychiatric treatment of children was initiated through the court system, later becoming community based. This classic team approach is still utilized widely, in which a therapist sees the child, a psychologist does the testing, and a social worker works with the family, in addition to coordinating community resources.

The multidisciplinary team approach in the practice of child psychiatry has its parallel in theory. Theory remains a "mixed bag," pulling from a wide variety of frameworks, yet having no theory unique unto itself. Despite the criticism imbued by so-called purists, there remains the fact that no one method of treatment has been of help to all children in need of psychiatric intervention. Consequently, the field of child psychiatry continues to be the product of psychology, education, psychiatry, and social work.

Child psychiatric nursing practice

Nurses entered the field of psychiatry initially as custodial caretakers. Then with the advent of the somatic therapies between 1930 and 1940, some effort was placed on educating nurses in psychiatry to improve the care of psychiatric patients. The second half of the twentieth century has seen nurses functioning in ever-expanding roles, their advanced training mandated by federal legislation. The National Mental Health Act of 1946 provided funding for advanced training of psychiatric nurses (among other professionals) in undergraduate and graduate nursing programs. This became the stepping stone to recognizing that psychiatric nurses needed specialized training. Within the next decade Boston University had a graduate program for child psychiatric nurses. In 1955, Mental Health Law 182 charged the Joint Commission on Mental Health and Illness to conduct a study of mental illness and ways to prevent it. Significant among the findings was the recommendation that nurses be utilized more efficiently to provide mental health care in the face of a shortage of manpower.[20]

Scope of practice

Presently there are two levels at which child psychiatric nurses practice: generalist and specialist. Educational preparation differentiates the two levels. The registered nurse is considered to be a generalist and may intervene independently to provide care for nursing problems or dependently, through physicians orders, for medically diagnosed problems. A generalist may assume the role of therapist with qualified supervision.[1] The child psychiatric nurse specialist has earned a master's degree and has a clinical background in child psychiatric nursing. With successful completion of certification by the American Nurses' Association, the specialist may choose to engage in private practice. When employed by a health care facility she may assume indirect and direct care duties specified by the current state nurse practice act.

The American Nurses' Association has established standards of practice for psychiatric–mental health nursing. They list the following nursing activities as within the scope of practice[1]:

1. Providing a therapeutic milieu
2. Working with patients concerning the here-and-now living problems they confront
3. Accepting and using the surrogate parent role
4. Assuming the role of social agent concerned with improvement and promotion of recreational, occupational, and social competence
5. Providing leadership and clinical assistance to other nursing personnel

Roles are delineated for both direct and indirect

functions. Direct role functions include individual, group, family, and sociotherapist. Indirect role functions include administration, clinical supervision of nursing or other personnel, education, consultation, and research.

Another professional organization, Advocates for Child Psychiatric Nursing, Inc., has provided a position statement on the education of a child psychiatric clinical nurse specialist, which concurs with the American Nurses' Association definitions of the specialist.[8] In addition, they specify the need for a nursing framework and a theory of human behavior to apply to practice. They see the specialist as a therapist who demonstrates her competence through the certification procedure and maintains her competency by continued formal and informal educational experiences.

Practice settings

The nurse in child psychiatry may assume positions in primary, secondary, or tertiary prevention settings. In primary prevention settings, the aim is to prevent emotional problems. Nurses with knowledge in child psychiatry may provide services to prenatal clinics, day care centers, nursery schools, and other child care programs. Preventive care includes health education in the areas of infant and child development, child rearing and parenting, and counseling for life stresses such as divorce, death, or chronic illnesses. The child psychiatric nurse specialist may provide consultation to day care centers, nursery schools, and pediatric floors in hospitals.

Secondary care settings are geared toward early intervention in mental illness to minimize its disabling effects. Examples of such settings in child psychiatry include outpatient clinics and partial hospitalization programs. The nurse-therapist in this setting may use a variety of therapeutic modalities to help children and their families cope with high levels of stress. During crises the nurse may be called on to consult with schools to provide coordination of services and disseminate information relative to the child experiencing emotional difficulties.

Tertiary prevention settings provide rehabilitation to reduce the severity of mental illness. Common settings include child psychiatric inpatient units of general hospitals, residential treatment in psychiatric hospitals, transitional care settings, such as day care and group homes, and outpatient clinics. The child psychiatric nurse in such settings serves predominately as a milieu therapist. She provides therapeutic experiences by helping the child deal with daily life occurrences and providing a healthy adult-to-child relationship and role model.

Development of the school-age child

The latency period

The school-age child from ages 6 to 12 years has become quite an independent human being. When compared to earlier stages, he is competent in many areas. He is able to leave his parents for the 6-hour school period and consequently comes under the influence of a complex world of teachers, peers, and other adults. He has established gender identity and is increasingly concerned with measuring up to his peers' accomplishments. Cognitively, he is able to reason, based on the perception of his senses. Emotionally, he has the potential of reaching "latency," which is, according to Sarnoff, "... the ability to achieve a state of calm, educability and pliability, using an age-appropriate organization of defenses."[24] The child achieving latency has an ego developed sufficiently to exercise control over his impulses; therefore he is able to behave appropriately to the situation. In the classroom, he may sit in a seat for several hours and attend to intellectual tasks, provided that he is able to release pent-up energy at intervals on the playground.

Erikson describes the task of latency to be that of the achievement of a sense of competency.[11] The 6-year-old is aware of his "inferiority" to adults and sets about with "industry" to learn the many skills and attain the necessary knowledge to achieve a feeling of competency. Originally the latency period was conceptualized by Freud, who believed that during this phase of psychosexual development the sexual impulses of the id were quiescent or repressed. The ego psychologists concentrated their efforts on explaining the developing ego and less on the role of the id. Consequently, theorists such as Erikson, Mahler, Chess, and others have posed explanations for psychopathological conditions based on deficits in ego strength. Disturbances of the ego are believed to be caused either by organic defects, as in the case of autism, or by some distortion of the experiential history within the family during the child's development, as in borderline states.[7] It is less clear which is causative in childhood schizophrenia, and both organicity and family environment are believed to play a role.

Functions of the ego

The cognitive domain of the ego is the seat of thought, sensory perception, memory, and language. Piaget, in his cognitive developmental theory, calls the school-age years the *concrete operations stage* and notes that here begins the "age of reason." A concrete operation is a thought process based on a concrete (as opposed to abstract) point of reference. The ability to perform concrete operations moves the school-age child beyond the magical thinking of preschool years. Learning is enhanced by the cognitive developments in this age range as is the skill of relating to others. Cognitive growth and its affective correlates that occur during the concrete operations stage as described by Piaget are presented in Table 26-1.

Another function of the ego is that of defend-

TABLE 26-1. **Cognitive processes of the ego in Piaget's concrete operations stage**

Ego function	Cognitive process	Affective correlate
Sensory perception	Takes in information more rapidly Organizes perceptions	Perceives reality in organized way
Thought	Demonstrates cause and effect thinking Problem solves and reasons Can follow rules	Learns and profits from formal education Behaves appropriately to given situation
Language	Knows basic rules of grammar Vocabulary increases Comprehension increases	Engages in meaningful communication and becomes more social
Memory	Mental representations are symbolic of objects, thus has increased ability to store and retrieve information	Establishes interpersonal relationships based on past events that give relations value

ing against instinctual drives using defense mechanisms. Sarnoff believes a major defense during latency is reaction formation. The anxiety of the oedipal period is harnessed during latency by converting one's drive to disorder into a desire for order and neatness. An example of this is the enthusiasm with which many children engage in collections of baseball cards, stones, small model cars, and the like.

Fantasy plays an important role in reducing anxiety for the child achieving latency. When able to engage in fantasy, much of the impulsiveness may be eliminated without it actually being acted out. Reading fairy tales performs this function, as does the fantasy material that occurs in spontaneous play.

The ego also functions to provide an individual with a sense of identity. Mahler has developed a theory whereby the child must separate from the mother and "individuate" in order to develop a sense of self.[17] Between birth and 6 months of age, the mother and infant are partners in a symbiotic relationship. Mahler postulates that the infant's awareness of self is limited to physical sensations from his body. He has no external reality and therefore mother and infant are fused into one amorphous unit.

In the latter half of the first year of life the infant begins the transition into Mahler's *separation-individuation phase*. His ability to locomote allows the external world to broaden under his control. His improved visual apparatus and memory help him realize he has one mother. During the following months the infant will continue to apply his physiological and cognitive growth to experimenting with leaving his mother. The crisis occurs between 18 and 24 months when the walking toddler realizes that he is separate from his mother, and, more important, has no control over her.

The reality of separating provides a benefit to the child in the form of increased ego strength. Mother's former help in the areas of impulse control, frustration tolerance, and reality testing are now part of the child's own repertoire of ego functions.[18] Mother encourages and supports the child's attempts to achieve autonomy and so cushions him from being overwhelmed by a sense of abandonment. Successful resolution of the rapprochement, or crisis, subphase in the separation-individuation process results in mother and child forming a reciprocal partnership, known as object relations, trading gradual

maturity of the child for ego support from the mother.

Implementing the nursing process

In the specialty of child psychiatry the nurse may be called on to intervene with children who have insufficient ego strength to function outside of the inpatient setting. Many theorists contend that this is because of a lack of differentiation among family members and especially a failure of the separation-individuation phase to progress according to Mahler's formulation. Consequently, the child is unable to function when he reaches school age and must leave the comfortable hub of his family. The anxiety of separating, coupled with a fear of abandonment, inhibit the calm period of latency that should allow the child to take his place in the school environment. Manifestations of this poor sense of identity, or lack of ego strength, are diverse and many have biological and organic overlays. Examples of psychiatric conditions from the DSM-III that may be seen among some children are attention deficit disorder, conduct disorder, infantile autism, and childhood onset pervasive developmental disorder.

In the remainder of this chapter a nursing process orientation is presented to the treatment of the child with deficits in ego strength. The practice setting to be explored is an inpatient setting, such as in a psychiatric or general hospital, residential treatment center, or group home. The nurse is an integral part of a multidisciplinary team, comprised of professional and paraprofessional staff members, all of whom are involved in the treatment of the child with severe ego deficits.

Data collection

A child may be found in an inpatient child psychiatric setting for several reasons. At times the primary consideration in the decision to admit the child is that an accurate and thorough diagnostic evaluation has not been possible with the child as an outpatient. Other times, outpatient therapy has not been helpful to the child, and his behavior threatens to deteriorate further. In this case it is hoped that hospitalization will minimize regression, as well as rehabilitation time. Moreover, the child's behavior may have become bizarre and irrational, making the child difficult to manage in the home setting or at school.

Yet another criteria for inpatient admission is to protect the child from a severely pathological or abusive family. When this is the case, it might be helpful to admit the child to an inpatient facility to serve as a transition to foster home placement. Finally, "any child lacking the ego strength to control drives and instincts sufficiently enough to engage in the tasks of mastery and growth, and being unable to establish interpersonal relationships in the home, school or community for psychosocial development is a candidate for inpatient admission."[23]

The assessment phase of nursing care begins as the child is admitted to the unit. It is often useful to bring the child in to visit and become orientated before admission to alleviate a traumatic separation whenever possible.

The nurse will begin to collect data to formulate a picture of the whole child, including his areas of strengths and weaknesses. The first data obtainable are his response to the admission procedure and presenting symptoms. Does he separate easily from his parent or significant other? If his separation is difficult, does he react by demonstrating feelings of abandonment or by masking his feelings with a violent and aggressive explosion? Lack of affect or a disinterested attitude will also give the nurse data relative to the child's relationship with his parents.

Mental status

The psychiatric hospitalization of the child enables the nurse to gather information relative to several areas. The first area is the mental status of the child. A mental status examination produces a picture of the ego functioning of the child and may be used to document the functioning of the child during a single contact or over a longer period of time. When focusing on a narrow time frame, however, one must bear in mind that generalizations and conclusions about the child are limited only to that time being considered. Its greatest value is in comparing the child's behavior and level of functioning from one time to another.

The mental status of a child should ideally be assessed over a period of time, and there should be a relaxed atmosphere with minimal stressors. The use of play materials is valuable in displacing focus from the child (which is anxiety provoking) to an imaginary doll or character. Data should be recorded as observable behaviors to maximize the objectivity of the assessment, and impressions, feelings, and opinions should be labeled as such. A list of areas that are commonly

covered by the mental status examination with a brief explanation of each part follows:

appearance Description of the physical size, manner of dress, hygiene, posture, and any obvious handicaps.

defense mechanisms Description of major defenses the child uses to cope with anxiety.

neuromusculature Description of the child's ability to locomote in a coordinated fashion and execute gross and fine motor movements.

thought processes Description of the child's thoughts (verbalized). Are they logical, cohesive, and secondary process, or are flight of ideas, loose associations, and primary process thoughts present? Is the child preoccupied or having hallucinations or delusions?

fantasy Description of the child's ability to fantasize and know the limits of fantasy. This gives data relative to wish fulfillment, dreams, etc.

concept of self Description of the child's level of self-esteem, self-image, and self-ideal.

orientation Description of the child's concept of time and ability to perceive who and where he is.

super ego Description of the child's value system, ability to discern right and wrong, and ability to respond to limit setting.

estimated IQ Description of the child's general fund of information for his age and other age-appropriate tasks.

A more detailed explanation of mental status and children can be found in Simmons's book.[25]

Interpersonal relationships

Observations relative to how the child relates to peers are important in assessing the child. Knowledge of age-appropriate behaviors for peer relations will help the nurse know what she is looking for. The following are a few of the many questions one should bear in mind:

■ Are the relationships formed with those of the nearest age to the child? With the same or opposite sex?

■ What is the child's position in the power structure of the group?

■ How good are the child's social skills in approaching other children and getting along with them?

■ Does the child have a "best friend"?

The child's ability to relate to adults is also of great importance. The child's comfort and skill in forming these relationships is of interest. Also the age and sex of the adults sought out will reflect his needs for role models and nurturance. Does the child use adults for support or see them as hostile enemies? Is he able to sublimate sexual interest? Is he able to accept limits from adults?

Activities

Another information source is found by observing the child's response to activities. Observations relative to the type of activities the child enjoys and in which he or she does well, the energy level and response (bored, excited), and the ability to engage in solitary, as well as group pastimes, should be noted.

Background information

In addition to observing the child's behavior in the inpatient setting, the nurse should familiarize herself with the child's background. A thorough history, including the precipitating problem, history of symptoms, growth and development, family life, school adjustment, and medical status is usually compiled by one or more members of the multidisciplinary team. This information serves as a backdrop against which the child's current functioning appears. It provides the nurse with an understanding of the child's behavior and helps in setting goals for treatment that are realistic and achievable. For example, the treatment goals of a child who has had several foster home placements would differ with reference to adult relationships from goals for a child growing up in a traditional home environment.

As the picture of the child approaches completion, the data must be analyzed to make a diagnostic formulation. The diagnostic formulation serves as the basis for planning further treatment for the child. In some instances inpatient treatment ceases at this point. For the child with severe ego deficits, however, a comprehensive long-term treatment program usually is recommended.

Nursing diagnosis

Children with severe ego deficits fall into three major categories and comprise the majority of child psychiatric inpatient admissions. They are, according to Rinsley,[23] the autistic-presymbiotic group, the symbiotic-psychotic group, and the borderline group. These diagnostic categories are by no means the quintessence of psychi-

atric thought. There is still much blurring of syndromes and division among theorists and researchers as to diagnosis and etiology of these disorders. Consequently, each category will be explained as it is to be used in this context. It should also be noted that these are general groupings based on underlying psychodynamics. Within these broad groupings it is possible to identify more specific medical and nursing diagnoses. DSM-III, for example, classifies disorders usually first evident in infancy, childhood, or adolescence. These psychiatric disorders can be separated into five major groups on the basis of the predominant area of disturbance as follows:

1. Intellectual
   a. Mental retardation
2. Behavioral (overt)
   a. Attention deficit disorder
   b. Conduct disorder
3. Emotional
   a. Anxiety disorders of childhood or adolescence
   b. Other disorders of infancy, childhood, or adolescence
4. Physical
   a. Eating disorders
   b. Stereotyped movement disorders
   c. Other disorders with physical manifestations
5. Developmental
   a. Pervasive developmental disorders
   b. Specific developmental disorders

In addition, DSM-III notes that a variety of other diagnostic categories will often be appropriate for children and adolescents, such as schizophrenic disorders, substance abuse disorders, psychosexual disorders, and adjustment disorders.

Diagnostic categories

The autistic-presymbiotic group constitutes the following medical diagnostic labels: nonremitting schizophrenia, infantile psychosis, pseudoaffective schizophrenia, nuclear or process schizophrenia, and early infantile autism. The onset of symptoms is 3 to 5 months of age, and symptoms are pervasive. The child is considered fixated in the presymbiotic phase of development according to Mahler's theory. The child does not achieve a symbiotic relationship to the mother and does not differentiate self from mother. The symptoms include failure to learn, communicate, and form relationships. Consequently, these children are often mistaken as mentally retarded. It must be mentioned that there is approximately an equal split among those attributing the cause to emotional or organic causes.

The symbiotic-psychotic group is differentiated from the autistic-presymbiotic group by age of onset of symptoms, which usually appear between ages 3 and 4 years. These children are fixated in the symbiotic phase and are poorly individuated from their mothers. This group of disorders is characterized by disrupted and distorted body image and boundaries, pananxiety, fluctuating hyperactivity and withdrawal, delusions, distorted perception, and cognitive, adaptive, and coping failure.[23] In adolescence this group takes on the classic picture of adult-onset schizophrenic thought disorder.

The borderline group, like the autistic-presymbiotic group, consists of several medical diagnostic labels: character disorder, adjustment reactions of childhood or adolescence, delinquency, and conduct or behavior disorder. Onset of symptoms usually occurs at about 10 to 12 years. In this disorder, the child is believed to be fixated in the separation-individuation phase of development according to Mahler. The mother of the borderline child is also fixated in this phase and therefore is unable to provide the child the support he needs to separate from her. Consequently, he has the biological drive and emotional need to separate from the mother but cannot do so without an overwhelming fear of abandonment and ensuing depression. The depression is characterized by feelings of rage, fear, passivity, helplessness, and emptiness.[18] Clinically, the borderline child or adolescent uses acting out as a defense against the abandonment depression.

Psychodynamics

The children in all three groups may be commonly characterized as having deficits in ego strength. These deficits are because of organic causes or developmental arrests during critical periods of early childhood. The period in which the child becomes fixated will determine the extent to which his ego functioning will be impaired; the earlier the fixation, the more likely the child will appear psychotic.

Pioneers in the topic of the ego functioning of emotionally disturbed children were Fritz Redl and David Wineman.[22] Their description of the "ego that cannot perform" was derived from work in a Detroit group home for boys and for the next 20 years was virtually unchallenged as

far as literature dealing with understanding and treating the aggressive child.

The first problem a child has with a poorly functioning ego is controlling his impulses. The child cannot stand even minimal frustration and insists on immediate gratification. Furthermore, when faced with a frustrating situation, panic overwhelms the child, and he becomes aggressive and destructive. The child is extremely susceptible to temptation; mere accessibility lures the child into the forbidden. The excitement of the forbidden then quickly spreads to the whole group of children. This "group intoxication" presents problems in many areas as ego boundaries blur and the atmosphere thickens with the excitation of aggressive impulses. The children show limited ability to use play materials for their intended use and destroy them, unable to see that this prevents the pleasure of future use.

New situations are frightening and overstimulating to the child with a poorly functioning ego. They may be the stimulus for a paranoid distortion, or the newness may be denied to squelch the anxiety of confronting the new experience honestly. Buffoonery and ridicule, as well as overly rough manipulation of materials, are used to master new situations, however maladaptive the results may be.

The child's social savvy is virtually nonexistent, and his presence in public places is painfully obvious. He is insensitive to feelings of others and cannot read the code of the informal social structure or abide by its mores. In fact, rules are often perceived as persecuting and, without external control, are all but forgotten by the child.

The child's ability to see his role in problems and bad experiences is severely limited. The few times when guilt feelings are predominant, the anxiety-panic-aggression cycle is triggered once again. The child does not have the capacity to learn from his mistakes or the mistakes of others, something that is taken for granted in the normal child. Normal doses of challenge, success, or failure totally disintegrate the fragile hold of the ego's control.

Perhaps the most devastating problem posed by the child with deficits in ego functioning is his resistence to forming relationships with mature and emotionally healthy adults. The very need they have for a nurturant role model sets off feelings of mistrust and fears of rejection.

TABLE 26-2. Some psychodynamics and nursing diagnoses applicable to children with severe ego deficits

Psychodynamic	Possible nursing diagnosis
Failure of normal repression	Sexual acting out
Persistence of primitive defense mechanisms	Extreme use of denial and projection
Pervading anxiety	Severe level of anxiety
Failure of ego to synthesize perceptual, cognitive, and motor functions, thus disrupting child's relationship to environment	Impaired ability to test reality
Lack of basic trust	Withdrawn and self-isolating behavior
Impaired object relations	Inability to establish intimate relationships
Persistence of narcissism	Lack of insight into own problems
Persistence of primary process thinking	Hallucinations
Failure of sublimation of impulses	Aggressive and destructive behavior
Various degrees of impairment of self-mother differentiation	Negative self-concept

Communication is hampered by the child's secretive, guarded, and aloof nature. The usual social reinforcers the adult uses to show he is willing to form a relationship with a child, such as smiles, praise, or attention, are met with indifference.[27] Consequently, many therapists believe that the classic one-to-one relationship is ineffective and even contraindicated when working with such children initially.

Table 26-2 summarizes some of the psychodynamics occurring in children with severe ego deficits.[9] From an understanding of the child, his stressors, and environment the nurse can arrive at an appropriate nursing diagnosis.

Family psychopathology

The child experiencing severe emotional problems is usually considered to be a "symptom bearer" for the larger family unit. Over the past 30 years attention has been increasingly placed on a systems theory view of psychopathology. In other words, the "problem" does not necessarily lie entirely within the identified patient, rather, the patient is one part of the problem. Certain children seem to be set up to have emotional problems, particularly those having special meaning to their parents at birth, such as the first born, the only child, or the child with a chronic illness or handicap. Parenting begins under anxious conditions and the child responds anxiously, eventually manifesting symptoms.

Along these same lines, parents who have been inadequately parented themselves are impaired in their abilities to parent. Winnicot's concept of the "good enough mother" requires that she be able to respond to the child's cues to separate and individuate with support and encouragement.[18] If she experiences the growth process of her child as abandonment, she will be unable to facilitate the process without becoming depressed herself.

Another phenomena of the pathological family is the double-bind communication pattern described by Bateson et al.[2] The double bind is a pattern of communicating between two people in which there are two conflicting messages, from which there is no escape, and when repeated over time are not even recognized as conflictual by the victim. It is believed that the anxiety caused by this distorting experience can lead to schizophrenia.

A final family phenomenon is the blurring of ego boundaries. This is manifested in several ways. Roles may overlap or be reversed, such as a child being expected to parent his parent. Feeling states may be blurred, such as when a mother projects her feelings onto the child. Yet another example is the way in which the family handles anxiety. High levels of anxiety in one family member may be easily picked up by other members, causing confusion and disorganization.

Perhaps the most interesting family discovery was made in the research of Bowen.[4] He found that all of these faulty mechanisms occur to some extent in most every family. The ability to improve family adaptation rests on learning to separate and differentiate from other family members in a nonreactive and emotionally mature way. He believes that the symptomatic child in a family is representative of a family having a poor capacity to tolerate differentiation of family members.

Planning

Once a thorough assessment is completed and the child's major problems have been identified, a comprehensive treatment plan must be formulated. The nursing responsibility is generally for milieu therapy, but her involvement is not confined to that area entirely. The nurse may take an active role in other therapeutic modalities, such as group therapy or family therapy, depending on her level of practice and specialized training.

The inpatient setting provides various functions for the child psychiatric patient. First, the inpatient admission may be merely intended for diagnostic and evaluative purposes, and treatment will be carried out elsewhere. A second function is the case finding of children who could most benefit from a residential treatment center. The inpatient setting makes possible a comprehensive treatment plan in which individual, milieu, group, family, drug, occupational, and recreational therapies are all readily available. Finally, it provides a setting and stimulus for family treatment of pathogenic relationships.[23]

Goals

Based on the identified problems, goals should be set that are individualized to the child's needs. Treatment goals usually include intervening in one or more of the following areas: modification of intrapsychic processes, altering peer group interactions, altering interfamily functioning, modifying the child's adjustment to school, and changing the child's environment.[29] Wilson and Kneisl[29] have formulated the following common goals for child psychiatric inpatients:

1. To meet the child's needs so tension will be reduced and the need for defensive behavior will be decreased
2. To help the child form a relationship with another person
3. To help the child develop a sense of self-identity
4. To offer the child an opportunity to regress and relive previous developmental stages that were unsuccessfully resolved
5. To help the child learn to communicate effectively
6. To prevent the child from hurting self or others
7. To help the child maintain physical health
8. To help the child form relationships with others
9. To promote reality testing by the child

In addition, most hospitalized children will need to develop internal impulse control to some degree.

Once goals are set, the appropriate therapeutic modalities must be chosen to help the child reach the goal. One must be reminded again of the "mixed bag" nature of child psychiatric treatment and the useful combination of various therapies. The practice of the following psychotherapies are fully explained in other chapters in this text. A few highlights specific to child psychiatry are appropriate to mention here.

Family therapy

Ideally, each child's family should be involved in family therapy (Chapter 25). From a systems perspective, expecting a young child to assume responsibility for changing when the family system opposes those forces toward change (in hopes of maintaining homeostasis) is absurd. Consequently, parents should be involved from the outset and slowly be educated as to their role in the problem and responsibility for change. The family must be dealt with carefully, since they are being asked to give up their symptom bearer (the hospitalized child) and are often overwhelmed by the task of changing their viewpoints. On the other hand, parents who are allowed to view their child as the only problem will be ill prepared to deal with him as the hospitalization reaches termination and, often, they become willing to abandon their problem (the child) after a significant time lapse has occurred. Some families will resist adopting a systems perspective, a phenomenon discussed by Bradt and Moynihan.[5] In such cases, special techniques are offered to avoid alienating families from involvement in treatment.

Group therapy

Group therapy (Chapter 24) is often a useful adjunct to inpatient milieu therapy. It may take the form of an activity group or a talking group. It is helpful in promoting reality testing, impulse control, self-esteem, growth, maturity, and social skills. The group therapeutic environment allows members to form relationships and experience a positive social situation in a controlled environment, which hopefully will be transferred to the outer world environment over time.

Drug therapy

Drug therapy (Chapter 15) is a controversial issue in the field of adult, as well as child, psy-

TABLE 26-3. Child psychiatric symptoms and drugs and dosages most widely used

Symptom	Drug	Dosage
Hyperactivity	Methylphenidate (Ritalin)	5 to 40 to 60 mg in two or three divided doses
Enuresis	Imipramine (Tofranil)	25 to 75 mg at bedtime
Anxiety	Thioridazine (Mellaril)	10 mg two or three times daily
Depression	Imipramine (Tofranil)	20 to 75 mg in divided doses or at bedtime
Childhood psychosis	Chlorpromazine (Thorazine) Trifluoperazine (Stelazine)	10 mg three or four times daily 1 mg two or three times daily

chiatry. However, when used under a physician's supervision and the appropriate guidelines are followed, they often are helpful in decreasing symptoms sufficiently for other therapies to be of increased value. Drugs should be chosen based on a target symptom, rather than a diagnosis. Dosages are prescribed on the basis of an effective *range,* rather than by body weight, because of the variability of response. Symptoms that have been most successfully treated with drugs to date are hyperactivity, aggression, impulsivity, and anxiety.[28] Table 26-3 includes common child psychiatric symptoms with the drug of choice and dosage most widely used.

Individual therapy

Individual psychotherapy in latency usually makes use of play equipment appropriate to the child's age. A variety of individual therapies exist, including psychoanalytical play therapy, psychoanalytically based psychotherapy, experiential play therapy, and various eclectic approaches. Play therapy provides a controlled stable environment for the child to work through conflicts and master phase-specific developmental tasks with the aid of an adult therapist. Play serves as a tool for communication with the inner self and with the therapist and as a way to master past experiences that have been problematic to normal adjustment and development. In the older latency age child, play often serves as a diversion that is employed to help the child express anxiety-provoking thoughts and feelings, such as in artwork or board games. The relationship between the child and the therapist provides the opportunity for experiencing a positive adult

relationship tempered with judicious amounts of nurturance and reality testing.

Milieu therapy

This occurs in an inpatient setting (Chapter 18). The milieu is the actual background of daily events and interactions occurring in the unit or ward. A therapeutic milieu is present when the daily life events are exploited to provide learning experiences to the patients. Just how this is managed will be the major topic explored in the discussion that follows.

Intervention

Inpatient treatment in child psychiatry usually comprises three major components. The first is the life space interview, a group of techniques used to manage the behavior of children with weak ego strength. The second is some form of token economy that serves as a sanction for positive behavior. The third component is the establishment of one-to-one relationships that are therapeutic.

Treatment is best provided by professionals who have a genuine interest and concern for children. They need to have the capacity to withstand the multiplicity of moods and emotional outbursts that occur in these children. In other words, the nurse and her co-workers must have sufficient ego strength to cope with a fairly high level of anxiety in the emotional atmosphere. The nurse's role as a good parent demands that she be able to provide an environment with open honest communication and clearly delineated adult-child boundaries that are free from pseudointimacy.[23] The therapeutic milieu should provide the child with sanctuary from the pathological family dynamics that were detrimental to growth prior to hospitalization.

Phases of treatment

A comprehensive treatment plan for the child with weak ego strength can be expected to be of considerable length, as long as 3 or 4 years. Treatment usually procedes in three phases.[23] The first phase is the testing, or resistance, phase. In this phase the child is orienting himself to the setting and "casing it" for the purpose of finding out who is in charge and with whom he may align. After this brief honeymoon, the pseudocompliant front falls away and the child begins to test limits and demonstrate his problem with ego functioning. This entails negativism, reluctance to follow the program or form relationships, and destructiveness. The message is, "There is nothing wrong with me. I don't need to be in this place." The phase may last as long as 1 year.

The second phase is termed the definitive, or working-through, phase. During this time the child drops his resistance and begins to face his problems. There may be a significant regression during this time that often scares the child's family enough to withdraw him from treatment. However, the stormy phase gives way to therapeutic work toward separation-individuation, and the child begins to show improved ego functioning. This phase usually lasts 1 or 2 years.

The final phase, resolution or separation, hallmarks the child's successful achievement of object relations. The rapprochement crisis is resolved, and the child is able to move toward age-appropriate relationships with significant others. The child is able to handle extra privileges, visits home, and working through termination with the staff and other patients. This can also last up to a year.

Therapeutic milieu

The concept of a therapeutic milieu is built on daily events in the child's life. In the inpatient setting this comprises a daily routine of meals, school, sports, group and individual activities and pastimes, outings, and bedtime. Trieschman[27] delineates the various ways in which deficient egos are supported by the milieu. One way is through *shared ego,* in which the child behaves appropriately to please those persons with whom he has positive relationships. The group of children and adult workers in an inpatient setting makes up a *group ego* to which conformity is exchanged for acceptance and a feeling of belongingness. The culture of the institution is made up of rules and routine, as well as tradition, which serves as an *external ego* that guides the children's behavior. Finally, the milieu therapist, through careful assessment, is able to pick out the *ego pieces* or functions the child has in the here and now and find ways for the child to use them in managing his own behavior.

Types of interventions

With the daily routine, experiences arise that prove problematical to the child with inadequate ego strength. The nurse, as milieu therapist, extracts these problematical events as they take place and chooses one of two basic types of interventions to manage them: ego supportive or ego interpretive. A supportive ego intervention serves as a method of easing the child who is about to lose control, out of his panic-aggressive cycle and back into control, so that he may continue with the daily activity. These interventions serve to maintain the child at his current level of ego function through external control and over time set the stage for improving ego function. When conditions are ripe, the nurse is able to use interpretive ego interventions, which help the child to gain insight into his problematic behavior and use this insight as a basis for change, thus internalizing ego control. These two types of interventions were first described by Fritz Redl and are collectively known as *life space interview techniques.*[21] The life space interview is an interaction that takes place outside the context of individual therapy. It occurs between the child and the adult involved in the situation. The focus is on improving the child's sense of self-identity and ego functioning within the developmental process.

EGO SUPPORTIVE TECHNIQUES. This group of techniques can also be called "emotional first aid on the spot."[21] When the child inpatient confronts a developmental challenge or a demanding life situation, the milieu therapist may need to assist the child in coping with it. One technique for this is draining off the overwhelming frustration, caused by an interruption in the child's fun or routine, by communicating sympathy for the child's frustration and inconvenience. During periods when the child loses control and slips into his panic-aggressive cycle, it is important that the adult show support by staying with the child. This provides a sense of security and also affords the adult the opportunity to talk the child back into the daily routine after the stormy period wanes.

Often the child withdraws from relationships in times of emotional turmoil. To prevent this, Redl advocates dropping the issue that is being confronted in an endeavor to keep the child engaged, however trivial the subject may be. This prevents the phenomenon of "winning the battle, but losing the war" from occurring.

The milieu therapist also functions as a police officer in regulating and enforcing the social behavior of the children. This entails the act of benign and neutral reminding of rules and routines. "Enforcing the law" serves as an external booster to the children's ego at times when behavior is on the verge of slipping from the established norm. Along this same line the presence of an umpire is often necessary in settling arguments. A neutral outsider prevents breakdown in fair play or "petty swindling" in the children's transactions.

EGO INTERPRETIVE TECHNIQUES. The real therapeutic gains the child makes in ego strength occur as a result of self-examination and learning alternate behaviors to those which pose difficulty. In working with children who are prone to distorting and misinterpreting their experiences, insight may never be reached without a "reality rub in." This technique involves repeated confrontation with the reality that the child plays a part in his own self-defeating transactions.

Another intervention strategy is symptom estrangement. This interview situation focuses on enlisting the child to see his symptom as problematical, rather than as a tool that is used to manipulate and control. Symptom estrangement is accomplished by piling up evidence from past life events which provides proof that the symptom costs more than it pays to keep it.

Appealing to a sense of fairness and equality is helpful in awakening a value system in the children. The importance of developing an internalized standard for behavior may begin by this initial adherence to a code of fair play.

The technique Redl calls new-tool salesmanship has been enlarged on by Trieschman who calls it learning alternative or new behaviors.[27] This new behavior improves the child's coping ability, adaptation, and social acceptability as well. Selling a new way to handle frustration or guilt takes time and is often a by-product of a one-to-one relationship the child has with an adult. Substituting a mature behavior, from the adult model, for the old self-defeating behavior provides a step toward increased ego functioning.

The inclination to group contagion that many child psychiatric inpatients possess must eventually be countered. The life space interview in this situation focuses on increasing the child's boundaries so that he may withstand the group's atmosphere of excitement. In this way the child is educated as to how the process works and helped to remain outside the lure of misbehavior.

In summary, the clinical exploration of life events offers the opportunity to learn new behaviors and gain insight into the futility of old ones. The process of change takes time and often the stage must be set first through the use of ego supportive techniques.

Behavior modification as a tool in behavior control

Many inpatient settings utilize some behavioristic principles (Chapter 21) to manage the aggressive and limit-testing child. This is usually in the format of a token economy, in which socially acceptable behavior is rewarded or reinforced with points or tokens. The tokens are redeemable for extra privileges, such as an extended bedtime, a favorite food, or a special outing.

Maladaptive behavior is either ignored or punished by the use of time out. A time out requires that the child spend a brief period away from the group following acting out behavior. This serves as a time for the child to gain self-control and talk to an adult about the difficulty and also inhibits the spread of the child's acting out to other group members.

Yet another behavioristic program is contingency management. In this system, the milieu schedule promotes the use of positive or "on task" behavior with naturally occurring reinforcers, such as meals, free time, and outings. This is simply a variation of "grandma's law," which states, "If you want to eat dessert, you first must eat your peas."

All of these intervention strategies may be

used together or singly with excellent results. One principle, however, should be kept in mind. The focus is on the positive, self-esteem enhancing aspects of the program. The nurse and her co-workers should avoid slipping into a negative or threatening attitude by emphasizing that points are earned by the child, rather than taken away by the adult. Target behaviors should be clearly understood by the children and, whenever possible, positive reinforcement used instead of punishment.

A problem encountered in some behavior programs is that the child, after many acting out episodes in one day, has so few tokens that he gives up and completely decompensates. A way to provide further incentive to regain control is to build into each program a way in which the child can make up a portion of the points he has not earned. In doing so, he may not be able to reach the highest privilege status, but he will be able to rise above the lowest with some additional effort.

Also important to bear in mind is that the end point of behavior management is to internalize or learn self-control. Therefore it is hoped that social reinforcers such as praise will be paired with the token or extrinsic reinforcers so that the child eventually will reward himself for good behavior by feeling good about himself.

Establishing relationships

Children with deficits in ego strength have great difficulty forming relationships with adults. They are often distrustful because of their past experiences and, unable to discriminate a trustworthy adult, they withdraw from everyone. Therefore some special effort is usually required on the nurse's behalf to seek out and work toward the establishment of contact with the child.[19]

In the early stages of a relationship small talk is usually all that can be tolerated. Topics such as the child's reason for admission and other psychotherapeutic issues will actually hinder the child's ability to view the nurse positively in the milieu setting. Instead, the child should be approached casually, for the purpose of becoming acquainted with his interests and reactions to various situations or activities in the milieu. Exchanges should be short to avoid provoking the child's suspicious nature.

The adult working in this setting walks a precarious tightrope between appearing unapproachably square and disrespectfully "hip."

It is important for the child to view the nurse as an adult to promote his sense of security. Therefore gossip and off-color humor should be avoided, since they are tests of the adult's ability to abide by the rules of socially correct behavior. On the other hand, current fads in music, television, or movies may provide openings for conversations that demonstrate the adult's genuine interest in the child's world.

The adult will maximize his attractiveness to a child if he is able to find a common interest or skill to share with the child. This allows for many hours of diversional activity that serves as a backdrop for conversation in later stages of the relationship. It is important for the adult to demonstrate his inability to be manipulated. Since these children need external control, they will be unable to trust someone they are able to con.

Another important consideration in establishing and maintaining relationships is minimizing adult aversiveness.[27] One way in which this is accomplished is by staying out of power struggles. Sometimes potential altercations may be avoided merely by the adult failing to pick up a challenge. For instance, the child is asked to take a seat and responds by saying, "Make me!" The adult immediately picks up the child's cue and counters with "All right, I will." Avoiding a power struggle might be the answer here and the response could be, "For those who are seated, let's begin to clean up for a snack." The child is left to stand if he pleases while the rest of the group moves on with their activity. It is not always possible to avoid power struggles, but a concerted effort should be made at least in the case of minor or petty squabbles.

The nurse must actually prove her own trustworthiness to the child. One way she does this is by being as open and honest as possible with the child at all times. Being able to admit mistakes to a child communicates one's humanness and should be a firm operating principle. One can demonstrate increasing trust of the child by offering him small amounts of responsibility.

Once a positive relationship has been formed with the child it becomes more natural and the adult does not need to pursue the child quite so intensely. Topics will be centered around daily activities. The techniques outlined in the life space interview should then be incorporated into the adult-child interaction.

Evaluation

Most treatment facilities for child psychiatric patients have programs designed for specific periods of time. The brief hospitalization is usually 3 or 4 weeks in length and is planned for diagnosis and evaluation, crisis intervention, and comprehensive case planning. Therefore when the presenting symptoms have receded sufficiently, the clinical picture of the child is completed, and a long-term plan has been formulated, the child will be discharged.

The success of brief hospitalizations in terms of patient outcome is determined mostly by the patient's follow-up care. Consequently, the ability of the multidisciplinary team to formulate a plan that is mutually agreeable to the child and his family will be vital. Emphasis on the parent's responsibility to comply with the treatment plan for any persistent long-term gain should be made to the parents in the earliest contacts.

Long-term hospitalizations are more complicated in terms of determining readiness for discharge. Generally, the nurse's observations focus on basic changes in the child's behavior. The child should hopefully demonstrate some insight and understanding of himself through self-reflection and increase his ability to make rational decisions. Behavior should become less impulsive and drive ridden. Instead, the child should begin to live adaptively in his surroundings.

When the child's behavior has become more socially acceptable to the inpatient setting, it is important to begin expanding his or her environment to the community. The use of the public school system provides an excellent opportunity for the hospitalized child to stay "tuned in" to the outside world and also to demonstrate his ability to handle his environment prior to discharge. The child should be given home visits or visits to wherever it is that he will be placed after discharge. This also broadens the child's environment and tests his ability to internalize ego control. Social outings into the community should be ongoing in the course of treatment and should be handled age appropriately prior to discharge. In this way institutionalization is avoided.

When evaluating the child's overall therapeutic gains, it is important to examine the problems or symptoms, goals, and interventions on a regular basis. The treatment plan is kept up to date, and, as problems resolve, the lower priorities may be integrated into the plan. Sometimes the original goals must be reconsidered or interventions do not work so alternatives must be found. The use of team planning conferences is often helpful in the ongoing process of evaluation. Aspects of the treatment plan that need special scrutiny include the following:

1. Effectiveness of interventions in managing behavior
2. Ability to relate to peers, adults, and parents appropriately
3. Ability to carry out self-care and care of possessions
4. Ability to utilize program activities in recreation and learning (including school)
5. Response to limits, rules, and routines
6. Development of insight into problems and willingness to change
7. Overall mental status as outline earlier
8. Discharge coordination and planning

Termination

Terminating a therapeutic relationship is difficult for many nurses. This is in part because of the universally experienced feeling state of emptiness described by Fogarty.[12] Many people "use" relationships, albeit unconsciously, as a mechanism to avoid the empty feelings of loneliness, abandonment, and incompleteness. Termination stirs up these feelings within oneself and causes discomfort. Unfortunately, one must acknowledge these feelings to allow the termination to proceed therapeutically with the child.

The child has problems in leave taking as well. Behavior often regresses as the hospitalization draws to an end and a discharge date has been set. It is as if the child wants to prove that he still needs the hospital and its staff.

Some guidelines are helpful in terminating with children. Introducing the idea that there is an end point should be done early in treatment and stressed again when discharge nears. This allows ample time for the child and staff to experience the concomitant feelings and talk about them. Positive aspects of the termination process can be pointed out, such as the fact that discharge into family and community means the child is moving into a new phase of life where new relationships will be established in place of the old. Enumeration of the child's gains from hospitalization increase the child's confidence in facing a new environment. Finally, it is a valuable experience for the child to learn that one does not have to be mad or hurt to end a relationship, and a successful positive termination will be achieved when the child is able to grasp this.[7]

The use of ritual is a helpful method of handling "last days." Parties or special activities may be planned in the departing child's honor. Children sometimes enjoy autographs with special messages written to them from staff and other patients. All of these suggestions are merely aids to soften the finality of terminating, a painful fact of life for all people.

Follow-up and discharge

The discharge of a patient should occur only when the health teaching plan has been completed. The child and his family should have information relative to the nature of the child's illness and his status at discharge, including the family's role in the pathological condition. They should also know how stress relates to emotional illness and ways to cope more effectively with it. In addition, anticipatory guidance is often helpful in forewarning parents and children about future developmental or situational stressors that might have deleterious effects on the child's or family's functioning.

If the child is discharged and will be receiving drug therapy, it is extremely important that the child and family know the reason for the drug's prescription, the dosage, times of day it is to be given, and side effects that should re-

ceive medical attention. This cannot be overemphasized because of the common experience of many nurses with well meaning parents who do not understand the way in which many psychoactive drugs build up in the body. The layman's perception that the drug works much in the same way as an "aspirin stops a headache" may lead to the drug being ineffective or abused.

Follow-up care usually consists of some type of ongoing psychotherapy, whether it be individual, group, or family. Medication monitoring is carried out according to the specific indications of the prescribed drug. Sometimes vocational and school placements are part of the posthospitalization plan. Dispositions are made to the family of origin whenever possible. If this cannot be accomplished, placements with extended family members, boarding schools, and foster homes or group homes are considered.

Suggested cross-references

Behavior modification is discussed in Chapter 21. Group therapy is discussed in Chapter 24. Family therapy is discussed in Chapter 25.

SUMMARY

1. Child psychiatry evolved from the fields of psychoanalysis, education, psychology, and social welfare.

2. The child psychiatric nurse functions in a therapeutic role as a milieu therapist. Her expanded role as an independent practitioner requires advanced study at the Master's level. Care settings in child psychiatry are diverse and vary from primary to tertiary prevention.

3. Latency has a potential for growth that is reached by the school-age child by sublimating basic instinctual drives to reach a calm and educable phase. Cognitive ego functions facilitate the child's emphasis on learning so that he develops a sense of competency about self. Children with ego deficits are believed to have developmental delays in differentiating from their mothers and developing object relations. The-

orists differ in their views of the etiology of weak ego states.

4. The data collection phase involves the development of a profile of the child that includes presenting symptoms, mental status, interpersonal relationships, activities and behaviors in the inpatient setting, and background information. Brief hospitalizations are often used for diagnostic purposes.

5. Nursing diagnoses are devised from the psychodynamics specific to each child's problems. Common problem areas include faulty impulse control, negative self-concept, impaired reality testing, poor interpersonal relationships, and lack of insight.

6. Children hospitalized in child psychiatric inpatient settings fall into three main categories of diagnostic labels: autistic-presymbiotic, symbiotic-psychotic, and borderline. Families of such children are often found to have faulty communication patterns, poorly defined ego boundaries, and difficulty identifying their role in the child's problem.

7. Helping children with deficits in ego strength requires a comprehensive treatment plan and specific nursing care goals. Residential treatment programs serve as therapeutic milieus in which daily living experiences are used to help children learn more adaptive behaviors and gain a stronger sense of self-identity.

8. Interventions such as the life space interview, behavior modification programs, and one-to-one relationships are helpful in facilitating the child's growth and development, and therapeutic modalities have an impact on the child in residential treatment. Individual, group, family, drug, special education, and recreational therapies are a few.

9. The child who has been hospitalized on a long-term basis should achieve some measure of insight into his problems, impulse control, and reality testing prior to discharge. Termination may bring about temporary symptom recurrences, but can be handled through adequate communication and cultural ritual. Health teaching and follow-up care have important prognostic value on the child's outcome after discharge.

References

1. American Nurses' Association, Division on Psychiatric and Mental Health Nursing Practice: Standards of psychiatric–mental health nursing practice, Kansas City, Mo., 1976, The Association.
2. Bateson, G. et al.: Towards a theory of schizophrenia, Behav. Sci. **1:**1, 1956.
3. Binet, A., and Binet, S.: The development of intelligence in children, Baltimore, 1916, The Williams & Wilkins Co.
4. Bowen, M.: Theory in the practice of psychotherapy. In Guerin, P., editor: Family therapy, New York, 1976, Gardner Press, Inc.
5. Bradt, J.O., and Moynihan, C.J.: Opening the safe: a study of child-focused families. In Bradt, J.O., and Moynihan, C.F., editors: Systems therapy, Washington, D.C., 1972, Groome Child Guidance Center.
6. Catell, J.M.: Mental tests and measurements, Mind **15:** 373, 1890.
7. Chess, S., and Hassibi, M.: Principles and practice of child psychiatry, New York, 1978, Plenum Publishing Corp.
8. Child psychiatric–mental health nurse clinician, position statement, Chicago, 1980, Advocates for Child Psychiatric Nursing, Inc.
9. Ekstein, R.: Psychoanalysis. In Noshpitz, J., editor: Basic handbook of child psychiatry, vol. 3, New York, 1979, Basic Books, Inc.
10. Elkind, D.: Children and adolescents: interpretive essays on Jean Piaget, London, 1974, Oxford University Press.
11. Erikson, E.H.: Childhood and society, New York, 1950, W.W. Norton & Co., Inc.
12. Fogarty, T.F.: On emptiness and closeness. I. The Family 2(1):22, 1975.
13. Freud, S.: Sexual enlightenment of children, New York, 1963, Macmillan, Inc.
14. Gisell, A.L.: Infancy and human growth, New York, 1928, Macmillan, Inc.
15. Halpern, W.I., and Kissel, S.: Human resources for troubled children, New York, 1976, John Wiley & Sons, Inc.
16. Healy, W.: Twenty-five years of child guidance, Chicago, 1934, Institute for Juvenile Research.
17. Mahler, M.: The psychological birth of the human infant, New York, 1975, Basic Books, Inc.
18. Masterson, J.F.: Intensive psychotherapy of the adolescent with a borderline syndrome. In Caplan, J., editor: American handbook of psychiatry, ed. 2, New York, 1974, Basic Books, Inc.
19. Meeks, J.E.: The fragile alliance, Baltimore, 1971, The Williams & Wilkins Co.
20. Middleton, A.B., and Pothier, P.C.: The nurse in child psychiatry—an overview. In Fagin, C., editor: Readings in child and adolescent psychiatric nursing, St. Louis, 1974, The C.V. Mosby Co.
21. Redl, F.: Life space interview, Am. J. Orthopsychiatry **1:**1, 1957.
22. Redl, F., and Wineman, D.: The aggressive child, Glencoe, Ill., 1957, Free Press.
23. Rinsley, D.B.: Principles of therapeutic milieu with children. In Sholevar, G.P., editor: Emotional disorders in children and adolescents, New York, 1980, Spectrum Books.
24. Sarnoff, C.A.: Latency-age children. In Sholevar, P. et al., editors: Emotional disorders in children and adolescents, New York, 1980, Spectrum Books.
25. Simmons, J.E: Psychiatric examination of children, ed. 2, Philadelphia, 1974, Lea & Febiger.
26. Sully, J.: Studies of childhood, London, 1903, Longman Group.
27. Trieschman, A.E., Whittaker, J.K., and Brendtro, L.K.: The other 23 hours, New York, 1969, Aldine Publishing Co.
28. White, J.H.: Psychopharmacology in childhood, Psychiatr. Clin. North Am. **3:**443, 1980.
29. Wilson, H.S., and Kneisl, C.R.: Psychiatric nursing, Reading, Maine, 1979, Addison-Wesley Publishing Co., Inc.
30. Wingfield, A.: Human learning and memory: an introduction, New York, 1979, Harper & Row, Publishers, Inc.

Annotated suggested readings

Arnold, E.L., editor: Helping parents help their children, New York, 1977, Brunner/Mazel, Inc.

This book discusses general principles of parent guidance and offers advice for helping parents of children with specific problems. It is an excellent reference for people working with children and families.

Axline, U.M.: Play therapy, Boston, 1947, Houghton Mifflin Co.

This classic work describes the author's unique art and style of play therapy.

Bradt, J.O., and Moynihan, C.J.: Opening the safe: a study of child-focused families. In Bradt, J.O., and Moynihan, C.J., editors: Systems therapy, Washington, D.C., 1972, Groome Child Guidance Center.

This is highly recommended to the student interested in viewing the child psychiatric patient from a systems theory perspective.

Chess, S., and Hassibi, M.: Principles and practice of child psychiatry, New York, 1978, Plenum Publishing Corp.

This is a comprehensive text with its main emphasis on etiology and description of syndromes. It is an excellent review of current research.

Elkind, D.: Children and adolescents: interpretive essays on Jean Piaget, New York, 1974, Oxford University Press, Inc.

For the student interested in cognitive developmental theory, this book is a readable interpretation of the extremely technical writing of Jean Piaget.

Fagin, C.M., editor: Readings in child and adolescent psychiatric nursing, St. Louis, 1974, The C.V. Mosby Co.

This book provides the child psychiatric nurse with an interesting look at her beginnings and also provides a variety of intervention techniques for use in specific situations.

Freud, A.: The psychoanalytic treatment of children, New York, 1965, International Universities Press, Inc.

This classic in the field of child psychoanalysis is highly recommended to the nurse interested in advanced study.

Gordon, T.: P.E.T.: parent effectiveness training, New York, 1970, Wyden Books.

The author presents an alternative approach to child-rearing based on Rogerian communication techniques. It is helpful for parents as well as professionals.

Guerin, P.J., editor: Family therapy theory and practice, New York, 1976, Gardner Press, Inc.

This book is the bible of the family systems therapist, offering many valuable chapters on theory and technique. It provides in-depth knowledge about the child as a symptom bearer of family problems.

Noshpitz, J.D., editor: Basic handbook of child psychiatry, vols. 1-4, New York, 1979, Basic Books, Inc.

These volumes represent a wealth of information for the advanced student. Subjects included are child development, assessment, deviations and syndromes, therapeutic interventions, and community mental health. An excellent, if somewhat costly, addition to the child psychotherapist's library.

Redl, F.: The life space interview, Am. J. Orthopsychiatry **1:**1, 1959.

The author presents his classic work in concise form.

Redl, F., and Wineman, D.: The aggressive child, Glencoe, Ill., 1957, Free Press.

This book is required reading for milieu therapists because it describes the ego pathology of the aggressive child and delineates the life space interview techniques. It is replete with clinical examples.

Schaeffer, C., editor: The therapeutic use of child's play, New York, 1976, Jason Aronson, Inc.

This is a compilation of individual and group approaches to treating the child. Psychoanalytic and humanistic theory and clinical applications predominate.

Simmons, J.E.: Psychiatric examination of children, ed. 2, Philadelphia, 1974, Lea & Febiger.

Simmons offers a compact and concise paperback manual explaining mental status and psychiatric examination of children. A case study and suggested format are included.

Trieschman, A.E., Whittaker, J.K., and Brendtro, L.K.: The other 23 hours: child care work with emotionally disturbed children in a therapeutic milieu, New York, 1969, Aldine Publishing Co.

Many aspects of milieu therapy are included in this book which is available in paperback. The concept of milieu therapy, therapeutic relationships, program development, and recording are covered to make a basic text for beginning practitioners.

I'm so mixed up and lonely
Can't even make friends with my brain.
I'm too young to be where I'm going
But I'm too old to go back again.

John Prine, *Rocky Mountain Time**

*Song from album "Diamonds in the Rough," 1972.

CHAPTER 27

ADOLESCENT PSYCHIATRIC NURSING

AUDREY REDSTON

Learning objectives

After studying this chapter, the student should be able to:

- *state the scope and function of adolescent psychiatric nursing practice.*

- *list the developmental tasks of adolescence.*

- *compare and contrast the following theoretical views of adolescence —biological, psychoanalytical, intellectual, and cultural.*

- *identify the major categories of data that should be collected by the nurse with regard to the adolescent's health status.*

- *discuss common areas of conflict for adolescents and the implications of them.*

- *describe the nursing diagnosis relative to specified problematical adolescent behaviors.*

- *analyze the indications for and implications of the use of family, group, and individual therapies by the nurse working with adolescents.*

- *assess the importance of evaluation of the nursing process when working with adolescents.*

- *identify suggested readings for future study.*

Adolescence is a time of transition—an age when one is not an adult and not a child. Yet the issues reflected in the adolescent experience are central to one's development as a person. Of profound proportion in adolescence, they are often recapitulated later in life. The intense feelings during the teenage years are perhaps the most meaningful of any experienced in a lifetime. Assisting adolescents during this conflictual period of development can be an enlightening and rewarding experience.

In this chapter an attempt is made to understand adolescent behavior and the nurse's role in facilitating growth during this developmental phase. An overview of various theoretical models is presented to illustrate a number of diverse perspectives of the adolescent experience. In addition, areas of conflict such as identity, social role, sexual behavior, independence, and body image are examined. The "normal" behaviors of adolescents result from these conflicts and are experienced by virtue of the biological and subsequent psychological growth that occurs.[8] An exploration of these conflicts and resulting behaviors is presented to help the nurse in assessing the adolescent and his functioning. When these conflicts are intensified, certain maladaptive coping patterns may be seen, and a nursing diagnosis of the adolescent's problem can be made. These maladaptive behaviors and nursing diagnoses, such as delinquency, hypochondriasis, weight problems, sexual promiscuity, and drug abuse, are discussed here as well. These lead to the formulation of a plan of action that aids the nurse in assisting the adolescent in productive movement on the developmental continuum.

This chapter attempts to provide the nurse with the assessment skills necessary to formulate therapeutic interventions. The collection of data in an organized fashion is reviewed to facilitate diagnosis and action. Finally, various therapeutic modalities are reviewed. Concrete suggestions for the implementation of these techniques are presented to provide the nurse clinician with some of the skills required to initiate and follow through on a productive therapeutic experience with adolescents.

Role of the adolescent psychiatric nurse

Adolescent psychiatric nurses are prepared in psychiatric–mental health nursing and are characterized by specific interests in meeting the needs of this age group. They focus on adolescents as they develop toward adulthood—considering social, emotional, and physical aspects of their adjustment in their family, school, and peer groups. These nurses concentrate on facilitating the adolescent's successful movement in the growth process toward adulthood. Adolescent psychiatric nurses become experts in identifying deviations or stalls in the developmental process and work closely with the adolescent's support systems to further enhance the growth process. This is in contrast with adult psychiatric nurses, who work with people who have attained some level of maturity and often need a reeducative experience to correct deficiencies in developmental areas.[4]

The scope of adolescent psychiatric nursing practice encompasses direct and indirect care in the areas of prevention, intervention, and rehabilitation. Direct nursing functions focus on actions toward the particular adolescent and include the following:

1. Psychotherapy (individual, family, and group therapy)
2. Intake screening and evaluation
3. Home visits (or substitute dwellings)
4. Provision of therapeutic milieu
5. Counseling (time limited on a specific problem)
6. Health teaching (role model and didactic teaching, usually on sex and health)
7. Support and medication surveillance
8. Community action (resource person to others dealing with adolescents; help formulate programs needed)

These functions attempt to alleviate emotional difficulty and discourage maladaptive relating patterns.

Indirect nursing functions focus on actions taken to assist another person who actually carries out the care given to the adolescent. These functions are usually done by an adolescent psychiatric nurse specialist in the following roles[4]:

1. Educator
2. Administrator
3. Clinical supervisor
4. Consultant
5. Nurse researcher

Developmental stage of adolescence

Adolescence is a unique and distinct stage of development that, although often seen in the context of contemporary social change, has great significance in the understanding of human behavior. A look at human development reveals a progression of movement from one stage of life to the next, from infancy through old age. The common age range for adolescence (11 to 20) indicates that during that time period a shift in the developmental and learning process occurs. It is more accurate to view this progression as continuous in which each stage overlaps the next. Goals and tasks within the specific stage of adolescence, and the way each stage of life moves into the succeeding ones, have been studied by various theorists.

The new developmental tasks that emerge during adolescence stress the individual's defenses and can either stimulate growth in the form of new ways of coping or lead to regression and disorganization from failure to cope. Long-standing difficulties from the past may contribute to disorganization, and the current environment may help or hinder the adolescent's attempt to deal with these issues. Beginning at infancy, development is often marked with episodes of disintegration at the onset of learning a new skill, with movement toward integration as the new skill is acquired. The pattern of dealing with developmental stress contributes to how the adolescent will cope with current anxieties. Skills established during latency do little to ward off anxieties associated with changing body image and new instinctive feelings. Past coping skills, if integrated with success, can assist toward healthy integration of adult functions.

During adolescence major events are encountered and attempts to resolve these events are made. These result in behavior uniquely "adolescent."[24] Havighurst delineated tasks that should be accomplished during adolescence[15]:

1. Achieving new and more mature relations with age mates of both sexes
2. Achieving masculine or feminine social roles
3. Accepting one's physique and using the body effectively
4. Achieving emotional independence from parents and other adults
5. Preparing for marriage and family life
6. Preparing for an economic career
7. Acquiring a set of values and an ethical system as a guide to behavior and developing an ideology

Different theoretical concepts of adolescent development have evolved in conjunction with how these developmental tasks are encountered and resolved to produce an adolescent moving toward adulthood.

Theoretical views of adolescence

Biological theory

Gesell, Ilg, and Ames[13] believed that biological influences are the major determinants of adolescent development. They studied humans from birth to age 16, placing great emphasis on observable behaviors of the child and adolescent and the role of environmental influences on adolescent development. They believed that growth patterns followed certain principles of maturation. Through maturation and environmental influences a person learns how to adjust. Behavior is therefore a conscious growth experience. Gesell and associates described adolescent development as consisting of intense physical growth changes which are so dramatic that they affect all aspects of the human being. He presented a normative theory, categorizing through his observation certain behaviors that occur at particular points in the maturational development of most adolescents. Gesell's specific normative data consist of feelings, thoughts, and behaviors seen at each age. He indicated differences in equilibrium ranging from stormy disequilibrium to calm equilibrium and maintained that these changes are caused by maturational states which cause the adolescent to grow.

Psychoanalytical theory

Freud also believed that human development was biological and was marked by stages. He put more emphasis on the first year of life, concluding that adolescence and adulthood have their roots in the resolution of childhood developmental stages. These stages originated in the sexual instinct he called the id, which he viewed as a primary factor in determining an individual's successful personality development. The rational, reality-based part of humans he called the ego, which helped control and modify the id and created coping mechanisms to deal with the environment. The superergo was described as the conscience, which assisted the ego in establishing socially acceptable behaviors and attitudes. Freud constructed five stages of development from birth to adolescence: oral, anal, phallic, latency, and genital.

During puberty (ages 13 to 18), which is Freud's genital stage, there is a reawakening of sexual interest. The adolescent with new sexual urges looks for gratification outside the home. This renewal comes from physiological maturing. The genitalia mature, and there is an increase in the release of sex hormones. Sexual exploration and maturation often occur. Freud stressed that the first years of life were important in establishing traits that become permanent in adolescence.[11]

The more modern psychoanalytical theories of today are the most descriptive in defining adolescence. Classically, they, as did Freud, define it as the stage between childhood and adulthood correlated with the biological changes of puberty. Adolescence is described by Josselyn[17] as the psychological development that attempts to deal with pubescent changes and is therefore initiated by them. The biological changes of puberty upset a balance that previously existed between the ego and id during latency. Increased drives or impulses initiated by the greater hormonal secretion cause a personality reorganization in adolescents as they attempt to adjust to their new physical status. These increased impulses confront a relatively weak ego. Most evident at this time is a resurgence of the oedipal complex, which brings along with it derivatives of pregenital drives, oral and anal impulses, and aggressive drives. Adolescents therefore return to earlier modes of adaptation in an effort to reevaluate and reestablish mastery over the environment. Many solutions to problems caused by instinctual pressures are tried.

Psychoanalysts believe that sexual development does not begin with puberty but that new avenues for dealing with drives and the growth spurt come to the forefront in adolescence. The simple solutions of drive satisfaction that a child used no longer work, and efforts toward new solutions are made. The ability to make these adjustments comes about by the ego's capacity to renegotiate between the id, the superego, and the environment. The groundwork for this is laid earlier in development. If there has been inadequate accommodation in earlier stages, this is often reflected by difficulties in adolescence. Adolescence is a developmental maturational process in which the individual attempts to work through his life experiences to achieve maturity. Related to the oedipal conflict is the adolescent's task of freeing himself from dependency on parents. This detachment from incestuous objects can be evident in rejection, resentment, and hostility toward parents and authority. For this reason Blos[9] calls adolescence a "second stage of individuation," the first occurring during the oedipal period.

The classical psychoanalytical description of adolescence has been modified by Erikson, Fromm, Horney, Sullivan, and others who emphasize the effect of social factors on these developmental processes. Erikson[12] speaks about ego identity, or the relationship between what a person seems like to others and what the person himself thinks he is. To Erikson, adolescence represents an attempt to establish an identity within the social environment. This search is described as a "normal adolescent identity crisis." Erikson outlined this in the theoretical framework of his eight stages of human beings. He called the stage of adolescence "identity vs. identity diffusion," which is followed in young adulthood by the stage of "intimacy vs. isolation." He stressed that identity must be established before intimacy can occur.

Intellectual development theory

Cognition was most completely described by Piaget.[22] By gradually internalizing actions, one evolves a system of thought processes. A child learns to reason by a process he described as "concrete operations," based on concrete objects. Adolescence was defined as an advanced stage of cognitive functioning in which one is able to reason beyond concrete objects to symbols or abstractions, or what Piaget called "formal thought." Piaget believed the adolescent has the ability to deal with propositional logic, to grasp metaphors, and to reason about thought. This develops in a continuous fashion from the concrete thinking of childhood to (at about age 12) a rapid progression toward free reflection. This Piaget called the "formal operational period." The concern with realities and tangible objects manipulated toward real action is transferred to an ideational plan, permitting one to draw conclusions and reflect in the absence of the object. This ability he called "logic of operations."

Cultural theory

Anthropologists who studied adolescent behavior concluded from studies of adolescents in different cultures that primitive cultures had less stressful periods than those experienced by American teenagers. Mead[20] concluded that the experience of adolescent rebellion was culturally determined by the changes in generations and not biologically based. Anthropologists believe adolescence is a period when the person feels he deserves adult privileges that are not given to him, and it ends when the full power and social status of an adult are delegated to him by society. Anthropologists see growth as a continuous process and a cultural phenomenon, with individuals reacting to social expectations. The more clearly defined these expectations are, the less stressful and ambiguous the adolescent period. The more the culture has changed, the greater the generation gap.

Today's adolescents have the culture of the 1980s to cope with, which can exacerbate conflicts awakened by increased drives and changes in body image. Several issues in the complex and changing American society bear mentioning, since they directly influence the support an adolescent is able to obtain from the environment. Blurring sexual roles is one phenomenon affecting contemporary adolescents. Women today have less traditional attitudes, expectations, and behaviors. Men are increasingly aware of women in changing and evolving roles, and they are consequently more involved in functions that were previously believed to be predominantly in the woman's domain and vice versa. The anxiety associated with these role changes has begun to be identified and explored.

The current economic reorientation from abundance to conservation brings a new focus on such issues as economic stability, restraint, and budgeting. There are fewer jobs, particularly for adolescents, and the cost of higher education has increased dramatically. In the 1980s women are also developing careers and entering the work force, which requires a new perspective on two-parent working families, as well as an increase in divorce and single-parent families. The results of these changes can only be speculated on; however, it is obvious that these issues increase the complexity of society and add new pressures to adolescents who are becoming adults and attempting to define their role in today's cultural milieu.

Data collection

Collection of data through clinical observations, which are based on theoretical knowledge, is an important aspect of the nursing process model. It involves observation and interpretation of behavior patterns in an organized way, which may indicate a need for growth-promoting relationships. The collection of data about the ado-

lescent's health status is often referred to in other disciplines as the developmental history. It specifically includes the following information:

1. Growth and development (including developmental milestones)
2. Biophysical status (illnesses, accidents)
3. Emotional status (relatedness, affect, mental status)
4. Cultural, religious, and socioeconomic background
5. Performance of activities of daily living (home, attending school)
6. Patterns of coping (ego defenses such as denial, acting out, withdrawal)
7. Interaction patterns (family, peers)
8. Adolescent's perception of and satisfaction with his health status
9. Adolescent's health goals
10. Environment (physical, emotional, ecological)
11. Available and accessible human and material resources (friends, school and community involvement)

These data are collected from adolescents, their families, and other significant persons, such as school personnel and the physician, by interviews, examinations, observations, and reports.

The importance of detailed information on the psychological development of adolescents has been challenged by many, since it places an emphasis on past occurrences. Data collection by the nurse is based on current, as well as past, functioning in all realms of adolescent life. It helps to give a view of the adolescent experience and aids the nurse in assessing the success of the adolescent's attempts to complete the prescribed tasks.

An examination of the common behaviors that adolescents display reveals that adolescence is a time of anxiety and conflict. Conflictual issues such as body image, identity, independence, sexuality, social role, and social behavior are the most common. These conflicts can produce adaptive or maladaptive behaviors in an attempt to master the tasks at hand. The extent of these conflicts, or the qualitative response of the adolescent's attempt to master and move toward adult functioning, is the key to the necessity of intervention with conflicted adolescents.

Body image

Chronological age is not a valid guide for physical maturation, since growth often occurs in spurts and there are individual differences. Since the grouping of adolescents is usually done chronologically, the adolescent must face being with others who vary greatly in physical development and interests. This explains the predominance of imitative behavior resorted to in adolescence as an effort to keep within the expected range of conduct and be compatible with peers. The greater the divergence from the rest of the group, the greater the adolescent's anxiety. The lack of uniformity of growth often puts great demands on physical and mental adaptability. Growth being uneven and sudden, rather than smooth and gradual, causes a change in body image.

Adolescents reevaluate themselves in light of these physical changes, particularly the onset of primary and secondary sex characteristics, which are so pronounced. They tend to compare themselves and their physical development to that of their peers. They are very concerned about the normality of their physical status. The absence of clear-cut norms only adds to this uncertainty. The physical changes of puberty cause adolescents to be self-conscious of their changing bodies. Often they are reluctant to have medical examinations because they fear abnormalities will be found. Examinations may intensify masturbatory conflicts, sexual fantasies, and guilt feelings. Extreme concern with body changes may lead to deviant behaviors such as hypochrondriasis, in which physical complications are the focus of underlying conflicts.[8]

Identity

In an attempt to adjust to the physical changes of puberty, adolescents experience a surge of excitation and tension. Methods of gratification and defenses against these feelings that were used in infancy and childhood are renewed. This mixture of previous infantile solutions, plus new adult attempts at mastery, accounts for the often bizarre and regressive nature of adolescent behavior. As they attempt to cope, adolescents sometimes act as adults and other times as children.

They can be seen to be experiencing a second individuation process, similar to the first one noted at about age 2. Blos[9] equates the characteristic "no" predominating in the 2-year-old's effort to differentiate between self and nonself with the rebellious and oppositional behavior of the adolescent. Adolescents exhibit behavior marked with experimentation, testing the self by going to extremes. This has a usefulness in the establishment of self-identity. The rebelliousness or negativism shows a movement toward

individuation and autonomy that has greater complexity but also elements similar to the 2-year-old's "no." Adolescents assert themselves in affirmation of their self-identity by being negative to parents and other authority figures whom they feel are not allowing them to be separate and unique, as illustrated by Clinical example 27-1.

CLINICAL EXAMPLE 27-1

David, although an avid football fan for several years, suddenly switched his interest to basketball. He quit his local football team despite his father's urgings to continue. His father, also a football fan, could not understand David's sudden negative attitude toward football and newly found interest in basketball.

The individuation process is accompanied by feelings of isolation, loneliness, and confusion, since it brings childhood dreams to an end and attributes them to fantasy. This realization of the end of childhood can create intense fears or panic. Many adolescents therefore attempt to remain in this transitional stage. The awakening of emotional ties with the family also occurs in the establishment of new, more interdependent relationships. This fearful, yet exciting, entrance into adulthood is a profound personal experience that is not totally resolved in adolescence but is dealt with throughout the course of one's lifetime. Adolescents mourn the loss of childhood, and the feelings of loneliness and isolation that accompany this loss establish an intense need for closeness, love, and understanding. If they are unable to obtain support during this struggle, an intense nontransient depression may result.[8]

Independence

There is an unconscious longing by adolescents to give in to their dependency needs. It is also a time of profound movement toward independence. Adolescents reveal this ambivalence by responding to petty annoyances and irritations with outbursts more intense than seem warranted. They see the process toward independence as being free of parental control. They do not view attainment of independence as a gradual learning process but as an emancipation accomplished by acting "differently." If one acts adult, then one is adult. Therefore they expose themselves to situations beyond their capabilities and then become overwhelmed and frightened. They seek reassurance in an attempt to alleviate their anxiety by returning to childlike ways and being dependent on those with whom they feel most secure, usually their parents. This accounts for the inconsistency of adolescent behavior.

Well-adjusted adults usually use a problem-solving approach and do not feel as threatened when inexperience requires dependency on others. Adolescents, however, already tempted to give in to dependency needs, feel as if they are regressing to childhood, which deflates their self-esteem. They must deny their need for their parents. Sometimes they will criticize their parents for treating them as a child and not allowing them freedom and then remark that their parents are not helpful enough. When adolescents seem to be rebelling against their parents, they may be rebelling against their own childhood conscience or superego. They project their ambivalence onto their parents, since they were the original source of restrictions. This projection actually reveals a movement toward a more mature standard and also indicates their insecurity about relinquishing childhood standards. By blaming their parents for their childish actions, they can avoid blows to their fragile self-esteem and protest that their actions result from parental demands, not their own.

Sexuality

Most adolescents accept the sexual mores of our culture, which dictate that sexual feelings be directed toward persons of the opposite sex. This is not achieved without confusion, since the adolescent is capable of a greater depth of emotional experience than the child. The biologically induced sexual feelings that are intensified during adolescence go along with intensified emotional feelings. The fusion of sexual impulses with love means that sex is the usual mode of discharge of feelings of deep affection. The strongest emotional ties are felt toward the parents, but the channeling of these sexual impulses creates a conflict. The adolescent interprets love for the parent of the same sex as suggestive of homosexuality. At the same time, feelings of love toward the parent of the opposite sex are equally conflictual, since they are viewed as incestuous. Movement toward independence complicates this issue, necessitating defensive activities toward these new emotions.

Rejection of parents, so frequently expressed by adolescents, can also be seen as a defense to diminish ties to the parents and therefore avoid sexual arousal. Efforts to resolve this conflict can be seen in experimentation through heterosexual and sometimes homosexual relationships. Ambivalence is apparent, since adolescents are often flirtatious one moment and rejecting the next, and parents may find these flirtations enjoyable. Clinical example 27-2 is an example of this ambivalence.

CLINICAL EXAMPLE 27-2

Debbie, at age 13, would not let her father kiss her. She was often snotty and aloof when he attempted closeness. In contrast, she was often teasing and flirtatious, often remarking about his muscular body structure.

Social role

Adolescents respond to persons and events with great intensity. They may be totally invested in one interest and then suddenly change to something different at a moment's notice. This intensity of feelings and lack of stable identity can account for their extreme sensitivity to the response of others. They are easily hurt, disappointed, and fearful of others. There is a tendency toward "hero worship" and "crushes," but with poor discrimination in evaluating the individuals to whom these feelings are directed. Adolescent relationships serve many functions. Frequently adolescents relate to a chum as if neither person were a separate individual. They often mimic each other's dress, speech, language, and thoughts. These relationships help in the development of self-identity and establishment of a social role.

The peer group is of extreme importance to adolescents, since within the security of the peer group, adolescents can attempt to resolve conflicts. They can relate to peers in a way in which they cannot relate to others, and with peers they can test out their thoughts and ideas. Their thoughts may be different from their peers, but through mutual sharing, they can attempt to find an answer. The peer group explores more autonomous ways of dealing with problems in life. A peer group that shares these explorations offers its members companionship, protection, and security, with acceptable elements of dependent gratification. In the peer group, adolescents can accept dependency, not as a child but as one of the gang, testing out ideas and trying new values. Within the safety of the peer group they can observe, comment on, and evaluate the activities of other peer groups. Adolescents usually are very loyal to their group of friends. Sometimes group security is so important that it is necessary at all costs. Then destructive experimentation may occur to preserve acceptance in the group.

Adolescents often test out ideas pertaining to values. They either eventually abandon them or incorporate them gradually into their adult personality. They react to many stimuli and drain off the tension created by new drives and impulses by investment in many interests. They do this with great intensity, and that is why adolescents are susceptible to many brief fads. This is often seen in their dress, love for music, or hobbies.

Close relationships with the opposite sex provide adolescents with security (often by "going steady") and a person with whom to discuss problems and evaluate solutions. Often the partner may take on similar characteristics. This reciprocal relationship enhances self-esteem by demonstrating sexual attractiveness to the self and to the world, and it indicates that one is lovable. It also allows for bisexual expression, since the girl expresses her partner's feminine parts and her boyfriend represents her masculine parts. It is frequently observed that people tend to marry someone resembling the parent of the opposite sex. However, adolescents may purposely choose someone different to free themselves of their ties to their parents, which are sexually tinged, or may choose someone who is an acceptable substitute for parents.

Sexual behavior

Fantasy is used by adolescents to discharge tension meant for sexual play. Secretly they can be participant and observer and try out means of direct sexual discharge. They may, however, feel guilt and shame about sexual feelings, or they may experience the incompatibility of their fantasies with their ideal of themselves. Fantasies usually are an attempt to find solutions and evaluate consequences. Most adolescent fantasies are of a problem-solving nature. They may indicate a disturbance if they continually occupy the adolescent's thoughts, are not converted into constructive actions, or are not modi-

fied by reality. Then they may disrupt other activities that are important to adolescent functioning and indicate a withdrawal from reality.

Masturbation is also a frequent mode of discharge of tension for adolescents, particularly when alone, unhappy, or frustrated, and it serves to fuse psychological and physical sexuality. It is not always associated with sexual fantasies. The value of masturbation may be lessened by the shame and guilt that accompany it. Male adolescents often fear discovery of evidences of ejaculation and females often fear changes in their genitalia as a result of masturbation. Fears are not limited to discovery by others but also are caused by the expansive experience of orgasm, with the resulting feelings of loss of ego boundaries. If masturbation is used as a continual source of comfort or with inappropriate exposure (exhibitionism), it is indicative of disturbance.

Mutual masturbation can also serve the purposes of tension release and fusing of identity. If mutual masturbation is the primary focus of the relationship, without the enrichment of other aspects of a relationship, then it may be maladaptive. Mutual masturbation is often acceptable to adolescents as long as it does not lead to intercourse. It can help to dispel anxieties about sexuality by assuring adolescents that they are sexually adequate.[17]

Nursing diagnosis

Behaviors that cripple growth and development may warrant nursing intervention. The nurse should consider the degree of destructiveness and the nature of the defense and regression that the adolescent experiences. If the difficulty is predominant and not transient, it may mean intervention is needed. These destructive behaviors become the basis for the identification of specific problem areas.

Sexually active adolescent

The sexual behavior of adolescents is often not as much an outlet for sexual passion as a desire to achieve closeness with another individual. The sexual expression seems to fulfill needs of love and security. Adolescents tend to use their sexuality to sublimate other needs. Josselyn[17] mentions some of the common interpretations sexual relations may have:

1. Finding an alternative choice to replace incestuously laden parental object of the opposite sex
2. Identifying with the parent of the same sex and trying to do what they do
3. Attempting to camouflage homosexual feelings
4. Expressing anger or hostility toward the parent of the opposite sex

Personal anxiety about sexual adequacy and peer group pressure also seems to add to the possibility of using sexual relations inappropriately. Some adolescents use sexual relations in a self-destructive way as a means of punishing themselves. Their promiscuity elicits external control and condemnation from others. This is apparent when there is an exhibitionistic quality, and subtle efforts to "get caught" are seen. Periods of extreme prudery may alternate with periods of extreme sexual activity. Adolescents often attempt to have the nurse take a stand against their behavior and thereby avoid the underlying conflictual issues.

Meeks[21] suggests exploring the meaning of sexual behavior in adolescents by asking the following questions:

1. Does the adolescent desire sexual gratification for punishment?
2. Do the adolescent's goals match the situation or is he deceiving himself?
3. Is he demanding adult privileges while acting irresponsible and dependent?
4. To what extent is the behavior a defense for depression, anger toward others, or exploratory experimentation?
5. Is the behavior to avoid anxiety-producing fantasies?
6. How close is the relationship to a mature one?

Clinical example 27-3 illustrates inappropriate use of sexual activity.

CLINICAL EXAMPLE 27-3

Janet, a 14-year-old adolescent, had apparently been sexually active since age 12. She was brought to the clinic by her parents when they had been told by a neighboring friend of Janet's exploits. Janet had bragged to the neighbor of her sexual ventures. Two years before referral her parents had placed Janet in a more controlled parochial school because they were concerned she was "acting wild." It became apparent that Janet had wanted her parents to know about and put limits on her behavior. She admitted to not enjoying sexual intercourse very much. She seemed to

be trying desperately to get approval from her distant and punitive mother. Her father, who was a policeman, was what she described as "a hopeless case," secretly wishing that he would be a better policeman for her.

Pseudohomosexuality

Adolescents who are uncertain of their sexual identity often misinterpret certain characteristics as being masculine or feminine. The anxiety that results can precipitate a fear of homosexuality. This triggers additional feelings of depression and anxiety that exaggerate the initial ones. This is common in males who see characteristics such as passivity as castrating and diminishing their maleness. Their fear of homosexuality increases their anxiety, causing them to withdraw into a cycle of failure. They may then feel dependent, have trouble asserting themselves, and respond by "acting out." It is important to differentiate between deviant behavior and defects in socialization skills in this regard. Defects in socialization skills causing a pseudohomosexual response may result from the absence of an adequate male figure, the mother or father's expressed fearfulness of aggressiveness, physical disabilities, seduction by an older adult, or a personality temperament of passivity.[21]

Overt homosexual activity in adolescence

During adolescence, when identity is unclear and much experimentation occurs, the individual may have both homosexual and heterosexual experiences. This does not mean that the adolescent is homosexual or bisexual.[18] If he is not severely conflicted either in his experimentation or in his regular homosexual relationships, he probably will not reach the nurse therapist. If he does, it may be to appease a conflicted family. Sometimes, however, homosexual relationships may interfere with establishing an adequate sexual identity. In this case homosexual behavior may be indicative of anxiety about heterosexuality. Because it is usually complex, the meaning of continued homosexual behavior must be assessed individually. This is evident in Clinical example 27-4.

CLINICAL EXAMPLE 27-4

Joanne, age 15, was engaged in homosexual experiences with an 18-year-old girl. She claimed she enjoyed sexual experiences more with girls than boys.

She had poor sexual experiences with boys because she believed boys wanted girls for their sexual exploits. This was understandable because her history revealed that she was sexually abused by her paternal grandfather several times and once by her father at about age 5. She had painful experiences and minor medical complications with her menstrual period. This, in addition to her early traumatic experiences, caused Joanne much confusion about her sexual identity. Her mother experienced sexual confusion of her own and related better to the boys in the family. Joanne always wanted to be close to her mother and gain her approval. Joanne, in her confusion, assumed that if she could be a boy (male counterpart of homosexual relationship), she could do to women what had been done to her (express her anger about early sexual traumas by identifying with the aggressor), could get her mother's approval (being a boy and not having sex with Daddy or boys), could gain closeness (sex with a girl), and could avoid mother's anger (for sex with Daddy). In her attempt to gain a comfortable sexual identity, she was trying out a homosexual identity because it seemed the least threatening.

Unwed motherhood

The meaning of pregnancy in adolescence is a complicated issue because there are social, as well as intrapsychic, factors involved. Some adolescent girls fear inadequacy of their femininity. These fears may stem from dependent attachment feelings toward the mother, which are frequently experienced during regressive periods and mistaken as signs of homosexuality.[8] To ease these fears, the adolescent girl may become pregnant. Sometimes pregnancy is an effort to escape a difficult family situation or to force the parents to agree to a marriage that may be inappropriate, as shown in Clinical example 27-5.

CLINICAL EXAMPLE 27-5

Susie, a 16-year-old adolescent, had run away for the second time, only to return home to the same chaos. She had tried to run away with her boyfriend. Her alcoholic mother and psychotic 19-year-old brother were making life unbearable. Her mother was surprised to learn about 3 months after her return that Susie was pregnant. Susie was delighted because she had hopes that now she could get out of the house, knowing her mother would now approve of her marriage to her boyfriend Jim.

Occasionally, emotionally deprived adolescents hope to give their child what they feel they have never received (or, probably more accurately, get from the child what they have not gotten). Sometimes pregnancy appears to be a device to allow parents to relinquish parental responsibility for the adolescent. In some cases the adolescent has lived out a scapegoat role as the bad one in the family, thereby justifying parental neglect and hostility. The pregnancy can then improve family relationships because, with the adulthood the pregnancy implies, parents may be freed of guilt and may then not need to encourage the adolescent to do things that make her unlovable.

Pregnancy in adolescence may have other origins. It can occur accidentally after sexual exploration. The adolescent may not be aware of contraceptive methods. Pregnancy in an unmarried adolescent is often associated with sexual promiscuity, and, if it is, the girl may be ostracized. Sometimes pregnancy occurs from a close interpersonal relationship. Both the circumstances and the adolescent's level of maturity need to be assessed. Peer groups can be supportive to a girl who becomes pregnant as a result of a meaningful relationship yet intolerant of one whose pregnancy is the result of promiscuity. In some cultures out-of-wedlock pregnancies are an accepted part of adolescence.

The decisions involving abortion, placement of the baby, and marriage are difficult ones. Attitudes and laws influencing these decisions are diverse. Many believe that to force the adolescent to have the baby and then give it up is more traumatic for her than abortion. Others believe that abortion can be more disturbing. Marriage is another alternative. Forcing a marriage to avoid societal condemnation usually adds to the adolescent's problems, but a mature couple might do well in marriage. All the alternatives should be presented to the adolescent with the consequences clearly stated. The adolescent should come to her decision with the aid and support of her partner, her family, the nurse, and other involved health care professionals.

Adolescent suicide

The most common factor in adolescent suicide is lack or loss of a meaningful relationship.[16] Many researchers think suicide is an attempt for attention and does not necessarily represent a true desire to die. Regardless, it is a bid for help that must be recognized. Subtle references, as well as attempts, should always be taken seriously and explored. Suicidal gestures are more often seen in girls, with boys expressing their depression by bravado that results in accidents,[23] as in Clinical example 27-6.

CLINICAL EXAMPLE 27-6

John, a 12-year-old depressed adolescent, had just gotten a small dirt bike. Six months earlier John's grandfather, his only friend, had died. John's father had died when he was 2 years old, and he had lived with his mother and grandparents ever since. John, feeling hopeless, had ridden his bike into a car. Luckily, after medical treatment for his broken arm and rib and multiple bruises, John was able to come to therapy. He described feeling helpless and lonely, especially without his grandfather.

The adolescent may be prevented from acting on suicidal feelings by parental concern and the establishment of new relationships. Adolescents may avoid the depression triggered by separating from their parents by expressing it through delinquent behavior. This behavior serves as a defense against self-destructive impulses that accompany feelings of self-loathing. The attempt to manipulate parents, which can motivate the runaway as well as the suicidal adolescent, often has secondary gains that are less important then the internal conflict causing this manipulation. Feelings of helplessness and worthlessness can be initiated by threatened abandonment, being asked to take the adult role, and lack of opportunities to be dependent. Sometimes these adolescents perceive themselves to be expendable because the family unconsciously wishes them dead.

In working with suicidal adolescents, the nurse should explore the following areas:
1. The seriousness of the attempt (What are the chances of rescue?)
2. The mental status of the adolescent (Was he psychotic?)
3. The extent of environmental stress—especially family disintegration
4. The adolescent's wider social environment and the strength of his support systems (social isolation, school performance, parental loss, disruption of friendship or romantic alliance)
5. The likelihood of repeated suicidal attempts (especially if conditions remain the same)

Clinical examples 27-7 and 27-8 illustrate suicide attempts by adolescents.

CLINICAL EXAMPLE 27-7

Maria, a 15-year-old girl, was referred to her local community mental health center from the neighborhood emergency room after ingesting pills. Maria had taken five of her mother's "arthritis pills" after an argument with her father about her 17-year-old boyfriend, José. Her father, who came home only on weekends, told her to stay away from him. After he left, the other family members noticed Maria had become sleepy while playing cards in the living room. Maria admitted to taking the pills and was rushed by her mother to the emergency room. Maria claimed she would never do it again. She had clearly wanted to be rescued, not really wanting to die. She had had poor school performance for the last year since her father had left the family. She had many friends and had been dating José for the past year. Maria had always been her father's favorite. When she reached puberty at age 13, that relationship changed a great deal. Maria's position as her father's favorite was delegated to a younger female sibling, causing Maria to feel angry and rejected. Her father left the family a year later and returned for weekend visits, during which he mainly disciplined the children. Maria's attempt to get close to José as a replacement for her father was sabotaged by her father as well. Her only recourse was to elicit her father's caring and concern through a suicide attempt. Maria and her family are currently in outpatient treatment.

CLINICAL EXAMPLE 27-8

Donald, age 13, was brought to the emergency room after cutting his wrists one evening when he thought his family was asleep. His mother had awakened and found him bleeding. She rushed him to the local emergency room where he received medical treatment. It was then revealed that this was Donald's second suicidal attempt. The first attempt occurred a year ago when he had ingested pills. Donald had received therapy for about a month. It was then discontinued because of the family moving to a new location, despite recommendations to continue with a new therapist. Donald was always an isolated child. He was never very close with anyone but had two friends. Since the move he had become more withdrawn. He had done well in school in the past but now had given up and was failing almost every subject. The youngest of nine children, Donald had little relationship with his siblings, who were all older than he and not at home much. Donald's parents, both approaching old age, seemed not to notice that he had become increasingly upset. Donald was hospitalized, since the risk of his attempting suicide again was high. He was an isolated and depressed adolescent, seeking refuge from loneliness and defeat in death. He had not wanted to be rescued. The last year, especially, revealed many unsuccessful attempts to find meaningful relationships.

Adolescent runaways

Adolescents attempting to free themselves from an unbearable living situation may run away. The exit can indicate unconscious conflicts, and the running away usually points out difficulties between the parents and the adolescent. Parental rejection is often experienced from birth, and the parent may alternate between extreme punitive measures and a "laissez-faire" attitude toward the adolescent. Adolescent runaways are often conflicted, especially regarding dependency-independency, and feel embarrassed, helpless, and defeated by their dependency wishes. This can result in a panic that motivates running away to prove autonomy and escape painful circumstances. They usually run away from disappointment toward something viewed as favorable and supportive. Parents often feel guilty and ashamed and have difficulty acting on practical issues, although some, relieved of their responsibility, are secretly pleased. Frequently the adolescent becomes involved in dangerous activities after running away. Most runaway adolescents want to return home if they believe their parents really want them.[21] Clinical example 27-9 illustrates home conditions that may lead to an adolescent's running away.

CLINICAL EXAMPLE 27-9

Karen, age 14, ran away from home to a friend's house. Her mother had often expressed a desire to leave; in fact, she had once left the family to the charge of Karen's father when Karen was 9 years old. Karen's mother had suddenly told her she could not see her boyfriend for a month because she had come in late the night before. This caused a tremendous scene because Karen had been out late every night the week before without her mother even noticing. Karen's friend's mother was different. She spent a lot of money on her children, talked to them, and never limited their activity; thus the friend's home appeared attractive to Karen.

Juvenile delinquency

Delinquent adolescents often experience poor parent-child relationships. Antisocial acts enable

the adolescent to express anger toward parents, who are punished for the adolescent's acts. Parents are often scapegoated because the child is seen as a helpless victim. It is important to keep in mind that some parents are not effective with some adolescents. Children are socialized mainly by the parents and, hopefully, learn from the parents acceptable behaviors that become part of the internalized self or conscience. A good relationship between parent and child facilitates this process. However, adolescents learn not only from their parents but also from others in their environment. The school and peer groups are influencing factors, as are the social, economic, and cultural environments. The self-destructive behaviors seen in delinquent adolescents may be indicative of need for punishment, anger at the family, peer group pressure, depression, feelings of self-defeat, a search for opportunities to take what they feel emotionally deprived of, and testing omnipotence through exciting experiences. Alignment with delinquents gives a defeated adolescent a feeling of self-respect and companionship through a sense of belonging to a subculture.[17]

A classical work on juvenile delinquency, *Wayward Youth,*[3] was written by August Aichhorn in 1935 and revised several times, most recently in 1966. This is a classical Freudian look at juvenile delinquency and attempts to apply psychoanalysis to the treatment of delinquents. Aichhorn continues and extends his classical understanding of delinquency in a more recent work entitled *Delinquency and Child Guidance,*[2] in which he applies these principles and explores how the court and other systems handle these problems.

Clinical example 27-10 of an adolescent who steals illustrates the many factors that may lead to adolescent delinquency.

CLINICAL EXAMPLE 27-10

John, 13 years of age, was referred by the juvenile court for psychotherapy because he had been picked up for the second time after breaking into a store with another boy. John's parents were separated for the past 2 years after John's father had served a sentence in jail for tax evasion. John, very attached to his father, was extremely upset when his parents separated and rarely saw his father. His antisocial acts caused his father to become more involved with him, since his father claimed he did not want John to go through what he had experienced in prison. John gained his father's attention during these times, even though his father was angry. His delinquent actions therefore enabled John to express his anger at his father's leaving, as well as to fantasize about having his father return.

John's actions illustrate that adolescents may not differentiate between their stealing and their parent's business dealings. Stealing may also be an effective way to rebel against parents. Adolescents may perpetuate childhood through stealing by indulging in immediate gratification rather than maturely working for things. Sometimes adolescents steal in hopes of getting caught and obtaining help. Parents may consciously or unconsciously condone stealing. Adolescents may act out their anger with the justification that they deserve the stolen items. The reasons for stealing must be established for the individual adolescent, since causation may be diverse.

The conflict of dependence vs. independence can be expressed in poor school adjustment. Some adolescents view teachers as parental surrogates who do not help or who merely apply rules of attendance and homework. Dependent feelings are sometimes elicited by these rules, and adolescents, in proving their independence, may become negative about learning. They may think that schoolwork is secondary to other more important things that they are attempting to master. Daydreaming may interfere with schoolwork as adolescents concentrate on and fantasize about achieving an independent identity.

Adolescent students may drop out of school for practical financial reasons, or they may be rebelling against education laws. The adolescent may be part of a peer group that denounces school attendance and involvement. Parents may overtly or covertly discourage education. This is conveyed through lack of support and approval for education or by their making it difficult for the adolescent to follow through with school expectations, as illustrated by Clinical example 27-11.

CLINICAL EXAMPLE 27-11

Debbie, a 15-year-old adolescent, dropped out of school after several years of poor school performance and truancy. She would occasionally go shopping with her mother on a school day. Her mother never knew the names of her teachers or guidance counselor, and no provisions for a place or time to study were made.

Violent adolescents

Most adolescents displaying aggression have experienced frustration and observed violent models during their childhood. It seems appropriate to speculate that aggression is a human impulse which must be channeled constructively by a learned process that occurs within a supportive loving relationship. Under favorable conditions a child learns the healthy expression of aggression by involvement in activities that result in pleasure and active problem-solving attempts. Under less ideal conditions the expression of aggression can occur in destructive activities that are harmful to self and others. In adolescence, when aggressive as well as sexual impulses are increased, the energy that strengthens these impulses also strengthens the adaptive and defensive aspects that go along with aggression.[5]

Much anxiety of adolescents is therefore related to the fear that they may be unable to control their destructive aggression. Adolescents often have violent dreams and fantasies that they express in threats, even though in some the potential for violence is minimal. Pointing out the harmlessness of these thoughts is helpful to adolescents, since it is instrumental in showing that these thoughts are not as powerful as they fear. Some adolescents, however, are genuinely fearful that they will be unable to stop their thoughts from becoming actions. They require the recognition of their fear and the reassurance of the existence of external limits. Pointing out to the adolescent the necessity of self-responsibility and control is paramount. Their defenses against aggressive outbursts should be reinforced and supported. Focus should be on the behavior and feared loss of control, not on the roots of the anger.[21] Clinical example 27-12 is an example of management of a violent adolescent.

CLINICAL EXAMPLE 27-12

Ricky was a 15-year-old boy referred for treatment for violent outbursts at home. When frustrated, he would break and destroy objects in his path. Ricky was an only child, adopted shortly after birth by a couple in their forties who were unable to have children. Now Ricky's parents, who were about 55 years of age, were increasingly frightened by his aggressive outbursts. They had also felt powerless with his childhood temper tantrums and had consistently responded to outbursts by attempting to limit frustrating situations. They felt guilty and inadequate about his being an adopted child and continually made attempts to reassure Ricky of their love for him. They consequently reinforced his lack of control by assuming these outbursts were results of his fear of being unloved and would offer peace offerings of gifts and rewards. Ricky assumed he was omnipotent, successfully controlling his parents, but was fearful that he could not control his anger. Acknowledging Ricky's fear of loss of control, applying external controls, and pointing out areas of Ricky's ability for responsibility and control resulted in a gradual decrease in outbursts. First the outbursts became more limited as Ricky began breaking specific things that he did not value. Then he progressed to an elimination of violent outbursts.

Most adolescents fear violence; others pose a real risk. Adolescents who have committed extreme acts of violence, or homicide, are often from families in which violence is the norm. These adolescents may have experienced physical abuse, and, if not, they may have witnessed it between their parents. Behavior toward them has often alternated between seductiveness and physical brutality, adding to the adolescent's confusion and arousing intense frustration. Many times these adolescents are encouraged to be violent, since their outbursts are not firmly limited. Sometimes parents can predict the adolescent's ability to injure or kill. Frequently there is a history of dangerous assaults on family members and pets. In severely violent adolescents, violent acts can be followed by a calmness and lack of sorrow or guilt, since they claim that outside forces provoked them. Many homicidal adolescents will freely discuss their violent plans or fears. These should be explored and homicidal intent evaluated. Does the adolescent have a victim, weapons, or plan? This information, along with the history, shows the level of success or failure in controlling feelings and delaying gratification. Poor rapport with the therapist and evasiveness may indicate disturbing paranoid tendencies, revealing a greater potential for violence.

Adolescents and drugs

Adolescents may turn to drugs for relief of tension when pressures are intense. Meeks[21] and other theorists have spoken of the following types of drug users:

1. *Casual users—"the experimenters."* These adolescents use mostly marijuana in small quantities to substantiate their position in the peer group and to decrease the anxieties experienced because of their movement away from the family. Alcohol has often been used this way in the past, and there currently seems to be a return to alcohol for this purpose.

2. *Sociological users—"the seekers."* These adolescents are very aware of social realities, and they want to be active participants in the social process. They believe society's shortcomings to be their own inadequacies. They tend therefore to form separate communities in which they idealistically attempt to create a society of their own free of social conventions. Many seek relief from boredom through drugs and membership in this society. They lack the ability to express their inner feelings and tend to deal with their loneliness through mystical revelation and the group connection, with the hope of a conflict-free life with others.

3. *Sick users—"the heads."* Adolescents using drugs for cultural or neurotic reasons must be differentiated from those who use drugs to mask or correct maturational difficulties. This distinction is difficult to make. Those with serious interpersonal difficulties often are in a group that is bonded together by a high frequency of drug usage. They turn to drugs in times of stress and prefer drug-induced pleasures to those arising from interpersonal relationships and competitive efforts. This group also includes those who are socially critical and use the drug group as a personal justification rather than with any real social concern.

There are social implications connected with drug usage that must be considered. Our "pill relief" society gives a backdrop for pharmacological abuse. Drug abuse can reflect a general discontent with society's shortcomings in values and organization. The awakened interest in magic and mysticism also adds the potential of drug-induced exploration of life.

The meaning of drug usage in adolescence is a difficult and complex question. The adolescent's individual motivation must be explored, the nurse keeping in mind that it may be an expression of rebelliousness with support of a peer group, as well as a way of obtaining gratification of instinctual needs at a regressed level.

It may also indicate an effort to come to grips with feelings of vulnerability and inner emptiness.

Adolescents often report a wish for closeness that is satisfied by sharing a drug experience with friends. Drug users can experience an illusion of closeness because drugs decrease anxiety and users can share anticipation of use of the drug. Some adolescents fill the void of isolated loneliness with drugs and would otherwise feel suicidally depressed. Drugs can be crippling and delay healthy maturity by promoting the avoidance of the development of an adult identity in a real world, as illustrated in Clinical example 27-13.

CLINICAL EXAMPLE 27-13

Tommy was a 16-year-old adolescent boy who had been school phobic since age 10. He had been on home instruction since that age and was referred for a yearly assessment to get approval for a continuation of home instruction services. Tommy proudly spoke of his drug episodes. He and his small group of friends were close and had a repertoire of exciting experiences induced by various hallucinogens and amphetamines. Tommy had little support in the real world, since he had been isolated at home and experienced interpersonal relationships primarily in terms of obtaining and experiencing the effects of drugs.

It is rare that adolescent drug usage precipitates difficulties when the adolescent was previously well adjusted. This is especially true with soft drugs such as marijuana. Adolescents have been known to become psychotic, panicked, and assaultive after drug ingestion, especially of harder drugs. PCP, or "angel dust," has been noted to produce violence and incoherence. Sometimes "angel dust" is mixed with marijuana and other drugs without the adolescent knowing it. Bad trips have been reported with hallucinogens, as well as belladonna and opiate drugs. Often friends help to deal with upsetting reactions, but occasionally medical care is sought. Amphetamines have been known to produce psychosis. Belladonna can produce acute maniclike psychotic states accompanied by hallucinations.

Alcoholism among teenagers is currently on the rise and seems to be similar to drug abuse dynamically. Addeo and Addeo[1] have suggested some possible origins for alcoholism in adolescents, including parental and social influence, peer pressure, and emotional disturbances. Many researchers believe teenagers are currently switching from drugs to alcohol and alcoholism is the greater social problem.[10]

Hypochondriasis

Adolescents are preoccupied with their bodies and body sensations. There are many reasons for this concern and preoccupation. Adolescents are uncomfortable with their bodies because of the rapid changes in size, contour, and functioning. In an attempt to establish their identity, adolescents try to become familiar with their changing bodies. They respond to sensations with increased intensity. When an adolescent appears overly concerned, it may indicate underlying difficulties in the formation of a self-image.

Hypochondriasis occurs when the adolescent has intense anxiety about his health. This anxiety may be diffuse or directed toward one specific area. Focus on the body may conceal vague fears of catastrophe. Adolescents' concerns that their bodies are inadequate, that they will be rejected by others, or that they are unable to reach adulthood may predominate. Hypochondriasis may be a way of avoiding activities that expose these and other stressful fears. Fears such as inadequacy at school, either socially or in schoolwork, may be a projection of general fears of inadequacy. Lack of knowledge of the normality of body changes may be a simple precipitating factor. This can be tackled by reassurance that these changes are normal. If reassurance does not alleviate anxiety, then it is possible that other more intense fears are involved.

Reassurance and support can frighten the adolescent who uses body concern to mask an intense conflict. This is important to consider—the adolescent may then have no means to discharge the pressures of the basic anxiety, since the defense is removed. Support may imply to adolescents that the nurse or parents do not care for them. It is important to communicate to adolescents that people are aware something is wrong and that their concerns will be taken seriously until the core difficulty is alleviated. Intense body concern is a signal that something is not right and help is needed. Physical status must be assessed first before a psychological basis for concern is assumed. Sometimes body preoccupation is an effort to recreate infantile dependency by eliciting care giving. This is particularly seen in adolescents who experienced early emotional deprivation.[17] John in Clinical example 27-14 is an interesting example of this.

CLINICAL EXAMPLE 27-14

John, age 12, was referred for treatment from the local hospital after having been seen for chest pains. The physician found no medical problems. John was embarrassed and angry about the episode, insisting that the physician was wrong. The chest pains had disappeared, but he now had injured his arm. He also was often plagued by genuinely uncomfortable attacks of tonsillitis and middle ear infections. John had experienced early emotional deprivation because he was often moved around in his living arrangements. He was born out of wedlock and lived occasionally with his mother, often with his maternal grandmother, and infrequently with his father. He generally had the feeling that no one really cared for him. Further exploration revealed that John's body concerns were to precipitate care giving by those around him, who he feared really were not there for him. He performed well in school and had friends, but none of these compensated for his feelings of inadequacy.

Weight problems

Another disturbance often seen in adolescence is anorexia nervosa, or loss of appetite and refusal to eat, leading to emaciation. This life-threatening behavior often appears to be similar in psychodynamics to obesity or overeating. Many authors suggest that the underlying conflict in both syndromes is sexual. A denial of a wish to be sexual is expressed by the unattractiveness of being extremely thin or the camouflage of feminine or masculine characteristics with childlike heaviness. Often heaviness is equated with pregnancy, which represents sexuality. Another speculation is that anorexia nervosa is a reaction formation to the desire to be gluttonous, whereas excessive eating is the symbolical taking in of love. Extreme restraint of gluttonous wishes or giving in to these wishes represents a desire to return to infantile dependency, often precipitated by emotional deprivation. The possibility of a physical origin must always be considered and ruled out before the syndrome is attributed to psychological determinants. Obesity or loss of weight may be the result of abnormal glandular functioning.

Clinical example 27-15 illustrates the development of anorexia nervosa in a young girl.

CLINICAL EXAMPLE 27-15

Janet, age 15, was admitted to the hospital because it was feared that her extreme loss of weight was endangering her life. Exploration revealed that Janet was petrified of her sexual feelings and the response of others to her budding sexuality. Her father, provocative and teasing toward Janet, was continually kidding her about her oncoming sexual attractiveness and implied that he really preferred her to her mother. This created panic and Janet refused to eat. She liked her thinness, which was protection from sexual desires. In the hospital, the area of concentration was not the behavior of not eating, but rather the underlying panic feelings about her sexuality and her relationship with her father. This provided freedom for normal sexual growth and development.

School phobia

School phobia is an example of neurotic anxiety often seen in adolescence. Some school dropouts may be suffering from undiagnosed school phobia. This differs from other disturbed behaviors in that school represents the focus of their fears. The parents (most often the mother), although verbalizing the wish for the adolescent's maturity, often unconsciously want the adolescent to remain at home, limited in opportunities to move toward adult development.[17] Other possible causes may be fears experienced by the adolescent concerning maturing and leaving childhood protection, the meaning of new knowledge, exposure to feelings and wishes stimulated by close relationships with peers and adults, and failure to meet the adolescent's idealized self-image.[7]

Adolescents may use destructive means of obtaining attention, demonstrate their poor conception of themselves, or hide from dealing socially with the opposite sex by remaining at home. Clinical example 27-16 is an example of school phobia.

CLINICAL EXAMPLE 27-16

Donna, a 13-year-old girl, had always been shy with others. She was referred for therapy after the third week of classes in her new junior high school because she was not attending school on account of illness. Her mother claimed that despite her efforts to get Donna to school, she would return home with an upset stomach or headache. Her mother had taken her to school the 2 days she had attended, only to have her return home 3 hours later. A medical work-up provided no medical basis for her stomach and head pains. As the evaluation proceeded, it became clear that Donna had an extraordinarily close relationship with her mother. In the past her mother had worked as a teacher's helper at the elementary school Donna attended. Treatment dealing with the mother-daughter dyad was instituted.

Planning and implementation of nursing interventions

When dealing with the adolescent, it is advisable whenever possible for the nurse to have an initial contact directly with the adolescent. Many adolescents are concerned that the nurse therapist is aligned with the parents. Other adolescents take a passive role, letting the adults straighten things out for them. By initiating contact with the adolescent, an alignment is made with the independent mature aspects of the adolescent. Parents asking for advice on how to present coming to a therapist to the adolescent should be advised to be honest, stating the true nature of the visit and their reasons for requesting it. Many agencies and institutions use a child guidance approach, seeing the parents first to get a full developmental history. Family sessions have also been used in the diagnostic evaluation, helping to reveal family interaction and later being helpful in establishing family support.

Family therapy

Family therapy is particularly useful to an adolescent when chronic disturbed family interaction is seriously interfering with the adolescent's development. Sometimes a series of family sessions may be enough, and the adolescent may benefit from either individual or group approaches to offer greater support to his effort to separate emotionally from his family. Occasionally, after a few family sessions, it may become clear that the adolescent may not need the intervention directly. Engaging the parents may free the adolescent to progress on the developmental continuum.

The techniques used in family therapy are reviewed in detail in Chapter 25. Whatever modality is selected in working with the adolescent,

a family orientation and the adolescent's attempt to separate from his family and become an independent adult should be considered.

Group therapy

Group therapy uses adolescents' propensity to gain support from their peers. The conflict of dependence-independence with adults becomes somewhat diluted by the presence of other adolescents. Conflicts, especially about authority, can be detected by peers rather than adults, making this modality particularly desirable for adolescents. Many nurses use group therapy as a catalyst and combine it with individual therapy. It is a valued modality in teaching skills in relating and dealing with others. It helps fulfill the adolescent's need for a positive, meaningful peer group for ego identity formation.

Adolescent groups, in contrast to other groups, are difficult in that many adolescents turn to peers in a defensive and tenuous connection. Sibling rivalry often disrupts group cohesion. Many groups suffer from poor attendance, a high dropout rate, antisocial behavior, and a lack of group cohesion. However, group therapy with adolescents has proved to be successful in many community mental health centers, outpatient clinics, and hospital settings.

Coed groups are generally the best, when possible. Berkovitz[6] believes that coed groups decrease homosexual anxiety and anxious disruptiveness. Often, beginning groups with some activity helps to provide a stabilizing factor for young adolescents. The number of members to include in the group depends on the type. For example, it may not be feasible to limit an outpatient "drop-in" group. Because of the age spread among adolescents, it is usually preferable to form at least two groups. A possibility is an early adolescence group consisting of 13 to 15 year olds who have conflicts of separation from parents as well as homosexual and incestuous anxieties. An older adolescent group, age 15 to 17, would probably consider issues such as the further establishment of identity, the beginning of dating or exploration of relations with the opposite sex, experimentation with drugs, handling money, responsibilities of driving, and vocational plans. Mixing the two age-groups with varying concerns may not be productive.

The most ideal situation is to have male and female co-therapists; however, this is not always feasible. If there is a single therapist for an unmixed group of the opposite sex, anxiety of group members may be shown by disruption or flight. Conflict between therapists, if there is an open and honest discussion, can provide a corrective experience because adolescents can see adults disagree without devastating consequences. If therapists are of the opposite sex, a parental similarity is often apparent and members often play on the therapist's feelings and try out tactics as they would with their own parents. Even if both therapists are of the same sex, one is usually more active, and a member may project a good or bad image onto each therapist that corresponds with his view of his parents.

Group process with adolescents is often similar to that with adults, and specific aspects of group therapy are reviewed in Chapter 24. Resistances such as silence, passivity, disruptiveness, and intellectualization are often seen with adolescents, since they tend to act out rather than verbalize anxiety. Differences among various types of groups, for example, residential groups vs. outpatient groups, must be considered.

Individual therapy

Individual therapy done by the psychiatric nurse specialist can consist of brief goal-directed therapy, behavioral therapy, or insight therapy. A description of insight therapy is presented here, since the principles are helpful in other types of individual therapy as well. Once the decision to engage in individual therapy is made, a pact or contract between the therapist and adolescent is established, depending on the approach and type used. This contract in insight therapy is described by Meeks[21] as a "therapeutic alliance" in which the nurse aligns herself with the healthy, reality-oriented aspect of the adolescent's ego and moves toward an honest and critical understanding of the adolescent's inner experience. This alliance is created through the orderly interpretation of the adolescent's feeling states and defensive behavior, especially toward the nurse.

The alliance in dealing with adults differs from that with the adolescent in that with adults there is a promotion of a regulated and controlled regression. This is not useful for the adolescent. Adolescents' alliances are focused toward links between their feelings and behavior in the present. Brief regressions occur anyway, and focuses usually are aimed at efforts to recover from regressions and at reinforcing and supporting progressive development. The alliance is a central aspect of individual therapy, and, once it is established, a feeling of working together is ap-

parent. Meeks[21] mentions helpful specific hints to establish and maintain this alliance:

1. Point out that behavior is motivated by feelings. Often, early in treatment, adolescents may express feelings of impatience, helplessness, and failure at having to see a therapist. Defenses are often seen in rebelliousness, passivity, shyness, negativism, and intellectualization. Adolescents generally have a propensity to act and avoid feelings.

2. Limit acting out by pointing out how it interferes with the therapeutic process and that it must be controlled to proceed. Maintain a neutral but interested attitude toward all behavior.

3. Point out the adolescent's tendencies to be judgmental and self-critical. This is supportive and helps to encourage the adolescent to look for sources of behaviors, attitudes, and feeling states.

4. Establish that the adolescent's behavior is the end result of many inner feelings. Some of these unknown feelings sabotage freedom. This knowledge strengthens motivation for therapy and maintains an alignment with the adolescent's wishes for autonomy. Encourage therapeutic efforts as a means to alter rebellion into true self-direction and freedom.

5. Point out the adolescent's propensity to see things in extremes; the desire to be complete master opposes the feelings of total helplessness. Reveal areas of strength and competence that are often unrecognized. Avoid focusing exclusively on problems and weaknesses. This shows neutrality and is supportive. Giving the adolescent as much information as possible to be prepared to make his own decision helps the adolescent work toward self-direction.

6. Distinguish between thought and action, discouraging impulsiveness. Encourage open expression of strong feeling but not strong action. For example, anger does not mean killing; sexual feeling does not mean intercourse. Adolescents sometimes confuse discussion with permission to experiment with action, especially with sexual issues.

7. Encourage real emotion in sessions by expressing interest in and acceptance of feeling states appearing in relation to the nurse and feelings expressed in description of events outside the session. Point out the importance of feelings.

8. Watch out for the defenses of denial and reaction formation. Maintain neutrality and encourage objectivity without directly assaulting

essential defenses. Adolescents will resort to pathological defenses when threatened by emergencies.

9. Adolescents often act provocatively to get important adults to delegate punishment. This puts the nurse in alignment with the self-hatred aspect of the adolescent's conscience and should be avoided. The nurse is supportive by continuing therapy even during these difficult periods.

The work of the nurse therapist is to recognize the adolescent's anxiety and try to assist him in finding ways to deal with emerging impulses. Defenses suggested by the nurse are rarely useful, but pointing out, supporting, and accepting any healthy defense of the adolescent strengthens his sense of ego mastery. Adolescents often have wishes that they regard as crazy and frightening. Open discussion of fears of homosexuality, incest, or homicide helps adolescents realize these feelings do not lead to psychosis and are uncomfortable but harmless thoughts.

Transference, as with the adult patient, is an important aspect of adolescent treatment. Pointing out that these irrational projections originate in the adolescent's mind and not in reality and that they usually represent a meaningful person such as a parent is necessary. It is often good to point out the commonality of this response. Transference is interpreted to diminish its impact on the therapeutic situation. Several common transference patterns have been identified[21]:

1. *Erotic-sexual*—especially if the nurse is young and of the opposite sex. Usually, this transference is shown by awkward blushing and agitated confusion by the adolescent. It is usually best to emphasize value in the mutual work of emotional growth while establishing, tactfully, the nurse's unavailability as a sexual object. Focusing on origins or encouraging elaboration of these feelings is not helpful and is anxiety provoking.

2. *Omnipotent*—expecting the nurse will have the answers to all questions. It is easy for the nurse to drift into this pattern, since often the adolescent appears to be a helpless cripple. The adolescent's secret desire for personal omnipotence is somewhat fulfilled by granting it to the nurse. The nurse then serves as a front, hiding the adolescent's fear of confronting reality without magical powers.

3. *Negative transference*—usually intense and pervasive. Negative feelings toward the nurse usually represent a negative attitude toward all adult authority figures. This transference is often defensive to cover feelings of shame, inadequacy, and anxiety, and it disappears as the adolescent respects the nurse's feelings. The adolescent tries to force the therapist to reject him. Open discussion to explore these feelings objectively and establish their origin is beneficial. Sometimes interpretations arouse anger toward the nurse because of the anxiety they create. These are reactions to the realities of therapy and are not to be confused with negative transference.

A true negative transference occurs when situations reactivate early experiences in which negative feelings toward important others predominate. The nurse is seen as a frustrator whenever she, representing reality, opposes gratification of impulses and ego drives. Negative transference tends to appear whenever the nurse refuses to gratify needs that the adolescent feels are important and legitimate. The nurse unavoidably will frustrate the adolescent, who often has trouble delaying gratification to reach long-range goals. The nurse should point out the true motive behind activities that express anger. Clarifying hidden hostile feelings frees them for expression toward the nurse, and irrational expectations may then be revealed. Negative transference is dealt with as any other resistant behavior through objective exploration, which includes seeking causes of anger and pointing out irrationality. This is often followed by an expected period of regression and depression. Empathic understanding that the adolescent is mourning a loss is helpful, but it should be emphasized that what was lost was an illusion.

Another negative transference occurs when the adolescent sees the nurse as his superego. Projecting his superego onto the nurse may cause all interventions to be seen as superego sanctions. Adolescents have trouble understanding the rationale for foregoing gratification of an impulse. It is important to point out that these are the adolescent's own taboos and to encourage open confrontation with these taboos rather than avoidance. A common occurrence is for an adolescent to rebel against his conscience and then respond to guilt through self-destructive behaviors. Pointing out this pattern helps the adolescent to eventually become aware of this.

Termination of therapy is an integral part of the therapeutic process. Often, leaving therapy symbolizes the process of loosening bonds to parental images, relinquishing accompanying desires to be passive and expectations of the omnipotence of these figures. One therefore expects defensive and regressive behaviors as the adolescent attempts to deal with the anxieties related to the termination process. This can mean the recurrence of emotional crises, symptoms, self-destructive fantasies, and even dependency behavior to provoke rescue.

Termination should be flexible and correctly timed. The decision should be made in line with adolescent norms, not adult ones. Often adolescents will verbalize appropriate interest in termination. When this occurs, it is often helpful to open it to discussion without commitment to a set time. This implies that further work needs to be done in a definite time span, and it maintains a focus on the adolescent's responsibility to finish. Gradually supporting and approving of the adolescent's independence and mature functioning prepares for a positive termination. Some adolescents leave therapy to return later. Some can never leave forever, seeing termination as a rejection rather than a vote of confidence. Gradual reduction of sessions without pressing for final termination may help as long as the overall situation is reviewed occasionally.[14]

Sometimes terminations occur prematurely because of either the lack of success in establishing an alliance or some external events. Occasionally terminations are forced because of a nurse's change of location, death, or illness. The adolescent will express anger at the new therapist until the feelings about the lost therapist are accepted and resolved. In working out this attachment, a new therapeutic alliance can be established.

Talking with adolescents

Adolescents are different from adults and children, and often interactions pose difficulties not as apparent with other age-groups. Following is a discussion of some important considerations in communicating with adolescents.

SILENCE. Silence is often effective with adults but frightening to the adolescent, especially in the beginning stages of treatment or evaluation. This anxiety often is reflecting the adolescent's feelings of emptiness and lack of identity. Brief silences can be creative and productive when the adolescent is engaged in treatment, and, when the adolescent is able to tolerate them without anxiety, it indicates growth in self-confidence and acceptance of inner feelings. More often, however, silence is used defensively by adolescents to avoid discovery of hostile feelings or fantasies that might appear. Older adoles-

cents may tolerate interpretative remarks, but with younger adolescents it is usually helpful to suggest an activity to help facilitate discussion and establish a relationship. For some adolescents silence is a characterological defense of inhibition and withdrawal, since they have never learned to communicate in a positive way. In these cases the therapist must carry the burden of responsibility for dialogue.

CONFIDENTIALITY. Confidentiality is a concern to many, but especially to the adolescent who is fearful of the nurse reporting to his parents. A blanket promise to tell nothing to the parents is not advised, since the nurse may need to contact the parents if the adolescent reveals suicidal or homicidal behavior or the use of illegal drugs. It is usually best to tell the adolescent that the nurse will not divulge any information without informing the adolescent of the intention to do so in advance. It is also helpful to explain that feelings are confidential but that actions considered dangerous to the adolescent or others may need to be shared.

NEGATIVISM. Negative feelings are often expressed by adolescents, especially initially, because they are frightened of the implications of coming for treatment. The young adolescent's lack of objectivity and upsurge of instinctual impulses, as well as the tendency to confuse fantasy and action, make the discussion of feelings threatening. Usually, gently noting in a supportive way defensive techniques the adolescent uses during the session helps to gain cooperation.

RESISTANCE. Often adolescents begin by testing the nurse to see if she will be another authoritarian figure. The rebellious adolescent may claim he does not need therapy or help. If the adolescent appears anxious, it is best to be supportive and sympathetic, expressing interest in getting to know the adolescent and then discussing a neutral area. A more angry, rebellious adolescent may require a direct approach, with the nurse saying openly that she feels the adolescent is opposing the visit because he believes no help is needed. This can lead to a further discussion of feelings about the visit, for example, parental coercion to come to the session. A productive discussion of feelings about authority may then ensue. Some adolescents are just baiting and testing to see if the nurse is an anxious

and defensive adult. If so, it is best to ignore
their comments about not wanting treatment
and move on. Often adolescents with an angry
facade depend on their omnipotent control of
the environment and are often successful in
manipulating their families. They are angry at
attempts to disturb this power, and the anger
is expressed in their lack of cooperation in the
session.[19]

ARGUING. Adolescents always argue and, although they do not admit it, learn from arguments. Often the adolescent goes against the
viewpoint of the nurse and then in the next session states her opinion as his own. It is best not
to comment on this and accept it as a harmless
defense. If the nurse admits having areas of ignorance, it is productive to the adolescent, who
may fear that he must be perfect.

TESTING. Adolescents often need and want
limits. They are confused and cannot set their
own limits. They experiment by trial and error
to find a self-concept. Often an adolescent will
test the nurse to see how firm and consistent
she will be. Controls frequently are effective if
there is a basic positive relationship with the
nurse. Limits should be set only when they are
essential for current and future well-being, and
the adolescent will value the security they provide. The nurse represents a substitute parental
figure allowing independence. Adolescents will
dare to be independent if it is conveyed that
the nurse will serve as a control against carrying independence too far.

DREAMS AND ARTISTIC CREATIONS. Adolescents are often creative, and a lot can be learned
from studying their productions. As long as the
discussion is relevant to achieving ego synthesis,
it can be a productive source for exploring inner
feelings that, along with dreams, can reveal
valuable information about their real concerns,
even when attempts are made by the adolescent to avoid them. The nurse must be careful
not to engage in intellectual discussion irrelevant to the adolescent's inner life. ·

BRINGING FRIENDS. The adolescent who brings
a friend to a session may be attempting to
avoid the seriousness of therapy. There is some
benefit in sharing the experiences with the peer
group, since this lowers anxiety. Telling the adolescent that bringing friends is not allowed may

not be successful because the nurse cannot always enforce such a rule. The reason for bringing friends may vary, but the action should be
seen as communication to be explored and understood. Sometimes adolescents want to refer
friends. This may be positive but may also focus
attention away from the original adolescent. The
nurse should insist on exploring motives behind
the referral before accepting the new patient,
since the adolescent may feel that the nurse's
acceptance of another is a betrayal of loyalty. If
the friend clearly wants and needs therapy,
referral to a competent colleague is usually best.
If a friend is brought late in therapy, it may
mean the adolescent is getting ready to terminate.

EMBARRASSMENT ABOUT BEING IN THERAPY.
Embarrassment may occur in any age group, but
it is prominent in adolescents, especially during the early stages of treatment. It also can
become an issue as therapy progresses because
it often reveals the adolescent's embarrassment
about his wishes for dependency. Therefore adolescents may become uncomfortable in the therapeutic relationship. This is usually dealt with
effectively by indicating the normalcy of these
types of feelings. Behind the fear of accepting
help is the wish for care, and this can be dealt
with by pointing out the adolescent's strengths
and areas of independence. The nurse can then
reveal that any wish or thought of care or dependency is thought by the adolescent to represent
total dependency. This helps the adolescent to
be more tolerant of his wishes, seeing them realistically as wishes that all people have.

Some adolescents, by expressing embarrassment about being in therapy, are actually revealing a fear or social stigma that they have heard
from their parents. The adolescent who has feelings of inferiority often focuses these on the
therapeutic process, blaming therapy for discomfort. It is best to encourage and be supportive to the adolescent, gently refusing to accept blame for this discomfort. The issue of
whether to tell friends should be explored dynamically.

REQUESTS FOR SPECIAL ATTENTION. Some adolescents can develop intense dependency ties to
the therapist. They reflect this in requests for
additional appointments, extra time in appointments, frequent telephone calls, or social contact outside the therapeutic sessions. Late in
therapy there is little advantage to meeting these
primitive needs. The regressed adolescent needs
an undemanding nurse who allows him to ex-

perience inner feelings of emptiness. The therapist cannot fill this emptiness and should avoid false promises. Focus should be on the exploration of feelings of inner emptiness, deprivation, and incompleteness.

Parents of the adolescent

If group or individual treatment is selected for the adolescent, the nurse must still consider the family. Many parents overtly claim desire for their adolescent's maturity and independence but unconsciously need to maintain him as a child and covertly undermine growth. Parents may sabotage the adolescent's treatment if they are not helped to understand and accept it. It is possible to work with the parents without revealing confidential material.

Adolescents frequently try to avoid limits by playing parents against the nurse. If parents are angry with the restriction of their involvement in their child's therapy, there is a greater potential for this. The nurse can encourage healthier aspects of the parent-adolescent relationship and sympathetically accept parental anxieties and needs.

Not all parents of adolescents need treatment. Many adolescents do well despite parental difficulties. It is helpful for parents to have treatment if the adolescent is asked to assume an inappropriate destructive role at home, since this interferes with the therapeutic role. If the parents are resistant, the nurse must usually begin with the adolescent until the parents are more receptive.

Telephone contact is a helpful way to ensure cooperation and support by having the parent call when necessary. Parents should tell the adolescent when they call. Parents should be told of normal adolescent behavior they should expect. The nurse should avoid advising the parents about specific actions and focus on attitudes and feelings, especially concerning discipline. Parents can be helped with understanding the purpose of limit setting. Some parents exclude themselves entirely from their adolescent's life. They have brought the adolescent to treatment to assuage their guilt by doing all that is possible. They may often want the nurse to take over parenting functions. This should not be permitted, especially during crises. If the adolescent is suicidal or homicidal, the parents are informed and must take the responsibility for action with the nurse's help.

Adolescents often need help in dealing with their parents. At times, late in therapy, it is helpful to verify parental pathological behavior. If done too early in treatment, it can cause the adolescent to see himself as the victim. Later, well into the therapeutic alliance, it permits the adolescent to see his parents realistically, to forgive them, and to work on his own strengths and limitations. Parents should be discussed in an open exploratory manner, with emphasis on the fact that they have their own feelings on which their actions are based.

Adolescents can be helped to realize that if their parents are being controlling, adolescents must be free to reject or accept parents' goals according to their own needs and abilities, rather than merely rebelling. Even if the parents treat the adolescent as a child, that does not make him a child. The danger is the adolescent's own childlike wishes.

Sometimes adolescents want to leave home because they hope they will feel more adult away from their parents. It is usually best to support the wish to leave, emphasizing that it must be done in an adult way. If leaving is an impulsive thought with no feasible plan, it will ensure failure, parental rescue, and continued dependency. This is often recapitulated in termination from therapy if the adolescent quits early to avoid the pain of separation that a planned termination would bring.

Evaluation

Problems presented by adolescents, more frequently than those of any other group, activate the nurse's own unresolved conflicts. This countertransference reaction decreases her usefulness because of her anxiety and confusion. Alignment with either the parents against the adolescent or the adolescent against the parents should be watched for. Most adults are resistant to reexperiencing the feelings of adolescence and have repressed these experiences. As a result of anxiety, the nurse occasionally may have trouble listening or may encourage the adolescent (for her own unrecognized wishes) to do what the nurse herself never dared do. The adolescent may be acting as the nurse did during her own adolescence. The nurse, in an effort to deny this, may see this adolescent behavior as nondeviant. Identification of the nurse with the adolescent can contribute to delays in exploring areas important for psychological growth. The nurse may relate well to the adolescent but because of unresolved, unrecognized conflicts or resentment toward her own parents, may be locked into her own adolescent rebellion. She may overtly or covertly encourage the adolescent to express rage toward his family. Both the adolescent and the nurse then avoid facing the reality of adult burdens. It is easier for the nurse to do this if the adolescent's parents are indeed hostile, rejecting, and irresponsible.

Adults often have motives for emphasizing the inadequacies of adolescents, which can lead to an underestimation of the adolescent's abilities. These motives are often seen in protective or competitive attitudes of varying degrees that make it difficult for the nurse to let the adolescent do things on his own. In terminating with an adolescent, as with any valued human relationship, the nurse often has feelings of being abandoned and unappreciated. Many adolescents therefore often seem guilty and apologetic about their wishes to terminate and deal with things on their own. Just as many nurses hold on to adolescents too long, many times, unconscious hostile feelings on the part of the nurse can cause her to claim exaggerated progress. This allows her to disguise her unconscious angry rejection and avoid waiting for appropriate termination. Often the nurse's need to achieve quick success causes a superficial handling of necessary therapeutic work. Pressures from the family with financial troubles can hurry an insecure nurse. Fears of erotic feelings stirred up by closeness with the adolescent can lead her to a panicked withdrawal and termination motivated by self-preservation.

Nurses owe it to themselves and the adolescents they treat to be honest and rely on intellectual and emotional strengths, using the same exploratory attitude with themselves that is required and encouraged with the adolescents they treat. It is unavoidable that errors will occur. Doing therapy should provide growth experience for the nurse as well as the adolescent. Critical self-evaluation and reassessment of effectiveness of nursing actions, as well as assessment of the client's progress, is paramount in the treatment of any human being of any age group. Supervision provides an opportunity to objectively explore and evaluate the therapeutic process with an experienced colleague and is a necessary tool to encourage and facilitate this process. Supervision is a necessity for all therapists, no matter how much experience they have, because of the highly emotional nature of the work in treating adolescents.

Suggested cross-references

Issues of identity and self-concept are discussed in Chapter 8. Suicide and other forms of self-destructive behavior are discussed in Chapter 10. Problems with the expression of anger are discussed in Chapter 12. Substance abuse is discussed in Chapter 14. Group therapy is discussed in Chapter 24. Family therapy is discussed in Chapter 25.

SUMMARY

1. The adolescent psychiatric nurse was defined as a person who assists adolescents in their growth toward adulthood. Nurses take on roles as therapists, evaluators, educators, community consultants, and administrators in attempting to assist adolescents with their struggles.

2. Adolescence, as a developmental stage, was identified as movement on a life continuum between the ages of 11 and 20. During this time, shifts in past developmental and learning processes occur. Tasks accomplished during adolescence were presented.

3. Various theories explaining the adolescent's resolution of these tasks were presented. The biological theory consists of Gesell's beliefs that adolescence is biologically determined by physical growth changes. The intellectual development theory bases

adolescence on cognitive development and was conceived by Piaget. Psychoanalytical theorists, whose beliefs are based on the theories of Freud, were reviewed. Josselyn sees adolescence as the psychological consequence initiated by the hormonal changes of puberty. The increase in sexual and aggressive impulses causes a psychic restructuring. Blos described adolescence as the second individuation process. These analytical theories were modified by Erikson, Sullivan, and others. Erikson speaks of adolescence as a normal crisis with a great growth potential in facilitating adjustment to the new environment. Cultural theorists consisting of sociologists and anthropologists view adolescence as a societal phenomenon induced by society's lack of formal structure for passage into adulthood.

4. Areas explored in data collection reflect an understanding of the adolescent's experience and health status and include factors such as growth and development, physical status, emotional status, socioeconomic background, environment, daily activities, and support systems.

5. An understanding of normal behaviors seen in adolescents reveals basic conflicts adolescents experience. Conflicts considered were those involving body image, identity, independence, sexuality, social role, and sexual behavior. Body-image conflicts reveal behaviors such as self-consciousness, imitativeness, and body concerns. Conflicts concerning identity reveal regressive characteristics, rebelliousness, negativism, confusion, isolation, and depression. Independence vs. dependence conflicts lead to behaviors such as independent strivings, inconsistency, intenseness, and defensiveness. Sexuality conflicts produce behaviors attempting to deal with sexual impulses, such as heterosexual relationships, homosexual relationships, and parental rejection. In establishing a social role, adolescents exhibit behaviors involving hero worship, chums, crushes, peer group importance, and acting out. Fantasies, relationships with the opposite sex, masturbation, and homosexual activity reveal sexual behavior conflicts.

6. Various problem areas were described, including the sexually active adolescent, the unwed mother, the pseudohomosexual, the overt homosexual, the suicidal adolescent, the runaway, the juvenile delinquent, the violent homicidal adolescent, the drug abuser, the hypochondriac, the adolescent with weight problems, and the school phobic adolescent. The planning and implementation of various techniques of intervention were presented.

7. Family therapy and group therapy, with its particular advantage to adolescents who can supportively use the peer group, were briefly explored. Individual treatment, which focuses on establishing an alliance, dealing with transference, and reviewing termination aspects, was presented in an attempt to provide the framework for a productive, growth-producing, therapeutic relationship.

8. The special difficulties in dealing with adolescents, including silence, confidentiality, negativism, resistance, limit setting, power struggles, requests for special attention, embarrassment about therapy, bringing friends, and artistic creations, were discussed.

9. Dealing with the adolescent's parents is often a difficult task for the nurse, and some suggestions to facilitate parental support without sabotaging the therapeutic relationship with the adolescent were presented.

10. Evaluation of the nurse's intervention is a necessity. Adolescents arouse feelings within the nurse that must be dealt with if a therapeutic relationship is to be established. Supervision of the nurse is important to promote the evaluation process.

References

1. Addeo, E., and Addeo, J.: Why our children drink, Englewood Cliffs, N.J., 1975, Prentice-Hall, Inc.
2. Aichhorn, A.: Delinquency and child guidance, selected papers, New York, 1964, International Universities Press, Inc.
3. Aichhorn, A.: Wayward youth, New York, 1966, The Viking Press.
4. American Nurses' Association, Division of Psychiatric Mental Health Nursing Practice: Statement on psychiatric and mental health nursing practice, Kansas City, Mo., 1976, The Association.
5. Bandura, A., and Walters, R.: Adolescent aggression, New York, 1959, Ronald Press Co.
6. Berkovitz, I.: Adolescents grow in groups. On growing a group: some thoughts on structure, process and setting, New York, 1972, Brunner/Mazel, Inc.
7. Bhoyrub, J.P.: School phobia, in-patient involvement, Nurs. Times **73:**1388, 1977.
8. Blos, P.: On adolescence, New York, 1962, The Free Press.
9. Blos, P.: The second individuation process of adolescence, Psychoanal. Study Child **22:**162, 1967.
10. Bragg, T.: Teenage alcohol abuse, J. Psychiatr. Nurs. **14**(12):10, 1976.
11. Brenner, C.: An elementary textbook of psychoanalysis, New York, 1974, Anchor Press.
12. Erikson, E.: Childhood and society, ed. 2, New York, 1963, W.W. Norton & Co., Inc.
13. Gesell, A., Ilg, F., and Ames, L.: Youth: the years from ten to sixteen, New York, 1956, Harper & Row, Publishers, Inc.
14. Harley, M.: Analyst and adolescent at work, New York, 1974, Quadrangle/The New York Times Book Co., Inc.
15. Havighurst, R.L.: Developmental tasks and education, ed. 3, New York, 1972, David McKay Co., Inc.
16. Jacobs, J.: Adolescent suicide, New York, 1971, Wiley-Interscience.
17. Josselyn, I.: Adolescence, New York, 1971, Harper & Row, Publishers, Inc.
18. Kappelman, M.: When your teenager needs you the most, Fam. Health **9:**44, Aug. 1977.
19. Marshall, R.: The treatment of resistances in psychotherapy of children and adolescents, Psychother. Theory Res. Prac. **9**(2):143, 1972.
20. Mead, M.: Culture and commitment: a study of the generation gap, New York, 1970, Basic Books, Inc., Publishers.
21. Meeks, J.: The fragile alliance, Baltimore, 1971, The Williams & Wilkins Co.
22. Piaget, J.: Six psychological studies, New York, 1968, Vintage Books.
23. Reuben, R. et al.: Adolescents who attempt suicide, J. Pediatr. **58:**636, 1977.
24. Thornburg, H.: Development in adolescence, Monterey, Calif., 1975, Brooks/Cole Publishing Co.

Annotated suggested readings

Alissi, A.S.: Concepts in adolescence. In Neubauer, P., editor: Process of child development, New York, 1976, The New American Library, Inc.

This article gives an overview of the concepts of the adolescent developmental stage. Cultural and sociological factors are included to indicate that development must be understood within the context of the environment.

Blos, P.: The young adolescent, New York, 1970, The Free Press.

Peter Blos gives two case studies, one female and one male, to explain through clinical observation and theory the development of adolescence. The successful treatment of Susan and Ben gives an understanding of insight analysis during this developmental stage.

Brandes, N.: Group therapy for the adolescent, New York, 1973, Jason Aronson, Inc.

This is a good primer for beginning group therapists dealing with adolescents.

Chaiklin, H. et al.: Delinquency and health status, Health Soc. Work 2(3):24, 1977.

This article gives a good description of delinquency in adolescence and its effects on healthy development.

Danziger, S.: Major treatment issues and techniques in family therapy with the borderline adolescent, J. Psychosoc. Nurs. 20(1):27, 1982.

This excellent paper focuses on five major issues in the treatment of the borderline adolescent and his family: separation-anxiety, lack of control, poor ego boundaries, inability to express feelings, and borderline defense mechanisms. Treatment techniques are suggested for each.

David, P.: International trends . . . pregnancy and the unmarried girl, J. Psychiatr. Nurs. 15:40, Feb. 1977.

This article addresses itself to the unmarried pregnant teenager. Difficulties such as isolation caused by fear of communicating with parents and the various consequences of the possible alternatives are discussed. There is a call for more education for teenagers and their parents.

Duffey, M.: Factors contributing to the development of a cohesive adolescent psychotherapy group, J. Psychiatr. Nurs. 17:21, Jan. 1979.

A nurse describes her experiences in setting up an adolescent group. Goals, guidelines, and a group contract are presented in this informative article.

Fagin, C., editor: Readings in child and adolescent psychiatric nursing, St. Louis, 1974, The C.V. Mosby Co.

This is an excellent view of the role of the nurse with adolescents. Case studies are given (e.g., a nurse organizing and running an adolescent girls group.)

Feinstein, S.C., and Giovacchini, P., editors: Adolescent psychiatry, vols. 1-3, New York, 1971, 1973, 1974, Basic Books, Inc., Publishers, vols. 4 and 5, New York, 1976, 1977, Jason Aronson, Inc.

This is a collection of works that acts as a guide to present-day adolescent psychiatry. Numerous outstanding contributors present past and current developments in the field. Basic theoretical notions plus clinical findings are included.

Fox, K.: Adolescent ambivalence: a therapeutic issue, J. Psychiatr. Nurs. 18(9):27, 1980.

Through clinical examples the dynamics of adolescent ambivalence are explored and related nursing interventions are suggested.

Gamage, J.R., editor: Management of adolescent drug misuse: clinical, psychological and legal perspectives, Beloit, Wis., 1973, Reash Press.

This book contains articles on various drug issues, such as college students' perspectives of their parents' attitudes and practices regarding drugs, toxic reactions to marijuana, management of emergencies, long-term treatment of adolescent drug abuse, and drugs and the law. It is a good overview of various aspects of adolescents and drugs.

Group for Advancement of Psychiatry, Committee on Adolescence: Normal adolescence: its dynamics and impact, New York, 1968, Charles Scribner's Sons.

This paperback provides a good overview of normal adolescence, including physical, psychological, and environmental factors.

Guest, J.: Ordinary people, New York, 1976, The Viking Press.

This novel relates the story of an adolescent boy after his discharge from the hospital after a suicide attempt. It is sensitively written, with realistic views of his family and therapy.

Haley, J.: Leaving home: the therapy of disturbed young people, New York, 1980, McGraw-Hill, Inc.

This famous family therapist discusses ideas that plague therapists in dealing with adolescents. Using a family focus, he describes in detail specific issues using actual dialogue that provides easy, informative, and enjoyable reading. He discusses the therapist's support system, co-therapy, supervision, and the stages of therapy.

Holmes, D., Holmes, M., and Appignanesi, L.: Language of trust, New York, 1971, Science House.

Issues discussed include the contemporary adolescent, the contemporary parent, and drugs. There are examples with actual dialogues.

Jones, V.: Adolescents with behavior problems: strategies for teaching, counseling and parent involvement, Boston, 1980, Allyn & Bacon, Inc.

This is a good overview of dealing with problematic adolescents. Issues such as talking to adolescents, understanding their behavior, working with parents, understanding school difficulties, and developing strategies to promote productive behaviors are considered.

Lewis, D., and Balla, D.: Delinquency and psychopathology, New York, 1976, Grune & Stratton, Inc.

The authors give psychiatric and social viewpoints of delinquency. The focus is on diagnostic evaluation of abused children, sociopaths, and the delinquency and the delinquent child with CNS dysfunction. Social issues and their important influence on delinquents are examined psychodynamically.

Long, B.L., and Krepick, D.S.: Symposium on the young adult in today's world: new perspectives on drug abuse, Nurs. Clin. North. Am. 8:25, March 1973.

This article is a view by nurses of the drug problem with adolescents.

Marohn, R.: Juvenile delinquents: psychodynamic assessment and hospital treatment, New York, 1980, Brunner/Mazel, Inc.

This is a discussion of adolescent behavior describing developmental and psychodynamic theory. A description of their philosophy of treatment with disturbed teenagers who stayed on their unit follows with specific exploration of dynamics, environment and modes of intervention with case examples.

Masterson, J.F.: Treatment of the borderline adolescent, New York, 1972, Wiley-Interscience.

This book is a description and treatment of adolescents diagnosed according to the medical model as borderline.

Masterson, J., and Costelle, J.: From borderline adolescent to functioning adult, New York, 1980, Brunner/Mazel, Inc.

This is a follow-up report of Masterson's Treatment of the Borderline Adolescent.

McKuen, R.: Finding my father: one man's search for identity, New York, 1977, Berkley Publishing Corp.

This famous poet writes of his lifelong search for the father he never knew. Like the adolescent, he searches not just for his father but for his identity. This is an account of a lonely boy approaching manhood and looking for a caring and loving father of each boy's dreams.

Mellencamp, A.: Adolescent depression: a review of the literature with implications for nursing care, J. Psychosoc. Nurs. **19**(9):15, 1981.

This article is true to its title. It treats this important problem in a scholarly and thorough way with clinical application to nursing care. Highly recommended.

Meyer, A.: School phobia: care in the community, Nurs. Times **73**:1393, Sept. 1977.

This is a description of a nurse's successful work in the community with a 15-year-old adolescent boy who was school phobic for more than 12 months.

Miller, D.: Adolescence: psychology, psychopathology and psychotherapy, New York, 1974, Jason Aronson, Inc.

This is a good overview of adolescence that discusses theory, psychodynamics, and treatment.

Miller, D.: Development of psychiatric services for adolescents. In Schoolar, J., editor: Current issues in adolescent psychiatry, New York, 1973, Brunner/Mazel, Inc.

This chapter contains a helpful description of psychiatric services needed to treat adolescents and a projection of ideal settings to meet their unique needs.

Nakashima, L.: Teenage pregnancy—its causes, costs and consequences, Nurs. Practit. **3**:10, Sept.-Oct. 1977.

The issues involved with teenage pregnancies are reviewed. Possible origins of teenage pregnancy and the consequences of alternative solutions are discussed.

Novello, J.: The short course in adolescent psychiatry, New York, 1979, Brunner/Mazel, Inc.

This is an overview of a 2-day symposium at the Psychiatric Institute Foundation in Washington, D.C. It is a good encapsulated discussion of adolescent development, evaluation, diagnosis, and treatment.

Offer, D.: The psychological world of the juvenile delinquent, New York, 1979, Basic Books, Inc., Publishers.

The findings of a 5-year research project are presented in which juvenile delinquents were treated in a hospital setting.

Ottenberg, P.: Delivery of adolescent services, In Schoolar, J., editor: Current issues in adolescent psychiatry, New York, 1973, Brunner/Mazel, Inc.

This article reviews the various programs available to adolescents and discusses the specific needs of adolescents needing services.

Robichow, H., and Sklansky, M.: Effective counseling of adolescents, Chicago, 1980, Association Press.

This is a complete overview of adolescent stresses, ego, defenses, and regressions. Treatment is described with discussion of assessing treatability, engagement and continuing treatment, and termination.

Schlesinger, B.: From A to Z with adolescent sexuality, Can. Nurse **52**:34, Oct. 1977.

In this article an attempt is made to understand adolescent motherhood. Schlesinger uses an alphabetical listing to discuss such issues as the double standard for the sexual act (girls responsible, boys not); including fathers in programs; limit setting with adolescents; adults being models, not judges; women's rights; and possible origins for teenage pregnancies.

Sorenson, R.: Adolescent sexuality in contemporary America, New York, 1973, World Publishing.

A valuable overview of sexual behavior is presented in this text. Every aspect of adolescent sexual behavior is explored from homosexuality and unwed pregnancy to sexual attitudes and uses of sexual behavior.

Spicer, F.: Aggression in the home, Nurs. Mirror **45**:45, Dec. 15, 1977.

This article discusses violence in the home and adolescent and parental involvement.

Stoke, J.: Drugs, youth and society, N.Z. Nurse, **70**:3, July 1977.

This article is a general discussion of teenagers and drugs Societal influence on adolescents and their use of drugs is also discussed.

Stone, J., and Church, J.: Childhood and adolescence, New York, 1973, Random House, Inc.

A good review of normal growth and development, this book has been revised several times and brings a concise and contemporary view of normal behavior and age-specific guidelines. The combination of theory and observable behaviors makes this reference a must for beginners.

Thornburg, H.: Adolescence: a re-interpretation. In Neubauer, P., editor: Process of child development, New York, 1976, The New American Library, Inc.

A good description of adolescence, this book also defines and interprets in detail Robert Havighurst's developmental tasks in adolescence.

CHAPTER 28

NURSING INTERVENTION IN FAMILY ABUSE AND VIOLENCE

Theresa S. Foley

When I was a laddie
I lived with my granny
And many a hiding my granny di'ed me.
Now I am a man
And I live with my granny
and do to my granny
what she did to me.

Traditional rhyme, anonymous*

Learning objectives

After studying this chapter, the student
should be able to:

- *define family violence, incorporating the concepts of abuse and violence.*

- *state a general description of the "abuser" and "victim" using known demographic data.*

- *describe 12 characteristics of violent family systems.*

- *analyze the stress reaction process in abusive and violent families.*

- *identify types of violent behavior, motives of the abuser, and targets of violent behavior.*

- *relate current data on the incidence of family violence.*

- *compare and contrast present theories on the etiology of family violence.*

- *identify possible sources of data for the nursing assessment of violent families.*

- *utilize the epidemiological model to identify the data that should be collected by the nurse who is working with a violent family.*

---

*From Davidson, J.L.: Elder abuse. In Block, M., and Sinnott, J., editors: The battered child syndrome: an exploratory study, College Park, Md., 1977, The University of Maryland Center on Aging.

- *formulate individualized nursing diagnoses for violent and abusive families.*

- *develop long-term and short-term individualized nursing goals for violent and abusive families.*

- *describe nursing interventions in secondary prevention appropriate to the needs of violent families utilizing various treatment models.*

- *describe nursing interventions in tertiary prevention appropriate to the needs of violent families.*

- *describe nursing interventions in primary prevention directed toward preventing family violence.*

- *assess the importance of the evaluation of the nursing process when working with violent and abusive families.*

- *identify suggested readings for future study.*

Family violence is an extremely unpleasant topic, one that most people do not bring up in public or social conversation. If the topic is introduced it often is met with complete silence or failure to pursue a discussion about violence and abuse. Nurses need to be aware of the problem of family violence because they work with children, their families, and society at all levels of prevention. Family violence is more than a family problem. It is a reflection of a sick society that fosters and sanctions violent behavior as a norm in response to the stressors of daily life. As a learned behavior, the cycle of violence is frequently passed from generation to generation—the child victims later resorting to violence with their own mates or children and perhaps again experiencing victimization as elderly persons by those whom they had previously abused. The statistics on the incidence of family violence are staggering, and projections of future trends indicate that it is likely to increase. Because of the many settings and roles nurses work in, they are in an ideal position to contribute to the prevention, identification, treatment, and eradication of family violence.

Abuse and violence are two closely related concepts. Often the terms are used interchangeably in the literature; lack uniform definitions or parameters across research studies or social values, limiting generalization of the findings; and are subject to a wide variety of theoretical propositions to explain the phenomena. *Abuse* is generally defined as an act that "deceives, puts to wrong or improper use so as to injure, damage, maltreat or corrupt,"[46] whereas *violence*

is defined as an act "marked by extreme force or sudden intense activity to the point of loss of self-control."[46] Acts of physical injury and death are often contained within the definitions and use of the terms. For example, child physical abuse usually refers to overt, active, physical violence by an adult against a child, which causes injuries ranging from bruises and burns to fractures and death, or covert violence through neglect, which may have the same outcomes. Although child sexual abuse generally involves coercion to gain the victim's compliance, the phenomenon creates a condition of psychological violence that has long-term effects on the family system yet is not as easily detected or measured as physical signs of injury. This offense is primarily described in terms of abuse, yet it is not uncommon for a sexually abused child to also be subjected to physical violence by the parents or siblings.

Furthermore, a fine line exists between what one considers abuse as opposed to violence. There is, for example, a questionable distinction between corporal punishment and physical violence; the definition usually is determined by the parent or guardian. The situation is further complicated in that the abusive/violent family does not perceive their behavior as abusive or violent; the members tend to deny and discount the existence of the problem as do many professionals who have an awareness of or reason to suspect that a case exists.[28,31,43] For the purposes of this chapter the term *family violence* is used to refer to all forms of family abuse or violence and is defined as the physical, psychological, sexual, material, or social violation of a person by a family member or their delegate.

Most of the literature discusses family violence according to the way in which the dysfunction is expressed: child physical abuse, child sexual abuse, sibling violence, spouse abuse, or elder abuse. This chapter attempts to examine what is common across categories of family violence, that is, what is common to violent family systems rather than to a specific form of family violence. The nature and scope of the problem, theories on the etiology of family violence, and treatment issues within a nursing process model will be analyzed in this chapter. Books and monographs have been written on each form of family violence, thus the following discussion is necessarily and intentionally limited in scope. It is assumed that the reader has a working knowledge of family theory and concepts as discussed in other chapters of this textbook and family therapy (Chapter 25), permitting fuller attention to the application of theory and concepts to intervention in family abuse and violence.

Defining the problem of family violence

The problem of family violence can be defined and described in a variety of ways. *Family violence* is the physical, psychological, sexual, material, or social violation of a person by a family member or their delegate. Questions frequently asked include the following: Who is the abuser? What is this person like? Who is the victim and what is he or she like? Who could ever marry or live with such a person? How does family violence get started and perpetuated? What do the abusive/violent behaviors consist of?

Demographic data

It is known that family violence is evident at all socioeconomic levels, in all educational, racial, occupational, gender and religious groups, and regions in the United States. Table 28-1 presents a profile of the violent family, reporting data specific to each form of family violence. Data presented in Table 28-1 suffer from difficulties common to the field of victimology: the statistics are derived from a variety of sources (police files, hospital records); collection methods have not been uniform; definitions of terms differ; disadvantaged families are identified through care delivery systems, whereas middle and upper class families often escape detection and reporting; and unreported cases (estimates ranging from 10 to 20 unreported for every reported or founded case) ultimately skew a clear profile of the violent family.

These data do, however, offer a starting point in recognizing individuals who have most frequently come to the attention of authorities and professionals. Generally, the *abuser* ranges in age from a toddler to about 60 years; is male, married, and living with a spouse or partner; is

TABLE 28-1. Profile of the violent family*

Identifying data	Child physical abuse		Child sexual abuse	
	Abuser	Victim	Abuser	Victim
Age	Mother, average age = 26; father average age = 30; all ages	Most under 2 years; average age = 4 years; all ages	All ages; 21 to 30 years old most often; 11 to 20 years old next often	All ages; 6 to 9 years old at onset; 12 years old when disclosed; mean age = 7.9 years
Sex	Male and female; father more often than mother, but mother more violent	Not a factor	Male; accomplice sometimes female	Male and female; most reported cases are female (7 females to 1 male); in females, 63% are younger than 12 years old; in males, 64% are older than 12 years old
Relationship	Father or stepfather; not a stranger most often, e.g., babysitter or guardian	Acquainted or known; oldest/youngest daughter or only child most often	Father more often than mother	Son/daughter or stepchild
Marital status	Married and living with spouse	Single	Married and living with spouse	Single

*Data from references 8, 12, 16, 20, 22, 25, 37, 41, 45.

frequently not fully employed and has a semiskilled job; has completed high school; is likely to have been a victim of childhood physical or sexual abuse; is of a minority religion or does not share the same religion as other family members; and can reside anywhere in the United States. The *victim* is generally a female; ranges in age from newborn to old age; is related to and living with the abuser; is not employed, has not developed an occupation, or has retired; does not have a high school diploma; can reside anywhere in the United States; and is usually in a captive position within the violent family as a result of emotional or economic issues in the system.

The violent family system

The question that continues to be explored by family therapists is: Why are some families violent and others not? Some families that come for therapy have the same characteristics as violent families but are not violent. What clinicians and researchers do agree on is that there are a number of characteristics which describe what

a violent family is like, and yet these same characteristics can be found in nonviolent families with the dysfunction expressed in an alternative form (e.g., one member may be diagnosed as a schizophrenic).[17,44] *Family violence is, then, the mode by which a given family system expresses its dysfunction.* Why family violence is elected rather than an alternative form, such as schizophrenia, remains to be researched. Thus emphasis is placed on genetics and the context in which any given set of variables is present as important factors in determining violent behavior. Some researchers and clinicians believe that a healthy family system, if subjected to the right combination of stressors, could develop violent interactions. The concept of family violence therefore focuses on the system, not the individual members, as being "self-destructive." For example, in a violent family the individual members are usually at a low level of differentiation, but emphasis is placed

Spouse abuse		Sibling abuse		Elder abuse	
Male	**Female**	**Abuser**	**Victim**	**Abuser**	**Victim**
Often 17 to 30 years old at disclosure; all ages; seen in abuse of elders		All ages; most reported cases are 17 years old or less; rate decreases as age increases		40 to 60 years old	60 years old and older
Male and female; most reported cases have female victims		Male most often; higher incidence in all male–sibling families	Male most often; higher incidence in all male–sibling families	Female	Not a factor; more elder are female
Spouse or partner		Brother to brother as victim most often; brother to sister as victim next often		Son/daughter, relative, or caretaker	Parent of abuser most often
Married most often; living together next often		Single	Single	Married	Widowed

Continued.

Table 28-1. **Profile of the violent family—cont'd**

Identifying data	Child physical abuse		Child sexual abuse	
	Abuser	Victim	Abuser	Victim
History of childhood physical/sexual abuse	60% of cases	Repeated multiple victimization or neglect	70% of cases	Repeated multiple victimization
Socioeconomic status (SES)	Evident at all SES levels; rate twice as high in reported cases of families under the poverty line ($5999) as in families of $20,000+ income		Evident in all SES levels; founded cases most often lower SES	
Occupation	Reported cases most often skilled or semiskilled	Student	Founded cases most often professional, skilled, or semiskilled	Student
Employment status	Unemployment not disproportionately prevalent; abuse twice as high if father is employed part time	Not employed	Employed; higher rate if part time or un-employed	Not employed
Race	Blacks and minorities inaccurately represented; all races	Same as abuser	Not a factor	
Religion	Highest, one or more parents of minority religion; lowest, Jewish	Mixed religious background	Highest, highly religious family, rigid inflexible belief system; lowest, realistic balance of religion in family belief system	
Education	Most violent, high school diploma for both men and women; least violent, grammar school dropout or some college education	Mostly preschool; if in school, performance may be poor (stress symptom)	Inaccurately presented Often high school and some college	Grammar and high school student; performance may be poor (stress symptom)
Residence	Large city most often; not Southern phenomena Evenly distributed in United States		Evenly distributed in United States	

Spouse abuse		Sibling abuse		Elder abuse	
Male	**Female**	**Abuser**	**Victim**	**Abuser**	**Victim**
Most were subject to repeated victimization as children		Live in abusive/violent home; often victims of parent/guardian as well		Data not widely available; positive history in some cases	Positive history in some cases; repeated victimization
Evident at all SES levels; five times more common in families at or below poverty line than in families over $20,000 income in reported cases		Evident at all SES levels		Not a factor; evident at all SES levels; founded cases mostly lower to middle class and found through health care systems	
Reported cases skilled or semiskilled most often		Childhood (or history of delinquency)		Professional or semiskilled	Not employed
Violence two or three times higher if man is unemployed or has part-time employment		Not employed		Least violence in homes of retired men; victim often physically/mentally impaired	
All races; reported most by minorities; black more than whites (2:1)		Highest, racial minorities; lowest, blacks		Highest, American Indians, orientals, minorities; blacks = 12%, whites = 88%[8]; also reported as no difference[40]	
Highest, minority religions and Jewish women; lowest, Protestants and Jewish men		Highest minority religions (excluding Jewish, Catholic, or Protestant)		Protestant	
Victim more often without high school diploma and less often with college education		Most violent if father/male highly educated and mother/female high school diploma or some college education		High school diploma or some college	
Most violent husbands, high school diploma; least violent, grammar school dropout or some college	Most violent, wives without high school diploma				
Evenly distributed in United States	Abused by male in large city or rural area; rate decreased by half in suburbs	Higher rates in rural area and large cities Not Southern phenomena		Limited data, evenly distributed with more reports in large cities Not Southern phenomena	

on the fact that the entire system is undifferentiated. What is important is that these individuals formed a group but were unable to meet their own or others' needs, thereby setting up a context in which family violence is the outcome of dysfunctional relationships and emotional processes.

Because so much of the literature focuses on a specific type of family violence, a tremendous volume of data must be synthesized and ordered if one is to begin to understand the nature of a violent family system. This requires knowledge of both the characteristics of the violent family system and the stress reaction process involved in family violence. Both of these aspects are illustrated in Clinical example 28-1.

CLINICAL EXAMPLE 28-1

Mr. F came home from work after a "terrible day." The boss rejected a request for a salary increase yet hired a new employee, and arguments with co-workers had escalated. All Mr. F wants is a little love, attention, and nurturing. He feels lonely, depressed, and unappreciated. He handles his conflicts by pursuing companionship and shutting out the outside world.

Mrs. F had a hectic day with the three children, and the last thing she needs is to mother another person. She just wants to be left alone and feels depleted from giving to others. Mr. F's depression leaves her feeling angry and frustrated. She feels hopeless about things ever being any better in their relationship but ignores that feeling in trying to make it from day to day. Mrs. F handles her frustration by withdrawing from her husband and the family; she reads books for days at a time, goes on spending sprees to lift her mood, and plays bridge at least two evenings a week.

Mr. F started drinking after work to "get rid of his troubles" and followed his wife around until she exploded, telling him what a "no-good drunken provider" he is. An argument ensued, and Mrs. F left the house to play bridge with her friends. Mr. F retreated to the bedroom and drowned his misery by leafing through pornographic literature but continued to feel intolerably depressed and lonely. He was angry that he could not control his wife's activities so she would be exclusively with him.

The oldest daughter, Sue, entered the bedroom to inform him that the younger children needed to have dinner and be helped getting to bed. Mr. F picked a fight with her. He stormed out of the bedroom to take care of the children and dragged her by the arm downstairs to "teach her" how to be a "mother." Feeling intense irritation with his wife, he continued picking and nagging at Sue over little things—the way the table was set, which dishes were used, what food items were selected, and so forth—and eventually hit her. She cursed at him and ran to her bedroom.

The other children ran to the other room to escape the frightening situation. They played with toys but did mean things with them like hit them and pull their hair. The television was on and is their best friend most of the time. They watch more violence on television and learn that violence is a norm for solving tension in daily living, just like in their house.

Mr. F then tried to handle his frustration by pursuing closeness with his daughter. He'll "be damned" if he'll "let her get the best of me." He's determined to prove that *he* is right; he can't stand feeling powerless. He already felt like a miserable creature and wouldn't allow her to have power over him. He felt kind of rotten for having hit her and was determined to see that she kept that a secret from mom. Mr. F entered the bedroom, apologized to Sue for having hit her, but told her it was for a good reason given her "mouthy disrespectful behavior and attitude." He insisted that she talk the conflict out with him and began to rub her back. Sue started to tell father how she felt; Mr. F listened and soothed her and gave her a back rub. Sue appreciated the attention because she was feeling worthless after her father's demeaning verbal assault earlier. Mr. F's back rub gradually progressed to her genitals, and he convinced her that he should "teach her about sex." He taught her about oral sex and used his pornography to show her other sexual behavior he wants to teach her about. He told her about all the terrible things that would happen to her and the family if she ever tells anyone about tonight and that he wouldn't want that to happen because he truly loves her, sometimes more than mom. Mr. F felt relieved but left Sue's room because he was nervous about his wife returning to discover him.

Mrs. F returned from her evening out, her frustration temporarily relieved after having withdrawn from the family. Mr. F argued with her (wanted to know why she was home so early, why she didn't get the food at the all-night store as he had asked), and she gave him "the silent treatment," going to bed for the night with a book. Mr. F retreated to the living room to drink a few beers and watch the late show but found that he was, instead, obsessively preoccupied, recalling highlights of the tantalizing sexual intimacies with Sue.

This situation could have had any number of different transactions and reactions. For example, Mr. F could have insisted that Mrs. F stay home (jealousy and possessiveness) and beat her up for even thinking about leaving him. Sue could have complied and been submissive with every verbal assault from her father but physically beat the younger siblings while putting them to bed. Mrs. F could have stayed home and gone on a spending spree the next day to lift her mood and get away from the hassle of the kids and use up money set aside for support of her elderly mother who now must do with little or no food until the next payday. The point of this clinical example is to illustrate the interlocking nature of individual members' conflicts within the family system.

CHARACTERISTICS OF THE VIOLENT FAMILY AS A SYSTEM. Although specific forms of family violence may differ somewhat on family system characteristics, the literature and clinical practice suggest some general patterns. First, violent families have *boundaries* that seem impermeable to outsiders. Until disclosure, no one is aware of what is going on in the family, often including other members of the family. In therapy the family is extremely resistant to being opened up for change to occur. When "in trouble" (for example, when charges are pressed and the family is facing separation by legal authority) the system will usually loosen its boundaries, if forced or pressured to do so, and become more permeable to the degree that people or agencies are believed to further the family system's direction and can be co-opted (for example, by obtaining home-care aids or professionals who will testify in their behalf). When outsiders attempt to permeate the system's boundaries, the action is felt to be an invasive assault, and the family becomes more firmly entrenched, cutting off contact with the outside world, which is a perceived threat. It is not surprising therefore for the abuser* to assert and believe that his own assaultive behavior within the system was justified, given his intent of preserving the family, and for him to ignore the reality of the destruction his violence creates. In Clinical example 28-1, the father ensured that boundary lines would be maintained by convincing the daughter to keep the violence a secret; the system was sealed off by a conspiracy of silence. In addition, the father crossed over generational boundaries by seeking companionship with the daughter and excluding the mother. Finally, in terms of boundaries, it is found that violent families are socially isolated; they have few friends and little contact with helping persons. The family is "roped off" from the outside world, which only

serves to create a pressure cooker within the system that eventually explodes in violence.

The *mood,* or *feeling tone,* in such families is one of pain and desperation. The members compete for affection, caring, attention, and nurturance as if the supply were insufficient and limited and generally ignore the needs of the other members. When two adults with low self-esteem who are unable to meet their own needs merge, the relationship system can be potentially explosive. No one person can possibly meet all the needs of another person, yet that is often what violent couples expect of each other. The violent couple have frequently married or moved in together when quite young and have many unresolved separation-individuation issues that get transferred onto their new relationship. Cutoffs or fusion with the family of origin are also quite common. When marriage fails to resolve these residual developmental issues, the couple becomes disillusioned, and disappointment with the mate creates tension that explodes in family violence. Add elderly persons or children to that system and the situation becomes even more volatile. The child or elderly person is expected to meet the adult's needs, and his or her needs for care and love place an intolerable burden on an adult already stressed by demands made by a mate. The elderly person or child then becomes at high risk as a target for physical or sexual violence by adults who focus only on gratifying their own needs while disregarding, denying, and discounting the needs of the developing child or elderly person. In the clinical example the mother was unable to meet the father's needs for empathic listening because of her own need, withdrew from his intense unhappiness, and the tension was subsequently released between the father and daughter through physical and sexual violence.

Another characteristic of violent families is their lack of *autonomy,* or *differentiation.* Unlike adequately functioning families, violent families tend to be characterized by low levels of differentiation and fusion with others to attain a sense of self. Family members operate on an emotional level and are threatened by the individuation of other members.

A characteristic related to lack of autonomy is the violent family's inability to *trust.* Usually violent adults have experienced a history of one or more premature separations, neglect, or episodes of childhood physical and sexual vio-

---

*Since most reported abusers are men, the abuser is referred to by the male gender here, but I acknowledge that women also fall into this category as the identified patient, signaling the system's distress and dysfunction.

lence. The violence experienced in childhood is a predisposing factor to violent behavior in adulthood in response to high levels of stress. It emerges as difficulty with object loss or separation from those emotionally depended on. No matter how terrifying the family environment is, the members desperately work to keep the system intact rather than lose another member; hence the fusion of spouses with their families of origin, each other, or one of the children. Staying together is a painful rather than joyful process, with an absence of humor, flexibility, caring, genuine empathy, excitement in exploring an adventuresome world, recognized productivity, and clear communication. The result is that violent families have no real intimacy, only a pseudointimacy. The violence can thus be viewed as a misguided and desperate attempt by the system to gain closeness and companionship and provides a release for accumulated frustration. It is also a way of coping with a world that is viewed as threatening, demanding, unrewarding, and problematical. Through repetitive episodes of family violence, the family ignores and denies a multitude of daily living problems, and members experience an absence of empathy, traumatic loneliness, and a high degree of both overt and covert conflict.

Conflict is expressed overtly through violent aggression and covertly through constant power struggles, depending on the motive of the abuser and the needs of other members in the system. In some families, conflict is the way in which closeness is expressed or communicated. It is as if the message communicated in the system is, "I only know that you care about me when you are really (violently) upset." The result is a confusion of closeness and caring with violence. Many professionals hypothesize that it is at this point that sexuality and aggression become confused and fused, resulting in rape within domestic violence and marriage. Although colleagues discuss that viewpoint in their clinical work, the question has yet to be researched. What is known about conflict in the family system is that the release of frustration and accompanying relief is only temporary. The emotional cycle rebuilds gradually, arguments are frequent, and relief is again sought through violent behavior. Violent behavior thus becomes a learned mode of response to reduce stress or tension, and the relief felt from the violent behavior acts as a positive reinforcer to the maladaptive coping style.

Conflict resolution in families is closely related to their *regulation of duties,* such as aggression and sexuality. Violent families are characterized by a lack of impulse control and self-discipline and a reduced capacity to delay gratification. With inadequate internal controls and limit setting, they tend to "act out" their needs without regard for others. Their very acts of abuse and violence speak to their lack of ability to tolerate frustration and regulate drives.

The violent family thus focuses on getting their needs met in the present—for example, decreasing an immediate state of loneliness or low self-esteem. The result is that an awareness of past, present, and future, known as *time binding,* is poor or minimal. However, an awareness of the passage of time surfaces acutely when the victim begins to physically separate from the system or becomes less available as a target of emotional release, such as in puberty and adolescence when peer relationships are built and separation from the family system is in process. Another instance of the awareness of the passage of time is when the system's direction is impeded, as when an elderly person is brought into the family home and home care responsibilities interfere with the wife's ability to achieve career goals. The members define time, then, in terms of the narcissistic self rather than the family system, and the nurse will note that the violent family is unable to tolerate interference with need gratification. Thus long-range goal-directed behaviors that often interfere with need gratification (for example, years of education prior to gainful employment and a successful career) are often absent or weak.

This leads to problems with *task performance,* which can affect all aspects of the family's life. Frequently, members have difficulty obtaining and retaining jobs. If employed, they may experience job dissatisfaction and interpersonal problems with co-workers. Financial problems are recurrent. Problems also spill over into parenting and social situations. There may be early or forced marriages, unplanned children, lack of parenting skills, and the generalized inability to problem solve effectively. The adults tend to have unrealistic and magical expectations of other members of the family system, and conflicts around discipline and child rearing or care for an elderly parent are quite high. The problem is further escalated in that the system is cut off from the outside world, which could provide inputs to reduce the tension. For example, they do not discuss their problem child with "outsiders" and therefore do not hear others say, "That's normal behavior for a 3-year-old.

Yes it does drive you up a wall, but it will pass. . . . What I did when my kid was that age was. . . ." Violent families have a need to learn not only normal aspects of growth and development, but also how to meet their needs through their own resources and the resources available outside the family. This is a significant area for preventive interventions by nurses and other health professionals.

Communication in violent families is characterized by mixed or double messages, an emphasis on nonverbal messages, and an absence of direct communication that is believed to be intolerably threatening. Communication is frequently used to keep the family cut off from the outside world. For example, the victim is told not to tell anyone about the violence or she will be responsible for the family being dissolved and broken up or the father going to jail. The victim thus learns to subject her own needs to the violent system, feels like an object that is used and discarded or is valued by the violent system only as a target for discharge, and may have long-term conflicts because of the sense of worthlessness conveyed by the system. Communication can also be quite threatening and intimidating to gain the victim's compliance. For example, an elderly person may be threatened with being abandoned to a nursing home or losing control over his will and inheritance unless certain demands by the family system are met. Food, clothing, and other necessities may be denied or used in barter as a trade-off or payoff. Meanwhile the terror and rage felt in response to the violence continues to be denied, ignored, or discounted.

This denial process contributes to a faulty *belief system* and perception of reality. The family system may believe that violence is what happens in all families, violence is a norm, the victim is responsible for the assault, or violence is the way to solve problems. The family system can teach its members faulty or impaired cognitive processes in coping with daily stressors. In Clinical example 28-1 Mr. F taught Sue that she was responsible for the violence because of her "mouthy disrespectful behavior" and thus taught her to discount the reality that his violent behavior was out of bounds.

Distorted perceptions and communications may also be used by the abuser to maintain an imbalanced *power ratio* in the system, giving the abusive person an advantage over the other members. For example, the abusive person may tell the members they are worthless for any number of reasons, which may or may not be rational; have them convinced of their worth-lessness, powerlessness, helplessness, and hopelessness; and keep them from reaching out to others for help or taking any assertive action in their behalf. Or the abusive person may tell the victim that the violent behavior was justified given the victim's behavior and have the victim attribute the fault to himself, thereby excusing the violent member for the abuse. Essentially, the abusive person has learned to be a master "con" artist who can talk almost anyone into believing his point of view. The net effect is that the members in the system learn to abuse power; use people to achieve personal or narcissistic aims with a disregard for the individual being abused; use manipulation, lying, and deceit as coping mechanisms and use covert passive-aggressive power to control relationships that can ultimately result in the development of mental illness, psychophysiological stress reactions, and characterological behaviors, such as prostitution and drug and alcohol abuse. Thus the covert use of power is ultimately self-destructive, with the victim perpetuating the victim role as a scapegoat for the family system's focus of attention (for example, an adolescent's drug habit is of more concern than the factors contributing to it).

Competition and the abuse of power was evident in Clinical example 28-1. The mother was powerful by withdrawing and refusing to give empathy to father; the father was powerful in hitting the daughter, insisting that the daughter talk with him and winning her closeness; the daughter was powerful in fleeing from her father, refusing to interact with him, and granting or denying him satisfaction of aggressive and sexual drives; the siblings yielded power by removing themselves as potential scapegoats and by making demands on the system for care and attention. The power ratio is also evident in the structure of relationships within the system so that the abusing person usually assumes a dominant role, the victim a passive and submissive role, and the other members silently collude in the abuse if only to escape the scapegoat position in the system. The members often have good reasons to be frightened of the one holding the power and do not challenge that person.

The clearest example of power inherent in a relationship structure is seen in the family's *role stereotyping* and belief system, which is quite rigid, absolute, and traditional: a women's work is at home taking care of everyone else, chil-

TABLE 28-2. Characteristics of abusive and violent family systems*

Criteria	Assessment data
Boundary	Impermeable to outsiders; generational boundaries are crossed over, blurred, nonexistent; others' boundaries are intruded; system is socially isolated; permeation felt as invasive assault
Mood/feeling tone	Pain; depression; competition for caring, affection, and nurturance; longing for closeness but allergic to it; intense tension and anger; fear; great intensity, force, and fusion; lack of empathy; constant crises; extreme deprivation and neediness; helplessness and hopelessness
Autonomy/differentiation	Nonexistent autonomy or pseudoautonomy; low level of differentiation; threatened by separation-individuation of members; own needs subjected to those of the family system; fused with others for a sense of self; members propelled by feelings; intergenerational transmission process (over one or more generations)
Trust	Absent or shattered sense of trust; history of premature separations/neglect; high-level denial and discounting of problem; pseudointimacy; fear of authority figures; inability to trust self or others in or outside system; no reaching out to others; staying together is a painful process
Conflict	High level of conflict that is overt and covert; conflict exacerbated by drug/alcohol abuse; may be either denied or condoned; intense triangulation; closeness and caring confused with abuse/violence; learned behavior to reduce stress
Regulation of drives (aggression/sexuality)	Little or no impulse control; low frustration tolerance; acts out drives without regard for others; abuse of alcohol/drugs; projection and acting out of self-hatred on scapegoat (victim); inadequate limit setting; reduced capacity to delay gratification
Time binding	Ignored or minimal awareness; focus on self and daily crises; awareness emerges as victim escapes field or is less available; panic sets in to locate replacement for gratification/discharge of tension; time defined in terms of narcissistic self vs. family system; long-range goal-directed behaviors are absent or weak; severe stress reaction to loss
Task performance	Inefficiency; high unemployment and conflict with co-workers/family system around tasks; child/adult role responsibilities reversed; discipline problems; dysfunction may be expressed as "workaholic"; high-level job dissatisfaction; recurrent financial problems; ineffective problem-solving skills; unrealistic and magical expectations of others
Communication	Poor communication; double messages; mixed nonverbal messages; threatened by direct messages; discounts problems and people affected; threatening or fear inducing; incongruent; abusive; blaming; confusing; demeaning; failure to talk and share with others; unkept promises
Belief system	Faulty perception of reality; family's view not congruent with assessment by outsiders; members taught faulty or impaired cognitive processes
Power ratio	Imbalance in power ratio; usually male dominated; struggle for power and dominance acted out; self-esteem determined by power wielded in system; need for constant refueling through abuse/violence; abuse of power often maintained by distorted communication; master con artists; members are impersonal objects to achieve narcissistic aims; power often maintained through lying, deceit, manipulation, and passive-aggressive behaviors; members learn and perpetuate victim roles.
Role stereotyping	Traditionalist; absolute; rigid rules; serves to control the system; departure from prescribed role can precipitate violence; members growth and development restricted; members feel unable to leave or separate; parental coalition is nonexistent or in shambles; adults role model is of abuse/violence; role confusion and reversal

*Data from references 8, 12, 25, 30, 41, 43, 45.

dren are to be seen and not heard, older siblings have the right to discipline younger ones with physical punishment, elders are seen as having nothing to contribute to the family or society and are best left alone, and so forth. Any departure from a prescribed role can precipitate violence (for example, if a woman decides to get a job, if a younger sibling challenges an older sibling's authority, if an elder refuses to turn over a savings account to the family and become dependent on them). Rigid roles control the members by keeping them from growing or developing and reduce the threat of system dissolution, since the members feel unable to leave or separate. Finally, in relation to this issue, it is common to observe that the parental coalition is absent or in shambles. In the clinical example the father and mother were not allied in their parenting responsibilities. They were, in fact, emotionally oppositional. The father fused with the daughter to meet emotional needs and excluded the mother, while the siblings fled the frightening situation.

Table 28-2 summarizes these 12 characteristics of violent family systems. They are common aspects of all violent families, regardless of the form in which the system dysfunction is expressed. However, as summary sketches, the nurse needs to realize that not all characteristics will apply to each family. Rather, they describe background dimensions that can be useful in working with these families.

Stress reaction process

Effective intervention in family violence requires that the nurse understand the interactional sequence of events leading up to the system's explosive dysfunction. In therapy the members demonstrate their individual reactivity to problems in the family that fuel the dysfunctional process. Ultimately a composite of the interlocking variables may be worked out, with the family actively contributing to developing cognitive awareness of the process. Fig. 28-1 depicts an overview of the stress reaction process in abusive and violent families.

Forms of family violence

Forms of family violence are described in three ways: (1) the types of violent behavior, (2) the predominant motive expressed by the violent behavior, and (3) the target of the violent release of tension. *Types of violent behavior* include psychological, physical, sexual, material, and social acts as follows:

1. *Physical violence:* Beating; withholding personal care, food, and medical care; lack of supervision; bruises, wounds, cuts, punctures, and bone and skull fractures; sprains and dislocations, abrasions, and lacerations; an environment of dirt and vermin in the house, an odor of urine, or inadequate heat[8,28]
2. *Psychological violence:* Verbal assault and threats, provoking fear, and isolation; disturbed communication patterns and cognitive processes[8,28]
3. *Material violence:* Theft of money or property; misuse of money or property[8,28]
4. *Social violence:* Violation of rights, such as forceful eviction from one's residence and relocation in another setting,[7] being locked out of the refrigerator or one's home,[7] being restrained from seeing one's friends or helping persons, being pressured or forced into isolative behaviors
5. *Sexual violence:* Pressured or forced sexual activity or stimulation that "includes physical acts of kissing, fondling of genital areas, mutual masturbation, fellatio or cunnilingus, sodomy, attempted or actual coitus, and nonphysical activity or stimulation which includes acts of exposure of the genitals, use of pornographic materials, voyeurism and verbalized sexual fantasies"[10]

The family system will respond differently to violence depending on the predominant *motive* of the abusive/violent person throughout the episode. For example, the system responds to extreme aggressive violence with high levels of anxiety and fear for physical safety and survival, whereas power violence tends to generate responses of guilt, repressed anger and hostility, reactive depression, and an impaired ability to trust.[22] Although family violence may contain elements of both aggressive and power motives, usually one of the two elements will be predominant. If the violent behavior is *aggressive*, it is characterized by an extreme use of force, causing physical injury to the victim. It is episodical, unplanned, and often impulsive. The language tends to be abusive with the use of obscenities and swearing. The abusive person's mood is one of depression and rage over unmet needs and perceived wrongs, injustices, or "put downs," and the assault is usually of a short duration.[22] The most frequently identified forms of aggressive violent behavior are families of

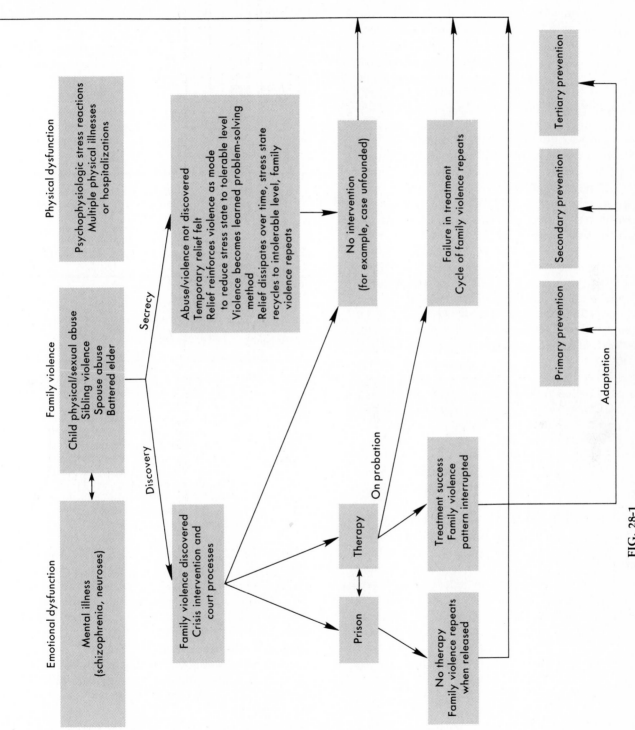

FIG. 28-1
Flowchart depicting stress reaction process in family abuse and violence.

domestic and sibling violence and child physical abuse.

In contrast, if the violent behavior is a result of unresolved *power* issues, it is characterized by anxiety because of intolerable feelings of inadequacy, insecurity, loneliness, and low self-esteem. Force is used only to subdue, dominate, or gain the victim's compliance. The language is inquisitive or instructional and demanding to control the victim's and other family members' responses. The victim is usually not harmed but may be held captive for long hours while the abusive person attempts to relieve stress. The assault is usually premeditated and planned with "props" or fantasies that are acted out as part of "the act," and the behavior tends to be repetitive and increase in violence over time as the abuser's needs continue to be unmet and his sense of desperation intensifies to relieve pent-up stress.[22] The most frequently identified forms of power violence include child sexual abuse and elder abuse.

Last, the form of family violence is defined by the *scapegoat,* or *target,* of released aggression or unresolved power issues within the emotional and relationship subsystems. Forms of family violence defined by aggression and unresolved power issues include the following:

1. *Child physical abuse:* Any mistreatment, physical or mental, brought about through acts of commission or omission by parents or other care givers[31]
2. *Child sexual abuse:* The forced or pressured sexual contact on a child or adolescent by another person[20]
3. *Spouse abuse:* The physical, social, psychological, material, or sexual violation or injury of one's mate/partner
4. *Sibling abuse:* Violence between and among siblings that includes physical, psychological, material, social, or sexual acts
5. *Elder abuse:* The physical, psychological, material, medical, social, or sexual abuse or injury of a person 60 years of age or older who resides in the home of a son, daughter, or other relative or with a caretaker[43]

Incidence

Given an understanding of the nature of family violence, the question that remains to be addressed is: How serious is the problem of family violence? Statistics are, at best, only estimates of the incidence of family violence and fail to

TABLE 28-3. Incidence of family violence

Category	Statistics
Child abuse	
Physical	3 in 5 families[41]; 500,000 to 2.5 million cases per year[23]; 100 unreported for every reported case[13]; 2000 die and 6000 have permanent brain damage, 60,000 have significant injuries[13]; every other household has abuse at least once a year[41]
Sexual	1 in 4 women before the age of 18[21]; 150 per million per year in the United States[27]; 200,000 to 300,000 per year in the United States (of females)[13]; 20 unreported for every reported case[26]
Sibling abuse	Most prevalent form of family violence[41]; 4 in 5 children (3 to 17 years old) experience sibling violence once a year[41]; 36.3 million children are 3 to 17 years old[45]; 29 million children commit one act of violence per year[45]; affects 1 in 6 families[41]
Spouse abuse	
Wife	Over 2 million cases per year[41]; 50% are abused some time during their marriage[45]
Husband	Over 2 million per year[41]
Elderly abuse	Estimated incidence of between 1 and 2.5 million cases per year[21a,24a]; 9.6% of elderly clients are seen by an agency[28]; in 55% of 183 cases, there was one incidence or more within 18 months[28]; 13.43% of 134 professionals surveyed reported a case[8]; 87% of service agencies, professionals, or elderly do not report suspected cases of abuse[8]; 4% of 73 elderly reported abuse[8]; 62.3% (151 of 228) service agency personnel report experience with elder abuse cases[18]

even begin closing the gap on reliable figures of prevalence. For a variety of reasons common to the problems of conducting any valid and reliable research study, as well as to the taboo and secret nature of the topic in our society, the statistics on family violence are limited. In the United States people would prefer to ignore both that it does exist and that it is as prevalent as it is. Table 28-3 presents current data on the incidence of family violence.

Theories on the etiology of family violence

Theories on the causation of family violence are abundant, overlap with each other in explaining determinants of family violence, and are incomplete in explaining family violence when standing alone. The greatest focus of debates on the etiology of family violence centers around whether the behavior is the outcome of external pressures or internal intrapsychic conflicts. It is important for nurses to be aware of theories on causation of family violence because the nurse's theoretical framework will affect the treatment approach implemented. Several theoretical models explaining family violence will be discussed briefly.[25]

Psychodynamic theories assert that the abuser was deprived of the necessary nurturance and mothering in childhood to be able to give to and nurture his own family as an adult. The focus is at the individual level on the abusive person's potential for abuse, and history of physical or sexual abuse as a child is recognized as a contributing factor. Attention is given to impaired trust and unrealistic expectations of others, a nonsupportive relationship with a mate, and a tendency toward emotional and social isolation. Within the psychodynamic theories are contained theories about the characterological structure of the abusive person's personality. In particular, emphasis is placed on antisocial behaviors, drug and alcohol abuse, evidence of a criminal record, and lack of impulse control.

Many people are inclined to believe that the violent family and the abusive member in particular are *mentally ill.* Researchers and clinicians agree that family violence is the result of personality and system dysfunction; however, they disagree on whether that dysfunction constitutes mental illness. According to the DSM-III, a mental disorder is a "clinically significant behavioral or psychological syndrome or pattern that occurs in an individual typically associated with a painful symptom or impairment in one or more areas of functioning."[4] According to the earlier discussion on the nature of the problem, family violence does fit the definition of mental disorders. Antagonists of the mental illness theory of family violence caution that the proponents of the theory tend to excuse the perpetrator's behavior as "sickness," rather than viewing it as irresponsibility and poor impulse control, for which the perpetrator is held responsible. Theories about mental illness focus on individual intrapsychic dynamics and thus fit under the category of psychodynamic theories of family violence.

Social learning theory emphasizes the absence of healthy role models of parenting and problem-solving in childhood, which impairs a person's knowledge of and ability to provide parenting to others as an adult. Attention is given to behavior as a learned process that can be unlearned if the sequence of behaviors, precipitants, and preceding events are clearly identified.[5,36] Complementing social learning theories are *psychosocial theories,* which account for the influence of socialization processes, cultural scripting in society, social class, the community, and a variety of stressors such as unemployment, unwanted or too many children, or a "problem" child or elderly family member.

Environmental stress theories emphasize stress as the determinant of family violence. Proponents of environmental stress theories set up social programs to remove stress that results from poverty, poor education and occupational skills, and economic conditions that contribute to unemployment and poverty.

Family structure theories assert that violence is the result of problems around the system's enmeshment and disengagement, alliances, coalitions, boundaries, and role relationships.[33] It is believed that violence results from a faulty structure in the family system and that the behavior can be stopped by a reordering of structural properties among the members. Structural reorganization of the family system is believed to provide the members with a new emotional and relationship experience in a context different from that which caused the violence.

Family systems theories complement structural theories and incorporate many of the same formulations. It is believed that violent family members are at a low level of differentiation and are driven by feeling states (anxiety, low self-esteem, inadequacy, loneliness, depression, and so forth) to seek relief. Relief is sought by fleeing oneself and fusing with another person. This process creates intolerable tension, which is released through family violence in one or more dysfunctional processes: triangulation; marital conflict; dysfunction in a spouse, child, or elderly member; physical illness or psychophysiological distress; or emotional illness of a member. Treatment is directed toward helping individual members achieve higher levels of differentiation, ideally resulting in a family system that is more differentiated. The differentiation process requires changes in the members' emotional and relationship processes that result in higher and more adaptive functioning. It requires that family members gain an awareness of certain processes which operate in their family, for example, feeling states that drive individual members' behaviors and how other mem-

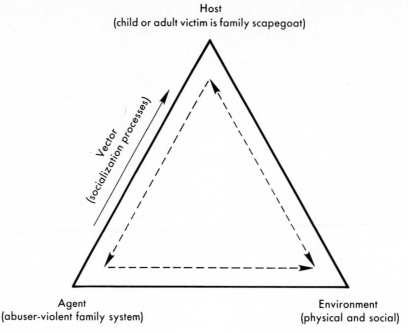

FIG. 28-2
Epidemiological model of family violence.

bers in the system respond to them or fuel the process. Thus the system is taught to acquire impulse control; to stop, look, and observe instead of reacting to every stressor; and to "ride the wave" of stressors in a manner that puts self, and ultimately the family system, in command. Working on "self" in the system puts individual members in charge and in control of self, bringing the system into balance with a different form of equilibrium than that maintained by family violence. Feedback processes result in higher levels of self-esteem that reverberate throughout the family system, resulting in a wide range of positive outcomes, including higher levels of functioning, goal-directed behaviors, reaching out to others, and a realistic world view.

Epidemiological theories incorporate all of the foregoing theories as they take into account the following: the agent (abuser, violent family system), environment (social and physical dimensions), hosts (child or adult victims, family scapegoats), and vector (socialization processes, cultural scripting in society). Epidemiological theories are the most comprehensive in attempting to explain family violence. Treatment is multifactorial, since no single factor is believed to exist in isolation from the others in causing fam-

ily violence. Fig. 28-2 depicts an epidemiological model that incorporates two psychosocial systems: the family system and the larger systems of environment, agent, vector, and host.

Nursing assessment

Self-awareness

Self-awareness is the beginning of a nursing assessment. The moment the nurse comes into contact with a violent family, personal or subjective responses are elicited. It is particularly important for nurses to be aware of and in control of such responses. Violent families have a history of mistreatment that makes them extremely sensitive to any potential present mistreatment. They anticipate abuse and mistrust helping persons or authority figures. If the nurse unleashes a strong negative emotional reaction on the family she is only continuing to fuel the maladaptive emotional climate and dysfunctional family processes. The family can then be expected to become more entrenched and impermeable, closing off the nurse, and thereby becoming resistant to therapy, since the nurse cannot impact on the system as a change agent. Also, if the nurse is not aware of and in control of herself, she is not in a position to provide objective and competent nursing interventions. In effect, the nurse will have fused with the violent family system. Negative feeling responses that violent families elicit in nurses include, but are not limited to, the following:

Anger   Intimidation
Betrayal   Mistrust
Disgust and revulsion   Powerlessness
Fear   Sadness
Frustration   Sympathy
Hopelessness

Violent families can also elicit positive feeling states in nurses, such as humor, warmth, laughter, and pride in their achievements. These are responses that foster family healing rather than having destructive consequences.

Violent families also elicit a number of cognitive, attitudinal, and behavioral responses in nurses such as, but not limited to, the following:

Blaming the abuser, victim, or family members
Believing that change is hopeless
Commitment to prevention and eradication of family violence
Memories of personal experiences with abuse or violence
Research and publication of findings
Search for intervention methods that are effective
Social action

The nurse's thoughts and attitudes will affect what she does in response to family violence as a social problem and in therapy with violent families. Effective mental health therapists working with violent families believe that change is possible; the violence can and will stop. They refuse to give up on the family or feel hopeless and continue to search for, research, and report effective intervention methods. They also support social action that reduces or eliminates psychosocial environmental stressors which contribute to family violence.

Clinical assessment

Clinical assessment of the violent family incorporates all that is known about the nature of such a family discussed earlier in this chapter. Data are collected from these sources[22,39]:
1. Face-to-face interviews with the complainant, the victim, the mother or adult ally for the victim, the perpetrator, and collateral interviews
2. Physical evidence and medical examination
3. Behavioral observation
4. Field investigation

5. Documents
6. Referrals
7. Psychometric tests
8. Physiological measurements

Not all of these data sources are utilized in every case. However, the more comprehensive the assessment is, the more able the clinician is to be "on target" with an effective intervention. Knowing what nursing action to implement requires a solid understanding of the family system. The nurse can complete an assessment of a violent family by applying an epidemiological model as follows.

AGENT. The agent consists of the family members both as a system and as individuals contributing to the functional state of the family. Thus an assessment is made of the family system and of the individual members, and treatment plans are ultimately developed to intervene in the dysfunctional state of both the family as a system and its members. Characteristics of the family system as described in Table 28-2 should be assessed, as well as the following:

1. Boundaries
2. Feeling tone
3. Autonomy/differentiation
4. Trust
5. Conflict
6. Regulation of drives
   a. Alcohol and/or substance abuse[35]
   b. Aggression
   c. Sexuality
7. Time binding
8. Task performance
9. Communication
10. Belief system
11. Power ratio
12. Role stereotyping
13. Relationship and social skills[35]
    a. Intrafamily interpersonal: Husband-wife, father-child, mother-child, child-child, adult-elder, child-elder
    b. Adult sexual: Relationships between adults, between adults and children
    c. Child sexual: Relationships with adults, peers, younger children
    d. Interpersonal/social: Outside of family, larger external systems
14. Health problems of any family member[35]
15. Form of family violence[22]
    a. Type of acts committed
    b. Motivation for the offense
    c. Style of attack
    d. Selection of the victim

e. Response to attack by perpetrator and family members
f. Safety or protection issues: Presence of functioning adult ally for the victim or history of threats, use of force or violence

A descriptive statement should be made for each factor as illustrated in the following example:

Criteria	Example
Boundaries	Mr. and Mrs. X are closed to outsiders and helping persons. The family is socially isolated, and they have few friends.
Feeling tone	The family is engaged in intense competition for caring, attention, and nurturance. The mood is one of depression and pain, with members lacking empathy for each other.
Autonomy/ differentiation	The children demonstrate precocious maturity and responsibility for the family. The elders depend on the family because of impairments from aging. The mother is fused with her family of origin, which creates marital conflict with her spouse.

Completing such an assessment gives the nurse data on the nature of the family as a system, and areas requiring intervention are specifically identified. The family is, although seemingly impermeable, also affected by environmental factors. It is important for nurses to be aware of factors external to the family that add to tension within the family system.

ENVIRONMENT. Assessment of environmental factors takes into account physical and social variables. In making an assessment of the family the nurse evaluates the following stressors[22,25,45]:

1. Employment
   a. Present status part time, full time, unemployed
   b. Pattern of employment
   c. Job satisfaction
   d. Self-actualization
   e. Number of members employed combined with role stereotyping
   f. Marketable skills
2. Financial status
   a. Management techniques
   b. Recent increases or reductions in income
   c. Type of occupational preparation
   d. Resources
3. Housing
   a. Adequacy
   b. Crowded conditions
   c. Cleanliness, order, upkeep

4. Transportation
   a. Use of a car
   b. Use of public transportation
   c. Financial burden
   d. Refusal to use available means or social mobility
5. Support services
   a. Nature of relationship with extended family
   b. Relationships with neighbors, friends, or church affiliates
   c. Use of social service agencies
   d. Perception of resources and support systems
6. Criminal justice system
   a. History of criminal/delinquent offenses
   b. Current probation status
   c. Present and past status of criminal charges

An attempt is made to identify stressors that contribute to family violence. Frequently cited stressors include unemployment or part-time employment, limited education and support systems in achieving career goals, and financial difficulties. No single factor is believed to be causative of family violence, but rather it is the accumulation of multiple stressors that cannot be accommodated or dissipated within the family system that leads to violence. The family is also impacted on by less obvious factors that are contained within culture and society and defined as the vector.

VECTOR. The vector is the mode by which cultural scripting and socialization processes are communicated to and within the family system. Cultural variables that the nurse assesses include, but are not limited to, the following[22,25,45]:

1. Attitudes
   a. Toward the family and individual members
   b. Toward outsiders, support services, and helping persons
   c. Toward the use of physical punishment
   d. Toward sex and sexual relationships
2. Value systems
3. Sex-role stereotyping
4. Way of life
5. Language
6. Ethical positions

Cultural scripting often includes positions that uphold the sanctity and privacy of the family and view outside help as interference in the private domain of the family. The family is likely to report a belief in traditional sex roles and sanction the use of physical punishment in "disciplining" its members.

Professionals and social activists focus on the means by which cultural scripting is communicated, such as the way in which mass media portrays and sanctions violence as a way of life or solving problems. Intervention then focuses on altering learned attitudes, value systems, and behaviors and is often combined with teaching the family members different or alternative attitudes and behaviors, such as more effective child-rearing practices. The final factor to consider is that of the victim and the impact of family violence on that person.

HOST. The host is defined as the scapegoat, or target, of family violence. Agents of family violence include children, adults (parents/spouses), and the elderly. Data are collected in relation to each member, including the agent, or abuser, and problems specific to individual family members are identified. Data on individual members include the following:

1. Developmental life stage
   a. Tasks accomplished
   b. Tasks not accomplished
2. Feelings about self
3. Power
4. Relationships
5. Intrapsychic conflicts
6. Regulation of drives
7. Boundaries
8. Psychosocial values/belief system
9. Coping style
10. Skills/task management
11. Family background
12. Crisis state

PROTOCOL FOR CLINICAL ASSESSMENT OF THE OFFENDER'S (SEXUAL) BEHAVIOR*

Obtain the offender's account of the current sexual offense and any other sexual offense committed by him and explore the following aspects of each:

1. Premeditation
   a. Intentional
   b. Opportunistic
   c. Spontaneous
2. Victim selection
   a. Age
   b. Race
   c. Sex
   d. Social relationship
   e. Situation
   f. Physical characteristics
3. Style of attack
   a. Exploitation
   b. Threat
   c. Intimidation
   d. Incapacitation
   e. Physical force
   f. Violence
4. Accompanying fantasies
   a. Content
   b. Development
5. Role of aggression
   a. Establishing control
   b. Reactive aggression
   c. Discharging anger
   d. Erotic aggression
6. Conversation
   a. Hostile
   b. Instructional
   c. Inquisitive

7. Sexual behavior
   a. Sexual conduct
   b. Duration
   c. Sexual dysfunction
   d. Sexual response
8. Mood state
   a. Feelings
   b. Change
   c. Subjective reaction
9. Contributing factors
   a. Precipitating stressors
   b. Compounding conditions
   c. Release mechanisms
10. Responsibility
    a. Full admission
    b. Qualified admission
    c. Denial
11. Recidivism
    a. Onset
    b. Frequency
    c. Intervention
    d. Progression
12. Deterrence
13. Sexual development
    a. Sex education
    b. Conventional sexual behavior
    c. Unconventional sexual experiences
    d. Marital relations
    e. Sexual life-style
    f. Sexual fantasies
    g. Sexual concerns
    h. Sexual traumas

*From Adleman, C.S.: Los Angeles, Victimology Program, 1980, Wright Institute; modified from Groth, N.A., and Birnbaum, J.: Men who rape: psychology of the offender, New York, 1979, Plenum Press.

TABLE 28-4. Guidelines for assessment and treatment of the sexual offender*

Information	Clinical significance	Target areas
Identifying information Name, address, date of birth, age, race, religion, marital status, physical characteristics	In addition to identifying the offender, there may be clinical significance to some of the data, e.g., if offender was powerfully built, he may be very intimidating to others	Determine if issues raised are supported by other information
Family background Parents, siblings, birth order, nature and quality of intrafamily relationships, intactness, stability of early family life	Formation of personality by significant role models; development of attitudes, values and behavior, family crisis, disruption, trauma, etc., that interfered with ability to negotiate life demands and manage activities of daily living.	Abandonment, death, divorce, separation, etc., poor or ineffective parenting, abuse, family violence, alcoholism
Medical history Previous and current physical and mental problems; prenatal care, delivery, and neonatal development; illnesses; handicaps; operations; hospitalizations during childhood, adolescence, or adulthood; drinking or drug abuse	Effect on his self-image, vulnerability, and perception of the world as dangerous place; anxieties that have been created; relationship to impulse control, feelings of inadequacy	Major illness or accidents, serious disabilities, impairments or handicaps, hyperactivity, enuresis, venereal diseases, suicide gestures, mental illness
Educational development School adjustment and academic performance; level of intellectual functioning and cognitive skills; scholastic interests, aptitudes, abilities, and achievements; attitude toward teachers, administrators, and peers	Indication of ability to persist with reality oriented, long-range goals, or signal of early psychological concerns that interfered with self-discipline, handling responsibilities, and mastering life tasks	School phobias, learning problems, dramatic changes in I.Q. scores or grades, behavior, or discipline
Interpersonal development *Social.* Nature and quality of interpersonal relationships, types of friendships with persons older, younger, peers, etc., basis for friendships	Does he regard others as objects? How does he value people? Can he successfully negotiate friendships? Are relationships based on power and control? Is he a loner? How stable are relationships?	Social isolation, unstable relationships, self-centered, uses others
Sexual. Nature and quality of sexual development and experiences, types of sexual encounters, types of partners, fantasies, attitudes, values, sexual performance, frequency	Does he achieve sexual relationships through negotiation and consent, pressure and exploitation, force and assault? How conservative are his sexual attitudes and values? How comfortable is he with his sexuality; is sex a positive (affectional) or negative (hostile) act? Why has sexuality become the symptom of his psychological dysfunction?	Sexual trauma of victimization, pathological sexuality within the family, sexual dysfunction, sexual offenses, unconventional sexual interests and behaviors (sadomasochism, obscene phone calls)
Criminal history Antisocial behavior and problems with the law, arrest record, age at time of first offense, types of crimes committed, disposition, institutional adjustment, probation or parole record	Criminal history can help differentiate sexual offender whose offenses are one of many expressions of criminal personality from offender whose sexual crimes constitute change in behavior; criminal behavior can be viewed as symptomatic of personality defects; criminal record may indicate dangerousness and failures of offender and his inability to lead responsible and adaptive life	Preadolescent delinquent behavior (stealing, property damage, firesetting, cruelty to animals, children), crimes against the person, crimes of violence (arson, murder, sexual assault, prostitution, pornography, recidivism)

*From Adelman, C.S.: Los Angeles, Victimology Program, 1980, Wright Institute; modified from Groth, N.A., and Birnbaum, J.: Men who rape: psychology of the offender, New York, 1979, Plenum Press.

Assessment of individual members tends to be specific to the form of family violence and can be quite comprehensive. For example, Groth and Birnbaum have developed guidelines and a protocol for the assessment of a sexual offender (p. 815 and Table 28-4). They have been used to assess patients who exhibit other forms of family violence as well. Most of the clinical assessments reported in the literature tend to focus on the agent, or abusive/violent member. This is in keeping with the fact that many health care settings and therapists focus on the violent member rather than the entire family as a system. As more care providers take a family approach in treating family violence, more tools will be developed, reflecting the dysfunctional state of the other members in the system. The results of a careful assessment are utilized to formulate a nursing diagnosis of the problems requiring intervention.

Nursing diagnosis

A comprehensive diagnosis of family violence includes the *family's presenting problem* and *related stressors*, as well as the *family assets and resources*. These assets or resources are then used in planning interventions related to the family's problem areas or stressors. For example, the nurse could emphasize that the family is able to "get done those things which need to be done," such as housework, or that they are a good team together. Such a family has the skill to solve the dilemma around who does what in the house. They may reverse roles to get the work done by having the daughter do the laundry, cooking, and cleaning instead of the parents. The nurse emphasizes that the family's asset is one of management skills whereas its liability is in functioning as a group related to the assumed or assigned responsibilities and tasks. Or the nurse might assess and emphasize that the family members have a sense of humor, which decreases tension in the family. The family has the ability therefore to respond with warmth and empathy to each other. However, its liability is in their use of humor to discount serious problems, such as financial difficulties. The nurse role models how to talk about stressful topics (financial difficulties), while using humor to balance working out the problem operationally. The asset identified by the nursing diagnosis is thus used to the family's advantage in making changes in the system's dysfunctional patterns and interactions. Family assets and resources related to these nursing

diagnoses and problem areas should also be included in the assessment of a family.

Finally, after a list of nursing diagnoses is compiled, these can then be grouped into categories that more clearly conceptualize the problem areas and related stressors.[1] Selected nursing diagnoses which reflect problem areas that frequently arise in working with violent families are depicted in Table 28-5.

One nursing diagnosis can apply to one or more problem areas. The effect of such an outcome is to conceptualize a cluster or pattern in which certain problem areas or assets are more severe or prevalent than other areas and thus guide the nurse in planning interventions in the most dysfunctional aspects of the family's functioning while capitalizing on the family's assets.[1]

The nursing diagnosis is best completed with the family participating in the process. However, at this time, the majority of violent families do not acknowledge that a problem exists and often are in treatment only as a result of a court order. Developing a collaborative relationship with the family in involuntary treatment is often a major task of the nurse in the first phase of therapy. Despite these limitations, the nurse needs to make every effort to formulate a nursing diagnosis and treatment plan with the family.

Planning and implementation of nursing interventions

Goal setting and formulating a treatment plan

The general goal of the nurse working with a violent family is to help them achieve a higher and healthier level of functioning. Goal setting is directed by the following:

1. The nursing diagnosis, specifically, the presenting problem (e.g., family crisis related to disclosure of elder abuse)
2. The intensity of the problem or level of illness (e.g., compulsive acting out of violent behavior in contrast to obsession with violent behavior)
3. The form of family violence
4. The role, setting, and point in time at which the nurse sees the family (e.g., general nursing care, family therapy, follow-up care, or prevention program)

Most violent families come to the attention of professionals when the violence is initially dis-

TABLE 28-5. Nursing diagnoses and assessed problem areas in abusive/violent families*

Nursing diagnosis	Problem areas			
	Personal factors of family members	Style of interaction on average daily basis	Historical or developmental factors	Social factors
Denial of violent behavior related to extreme emotional deprivation and low self-esteem	X	X	X	X
Compulsive acting out of violent behavior related to failure of family to disclose the act and of society to respond	X	X		X
Obsessive fantasies of violent acts and accompanying behaviors related to loneliness and low self-esteem	X			
Impaired ability to trust related to violation of rights and lack of physical safety	X	X	X	
Poor social skills related to social isolation of family	X	X		X
Inadequate ego strength and emotional deprivation related to childhood neglect and violence	X		X	
Inadequate controls and limit setting related to severe low esteem	X	X	X	
Magical expectations related to coping style of denial and discounting	X	X		
Fear of authority related to violence by authority figures	X	X	X	
Depression related to self-hate and lack of achievements	X	X		X
Blurred role boundaries and role confusion related to reversal and family coalitions		X		
Repressed anger and hostility related to abuse of power and poor communication patterns	X	X		
Lack of empathy related to competition for nurturance and attention	X	X		
Isolation related to feelings of inadequacy, low self-esteem, and fear	X	X		X
Repetitive violence related to denial, discounting, and low self-esteem	X	X	X	
Pseudomaturity coupled with failure to accomplish developmental tasks related to role reversal, family coalitions, and boundary violations	X	X		
Guilt related to participation in violence with failure to resist or disclose it	X	X		
Negative self-concept related to negative appraisals by family system and outsiders	X	X	X	X

*Family assets and resources should also be assessed for each individual family and related to the identified nursing diagnoses and problem areas.

closed or reported. Short-term goal planning at this time requires that three key questions be answered[22]:

- How probable is it that this family will behave in a way that will jeopardize the safety of another person?
- Under what psychosocial conditions is such behavior most likely to occur?
- What is the likelihood that these psychosocial conditions will prevail?

The treatment plan will be different, depending on whether or not it is probable that the family violence will be repeated and whether the conditions that contribute to the violence are removed. Initial plans address the following management areas[22,38,45]:

1. Report to authorities
   a. Police
   b. Child welfare
   c. Center for victims
2. Safety
   a. Physical: Is behavior repetitive?
   b. Social: What environmental stressors are present?
   c. Psychological: Denial of violent behavior, acknowledgement of violent behavior, use of threats or force, concern for impact on the victim and family.
3. Medical examination and evidence collection
4. Decision regarding separation
   a. Abuser from victim and family
   b. Victim from abuser and family
   c. Family from victim and abuser
5. Treatment decisions
   a. Outpatient therapy: Individual, group, family, community
   b. Residential treatment
   c. Incarceration
6. Essential life-support, therapeutic, and social services
7. Anticipatory guidance
8. Preparation for court

Once initial management decisions are made, the family is usually in treatment. The planning phase then reflects the type of therapy being implemented to eradicate target behaviors and processes, as well as to learn new behaviors and processes in the family system. For example, the work done in crisis intervention (removal of the abuser from the home and placement of children in a shelter is very different from the work done in family therapy (restructuring role and emotional relationships in the system) or group therapy (individual members working on their own ability to identify feeling states, triggers, tools, sequences of behaviors, outcomes, and reinforcers as interplayed with the family system dynamics). The problems identified in the nursing diagnosis become the target areas for formulating goals of treatment and areas for nursing intervention. Such intervention may include short-term and long-term treatment at the secondary and tertiary levels of prevention. Several treatment models currently being implemented in therapy with violent families will now be presented.

Interventions in secondary prevention

The discussion of intervention in family violence will begin with secondary prevention, that is, the point in time at which the violence comes to the attention of authorities, and outside help

is legally brought to bear on the family system. It is at this time that a nurse with a master's degree in psychiatric–mental health nursing might see the violent family for therapy. Furthermore, given the staggering statistics on the incidence of violence, it is expected that nurses in all fields of practice will see members of violent families for their various health needs.

CRISIS INTERVENTION MODEL. Crisis intervention is the first model of care that can be implemented with violent families. A *crisis* is defined as an upset in a steady state when, temporarily, a person's usual mode of coping is ineffective and results in dysfunction, decompensation, or disorganization.[2,14] Crisis intervention theory (Chapter 20) asserts that if a person's perceptions of an event, coping mechanisms, and support systems are kept in balance, a crisis state can be avoided or reversed.[2] Usually when violent families come to the attention of authorities, all three balancing factors are separately and together in imbalance; for example, the family is no longer allowed to perceive violent behavior as tolerable or acceptable because of society's sanctions. The coping mechanism (violence acted out) is no longer effective if only because the violence is disclosed and the family's boundaries (secrecy) are permeated. Support systems are usually absent or cut off because of the family's maladaptive social isolation prior to disclosure of the violence and to society's stigma and social rejection of families involved in such violence. The violent family is thus in a severe crisis state. Given the extreme imbalance in the family's steady state, the system is particularly open to therapeutic intervention at this time. Unfortunately, the family is not often in therapy at this point but rather is dealing with separation and prosecution. It is more often the case that the family will be seen by a therapist 3 to 6 weeks after disclosure of the violence, when the family is already beginning to "seal off" outsiders and is more entrenched in protecting itself from invasion.

Crisis intervention in family violence is well documented and discussed in the literature.[2,38,45] The reader is referred to these writings because each form of family violence has procedures and protocols that are varied, yet comprehensive. Intervention that can be provided is also influenced by legislation in the nurse's state of residence and other factors, such as the decision of the judge and the testimony of professionals or other witnesses. This is illustrated in Clinical example 28-2.

Clinical example 28-2 reflects the importance of professionals and legal officials working together in making decisions that affect therapy with violent families. It is particularly important that professionals arrive at a level of agreement about such cases before testifying in court. If not, they may act out the family's dynamics around power plays, a game the family is quite good at playing. The person who ultimately suffers is the victim who lives on a daily basis with the constant terror of abuse and violence.

CLINICAL EXAMPLE 28-2

Hearing: A hearing was held before a judge to determine whether it was safe for two children to be returned to the home of a child sexual abuser.

Accused abuser: Charges had been dropped against the abuser by his wife 2 weeks after the petition for prosecution. She "could not live without him." The accused denied ever having committed the crime, the charges were dropped, and no legal record reflecting conviction was "on the books." The accused and his wife wanted the children returned home. The accused stayed in therapy with the two co-therapists and a family therapist.

Co-therapists: Both testified that the accused was not in control of himself, that he was not working in therapy on himself, and that the children were at risk for sexual abuse if returned home. They recommended that the wife could care for all the children and the accused should be removed from the home or that all the children remain out of the home at this time until the accused, through work in therapy, was safe in the home.

Wife: Testified that their relationship had changed since the disclosure. She had assumed mothering responsibilities and their sex life had improved. She wanted her family together and would kill herself if she had to choose between her children and her husband. She cried on the stand.

Family therapist: Testified that the family relationships had been restructured with parents in their appropriate roles (Menuchin model). The accused had become less domineering in the home and was respected by his peers at church. He believed the accused was safe in the home and the children should be returned home, but he admitted that he never had dealt with the accused's sexually abusive behavior or dynamics. (The family therapist was from a different agency than the co-therapists.)

Children and youth services: Testified that they could not safely recommend that the children be returned to the home.

Grandmother: Testified that the children were not safe in the home. (The accused and wife testified that they thought the grandmother, who was currently caring for the children, was trying to split them up.)

Judge's decision: Return the children to the home.

During crisis intervention the following steps are usually implemented[42,45]:

I. Police/legal intervention
   a. Receiving the complaint
   b. Arriving at the scene
   c. Gaining entry
   d. Establishing control
   e. Protecting the victim
   f. Interviewing the victim
   g. Interviewing witnesses
   h. Interviewing the assailant
   i. Gathering evidence
   j. Arrest
      1. Prosecution
      2. Charges dropped
      3. No petition to prosecute
      4. Separation of the perpetrator from the family
II. Hospital intervention
   a. Treatment of injuries
   b. Collection of evidence according to protocol
III. Children and youth services
   a. Complaint filed with police
   b. Investigation of complaint
   c. Interviews with the victim, accused, family members
   d. Collateral interviews
   e. Assessment of the home situation and environment
      1. Welfare assistance as needed
      2. Homemaker services
   f. Separation of the victim, accused, or family as necessary
   g. Shelter, group home, or residential treatment
IV. Psychological intervention
   a. Hotline crisis counseling
   b. Therapy
      1. Specific to form of violence, e.g., Parents United/Parents Anonymous; Rape Crisis Center
      2. Community mental health center
      3. Private therapist
   c. Referral for long-term therapy with the same or a different agency
V. Community linkages initiated
   a. Medical institutions
   b. Social service agencies
   c. Criminal justice agencies
   d. Legal aid
   e. Vocational rehabilitation
   f. Support or self-help groups

Crisis intervention with violent families usually merges with and extends into longer term therapy, counseling, and social service intervention. It is this phase of therapy that is the least described or discussed in the literature. The following discussion presents some models currently being implemented in therapy with violent families. The extent of their effectiveness remains to be researched.

TRANSACTIONAL ANALYSIS MODEL. The transactional analysis model of treatment has been well developed and discussed in the literature over the last 15 years.[6,7] Application of the model in the treatment of violent families has been most thoroughly described by Justice and Justice[25] in their work with physically abusive families. In the transactional analysis model all three spheres of a person's functioning—cognitive, behavioral, and affective—are engaged in the treatment process. Justice and Justice treat the physically violent family by seeing the couple in group therapy with other couples who have the same problem; children do not attend these group therapy meetings.

Group treatment of the physically violent family involves the implementation of goals that arise out of the nursing diagnosis. In transactional analysis models of therapy the patients make a contract with the therapist to work on specific behaviors or problems, and goal achievement is specified by behavioral outcome statements. For example, a behavioral goal might be, "At the end of 1 week Mrs. X will have made one new friend" for the nursing diagnosis of "Severe social isolation related to feelings of inadequacy and worthlessness." Measurement of goal achievement is a way of systematically quantifying and measuring progress in and long-term effectiveness of the treatment. Beyond the goals worked on in therapy, Justice and Justice also work on the following family system processes with physically abusive families. Behavioral outcomes are specified for each[25]:

1. *Symbiosis.* Shifting symbiotic relationship processes will be dissolved.
2. *Isolation.* Social and emotional isolation will be reduced.
3. *Talking and sharing with mate.* The couple will be able to talk and share with one another, intimately and superficially.
4. *Impatience/temper.* The family will demonstrate alternative nonviolent coping styles for working through frustrations.
5. *Child management.* The family will be knowledgeable about child growth and development and nonviolent child-rearing practices in parenting.
6. *Employment.* At least one spouse will obtain gainful employment within 3 weeks of entrance into treatment.

The behavioral outcome goals are then further operationalized for measurement. For example, dissolving the shifting symbiotic processes might include the following behavioral outcomes:

■ Makes all or most decisions on one's own.
■ Offers suggestions to others when asked.
■ Takes responsibility for children when asked.

These specific behavioral outcomes are then measured on a goal attainment scale (Table 28-6) that predicts the level of attainment on a five-point Likert scale of (1) most unfavorable outcome thought likely, (2) less than expected success, (3) expected level of success, (4) more than expected success, and (5) most favorable outcome thought likely.[25] The specific behavioral goals filled in are unique and individualized to each family's needs. The scale can then be used to monitor the family's progress in therapy.

In implementing goals of treatment, the transactional model of intervention utilizes the following approaches: (1) structural analysis of personality, (2) teaching about siamese-twinning life scripts, (3) relaxation and hypnosis therapy, and (4) gestalt and confrontation techniques.[25]

Structural analysis. As part of the work in helping patients gain a cognitive understanding of their difficulties, couples are taught in group therapy sessions how to structurally analyze their personalities. The couples come to recognize their Parent, Adult, and Child ego states involved in particular transactions. The couple also learns about the interlocking nature of their ego states. For example, the husband typically acts as if he has no Child ego state (exemplified by feeling states such as sadness, gladness, or fear), and the wife interlocks with the husband's ego states, acting as if she has no Adult or Parent ego states (exemplified by an absence of care taking behaviors, decision making, and judgment capacities).[25] The "shifting symbiotic" relationship structure of the physically violent family who relates in this way is depicted in Fig. 28-3.

Siamese-twinning life scripts. The couple is taught about their interlocking symbiotic relationship structure as they learn about life

TABLE 28-6. Goal attainment scale follow-up guide for a physical child abuser*

Goal headings	Level of predicted attainment				
	Most unfavorable outcome thought likely (−2)	Less than expected success (−1)	Expected level of success (0)	More than expected success (+1)	Most favorable outcome thought likely (+2)
Symbiosis	Talk, think, act for spouse; turn to children to be cared for		Do no talking, thinking, acting for spouse; seek no nurturing from children		Meet own needs, give support when requested to spouse; support two children
Isolation	Stay in house all day; visit no one; call on no one for help		Get out of house each day; visit neighbors; call on them or friends in crisis		Get out of house each day; go somewhere with a friend; go out with husband; call people in crisis
Talking and sharing with mate	Criticize and nag spouse; give no positive strokes		Give positive strokes instead of nagging and criticism to mate while talking and sharing for at least 10 minutes		Give positive strokes to mate while talking and sharing for at least 15 minutes
Impatience/ temper	Outbursts of temper and impatience at husband, children, and persons outside the home		No outburst of temper or impatience at children or husband		No outbursts of temper or impatience in home or elsewhere
Child development and management	Continue present disciplining; learn no child development or management techniques; children not allowed to be children		Learn developmental needs; use "I messages" and reinforcement techniques; let husband do any physical disciplining; children allowed to be children		Learn developmental needs; use "I messages" and reinforcement techniques; leave off yelling at kids
Employment	Continue to remain idle at home and demonstrate "job phobia"		Overcome "job phobia" by getting and keeping job at least 3 months		Overcome "job phobia" by getting and keeping job at least 6 months

*Modified from Justice, B., and Justice, R.: The abusing family, New York, 1976, Human Sciences Press, Inc.

FIG. 28-3
Shifting symbiotic relationship structure that may characterize physically violent families. (From Justice, B., and Justice, R.: The abusing family, New York, 1976, Human Sciences Press, Inc.)

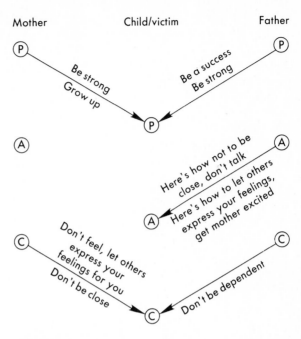

FIG. 28-4
Siamese-twinning script matrix of a child abuser's partner. (From Justice, B., and Justice, R.: The abusing family, New York, 1976, Human Sciences Press, Inc.)

scripts: how these were communicated to them; how they fit with their spouse's life scripts in a complementary and reciprocal manner, and how they communicate the same life scripts to their children. Siamese twinning is explained as a process in which one spouse cannot act without the other going along with the action or direction either by doing nothing or failing to change the course of action.[25] Life-script messages are usually communicated verbally from Parent to Parent ego states, nonverbally from Child to Child ego states, with strong influences on later feelings and behaviors in life, and behaviorally from Adult to Adult ego states when the implementation of a life script is demonstrated or role modeled. Fig. 28-4 depicts a siamese-twinning script matrix of a child abuser's partner. It shows the way in which the physically abusive family is fused around transactional processes.

Most of the literature focuses on the abuser, whereas this model focuses on the family as an interlocking system. The dynamic processes are the same in the physically abusive family as in the sexually abusive family. Tension builds in one member until it can no longer be contained, and the feelings are relieved by the physically or sexually abusive act. Usually the nonabusive partner emerges from the violent episode "smelling like a rose," since the focus is typically on blaming the abusive or violent member for the system's dysfunctional processes. The nonabusive spouse family member generally colludes in the violence by doing nothing to relieve or prevent high stress levels that build to a violent release, and, after the violence, takes care of the crisis calmly as if in command of the entire situa-

tion. Both adults have learned not to ask outsiders for help or show feelings, which "seals off" the family system from potential therapeutic intervention. This transactional interactional process is brought to the couple's awareness in therapy by visually diagramming the process on paper or a blackboard (Fig. 28-4). In this way, the transactional model implements the goal of helping patients gain control of themselves in transactions with others.

Relaxation and hypnosis therapy. Relaxation and hypnosis therapy use behavior modification strategies to teach patients how to relax in tense situations and to prevent accumulation of tension to explosive levels. They are thus taught how to respond differently to stressful stimuli. The reader is referred to Chapter 1 and the literature for detailed discussion of these two approaches in treatment.[36]

Gestalt and confrontation strategies. Gestalt techniques are used to give members "permission" and "protection" in disclosing painful feelings (sadness, depression, loneliness) and intense feelings (love, hate, jealousy, rage, fear) in a safe environment of people who care about each other.[25] Caring is communicated verbally through empathic remarks that reflect the therapist's and members understanding and appreciation of a family's painful existence and struggle for healthier functioning.

The strongest confrontation strategy is to insist that the violence and abuse stop and may include close monitoring of the family.[25] In terms of a behavioral goal, the patient might be told, for example, that "under no circumstances is he or she to be left alone in the house with the child or elder." Confrontations are used throughout group therapy, such as when group members confront each other on denial, blocks, destructive communication, and responsibility for self.

INDIVIDUAL PSYCHOTHERAPY APPROACH. Generally, violent family members are not in individual psychotherapy as the primary mode of therapeutic intervention. Individual psychotherapy is more often used as an adjunct to group or family therapy. It is believed by experts in victimology that the character structure and lifestyle of the family members is not conducive to traditional or classic psychoanalytical psychotherapy. The level of denial is so severe that family members are extremely resistant to therapeutic change by classic methods. Another reason violent families are not seen primarily in individual therapy is that they desperately need to experience the curative factors that group therapy has to offer. The family needs to decrease social isolation and make new friends, have "input" from a variety of sources to open up their closed system, develop social skills, feel wanted and a sense of belonging, and feel accepted and cared about.[25]

Basically individual therapy reinforces the work done in group or family therapy. Patients might work on other problem areas, such as getting themselves out of financial difficulties or pursuing career goals, in individual therapy. What seems consistent across problem areas is the "powerless to power" dynamic, regardless of the issue being worked through or the approach to treatment.

FAMILY THERAPY APPROACH. Controversy characterizes the issue of using family therapy as the primary approach in treatment and whether it should precede or exclude other forms of intervention, such as individual counseling of victims. The family therapy approach most frequently reported in work with violent families is Menuchin's structural therapy.[32] Generally, it is agreed that all of the factors characterizing violent families (Table 28-2), if present in a given family system, are in need of intervention. Thus one would see a family therapist work toward a variety of goals such as the following[15,34,39]:

1. Rebalance the power bases in the system (put mom in charge, establish rules)
2. Build the relationship between the mother and daughter (through a shared activity) and break the closeness between father and daughter related to the sexual abuse
3. Open communication between the spouses (assign mom and dad to plan a picnic, talk about finances or the wife going to work)
4. Stimulate members' efforts toward independence and autonomy (family is assigned the task of dividing up household chores, teenage daughter is made responsible for mothering 2-year-old out-of-wedlock child, wife is instructed to learn to drive a car)

The effectiveness of traditional family therapy methods in treating violent families remains to be widely reported in the literature. Vasquez[44] recently completed a federally funded family therapy research study (Menuchin model) assessing and intervening with physically and sexually abusive families. His findings are currently being analyzed and have yet to be reported.

The family therapy that is accomplished is often achieved through group therapy approaches. As members work on their individual identities, the family system processes are gradually restructured and altered, changes are slowly created in emotional and relationship systems, and over time higher levels of differentiation are achieved. The preference for group approaches largely arises out of the resistance of the family to change by other treatment approaches. Work begun in secondary prevention takes a long time to complete and is supported by tertiary prevention interventions.

Interventions in tertiary prevention

Tertiary prevention consists of interventions implemented after adaptation has occurred. Efforts are directed toward helping the family system stabilize, adapt, become educated, or be maintained at a desired level of healthy functioning. Furthermore, interventions are directed toward reducing the possibility of further episodes of violence in the family. A variety of tertiary prevention activities implemented with violent families are briefly described. Many of these activities, because of present governmental policies of budget cuts and financial constraints, will no longer be funded or available to many violent families as tertiary or primary prevention interventions.

THERAPEUTIC EDUCATION. Part of preventing repetition of family violence depends on the family becoming educated (1) with more information and teaching strategies that foster learning about the nature of their dynamic processes and (2) by achieving academic advancement through completing diplomas, certificates, and college. The family, staying in therapy at this time, learns how to restructure their lives so as to achieve positive and satisfying goals in their lifetime. Children also need to be educated about family violence because if they are made aware of the problem they will usually report it to a "grown-up." In this way children learn that they do not have to be victims of violence and become community monitors on the welfare of the family within its private inner sanctum.

The family needs to see how the abuser uses his attitudes and emotional states just prior to a violent episode. Tertiary prevention begins when the abuser is in control of his behavior and when the therapeutic focus can turn more deeply into the system's dynamic processes. For example, the wife of an abuser needs to see that she is not responsible for his feelings. However, then the wife needs to recognize the abuser's feeling states by which he calls attention to himself, indicating "where he is at." The message from the therapist to the abuser's wife is, "If you care at all about your husband you will see to it that he doesn't repeat the violence. And, to do that you need to deal with yourself. You need to deal with your dynamics because you accepted this situation all these years. Therefore you need to get to know yourself better if you're going to help your husband. It doesn't have to happen again."

In the final phase of therapy the family continues to deal with the issue of powerlessness-to-power as a dynamic in their transactions and enmeshment.[24] The members need to learn to differentiate and discriminate affection from power because in the act of abuse or violence, affection and power are often fused and confused. Becoming aware of oneself and the family system, a learned behavior by this point, then generalizes to objectively assessing transactions outside the family. It becomes obvious to the violent family, depressingly so at times, how the powerlessness-to-power dynamic is "played out" in every aspect of their lives. It is often not confined or limited to the physically or sexually abusive or violent transactions. Awareness of the pervasiveness of the powerlessness-to-power dynamic, combined with awareness by patients of the tendency to fuse affection with power, is a sobering moment. It can be the turning point in therapy for making changes to replace faulty maladaptive processes. It can also be so painful that patients reactivate old coping patterns, such as denial and discounting, to flee acknowledging and accepting themselves. When families are able to be open and accepting of themselves, admit or acknowledge that changes are needed, and work continuously in therapy to achieve these changes, then the system is generally demonstrating a healthier level of self-esteem and reality testing.

Another area that is explored at this time is the relationship of the therapist with the family. Often the family's dynamic conflicts are worked through around the therapeutic relationship. One of the important relationship issues in this regard is the *power dynamic*.[17,24] For example, the therapist is caring, attentive, and committed to helping the violent family stop the violence. The family usually interprets this as, "That person genuinely cares about us," or "I have good feelings about that therapist because she cares enough to care about me. Even when I have temporary setbacks she sticks by me, expects me to change, and doesn't give up hope that I can and will change." At some point the family may test out the limits of their relationship with the therapist, who then needs to redefine that this is a therapy relationship. Exactly how families work through this power issue is quite varied and unpredictable. The only factor that is predictable is that the power dynamic in the relationship with the therapist does come to the fore and needs to be attended to. This can be seen in Clinical example 28-3.

━━━━━━━━━━━━━━━━━━━━━━━━━━━

CLINICAL EXAMPLE 28-3

Joe, a 30-year-old father of five, was convicted of sexually abusing his two stepdaughters. Joe claimed he did not commit the act because he does not remember doing it; he was drunk at the time. The judge ordered Joe out of the family home and to therapy. Since Joe has been living alone, the children have become physically and psychologically violent at home with each other, and their mother has not stopped the violent behavior. An uncle came from California to visit, and while he was there he sexually abused the daughters. The father moved back into the home, knowing he was breaking his parole regulation. The mother did nothing to stop the father from moving back into the family home. The two daughters, in group therapy with other adolescent victims, were very distressed and acted "strange," but it took a month before they found the situation intolerable and disclosed the events.

The therapist had to do something about the situation presented in Clinical example 28-3. To not act would have meant she had been co-opted by the family system into permitting the violence to continue and ignoring it as a reality. The two daughters were placed in a shelter, and the father was returned to prison for parole violation. The mother was court ordered to not only attend, but to participate, in therapy as indicated by the therapist's progress report in 2 months. The mother was confronted with the dynamic way in which she contributed by default to the father's lack of control. In this situation, the power dynamic was played out around the following questions: Would the therapist find out about the parole violation or rule-breaking behavior? Would the therapist do anything about it after the act was discovered? Did the therapist have any power to do anything about the violation? It is precisely at this point that the violent family translates and misconstrues the therapist's adult/responsible behavior of reporting and testifying in court as "not caring" about them, being "out to get us, to split up the family," and being "on a big ego trip." The issue then becomes, in some cases, the turning point at which reality is reevaluated, "I care about you because I won't let you continue to be violent and abusive." Caring and affection are gradually seen as mature adult behaviors, and gradually the therapist's intervention can be seen as caring rather than as a power trip. And so the family learns to separate caring and affection from power in the therapeutic relationship and is helped to generalize that learning experience to other relationships, particularly with authority figures, such as employers or supervisors. It is clear at this point that therapeutic intervention with violent families continues for an ex-

tended period of time, and discussion is in terms of control rather than cure. Therapy must necessarily be supported by the use of programs in the community.

COMMUNITY LINKAGES. Since the beginning of the community mental health movement and federally funded social programs in the 1960s, many programs have been developed that offer both tertiary and preventive interventions to violent and highly stressed families. These programs are currently being reduced or eliminated because of cuts in the federal budget and the austere economic condition of the nation. This is a sad commentary because by eliminating such services one can predict that the level of family violence will increase in this nation, and agencies offering support after secondary intervention will no longer be as available to clients. In times of stress, healthy families usually become more permeable and activate extended family contacts. However, violent families do not act in this manner, and, when they do, usually at the encouragement of professionals, the family is exposed more intensely to family processes that are dysfunctional and intensify the family pathological conditions. Experts generally do not advise putting the victim with grandparents, since grandparents often violated their own children and may do the same with the victimized grandchild, or otherwise perpetuate the family's violent dynamic processes. Thus, for a variety of reasons, community programs have been an important mode of intervention in work with violent families. The following is a brief listing of some programs that have been available.

Foster grandparent programs or lay therapy. These programs are usually comprised of people willing to give of themselves to others. Foster grandparents can give to (and receive from) children a lot of love and attention; often the very kind of nurturing the child needs but the parents feel unable to provide. Lay therapists are usually viewed as adults who give to adults, one couple to a family, and provide the needed nurturing, attention, and caring that violent families so desperately seek.[25] As a peer experience it is particularly valuable for adults who have lacked the experience of intimacy with peers during adolescence, or the ability to give of self to another. As outsiders, the input into the violent family system of new experiences, perspectives, and feeling states, is particularly powerful. Professional therapists can strategically work with foster or lay therapists to create changes in a violent family system. However, the team must guard against arguing and fighting among themselves, playing out their own power dynamics, and, ultimately, diverting attention away from a concentrated multimodel approach in treating the violent family.

Support services. Support services consist of programs or services available in the community that, when used by the violence-prone family, will help prevent repetition of family violence. Thus support services are a tertiary intervention and also a primary intervention. Some of the support services available in the community include the following[25,45]:

1. Visiting or public health nurses
2. Homemaker services
3. Cooperative nurseries
4. Crisis nurseries
5. Day care centers/nurseries
6. Foster home care
7. Classes on child and elderly development and management.
8. Telephone hotline services for violent families
9. Classes about personality and family dynamics
10. Transportation car pools or taxies
11. State and national hotlines for information and reporting
12. Self-help groups, such as Alcoholics Anonymous, Al-Anon, Al-Teen, Abusers Anonymous, Parents United/Parents Anonymous, and Daughters and Sons United
13. Financial assistance programs
14. Suicide hotlines and crisis intervention teams
15. Peer counseling (women's centers, rape crisis centers)
16. Assertiveness training
17. Divorce counseling

Many families need supportive follow-up care while establishing healthy network systems, and nurses are in a unique position to (1) provide the service, (2) monitor the family's adaptation, and (3) intervene to prevent future violence.

Interventions in primary prevention

The aim of primary prevention is to reduce the incidence of and, ideally, eradicate family violence. Primary prevention focuses on promoting optimum health and uses measures that will prevent maladaptation or disease. Research is directed toward identifying possible risk factors and associated stressors that place a family at high risk for violent transactions. Interventions are then directed at identifying those families at high risk and intervening to prevent the violence from happening. Primary prevention also strengthens current adaptive coping mechanisms of patients, and interventions are directed toward preventing dysfunctional de-

compensation. The following discussion briefly outlines a variety of primary prevention programs that have been or could be implemented.

VALUE EVALUATION. By the time professionals become actively involved in primary prevention programs, the gravity of the problem of family violence has been fully realized. It is no longer sufficient to stop the violence; the professional becomes committed to preventing its occurrence based on an awareness of the destructiveness and devastation it creates. That process is a gradual experience over time, culminating in a full value clarification process with commitment to action. This process is called a *value evaluation process*. It is very similar to a self-awareness, philosophical-meditative, self-exploratory process in which the professional comes to terms with what one thinks and feels about the problem of family violence and what action or inaction is taken as a result.

Value evaluation requires that the nurse take a value position about the problem of family violence. For example, if the nurse believes the problem of family violence is of epidemic proportions, there is greater likelihood that action will be taken to eliminate it. What one does about a problem is directly related to what one thinks about that problem or even if it is classified as a "problem."

At this point, it appears that not many professionals are involved in primary prevention activities.[25,45] Community and public health nurses could make an excellent contribution in primary and secondary prevention through case identification, referral, education, and agency collaboration. Nurses in every field of practice could contribute in similar fashion. At present most of the professionals working with violent families are providing secondary prevention services, and few people are qualified to do such work. It is only when the problem becomes epidemic in proportion that there is a massive, often federally funded, program to reduce or eradicate the epidemic, whereas prevention would have been less costly and destructive.

The people of this nation appear to value secondary prevention more than primary prevention.[25,45] Otherwise, more health professionals would be involved in clinical work to prevent family violence, and more social resources would be allocated to that end. Progress in that direction, however, is slowly occurring. For example, the American Nurses' Association

---

RESOLUTION ON VICTIMOLOGY*

Whereas, The number of reported cases of abused victims of all ages is increasing; and

Whereas, Abuse victims present themselves in all settings where registered nurses practice; and

Whereas, Comprehensive nursing care of abused victims requires a definite knowledge base in family dynamics, human sexuality, and victimology; and

Whereas, Registered nurses providing primary, secondary, and tertiary intervention generally are not prepared in victim health care; and

Whereas, This knowledge can be assured only with an adequate cadre of clinicians and faculty prepared in victimology; and therefore be it

Resolved, That the Council of Specialists in Psychiatric and Mental Health Nursing encourage universal inclusion of victimology in the curricula of basic nursing education programs; and be it further

Resolved, That the Council of Specialists in Psychiatric and Mental Health Nursing encourage graduate programs in psychiatric and mental health nursing to **assure adequate numbers of faculty to teach victimology and victimologist researchers to expand the scientific base for psychiatric and mental health nursing practice with victims; and be it further**

Resolved, That the Council of Specialist in Psychiatric and Mental Health Nursing encourage clinicians who care for abused victims to write and report their information concerning clinical practice.

---

*From American Nurses' Association, Council of Specialists in Psychiatric and Mental Health Nursing: Resolution on victimology, Kansas City, Mo., 1980. Reprinted by permission.

Council of Specialists in Psychiatric–Mental Health Nursing recently passed a resolution on victimology (above).* In passing that resolution, the council members made the following public commitment:

To include victimology in the curricula of basic nursing education programs, to encourage graduate programs in psychiatric–mental health nursing to assure adequate numbers of faculty to teach victimology and victimologist researchers to expand the scientific base for psychiatric and mental health nursing practice with victims, and to encourage clinicians who care for abused victims to write and report their information concerning clinical practice.[3]

A second nursing activity at the national level endorsing victimology as a legitimate field of practice has been the endorsement of a subspecialty interest group in victimology by the Council of Specialists in Psychiatric–Mental Health Nursing, and nursing research groups

*From American Nurses' Association, Council of Specialists in Psychiatric and Mental Health Nursing: Resolution of victimology, Kansas City, Mo., 1980. Reprinted by permission.

such as the Midwest Nursing Research Society. These activities reflect a beginning, but much remains to be done. Specific strategies in primary prevention are clearly planned interventions aimed at a specific problem area. A number of different specific strategy programs exist, and six of them will now be discussed.

HIGH-RISK IDENTIFICATION. Programs aimed at high-risk identification teach people how to identify cases that have a high risk or potential to become violent and then provide primary prevention to prevent an occurrence of violence.[9] For example, community health nurses might be alert to elders who are at high risk for family violence according to current, although rather limited, research findings, which suggest the following characteristics of families of abused elders:

1. A middle income family in which their dependency stresses a high-achieving, career-oriented family beyond its limits, with a son (daughter or relative) striking out in violence

2. Unemployment

3. Financial difficulties
4. No relief from the responsibility of care taking
5. A stressed economy

TRAINING PROGRAMS IN VICTIMOLOGY. The field of victimology is expanding at an exponential rate. It is difficult to keep up with all the literature that is being published on each form of family violence, as well as data on cases in which more than one form of family violence exists. Enough information exists at this time that it could legitimately be "institutionalized" by a training program.[11] Such a program would address issues such as the following:
1. Case identification for every form of violence
2. Crisis intervention in family violence
3. Therapy with violent families
4. Therapy with prisoners in prison systems who have been abusers, victims, or both of family and other violence
5. Programs to eradicate family violence that have been or could be developed
6. Workshops that teach self-defense
7. Therapy with schizophrenics who have episodes of violent behavior

This list is a small sampling of content that could be included in a training program. The programs that are currently being offered at a national level have been federally funded programs and generally have not been sponsored by nurses.

PROFESSIONAL EDUCATION. Curricula in schools of nursing need to include more content on all forms of family violence than is currently included in most existing curricula.[11,19,20] All professional schools need more content on family violence and intervention in their curricula. The educational process needs to be extended as well through continuing education and community speaking activities as a way of reaching professionals and laypersons in what could become a "common cause," and, at a minimum, meet their educational needs.

LAY EDUCATION.[31,45] Violent families are sorely lacking in knowledge in many fields of information. A prevention program could set up educational classes to provide people with information they need to achieve their developmental tasks with a minimum of stress. Examples of such programs include educational courses on relationships and marriage, child-rearing practices and development, and anticipatory guidance.

Relationships and marriage. Adolescents have demonstrated a need for courses on relationships and marriage.[29] What are relationships all about? How do you handle all the strange and stressful things that arise in a relationship? Are there some people who should not get married or have kids? How does homosexuality fit into a relationship with someone? All kinds of other management and relationship questions should be examined: Who is in charge of the money or to what extent does that person have control over the funds? If there is a disagreement, who has the last word and is it the same person all the time? How do you get along with someone? Who is the family manager, plans the social life, meals, bedtimes, clothing, career schedule? These and many other questions are familiar to "elders" who have gone through more of life. They could be explored and discussed with the youth in this nation and hopefully help them achieve answers and emotional well-being.

Child-rearing practices and development. Violent families are often limited in their knowledge about child development and how to raise a child. Their paucity of information adds stress to an already stressed psyche. Nurses could preventively intervene by providing more families, particularly families at high risk for violence, courses on child development and child-rearing practices. Community health nurses entering family homes are in an excellent position to identify families who would benefit from such a nursing action.

Anticipatory guidance. In preventing a crisis from developing, one strategy that is often implemented is that of anticipatory guidance. The patients can be prepared for what is about to happen to them and their lives. The following are two important areas in which violent families could benefit from anticipatory guidance[38]:
1. *Therapeutic education.* The therapist talks with the patient about setbacks while in therapy and advises the patient to be on the lookout for clues or warning signals that indicate regression into a violent episode.
2. *The court process.* Patients undergo a painful process of having all the case data presented publicly, often in front of curiosity seekers who listen to court cases the way some people follow soap operas. The family needs to be prepared for what to expect, exactly what can happen, what some of the outcomes might be in the case, the consequences of any of those outcomes, and where to turn when they really

need someone to talk to about what they are experiencing. It is important for the professional to be steadfast with the family at this time, and it is even more favorable if the nurse could begin therapy with the family during this critical period, which is usually perceived as a crisis by most families.

COMMUNITY AWARENESS PROGRAMS. Community awareness programs are prevention programs that are offered through public speaking engagements and are designed to inform the audience about the nature of a problem, how it is treated, its causes, and how to prevent it. Rape crisis centers have actively sponsored community awareness programs. Nurses could offer such programs to the public and become publicly identified as someone to turn to before, or in the event of, family violence. Such programs need to be more widely offered in relation to all forms of family violence. Groups who could be addressed include parent-teacher associations, church groups, children in school systems or after-school activities, Rotary Clubs, and a wide range of men and women's groups.

PERSONAL GROWTH GROUPS FOR MEN AND WOMEN. Groups run by nurses could help men and women work through issues they confront in passing through life and prevent family violence by providing the opportunity for them to talk about such issues as:

■ How does one cope with problematical parents as they get older? Yurick and Nelson at the University of Pittsburgh School of Nursing have offered such a preventive group to children caring for their older parents, the children usually being middle-age couples.

■ What options are open to women and how do they decide what is best? Such groups can facilitate women talking to other women about women's issues throughout the life cycle, such as sexuality, marriage, and childbearing. They can serve as a support network that can be activated in times of crises. Women are raised with many myths that can be sources of stress in their personal lives. Growth groups, like those spearheaded by the women's movement, could help women and men work through developmental issues on a consistent basis and thus reduce the accumulation of tension

from such stressors into a family system until it explodes. Part of preventing violence is helping men and women work through issues that confront them at every stage of the life cycle.

OTHER STRATEGIES. Descriptions of prevention programs could be endless. They are only limited by the nurse's creativity and environmental influences, such as governmental policy, economic constraints, and manpower issues. The following list briefly identifies additional prevention programs nurses need to be aware of and can potentially offer as a service[25,45]:

1. Visiting or public health nurse programs provide support, aid, nurturance, and human contact to isolated individuals who are at high risk for violence.
2. Homemaker services provide teaching to parents who are poorly equipped or unable to perform functional tasks, such as doing the dishes or laundry, disciplining the children without corporal punishment, or cleaning house. These homemakers often become a friend of the family in the truest sense of a friend helping one out in a time of need.
3. Child care services offer care to children in crisis nurseries, emergency shelter care, cooperative nurseries, day-care centers, and foster care.
4. Transportation includes publicly organized car pool systems to help the disadvantaged, such as vans that chauffeur senior citizens around the city.
5. Telephone reassurance services consist of crisis hotlines available to people in times of crisis, such as Alcoholic Anonymous, Parents Anonymous/Parents United, and Suicide Crisis Intervention.
6. National networking is when persons concerned about victimology form a national group and stay in frequent contact with each other, such as members of the National Organization of Victims Assistance and nurses belonging to the council's special interest group in victimology.
7. Self-help groups of laypersons share a particular problem in common and meet to help one another cope with that problem.
8. Family planning programs provide individuals with contraceptive options and education.
9. Political action includes activities directed toward public policy and getting legislators and politicians to support programs for

preventing family violence. This is an area in which increased activitiy is needed by nurses and other health professionals.

Evaluation

In the 1960s physical abuse of children was brought to public attention, in the 1970s spouse abuse and sexual abuse of children became important social issues, and in the 1980s it is expected that abuse of the elderly and sibling violence will come to greater public attention.[43] At this point, however, little is known about the effectiveness of treatment and even less is known from a strict empirical position. Professionals are only beginning to widely report treatment interventions (as opposed to assessment factors) with violent families. Most of these reports are descriptive and are clinical research studies that evaluate the effectiveness of a given treatment approach. The secondary interventions discussed in this chapter were presented as currently reported treatment strategies with violent families. However, much remains to be researched about these descriptive clinical impressions.

Research is even less available on primary and tertiary prevention programs. It is known that a certain cluster of variables (unemployment, limited education, and emotional deprivation) are high-risk factors for family violence; however, it is difficult to measure the effectiveness

of any prevention program. That fact continues to present nurses in all fields of practice difficulty in designing primary prevention research studies. In terms of tertiary interventions, there are many influences, and it would require factor analysis to determine which variables were contributing to preventing further episodes of family violence. Research is also lacking in studies reporting longitudinal therapeutic work with violent families and follow-up assessment. Much remains to be done in the treatment and prevention of this mounting social problem.

Suggested cross-references

The transactional analysis model of communication and self-awareness of the nurse are discussed in Chapter 3. Primary prevention activities are discussed in Chapter 5. Rehabilitation activities are discussed in Chapter 6. Relaxation techniques are discussed in Chapter 7. Crisis intervention is discussed in Chapter 20. Group therapy is discussed in Chapter 24. Family therapy is discussed in Chapter 25. Interventions with victims of rape are discussed in Chapter 26.

SUMMARY

1. Family violence is the physical, psychological, sexual, material, or social violation of a person by a family member or their delegate. Family violence is often described in terms of abuse or violence, and both acts can exist in the same family.
   a. Abuse is defined as an act that deceives or puts to wrong or improper use so as to injure, damage, maltreat, or corrupt.
   b. Violence is defined as an act marked by extreme force or sudden intense activity to the point of loss of self-control.
2. The problem of family violence was defined in terms of demographic data, the violent family system, the stress reaction process, forms of family violence, and the incidence of the problem.
   a. The following 12 characteristics by which violent family systems differ from competently functioning families were described: boundaries, mood/feeling tone, autonomy/differentiation, trust, conflict, regulation of drives (aggression/sexuality), time binding, task per-

formance, communication, belief system, power ratio, and role stereotyping.
   b. Types of violent behavior include physical, psychological, sexual, material, and social acts that violate another person. Motives of the assailant and colluding members include power and aggression. Both motives may be present throughout the assault. Targets of released aggression and unresolved power issues in violent/abusive families were defined as child physical abuse, child sexual abuse, spouse abuse, sibling abuse, and elder abuse.
   c. Incidence of family violence was reported in terms of founded cases. These are believed to be only estimates of the prevalence of the problem because of problems in conducting reliable and valid research studies, as well as the taboo nature of the topic in society.
3. Theories on the etiology of family violence are abundant, overlap with each other, and when considered alone are incomplete in explaining the phe-

nomena. Theoretical models used to explain family violence include psychodynamic theories, social learning theories, psychosocial theories, environmental stress theories, family structure theories, family system theories, and epidemiological theories.

4. The nursing process model is used in assessing family violence and identifying ways in which to best intervene in the problem. Self-awareness by the nurse is essential. Clinical assessment of the violent family includes all that is known about the nature of such a family and can be completed by applying an epidemiological model which assesses the hosts, environment, vector, and agent. Assessment of individual members tends to be specific to the form of family violence and is usually quite comprehensive.

5. The formulation of a nursing diagnosis includes the family's presenting problem and related stressors, as well as the family's assets and resources. It is best completed with the family participating in the process.

6. The planning phase of the nursing process includes the general goal of helping the family achieve a higher and healthier level of functioning. Goal setting is directed by the nursing diagnosis, the intensity of the problem or level of illness, the form of family violence, and the role, setting, and point in time at which the nurse sees the family. Short-term goals require an assessment of potential repetition of the abuse or violence and victim safety, as well as initial management plans. Short-term goals merge with longer term goals in treatment and are directed by the type of therapy being implemented.

  a. Interventions in secondary prevention include crisis intervention, group therapy that applies a transactional analysis model, individual therapy as a complement to group therapy, and family therapy that applies both family structure and family systems theories.

  b. Interventions in tertiary prevention include therapeutic education and community linkages that offer support after secondary intervention.

  c. Interventions in primary prevention include value evaluation and programs directed at high-risk identification, training programs in victimology, professional education, lay education, community awareness programs, and personal growth groups for men and women.

7. Evaluating the long-term effectiveness of different treatment modalities has yet to be implemented as a strict empirical process. Nurses can make a significant contribution in this area. The problem of family violence is believed by experts to be the result of a dysfunctional family system in response to predisposing and precipitating stressors, including cultural and socialization processes, values, attitudes, and belief systems. The problem of family violence and its generational repetition/transmission will be eradicated only to the extent that such families are helped to achieve higher levels of differentiation and healthy functioning.

References

1. Abraham, I.: Personal communication, Nov. 1981.
2. Aguilera, D., and Messick, J.: Crisis intervention: theory and methodology, ed. 4, St. Louis, 1981, The C.V. Mosby Co.
3. American Nurses' Association, Council of Specialists in Psychiatric and Mental Health Nursing: Resolution of victimology, Kansas City, Mo., June 9, 1980, The Association.
4. American Psychiatric Association: Diagnostic and statistical manual of mental disorders (DSM-III), Washington, D.C., 1980, The Association.
5. Beck, A. et al.: Cognitive therapy of depression, New York, 1979, The Guilford Press.
6. Berne, E.: Games people play: the psychology of human relationships, New York, 1964, Grove Press, Inc.
7. Berne, E.: Principles of group treatment, New York, 1966, Oxford University Press, Inc.
8. Block, M., and Sinnott, J., editors: The battered elder syndrome: an exploratory study, College Park, Md., 1979, The University of Maryland.
9. Blumberg, M.: Treatment of the abused child and the child abuser, Am. J. Orthopsychiatry 31(2):204, 1977.
10. Brudnak, L.: Self-esteem levels, sexual knowledge, and sexual attitudes of male child sexual abuse offenders, master's thesis, Pittsburgh, 1981, The University of Pittsburgh School of Nursing.
11. Burgess, A.W.: Personal communication, Oct. 1981.
12. Burgess, A.W. et al.: Sexual assault of children and adolescents, Lexington, Mass., D.C. Heath & Co.
13. Burns, R.: In Fontana, B.J.: Somewhere a child is crying, New York, 1973, Macmillan Publishing Co., Inc.
14. Caplan, G.: Principles of preventative psychiatry, New York, 1964, Basic Books, Inc.
15. Coleman, P.: Incest; family treatment model. In Holley, K.C.: Sexual misuses of children: tools for understanding, Tacoma, Wash., 1979, Pierce County Rape Relief.
16. Davidson, J.L.: Elder abuse. In Block, M., and Sinnott, J., editors: The battered elder syndrome: an exploratory study, College Park, Md., 1977, The University of Maryland Center on Aging.
17. Davis, B.: Personal communication, Oct.-Nov. 1981.
18. Douglass, R., Hickey, T., and Noel, C.: A study of maltreatment of the elderly and other vulnerable adults, Ann Arbor, Mich., 1900, The University of Michigan School of Public Health.
19. Foley, T.: The development and evaluation of an instructor's manual on nursing care of victims of rape, doctoral dissertation, Pittsburgh, 1979, The University of Pittsburgh School of Education.
20. Foley, T., and Davies, M.: Rape: nursing care of victims, Soc. Probl., 1978.
21a. Geriatric Nursing 1:153, Sept.-Oct. 1980.
21. Gagnon, J.: Female child victims of sexual offenses, J. Soc. Probl. 1978.

22. Groth, A.N., and Birnbaum, J.: Men who rape: psychology of the offender, New York, 1979, Plenum Press.

23. Harbin, H.: Episodic dyscontrol and family dynamics, Am. J. Psychol. **134**:1113, 1979.

24. Hayes, P.: Personal communication, 1981.

24a. Journal of the American Medical Association **243**:1221, 1980.

25. Justice, B., and Justice, R.: The abusing family, New York, 1976, Human Sciences Press, Inc.

26. Justice, B., and Justice, R.: The broken taboo, New York, 1979, Human Sciences Press, Inc.

27. Kempe, R., and Kempe, C.: Child abuse, Boston, 1978, Harvard University Press.

28. Lau, E., and Kosberg, J.: Abuse of the elderly by informal providers, Aging **12**:299, 1979.

29. Lidz, T.: The person, New York, 1968, Basic Books, Inc.

30. Martin, E.J.: Types of families continuum, Pittsburgh, 1981, The University of Pittsburgh School of Nursing.

31. McNairy, D. et al.: A community approach to child abuse and neglect, Popular Government **41**:10, Spring 1976.

32. Menuchin, S.: Families and family therapy, Cambridge, Mass., 1974, Harvard University Press.

33. Papp, P.: Symposium on strategic-structural family therapy, Ann Arbor, Mich., Oct. 16, 1981, Ann Arbor Center for the Family.

34. Porter, F.S., Blick, L.C., and Sgroi, S.M.: Treatment of the sexually abused child. In Sgroi, S.M.: A handbook of clinical intervention in child sexual abuse, New York, 1981, Garland Publishing, Inc.

35. Research Division of Child and Family Services of Connecticut, Inc.: Child sexual abuse problem categories.

36. Rimm, D., and Masters, J.: Behavior therapy: techniques and empirical findings, New York, 1974, Academic Press, Inc.

37. Sexual abuse of children, San Francisco, 1976, Queen's Bench Foundation.

38. Sgroi, S.M.: An approach to case management. In Sgroi, S.M.: Handbook of clinical intervention in child sexual abuse, New York, 1981, Garland Publishing, Inc.

39. Sgroi, S.M.: Family treatment issues in parental incest families. In Sgroi, S.M.: Handbook of clinical intervention in child sexual abuse, New York, 1981, Garland Publishing, Inc.

40. Stevens, D.: Personal communication, July 7, 1981.

41. Straus, M., Gelles, R., and Steinmetz, S.: Behind closed doors: violence in the American family, New York, 1980, Anchor Books.

42. Training Key No. 246: Investigating wife beating, Gaithersburg, Md., 1976, Police Management and Operations Divisions of the International Association of Chiefs of Police, Inc.

43. U.S. Department of Health and Human Services: Elder abuse, Washington, D.C., 1980, Office of Human Development Services.

44. Vasquez, J.: Child-abuse neglect, substance-abuse family therapy project, Ann Arbor, Mich., The University of Michigan. (Unpublished.)

45. Warner, C.: Conflict intervention in social and domestic violence, Bowie, Md., 1981, Robert J. Brady Co.

46. Webster's New Collegiate Dictionary, Springfield, Mass., 1977, G. & C. Merriam Co.

Annotated suggested readings

Anderson, L., and Shafer, G.: The character-disordered family: a community treatment model for family sexual abuse, Am. J. Orthopsychiatry 49(3):436, 1979.

An interagency model for treating sexually abusive families is presented. Inherent in the model is a view of the family as a set of character-disordered individuals who require, for successful treatment, a community approach for control of dysfunctional behavior, the use of many resources in cooperative concert, and more than one therapist. Each phase of treatment is described.

Ayoub, C., and Pfeifer, D.: An approach to primary prevention: the "at-risk" program, Child. Today 6(3):14, 1977.

The authors suggest that the "at-risk" program is a realistic approach to child abuse prevention. Described are three segments of the program: (1) inpatient screening of infants and children during the mother's pregnancy, when the child is born, or when a child is presented for hospitalization on a pediatric unit; (2) inpatient protocols and teaching programs on child and family health; and (3) the pediatric outpatient clinic at-risk population. Program goals and characteristics of families served are presented.

Barrett, D., and Fine, H.: A child was being beaten: the therapy of battered children as adults, Psychotherapy: theory, research and practice 17:285, 1980.

The authors discuss cultural and historical backgrounds of the battered child syndrome. Five case studies are used to demonstrate the way in which adults who were battered as children adapt, as well as various psychopathological disturbances that emerge as a result of traumatic childhood events.

Bavolke, S.: Primary prevention of child abuse and neglect: identification of high risk adolescents prior to parenthood, doctoral dissertation, Dissertation Abstracts Int. **39**: 3511A, 1978.

The author developed an instrument to assess parenting and child-rearing attitudes of adolescents. Abused adolescents scored significantly lower than nonabused adolescents on parenting and child-rearing attitudes. The instrument could be used by nurses to identify those adolescents who may be at high risk for becoming abusive parents.

Beck, A. et al.: Cognitive therapy of depression, New York, 1979, The Guilford Press.

The authors describe the application of cognitive-behavioral therapy in the treatment of depression. The method is also used in therapy with victims of violence and has adaptability for nursing interventions in family violence.

Blumberg, M.: Treatment of the abused child and child abuser, Am. J. Orthopsychiatry 31(2):204, 1977.

The author first describes the characteristics of a child abuser. Support is given to multidisciplinary work involving the court, social worker, child placement agent, and psychotherapist.

Burgess, A.W. et al.: Sexual assault of children and adolescents, Lexington, Mass., 1978, D.C. Heath & Co.

Burgess, A.W., and Holmstrom, L.L.: Rape: victims of crisis, Bowie, Md., 1974, Robert J. Brady Co.

Burgess, A.W., and Holmstrom, L.L.: Rape: crisis and recovery, Bowie, Md., 1980, Robert J. Brady Co.

Clinebell, H.: Growth counseling for mid-years couples, Philadelphia, 1977, Fortress Press.

This small paperback is chock-full of suggestions for interventions with midlife couples. Particular emphasis is placed on making the most of the midyears, enriching the midyears, revising priorities and values, spiritual enrichment and inner renewal, enhancing sex, creative parenting, and growth counseling. Nurses will find the practical suggestions useful in work with families.

Del Martin, M.: Battered wives, San Francisco, 1976, Glide Publications.

Denicola, J., and Sandler, J.: Training abusive parents in child management and self-control skills, Behav. Ther. **11:** 263, 1980.

The authors describe a research study in which parents were taught self-control techniques and given parent training with a two-variable withdrawal design. Parent training focused on inappropriate or punitive child management techniques. Cognitive-behavioral training focused on helping the parents cope with their aggressive impulses and feelings of anger and frustration.

Despert, J.L.: Children of divorce, New York, 1962, Doubleday & Co., Inc.

In this practical text for parents, the author concretely describes how divorce or its prospect affects one's children, what to do about it, and where to get help. Nurses will find the book useful in counseling parents, single parents, and those contemplating remarriage. As a tool, the book provides a means for parents and children to begin to talk about what they are, have, or are about to experience in relation to separation and divorce.

Elmer, E., Bennett, H., and Sankey, C.: A state-wide child abuse training program for public health nurses, Child Abuse Neglect 3(1):131, 1979.

The authors describe a program for Pennsylvania public health nurses addressing their needs in relation to roles and responsibility in child abuse cases. Problems in nurses' dual role in the community and reactions that inhibit responsible reporting of cases are discussed. The project can be used by nurses as a model in developing programs for each form of family violence.

Foster, P., Lanier, M., and Whitworth, J.: Expanding the role of nurses in child abuse prevention and treatment, J. Psychiatr. Nurs. **18**(21):24, 1980.

The authors describe a multidisciplinary program designed to meet family needs in times of crisis, help resolve problems that precipitate abuse, and coordinate with other agencies to plan longer term treatment as indicated. A case example is used to illustrate the multidisciplinary team's responsibility in assessment planning, and treatment. An outline identifying physical, emotional, marital, environmental, and safety problems, as well as treatment, is provided.

Freeman, J., editor: Women: a feminist perspective, Palo Alto, Calif., 1979, Mayfield Publishing Co.

Freize, I. et al.: Women and sex roles: a social psychological perspective, New York, 1978, W.W. Norton & Co.

Gelles, R.: Family violence, Beverly Hills, Calif., 1979, Sage Publications, Inc.

Important questions about family violence are addressed: violence toward children, marital violence, and family violence.

Gerontological Society of America: Gerontologist, vol. 21, Oct. 1981.

This special issue featured the program bulletin of the thirty-fourth annual scientific meeting of the Gerontological Society of American and the tenth annual scientific meeting of the Canadian Association on Gerontology, Toronto, Ontario, Nov. 8-12, 1981. The program bulletin has an abstract of every paper presented at the meeting. The papers covered a range of topics affecting the elderly, such as biological, physiological, psychological, societal, public policy, and economic issues.

Harris, T.: I'm ok—you're ok: a practical guide to transactional analysis, New York, 1969, Harper & Row, Publishers, Inc.

The author's work is an excellent guide for nurses in learning how to apply transactional analysis concepts in therapy with patients. The book is easy to read and complements Eric Berne's original work in the field.

Herr, J., and Weakland, J.: Counseling elders and their families, New York, 1979, Springer Publishing Co.

The authors present practical approaches based on theory for working out some of the problems of the aging and their families. Problems such as physical and mental health, income, and loneliness are presented clearly and sensitively.

Johnson, J., editor: Family violence, J. Fam. Issues, vol. 2, issue 4, 1981.

This special issue is devoted entirely to the many aspects of family violence. It reviews the most recent research and thinking on this problem area.

Miller, V., and Mansfield, E.: Family therapy for the multiple incest family, J. Psychiatr. Nurs. **19**(4):29, 1981.

The authors describe the incidence and types of family incest that are most prevalent. Note is made of five conditions that foster breakdown of incest barriers. A case example is presented, discussed, and evaluated using Bowen's theoretical framework of family functioning.

Murray, R., and Zentner, J.: Nursing assessment and health promotion through the life span, ed. 2, Englewood Cliffs, N.J., 1979, Prentice-Hall, Inc.

The authors introduce the reader to the person and his family throughout the life span. The text is an excellent resource for nurses in teaching families normal development, how to deal positively with behaviors, and what changes to expect in the future. Emphasis is placed on intervention measures that maintain health.

Nasjleti, M.: Suffering in silence: the male incest victim, Child Welfare **59**:260, 1980.

The author explores why the male incest victim remains silent and the special meaning of victimization to males. The author calls for society to reexamine role expectations of male children, and professionals' responsibilities in regard to the same are discussed.

Nix, H.: Why parents anonymous? J. Psychiatr. Nurs. **18**(10):23, 1980.

This article describes the formation of the self-help group of Parents Anonymous to help with preventing child abuse. The group's definition, structure, role, and processes are briefly described.

Norman, W., and Scaramella, T.: Mid-life developmental and clinical issues, New York, 1980, Brunner/Mazel, Inc.

The authors focus beyond the losses and deprivations of midlife to the potential for active fulfilling growth. Addressed are social and intrapsychic factors that affect perceptions of self and adaptational patterns, developmental challenges, options, and potentially problematical areas that are critical in the clinical setting. The book is useful to nurses in preventive interventions with midlife couples who may be caring for an elderly parent and may be more vulnerable to family violence.

Rathbone-McCuan, E.: Elderly vicitms of family violence and neglect, Social Casework **61**:296, 1980.

The author discusses noninstitutional aged persons as victims of nonaccidental violence. Intervention in this problem has been limited because of lack of community and professional awareness, absence of protective service legislation; manpower shortages among agencies; and restrictions on data availability.

Schmidt, A.: Adolescent female rape victims: special considerations, J. Psychosoc. Nurs. **19**(8):17, 1981.

This concise article describes the somewhat different strategies that the nurse should use to help the adolescent rape victim resolve the crisis effectively.

Sgroi, S.M.: Handbook of clinical intervention in child sexual abuse, New York, 1981, Garland Publishing, Inc.

Sharer, K.: Nursing therapy with abusive and neglectful families, J. Psychiatr. Nurs. **17**(9):12, 1979.

The author presents a thorough review of the problem of child abuse and neglect, including explanatory theories surrounding the problem. Types of interventions available to the nurse are discussed in terms of six subroles of nurses: mother-surrogate, technician, manager, teacher, socializing agent, and nurse psychotherapist. A case study is presented, applying the theoretical framework of the six nursing subroles.

Steinmetz, S.: Women and violence: victims and perpetrators, Am. J. Psychother. **34**:334, 1980.

The role of women as victims and perpetrators of violence is examined with a focus on violence within the family context. Violence against women is traced historically, and trends of increasing female criminal violence are briefly discussed. The author suggests that society's values and myths will need to be reevaluated as greater understanding of the processes and dynamics of family violence becomes known.

Tsai, M., and Wagner, N.: Therapy groups for women sexually molested as children, Arch. Sex. Behav. **7**:417, 1978.

The authors describe the results of group therapy with a total of 50 women. Problems treated included feelings of guilt and depression, negative self-image, problems in interpersonal relationships related to an underlying distrust of men, inadequate social skills, and difficulties in sexual functioning. The primary curative component was identified as a sense of identification and emotional closeness in an environment that is warm and supportive of persons who shared a common bond.

Victimology.

An international journal.

Walker, L.: The battered woman, New York, 1979, Harper & Row, Publishers, Inc.

Warner, C.: Conflict intervention in social and domestic violence, Bowie, Md., 1981, Robert J. Brady Co.

This is a collection of papers that includes theories about violence, its incidence, and suggestions for specific intervention techniques with victims and their families.

Widner, A., Greif, A., and Kelso, E.: Family therapy: the single parent family and the battered child, Fam. Ther. **3**(2):96, 1976.

The authors present research on child abuse and single-parent families. Boszormenyi-Nagy's concept of parentification is used to analyze a case study. Parental relief through role reversal is demonstrated.

Wolkenstein, A.: The fear of committing child abuse: a discussion of eight families, Child Welfare **56**(4):249, 1977.

The author describes a child abuse prevention program with eight families, five of whom were single-parent families and volunteered to participate in a program for potentially abusive parents. A life-line procedure was used so that staff were available to clients 24-hours a day, 7 days a week, for help as long as necessary. Four stages of treatment were described: emotional release, outbursts of rage at others in the family, denial of the initial problem, and integration and resolution of reality.

Yurick, A. et al.: The aged person and the nursing process, New York, 1980, Appleton-Century-Crofts.

Part one of the book addresses information nurses need to complete assessments. Part two applies the nursing process to the adaptive experience of the aged person: developmental tasks, cognition, sensory experiences, nutrition and elimination, activity, and body protection, including drugs. The text is an excellent reference.

CHAPTER 29

COUNSELING
THE VICTIM
OF RAPE

THERESA S. FOLEY

One summer's night I was digging and tripping
  around
I found myself drinking with an old friend,
Then getting pinned to the ground
This was an occasion when I first found my true
  identity with the cross,
As he pounded himself into me,
I lied motionless,
And to him it was a loss.
So yelling about God got me here.
But I trust Him so my day is near.
'Cause soon I'll be home and rid of this shit,
They will realize that I am a mere child of God
In the midst of a God-for-saken-fit.

A rape victim and mental hospital patient, The Nut That Put Me
Here[7]*

*Reproduced with permission of the Robert J. Brady Co.,
Bowie, Md. 20715 from its copyright work *Rape: Victims of
Crisis* © 1975.

Learning objectives

After studying this chapter, the student
should be able to:

- assess the extent of the problem of rape for women
  in the United States and the purpose of rape crisis
  centers.

- define rape and the three main types of rape according to the victim's lack of consent.

- critique some of the common myths about rape,
  the results of believing the myths, and the facts.

- describe three phases of response to rape and two
  emotional styles of response.

- relate the influence of a victim's age and life stage
  to her response to being raped.

- identify the variety of crisis and counseling requests initiated by victims of rape.

- discuss the importance of self-awareness, a support network, legal responsibility, crisis dimension, and the nursing contract in completing a
  nursing assessment of the rape victim.

- apply therapeutic nurse-patient relationship principles to planning the care of the victim of rape,
  based on her phase of response.

- analyze nursing interventions appropriate to the
  needs of the rape victim based on the setting in
  which she is seen and the three phases of the
  change process.

■ *assess the importance of the evaluation of the nursing process when working with the victim of rape.*

■ *identify suggested readings for future study.*

Nurses will see rape victims of all age-groups in every area of their practice, raising questions about rape prevention, nursing interventions, and long-term counseling of victims. This chapter is concerned with the adult female victim of rape. In 1979 the FBI Uniform Crime Reports[11] stated that 75,789 women *reported* forcible rapes, assaults, or attempts to commit rape by force or threat of force. When multiplied by estimates of *unreported rape* because of embarrassment, guilt, or fear of the assailant, the incidence of rape is considered by crime experts to be 10 to 20 times higher than the reported crime, or no less than 757,890 rapes per year. In 1979 the number of reported rapes was up 13% over 1978. Rape is the *highest* rising violent crime in the nation and the most underreported of all Crime Index Offenses. It quickly becomes apparent that western society reflects a culture of increasing violence and that the nurse can expect to see many victims of violence. For some victims the nurse may well be the first person encountered subsequent to the rape and may be the only advocate the victim will have throughout attempts to receive care. The treatment a rape victim receives immediately after the event has been noted to be a critical variable in later resolution of the crisis. It is therefore imperative that nurses utilize in their practice what is known about rape and rape counseling.

Historical perspective

Rape crisis centers are the structures developed by feminists "through which women can begin to take back control over our lives—control which is denied in part by the threat of rape."[24] Women recognized that they were more able to control what happened to them when they joined together to help each other after rape had occurred to obtain needed services, learn to protect themselves, and work to eradicate the crime. In the 1960s the women's movement recognized the political aspect of rape and raised the issue of victim treatment as part of a pattern of systematic abuse of women. Brownmiller[3] asserts that, like the lynching of blacks in the South, the intent of such random terrorizing is to keep all women "in their places."

In 1971 Germaine Greer was the first to interview a rape victim on national television. The New York Radical Feminists broke the silence of the crime by holding a "rape speakout," in which, for the first time in public forum, women began to tell of the horrors they sustained. The forum resulted in publication of a book, *Rape: the First Source Book for Women,*[10] exploring the reasons for rape, what a woman can do to protect herself, and how women can join forces toward resolution of rape as a problem. A movement against rape began throughout the United States with the joint efforts of dispersed grass roots groups. The basic unit of the antirape movement continues to be the local rape crisis center.

In 1972 there were three centers compared to more than 1500 today, most of which are in large cities or university towns. Rape crisis centers are located in a variety of settings ranging from the YWCA to rented office space and hospitals and function within varying organizational structures. Because of limited funding most centers are staffed by volunteers. Services provided generally include a crisis telephone line for immediate support, information, and short-term counseling of victims. Most centers also provide advocates to go with victims to the hospital, the police, and court proceedings. When long-term counseling needs arise, victims are generally referred to other social service agencies. Rape prevention and treatment for victims is one of the 13 services mandated by the federal government to be provided by community mental health centers. Professionals in community mental health centers are now being challenged to demonstrate the effectiveness of treatment received by victims referred to them.

Most often professionals are welcomed in antirape projects. Feminists noted the need for professional involvement in rape crisis centers if victims were to receive better care and more sensitive treatment from professionals. However, the tendency to defer to professional leadership, as happened in the development of suicide crisis prevention centers, is a current trend feminists caution against. Working as peers within the system, professionals offer skills and knowledge that are valuable resources in a project. Nurses have yet to demonstrate a significant impact on the opportunities available in this area of practice for using their expertise to open boundaries between themselves, victims of rape, rape crisis centers, other disciplines, educators, and the community.

Rape defined and described

The legal definition of rape is "forcible perpetration of an act of sexual intercourse on the body of a woman not one's wife."[3] Some states have recently omitted the last three words of the definition and thus accept the idea of rape within marriage. Legal definitions of rape generally exclude other forms of forcible sexual assaults such as oral or anal sodomy by males on females; however, the law varies among states, and nurses need to be aware of their state statutes when counseling victims. Many victims consider oral or anal sodomy to be more humiliating and traumatic than the limited legal definition of penile-vaginal attacks. A more contemporary definition of the crime would include these forms of forcible sexual assault.

The legal definition of rape has its origin in the property rights of man. Historically, man has protected his property, progeny, and inheritance rights. With woman as his property, he had complete, sole, and total access to a woman; she was barter in a trade. The rapist, when convicted, was punished for unlawful possession of property. The concept operating was that male rights of possession had been violated based on the bargain of marriage for the virginity, chastity, and sole consent to her person.

In 1974 Burgess and Holmstrom[7] categorized three main types of rape according to the victim's lack of consent:

1. Rape—sex without consent
2. Accessory to sex—inability to consent or not consent because of the victim's stage of cognitive or personality development
3. Sex-stress situation—sex with initial consent in which something drastically went wrong; usually the male exploited the initial agreement

The authors also reported two main styles of attack. The first is the *blitz rape*, in which the victim and assailant lack prior interaction, as described in Clinical example 29-1.

CLINICAL EXAMPLE 29-1

Susan is a 20-year-old college student attending a university and living in an apartment. Susan awoke suddenly to find a man had entered her apartment through a window in her kitchen. She screamed and tried to escape but was unsuccessful and the man raped her.

The second style of attack is a *confidence rape*, in which interaction between the victim and assailant generally occurs prior to the assault, and the assailant obtains access to the victim through the use of deceit, betrayal, or violence, as in Clinical example 29-2.

CLINICAL EXAMPLE 29-2

Cheryl is a 16-year-old high school student who attended a jazz concert at the civic center. She lost her friends and became confused by the building when the concert was over. Two men offered to show her where to go. They escorted her down a hallway and shoved her into a closet used for cleaning equipment. They threw Cheryl on the floor and raped her. Cheryl felt betrayed. She was afraid to tell her parents about the rape because they did not want her to go to the concert and were concerned about her safety.

In literature, myth, and culture, rape is sanctioned as an act of power intended to humiliate and degrade the person. Brownmiller defines the effect of rape as follows:

A sexual invasion of the body by force, an incursion into the private, personal inner space without consent. . . . In short, an internal assault from one of several avenues and by one of several methods. . . . [It] constitutes a deliberate violation of emotional, physical and rational integrity and is a hostile, degrading act of violence.[3:376]

For the woman, rape implies total loss of self, in which she is reduced from a person to an object and a function. She experiences total isolation and emptiness from herself and society. The net effect is to simultaneously destroy the sense of person and the sense of community, to depersonalize the woman by separating her person from her humanity. A woman's ability to maintain coping defenses is challenged by a rape because intense feelings of anxiety, guilt, and inadequacy are aroused. Rape is experienced as a loss, and thus the victim needs to be afforded all the rights and privileges of a period of mourning and grief.

Myth dimension

The myths that exist about the crime of rape are damaging to everyone involved. The victim will not be taken care of empathically when law enforcement and medical personnel subcribe to rape myths. The victim will find her claims doubted by family and friends. If the victim believes rape myths, as many do, she will have greater difficulty resolving shame and guilt. Finally, the crime of rape is fostered as society plays out the myths in different health care settings that continue to excuse or condone the act.[17] All myths have a similar function: they result in the victim blaming herself.

Before the nurse can effectively assist the rape victim, it is essential to be aware of biases held and the extent to which biases affect one's belief system about rape and nursing care of victims. Brodsky and Hobart[2] note that on the basis of assumptions about the nature and causation of sexual assault, treaters and researchers develop differing treatment plans and decisions and act on these assumptions within the treatment plans, whether or not they are aware of doing so. The authors define blame as "attribution of responsibility and focus of attention," which is put into operation in one of four blame models[2]:

1. *Offender blame model.* In the offender blame model sexual assault takes place when a person with *deficits* in aggressive/sexual behavior makes forcible sexual contact. "He had to be crazy."

2. *Victim blame model.* Under this model sexual assault takes place when a woman has in some way, obviously or nonobviously, consciously or unconsciously, allowed herself to be in an interpersonal or physical position that antecedes forcible sexual contact. "She deserved what she got."

3. *Situational blame model.* Sexual assault takes place when environmental and structural circumstances, transient factors in mood or place, and assault-vulnerable parties merge to generate a forcible sexual contact by one person or another. "She should not have gone to the party, concert, bar."

4. *Societal blame model.* Sexual assault takes place when accumulated cultural and societal attitudes are manifested through the forcible sexual contact of one person on another. "Men dominate and abuse women."

Blame models suggest levels at which prevention, education, and intervention can occur. Table 29-1 is a composite presentation of existing rape myths, the results of believing the myths, and the facts. There are many other myths not listed that need to be considered, for example, rape is not a serious problem for older women because they have experienced sex, or mental patients who claim rape cannot be believed and probably provoke rape. Nurses need to be aware of all rape myths.

Responses of the victim of rape

The tenet that the majority of human behavior is learned is now widely accepted. Behaviors develop as a result of one's interacting with the environment. We have learned to be the kind of person we are through relating with others who represent a significant source of rewards, punishment, and motivations. The person one grows into tomorrow is partly a result of relationships with people today. Our self-perception is largely determined by the way we are treated by people believed to be important. Significant others help the individual learn what and who he is. The self-structure incorporates the personal evaluations made by significant others and generally influences how one regards self. One's self-concept provides a screen through which everything else is seen, heard, evaluated, and understood. It is not surprising, then, that victims have difficulty resolving a rape experience when society defines and attributes fault for the crime based on the victim's sociodemographic characteristics, which have essentially nothing to do with the fact that she was raped. Such characteristics include whether she is of "respectable character" or is married, separated, or divorced. It is a difficult process for a rape victim to differentiate herself from society's blaming response and to sort out the thoughts, feelings, and behaviors that follow from the rape experience, particularly when she is in a vulnerable crisis state, and society has told her she is responsible for someone else's behavior.

Phases of response to rape

Sutherland and Scherl[23] reported follow-up interviews with a small homogeneous sample of 13 white female victims in which three separate phases of response to rape were identified. In phase 1, *acute reaction*, the victim feels dismay, disbelief, and shock. She may be volatile, incoherent, and agitated, or she may be unable to talk about the rape and the man who assaulted her. The initial shock and dismay are replaced by high levels of anxiety when the victim first addresses the consequences of being assaulted.

TABLE 29-1. Rape myths, results of the myths, and facts*

Myth	Result of myth	Fact
Rape is provoked by the victim; victims are responsible for their victimization either consciously or by default; all women really want to be raped	Blame is taken from rapist and responsibility for crime is shifted to victim; it fosters public statements incorrectly connecting sexual permissiveness with rape, such as that made by Judge Archie Simmons of Dane County, Wisconsin (since recalled from office)	About 80% of rapes are planned in advance by rapist; victim is usually threatened with death or body harm if she resists; rape is violent attack using sex as weapon; a woman does not ask for violence (rape) by accepting a date, acting polite, being friendly and cheerful, dressing and walking in socially defined attractive ways; no woman's behavior or dress gives a man the right to rape her; Federal Commission found only 4% of sexual assaults involved "precipitative behavior," which consisted of only a slight "gesture" in their definition
Only young beautiful women in miniskirts are raped; it can't happen to me; only other types of women get raped; only "bad girls" get raped; rape reflects demographic strain caused by sex–marital status imbalance in community; only promiscuous women get raped	Women deny rape could happen to them; belief in myth perpetuates unhealthy denial defense mechanism and lack of readiness for self-defense; rape is the only felonious, violent crime in which victim is held suspect and has burden of proof of innocence; women tend to blame themselves for crime, not report it or not seek support from others because of embarrassment, shame, and questions about where they can turn for empathy and help	Rapists choose victims without regard for age, race, or socioeconomic class; chances are 1 in 15 a woman will be raped in her lifetime; some cities report probability as high as 1 in 3; reported victims' age range is 6 months to 93 years; highest incidence is in women 15 to 24 years of age (target population)
Women are raped when they are out alone at night, primarily in dark alleys; if women stay at home, they will be safe	Belief is perpetuated that women are not raped by their husbands; it reflects a "just world" rationale, implying she would not have been raped had she been "in her place" or "undeserving"; it violates her right to freedom of movement by dictating self-defense strategies	Any woman can be victim of rape, regardless of social or economic class, appearance, age, or place of residence; woman's husband can rape her; half of all rapes occur in private residence and a third to a half of all sexual assaults are committed in victim's home; on October 5, 1977, Oregon was first state to amend its laws so that a women could prosecute her husband for rape
Sexual assault occurs only among total strangers; if I avoid strangers, I will not be raped	Women who are acquainted with the rapist tend to blame themselves more and are less likely to report the crime or prosecute the assailant; fault is attributed to woman for "leading him on"; women deny that their spouse/lover could be rapist; one will not believe victim if one believes this myth; women do not report rape for fear of repercussions if they are raped by acquaintance/friend; they wonder if they will be believed, how others will react, and if offender will seek revenge (a common threat to keep rape secret); marital conflict and divorce are kindled by belief in this myth	Amir[1] found 66% of *reported* rapes took place between strangers, yet in 34% victim and offender were acquainted; in 14%, rapist was member of family, friend of family, or close personal friend. It is important to note that these statistics reflect only reported forcible rape and that woman is more likely to report rape by stranger than friend or relative, as is often the case with adolescents; victims report that spouses and lovers do not believe them, blame them, and separate or divorce in many cases

*Modified from Keller, E., and Remus, S.: Statistics on sexual assault, Minnesota Program for Victims of Sexual Assault, 430 Metro Square Building, St. Paul, Minn. 55101; Travis, M.: The most common myths concerning rape—and the facts, *Brainerd Daily Dispatch*, May 15, 1976; and the collected publications of A.W. Burgess and L.L. Holmstrom.

TABLE 29-1. **Rape myths, results of the myths, and facts—cont'd**

Myth	Result of myth	Fact
Any woman could prevent rape if she really wanted to; no woman can be raped against her will; victims generally do not resist their attackers; any woman who resists her attacker will be killed	One who believes this myth expects victim to be brutally beaten because of her resistance and does not believe her in absence of bruises and cuts, although only victim can assess what resistance is possible if she cannot escape assailant; myth fails to recognize that immobility or "freezing" is psychological response to extreme fear; carrying this myth to its "logical" extreme, it is better to be dead than alive	Amir[1] found in a majority of cases, victim was threatened with death if she resisted; rapist carried weapon or threatened death in 87% of cases, manhandled in 30%, verbally threatened in 20%, used no force in 15% (usually with child victims); almost all victims reacted with fear for their lives; in view of known humiliation, fear of injury or death, and loss of control over her life and body, it is amazing this myth still exists; suicide is a documented behavior of victim response to rape
Rape occurs only in large cities	One who believes this myth is less likely to believe victim who reports rape that occurred outside large city	Sexual assault happens everywhere—rural, suburban, and urban areas; majority of reported rapes occur in urban areas; rural rape crisis centers report high incidence of the community believing rape myths and thus difficulty in obtaining adequate care for victims; both factors affect underreporting of rape in smaller communities
Most rapes involve black men and white women; blacks are more likely to attack white women than black women; all rapes are interracial	A woman who was raped by someone of her own race would not be believed by one who believed this myth; myth perpetuates racial prejudices that exist in society	Amir[1] found that rape was intraracial, especially between black men and women; FBI statistics cite 3% of rapes involve black women and white men; most rapes involve victim-offender of same race and socioeconomic class
Rape is impulsive, uncontrollable act of sexual gratification (i.e., a sexually frustrated man sees attractive young woman and "just can't control himself")	One will expect victim to be accountable for actions of rapist; one will not hold rapist responsible for his behavior and will excuse and condone his "need" rather than challenge his violent lack of impulse control	Amir[1] found 71% of all rapes were planned; rapist had it in his mind to rape specific woman or any woman; in 11% of cases, rapist took advantage of woman in more "vulnerable" position—drunk, walking alone at night, hitchhiking; only 16% were rapes with no prior intent to commit crime; rapists describe their motivation as hatred, conquest, humiliation, and degradation, not in terms of sexual gratification and report a lack of sexual gratification afterward; Groth and Birnbaum found 58% of 170 convicted rapists experienced sexual dysfunction during rape and often dysfunction increased assailant's rage toward victim
Rapists are abnormal perverts or men with unsatisfied sex drive; only "sick" or "insane" men rape women; primary motive for rape is sexual; rapist is sexually starved psychopath	One would not believe that normal-appearing and acting man could have committed rape; one may expect rapist to stand out in crowd, to have special identifiable characteristics; attire worn at jury trials to convey respectable character reference plays on public's tendency to believe this myth	Rapists generally exhibit "normal" types of behavior, are generally sexually active with spouse or partner, and have normal sex drive; their major difference is lack of impulse control seen in greater than average tendency toward expressing violence; rapist is assessed as having abnormal tendency toward being aggressive and violent; otherwise his personality appears within "normal" limits.

Continued.

TABLE 29-1. **Rape myths, results of the myths, and facts—cont'd**

Myth	Result of myth	Fact
It is easy to prosecute rapists; not to prosecute implies that woman is guilty of consent	One may believe that if woman was really raped, she will prosecute man; one fails to look at reasons she does not report or prosecute and work for change in those areas; one may have contempt for victim who does not win her case or who refuses to prosecute	Unless victim has "respectable character," filed prompt report with police, has eye witness to crime, is not acquainted with assailant, is assaulted by man of different race, is sexually inexperienced, and sustained physical injuries, case is unlikely to be taken to trial or receive conviction; Holmstrom and Burgess found that of 109 cases, 24 went to trial and 4 received convictions for rape; nationally approximately 3% of reported cases lead to conviction; this means conviction rate as low as 0.3% if estimates of unreported rapes are taken into account; many cases are lost because of jurors' tendency to believe myths, failure to interview and exclude jurors holding myths beliefs, and improper collection of corroborative evidence
Women frequently cry "rape"; there is a high rate of false reports	One will not develop or provide type of care victim desperately needs; one will be skeptical of anyone who reports rape or seeks care; victim who believes this myth will blame herself for attack; if she knows others believe myth, she may not report rape, fearing she will not be believed	False report rate for other kinds of felonies is 2%; rape has same rate
Rape is minor crime affecting only few women	One who believes this myth will act with disbelief when someone reports rape; one will not believe that sexual assault would occur in his area or to anyone he knows	Rape is the fastest rising violent crime in United States; in 1979 number of "founded" reported rape cases was 75,789; if this number is multiplied by factor of 10 to account for unreported cases, no less than 757,890 women were raped in 1979; these are epidemic proportions; it is estimated that chances are 1 in 15 that woman will be raped in her lifetime
Rape is predominantly hot weather crime; women provoke rape by their style of dress and behavior	One may believe that people who dress for warmer weather invite rape and are at fault for crime	Amir's[1] study found that thermic law of delinquency was not confirmed in his study; Denver Report found higher incidence of rape in summer months correlated to cold weather areas; person's dress style is not license for others to assault that person with impunity

The initial phase lasts from a few days to a few weeks. In phase 2, *outward adjustment*, which may begin a few days to several weeks after the rape, the victim resumes her usual pursuits at work, home, or school. The behavior conceals a faulty adjustment based on the denial and suppression of anxieties and fears deeply felt. The woman is not interested in talking about her experience or seeking help at this time for herself but may do so at the urging of a friend or relative. She often will cancel or not show up for appointments and may be misjudged as not needing further follow-up care because she is "doing just fine." In phase 3, *integration and resolution*, the victim develops an inner sense of depression and a need to talk. In this phase the victim integrates a new view of herself as she accepts the event as part of her history and realistically appraises her complicity in the assault. The victim also resolves her feelings about her relationship with the offender. She becomes aware of her feelings of resentment and anger, rationalizations for feelings, and doubts about responsibility in the assault. As one woman stated, "The scariest thing is that I stabbed him in the back. I don't trust myself anymore. I worry about being out of control for having done such a thing. . . . If they don't convict him, I'm afraid I'll murder him myself."

Burgess and Holstrom[6] analyzed 92 interviews in a heterogeneous sample of victims diagnosed as having a "rape trauma syndrome" and reported a two-phase reaction. In the acute first phase, *disorganization,* impact reactions were shown by the victim's expressed or controlled emotional styles. Somatic reactions included physical trauma, skeletal muscle tension, gastrointestinal irritability, and genitourinary disturbances. Emotional reactions included embarrassment, anger, humiliation, self-blame, fear, and desire for revenge. The primary feeling described was *fear* of physical violence and death. The long-term process of phase 2, *reorganization,* began at different times for victims and was affected by factors such as coping behavior regarding the rape, the way people treated them as victims, and social network support systems. This phase was characterized by four phenomena: motor activity such as changing residence or telephone number, turning to family members for support, nightmares and dreams of fighting off the assailant or wishing to do something but waking before acting, and traumatophobia or phobic reactions as a specific defensive reaction to the rape. Common phobic reactions included fear of outdoors or indoors, fear of crowds and of being alone, fear of people behind them, and sexual fears.

Psychological responses

Burgess and Holmstrom[4] also identified two emotional styles characteristic of victims in response to discussing the rape. The first is an *expressed style* in which the victim expresses feelings of anxiety, fear, or anger by talking, shaking, crying, smiling, muscle tenseness, and restlessness. The second is a *controlled style* in which victims mask feelings by a subdued, calm, or composed affect. Some women showed more than one response during the interview. The primary reaction was fear for their lives; the assault represented an act of violence. Other emotional reactions included anger, laughing to avoid cry-

ing, feelings of loss, and concern about how to cope with men in future relationships.

The authors further identified a *compounded reaction* with women who had a previous history of psychiatric, physical, or social difficulties. The compounded reaction was characterized by psychotic behavior, depression, suicidal behavior, psychosomatic disorders, and acting-out behavior (alcoholism, drug abuse, and sexual promiscuity) combined with difficulties in the previous history. Finally, the authors discuss management of the *silent rape syndrome* in which a woman has not told anyone about being raped, has not settled her reactions and feelings about the trauma, and carries alone a tremendous psychological burden. The authors' historical data indicated that many of the women in the sample had been previously raped or molested, often as children, and that the current rape reactivated unresolved responses and reactions to the previous experience.

Developmental responses

The influence of a victim's age and life stage in response to being raped has been noted in relation to expected task performance within varying stages of the life cycle.[8] For the grade school or adolescent victim, task disruption occurred in school performance and attendance. All victims enrolled in school experienced a disrupted school life, with 41% either changing schools or stopping abruptly. It was difficult for the school-age victim to return to school, and most missed an average of 2 to 5 days following the rape. When absence continued for more than a week, the symptoms of an acute phobic reaction were observed. In the sample academic difficulties were almost universally evidenced.

The adult victim experienced difficulty in three areas: parenting and housewifery, schooling, and employment. Most women regained their coping skills within the first week and gradually resumed their usual homemaking and parenting style within the home. Slightly over half quit or changed jobs within 6 months of the rape. Some women found it impossible to change jobs because of economic factors. Adult victims who were students sometimes faced a conflict over the need for a school degree and the need to make money. Flight or avoidance behavior was common for those who lacked a social network support system of authority figures or peers. In contrast to the child victim, the adult was more able to verbalize her needs when she experienced school difficulty. In assessing a victim's coping ability, the nurse needs to inquire about specific duties and functions of task performance. The woman often needs to be helped to see any progress she has made in completing task expectations. When task expectations are relegated to an insignificant role in therapy, they emerge with major significance in crisis counseling.

Notman and Nadelson[18] noted that the most frequently reported rape victim is the young single woman between ages 17 and 24. The rape may revive psychodynamic concerns about separation, independence, and the ability to take care of oneself. Temporarily obtaining help or relying on one's family may be misconstrued by the victim as unhealthy dependence vs. use of a support network in a crisis period. The victim wants reassurance and is concerned about the integrity and intactness of her body. For the divorced or separated woman, the rape may confirm feelings of inadequacy, especially since she is more likely to have her credibility investigated with questions about her life-style, character, and morality. She is particularly inclined to feel enormous guilt and may fail to report the crime or obtain aid. She worries about her adequacy as a mother and the implications for her and her children if the rape is known about in the community. Issues for the middle-aged woman include concerns about independence and the ability to have control. The midlife crises of husbands sometimes interfere with their ability to be responsive and supportive to their wife's emotional needs. A woman already concerned about her sexual adequacy cannot quantify the feelings of worthlessness, self-devaluation, and shame when faced with the common misconception that a woman who is past her most sexually active period, whether single or married, has less to lose than a younger woman.

On the basis of exposure to the elderly rape victim, Fletcher[12] proposed specific areas for consideration in counseling this victim. The older woman may demonstrate a greater fear of others' finding out about the rape because of social differences in upbringing. She may even exclude her family in working out the experience and thus drastically limit her supportive network. Her major concern is to maintain her reputation and respectability. The rape may pre-cipitate a major alteration in her life-style. The victim may go so far as to change cities, compounding her emotional reaction with the physical stress of moving. When pressured to move in with family, because of her own fear or family demands, problems may arise resulting from the exchange of her independent status for security. Increased feelings of helplessness may be experienced by the older woman. She may feel more vulnerable after being raped and thus experience increased feelings of hopelessness. Family members who feel guilty become overprotective and force her into the role of a "helpless old lady." The victim may experience a great deal of confusion about the assault. The feelings of "Why me?" and "How could I have avoided this?" are more common than the typical guilt reaction. The victim encounters the false assumption that her sexuality automatically terminates at age 60. Although feelings about her sexual identity may not be a major concern, these should not be ignored in the counseling process. Because of the process of aging, the older victim has a greater chance of becoming physically traumatized. Securing her physical well-being is instrumental in effecting her emotional well-being. There is sufficient evidence that the elderly victim's response is a valid area of concern with needs that should be met.

Crisis and counseling requests

In a study of 146 adult and pediatric victims of sexual assault, Burgess and Holmstrom[5] found that victims identified what they wanted or needed if the nurse listened to their direct verbal statements. The victim's self-care requests became the clinical guidelines for nursing interventions. They identified five categories of crisis requests:

1. *Medical intervention,* or "I need a physician." In this category the hospital staff and emergency room services were viewed in a traditional medical role with the physician explicitly asked to do something to alleviate the victim's fears of disease and pregnancy.

2. *Police intervention,* or "I need a policeman." Here the police were viewed as the first official authority to turn to because of their traditional role of supporting, protecting, and defending the community against crime. The victim within this category had a strong desire to retaliate against the assailant and did not view psychological and medical care as first priorities.

3. *Psychological intervention,* or "I need to talk to someone." These victims wanted to talk

with someone about the rape experience and viewed the hospital staff and emergency room services as providing both emotional support and medical care.

4. *Uncertain,* or "I'm not sure I want anything." These victims went to the hospital or police as a result of outside pressure or advice but did not necessarily view these persons as being able to help. In their ambivalence about what to do as a result of the rape, they tended to seek out and be emotionally propelled along by the thoughts and feelings of others.

5. *Control,* or "I need control." These victims were incoherent because of the use of alcohol or drugs, a psychotic state, or mental retardation, which aggravated the current crisis and their general inability to verbalize their wants or needs.

Counseling requests made by rape victims included the following:

1. *Confirmation of concern,* or "It's nice to know you are available." These victims volunteered minimal information, were polite, and answered routine questions but tended to be guarded and controlled. They were satisfied that the counselor was available and concerned should they need assistance.

2. *Ventilation,* or "It helps to get this off my chest." These victims were relieved to share the burden with someone. They felt burdened psychologically by the crisis and had much to say about their experience in a spontaneous manner with a strong focus on feelings.

3. *Clarification,* or "I want to think this through." These victims explicitly wanted to think through and settle the crisis for themselves by sorting out conflicting thoughts and feelings to put the crisis in a realistic perspective.

4. *Advice,* or "What should I do?" These victims explicitly asked about alternatives or what to do about physical, social, legal, or psychological problems related to the rape and viewed the counselor as having the information to suggest possible alternatives.

5. *Nothing,* or "I don't need the counseling services." These victims did not indicate a wish for follow-up counseling, gave a false phone number and address or none, and tended to seek police intervention.

A nursing process model

A victim of sexual assault confronts two areas of need. One is inner-directed, concerning psychological adjustments and emotional well-

being. The other is outer-directed in relation to the police, legal, and hospital systems. In both areas she enters seemingly hostile, foreign, and male-dominated systems. She faces medical examinations, possibly a long series of legal procedures that may be incomplete as much as a year later, and a long-term reorganization process. Fig. 29-1 is a flowchart summarizing the self-care decisions a victim of rape makes after a sexual assault.[21] Often these systems present the victim with fragmented services, inadequate information, and little emotional support at a time when she most needs competent care. In any health care delivery system the victim of rape has the following rights*:

1. To transportation to a hospital when incapacitated

2. To emergency room care with privacy and confidentiality

3. To be carefully listened to and treated as a human being with respect, courtesy, and dignity

4. To have an advocate of choice accompany her through the treatment process

5. To accurate collection and preservation of evidence in an objective record that includes signs and symptoms of physical and emotional trauma

6. To receive clear explanations of procedures and medication in language she can understand

7. To know what treatment is recommended, for what reasons, and who will administer the treatment

8. To know any possible risks, side effects, or alternatives to proposed treatment, including all drugs prescribed

9. To ask for another physician or nurse

10. To consent to or refuse any treatment even when her life is in serious danger

11. To refuse to be part of any research or experiment

12. To reasonable complaint and to leave a care facility against the physician's advice

13. To receive an explanation of and understand any papers she agrees to sign

14. To be informed of continuing health care

---

*Modified from Pittsburgh Action Against Rape: Patient's rights handout, 1976-1977, 211 S. Oakland Ave., Pittsburgh, Pa. 15213, and Westmorland Alliance Against Rape: Patient's rights, 1978, 102 W. Otterman St., Greensburg, Pa. 15601.

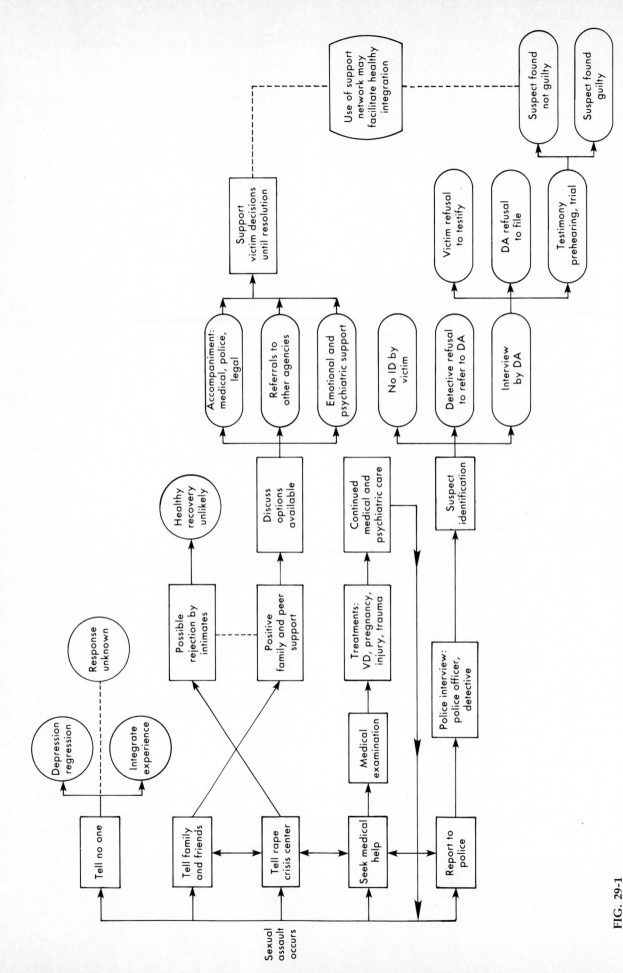

FIG. 29-1
Victim decisions following a sexual assault. (From Rape Crisis Services Division of the Greater Harrisburg Area YWCA, 215 Market Street, Harrisburg, Pa. 17101.)

needs after discharge from the emergency room, hospital, physician's office, or care facility

15. To receive a clear explanation of the bill and review of charges and where to apply for compensation to cover costs

Assessment

SELF-AWARENESS. Self-awareness is the beginning of a nursing assessment. Counseling the victim of rape can be emotionally fatiguing and raise many feelings within the nurse, particularly if the nurse is a woman. Effective nursing care emerges from working conditions that offer an arena in which feelings, experiences, problems, and cases can be freely discussed and provide the nurse with greater self-awareness.

In completing the assessment, a number of factors should be considered by the nurse[22]:

1. *Philosophy*. The issue of "Who owns the rape?" or who makes the decisions is the most important issue in counseling to ensure that the victim regains control over her life as soon as possible.

2. *Confidentiality*. All that the victim tells the nurse should not be passed on to others without the victim's explicit permission. Consultation can be obtained while the victim's identity is protected.

3. *Neutrality*. By maintaining a neutral position, the nurse facilitates the victim's making her own decisions from information on alternatives and from the chance to review advantages, disadvantages, and options.

4. *Intense feelings*. The nurse needs to allow the victim to lead the conversation, help her explore her feelings, and meet her level of intensity through empathic responses. Encouraging verbalization and ventilation is one means of helping her regain control.

5. *Silences*. If the nurse can allow long pauses without becoming alarmed, she can use the time to think about what is going on with the victim, the situation, and possible actions.

6. *Keeping the nurse's problems in the background*. Focus needs to be maintained on the victim's concerns rather than the nurse's own "causes," such as abortion, politics, or reporting.

7. *Keeping the nurse's agenda out of the discussion*. The use of "should" or "ought" is to be avoided, since they cut short an exploring dialogue, may irritate or alienate a victim, and usurp her decision-making right. One way for the nurse to help the victim clarify values is to be in touch with her own feelings and values.

8. *Searching for alternatives*. Instead of giving overhelpful advice, the nurse can assist the victim to assess all possible alternatives, examining the advantages and disadvantages of each.

9. *Avoiding "why" questions*. The nurse needs to support the victim without putting her on the defensive or making her justify her plans or what she did "Why" questions are for necessary information only, not curiosity.

10. *Recognizing the real issue*. The victim needs to be allowed to direct the conversation and decide what the real issue is, such as feelings vs. care system procedures.

11. *Message behind the statement*. The nurse can assist the victim in identifying a feeling position. The woman can then examine it, choose to keep it, reject it, or choose not to decide about it. Feelings that are identified and verbalized prevent long-term confusion.

12. *Hostility toward the nurse*. The nurse can avoid personalizing hostility when the care provided is competent. The nurse may be the first person the victim has come in contact with since the assault to whom she can safely express her rage. Finally, it is necessary for the nurse to be aware of the biases held, the myths believed, and their impact on nursing actions.

SUPPORT NETWORK. Advocates from rape crisis centers, hospital, or community mental health teams provide information, intervene, and support victims, particularly if the woman lacks assertiveness in meeting her needs within an authoritarian mystifying system. Advocates have specialized skills in helping victims, coordinate all systems with them, and are available for counseling long after the acute care is completed. They provide a needed support system and link in the continuity of care with victims. For this reason nurses are encouraged to welcome them when they accompany a victim. In communities lacking prevention and education programs, police officers and officials in the criminal justice system sometimes ridicule or otherwise respond to victims in a discourteous manner. Nurses in the emergency room can assess the police officer for his degree of supportiveness with victims and act as the victim's advocate. The victim may need more support if the attending officer is not supportive and believes or acts on any of the myths surrounding rape.

Family, friends, and groups can also be supportive to the victim. Who are the members of her family and which ones will she talk to or avoid? Which family members are important to her? Which friends at work or school will she talk with about the rape? Does she have a therapist, counselor, or minister? Is she aware of the pathological risks involved in keeping the event secret or not using support systems? What groups is she a member of or participating in within her community—church groups, women's groups, single-parent groups, self-defense groups? Discussion groups have proved an excellent support for victims. Often they are a first step in initiating long-term counseling with a professional. Victims cite a sense of universality, a decreased sense of isolation, a sharing of anger and pain, a catharsis in sharing their secret, an ability to do something constructive with feelings, a validation that intense feelings do not mean they are "crazy," and minimized feelings of guilt, depression, and suicide. A final factor in assessing a victim's support system is the provision of safe transportation to a place of her choice. She should not be released from the hospital alone unless she so requests.

LEGAL RESPONSIBILITY. Nurses need to be knowledgeable about the role they may play as witnesses in legal proceedings. Prosecution is difficult when medical data are not properly recorded, if the evidence is not gathered completely and quickly, and if the signs and symptoms of physical and emotional trauma are not cited. The victim holds the burden of proof beyond a reasonable doubt for all of the elements of the crime. The nurse therefore has a responsibility to carefully collect and preserve corroborative evidence. Victims have lost their case in court when evidence has not been properly collected, and the professional is then faced with counseling a person experiencing dual legitimate rage: (1) the rape experience, and (2) negligent medical and nursing care. As part of an official medical record a nursing assessment becomes an objective record corroborating evidence in court proceedings and has the potential to increase conviction rates.

Burgess and Laszloa[9] discuss four particular areas in their assessment instrument:

1. *Signs of physical trauma,* which describe specific physical findings.

2. *Symptoms of physical trauma,* which include the patient's verbatim statements about the nature of the attack. The types of sexual acts demanded are especially important to include here, as well as how they were carried out and in what order. Should the victim's accurate recall about this falter later, the objective account stands witness to a jury and clarifies misinterpretations of evidence submitted in a courtroom. The jury is likely to believe the written record. If the victim is in crisis, the nurse may have to ask what sexual acts occurred. These questions need to be carefully worded to obtain accurate facts, since the victim is under stress. Victims will also appreciate respect for their sensitivity at this time, as shown by the way the nurse asks questions about the interactive components of the sexual assault. It is important to convey one's intent to obtain information, not to judge the victim. This is especially important with sexual behavior other than vaginal intercourse. Avoid phrases that ordinarily connote lovemaking, those which the woman may not know the meaning of, such as fellatio or cunnilingus, and those which suggest that she took initiative in or precipitated the assault. The nurse could ask, for example, "Did the rapist put his penis in your mouth, vagina, or rectum?" Although the questions are more graphic, they suggest less than a passive reconstruction of the victim's behavior in the assault. In addition, such phrasing helps to defuse the victim's emotions and depersonalize the attack, which can serve as a healthy coping mechanism.

3. *Signs of emotional trauma* consist of the victim's behavior during the interview. Any precise, concrete signs should be recorded, such as withdrawn or quiet behavior, hyperventilation, signs of extreme anxiety, sobbing, or tears.

4. *Symptoms of emotional trauma* include the victim's verbatim statements about the method of force used and the assailant's threats. If a weapon was used by the assailant, this should be noted. The nurse's subjective impressions and opinions should not be recorded in the account. To try to discredit the victim or establish "character fault" by claiming that consensual intercourse occurred, the defense counsel will often use such subjective data.

CRISIS DIMENSION. Hilberman[15] points out that support during phases of a crisis prevents maladaptive stress responses in later resolution processes. However, the rape crisis differs from other stress reactions in that family and friends are often rejecting, not supportive. It is not surprising, then, that the anxiety response a rape victim endures is for a longer period than anxiety in other kinds of crises.

Assessing the crisis status of a rape victim follows the same guidelines presented in crisis intervention (Chapter 20). However, two balancing factors are particularly significant when assessing a rape victim's crisis status. The first is the victim's perception of the event. The crisis a rape victim experiences differs from other crises because of societal attitudes that are nonsupportive. The nurse can make this crisis more, or less, like other crises depending on the attitude and the way in which she works with the attitudes of others. When the victim has a distorted perception of the rape, perhaps from her belief in myths, there is diminished ability to recognize a relationship between the feelings of stress and the rape. It is important to consider what the rape means to the individual. How is it going to affect her future? Does she distort its meaning or can she look at it realistically?

The second significant balancing factor is the presence of situational supports. Appraisal by significant others tends to reinforce the victim's perception of herself. It is important to help the victim identify those persons who can be most supportive to her at this time. The nurse needs to recognize that those whom the nurse might automatically identify as supports, such as parents, may *not* be those whom the victim would have selected. With persons who support feelings of ego integrity and who diminish feelings of insecurity, a dependency relationship is more readily established and this is a critical variable in crisis resolution. This is a decision point for some crisis centers in referring patients for long-term counseling or moving them from individual to group or family counseling. If a rape victim continues to feel vulnerable, given a lack of situational supports, a state of disequilibrium and possible crisis will emerge.

The nurse's objectives in assessing crisis with a rape victim include the following:

1. To evoke present feelings and facts, helping the victim connect these to the crisis precipitant (the rape and the responses of herself and others).
2. To help the victim deal with the situation that she identified and is unable to resolve alone.
3. To provide the specific information the victim needs in problem solving. Autonomy is restored by presenting the victim with alternatives and supporting her in the way she chooses to handle the situation.
4. To refer the victim to persons best able to help her reach final resolution of the crisis.

This is done only when, in a nursing assessment, one is certain that the victim needs or will seek the help. In making referrals, the nurse must be aware that feelings of anxiety and rejection may be stirred up. Referrals need to be offered as several alternatives, leaving the decision to the victim. The nurse can also offer to assist the victim in initiating contact with a referral source.

5. To help the victim obtain immediate help when such is necessary.

NURSING CONTRACT. It is obvious that there are many factors for the nurse to consider in completing an assessment with a victim of rape. These areas are summarized in the following outline of nursing assessment guidelines for victims of rape. At the end of the assessment process, the nurse will describe her clinical impressions, formulate a nursing diagnosis, and identify the nursing services requested by the victim.

A. Self-awareness of nurse, including blame models
B. Myths believed
  1. Nurse
  2. Victim
  3. Others
  4. Impact or result thereof
C. Phase of response
  1. Acute phase
    a. Impact reactions
    b. Somatic reactions
    c. Emotional reactions
  2. Outward adjustment
  3. Integration and resolution
    a. Motor activity
    b. Family support network
    c. Nightmares
    d. Traumatophobia
D. Psychological responses
  1. Emotional style
    a. Expressed style
    b. Controlled style
  2. Compounded reaction
  3. Silent rape syndrome
E. Developmental responses
  1. Task performance disruption
    a. Grade school or adolescent
    b. Adult victim
  2. Life stage and age
    a. Young single woman
    b. Divorced or separated woman
    c. Middle-age woman
    d. Elderly woman

F. Crisis and counseling requests
  1. Crisis requests
    a. Medical intervention
    b. Police intervention
    c. Psychological intervention
    d. Uncertain
    e. Control
  2. Counseling requests
    a. Confirmation of concern
    b. Ventilation
    c. Clarification
    d. Advice
    e. Wants nothing
G. Patient record: assessment and formulation
  1. Signs of physical trauma
  2. Symptoms of physical trauma
  3. Signs of emotional trauma
  4. Symptoms of emotional trauma
H. Crisis status
  1. Perception of the event
  2. Response to the event
  3. Situational supports
  4. Coping mechanisms
I. Clinical impressions
J. Nursing diagnosis
K. Nursing services requested
L. Referrals
M. Nursing plans

After a victim recognizes a need for services, the nurse must decide if that service is within her domain of practice. The victim has to indicate a willingness to do something about the identified need and perceive the nurse as the appropriate professional to assist her with it. The nurse needs to obtain clarity about the implicit contract with the victim and the services requested by the woman.

Planning

Professionals, volunteers, and rape crisis centers urge that the victim be actively involved in her own treatment program. The position is based on Orem's self-care model with the philosophy of maintaining and restoring the victim's self-respect, dignity, integrity, autonomy, and self-determination. The intent is to help the victim regain control of events and so renew mastery over her own life. The overall frame of reference is that each person needs to be listened to so that her current status and what she is experiencing within her environment can be determined. The victim should not be fitted into discrete phases of response patterns. Response patterns overlap and are unique to each person.

Plans for interventions must reflect individualized needs. A few generalized guidelines, however, may be helpful in planning nursing care.

If a victim is experiencing the *acute disorganization of phase 1,* the goal is to restore emotional control so that feelings do not reactively determine actions or dominate judgment. The first step is for the victim to get in touch with her own feelings. The nurse's task is to assist the victim's process of self-exploration through listening to and understanding her feelings and communicating to the victim that she has been heard and understood. The focus of the conversation, based on crisis theory, is what the nurse and the woman can do together to make the situation better. The goal is to develop a relationship with the victim that will help her sort out her thoughts and feelings prior to making a decision and acting on it.

Included in the planning is the working through of seven issues by the victim: legal matters and police contacts, clarification of factual information, medical attention, notification of family or friends, emotional responses, current practical concerns, and psychiatric–mental health consultation. Sutherland and Scherl[23] suggest the use of anticipatory guidance, or forewarning the victim of responses she might experience in later phases. Others disagree with that approach, claiming it gives the victim a preset that could become a self-fulfilling prophecy or precipitate self-doubt if later phases are not experienced.

In a *medical model* the nurse will attempt to ensure adequate medical care for all victims and watch for gynecological problems or somatic disturbances. In a *social network model* the nurse facilitates the victim's active involvement with her extended family and social network. In a *behavioral model* the nurse attempts to decrease the victim's stresses, anxieties, and fears while increasing her self-confidence and self-esteem. The painful parts of the experience are neutralized by talking about them. Intensive counseling at this time has three goals: further identification and acceptance of feelings; reorientation of perceptions, feelings, attributions, and self-statements; and resumption of a normal regular life-style. The nurse identifies the ways in which a victim processes and attributes causality to events connected to the rape and how her daily behaviors are influenced by such processing.

If a victim of rape is demonstrating the *outward adjustment or pseudoadjustment of phase 2,* the goal is to remain available and supportive to her. Concrete problems can be further explored now that excessive emotionality characteristic of a crisis state has subsided. The nurse avoids challenging the victim's wish to forget the rape or get on with her life; she will resolve the event at her own readiness. The nurse can use energy to reflect back with greater clarity and in different words what it is the victim seems to be feeling and thinking. At this point different alternatives for solving the presenting problem are explored. In addition, the nurse can help family and friends of the victim evaluate their responses to the victim and the rape. If their responses are negative, nonsupportive, or rejecting, the importance and need for counseling increases.

If a victim of rape has moved in the *integration and resolution of phase 3,* the nurse's goals are to assist the victim in (1) exploring feelings about the assailant, (2) exploring feelings about herself, and (3) in making decisions for herself. Planning provides for the resolution of feelings of guilt, shame, and anger toward the assailant when these are experienced. Planning for an extended evaluation is indicated in the presence of one or more of the following: compulsive rituals such as cleaning or washing, sleeping or eating disturbances, or fears that have generalized. Finally, the nurse aims to help the victim make her own health care decisions and to achieve her goals in life. In a *psychosocial model* the nurse stresses three dynamic issues: (1) the need to be in control, which is approximated as the victim reorders her life, (2) the need to be cared about, which can be met by helping the victim with ways to tell people about her needs and by showing her ways to have more people concerned about her, and (3) the need to achieve, which can be channeled into such activities as enrolling in a self-defense course or working with the rape crisis center.

The overall goal is to help the victim acknowledge, face, and resolve the response she is feeling. Ultimately all planning will follow from the victim's crisis and counseling requests and the nursing assessment.

Implementation

The type of intervention implemented will follow from the planning and be partially determined by the setting in which the victim of rape is seen.

HOSPITAL SETTING–EMERGENCY ROOM. Rape victims arrive at the emergency room in vary-

ing degrees of emotional trauma. It is essential that careful and prompt treatment be provided. One recommended procedure for medical examination of victims of rape is given on pp. 852 to 853. Preferably, a comfortable and private waiting room should be available. When a private room exceeds pragmatic possibilities and the victim must wait with others, it is advisable to refer to sexual assault patients by name or a code such as Code R. A code call system sometimes avoids insensitive comments such as "Where's the rape?" The examination should be done in a private area located near the emergency room. If the police later interview the victim, a similar facility should be made available to them. It is recommended that medical care be provided in advance of any interviews with the police. There is no valid reason to interrogate or interview a victim in a public area or waiting room. To protect the woman's rights, no information should be released without her consent.

In many communities there will not be an advocate to go with the victim through the medical and legal systems. The nurse may be her only advocate during a physical examination and may be able to assist her with the beginning phases of crisis resolution. Whenever possible two nurses need to be available, one to assist with the examination and evidence collection and the other to provide direct care to the victim, especially in the absence of an advocate. If the nurse has a clear idea of how the woman feels about herself, her level of self-esteem, and whether it is important for her to be in control, the nurse will have the necessary data to act as an effective advocate with the victim during a physical examination and interview.

The nurse begins by listening to the victim's account of the attack in a warm and empathic way. The nurse needs to convey acceptance of the victim's description of the use of threat or force, that the assault involved penetration, however slight, and that whatever her response to the assault was, it was appropriate. The nurse needs to strive to get as clear an idea as possible of what the woman would like the nurse to do for her. The nurse needs to let the victim know that, although she just survived a trauma she has some strengths to cope with and get over this event. Thus to help her begin the resolution process the nurse will not speak for her unless it is clear she wants help in conveying her needs. The nurse can provide the victim with

MEDICAL EXAMINATION OF THE VICTIM OF RAPE*

History

A medical history should be obtained and a statement taken about the time and place of the event; relationship to the assailant, if any; nature of suspected physical and sexual acts; time lapse between assault and current examination; victim's physical state; and whether there have been any physical changes since the assault (e.g., if the victim bathed, douched, showered, urinated or defecated, changed clothes, used or removed a tampon, treated wound, etc., prior to examination)

Examination, treatment, and follow-up care

Equipment recommended for evidentiary material
1. Fresh-sealed package of microscopic slides with frosted ends
2. Eyedropper bottle with 0.9% saline
3. Six to twelve packages of sterile cotton swabs
4. Nine to twelve test tubes with stoppers
5. Urine container
6. Sterile new comb
7. Sterile scissors
8. Nail scraper—plastic or orangewood
9. Envelopes
10. Package of gummed labels
11. Glass-cutting pencil
12. Sterile gauze and envelope for saliva sample.

Complete physical and gynecological examination
1. Evaluate vital signs, general appearance, and mental status.
2. Identify and measure cuts, bruises, and scratches; record and photograph (black and white only admissible in court).
3. Take fingernail scrapings, particularly if nails are broken or victim scratched the assailant.
4. Examine for extragenital sexual trauma to mouth, breasts, neck, and other body parts. Take swabs and smears from mouth, throat, or anus in the case of sodomy to check for semen presence.
5. Do a baseline check for venereal disease (VD) and gonorrhea, followed 6 weeks later with another set of tests. Sometimes massives doses of penicillin are given to help prevent VD infection. The victim should understand what is being given and may refuse any medication.
6. Discuss with the victim her birth control practices, use of oral contraceptives, and intrauterine devices, and belief system surrounding abortion. A discussion of possible types of postcoital contraception with a full explanation of possible effects is indicated (diethylstilbestrol [DES] has been shown to cause cancer in daughters born to women who have taken it during pregnancy).
7. Discuss with the victim the sexual functioning of the rapist (impotence, retarded ejaculation, premature ejaculation, masturbation).
8. Pregnancy testing and information on abortion, location of free clinics, women's health services, and crisis and counseling centers in the community should be provided.
9. Pelvic examination should include the following:
   a. Observation for matted or free hair
   b. Combings of pubic and head hair to find any traces of assailant's hair and collection of pubic and head hairs from victim for reference
   c. Description of vulvar trauma, redness, lacerations, and bruises and photography in black and white
   d. Examination of condition of hymen

*Modified from The Hospital Association of Pennsylvania and the Pennsylvania Medical Society: Guidelines for treatment of suspected victims of sexual assault, Penn. Med. 79:73, June, 1976; Bragonier, R., and Nadelson, C.C.: Caring for the rape victim, in Interact: new perspectives for the clinical management of sexual problems, Chicago, 1977, G.D. Searle & Co.; and the collected publications of A.W. Burgess and L.L. Holmstrom.

MEDICAL EXAMINATION OF THE VICTIM OF RAPE—cont'd

Examination treatment, and follow-up care—cont'd

  e. Determination of parity
  f. Determination of date of last menstrual period
  g. Determination of date and time of last voluntary coitus
  h. Determination of condition of anus and rectum
  i. Vaginal examination with lubricated, water-moistened speculum
  j. Specimen of victim's blood for matching if she is bleeding
  k. Examination of adnexa for hematoma
  l. Swabs and smears from vagina, vulva, rectum, and thighs to check for presence of semen
10. Clothing should be checked for tears, blood, semen, and stains. Victim's clothing should be preserved, marked, photographed, and collected in a paper bag (never plastic).
11. Obtain 5 ml of blood for typing.

Evidentiary material

Evidentiary material should be gathered and held for release to the police. It should not be released without consent of the patient or guardian, except by subpoena or court order. Specimens should be gathered and handled as follows:

1. Take swab from the vaginal pool and from any suspicious area about the vulva and protect in dry test tube. These can be examined by a hospital or police laboratory for the following:
   a. Acid phosphatase test
   b. Blood group antigen of semen test
   c. Precipitin test against sperm and blood
2. Examine wet sample from fornix immediately for motile sperm. This examination should be performed only by an experienced person who understands the limitations of examining sperm material.
3. Take separate smears from the vulva.
4. Culture for *Neisseria* organisms in appropriate medium such as Thayer-Martin.
5. Comb pubic and head hair for free hairs; pull (do not cut) a minimum of 25 of the victim's pubic and head hairs.
6. Take fingernail scrapings.
7. Chain of evidence: laboratory specimens should be gathered by a physician in the presence of a witness and personally handed to a technician or pathologist. Slides and containers should be clearly labeled with patient's name. The victim should be advised that turning bloody, torn, or stained clothing over to the police may help their investigation and prosecution of case (if she chooses to prosecute). It is critical that a chain of evidence be established identifying all persons responsible for handling or keeping evidentiary material.

Follow-up care

The patient should be examined for lacerations, contusions, and other wounds. Retesting and examining for pregnancy, VD, and gonorrhea should be completed. Counseling to assess and prevent long-term psychological effects should be provided or made available.

Medical records

The medical record should contain complete documentation of the history, examination, and treatment provided. It should describe the physician's findings and what was done. It should state what evidentiary materials were given and to whom. Only the medical conclusions, opinions, and diagnosis should be in medical record. Above all, it must be legible, and preferably typed, to avert case dismissal in court proceedings. The medical personnel and record may be subpoenaed. Misinterpretations can be avoided if all data are exact and detailed. Negative findings are as important as positive ones and may assist in protection of all concerned parties.

adequate information about what her rights are and what she can expect from the hospital staff to reduce her sense of anxiety and helplessness. It is important to determine if the woman generally finds it easy or difficult to assert herself and whether she values that ability. Even a woman who is normally assertive may not ask what the physician is doing, given her emotional and physical pain. Later she may regret having been so passive in the examination and feel angry. Muscular tension is common during an examination for a victim of rape. The nurse needs to encourage the victim to let the physician know her response as the examination proceeds. The nurse needs to try to get an idea of the woman's values and give her the opportunity to express her feelings. The nurse needs to let her know that whatever she is feeling is valid and acceptable and that victims respond in a wide variety of ways. The woman needs to be assured that current feelings may change with distance from the attack and that she can remove distorted perceptions by reviewing the incidence when she is in a period of greater calm. The woman will resolve the crisis better if she finds the nurse supports her beliefs and her own value system.

The rape examination requires that the victim describe the kinds of sexual contact that took place. The nurse is often the person to conduct the interview and will find the process easier if the victim is given a rationale for the questions asked combined with empathy and good interviewing skills. Explaining the nature of and rationale for any tests done is a nursing action that can alleviate the victim's anxiety and fears. Since recall under high anxiety is minimal, it is recommended that these facts be given to the woman *in writing,* as well as in a packet of follow-up information. The nurse needs to also ask the woman how she feels about the morning-after pill (diethylstilbestrol [DES]), menstrual extraction, and abortion. The nurse can provide a full explanation of the use, side effects, and risks of DES. For more details *Our Bodies, Ourselves* and *Contraceptive Technology* are excellent resources.

Another area of nursing intervention is asking the woman if she is willing to answer questions that are nonmedical but which may be pertinent if she prosecutes the assailant. Valuable evidentiary material can be lost if she does not report the rape during the first 24 hours or few days, and she may also lose an opportunity for compensation or restitution. She can decide later about signing a release form and concentrate for now on acquiring medical attention; thus the victim is not pressed for a decision she may not feel ready to make. The nurse can inquire if she is willing to sign a medical release form and find out if there is any information to appear on it that she might not want released. Only information obtained through the physical examination and interview will be released, not her entire medical history. The victim may later want to share the whole, detailed, ugly event at least once with someone with whom she feels secure. The nurse can offer to be that person. The nurse can ask to provide follow-up care by calling the victim in a couple of days to see how she is doing or referring her to a specified follow-up team (rape crisis centers, community mental health centers).

Assisting the victim during the medical examination is very important. The nurse needs to ask the woman if she wants to know what is going on during the physician's examination. Without medical information some women feel powerless; with it they may feel more in control of what happens to them and more able to knowledgeably participate in the decision-making process. It will be helpful to explain in detail all medical procedures in advance of their implementation and assist the woman in coping with any discomfort caused by the physical examination. The woman needs to be reminded of the body's excellent healing capacity, its tissue elasticity, and its rich blood supply. Any bleeding or discomfort needs to be discussed, as well as measures she can take to facilitate healing. The victim may fear infection, verification of damage to her body, pain, and even being repugnant. Before the victim leaves, she needs to be given a card or packet with follow-up information, appointments, and telephone numbers of local crisis and counseling centers. The nurse emphasizes the importance of a follow-up check for venereal disease and pregnancy and asks permission to call in a day or two to see how she is doing.

TELEPHONE CRISIS COUNSELING. Crisis theory is applied in the process of counseling on the telephone. The nurse assesses the victim for the absence of one or more balancing factors. The functional strengths the woman possesses are conserved as a useful resource. The nurse assists the victim to view this crisis as an opportunity for personal growth and identify what ser-

TELEPHONE INTERVIEWING GUIDELINES WITH VICTIMS OF RAPE*

Date _____ Time _____

General information

Introduction: Hello. This is _____ from _____
    How can I help you?
Name of victim/caller _____
Phone number calling from _____
Address or general area _____
    Location/neighborhood of assault _____
    Why in the area _____
When did assault occur (date, time)? _____
Are you in a safe place? _____
Are you hurt? _____
How are you feeling now? _____
Time between assault and call to crisis line _____

Demographic data

Age of victim _____
Race and sex of victim _____
Marital status _____
Description of assailant:
    Who did it? _____
    Age _____
    Race and sex _____
    Acquainted with victim _____
        Describe relationship:

Crisis status

Perception of the event _____
Response to the event _____
Situational supports _____
Coping mechanisms _____

Type of assault

_____ Rape
_____ Attempted rape
_____ Involuntary deviate sexual intercourse
_____ Indecent assault
_____ Sexual assault of a minor
_____ Other degrading acts
        Describe:
_____ Use of weapon
        Type:
_____ Struggle by victim
        Feelings now about that
_____ Threats (describe)
        Verbal _____
        Physical _____

Services requested and questions to consider

1. Medical intervention (hospital): Has the victim had a medical examination? Encourage going to the emergency room for treatment of injuries and collection of evidence pending decision to prosecute.
   a. **If not examined:** If she does not want to go to the hospital, does she know about the importance of testing for VD, gonorrhea, and pregnancy now and later? Is she injured other than the sexual assault? What supportive network is available to her? Does she want/need an advocate to accompany her to a shelter/care facility? Give her information about the local hospital procedure and what to expect, her rights.
   b. **If examined:** How did she get to the hospital? What did she expect would be done for her at the hospital? Were tests for VD, gonorrhea, and pregnancy done? Did she change clothes or cleaned up before going to the hospital? Was medical evidence collected (what, where)? Was she treated for lacerations, abrasions, bruises? Is she taking any medications or DES? Specify these. Does she know their side effects and risks involved? Is she having any medical problems? Was follow-up care discussed/planned? How does she feel she was treated by the health professionals? What is her reaction to this experience? Did she decide to obtain help or did someone else pressure her to seek help?
   c. **Abuse:** Is there evidence of physical abuse to a child or elderly person or battered wife syndrome? Describe the data. Has the evidence been reported to the police, hospital, and/or child welfare office?

*Modified from Pittsburgh Action Against Rape: Crisis call form, 211 S. Oakland Ave., Pittsburgh, Pa. 15213, and Burgess, A.W., and Holmstrom, L.L.: Crisis and counseling requests of rape victims, Nurs. Res. 23:198, May-June, 1974.

Continued.

TELEPHONE INTERVIEWING GUIDELINES WITH VICTIMS OF RAPE—cont'd

Services requested and questions to consider—cont'd

2. Shelter and transportation intervention: Does she need emergency transportation?
   From _____ to _____ Date _____
   Time _____ Does she need emergency shelter? _____
   Contributing factors _____
   Length of time requested _____
   Accompanied (children) or alone _____
   Economic/financial concerns (describe) _____

3. Police and legal intervention: Has she reported to the police?
   a. **If not reported:** Does she want to report? Does she want the report kept anonymous? Does she want to press charges? Does she want to talk about the pros and cons of not reporting/ reporting? What feelings/factors are contributing to a no-report decision? Does she know about victim compensation-restitution (that she can be compensated for unpaid medical expenses if she reports the crime within 72 hours)?
   b. **If reported:** Does she understand the legal procedure and what to expect at the preliminary hearing, pretrial, trial? Is she aware of the possibility of a trial postponement and of a not-guilty verdict? To whom did she report (which police station and name of officer taking the report). Was a report taken? Was she encouraged or discouraged from prosecuting? What is happening with the police follow-up at this time? Is she aware of the procedures necessary to identify the assailant? Has the assailant been picked up by the police? Is the assailant in jail, out on bond? Is she being harrassed or threatened by him or others? Describe. Does she have any intent to retaliate against the assailant? Name of officer arresting the assailant and police station(s) he is assigned to? Who is the district attorney? How does she feel the police treated her? What is her reaction to the experience of reporting?

4. Psychological intervention.
   a. **The victim:** How did she feel at the time of the assault? And now? Does she feel the rape was her fault? Does she believe in the myths? Which ones and what impact are they having on her? Does she perceive anyone as able to assist her? Did she go or not go to the police/ hospital as a result of outside pressure/advice? Is she ambivalent regarding what to do? Describe. Is she seeking others' opinions? (Whose? What content? What action taken?) Was she or the assailant affected by the use of alcohol and/or drugs? (What ingested? When? Amount? By which party? Feelings about this?) Is she unable to verbalize her needs? Is she psychotic? Mentally retarded? History of social difficulties? History of physical difficulties? Hospitalized or under a physician's care now or previously? Mental status is (describe). What is the most painful part to recall/discuss? Has she been raped before? Is this her first sexual experience? What is her usual sexual style? What does this sexual assault mean to her? How did she react to sexual acts demanded (feelings, behaviors [e.g., compliance, resistance])?
   b. **Family and friends:** Who are her friends, relatives? Where do they live? Quality and frequency of contacts? Persons most and least in touch with? Does she have a therapist, minister? Does she attend any women's groups, any rap sessions? Does she want to talk with other victims of rape? Can she rely on her support systems if she wants to talk about the rape? Will they listen? How will she feel if they do not listen or reject her? How is her church community a support system for her? Has she decided to talk about the incident? (Discuss pros/cons of doing so and with whom—she is the best judge of her situation.) Who knows about the assault? Describe their response. Do family/friends want to talk with a counselor, or does she want a counselor to talk with them? Is the family responding with (1) caring for the victim's welfare, empathy, support, anger directed at the assailant, ability to give to the victim or (2) blaming the victim, caring for their own welfare (e.g., what others will think), recriminations, anger directed at the victim, blaming themselves?

TELEPHONE INTERVIEWING GUIDELINES WITH VICTIMS OF RAPE—cont'd

Services requested and questions to consider—cont'd

5. Narrative summary.
   Services requested _____ Medical
   _____ Police/legal
   _____ Shelter
   _____ Transportation
   _____ Advocate
   _____ Counseling (specify type)
   _____ Other

   Nursing diagnosis _____
   Plans _____
   Contacts made (e.g., police, hospital, name of person/agency)
   Referrals made or suggested _____
   Follow-up indicated and type _____
   Self-evaluation
   Describe feelings about the call, personal reactions, influence of biases/myths. List additional information/training that would help improve services. Delineate learning needs.

---

vices are needed. A set of recommended telephone interviewing guidelines for use with victims of rape is presented on pp. 855 to 857. Not all of the questions are covered in any one interview; these guidelines represent categories of information and helpful questions to explore. The nurse uses clinical judgment in deciding which areas to explore. The guidelines are an instrument from which to obtain data useful in assessing the victim and suggest questions to consider in relation to services requested.

COUNSELING. Professional literature on intervention in working with victims of rape recommends that nurses have a substantial working knowledge of theories of anxiety as they counsel victims. Anxiety is a response to a critical life transition, requiring that the nurse be familiar with means of working toward changes that are creative and positive. Since many victims experience a loss of self-respect, loss of virginity, threat of loss of one's life, and temporary loss of power, control, and autonomy, some experts in the field find it useful to perceive the victim's trauma in the context of a grief framework. The victim's response to rape closely approximates four interrelated feeling responses to loss or trauma

in a grieving process: denial, depression, anger, and resolution or reconstruction.

One recommended counseling model for helping victims of rape is called *active listening*. It is a method by which the counselor empathically responds to the feelings of another while being aware of the counselor's own thoughts and behavior. The model suggests that most people have difficulty understanding and responding to another's feelings at high levels of intensity that contrast to their thoughts or behavior. Growth of a person in counseling has been found to be related to certain dimensions present at high levels in the counselor. These core qualities are accurate empathy, respect for the other, objectivity, warmth, genuineness (self-disclosure), concreteness, and immediacy (Chapter 3). While implementing these core qualities through active listening, the nurse assists the woman through three phases of a change process: self-exploration, self-understanding, and action. Recognizing that something is "wrong" and coming for counseling must be joined with a commitment on the part of the woman to change and to do something about the situation or herself. If this essential motivation is lacking, the whole counseling process will have limited value. No one phase of counseling is discrete. The victim may revisit each phase of the counseling process based on what she is working through and may experience more than one phase within a given session.

The first phase of the change process is *self-exploration,* which "leads to a better understanding of concerns and a commitment to change which, in turn, makes possible a more successful course of action."[13] Here the problem is explored in depth by identifying feelings, thoughts, and behaviors. The approach is usually nondirective (Rogerian framework), and the primary focus of the nurse is on responding empathically to the feelings of the other. The nurse's role is to help the woman begin to understand what she can do to change the situation. Sometimes this phase is full of confusion. For example, the rape itself may be of minor significance for the woman, and something else (sexuality beliefs, her support system, society's response to her) may be more important. Clinical example 29-3 illustrates this self-exploration phase.

CLINICAL EXAMPLE 29-3

Gwen is a 17-year-old high school student who works part time at a shopping mall. She accepted a ride home from a teenager who frequented the mall and she casually knew. He talked her into a ride in his new jeep. Instead of taking Gwen home, he took her to a park where he raped her in the car.

During the self-exploration phase Gwen decided that she had been raped and betrayed and wanted to prosecute the assailant stating, "He's a real creep! He violated my body, even *I* don't do that. He deserves to be punished and has to be stopped from doing that to other women." A year later Gwen revisited self-exploration to gain understanding of homicidal feelings in response to a not-guilty verdict at the trial.

In the process of *self-understanding,* phase 2, identified feelings, thoughts, and behaviors are clarified, and causes and reasons are assigned by the victim to each as she explores her problems. The nurse assists her to make some sense out of the "pieces of the puzzle" when many nonspecific feelings arise by making these more concrete. The woman is then able to decide on what action she believes will resolve the difficulty and commits herself to a specific plan of action that is both reasonable and attainable. The nurse is more active at this time, sharing information such as how to contact the local crisis center. As a professional she knows how to help the woman with the services requested, such as learning how to be more assertive or referring her to where the service can be obtained. The approach tends to be more psychodynamic in nature. It employs analytical and conceptual thought processes as evident in the continuation of Clinical example 29-3.

CLINICAL EXAMPLE 29-3—cont'd

Gwen used counseling to understand many of her confused feelings and responses after the rape. She was able to see that she was not to blame for the rape and become more discriminating in trusting casual acquaintances. She shared the rape event with her parents when she felt herself enough out of a crisis state to cope with their response. She separated her own sexually active life-style from societal appraisals judging her as promiscuous and deserving of abuse. She understood her nightmares as an attempt to regain mastery over her life and make her life secure.

After the trial she saw the nurse counselor several times weekly because of homicidal rage. The nurse had to decide if Gwen would act on the feelings and if a temporary commitment for inpatient care was necessary. Gwen was able to graphically describe her rage: "I'd kill him without second thoughts. I'd like to maim him for life, hurt someone or something he cherishes." The nurse encouraged Gwen to fantasize and ventilate feelings of rage, for example, "I'd like to get a male prostitute to rape him so *he* knows what it's like." The nurse directed Gwen's rage in multiple areas to help diffuse overfocusing on the rapist; all the errors made by the police and medical staff in evidence collection were highlighted, and the insinuations of the defense attorney were recalled ("So after you *sobered* up. . . ."). Gwen gradually realized her anger was in more than one area.

In the process of *action,* phase 3, the woman decides precisely what she will do to accomplish life goals. Specific plans are devised from concrete and relevant information. In a facilitative position, the nurse acts on a philosophy that the victim's decision is her choice and includes a decision not to act. The nurse demonstrates objectivity and self-control by keeping her own agenda out of the counseling process. The action phase is identified by the woman's behavior, such as pressing charges, in contrast to her solely discussing what to do, which is characteristic of previous phases. This phase is emphasized within the counseling model. When a rape victim remains depressed, she does not gain mastery over the rest of her life. Although she was unable to control the external event of the rape, the nurse emphasizes that the victim does have control over internal intrapsychic events and her own behavior. Although unable to avert her own rape, a sexually assaulted woman sometimes acts to help herself and other victims of assault by working on a crisis hotline, by joining consciousness-raising women's groups, or by taking self-defense courses. For women who like to help others, this has been noted to be useful in helping a victim regain a sense of control over her life.

CLINICAL EXAMPLE 29-3—cont'd

Gwen realized that she did not have to kill the rapist as she had thought to dissipate her rage or prove to others that she was truly raped. Gwen went about making the rapist lose power over her life by living a constructive life: she finished high school, worked on making her relationship with her boyfriend satisfying, and was accepted for training in the police academy where she felt she could fight crime.

It may also be helpful to use behavior modification approaches at this time.[14] For example, cognitive restructuring techniques can be employed to stop the anxiety-producing chain of destructive self-statements. These include thought stopping, self-reinforcement, thought substitution, and the development of concrete plans. The nurse helps the woman consider her basic human rights and thus evaluate the legitimacy of self-blame attributions. In counseling, the nurse might ask, "Do you need to feel shame if you really did not have a choice of behaving in the matter?" Healthy anger directed toward the assailant replaces the victim's previous guilt-inducing statements, and negative self-evaluations tend to dissipate. Role playing and behavior rehearsal of such events as court proceedings or talking with one's family can help the victim develop the skills necessary to successfully implement a decision. When the woman experiences daily reinforcing events, the rape experience is more quickly put into proper perspective.

SOCIAL NETWORK. It is those closest to the victim and their responses which often influence how she resolves the attack. Rape crisis center staff report short-term counseling with families

on the request of the victim or family. The approach is crisis intervention and preventive education. One of the most devastating responses a victim encounters is denial by others who ignore the event or maintain secrecy about the rape. Appropriate nursing interventions when working with the family include emphasizing the importance of nonjudgmental support of the victim in making her own choices, which helps her regain control. It is important to emphasize to friends, relatives, and parents the understanding, compassion, protection, and warmth that a victim needs after such an intimately disturbing experience. Family are encouraged to put aside the desire to thrash the assailant in retribution and to direct their energy toward caring for the victim. She will need to be reassured, supported, soothed, comforted, and have attention to her immediate medical problems. Someone quiet and supportive is helpful while she resolves the event at her own pace.

An additional form of support is available through groups in rape crisis centers. Rape crisis centers are modeled after the Washington, D.C., center, which was an outgrowth of a feminist group that was attempting to open a women's center. Several members of the group had been raped and were dissatisfied with the treatment received. They formed a group to meet the needs of rape victims that they perceived were being unmet by the community. Their interventions on the behalf of victims are felt throughout the health care delivery system today. The justice system is also changing, as are the laws surrounding rape. Some judges fine the assailant to pay for damages suffered by the victim, and programs such as victim compensation-restitution are being implemented.

In rape crisis centers victims can request to meet with other victims or counselors. The structure of the group varies from a nondirective approach, which gives the victim space to focus on her concerns, to having members write down specific problems they would like to work on, such as sexuality, fears, or assertiveness. The leaders vary from professionals to volunteers who use active listening skills and facilitate the verbalization of feelings. Most groups evolve and dissolve spontaneously, usually at a time somewhat distant from the assault, when the victim has had time for reflection. Many of the crisis centers' programs extend into the realm of prevention and education within established groups, such as school systems, parent and church groups, and police and health care systems. Intervention in these programs is directed at changing societal attitudes and behaviors.

CASE EXAMPLES. To increase the effectiveness of one's nursing care, it may be helpful to role play some case situations.[19,20] One person can act out the role of the nurse applying the nursing process, and the other can play the role of the victim in the context of a person-to-person contact or a telephone call. Following are sample situations*:

- You are 25 years old and live alone. You dated a man you work with twice, and on the third date you invited him over for dinner. He forced intercourse on you. You did not tell anyone and have broken off all communication with the man. This happened 6 weeks ago. You now think you may be pregnant and do not know where to turn.
- You are a married woman, age 36. After a fight with your husband one night, you went alone to a bar. When you left, you were intoxicated. Your car would not start, and you accepted a ride from a man you knew only slightly. He drove to a deserted area and beat and raped you. You reported it, but no one really believes you, especially your husband.
- You are an 83-year-old widow. You were raped one night when you were sleeping by the 27-year-old man who rents a room from you. He cut the telephone cord, ripped your pajamas, and tried to smother you with a pillow. During the actual rape, you passed out. You are suffering from extensive internal bleeding. You want to prosecute.
- A woman was hitchhiking at midnight wearing a halter top and cutoffs. A black man picked her up, drove to a dark side street, and raped her at gunpoint. She was so exhausted, she sarcastically asked if she could have her ride home now and he gave it to her. You find out through the conversation that she is on drugs and has been in and out of therapy. How do you handle this?
- A woman was raped by an old acquaintance while out walking her dogs. She calls, feeling guilty and upset because she was afraid to fight and is afraid to be independent anymore. This incident has shaken her confidence in herself and her trust in people. What do you say?

---

*Modified from Rape Crisis Center of Madison, Wisconsin: Counselor's manual, 1976-1977, P.O. Box 1312, Madison, Wis. 53701, and Rape Crisis Center of Syracuse, Inc.: Training manual, Sept., 1976, 601 Allen St., Syracuse, N.Y. 13210.

Evaluation

There are no absolute counseling rules, since every situation has exceptions. Counseling does require a comprehensive knowledge base from which to make assessments, respond with compassion, plan appropriate interventions, and implement care effectively. The nurse can provide comfort and support in a time of need and assist the victim in the problem-solving process. The nurse is not responsible for the victim's choices or for her working or not working out problems. By maintaining a facilitative position, she can help the victim work through her own problems.

Research studies indicate that rape victim populations range from heterogeneous to homogeneous. There are also a variety of research methods, which include immediate interview and follow-up care, as well as a retrospective questionnaire and interview. There is a consensus that rape causes acute disorganization immediately after the trauma marked by fear and anxiety. The response to rape resembles most stress responses to other crises, and being raped sets in motion long-term reorganization processes.

The majority of research findings lack objectively measurable and quantifiable data. There are thus no systematical data regarding the long-term consequences of being raped or the impact it has on a woman's life. The various ways in which women respond to rape within the assault and the relationship of cultural, social, and personality variables is essentially unknown. Neither is it known how victims of rape differ from victims of other types of acute and chronic stress, such as battered women. As yet, long-term follow-up investigation is not well organized or implemented in many care systems in the nation. The professional literature needs to explore the work currently being done with nuclear and extended families and significant others in counseling.

Although counseling procedures have been described and implemented in various programs, they often lack internal and external evaluation with comparable treatment programs. Of particular relevance in the counseling of women is Bergin's challenge "that the effects of therapy are not uniform but that research should take into account which treatment by what therapist is effective for what client with what problem under what conditions."[16] Unfortunately, most authors that discuss rape counseling lack empirical evidence for the effectiveness of their treatment approaches. In the absence of such research, there is no scientific way to know if treatment programs are more effective than either no treatment at all or traditional treatments. In addition, there is no knowledge of the spontaneous remission of problems without treatment, changes from treatment, or the deterioration of problems and the client with treatment. Nurses are encouraged to develop a structure in their work setting to provide long-term follow-up care for victims, to scientifically investigate the effectiveness of treatment programs, and to open the dialogue about this area of practice on local, state, and national levels with colleagues and others in victim assistance programs.

CLINICAL EXAMPLE 29-4

Clair is a 15-year-old high school student who called the rape crisis hot line and talked with a nurse on call that day. She wanted to know if she had been raped and what to do next. Clair said she was out with her boyfriend, Dave, and he had been pressuring her for sexual relations. Clair said she reluctantly agreed after much pressure because she didn't want to lose him or continue to make him angry but then changed her mind before sexual intimacies "got underway" and told him this. Dave was enraged and forced sexual relations on Clair despite her screaming, crying, and pleading. Clair said she felt responsible for what had happened. She wanted to know if she could get pregnant from the rape. Clair said she couldn't tell her parents because they wouldn't understand; they would blame her, and she was calling the hot line while they were out of the house. She did not want to be called back, since it would divulge her secret. Clair said her best friend and only person she could confide in was out of town for the week on vacation. Clair cried during the phone call and said "I can't believe what happened. I didn't think anyone would ever do anything like that. I can't see him again, it's all over and so awful."

Assessment. The nurse assessed this situation as a confidence rape (style of attack) and a sex-stress situation (type of nonconsent). It was also agreed that Clair believed some of the rape myths (self-blame), that she was in a crisis state (without a support network, loss of boyfriend, not able to use customary coping mechanisms) but was able to express her stress (style of response).

Planning. The nurse provided crisis intervention and arranged for follow-up care.

Intervention. The nurse confirmed for Clair that she had been raped, the nature and type of rape, including the element of betrayal that was adding to her sense of stress and disbelief (phase 1 response). The nurse encouraged ventilation of feelings (crying, disbelief, anger, fears of falling apart, sadness over the loss of her boyfriend). The nurse refuted Clair's faulty perceptions (self-blame for the assailant's behavior) and encouraged Clair to talk with her parents, which she continued to refuse to do for fear of their response. The nurse provided her with information on where she could get free pregnancy and venereal disease testing and said the crisis center could send a taxi to pick her up. Since Clair was in the middle of her menstrual cycle, the nurse encouraged her to obtain follow-up care in 6 weeks. The nurse told her that the local women's health center was open Monday morning, and an advocate could go with her to get medical care. The nurse gave her the phone number of the health clinic and the crisis center and encouraged her to stay in touch during this difficult time.

Evaluation. Clair thanked the nurse for her help. She decided to wait until her girlfriend returned to take any action because she wanted her support. She said she felt better after talking out her feelings and shared her plans for an evening with other friends from school. Clair never called back and, to protect her secret, did not leave her phone number. Clair was a victim of rape.

Suggested cross-references

Therapeutic relationship skills and self-awareness of the nurse are discussed in Chapter 3. The phases of the nursing process and social support networks are discussed in Chapter 4. Crisis intervention is discussed in Chapter 20. Interventions with violent and abusive families are discussed in Chapter 28.

SUMMARY

1. Rape crisis centers are an outgrowth of the feminist movement and there are more than 1500 in existence across the United States. The contributions of professionals to these centers is currently being examined. Treatment of rape victims is a service that also must be provided by community mental health centers.

2. Rape is legally defined as the "forcible perpetration of an act of sexual intercourse on the body of a woman not one's wife." A more contemporary definition includes acts of oral and anal sodomy, which are often more traumatic for the victim and does not exclude marital rape. For the woman, rape implies a loss of self because she is reduced from a person to an object and a function.

3. The intent of rape is to degrade, humiliate, and defile the victim. It is an act of aggression and violence in which sex is the weapon, yet sexual gratification is not acquired, and many rapists experience sexual dysfunction. A vicious cycle is set up in which the offender repeats the act in an attempt to settle personality deficits. Many myths surround the crime of rape and all of them serve to place blame on the victim. Since many people believe these myths, they hinder the ability of the victim to receive adequate treatment in medical, legal, and sociocultural systems. Some of the facts related to rape include the following:

   a. Rape is the fastest rising violent crime in the nation, and among these it has the lowest proportion of cases closed by arrest and conviction.

   b. Chances are 1 in 15 a woman will be raped in her lifetime.

   c. The target population of victims is young women ages 15 to 24.

   d. By all appearances the offender is no different from the accepted norm of other men in our society except for an exaggerated tendency to express violence and aggression.

4. Victims of rape respond with feelings of fear, guilt, anger, self-blame, denial, disbelief, shock, depression, and isolation. They may also exhibit phobic reactions, sexual dysfunction, motor activity, nightmares, and disruption of task expectations. Victim response to rape is a function of the woman's life stage (adolescent, young adult, elderly), demographic status (single, married, divorced, widowed), and psychodynamic developmental process.

5. Three phases of crisis resolution for the rape victim were identified by Sutherland and Scherl[23]:

   a. An acute phase characterized by shock, disbelief, and dismay

   b. An outward adjustment phase characterized by denial of the event's impact and a desire to get on with her life.

   c. An integration and resolution phase in which the victim confronts her anger with the assailant and puts the event into realistic perspective

6. Burgess and Holmstrom[6] identified a "rape trauma syndrome," a "compounded reaction," and a "silent rape syndrome" among victims' responses. They noted two emotional styles: the "controlled style," and the "expressed style."[4] They also described five categories of crisis requests made by rape victims. These included medical intervention, police intervention, psychological intervention, uncertain, and control.[5]

7. The nursing process is used in assessing the victim's crisis and counseling requests and the ways in which to best facilitate meeting the victim's identified needs. Self-awareness by the nurse is an essential component of the assessment process. There are many factors for the nurse to consider in completing an assessment and it needs to be carried out with adequate knowledge of one's legal responsibility.

8. The planning phase of the nursing process requires the active involvement of the victim and reflects her individualized needs. Plans can be formulated on the basis of the victim's phase of response—acute disorganization, outward adjustment, or integration and resolution. Possible areas for intervention include medical care, emotional support, legal concerns, and social network. The overall goal is to help the victim acknowledge, face, and resolve the response she is feeling.

9. The type of nursing intervention implemented will be partially determined by the setting in which the victim is seen. If the woman appears in a hospital setting, the nurse can support her during the medical examination. The nurse can initiate counseling in a hospital setting or in a telephone contact. Counseling is focused on three phases of a change process: self-exploration, self-understanding, and action. Behavior modification is also an effective treatment approach for some victims.

10. Evaluating the long-term effectiveness of different treatment interventions has yet to be universally implemented. The existing research findings lack objectively measurable and quantifiable data. Nurses can make significant contributions in this area.

11. The problem of rape is a symptom of a dysfunctional social system with its attendant values, attitudes, beliefs, and socialization processes. It will be eradicated only to the extent that changes are effected in these areas. Brownmiller poignantly assessed, "Fighting back. On a multiplicity of levels, that is the activity we must engage in, together, if we women are to redress the imbalance and rid ourselves and man of the ideology of rape."[3:404]

References

1. Amir, M.: Patterns in forcible rape, Chicago, 1971, University of Chicago Press.
2. Brodsky, S.L., and Hobart, S.: Blame models and assailant research, Crim. Justice Behav. **5:**379, 1978.
3. Brownmiller, S.: Against our will: men, women and rape, New York, 1975, Simon & Schuster, Inc.
4. Burgess, A.W., and Holmstrom, L.L.: The rape victim in the emergency ward, Am. J. Nurs. **73:**1744, 1973.
5. Burgess, A.W., and Holmstrom, L.L.: Crisis and counseling requests of rape victims, Nurs. Res. **23:**196, May-June, 1974.
6. Burgess, A.W., and Holmstrom, L.L.: Rape trauma syndrome, Am. J. Psychiatry **131:**981, 1974.
7. Burgess, A.W., and Holmstrom, L.L.: Rape: victims of crisis, Bowie, Md., 1974, Robert J. Brady Co.
8. Burgess, A.W., and Holmstrom, L.L.: Rape: its effect on task performance at varying stages in the life-cycle. In Walker, M.J., and Brodsky, S.L., editors: Sexual assault, Lexington, Mass., 1976, D.C. Heath & Co.
9. Burgess, A.W., and Laszloa, A.T.: Courtroom use of hospital records in sexual assault cases, Am. J. Nurs. **77:**64, Jan. 1977.
10. Connell, N., and Wilson, C., editors: Rape: the first source book for women, New York, 1974, Lume Books.
11. Crime in the United States, 1979, Washington, D.C., 1980, Government Printing Office.
12. Fletcher, P.: Criminal victimization of elderly women: a look at sexual assault, April 28, 1977, Rape Crisis Center of Syracuse, Inc., 601 Allen St., Syracuse, N.Y. 13210. (unpublished).
13. Gzada, M., et al.: Human relations development: a manual for educators, ed. 2, Boston, 1977, Allyn & Bacon, Inc.
14. Heppner, M., and Heppner, P.P.: Rape: counseling the traumatized victim, Personnel Guidance J. **8:**78, Oct., 1977.
15. Hilberman, E.: Rape: the ultimate violation of self, Am. J. Psychiatry **133:**436, 1976.
16. Hill, C.E.: A research perspective on counseling women, Counsel. Psychol. **6:**53, 1976.
17. MacLean, J.: Rape: what's being done to stop it? In These times: a special report, Chicago, 1975, New Majority Publishing Co.
18. Notman, M.T., and Nadelson, C.C.: The rape victim: psychodynamic considerations, Am. J. Psychiatry **133:**408, 1976.
19. Rape Crisis Center for Madison, Wisconsin: Counselor's manual, 1976-1977, P.O. Box 1312, Madison, Wis. 53701.
20. Rape Crisis Center of Syracuse, Inc.: Training manual, Sept. 1976, 601 Allen St., Syracuse, N.Y. 13210.
21. Rape Crisis Services Division of the Greater Harrisburg Area YWCA: First night: flow chart—victim decisions following a sexual assault, 1977, 215 Market St., Harrisburg, Pa. 17101.
22. Rey, D.: Counseling tips, Marin Rape Crisis Center, May, 1976, P.O. Box 823, Kentfield, Calif. 94904.
23. Sutherland, S., and Scherl, D.J.: Patterns of response among victims of rape, Am. J. Orthopsychiatry **40:**503, 1970.
24. The Feminist Alliance Against Rape Newsletter: Professionalism, Fall 1975, P.O. Box 21003, Washington, D.C., 20009.

Annotated suggested readings

Alexander, C.: The responsible victim: nurses' perceptions of victims of rape, J. Health Soc. Behav. **21:**22, March 1980.

This is the report of an excellent research study conducted by a nurse on how judgments are made by hospital nurses regarding victim responsibility. A number of determinants of victim blame were evaluated, and an interesting finding was that psychological attributes of the nurse emerged as the strongest predictor of victim blaming.

Amir,, M.: Patterns in forcible rape, Chicago, 1971, University of Chicago Press.

This book presents a comprehensive empirical study of patterns of forcible rape over a 2-year period in Philadelphia based on the Philadelphia Police Department files. It considers ecological and demographic factors, and emphasis is given to the act of rape itself, the situations in which it is likely to occur, and to the victim/offender relationship. The author holds that the rapist is "normal" in a society that condones the offensive act. Prevalent myths associated with the crime of rape are attacked. The conclusions are specific within the context of the study.

Brodyaga, L., et al.: Prescriptive package, rape and its victims: a report for citizens, health facilities, and criminal justice agencies, Nov. 1975, National Institute of Law Enforcement and Criminal Justice, Law Enforcement Assistance Administration, U.S. Department of Justice.

From national surveys in 1974 the authors attempt to identify programs, techniques, policies, and procedures that are constructively innovative, especially effective, or otherwise valuable in coping with the crime of rape and that might be suitable for transfer or replication in other jurisdictions. The book is divided into four sections: "The Police Response," "The Response of Medical Facilities," "The Response of Prosecutors' Offices," and "The Response of Citizens' Action Groups." It also outlines suggestions for coping with problems that commonly hinder change.

Brownmiller, S.: Against our will: men, women and rape, New York, 1974, Simon & Schuster, Inc.

The author presents a well-documented, thorough scrutiny of the history of rape. From a historical perspective the author reveals rape as embedded in and supported by our culture. The myths, attitudes, and assumptions surrounding rape that obscure its nature and pereptuate it are challenged. Occasional generalizations without the necessary qualifications are sometimes made, yet the work remains an important and valuable contribution for anyone attempting to understand and eradicate the problem.

Burgess, A.W. et al.: Sexual assault of children and adolescents, Lexington, Mass., 1978, D.C. Heath & Co.

This book is designed as a handbook for persons who come into contact with either the victim or offender in their work. It attempts to provide some of the treatment answers in a manner that is easily understood and adaptable to both lay and professional counselors and their individual programs. Major themes are (1) the human dimension, (2) community program planning, and (3) interagency cooperation. It is recommended reading for all persons serving or involved with child and adolescent victims of sexual assault.

Burgess, A.W., and Holmstrom, L.L.: Rape: victims of crisis, Bowie, Md., 1974, Robert J. Brady Publishing Co.

The text presents a comprehensive analysis of a rape victim's counseling needs. Definitions of the act of both rapist and victim are given, and various types of rape are described. Two phases of victims' responses and a rape trauma syndrome are explained. Varying reactions of hospital staff, police, family, and community are presented. Crisis centers and their purpose are discussed. Methods in telephone and home counseling and crisis intervention are presented. Special needs of the victim who prosecutes, the prostitute victim, the child and adolescent victim, and the victim with prior psychosocial problems are presented. This is a highly recommended reading for all those serving or involved with rape victims.

Burgess, A.W., and Holmstrom, L.L.: Rape: crisis and recovery, Bowie, Md., 1978, Robert J. Brady Co.

The text contains a number of articles of the author's works from journal publications. It cuts across disciplines, addressing the nature of and reactions to rape, community, and forensic issues; crisis intervention, and counseling of victims, including long-term recovery.

DeFrancis, V.: Protecting the child victim of sex crimes committed by adults, Denver, 1969, The American Humane Association, Children's Division.

This report presents the results of a research project conducted under a child welfare research grant over a 3-year period in the late 1960s. It is based on a sample of 250 families. The study compared two boroughs in New York City, one with and the other without child protective services. It tested the hypothesis that added to the trauma of sexual assault are the impact of police investigations and the pressures and tensions of judicial proceedings to prosecute the offender. The study provides a comprehensive overview of the sexual abuse of children, cites 42 major findings, and suggests that the incidence is larger than the reported incidence of physical abuse of children.

Foley, T., and Davies, M.: Rape: nursing care of victims, St. Louis, 1983, The C.V. Mosby Co.

The text is directed toward the education of professional nurses with the goal of preparing practitioners competent in both physical and psychological management of rape and child sexual abuse victims. Theoretical frameworks that are most appropriate for understanding victim and societal response and providing nursing care are incorporated. Active learning exercises and annotated readings are helpful learning adjuncts in a text specifically designed to meet learning and clinical practice needs of nurses.

Gager, N., and Schurr, C.: Sexual assault: confronting rape in America, New York, 1976, Grosset & Dunlap, Inc.

Multiple dimensions of the crime of rape are presented in an informative, insightful, and thought-provoking survey. Legal, medical, and psychological aspects are considered. Attention is drawn to the "politics of rape" with description of how our society effectively predisposes men to rape and women to become victimized. The authors offer significant practical information and a comprehensive, consciousness-raising introduction to the problem. The book does not address the self-help mode of assisting victims in resolving their crisis.

Griffin, S.: Rape: the all American crime, Ramparts **10:**26, Sept. 1977.

This article offers a feminist analysis for the political meaning of rape as an aggressive act. Culturally rooted myths such as (1) rapists are insane, (2) women want to be raped, and (3) rape is an impulsive act are examined and refuted. Rape is described in the context of sexual domination of females by males and the act is regarded as a mirror image of our ordinary sexual folkways as opposed to a deviant act. The author concludes that the dissolution of patriarchy is the only means of ending rape.

Groth, A.N., and Birnbaum, J.: Men who rape: psychology of the offender, New York, 1979, Plenum Press.

The text presents 15 years of research with more than 500 sexual offenders. Examined are psychological and social factors that predispose one to react to situational and life events with sexual violence: developmental factors, life-style, and motivations. Diagnostical assessment and treatment of the offender are discussed in detail. Easy to read and nontechnical in style of presentation.

Halpern, S., editor: Rape: helping the victim—a treatment manual, Oradell, N.J., 1978, Medical Economics Books.

This text is a manual for use in emergency room and follow-up care with rape victims. Practical procedures, such as the medical examination, evidence collection, chain of evidence, and counseling of the family, are succintly outlined for ease in use.

Holmstrom, L.L., and Burgess, A.W.: The victim of rape: institutional reactions, New York, 1978, John Wiley & Sons, Inc.

The text describes how major institutions respond to rape victims and the often devastating effects of care received from hospital emergency wards up though court trials. Research findings substantiating the victim's plight are presented along with policy recommendations for change in institutional settings.

Katz, S., and Mazur, M.A.: Understanding the rape victim: a synthesis of research findings, New York, 1979, John Wiley & Sons, Inc.

An excellent reference book reporting and analyzing research findings and critiquing methodology across studies. The authors examine the facts about the victim prior to rape (risk factors, family and social background, personality, and sexual history), during the rape (setting, situation, transaction, reactions) and after the rape (reporting, prosecuting, counseling, and child sexual abuse) concluding with rape prevention and a summary of findings.

McCombie, S., editor: The rape crisis intervention handbook, New York, 1980, Plenum Press.

The text is a contributed work from experts in the field of victim care. It offers a practical handbook of treatment-oriented information for professionals working directly with victims and their families. Addressed are psychological, medical, and legal aspects essential in counseling rape victims.

Medea, A., and Thompson, K.: Against rape, New York, 1974, Farrar, Straus & Giroux, Inc.

This book describes rape as a culturally bound reflection of societal morals. It discusses the offender and his motivations, the victim and her psychological reactions to the assault, and methods of self-defense. It generally offers a good overview of the problem and a realistic evaluation.

National Association of Victim Assistance: Victim Programs Directory, 1977, Southern Station, Box 5127, Hattiesburg, Miss., 39401.

NOVA is a national organization aimed at the unification of scholars, students, professional members of the criminal justice system, volunteers, and lay citizens who are committed to the humanization of the criminal justice system through victim advocacy. The national directory provides a resource to contact persons identified by one or more of the following codes: victim service and victim advocate programs; restitution programs; rape programs; volunteer programs; educators, planners, administrators, legislators, and citizens interested in promoting victim programs; compensation programs; researchers of victimization survey and evaluation; author of articles or editor of journals, films, or books dealing with victims; child abuse programs; district attorney–victim-witness programs; elderly victim programs; spouse abuse programs; and persons involved with or interested in victim rights. To secure training manuals, conduct research, and collaborate to improve prevention and treatment programs, persons listed in the directory are an excellent resource.

Russell, D.: Rape in marriage, New York, 1982, Macmillan, Inc.

This is a report of a large-scale survey of San Francisco women that was supported by NIMH to try to ascertain the prevalence of marital and extramarital rape and other sexual assault. It is more accurately, however, a fearful experience and illumination of the human condition that has a compelling impact on the reader.

St. Louis Feminist Research Project: The rape bibliography: a collection of abstracts, St. Louis, 1976, St. Louis Research Project.

The book is divided into four areas: legal, medical, psychological, and sociological aspects of rape. A section entitled "Popular Press" covers all four major subject areas and is limited to works appearing in nonscholarly publications. Each major section is subdivided into "bibliography" and "abstracts." Abstracts include all scholarly books and articles written in English and published after 1970. Materials written prior to 1970 are included if the researcher determined they were of particular importance. Bibliography sections include a complete listing of all works written before 1970. In addition, there is a listing of pamphlets that have a wide circulation.

Schultz, L.G., editor: Rape victimology, Springfield, Ill., 1975, Charles C Thomas, Publisher.

This is a collection of lectures and essays drawn from law, social work, medicine, nursing, sociology, the feminist movement, and victims that speaks to various dimensions of the problem of rape. Special focus is given to the social aspects of rape. The child as a victim of sexual assault is also given attention. The anthology is wide in scope, providing a good introduction to the issue, and touches on some areas neglected in other similar efforts.

Selkin, J.: Rape, Psychol. Today **8:**71, 1975.

The author identifies a five-stage pattern in stranger-to-stranger rape: target selection, testing, threat, sexual transaction, and termination. Types of rapists are subdivided into two categories; however, no further diagnosis is included. The importance of immediate resistance at the onset of the attack is emphasized throughout the article.

Walker, M.J., and Brodsky, S.L., editors: Sexual assault, Lexington, Mass., 1976, Lexington Books.

This is a comprehensive compilation of scientific research, informed observations, and professional knowledge from recent addresses, essays, and lectures on diverse aspects of the problem of rape. The editors state that their purpose is to "raise the complex issues of causes and prevention of rape and to offer some preliminary answers to show the range of current developments in dealing with the victim and understanding rape" in a format that is readable and scientifically sound.

Weis, K., and Borges, S.S.: Victimology and rape: the case of the legitimate victim, Issues Criminol. **8:**71, Fall 1973.

This article discusses the relationship between victimology and rape and the origin of the legitimate victim. It describes ways in which socialization and sex-role learning exploit both males and females, producing both offenders and victims. Sociological, psychological, and legal reasons are cited as factors increasing victim trauma.

*What I ask for is absurd: that life shall have a
  meaning.
What I strive for is impossible: that my life
  shall acquire a meaning.
I dare not believe, I do not see how I shall ever
  be able to believe: that I am not alone.*

Dag Hammarskjöld, Markings*

*Hammarskjöld, D.: Markings, New York, 1966, Alfred A.
Knopf, Inc. (Translated by L. Sjoberg and W.H. Auden.) Re-
printed by permission of Faber & Faber, Ltd., and Alfred
A. Knopf, Inc.

CHAPTER 30

CARE OF THE CHRONICALLY MENTALLY ILL PATIENT

Ruth Wilder Bell

Learning objectives

*After studying this chapter, the student
will be able to:*

- *discuss the impact of deinstitutionalization on the
care of the chronically mentally ill.*

- *identify legal issues that have had an influence on
the treatment of the chronically mentally ill.*

- *describe the evolution of a chronic mental illness,
including the development of primary and secondary symptoms.*

- *assess the nursing care needs of chronically mentally ill patients based on data concerning problem
areas and strengths.*

- *compare and contrast the characteristics of chronically mentally ill young adults with those of older
patients.*

- *describe the elements of psychosocial rehabilitation
programs.*

- *analyze the role of the nurse caring for seriously
mentally disabled patients in community and acute
care settings.*

- *discuss nursing interventions based on the assessed needs of chronically mentally ill people.*

- *identify suggested readings for further study.*

Before the advent of phenothiazines in the 1950s, individuals with a chronic mental illness were relatively easy to locate. Primarily they were the residents of large public psychiatric hospitals that were located in rural areas, distant from the populations they served.

The identification and location of the chronically mentally ill and the nurses who care for them is more difficult in the 1980s. Since the CMHC movement of the mid-1960s, the resident population of state and county mental hospitals has decreased by two thirds.[2,5] Today it is estimated that of the 3 million persons in the United States suffering from serious mental illness, 1.7 million have a prolonged severe disability. Yet only 50% of these individuals with a severe disability of prolonged duration live in institutions such as nursing homes or hospitals. The other 50% are living in the community in a variety of residential settings.[16,31] Nurses care for them in a multiplicity of health care settings: hospital emergency rooms, community-based treatment programs, psychiatric units in general hospitals, nursing homes, home visits, and public psychiatric hospitals.

As the "careers" of the discharged chronically mentally ill unfold, there are likely to be periods when they cannot be maintained in the community, and rehospitalization is necessary. As the patients alternate between community-based and hospital-based care, nurses in both community-based and inpatient facilities share responsibility for care of the same group of patients. Knowledge of the special needs and characteristics of the chronically mentally ill as a population is important for all nurses who care for these patients, in whatever setting the care may be given.

Social perspective

Deinstitutionalization is the term used to describe the process of moving long-term mental hospital patients back into the community where they are to be supported by a "formal network of clinical, social, and vocational agencies, as well as by an informal network of family, neighbors, and local community resources."[18] Implicit in the concept, deinstitutionalization is the assumption that a network of community resources exists and is available to meet the needs of the chronically ill.

The move to develop resources needed to return the long-term or chronic psychiatric patient to the community was initiated by a 1961 report of the Joint Commission on Mental Illness and Health. Actual construction of facilities to provide community-based treatment for these patients was made possible by the enactment of the 1963 Mental Retardation Facilities and Community Mental Health Centers Construction Act. Policy statements by Presidents Kennedy, Johnson, and Nixon further supported the goal of community-based treatment for the mentally ill.

As health policy began to direct that there be alternatives to a lifetime in public mental hospitals, court decisions reflected increasing attention to protection of the rights of this patient population. The legal rights of psychiatric patients are discussed in detail in Chapter 16. Friedman and Yohalem,[15] however, specify five clusters of rights that most directly impact on the chronically mentally ill:

1. Civil commitment
2. The right to treatment and protection from harm in the least restrictive environment possible
3. The right to refuse treatment
4. Confidentiality
5. Employment

Civil commitment

Paternalism is the interference with the liberty of another or the controlling of another when such interference is justified in terms of what is ultimately good for the person being controlled. Paternalism reflects the attitude of a parent toward a child and is the concept underlying the state's right *(parens patriae)* to make decisions for those who are not able to make decisions in their own best interest. Involuntary commitment of the mentally ill is the paternalistic resolution of the conflict between the liberty of an individual and the consequences of his mental illness. Through the use of its *police power* to hospitalize mentally ill patients involuntarily, the state carries out its responsibility to protect its citizens from real or potential danger.[9,15]

In 1975 Donaldson, a patient who had been hospitalized involuntarily (committed) for 15 years without receiving treatment, challenged the state's right to hold him against his will. The court *(O'Connor vs. Donaldson)* determined that the state cannot "confine a nondangerous patient who is capable of living safely by himself or with the assistance of caring others unless treatment is being provided."[4]

With increasing attention to protection of individuals' rights, "dangerousness" (to self or another) rather than "need for treatment" is likely to be the condition necessary for commitment, or involuntary hospitalization. Although such a criterion provides for protection of the civil liberties of the chronically mentally ill, it makes it difficult for society to intervene paternalistically on their behalf.

The right to treatment in the least restrictive environment

In 1972 in a landmark decision (*Wyatt vs. Stickney*), the United States Supreme Court ruled that "mentally handicapped persons involuntarily confined to a state institution had a constitutional right to treatment."[15] The court identified treatment as including a humane environment, an individualized treatment plan, and adequate numbers of qualified staff to implement the individual treatment plan. In 1975 in the Willowbrook case, the court further ruled that not only did involuntary patients have the right to treatment but they had the right to protection from harm, including protection from "seclusion, corporal punishment, degradation, medical experimentation, and the routine use of restraints."[15]

Although courts have consistently upheld the right of involuntary patients to treatment, they also have upheld the right to treatment in the least restrictive environment. In a class action suit (*Dixon vs. Weinberger, 1975*) patients at the federally run St. Elizabeth's Hospital in Washington, D.C., sued for their right to treatment in community-based facilities. The court ruled that an individual has the right to treatment in the least restrictive environment and, as a result, directed the federal government to develop community-based facilities for patients who could be therapeutically maintained in the community.[15,32]

Court decisions such as these provided energy for the deinstitutionalization movement. Although increasing numbers of community resources are available and greater numbers of mentally ill are being treated in the community, concern has been raised that the quality of care and life of the chronically mentally ill has not changed. Concerned about the isolation and lack of treatment available to many chronically ill living in board and care homes, Bachrach[3] voiced the possibility that the back wards of public mental hospitals have merely been transferred to the board and care homes in the community. The right to adequate psychiatric care (*Wyatt vs. Stickney*) is ironically a right belonging to involuntarily committed patients. At present, in the United States voluntary patients have no guaranteed right to adequate psychiatric care.

The right to refuse treatment

To be valid, consent to treatment must be given by an individual who is knowledgeable about the nature and consequences of the choice being made, who is choosing voluntarily, and who is free to withdraw consent at any time without penalty. That is, the consent must be "competent, knowledgeable, and voluntary."[15] Nurses beginning to work with psychiatric patients often believe that the presence of mental illness negates the patient's competency to give informed consent. Involuntary commitment to a psychiatric hospital does not necessarily mean that patients cannot make informed and knowledgeable choices about their care. When patients are competent to give informed consent, they must be allowed a choice about their care. Given the intrusiveness of many psychiatric treatment interventions, particularly ECT and psychosurgery, it is imperative that patients are involved in deciding whether to participate in such treatments. Increasing evidence about the long-term side effects of psychotropic medications and the availability of long-acting intramuscular drugs, such as fluphenazine decanoate (Prolixin), has focused attention on the patient's right to refuse medication.[15]

If patients are not competent to make informed decisions about their care, they can be declared mentally incompetent by the court and a guardian appointed. The court-appointed guardian then participates in the informed consent process and makes knowledgeable decisions about the patient's treatment.

Confidentiality

As with civil commitment, the ethical and legal issues around confidentiality must strike a balance between the rights of the patient and society's right to protection from the consequences of the patient's illness. Additionally, insurance companies and health care professionals have legitimate needs for information from the patient's records. As the chronically mentally ill travel from agency to agency within the community, as well as between community agencies and psychiatric hospitals, the need for professional sharing of information about the patient increases. As a general principle, the patient's written consent must be obtained before health status information can be released or exchanged. At times agencies have patients sign a blanket permission for release of information on admission. This is not adequate protection of the patient's right to confidentiality. The patient has the right to know what information is being released, to whom it is being released, and for what purpose and under what circumstances it is being released. Such conditions require specific forms for each situation in which information is being released. As with other instances of informed consent, the patient has the right to withdraw consent, without penalty, at any time.[15]

At times, however, the right of society to information supersedes the patient's right to confidentiality. In *Tarasoff vs. Board of Regents of the University of California (1976),* the California Supreme Court ruled that the therapist is required to violate the confidentiality of the therapeutic relationship in circumstances in which the therapist "knew or should have known that the patient posed a danger of imminent physical harm to others."[15]

Employment

Issues surrounding the employment and pay of the mentally ill are not limited to employment in the community. In the past, large public psychiatric hospitals were largely self-supporting, with the patients providing much of the labor to run the hospitals' farms, bakeries, sewing rooms, kitchens, laundries, and housekeeping departments. Although work assignments were therapeutic at times, there were many instances of abuse: long hours, working conditions, and lack of monetary compensation provided for labor. The conditions under which patients worked often contributed to their sense of exploitation and worthlessness and limited the therapeutic potential of such activities.

An important ruling protecting patients from providing labor without adequate compensation occurred as the result of *Souder vs. Brennan* (1973). A federal district court ruled that provisions of the 1966 amendments to the Fair Labor Standards Act applied to institutional residents who provided labor. Residents were to receive minimum wages and overtime pay. Since the Souder decision, a consortium of states success-

fully challenged the right of the federal government to regulate the minimum wage in state-run institutions. Thus the federal requirement that institutions pay their residents minimum wages applies to private, not public, institutions.[15]

Employment is an even more critical issue once the mentally ill return to the community. It is one variable used to evaluate treatment program effectiveness. Federal regulations protecting the handicapped from discrimination apply to those with mental impairment, as well as those with physical impairment. Although the handicapped must be able to manage the essential features of a job to be hired, employers can be expected to make reasonable accommodation to special needs of handicapped persons. In job interviews the potential employer is prohibited from asking questions about the handicap and must limit questions to "specific abilities and talents." Furthermore, employers are prohibited from discriminating against the handicapped in terms of salary and benefits.[15]

The development of chronic mental illness

The chronically mentally ill are likely to have both primary and secondary symptoms of their illness. Primary symptoms are those associated with the intrinsic nature of the illness. For example, hallucinations, delusions, and inappropriate affect would be primary symptoms of schizophrenia, and elation and hyperactivity would be primary symptoms of manic-depressive illness. Secondary symptoms are a consequence of the illness process and are not only associated with the disability of chronic illness, but also perpetuate its existence. The progression from primary symptoms to secondary symptoms and ultimately the label "chronically mentally ill" is further understood by more specific examination of the interaction between an individual and his environment.

The behaviors of mentally ill individuals that are associated with the primary symptoms of psychiatric illness are likely to violate social norms and standards of proper conduct and may be considered deviant behavior. These deviant behaviors set in motion a social interactive process whereby society protects itself from the norm violation of the deviant. As this process unfolds individuals increasingly assume the self-identity "mentally ill" and relate to society more often in terms of this identity, rather than in terms of other available identities, such as wife, mother, husband, father, or worker. The ultimate acceptance of the deviant status mentally ill and adjustment to society in terms of this role are accompanied by the many secondary symptoms of chronic mental illness.

The process by which society and the individual interact to the end of conferring/accepting the role of deviant (chronically mentally ill) has been outlined by Lemert[20] as the following eight-step process:

1. Individual instances of deviant behavior; role and status are not defined at this time in terms of a deviant identity
2. Social penalties
3. Further deviant behavior
4. Stronger penalties and rejection of the individual with the deviant behavior
5. Further deviant behavior, perhaps with hostilities and resentment beginning to focus on those doing the penalizing
6. Crisis reached in society's tolerance quotient, expressed in formal action by the community stigmatizing the deviant
7. Strengthening of the deviant conduct as a reaction to the stigmatizing and penalties
8. Ultimate acceptance of deviant social status and efforts at adjustment based on an associated role

As Lemert's social interaction model demonstrates, the disability of chronic mental illness does not suddenly appear, but develops over a period of time as an exchange between individuals with deviant behaviors and the world within which they live. Similarly, through their attention to the "natural history" of chronic illness, public health epidemiologists view chronic illness not as a state or end point but as a process of progressive deterioration. According to the public health model, individuals with a chronic illness show increasing symptoms of functional impairment and disability as they move sequentially through the four stages of the "natural history" of chronic illness. The first stage, *susceptibility,* is a period of exposure to risk factors; the second stage, *presymptomatic disease,* is the period within which pathological changes begin; the third stage, *clinical disease,* is the period within which primary symptoms of the disease are recognizable; and the fourth stage, *disability,* is the period within which there are identifiable changes in both activity

TABLE 30-1. Stages of the natural history of chronic illness*

Stage	Characteristics
Susceptibility	Presence of environmental, biological, behavioral, and emotional risk factors
Presymptomatic disease	No overt symptoms of disease; pathological changes begin; risk factors intensify; behaviors increasing susceptibility solidify and become patterns
Clinical disease	Anatomical and functional changes occur; presence of recognizable disease symptoms
Disability	Disease symptoms increase; anatomical and functional changes produce reduction in activity; impairment of instrumental or expressive function

*Modified from Anderson, S., and Bauwens, E.: Chronic health problems: concepts and application, St. Louis, 1981, The C.V. Mosby Co.

level and role performance.[1] See Table 30-1 for a description of the characteristics of these four stages.

Description of the chronically mentally ill

Elaboration of the special characteristics of the chronically mentally ill portrays a population with difficulties with activities of daily living, maintaining interpersonal relations, lack of coping resources, and a need for long-term treatment.[9] Other characteristics influencing the course of their illness are their consistently low self-esteem and preoccupation with avoidance of failure rather than the achievement of success.[28] The chronically mentally ill, as a group, can be described not only in terms of the problems confronting the group but also in terms of the group's unique strengths and potentials. There is tentative evidence that the kinds of interpersonal strengths available to this population differ from those available to the general population.

Activities of daily living

When nurses refer to activities of daily living (ADL), they are usually referring to the complex of behaviors necessary to maintain independence in personal hygiene, dressing, and grooming. The use of the term when referring to the chronically mentally ill has an expanded meaning, referring to the skills necessary to live independently as an adult. At times professionals caring for the chronically mentally ill use the broader term *psychosocial rehabilitation* when referring to development of the many skills necessary for independent living.

If the premise that the chronically mentally ill relate to their world essentially in terms of the role "mentally ill" is accepted, it follows that these patients would have difficulty meeting the multiple functional requirements of an adult in the United States. Impairment in instrumental role performance is one of the characteristics of disability, the end stage of the progressive deterioration of individuals with chronic mental illness.[1] Individuals are considered legally disabled when they have impairment of instrumental role performance in at least three of the following areas: "self-care, receptive and expressive language, learning, mobility, self-direction, capacity for independent living, and self-sufficiency."[16]

Interpersonal relations

Over the years, patients in public mental hospitals have been described as apathetic, withdrawn, and isolated from other patients and their family. They have been described as possessing only the minimum of interpersonal skills. The process leading to impoverished interpersonal relations has been thought not to be a primary symptom of their mental illness, but rather a secondary symptom resulting from adaptation to life in a rigid and nonstimulating environment. The term *social breakdown syndrome* was coined to describe the progressive deterioration of the social and interpersonal skills of long-term psychiatric patients.[17] However, evidence is accumulating that chronically mentally ill patients who have spent most of their life in the community, with brief periods of hospitalization during acute crises, have the same deterioration of social and interpersonal skills as those who have had long-term hospitalizations. Studies of the social activities of the chronically mentally ill support the conclusion that these patients "lead an unusually barren and isolated existence."[21] Generalizing from a study of all non-hospitalized California residents who received social security because of a psychiatric disability, fewer than 50% were employed or had any structured activity around which to orient their lives.[19] The question must now be asked whether the social breakdown syndrome of the chronically mentally ill is in fact causally related to long-term hospitalization, or whether there might be another explanation for the syndrome's

appearing in patients cared for in both the hospital and in the community. Minkoff[21] wrote, "Those who tend to be more active socially, tend to be less chronic, married and employed and characterize a group of high functioning mentally ill whose lives stand apart from the more dreary existence of the rest."

Lack of coping resources

The social isolation, lack of support systems, and functional impairment of the chronically mentally ill leave them with minimal coping skills to use in dealing with stress. Social margin, as defined by Segal, Baumohl, and Johnson,[30] is the sum total of "all the personal possessions, attributes, or relationships which can be traded on for help in time of need." It is, in effect, the sum total of resources available to the individual. With a nearly nonexistent social margin, the chronically mentally ill are likely to respond to stress and the necessity for adaptation as a crisis. (See Chapter 20.)

Need for long-term treatment

Implicit in the concept, "chronicity" is the notion of illness over time. Federal policy makers acknowledge the need for long-term treatment in labeling patients as having a "chronic mental disability" when they have had either one episode of at least 6 months of continuous hospitalization within the past 5 years or two or more hospitalizations in a 12-month period.[21] Given the marginal existence of the chronically mentally ill living in the community and their vulnerability to stress, it is not surprising that within a year of their discharge from the hospital, 40% are expected to be readmitted.[3] Treatment factors that facilitate patients' maintenance in the community are the patient's compliance with a medication regimen and the patient's involvement in aftercare programs.[21] Because of their need for long-term treatment, whether in residential institutions or from community-based facilities, the proper focus of treatment for the chronically mentally ill is care and rehabilitation rather than cure.

Low self-esteem

Self-esteem is the feeling or sense of regard that accompanies individuals' self-perceptions.

It is "the personal judgement of worthiness that is expressed in the attitudes of an individual to himself . . . it indicates the extent to which an individual believes himself to be capable, significant, worthy."[10] As part of an extensive research project, Fitts[12,13] found the self-esteem of psychiatric patients to be lower, in all areas, especially in the areas of identity and behavior, than the self-esteem of the general population. The self-esteem of the chronically mentally ill parallels that of psychiatric patients,[6] and the chronically mentally ill suffer from the many perceptual and behavioral difficulties associated with low self-esteem. (See Chapter 8.) A description of the characteristics of an individual with low self-esteem is also a description of the chronically mentally ill individual:

Persons with low self-esteem . . . have come to believe they are powerless and without resource or recourse. They feel isolated, unlovable, incapable of expressing and defending themselves, and too weak to overcome their deficiencies. Too immobilized to take action, they tend to withdraw and become overly passive and compliant while suffering the pangs of anxiety and symptoms that accompany its chronic occurrence.[10:250]

Motivation

As described earlier, the chronically mentally ill have difficulty in achieving a level of psychosocial functioning that would allow them to live comfortably in the community. For many patients, success and greater competence are followed by increased anxiety and symptoms of regression, rather than by pride and the sense of improved well-being. Patients attribute their uneasiness with success to the fear that once they succeed, even more will be expected of them, and they may not be able to meet the new expectations.

Chronically mentally ill patients have experienced repeated failures. They have not met the expectations of family, friends, or society, but most important, they have not met their own expectations. New experiences, rather than being seen as opportunities for growth, are seen as opportunities for further failure. Studies of psychiatric patients, living both in institutions and in the community, support the observation that when compared with the general population, psychiatric patients are much more concerned with avoiding failure than they are with achieving success.[28] A pattern of motivation that is based on the avoidance of failure, rather than the achievement of success, not only produces resistance to involvement in new experiences, but also makes it difficult for the chronically mentally ill to acknowledge and assume responsibility for their personal achievements.

Strengths

Rehabilitation of the chronically mentally ill depends on the control of illness, as well as on the development of health potential by mobilizing patients' ego strengths. A strength is an "ability, skill, or interest" an individual has previously used.[22] Categories of individual strengths, as derived from work with assumed healthy nonpsychiatric patient groups are as follows:

Sports and outdoor activities
Hobbies and crafts
Expressive arts
Health
Education, training, and related areas
Work, vocation, job, or position
Special aptitudes or resources
Strengths through family and others
Intellectual strengths
Aesthetic strengths
Organizational strengths
Imaginative and creative strengths
Relationship strengths[23]

Although the assessment and description of patients' strengths is largely an individual matter and the profile of strengths will vary from patient to patient, there is initial evidence that the relationship strengths of the chronically mentally ill differ from those of a nonpatient population.

Concerned with the development of healthy interpersonal relationships, Porter[26] defined interpersonal strength as a "behavior trait . . . so employed as to enhance the production of mutual gratification between one's self and another person without violating the integrity of either person." According to Porter, interpersonal strengths cluster around three basic motivational patterns or orientations in interpersonal relationships. These are the "altruistic-nurturing" motivational pattern, the "assertive-directing" motivational pattern, and the "analytic-autonomizing" motivational pattern. Associated with each of the motivational patterns are positive goals in terms of interpersonal relationships. Individuals with strengths associated with the

TABLE 30-2. **Behind the weaknesses are strengths***

Altruistic-nurturing		Assertive-directing		Analytic-autonomizing	
Characteristic strengths	Risks	Characteristic strengths	Risks	Characteristic strengths	Risks
Trusting	Gullible	Self-confident	Arrogant	Cautious	Suspicious
Optimistic	Impractical	Enterprising	Opportunistic	Practical	Unimaginative
Loyal	Slavish	Ambitious	Ruthless	Economical	Stingy
Idealistic	Wishful	Organizing	Controlling	Reserved	Cold
Helpful	Self-denying	Persuasive	Pressuring	Methodical	Rigid
Modest	Self-effacing	Forceful	Dictatorial	Analytic	Nitpicking
Devoted	Self-sacrificing	Quick to act	Rash	Principled	Unbending
Caring	Smothering	Imaginative	Dreamer	Orderly	Compulsive
Supportive	Submissive	Competitive	Combative	Fair	Unfeeling
Accepting	Passive	Proud	Conceited	Persevering	Stubborn
Polite	Deferential	Bold	Brash	Conserving	Possessive
Adaptable	Without principle	Risk taking	Gambler	Thorough	Obsessive

*From Coopersmith, S.: The antecedents of self-esteem, Palo Alto, Calif., Consulting Psychologists Press, Inc. (1967), 1981.

altruistic-nurturing motivational pattern report their goal in interpersonal relations to be that of being genuinely helpful, with little regard for what they consequently received from others. Individuals having strengths associated with the assertive-directive pattern report their desire to lead others in a way that does not interfere with others' rights. The goal or desire behind the strengths associated with the analytic-auto-nomizing motivational pattern is to create order, becoming self-reliant and independent. The interpersonal strengths of the nonpatient population are evenly divided among those of the three motivational patterns and represent nurturing strengths, leading strengths, and analyzing strengths (Table 30-2).

Initial evidence supports the premise that the relationship strengths of the chronically mentally ill are not evenly divided among the three motivational patterns as are those of nonpatients. When interpersonal relationships are going well, the chronically mentally ill perceive themselves as mobilizing the nurturing strengths of the altruistic-nurturing motivational pattern. They feel good about themselves when they are genuinely caring for someone else, with little regard for what they receive in return. In conflictual interpersonal situations their strengths are those of the peacemaker. Aware of the personal cost of their peacemaking efforts, they will insist, probably explosively, that their rights be respected if harmony and peace cannot be restored.[6]

The young adult chronically mentally ill patient

The characteristics of the chronically mentally ill previously discussed describe the chronically mentally ill regardless of their age. However, researchers are beginning to describe the "young" chronic patient, generally between the ages of 18 to 35, as differing in important ways from the chronically mentally ill who are over 35 years of age. Many of the differences in the two groups of patients can be traced to the de-institutionalization movement and the development of community-based care as an alternative to hospital-based care.[24]

Generally, chronically mentally ill patients under 35 have not experienced lengthy psychiatric hospitalizations as have older psychiatric patients. For those under 35, recurrent short hospitalizations at times of crisis or during periods of acute exacerbation of symptoms have alternated with care in the community. The personal requirements for adaptation to long-term hospitalization are different from the requirements for adaptation to community life interspersed with short hospitalizations.

Patients who have spent years in psychiatric hospitals have been confronted over and over with their personal failure in terms of meeting their own, their family's, and society's expectations. In most instances older chronic patients have traded personal autonomy and adult functioning in roles such as father, mother, husband, wife, and employee for a life of personal dependence and the role of psychiatric patient. Through socialization into this role, chronic patients become compliant and nonassertive, and their social participation is likely to be limited to the social and geographical boundaries of the hospital or perhaps even the ward where they live. Although such adaptation may provide limited potential for growth, it does provide relief from the seemingly impossible demands of age-appropriate role expectations and continuing confrontation with failure.

Younger chronically ill patients do not have such protection from bombardment with messages as to their inadequacy and the resulting sense of failure. Alternating between hospital and community life, they compare themselves with others of their age and continue to expect of themselves behavior similar to that of their nonpatient peers. They expect that they should marry, have children and jobs, and perhaps even acquire advanced education. Given their failure in managing the role expectations of others their age and their limited ability to cope with the many tasks of community living, it is not surprising that the young chronically mentally ill are "acutely vulnerable to stress."[24] Generalizing from a study of nearly 300 patients, 42% of this population of young chronic psychiatric patients "present a risk of suicide for reasons that include the simple fact that they see no hope for the future."[24] They cannot see a future in which they will have the abilities to meet the ongoing demands of their daily lives.

Younger chronically mentally ill patients are not characterized by docile compliant behavior as are long-term hospital residents. They do not see themselves as mentally ill but as social casualties, unfortunate victims of social circumstances.[24] Not having been hospitalized for long periods of time, the younger chronically ill patient has not been socialized into the compliant nonassertive behavior associated with the older chronically ill patient. Their self-concept, ac-

companied by their particular symptoms, especially disorders of impulse control and disturbances of affect,[29] have important consequences in terms of supporting their marginal life-style.

Involvement in treatment

Because they do not see themselves as patients, there is little motivation to become involved in aftercare or treatment programs or to comply with a medication regimen. For example, a study of more than 100 young chronically mentally ill patients living in New York City found that only 17% complied with their aftercare plan.[8] Involvement in aftercare programs and maintenance on a medication regimen have been previously identified as critical factors for maintenance of the chronically mentally ill in the community.

Further interfering with their involvement in a therapeutic relationship is the general affective response of anger, which manifests itself in the sarcastic and argumentative manner in which these patients relate to the caregivers from whom they seek help. Caregivers report feeling frustrated and helpless when confronted by the many problems of this group of patients, and the manner in which they seek help. This behavior has been labeled "help-seeking–help-rejecting behavior."

Entry into the mental health system

Because their pathological condition interferes with voluntary involvement in treatment programs and ongoing participation in a therapeutic relationship, the younger chronically ill patient is likely to enter the mental health system through hospital emergency rooms or the legal system. Younger patients may seek help from emergency rooms either voluntarily or at the insistence of family or friends during times of personal or family crisis. Behavior resulting from their poor impulse control is often the precipitating event for the crisis. Schwartz and Goldfinger[29] reported that although suicidal threats and self-damaging acts are common, impulsive acts against others are less frequent. However, many of these patients enter the mental health system through involvement with the law for offenses such as "minor property damage" and "petty assault." Likewise, Caton[8] found the arrest rate of young chronically mentally ill patients to be eight times that of the general population in the areas in which the patients lived.

The symptoms and style of interpersonal relationships of the younger chronically mentally ill patients seem to interact nonproductively with present treatment resources. Further description of the special characteristics of this rapidly expanding subgroup must continue if programs suitable to their needs are to be developed.

Psychosocial rehabilitation: the Fountain House model

Ronald Peterson, a veteran of 10 years of residence in a state hospital, speaks poignantly of the loneliness and isolation he felt when he left the state hospital to live alone in a small hotel room. Since he had no job, knew no one, and lived on welfare, it never occurred to him that it could be any different. He said, "You take what you can get. There is no choice."[25] Now a staff member of Fountain House, a psychosocial rehabilitation program, Peterson speaks for many chronically mentally ill persons who are trying to adjust to community living when he describes their greatest need to be a place where they belong and are needed:

I think the greatest need is to have a place to go where you are expected each day, a place where you can be with people like yourself and do things that mean something to yourself and others . . . you have to remember that many of us did a lot of things in the hospital. If given a chance we can do lots of things in the community—if we have places to go and can be with people who need us to contribute, to take part, to help, and who notice when we're not present and do something about it.[25:41,42]

In making a judgment as to the effectiveness of any treatment program for the chronically mentally ill, the program's readmission and employment rates are compared with baseline readmission and employment data.[23] As a baseline it is expected that 6 months after leaving the hospital 30% to 40% of the patients will be rehospitalized. And, with regard to employment, 6 months after leaving the hospital it is expected that 30% to 50% will be employed. The percentage decreases to 20% to 30% after 12 months and to 25% after 3 to 5 years. Despite a lack of adequate follow-up studies of the fate of chronically mentally ill individuals returned to the community, it is generally believed that community-based treatment programs are inadequate.

One exception to this situation, Fountain House in New York City, has been described as an excellent program for assisting chronically ill psychiatric patients in making a place for themselves in the community and has been advocated as a model to be used in developing programs across the country.[7,32] For the first 5 years after returning to the community, Fountain House members have a 40% lower rehospitalization rate than the baseline percentage. After 9 years, Fountain House's rehospitalization rates are similar to the baseline rate. However, when hospitalization is needed, Fountain House members are hospitalized for only half the usual number of days.[11] Critical to Fountain House's success is attention to psychosocial rehabilitation, especially in terms of facilitating independence of living and employment.

Incorporating elements from the medical, rehabilitation, and social support models, psychosocial rehabilitation provides a variety of living and work opportunities to individually accommodate the needs and functional abilities of patients as they begin to live in the community. Staff not only help patients develop skills necessary to assume increasing independence in living and working, but they serve as buffers between the patient and the community, in a sense, by lending their own skills and competency to the patients until the patients can develop these skills for themselves. Compensating for patient's functional inadequacies while encouraging them to assume increasing responsibility, allows the patients to experience the pride of achievement rather than the pain and humiliation of failure. Basic to this rehabilitation process is focusing on the strengths of Fountain House members:

Fountain House attributes the state of isolation and alienation of its new members to the process of illness which initially brings the members to Fountain House—but it is the strengths and capabilities of each individual that validates his belonging and are the beginning of the discovery that he is worth something and may be able to achieve at least reasonably full participation in community life.[7:86]

Fountain House functions as a club in which patients are no longer patients, but members, and the usual hierarchical distinctions between staff (the healthy) and patients (the ill) do not exist. It is a place where members care about each other and pool their resources and abilities as they work toward increasing independence. Thus Fountain House combats loneliness and isolation while providing a variety of living and work situations that require differing levels of functional ability.

The first month at Fountain House is a residential phase, and residents are taught skills necessary for apartment living. Fountain House owns and leases apartments that have staff on call, although not in residence. These supervised apartments allow for a gradual transition to independent living situations in the community.

Fountain House runs several businesses itself and can provide work experiences in a protected environment in which patients can develop both self-confidence and transferable job skills. Progressing to a more complex work situation, Fountain House has creatively arranged for transitional employment placements, called TEPs. Recognizing that the job interview is a tremendously stressful experience for recently discharged psychiatric patients and is often seen as an obstacle that cannot be overcome, staff, rather than patients, seek out and contract with businesses for jobs. The jobs are assigned to Fountain House rather than to individual patients. Staff are then free to assign a patient to a transitional employment position for as long as needed. The employer is promised that if patients are unable to manage the job, or even portions of the job, or do not show up, Fountain House staff will cover for them. With such an arrangement, the dreaded employment interview is avoided. Fountain House members who share responsibility for a job with staff, can be delegated increasing responsibility as they are able to handle it, and a TEP can easily be transferred from one member who is ready for a more complex work experience to a member who needs a TEP. Furthermore, employers are satisfied because the quality of work is guaranteed by the staff. Again in the words of Peterson who tried a number of part-time TEPs:

> If you have the chance to go to work without having to pass a lot of hurdles first, you discover things. All of us found we could do parts of the job real well, but we couldn't do so well on other things. . . .[25:42,43]

Nursing care of the chronically mentally ill

Although there are many similarities in the needs of the chronically mentally ill, whether they are being cared for in inpatient units, community psychosocial rehabilitation programs, or emergency service, the health care setting in which the nurse cares for the chronically mentally ill influences the scope and priorities of nursing care.

Psychosocial rehabilitation programs

Nurses working in community-based psychosocial rehabilitation programs are ultimately concerned with assisting patients to achieve their fullest potential in terms of independent living and adequate interpersonal relations. In this situation nurses have the opportunity for long-term ongoing relationships with patients and the mutual setting of long-term goals. The nurses' functions will vary. For example, they may be on call for assistance to patients living in supervised apartments. Others may be active participants in a day treatment milieu, both creating situations for growth and serving as process observers to the patient so that he may benefit from analyzing his behavior as he functions in the therapeutic milieu. Nurses may also provide a formally structured educational experience, such as teaching patients about community resources, skills necessary for independent living, or self-care behaviors that facilitate health maintenance. They may participate in a variety of work programs with patients or may even be backing a patient up in a transitional work placement. If the nurse has had additional training and supervision, she may function in the expanded role of group leader or co-leader, conduct family meetings, or assume responsibility as the patient's primary therapist.

In most psychosocial rehabilitation programs the nurse works as a team member with other mental health professionals and nonprofessionals. Although the role and function of the nurse is always bounded by the nurse practice act of the state in which she is practicing, it varies from program to program, depending on the nature of the program and the available resources.

In some programs the nurse may be asked to function as "case manager" for a group of patients. This role cuts across professional boundaries and is based on two premises; that the chronically mentally ill have difficulty in establishing interpersonal relationships and that because of their many social, vocational, and health needs, services are likely to be needed from a variety of sources. At a minimum, the patient needs access or a link to family, friends, housing, and a source of income. Case managers are responsible for identifying, securing, and coordinating all the resources, from both folk and professional support systems, necessary for the patient's life in the community. When the patient is assigned a case manager, he does not have to independently negotiate relationships with the many individuals from whom services are needed. After an assessment process, the case manager is responsible for providing a 24-

hour plan with links to activities and services for coordinating the activities of those involved, monitoring both the quality of service provided and the patient's response to the 24-hour plan, and functioning as an advocate, intervening on the patient's behalf when necessary.

The case manager role and the role of primary nurse are similar in that both have accountability and responsibility not only for the development of a 24-hour plan of care but also for its implementation and evaluation. They are also similar in that it is easier for the patient, especially for a chronically mentally ill patient, to organize his requests for assistance around one person, rather than negotiating individual requests with a variety of persons. However, unlike the role of primary nurse, the case manager role, as generally conceived, is also concerned with the development of a social network, an area of responsibility typically associated with the social worker. A nurse fulfilling this function can enlarge the scope of the 24-hour plan to include a plan for meeting nursing and health care needs as well.

Acute care settings

Conceptualization of care of the chronically mentally ill as a shared responsibility between the community and residential inpatient facilities means that the focus of care is different in different settings. Because the chronically mentally ill are likely to disengage from community treatment programs, have ongoing difficulties in complying with a medication regimen, and are acutely vulnerable to stress, there may be periods of acute exacerbation of symptoms and the need for inpatient hospitalization. The goal of care in an acute treatment setting then becomes crisis resolution, with control of acute symptoms. The patient is helped to return to a pre-crisis level of functioning as quickly as possible so that he can return to the community, where he can continue to receive support and treatment in a less restrictive environment.

As with any acutely ill psychiatric patient, the nurse, after completing a nursing assessment, makes a nursing diagnosis and plans nursing interventions that help the patient cope with his behavioral responses to his illness. Given that chronically mentally ill patients are admitted to inpatient units for crisis intervention, the nurse working in such a setting must have a thorough understanding of the theory of crisis intervention and be skilled in its implementation. The specific factors to be assessed as the nurse attempts to understand the nature of the crisis and

its effect on the patient are those identified in Chapter 20. That is, assessment must be made of the precipitating event, the patient's strengths and previous coping mechanisms, and the nature and strength of the patient's support systems. Intervention may be in terms of any of the four levels of intervention: environmental manipulation; general support; generic intervention, especially in terms of what is known about grief work; and particularly in the area of individual intervention, which depends on an understanding of the meaning of the precipitating event to an individual at a certain moment in time and an awareness of the resources available to that patient at that point. An individual approach, by definition, is idiosyncratic in nature and depends on the development of a competent nurse-patient relationship for its implementation.

Primary nursing, one of several modalities of providing nursing care, has several advantages in terms of meeting the needs of chronically mentally ill patients hospitalized during periods of acute exacerbation of symptoms. The most obvious advantage is that once assigned a primary nurse, the acutely ill patient, who is likely to have difficulties establishing interpersonal relationships, knows who is responsible for his care and can focus his energies on developing a trusting relationship with one person who will look out for him and intercede on his behalf when necessary. And, because the chronically mentally ill patient is likely to have recurrent inpatient admissions, the same primary nurse can be assigned to him for each admission. Consistent assignment of patients to primary nurses for each admission has advantages for both patients and nurses. It is assumed that it would be easier for an acutely ill patient to feel safe when cared for by a nurse he already knows. Prior knowledge of the patient provides the nurse with a historical data bank of information about the patient, including the patient's past responses to particular nursing interventions. This should expedite nursing care on subsequent admissions; it certainly should facilitate family and community involvement in the patient's care in that the primary nurse, agency staff, and family members probably were involved with each other on previous admissions and already have working relationships established.

But perhaps an even more important consequence of primary nursing and consistency of assignment is the primary nurse's sense of the patient's progress over time. If the patient has been making incremental gains, however small, in a community rehabilitation program, the goal of crisis therapy during successive admissions would be return to a steadily increasing functional level. Thus rather than acknowledging only the repeated admissions of the chronically mentally ill, the primary nurse working in an acute care setting can document the successes and progress the patient experienced while in the community. These observations can then be used to combat the discouragement and sense of hopelessness occasionally experienced by both herself and the patient and find the energy needed to continue the rehabilitation process.

Developing patients' strengths and potentials

Rehabilitation has been conceptualized as the "process of actualizing the remaining potentialities and abilities of a handicapped person."[14] Psychosocial rehabilitation programs, such as Fountain House, attribute their success to focusing on the strengths patients bring with them. The rehabilitation model of care is as concerned with maximizing wellness as with the control of disease or pathological conditions. Nursing also accepts responsibility for the promotion of wellness and the improvement of patients' health status by the development of their health potentials. This view of nursing is consistently reflected in the models of nursing being developed by nursing scholars.

The following discussion focuses on nursing interventions that facilitate the development of patients' strengths and potentials, because of the importance of these interventions in the care of chronically mentally ill patients. Such interventions, however, do not occur in isolation, but as part of the implementation of the nursing process, with the development of an individual plan of care only after completion of a nursing assessment. The principles of developing and implementing nursing care plans for psychiatric patients, as described in this text, also apply in the care of chronically mentally ill patients.

The development of chronically mentally ill patients' strengths and potentials is important for several reasons. Nursing interventions that develop patients' strengths and potentials can help the chronically mentally ill develop their independent living skills, adequacy in interpersonal relationships, and coping resources and thus help meet their special needs. Such nursing interventions also help patients alter their motivational style, increasing their willingness to become involved in growth-producing situations. Ultimately the expected outcome of such interventions would be changes in the patient's self-concept and an increase in self-esteem.

Dr. Vallory Lathrop, a leader in forensic psychiatric nursing, remarked that she would be pleased to receive a nickel from every patient who, when asked to name one of his strengths, responded that he did not have any. The negative self-concept and low self-esteem that characterize the chronically mentally ill as a group interfere with their ability to experience themselves as individuals with strengths and potentials.

Rogers[27] wrote that a therapeutic experience was one in which experiences contradictory to the individual's self-concept were brought into awareness and accepted as part of oneself. Through environmental and interpersonal experiences of adequacy, self-concept can be altered and self-esteem increased. One nursing intervention that assists patients in altering their negative self-perceptions and thereby increases their health potential is to identify with patients their strengths as perceived by the nurse in the here-and-now experiences of patients' participation in the psychiatric milieu. Nursing interventions in which patients become aware of their strengths fall into two major categories: those which occur as a response to the patient's spontaneous participation in the milieu and those which occur as part of a structured intervention in which the nurse, or the nurse and the patient together, plan an experience in which the patient can mobilize his strengths and develop his potentials. The following clinical examples illustrate the nurse's use of two spontaneously occurring situations to increase a patient's awareness of her strengths.

CLINICAL EXAMPLE 30-1

During a 1-hour period a nurse made the following observations. Marie, a frightened 22-year-old young woman who was psychotic as the result of PCP use was sitting in the craft room. The nurse joined Marie. Janet, another patient, came in and heaped clothes that were still warm from the dryer in Marie's lap. (Janet had voluntarily done Marie's laundry when she noticed Marie having trouble with the dial on the washing machine.)

JANET: **Here are your clean clothes.**

MARIE: **Silence, continues drawing.**

NURSE: **Do you want some help folding these clothes? It looks hard to draw with such a full lap.**

MARIE: **No, I'm fine, except my head gets dizzy.**

JANET: **That's from your medicine. Didn't you just start on your medicine?**

MARIE: **Yes.**

JANET: **It'll get better soon. It takes a few days to get used to your medicine. You're drawing a Christmas picture. Merry Christmas and Happy New Year. You're thinking about wanting to be home for Christmas aren't you?**

MARIE: **Shakes her head yes.**

JANET: **Your picture sure makes me think of how nice home is at Christmas, except we don't have a fireplace. But having a fireplace doesn't make Christmas. Being home with a family you love does. (Janet continues showing the nurse other artwork that Marie has done, praising her ability.)**

Another patient and the recreational therapist came into the room. The therapist changed the music from soul music to a classical symphony. Both Janet and Marie disapproved of the new music. Marie began to look more tense. Janet put her arm around her and said, "Come on. Let's go walk in the hall." They left together.

Later, when the nurse saw Janet in the dayroom, the nurse shared with Janet that she saw her as having been very helpful to Marie. Janet grinned broadly and said "Yeah, I'm a real friend to her. It feels good."

Although the strengths identified in this sequence, caring and helping, are consistent with the altruistic-nurturing motivational pattern that is most characteristic of this population, they are not the only strengths which occur spontaneously in the milieu. Patients have many opportunities for demonstrating behaviors reflective of leadership strengths, strengths in problem solving, or in increased autonomy among others. A different kind of strength is evident in Clinical example 30-2.

CLINICAL EXAMPLE 30-2

A nurse walking down the hall saw a patient who had made a serious suicidal attempt 2 days earlier alone in the kitchen furiously cleaning out the refrigerator. The nurse joined the patient and began helping the patient clean the refrigerator. As they talked, the patient expressed concern that many of the feelings which led to the previous suicidal attempt were returning. She had initiated the cleaning project to attempt to control her feelings. The nurse defined the cleaning as a strength in that it was more adaptive than another suicidal attempt. As the nurse shared this observation with the patient the patient momen-

tarily looked surprised and then said, "I hadn't thought of it that way. Maybe I am better than I was before."

Nurses with general knowledge of the patients on a ward or in a psychosocial rehabilitation program can share with the patient their impression of his or her strengths, as they see them naturally occur. Nurses who have an ongoing therapeutic relationship with a smaller group of patients can reflect to these patients very individualized observations of strengths in areas that are uniquely relevant to these patients. These interventions may be in response to behaviors that occur spontaneously. They may also be in response to a structured growth experience that was arranged as an intervention for a nursing diagnosis which was formulated from a careful and thorough nursing assessment. The following structured nursing interventions occurred in a community-based psychosocial rehabilitation program.

CLINICAL EXAMPLE 30-3

Theresa, a woman in her 50s, had been in and out of psychiatric hospitals for 30 years and had been living in a supervised apartment in the community for 1 year. One of her nursing diagnoses was difficulty in dealing with interpersonal conflict because of her fear of her aggressive impulses. Theresa shared the apartment with two roommates. She was a talented musician and had her own baby grand piano. Despite her love for classical music, she only played the "oldies and goodies" her roommates preferred. She said that she didn't want to upset her roommates by practicing classical music. She was afraid that if she brought the issue out in the open she might get so upset she would hurt someone. She offered as evidence the numerous times she'd been placed in seclusion rooms for violent behavior. Clearly, keeping peace was her priority.

The nurse and Theresa discussed her strengths as a peacemaker, as well as ways in which she might calmly express her own needs to her roommates. The nurse offered to be with Theresa during the discussion. Declining the nurse's offer, Theresa said that even though she was somewhat anxious, she had a clearer understanding of the abilities she had to use in the situation, and she wanted to try to "stick up" for herself in a situation of interpersonal conflict. She carried out her plan and expressed surprise that her roommates accepted her need and quickly arranged 2 hours a day for her to practice. As she told of her success, Theresa smiled, saying she wondered what would have happened if she had tried expressing her needs many months earlier.

Cindy, in her early 20s, had recently moved into the supervised apartment with Theresa and one other roommate. One of Cindy's nursing diagnoses was difficulty in coping with stress related to low self-esteem and feelings of inadequacy. Cindy arrived at the day treatment program crying because she had had a seizure while at her nursing home job the evening before. She felt that in addition to having been embarrassed, she had failed to live up to the trust invested in her by the director of the nursing home. She had decided to quit her job.

The nurse explored with Cindy the meaning of these events in terms of her many strengths in caring for others. Her sensitivity to anticipated criticism and rejection from the director was related to the same sensitivity that allowed her to respond creatively to others' needs. Cindy, at this point, firmly stated that the job was important to her sense of being needed. The nurse encouraged her to call the nursing home, express both her embarrassment and sense of failure, yet, state that she wanted to continue working there. Cindy made the phone call with the nurse present for support. Her pleasure at finding out the job was still hers, that she was not viewed unfavorably by the director of nursing, and her sense of personal achievement at having taken a risk and won was so visible and contagious that the other patients staged an impromptu celebration.

An initial research project by Bell[6] provided some support for the premise that identification and education of the chronically mentally ill about their strengths increases their self-esteem. Another finding was that it is important for nurses to understand the meaning of observed behaviors to their patients, rather than making interpretations from the nurses' own outside perspective. For example, one woman who had been out of the hospital for 2 months, after having lived there 20 years, was seen as continually helping others. When the nurse shared this observation with the patient, the patient responded, "Helping's good, but what really counts is that when I say I'll do something to help someone else, I can count on myself to do what I say." The nurse then redesigned her nursing care plan to include more opportunities for development of the patient's autonomy and independence. As the patient's early efforts at independence and autonomy were acknowledged and supported by staff, the patient set increasingly complex goals for herself. As she

achieved these goals, she expressed how good it made her feel to be able to maintain herself in an independent living situation after so many years in a state institution.

The power of nursing interventions as described depends on the nurse maintaining her professional identity and setting priorities that include participation in the milieu with the patient. Within the context of a competent caring nurse-patient relationship, psychiatric–mental health nurses can make significant contributions to the care of the chronically mentally ill as they support them with one hand and with the other hand invite them to expand their horizons by involvement in growth-producing experiences. As Minkoff[21] stated, "It is only when rehabilitation is not attempted, that hope is truly lost."

Clinical case analysis

Clinical example 30-4 illustrates the "career" and development of increasing disability in a chronically mentally ill man. It focuses attention on several characteristics of chronically mentally ill patients: their low self-esteem, social isolation, involvement with the legal system as a consequence of the secondary symptoms of their illness, and poor coping resources. The example also provides a glimpse of the effect of his illness on his family. Particular attention is given to the nursing care he received when he was admitted to a state psychiatric hospital following a serious suicide attempt.

CLINICAL EXAMPLE 30-4

Abdul, the only son of a large and wealthy Middle Eastern family, came to the United States to pursue a graduate degree in engineering at a prominent university. He had been an outstanding student before coming to the United States but struggled all through his graduate education. He gravitated toward other international students and most of his social activities were with this group of people. He became involved with Ingrid, a graduate student from Germany. When Ingrid became pregnant, they married. Both Abdul and his wife described the discovery of Ingrid's pregnancy as a crisis, but by the time their daughter, Begum, was born, they had reconciled themselves to their situation and, in fact, were excited by the baby's arrival.

Despite the precipitous nature of their marriage, the early years together were pleasant with Abdul and Ingrid enjoying each other and their daughter. Both parents finished their graduate education, with Abdul finding work as an electrical engineer, and his wife finding employment as an assistant professor in the history department of a 4-year college.

By the time the baby, Begum, was 5 years old, Ingrid's parents were living in the United States; there was much visiting between the two families. Since Abdul had not yet introduced Ingrid and Begum to his family, they planned a trip to the Middle East the summer Begum was 5. Abdul's father had a sudden heart attack and died before Abdul and his family arrived. The visit home did not go well. Abdul's family expressed much disappointment in him. They were disappointed that he did not meet the family's standards for material wealth and were even more disappointed that he had not married a Moslem woman. Despite the family's disappointment in Abdul, they exerted much pressure on him to change his plans to return to the United States and remain in the Middle East to assume his proper role as the only son, now the head of the family. At the same time, Ingrid, who was experiencing both culture shock and a feeling of nonacceptance by Abdul's family, insisted on an immediate return to the United States. Abdul returned to the United States feeling disappointed in himself because he had not met his family's expectations and also because he had not been able to speak out in defense of his wife and American daughter.

Life began to deteriorate for Abdul and his family after their return to the United States. Abdul resigned from his engineering position because he believed he wasn't being promoted quickly enough. Although he soon found a position with another reputable company, his work record was increasingly spotty. Some days, Abdul just couldn't make himself get up and go to work. On other days, he'd set out for work, but by midmorning would call Ingrid and tell her he was going to a movie or a museum, followed by a visit to his favorite bar and grill. Abdul found alcohol comforting and began drinking more and more. As Ingrid pressured Abdul to be more responsible about working, Abdul increasingly withdrew and spent much of the time he was home, alone, watching television in his bedroom. Partly in response to her loneliness and sense of helplessness as she watched her husband change, Ingrid overate and began a rapid weight gain, which was accompanied by other physical problems.

After 7 years of university teaching, Ingrid lost her job because she did not meet the requirements for tenure. She began job hunting, but before finding another job, she was involved in a serious car accident and was hospitalized for several weeks. Tension between Abdul and Ingrid increased as a result of the accident. Abdul believed there had been a man in the car with his wife at the time of the accident and accused her of having an affair. This belief was never substantiated, yet Abdul held on to it tenaciously. While his wife was hospitalized, Abdul cared for 7-year-old Begum. However, the day Ingrid returned home from the hospital, Abdul took their car and left, not telling anyone where he was going. After 2 weeks of wandering across the United States, Abdul returned to find he had been fired.

Abdul made no pretense of looking for another job. Welfare funds became the family's sole income. He spent most days alone in his room "tinkering" with one invention or another, listening to Middle Eastern music, or sleeping. Increasingly he slept during the day and stayed up all night. Formerly a fastidious man, he paid little attention to his personal hygiene or nutrition and continued his alcohol consumption. Although he never again left home for any extended time, he periodically disappeared for 2- or 3-day intervals. He always took the family car and was arrested several times for driving without a license or for driving while intoxicated. Invariably Abdul called his wife to rescue him. Ingrid would somehow find money to pay his fine or post bail and would bring him home, where he would once again retreat to his bedroom.

Five years after his visit to the Middle East, Abdul became involved in an altercation with a policeman who stopped him for speeding. As a result of this altercation, Abdul was convicted of "assault" and served a brief jail sentence.

Ingrid was able to convince Abdul to seek psychiatric help after he was released from jail. He was admitted to an inpatient unit of a general hospital. He was given trifluoperazine (Stelazine), desipramine (Pertofrane), benztropine (Cogentin), and diazepam (Valium) and encouraged to participate in the ward milieu. He was not considered ready for discharge when his funds ran out 30 days later. At the encouragement of his psychiatrist, Abdul voluntarily admitted himself to the state mental hospital for continued treatment. Things did not go well for Abdul after his state hospital admission. Worried about Abdul's increasing nonresponsiveness to his environment, Ingrid supported and encouraged Abdul's leaving against medical advice after 3 weeks in the state hospital.

Abdul returned home still receiving medication. He was to attend a medication group at the local CMHC for regulation of his medication. However, he stopped taking his medication soon after he returned home because he did not like the side effects or the feeling that he was being controlled by the medications. He again withdrew to his room, lived a nocturnal existence, and occupied himself inventing electronic gadgets.

In the following year, Abdul made his first suicide attempt. He put a loaded gun into his mouth and pulled the trigger, but the gun didn't fire. He accused "men" who were always aware of his actions of coming into his house and making the gun nonfunctional by jamming it. Abdul was again hospitalized on a psychiatric unit in a general hospital in the community. He was once again given trifluoperazine (Stelazine), desipramine (Pertofrane), and benztropine (Cogentin) and was actively encouraged to participate in the ward milieu. After a month, his seclusive behavior had decreased enough that he was considered ready for discharge. The marital problems identified earlier had intensified sufficiently that couple group therapy was considered the aftercare treatment of choice, along with continuation of drug therapy. After discharge, Abdul unwillingly accompanied Ingrid to their appointments at the CMHC. He never actively participated in the sessions.

Ingrid occasionally sensed her husband's suffering and at those times felt compassion and caring for him. Generally, however, she felt anger toward Abdul and held him responsible for their predicament. She continued to deal with her frustrations by eating and now, because of her obesity, had difficulty getting around. She limited her trips outside the house to those absolutely essential. Because of health limitations and a general sense of despair about the family's situation, Ingrid became increasingly apathetic about the daily maintenance and upkeep of their home. Whenever possible, Begum, now 11, voluntarily accepted responsibility for family chores that her parents no longer performed. She cooked simple meals, did laundry, cleaned house, and cut the yard. The family received some support from the next-door neighbor who offered to help Begum with the heavy yardwork whenever he saw her struggling. Ingrid had long ago exhausted the support available from her friends and increasingly turned to Begum for companionship and emotional support.

In the next several years, Abdul and Ingrid were not involved in ongoing treatment. Ingrid would call a therapist at the CMHC at times of crisis, generally in response to her concern that Abdul was in physiological danger from not eating. In fact, during this 3-year time period, Abdul was admitted five times to general hospitals because of his extreme withdrawal that resulted in dehydration and other symptoms of malnourishment. Each time he was admitted because of these secondary symptoms, he also spent several weeks on psychiatric inpatient units where he received treatment for his withdrawal. Abdul's improvement after drug therapy with major tranquilizers or antidepressants was only moderate. Each time that Abdul was discharged with these medications, he immediately stopped taking them. Abdul, on discharge, would once again return to life in his bedroom and begin another sequence of isolation and progressive deterioration.

One of Abdul's discharge plans included a public health nursing referral. Home visits from the public health nurse helped monitor Abdul's condition but were ineffective in terms of helping him keep his appointments at the CMHC, comply with his medication regimen, and decrease his seclusive behavior. The public health nurse was helpful in arranging for health care for Ingrid and Begum, but was not able to help Ingrid alter her self-destructive behavior of using eating as a way of dealing with her own stress and frustration. By now Ingrid weighed over 250 pounds and was having serious health problems of her own.

The summer Begum turned 12, Abdul overheard a neighbor compliment her on her appearance. Abdul misinterpreted the neighbor's remark and accused the neighbor of making sexual advances toward his daughter. A loud argument followed. Abdul threatened his neighbor, telling him that if he ever saw him talking to his daughter again, he would come after him with a gun. As a result of this incident, Abdul and his family were ostracized and ignored by most of their neighbors. With no more help in outside home maintenance, Abdul and Ingrid's home, which was located in an upper middle class neighborhood, became increasingly run down. Abdul rarely went outside the house. Ingrid left home only to take care of essential errands and transport Begum. The years of impoverishment and dealing with chronic mental illness had taken their toll. Ingrid's world was that of her family, books, and television. No longer were there family outings or visits with friends. The concern had become that of getting through each day.

As she grew, Begum assumed more and more of the care of her parents. Yet, despite her many home responsibilities, Begum did well in school and talked of wanting to be a doctor when she grew up. Begum's physical education teacher took a special interest in her and helped her develop natural gymnastics abilities to the point where she applied for and won a scholarship to a first-rate gymnastics school. Begum quickly made friends with two girls who also attended her gymnastics school and developed strategies to spend time with her friends, away from her home.

The family's life followed much the same pattern until the Christmas Begum was 14. Ingrid and Begum planned to visit Ingrid's parents for several days. Although Abdul had been invited, he refused to accompany his family on their trip. Two days after Ingrid and Begum left, Abdul again made a serious suicide attempt. He cut both wrists and watched them bleed, as he waited to die. Several times, the blood clotted and he had to reopen the wounds for the blood to continue flowing. As he became weaker and started shaking, Abdul feared his suicide attempt would not be successful. He stated that he called the ambulance because he was too weak to hang himself. Abdul was taken to a general hospital for emergency treatment and, after his physiological condition stabilized, he was taken nonvoluntarily to the state psychiatric hospital that served his geographical area.

Immediately on arriving at the state hospital, Abdul was assigned to a nurse who would be his primary nurse for the period of time he was on the admission unit. After a first-level assessment, his nurse determined his immediate needs to be care of his bilateral wrist sutures, protection from further self-destructive behaviors, and maintenance of an adequate nutritional intake. Abdul was immediately given suicidal precautions, meaning he was always within arm's reach of a nursing staff member, except at night when he slept in an open seclusion room across from the nursing station. The primary nurse was able to spend the first hour of his suicidal precaution time with him.

She used this time to begin a relationship with Abdul, providing an initial orientation to her role as his primary nurse and to the ward, as well as finding out his immediate concerns. Abdul matter of factly expressed annoyance that measures such as suicide precautions were being used to keep him from trying to commit suicide. He stated he was disappointed in himself in that he had not succeeded in killing himself and was determined to succeed on his next attempt.

The nurse also discovered that Abdul had spoken with his wife, who was still out of state, only once since his suicide attempt. The nurse's offer to arrange a phone conversation between Abdul and his wife was met with a positive response and a slight smile from Abdul. Before the nurse left that evening, she had discovered that Abdul, who had barely touched his lunch, preferred several small meals to three large ones. In addition to leaving the nursing order that Abdul's nutritional intake be recorded, she requested that he be offered a snack at midafternoon and bedtime. The nurse also alerted the night staff to the possibility that Abdul might have difficulty sleeping because of his history of sleeping during the day and staying awake at night. If he did have difficulty sleeping, his primary nurse requested that staff stay with him and offer him hot chocolate or warm milk.

In the next few days, the primary nurse, in consultation with Abdul and the treatment team, developed a plan of nursing care for Abdul (Table 30-3).

When the nurse first began spending time with Abdul in an effort to develop a trusting relationship

TABLE 30-3. Abdul's abbreviated nursing care plan

Nursing diagnosis	Intervention	Expected outcome
Inadequate nutritional and fluid intake related to feelings of worthlessness and hopelessness	Monitor input; offer juices; offer snack at 3 and 9 PM	Independent maintenance of adequate nutritional intake
Inadequate personal hygiene related to isolation and feelings of worthlessness and hopelessness	Help patient shave; remind him to bathe; have clean clothes available each day	Independent maintenance of personal hygiene
Sleep pattern disturbance related to withdrawal and isolation	Involve patient in ward activities so he stays awake during day; provide at least one exercise period a day; decrease stimuli and offer bath and warm milk at bedtime	Sleeps at night; stays awake during day
Self-destructive behavior related to feelings of worthlessness and hopelessness	Observe patient closely; be alert for suicidal thoughts; offer hope that future can be different	Investment in future
Social withdrawal related to distrust of others and feelings of inadequacy	Establish therapeutic nurse-patient relationship; invite patient to participate in structured activities, such as cards, chess, walks; help him transfer learnings from nurse-patient relationship to other relationships	Development of relationships with staff and patients
Misinterprets meaning of events in his environment related to social isolation and inadequate feedback	Listen for disorders in logical thinking; matter of factly offer alternate interpretations of events; listen to meaning behind distortions and idiosyncratic interpretation of events	Decrease in idiosyncratic interpretation of events; independence in seeking feedback regarding his interpretation of events
Negative self-concept and low self-esteem related to failure in meeting own and others' expectations	Identify personal strengths with patient; offer alternate view of self based on experiences of patient in milieu; develop nurse-patient relationship to help patient explore his feelings of worthlessness and make choices about future	Self statements reflecting realistic sense of abilities and limitations; willingness to make more productive choices in future

he was unable to tolerate being in an office with her. He would either refuse to come into the office or, after 2 or 3 minutes, would become anxious and leave. The nurse, accepting him where he was, began sitting with him for periods of 10 to 15 minutes in the day hall. Sometimes they would work on a jigsaw puzzle together; sometimes they would carry on a conversation, essentially social in nature, and sometimes Abdul would use the time to sort out his reactions to living in a state hospital. Only rarely would he speak of his past life or personal concerns other than his adjustment to the hospital environment.

As Abdul began to trust the nurse, he accepted her invitation to meet at regular times in her office. Although he was only able to stay for 15 to 20 minutes before getting up and saying "I have to go now," he began to talk about his life and especially about his sense of humiliation at having failed in every area important to him. Despite the nurse's identifying growth he had made in the hospital, Abdul continued to believe there was no hope for the future, and suicide was the only alternative to a life as bleak as his.

Abdul had requested that he not be given medication. Because his history documented a poor response to psychotropic medication, the psychiatrist did not order medication. However, after Abdul had been hospitalized 6 weeks, he shared with his primary nurse his belief that during one of his hospitalizations, in a procedure that left no scars, an electrode had been implanted through his nostril into his brain. He believed that his behavior was controlled by laser beams from a radio tower 20 miles away. Because his behavior was under external control, he considered himself to be a robot and thus was not responsible for his behavior. Once the psychiatrist was aware of Abdul's delusional system, intramuscular fluphenazine decanoate (Prolixin) was ordered for him. Seven days after his first injection, Abdul showed significant differences in behavior. He began to initiate conversations with other patients, voluntarily attended ward activities, began to take care of his own hygiene, and expressed an interest in being able to go out for walks. His talk of suicide decreased, and he began to doubt he was controlled by laser beams.

As part of Abdul's treatment plan, the primary nurse and a psychiatric nurse prepared at the master's degree level met with the family weekly to help the family become more functional and again enjoy being together. Interventions were directed toward improving family communication and helping the family reorganize itself so that the parents would assume more parental authority and Begum would become more like the 14-year-old she was, rather than continuing to maintain her role as the third adult in the family.

Two critical incidents are shared as an illustration of the growth of Abdul, Ingrid, and Begum. The first incident occurred 3 months after Abdul's admission. In the family meeting, both Ingrid and Begum were speaking about the disrepair of their home. They focused on their inability, physically and financially, to maintain their home and their embarrassment that their home had become a neighborhood eyesore. Abdul told Begum he did not want her to undertake the heavy yardwork alone. He asked if he might return home to help with the yardwork and fix the plumbing. Although suicide precautions were only dropped recently and Abdul was not ready for a weekend pass, the primary nurse wanted to support Abdul's initiative in assuming family responsibility. Arrangements were made for the primary nurse and the family therapist to take Abdul home for an afternoon. A potluck supper was planned with both nurses and all three family members contributing to the effort. Abdul returned from the trip home with new-found energy and a feeling of self-worth that came from having been needed and the sense of a job well done. The primary nurse capitalized on this experience in that as she helped Abdul examine the sense of well-being, however fragile, that resulted from making a contribution, she suggested he become involved in the hospital work program. With much support, Abdul accepted her offer and began working in the hospital horticulture program.

The second incident occurred indirectly as a result of the home visit. After the potluck supper, Ingrid asked the primary nurse to look at some "sores" on her legs. The nurse was concerned not only about the large skin ulcers Ingrid showed her but also about the respiratory distress Ingrid was having. The nurse consulted a social worker who served as a liaison between the hospital and community, and, through the social worker, arrangements were made for Ingrid to be seen by a physician. After her appointment, Ingrid was hospitalized with pulmonary edema and skin ulcers. An old friend, with whom Ingrid had recently reestablished contact, was able to keep Begum for several days, but there was no one for Begum to stay with over the weekend. Abdul rose to the occasion and said he did not want his daughter home alone. He then marshalled his arguments and asked for a pass to go home and care for Begum. After much consideration, the psychiatrist and the primary nurse decided to let Abdul go home to be with Begum, provided the three following conditions were met: (1) the gun in Abdul's home was to be removed and brought to the hospital for safekeeping; (2) a written contract that specified activities and structure for the time Abdul was home was to be signed by Abdul, the psychiatrist, and the nurse; and (3) Abdul was to return to the hospital Monday morning on the bus. Abdul agreed to these conditions. He returned to the hospital grinning because the weekend had gone better than he had expected. He was especially proud that he had cooked dinner Saturday night and given Begum the best piece of meat.

Abdul's continued improvement was not without setbacks. However, after he had been hospitalized on the admission unit 5 months, he was transferred to an unlocked continued-care ward where rehabilitation would continue until he was ready for discharge. Abdul and his primary nurse met with the social worker who would be coordinating his treatment plan on the new ward to facilitate the transition. While Abdul was in the continued-care area, he worked with vocational rehabilitation and was judged capable of a sheltered workshop placement when he returned to the community. With an eye toward discharge and a desire to increase compliance with an eventual aftercare program, Abdul began making weekly visits home to attend family therapy sessions at the CMHC. On these visits home, he shared with Ingrid his fear that his life was destined to be one of limited functioning and recurrent hospitalizations.

On one of his last weekends before discharge, he had a longer than usual pass because he had a Monday afternoon appointment with the vocational rehabilitation center in the community. Tuesday morning, Ingrid called Abdul's primary nurse on the admissions unit. Abdul was dead. He had hanged himself the night before.

The primary nurse had her own personal grief to confront. Despite her caring and the best efforts of many professionals, the final choice was Abdul's. After struggling for many years, he chose the pain of death over the pain of life. The primary nurse was left with the hope that for a time, however brief, Abdul's life was less painful, that he had a momentary glimmer that life could be different, and that he had experienced the respect and positive regard she had for him. Out of her own grief, respect for Abdul, and continuing concern for his family, Abdul's primary nurse went to his funeral—and cried.

Suggested cross-references

The phases of the nursing process are discussed in Chapter 4. Tertiary prevention and rehabilitative psychiatric nursing are discussed in Chapter 6. Problems with self-esteem are discussed in Chapter 8. Legal issues, including commitment proceedings and patient rights, are discussed in Chapter 16. Crisis intervention is discussed in Chapter 20.

SUMMARY

1. Chronically mentally ill individuals no longer reside primarily in large public psychiatric hospitals. It is estimated that as a result of "deinstitutionalization," the process of moving long-term mental patients into the community to be supported by formal and informal resources, 50% of the chronically mentally ill are now living in local communities.

2. As health policy directed that long-term psychiatric patients have alternatives to life in a public mental hospital, court decisions reflected increasing attention to protection of the rights of this population. Of particular importance to the chronically mentally ill are issues surrounding civil commitment, the right to treatment and protection from harm in the least restrictive environment, the right to refuse treatment, confidentiality, and, employment.

3. Chronically mentally ill individuals have both primary and secondary symptoms of their illness. Primary symptoms are those associated with the intrinsic nature of their illness. Secondary symptoms develop over time as a consequence of the illness and perpetuate the illness's existence. Chronic mental illness, with its associated secondary symptoms is not a state or end point, but a process of progressive deterioration.

   a. Behaviors of mentally ill individuals are likely to violate social norms and standards of proper conduct and thus may be considered deviant behaviors. These deviant behaviors set in motion a so-cial interactive process in which society protects itself from these deviant behaviors, and the mentally ill person increasingly relates to society in terms of his deviant identity.

   b. According to the public health model, individuals with chronic illness show increasing symptoms of functional impairment and disability as they move sequentially through the four stages of the "natural history" of chronic illness.

4. Elaboration of the special characteristics of the chronically mentally ill as a population portrays a population with difficulties with activities of daily living, difficulties in maintaining interpersonal relations, a lack of coping resources, and a need for long-term treatment. Other characteristics influencing the course of their illness are their consistently low self-esteem and their preoccupation with avoiding failure rather than achieving success. As a group, the chronically mentally ill can also be characterized by their unique strengths and potentials.

5. The "young" chronically ill patient, 18 to 35 years old, differs from chronically mentally ill patients over 35 years old. Because of deinstitutionalization and the development of community-based treatment facilities, younger patients have not had to adapt to long-term residence in public psychiatric hospitals. They alternate between inpatient and community-based facilities and maintain age-appropriate role expectations for themselves. Not meeting these expec-

tations, they are continually confronted with their sense of failure. They are likely to enter the mental health system nonvoluntarily, are unlikely to follow through with aftercare plans, and have a high suicide rate. Present treatment resources are inadequate in meeting the needs of this group of patients.

6. Psychosocial rehabilitation programs that incorporate elements of the medical model, rehabilitation model, and social support model have demonstrated their effectiveness in meeting the needs of chronically mentally ill patients. Fountain House, a psychosocial rehabilitation program in New York City, has been used as a prototype for the development of other psychosocial rehabilitation programs. These programs offer their residents choices in living and work situations, but most important offer a sense of being needed and a place to belong. Basic to the rehabilitation process is focusing on the strengths of new members.

7. The role and function of the nurse in caring for chronically mentally ill patients is influenced by the setting in which the care is given.

    a. Nurses working in community-based psychosocial rehabilitation programs have the opportunity for long-term ongoing relationships with patients and the mutual setting of long-term goals. In these programs nurses may also be asked to function as "case manager," a role that cuts across professional boundaries.

    b. Nurses working in acute care settings often care for chronically mentally ill patients when they are in crisis. The goal of care is to return the patient to a precrisis level of functioning as quickly as possible so that the patient can return to the community to be cared for in a less restrictive environment. Nurses must be able to quickly establish relationships with acutely ill patients and be skilled in applying the principles of crisis intervention. Primary nursing, as a modality of nursing care, offers several advantages when caring for chronically mentally ill patients in acute care settings.

8. In all settings, nurses are responsible for improving their patients' health status by developing the patients' health potentials. Nursing interventions that develop the strengths and potentials of chronically mentally ill patients help them become more competent in meeting the demands of everyday life. Ultimately, the expected outcome of such interventions is a change in the patient's self-concept and an increase in his or her self-esteem. Nursing interventions in which patients are helped to become aware of their strengths fall into two categories:

    a. Those which occur as a response to the patient's spontaneous participation in the milieu

    b. Those which occur as part of a structured intervention in which experiences are planned to mobilize patients' strengths or develop their potentials

References

1. Anderson, S., and Bauwens, E.: Chronic health problems: concepts and application, St. Louis, 1981, The C.V. Mosby Co.
2. Bachrach, L.L.: Deinstitutionalization: an analytical review and sociological perspective, U.S. Department of Health, Education, and Welfare Pub. No. (ADM)76-351, Washington, D.C., 1976, U.S. Government Printing Office.
3. Bachrach, L.L.: A note on some recent studies of released mental hospital patients in the community, Am. J. Psychiatry **133:**73, 1976.
4. Baldwin, D.: *O'Connor v. Donaldson:* involuntary civil commitment and the right to treatment, Columbia Human Rights Law Rev. **7:**573, 1975-1976.
5. Bassuk, E.L., and Gerson, S.: Deinstitutionalization and mental health services, Sci. Am. **238:**46, Feb. 1978.
6. Bell, R.: The effect of interpersonal strengths identification and education on the self-esteem of psychiatric day treatment programs, doctoral dissertation, Washington, D.C., 1981, Catholic University of America.
7. Brown, B.: Responsible care of former mental patients. In New dimensions in mental health: report from the director, Washington, D.C., 1977, National Institute of Mental Health.
8. Caton, D.: The new chronic patient and the system of community, Hosp. Community Psychiatry **32:**475, 1981.
9. Chodoff, P.: The case for involuntary hospitalization of the mentally ill, Am. J. Psychiatry **133:**496, 1976.
10. Coopersmith, S.: The antecedents of self-esteem, San Francisco (1967) 1981, Consulting Psychologists Press.
11. Crossen, M.: Contemporary models in psychiatric care and rehabilitation: Fountain House, Hoffman-LaRoche Laboratories.
12. Fitts, W.: Tennessee self-concept manual, Nashville, Tenn., 1965, Counselor Recording and Tests.
13. Fitts, W.: The self-concept and psychopathology, Nashville, Tenn., 1972, Counselor Recording and Tests.
14. Fitts, W., et al.: The self-concept and self-actualization, Monograph No. III, Nashville, Tenn., 1971, Counselor Recording and Tests.
15. Friedman, P., and Yohalem, J.: The rights of the chronic mental patient. In Talbott, J., editor: The chronic mental patient: problems, solutions, and recommendations for a public policy, Washington, D.C., 1978, The American Psychiatric Association.
16. Goldman, H., Gattozzi, A., and Taube, C.: Defining and counting the chronically mentally ill, Hosp. Community Psychiatry **32:**21, Jan. 1981.
17. Gruenberg, E.: The social breakdown syndrome: some origins, Am. J. Psychiatry **123:**1481, 1967.
18. Krauss, J.: The chronic psychiatric patient in the community: a model of care, Nurs. Outlook **28:**308, 1980.

19. Lamb, H., and Goertzel, V.: The long term patient in the era of community treatment, Arch. Gen. Psychiatry **34:**679, 1977.

20. Lemert, E.: Secondary deviance and role conceptions. In Farrell, R., and Swigert, V., editors: Social deviance, New York, 1975, J.B. Lippincott Co.

21. Minkoff, K.: A map of the chronic mental patient. In Talbott, J., editor: The chronic mental patient: problems, solutions, and recommendations for a public policy, Washington, D.C., 1978, The American Psychiatric Association.

22. Otto, H.: The human potentialities of nurses and patients, Nurs. Outlook **8:**32, 1965.

23. Otto, H.: Guide to developing your potential, New York, 1967, Charles Scribner's Sons.

24. Pepper, B., Kirshner, M., and Ryglewicz, H.: The young adult chronic patient: overview of a population, Hosp. Community Psychiatry **32:**463, 1981.

25. Peterson, R.: What are the needs of chronic mental patients? In Talbott, J., editor: The chronic mental patient: problems, solutions, and recommendations for a public policy, Washington, D.C., 1978, The American Psychiatric Association.

26. Porter, E., and Maloney, S.: Strength deployment inventory: manual of administration and interpretation, Pacific Palisades, Calif., 1967, Personal Strengths Assessment Service, Inc.

27. Rogers, C.: Client centered therapy: its current practice, implications, and theory, Boston, 1965, Houghton Mifflin Co.

28. Ross, G.: Attribution retraining of the psychiatrically disabled, doctoral dissertation, Philadelphia, 1978, University of Pennsylvania.

29. Schwartz, S., and Goldfinger, S.: The new chronic patient: clinical characteristics of an emerging subgroup, Hosp. Community Psychiatry **32:**470, 1981.

30. Segal, S., Baumohl, J., and Johnson, E.: Falling through the cracks: mental disorder and social margin in a young vagrant population, Soc. Probl. **24:**387, 1977.

31. Talbott, J.: The national plan for the chronically mentally ill: a programmatic analysis, Hosp. Community Psychiatry **32:**699, 1981.

32. Turner, J., and TenHoor, W.: The NIMH community support program: pilot approach to needed social reform, Schizophr. Bull. **4:**319, 1978.

Annotated suggested readings

Bassuk, E.L., and Gerson, S.: Chronic crisis patients: a discrete clinical group, Am. J. Psychiatry **137:**1513, 1980.

This study of psychiatric patients who made repeated visits to an emergency room in a general hospital focuses on their nonproductive interaction with the caregivers from whom they seek help. The authors suggest interventions based on an understanding of their help-seeking–help-rejecting behavior.

Craig, A., and Hyatt, B.: Chronicity in mental illness: a theory on the role of change, Perspect. Psychiatr. Care **16:**139, May-June 1978.

General systems theory is used to explain the perpetuation of symptoms in the chronically mentally ill. Chronic mental illness is defined as a family systems problem rather than an individual problem, and interventions are related to the authors' theoretical position.

Crossen, M.: Contemporary models in psychiatric care and rehabilitation: Fountain House, Hoffman-LaRoche Laboratories.

The author provides an overview of the Fountain House program. Her report is based on interviews with Fountain House staff and members.

Donaldson, K.: Insanity inside out, New York, 1976, Crown Publishers, Inc.

This autobiography portrays Kenneth Donaldson's 15-year struggle to be released from a Florida state mental hospital. Donaldson describes his experiences as a patient and tells the story behind the landmark court decision (O'Connor v. Donaldson, 1975).

Friedman, P., and Yohalem, J.: The rights of the chronic mental patient. In Talbott, J., editor: The chronic mental patient: problems, solutions, and recommendations for a public policy, Washington, D.C., 1978, The American Psychiatric Association.

Five clusters of rights that greatly affect the quality of life for the chronically mentally ill are described. As court rulings are presented, the authors derive implications for this patient population.

Goldman, H., Gattozzi, A., and Taube, C.: Defining and counting the chronically mentally ill, Hosp. Community Psychiatry **32:**21, Jan. 1981.

These authors present the results of a national study with the purpose of identifying the chronically mentally ill, both descriptively and numerically. The findings provided a foundation to the development of the National Plan for the Chronically Mentally Ill.

Krauss, J.: The chronic psychiatric patient in the community: a model of care, Nurs. Outlook **28:**308, 1980.

The author, based on her experience of caring for chronically mentally ill patients in the community, describes the needs of this patient population and discusses nursing interventions useful in meeting these needs.

Minkoff, K.: A map of the chronic mental patient. In Talbott, J., editor: The chronic mental patient: problems, solutions, and recommendations for a public policy, Washington, D.C., 1978, The American Psychiatric Association.

The author provides a demographic overview of chronically mentally ill patients. The facts and figures presented supply information as to the scope and magnitude of the problems of this patient population.

Pepper, B., Kirshner, M., and Ryglewicz, H.: The young adult chronic patient: overview of a population, Hosp. Community Psychiatry **32:**463, 1981.

Based on a study of nearly 300 patients, 18 to 35 years old, the author provides a beginning description of the characteristics of this emerging subgroup of the chronically mentally ill.

Peterson, R.: What are the needs of chronic mental patients? In Talbott, J., editor: The chronic mental patient: problems, solutions, and recommendations for a public policy, Washington, D.C., 1978, The American Psychiatric Association.

Ronald Peterson, a veteran of 10 years in a state mental hospital, wrote this paper when he was a staff member of Fountain House, a psychosocial rehabilitation program. He provides an "insider's view" of the experience of leav-

ing a state hospital and adjusting to community life. The importance of programs like Fountain House in meeting the needs of the chronically mentally ill is highlighted.

Rubin, J.: The national plan for the chronically mentally ill: a review of financing proposals, Hosp. Community Psychiatry **32:**704, 1981.

The author summarizes and analyzes fiscal recommendations in the National Plan for the Chronically Mentally Ill.

Schwartz, S., and Goldfinger, S.: The new chronic patient: clinical characteristics of an emerging subgroup, Hosp. Community Psychiatry **32:**470, 1981.

The authors describe their impressions, based on 2 years' clinical work in a general hospital, of the characteristics of younger chronically mentally ill patients. They analyze the interaction of this patient group with present treatment resources and make recommendations for future development of treatment resources.

Sheehan, S.: Is there no place on earth for me? Boston, 1982, Houghton Mifflin Co.

This journalistic account of the life history of a chronically schizophrenic woman reveals the nature of the mental health care system, including changes initiated by the community mental health movement. The frustration of

the patient and her family as they try to find help is clearly communicated to the reader. This book would be particularly worthwhile to the nurse who has had limited contact with chronically mentally ill patients.

Talbott, J.: The national plan for the chronically mentally ill: a programmatic analysis, Hosp. Community Psychiatry **32:**699, 1981.

The author summarizes and analyzes the program recommendations in the National Plan for the Chronically Mentally Ill.

Toward a national plan for the chronically mentally ill, U.S. Department of Health and Human Services Pub. No. (ADM)81-1077, Washington, D.C., 1980.

This federal report, originally requested by President Carter's Commission on Mental Health, describes the needs of the chronically mentally ill, analyzes problems in the implementation of deinstitutionalization, and makes recommendations to improve services to this group of patients. Attention is given to fiscal considerations in meeting the needs of the chronically mentally ill.

Ulin, P.: Measuring adjustment in chronically ill clients in community mental health care, Nurs. Res. **30:**229, July-Aug. 1981.

This study examines the usefulness of the Psychological Mental Health Index (PMHI) in assessing the psychological well being of chronically ill psychotic patients being cared for in the community.

Youth is like a
fresh flower in May.
Age is like a rainbow
that follows the storms of life.
Each has its own beauty.

David Polis*

*From Susan Polis Schutz, editor: The best is yet to be: thoughts on growing old, Boulder, Colo., 1974. Copyright © Continental Publications 1974. Reprinted with permission. All rights reserved.

CHAPTER 31

GERONTOLOGICAL PSYCHIATRIC NURSING

BEVERLY A. BALDWIN

Learning objectives

After studying this chapter, the student
should be able to:

- describe psychiatric disorders associated with aging relative to the demographic characteristics of the population.

- identify the role and functions of the gerontological psychiatric nurse.

- critique the major biological, psychosocial, and personality theories of aging.

- assess the nursing care needs of the gerontological psychiatric patient.

- discuss the advantages and disadvantages of a variety of assessment tools that may be used by the nurse as one component of data collection.

- formulate nursing diagnosis consistent with observed patient behaviors and identified stressors.

- analyze the interrelationship between physiological and psychological stressors as they affect the behavior of the aging patient.

- compare and contrast several intervention strategies that may be implemented with gerontological psychiatric patients.

- identify opportunities to intervene in social support systems.

- describe areas of need for nursing research to evaluate the effectiveness of gerontological psychiatric nursing care.

- identify suggested readings for further study.

The fastest growing minority in the United States is the over-65 age group, now comprising almost 12% of the population. One in every nine Americans is 65 years of age or older; in the next half century, one in six or perhaps one in five Americans will be over 65 years old. By 2030 it is estimated that there will be 55 million persons over the age of 65, or 17% to 20% of the total United States population.[1] Stereotypes and myths surrounding this age group often portray a homogeneous profile of the elderly. To the contrary, the older adult represents the culmination of multiple interpersonal, developmental, and situational experiences. The complex and interactive nature of the needs and problems of old age is frequently underestimated and often understated. Mental health in later years depends on a number of factors, including one's physiological and psychological status, personality, social support system, economic resources, and prevailing life-style. It has been estimated that of the persons over 65, approximately 4 million have suffered moderate to severe psychiatric impairment secondary to either cerebral arteriosclerosis, senile dementia, functional psychosis, alcoholism, or other disease conditions. The elderly account for approximately 25% of the reported suicides; the highest rate occurring in white males in their 80s.[3] The extent of mental disorders in old age appears to be considerable; therefore nurses and other health care professionals will realize an increasing responsibility in the prevention and care of the older adult with mental and emotional health problems. Assisting the older adult to maximize his optimal potential can be a challenging and rewarding experience for the nurse. This chapter will address selected aspects of the psychiatric–mental health needs of the geriatric patient.

The problem of defining aging and the geriatric patient is complicated. Individual variations exist in how different people age, both psychologically and physiologically; therefore it is recognized that the chronological demarcation of age 65 is an arbitrary one. To provide a base for understanding the aging phenomenon and the impact of individual variations, an overview of selected theories of aging is presented. A format for applying the theories of aging is the examination of components of the mental health evaluation of older adults. Although it is acknowledged that the assessment of mental health status is but one aspect of assessment of the total person, for purposes of this chapter, emphasis will be placed on the mental and emotional evaluation. By integrating current research findings with the role of the nurse in the care of the geriatric patient, the purpose, criteria, and uses of standardized instruments for evaluating mental status are compared to functional and other behaviorally focused measures.

Data obtained from the mental status evaluation, along with a profile of the patient's general status, offer the nurse an opportunity to develop a working nursing diagnosis and plan intervention strategies. Memory loss, confusion, or disorientation may represent behavioral responses of the older adult to stress, whether originating from internal or external processes. Knowledge and skill are required of the nurse in determining the extent to which the stress is a negative or positive force in the observed behavioral responses of the patient. Comprehensive evaluation is the first step in making that determination.

The next step in the process of care is selection of intervention strategies to meet the needs of the patient. An overview of the current techniques being used in prevention and care of the mentally impaired (or potentially impaired) will focus on clinical research findings that indicate the effectiveness or ineffectiveness of selected interventions. The past two decades have witnessed a new interest in the treatment of the institutionalized geriatric patient on the part of health professionals. Once the predictable victim of widespread neglect, the geriatric patient is now viewed in a more favorable light. The discussion of these intervention strategies will focus on the role of the nurse in implementing and assessing the impact on the patient, whether in an individual or group setting context.

Evolution of the role of the gerontological psychiatric nurse

The sick elderly were found in general hospitals, their homes, and clinics, but the nurse attending them never thought of herself as a geriatric nurse prior to World War II. The passage of the Social Security Act of 1935 had profound effects on the status of the aged citizen in this country. Public assistance funds became available to the needy aged. It hastened the development of profit-making homes, since recipients receiving monthly stipends could not live in a public institution. Many of the retired and widowed nurses converted their homes into boarding houses and became, in practice, the first of our present day nursing homes.[13] Care in the boarding houses for the aged deteriorated as the clients became ill and their needs grew in number and complexity. After World War II each state established minimum standards for nursing home care, and licensing of homes was introduced. Many of the boarding house nurse-landladies became the administrators of the new federally subsidized nursing homes. With the increase in the number and needs of the patients, it became necessary to employ additional nursing personnel to provide the care.[14] The nurse administrator assumed the role of supervisor or manager of nonprofessional personnel, in addition to the duties of running the home.

The early practitioner in geriatric nursing experienced professional isolation from other nurses and felt a lack of prestige from physicians, nurses, and the general public. In fact, these nurses were completely outside the focus of concern in nursing's striving for professionalization. The usual avenue of continuing education for nurses was not available to geriatric nurses, and nursing literature on the care of the aged was nonexistent. As more nurses began to identify themselves with geriatric nursing, they sought to overcome their alienation by appealing to the American Nurses' Association.[6] In 1961, a committee within the association recommended the formation of a group whose main interest would be geriatric nursing. A year later, a conference called by this group became the forerunner of the Division on Geriatric Nursing Practice of the American Nurses' Association.

To meet criteria for constituting a separate nursing practice division, this group was charged with "providing evidence that a substantial number of nurses are practicing in a field with a well-defined and unique body of nursing knowledge and/or evidence that a significant health problem exists in which nursing is involved."[13] Certainly, there was sufficient evidence that the care of the aged was a major health problem involving nurses. In January, 1967, 1 month after the first meeting of the Executive Committee of the Geriatric Nursing Division, over 2000 nurses registered to become members of the division. The number of nurses identifying with care of the aged has continued to increase since the inception of the division. The division is charged with assessing the nursing needs of older people, planning and implementing nursing care to meet those needs, and evaluating the effectiveness of such care to achieve and maintain a level of health consistent with the limitation imposed by the aging process.[13] It was the first of the practice divisions to establish and publish standards of practice and to certify superior practitioners. The enthusiasm and momentum of this group merits attention from all areas of nursing. Although it is the newest of the practice divisions and probably the smallest, significant progress in upgrading nursing care in this area of practice has been made. The division voted, in 1974, to change the name to Gerontological Nursing Practice, to more accurately reflect the focus of this group. The term geriatric refers to the study of diseases of old age and gerontology refers to the study of the phenomenon of aging.[8] Since a primary function of the nurse is to assist the individual to reach and maintain optimum function throughout the process of aging, the term gerontological was considered to more appropriately reflect this function.

The prospects for the future of gerontological/geriatric nursing are encouraging for nurses seeking greater autonomy and control over their practice, in addition to increasing responsibility for decision making in the care of the aged. Several factors account for the potential for change within this field of nursing. Esther Lucille Brown,[5] in a study of nursing practice in hospitals, extended care facilities, and nursing and retirement homes, notes that except for a few specialists in geriatrics and chronic diseases, the medical profession is largely uninvolved in the problems of aging and care of the older patient who cannot be cured. The functional requirements of physicians in institutions devoted to chronic disease and rehabilitation are minimal. Most of the needs of the elderly in these settings, and in community and home care settings, are a result of chronic disability with multiple etiology. It is in these settings that the nursing domain may develop and expand.

Internally, the field of gerontological/geriatric nursing is changing rapidly. Stone[38] predicts this specialty promises virtually unlimited progress for the nurse in the future. Furthermore, she suggests five major roles for nurses specializing in care of the aged: (1) patient-care managers in nursing homes; (2) health assessors with a focus on the physical, mental, and functional assessment rather than medical assessment; (3) primary care providers in both institutional and community agencies; (4) independent practitioners in private or group practices with other nurses or other health professionals; and (5) researchers, involved in both nursing and interdisciplinary clinical studies.

As the role of the gerontological/geriatric nurse continues to expand and grow, the educational preparation for this specialist must expand. Presently, there are 26 graduate programs in nursing offering a concentration or specialty in this area. Preparation at the graduate level includes clinical specialization, administration, education, and nurse practitioner. Included is preparation of the beginning nurse researcher, the first in the step toward preparation at the doctoral level. Increasingly, faculty are including more content on gerontological/geriatric nursing in undergraduate curricula. Recognition of the need to prepare nurses to care for the aged continues to grow, with the recognition of the growing number in the older age groups. It is estimated that even in acute care settings, the number of patients over the age of 65 may range from 20% to 60%.[4]

In the spring of 1979 the Council of Nursing Home Nurses was established within the American Nurses' Association. Recognition of the needs of this group within the field of gerontological/geriatric nursing demonstrates the growing interest of nursing in influencing and directing the care of the aged. Some of the areas of involvement for the new council include enhancing the visibility and influence of the nursing home nurse, influencing the quality and delivery of nursing care in the nursing home at the local, state, and national levels and promoting effective utilization of gerontological nursing concepts to the consumer and health care community.[2]

Theories of aging

Approaches to defining aging and explaining the causes and consequences of the aging process constitute the basis for the numerous theories of aging. Theories are proposed based on two major conceptual approaches to aging: the causes of the biological and psychological process of aging or the psychosocial results of aging. It is clear that there is little consensus among gerontologists regarding the etiology and adaptation to aging, and it is unlikely that consensus will be sought. No one theory can take into account all of the variables that influence aging and the individual's response to it, which include cultural and ethnic factors, genetic make-up and heritage, physiological conditions at conception and birth, growth and maturation, the environment, the family system, and relationships to significant others. Theories of aging are difficult to differentiate from changes over time that are considered to be secondary to the aging process. Distinctions between stress, disease processes, and specific age-related changes in relation to individual variation and uniqueness are tentative and will probably remain so for a long time to come. Selected theories will be discussed from the perspective of increasing understanding of the interaction of biopsychosocial manifestations of later life. Explanations for aging may further enhance knowledge of the physiological and mental changes experienced by the geriatric patient with whom the nurse will work.

Psychobiological theories

DELIBERATE BIOLOGICAL PROGRAMMING. Deliberate biological programming is one theory of aging that has received considerable attention over the last two decades. This theory holds that the memory and capacity for terminating the life of a cell is stored within the cell itself. Through laboratory studies, Hayflick et al.[23] demonstrated that normal human fibroblasts, when cultured, underwent a finite number of population doublings and then died. The number of doublings is not different in male and female cells. The theory of man's biological clock represents an entropic approach to the explanation of aging. The decline of biological, cognitive, and psychomotor function is viewed as inevitable and irreversible, even though modification of diet and prolonged hypothermia may slow up the terminal process. The notion of programmed aging, while answering some of the questions regarding longevity, does not address questions regarding the intrinsic and external influences on individual variations in aging.

THE WEAR-AND-TEAR THEORY. The wear-and-tear theory suggests that structural and functional changes occur which may be accelerated by abuse and decelerated by care.[33] From a physiological standpoint, aging is viewed ontogenetically, beginning with conception and leading to decline and death. The pathological consequences of aging are the result of an accumulation of stress, trauma, injuries, infections, nutritional inadequacies, metabolic and immunological disturbances, and prolonged abuse. Although less popular than some of the current theories, it illustrates the decremental model of aging, leading to irreversible decline. This concept of aging is often popularized by widely accepted myths and stereotypes regarding the aged, as noted in phrases like, "He is doing well for his age" or "What can you expect at that age?" Newer research on the value of exercise and cognitive stimulation in later years refutes the basic premise of this theory in that the body and mind might benefit from use and stimulation.

THE STRESS-ADAPTATION THEORY. The stress-adaptation theory suggests the positive and negative aspects of stress on the physiological and psychological development of the individual. Eisdorfer[18] points out that stress is not always a negative experience, as is usually implied in many of the writings on the subject. Stress may stimulate a person to try new and more effective ways of adapting. Although it is presumed by some that stress actually accelerates the aging process, there is little evidence to substantiate that conclusion. Stress may deplete the reserve capacity of individuals, either physiologically or psychologically, thereby placing them in a vulnerable position for illness or disability to occur. Some of the assumptions regarding stress and adaptation are important for the understanding of the nature of emotional and mental problems in the aged. Although the link between stress and the development of mental illness is unclear, the effect and perception of stress by an individual plays a major role in his ability to cope and remain flexible in adverse situations.

Psychosocial theories

DISENGAGEMENT THEORY. This controversial theory evolved from studies conducted by the University of Chicago Committee on Human Development.[12] It postulated that older adults and society mutually withdrew from active exchange with each other as part of the normal process of aging. The withdrawal was assumed to be characterized by psychological well-being and adjustment on the part of the elder. This theory did not take into account heterogeneity of the elders and the personality variables important to coping with change. Stereotypes reinforced by this theory include the notion that older people enjoy the company of their own age exclusively and that retirement facilities should promote homogeneous age cohorts and prohibit intergenerational living arrangements. Although

many elders may desi
ment, others find them
the mainstream of soc

ACTIVITY THEORY.
ity of the disengagemen
velopment of the current and preva
that activity produces the most positive psychological climate for older adults. The activity theory[30] developed as a reaction to the negativistic perspective of disengagement. Many gerontologists champion the notion that aging is but one phase in the developmental process; others contend that old age is only an extension of the middle years and can be modified or abolished by increased activity levels. The activity theory maintains that the aged should remain active as long as possible. When work and community activities and affiliations must be curtailed or given up, substitutes should be found. The positive influence of activity on the older person's personality, mental health, and satisfaction with life are heralded, expressing the value of an active vs. a passive role in relationships and in society.

THE LIFE REVIEW. The life review was postulated in 1961 by Robert Butler.[7] Reminiscence in the aged is viewed as part of a normal life review process brought about by the realization of approaching dissolution and death. Characteristic of the life review is the progressive return to consciousness of past experiences and the resurgence of unresolved conflicts that are examined and reintegrated. Successful reintegration can give meaning to one's life and prepare one for death by alleviating anxiety and fear. This process is believed to occur universally and represents a functional preparation for the final stage of life. Although seen in all age groups to a certain degree, the emphasis and focused concentration is evidenced more in the later stage of life. The aged appear to have a vivid memory for past events and can recall early life experiences with clarity and imagination. The person appears to be reviewing and sorting previous life events to better understand his present circumstances.

The life review process may result in either positive or negative consequences. Anxiety, guilt, fear, and depression may surface if the person finds himself unable to deal with, resolve, or accept unchanged old problems. On the other hand, the righting of earlier wrongs can aid in

...e establishment of a sense of serenity, pride in ...working through old conflicts, and acceptance of mortal life. Reflective activity becomes a positive approach to aging. In addition to offering an explanation for the consequences of aging, reminiscence and the life review have potential for psychotherapeutic intervention. Further discussion of this process will be found in the section on strategies for intervening in the mental health problems of the older adult.

Personality theories

ERIKSON'S STAGE OF EGO INTEGRITY. Erikson's eight stages of man[19] delineate specific developmental stages and tasks present at each age, based on Freudian dynamics. The last stage of life that provides a point for reflection on one's life and accomplishments is one of ego integrity. Erikson maps out a predetermined structural order to development and maturation, progression by critical or crisis periods, and dependence on chronological timing and sequence. The rationale for the progression from one stage to the next is unclear; one must assume that there are biological or psychosocial forces that initiate and propel the movement. The concept of ego integrity leaves unanswered many questions regarding the consequences of fixation at one stage of development and the individual variation in the complex process of development and maturation.

STABILITY OF PERSONALITY. Costa and McCrae[17] contend that personality is established by early adulthood and remains fairly stable thereafter. Stability of personality has been observed in longitudinal studies of aging individuals at the National Institutes of Health Gerontology Research Center in Baltimore (the intramural research center for the National Institute on Aging). Usually no decline or change in personality, compared to other cognitive changes, is evident. If radical changes in personality do occur among older individuals, it may be indicative of brain disease. Drs. Costa and McCrae found that periods of psychological crisis in adulthood do not occur at regular intervals, contradicting some theories, such as Erikson's, regarding the constancy and stability of stages of adult development. Individuals with a long history of emotional instability are therefore more likely to encounter more crises. These investiga-

tors refute the conclusion that, according to their theory, individual's remain firmly locked into rigid behavior patterns. They note, to the contrary, that changes in roles, attitudes and situational demands create the need for new behavioral responses and the majority of elderly persons in their studies appear to adapt effectively to those demands.

Nursing assessment

The assessment process offers an opportunity for the nurse to collect data essential to the development of a nursing diagnosis. The interview and health history constitute a first step in the process. The use of selected standardized assessment tools augments the data obtained through interviewing the patient or family.

The interview

Establishing a supportive and trusting relationship is essential to a positive interview with the geriatric patient. Since the first encounter between the nurse and patient may produce discomfort in the patient, the nurse must make every effort to put the patient at ease and offer reassurance and positive feedback. It may take repeated contacts and frequent explanations to allay fears and reduce anxiety. The geriatric patient may feel uneasy, vulnerable, and confused in new surroundings or in the presence of strangers. Patience and attentive listening promote a sense of security for the patient. The more comfortable the patient, the better able he will be to respond to the purpose and direction of the interview. Respect should be acknowledged by addressing the patient by his last name. The nurse opens the interview by introducing herself and describing in a short concise manner the purpose and length of the interview. The patient will respond best when he feels the nurse is interested and concerned about his welfare. The patient should not be rushed or pressed for answers. Direct questions may have to be rephrased or asked in a more indirect less intimidating manner.

Specifying the time allotted and the topic to be discussed at the beginning of the interview orients the patient to the purpose and scope of the interaction. Reinforcing the amount of time remaining in the interview may facilitate redirection of wandering discussion and give the patient the security of knowing the nurse is in control of the situation. Older persons may be slow in responding to questions, since their reaction time to verbal stimuli is lengthened with age. It is important to give the patient sufficient time to formulate a response. Assuming the patient does not know the answer to a question, does not remember, or does not understand because he does not respond immediately can lead the interviewer to false conclusions regarding the patient's status and mental capabilities.

The manner in which the patient is questioned is important to the outcome. Older persons often have their own vocabulary and may not be familiar with new words, slang, or contemporary colloquialisms. Avoid medical abbreviations, terminology, or jargon. Ask short concise questions, particularly if the patient indicates that he has difficulty with abstract thinking and conceptualization. Techniques such as clarification and summarization are important in validating information. Rephrase a question if the patient fails to answer appropriately or hesitates when answering.

Concentrated verbal interaction may be uncomfortable for the older person. The nurse demonstrates interest and support in giving nonverbal cues and responses, such as direct eye contact, sitting close to the patient, and using touch appropriately. Touching the shoulder, arm, or hand of the patient in a firm purposeful manner conveys support and interest. Avoid stroking or patting the patient, since alterations in tactile perception and cultural orientation may result in misinterpretation.

The ability of the nurse to elicit useful relevant data in the assessment interview will depend, to a great degree, on her comfort and ease in the interview situation. The nurse's negative stereotypes and bias regarding the aged will surface in the interview setting. Older people are sensitive to others' disinterest and impatience.

Although older persons differ in their willingness to reveal life histories and personal experiences, most geriatric patients greatly desire relationships with others and are anxious to share information with interested persons. Elderly patients have much to tell and may offer more information than the nurse needs at a particular time. Reminiscence is common and should be reinforced and encouraged when possible. The patient is concerned with life review or integration of past events with current situations. The life review process may serve as an excellent source of data relevant to the patient's current health problems and support resources. Reminiscence and life review may present problems in keeping the patient focused on the topic at hand; however, it provides an opportunity to assess subtle changes in the patient, such as long-term memory, decision-making ability, judgment-making patterns, affect, and orientation to time, place, and person.

Many geriatric patients are aware of changes in their physical or psychological functioning; however, they may be hesitant to have some of their fears confirmed. Consequently, they may minimize symptoms or ignore them entirely, assuming they are age related and not relevant to current problems. Denial in changes in one's ability to function, remember, concentrate, or attend to personal needs is a common reaction among some older persons. Many geriatric patients consider alterations in functional ability, cognitive function, or emotional stage concomitant with aging and unimportant to maintenance of health and well-being. Often these misconceptions are reinforced by myths about aging and the false assumption by many health professionals that many of the presenting problems of the older person are irreversible or untreatable.

Contrary to popular myths, most older people do not dwell unrealistically on their health and usually have a physical problem when describing their health as poor. However, some older persons are preoccupied with their bodies and will dwell on the physical decline occurring with progressing age. It is essential that the nurse observe and listen carefully to clues that indicate the extent to which the patient's perception indicates individual personality factors developed over a lifetime of experience or represents a current distress.

The geriatric patient may misunderstand the purpose of the nurse's questions and fail to see the relevance to current health status of questions regarding habits, previous life experience, or social supports. Careful and repeated explanations are necessary if the patient is to cooperate with the nurse. Never assume the patient understands the purpose or protocol for the assessment interview. It is wiser to overstate than to increase the patient's anxiety and stress by omitting information. The nurse takes her cues from the response of the patient: listen carefully and observe constantly.

The unfamiliar or new surroundings of the hospital setting or outpatient clinic may impede the progress of the initial interview by distracting the patient and increasing his fear of the unknown. The physical environment should be altered as much as possible to promote comfort. Many older persons are unable to sit for long periods of time because of arthritis or other joint disabilities. Chairs should be comfortable and the patient encouraged to move about as much as he needs. Changing positions and range of motion exercises stimulate circulation and prevent stiffness because of limited mobility.

Most older persons experience some form of sensory deficit, particularly diminished high-frequency hearing and changes in vision, a result of cataracts or glaucoma. The environment should be modified as needed to decrease the impact of those deficits. The setting for the interview should be quiet and away from peripheral noises. The patient, already under a great deal of stress, may be easily distracted and annoyed by extraneous stimulation. The nurse should address the patient in a slow low-pitched voice. Shouting raises the pitch of the noise and makes hearing more difficult. Since fatigue may contribute to diminished mental functioning in the elderly, the morning is the best time for the interview. Patients not only experience fatigue as the day progresses, but may experience a phenomenon known as *sundown syndrome*[9] in which cognitive ability diminishes in the late afternoon or early evening. Some patients become disoriented, confused, or apathetic.

The reliability of the data obtained from the assessment interview should be carefully evaluated. If the nurse questions some aspects of the patient's responses, family or others knowledgeable of the patient should be consulted. Consideration should be given to the physical condition of the patient at the time of the interview and other variables that may influence his status, such as medications, nutritional state, or level of anxiety.

Functional assessment

Functional assessment of the gerontological psychiatric patient is not limited to parameters of mental health. Rather, the ability to function emotionally and cognitively depends, to a great degree, on the older person's overall functional capability. Although not considered in this chapter, a comprehensive assessment is considered necessary for an accurate diagnosis. The present discussion emphasizes the aspect of the functional assessment that has the greatest potential for determining present mental and/or emotional status.

The loss of mobility and independence are real fears among the elderly. The degree to which the gerontological psychiatric patient can move about unassisted should be determined early in the assessment process. Restriction of joints may limit ambulation. A plan for range-of-motion exercises or other activity may be needed to assure that the activity level of the patient remains functional. Patients in wheelchairs and/or walkers need assistance in moving from the bed or chair to standing or walking positions. Orthostatic hypotension is a possibility when patients move rapidly from a lying to a standing position. Secure footwear should be provided for the patient while ambulating since gait may be unsteady and perception of spatial limits altered because of visual impairments.

In addition to changes in functional ability because of changes in physical and/or psychological status, many of the medications routinely taken by geriatric patients may alter perception and make ambulation and mobility difficult. Of particular significance are the sedatives/hypnotics, tranquilizers, and cardiovascular, and hypertensive drugs. Patients should be cautioned about side effects of the medications and encouraged to take plenty of time when ambulating and moving from one position to another. Many falls in the elderly occur because the patient did not have enough time to accommodate to changes in the physical environment (e.g., lighting, texture, or grading of the floor or sidewalk).

Many geriatric patients remain self-sufficient and do not require assistance with eating or in identifying nutritional needs. However, some of the psychosocial problems encountered in the gerontological psychiatric patient that precipitate the need for assistance in eating and monitoring of nutritional intake include (1) patients who are depressed or lonely, with a consequent decrease in appetite; (2) patients experiencing changes in cognitive function, such as confusion or disorientation; (3) patients who are suicidal; (4) patients removed from their familiar ethnic/cultural patterns of eating; (5) patients fearful of hospital routines or procedures. The range of physical problems vary greatly from individual to individual, but some of the areas to be assessed include: (1) the degree of mobility and strength to open cartons of milk, cut meat, handle utensils; (2) the presence of neurological deficits or joint conditions that interfere with hand and/or arm coordination; (3) the presence of visual problems; (4) edentulousness and other losses of chewing ability; (5) problems in swallowing or shortness of breath; (6) the presence of ulcerations in the mouth or on the tongue; (7) periodontal disease; and (8) dry mouth because of side effects of medications. Careful evaluation of the needs of the patient in eating should be made routinely, since nutritional needs of the elderly present one of the most significant problems in institutionalization and can precipitate other problems, such as skin breakdown, inadequate absorption of medications, and diminished wound healing.

The assessment of self-care needs and activities of daily living is essential for establishing baseline data on the patient's potential for independence. Activity may be limited because dysfunctional physical status or psychosocial impairment. ADLs include preparing meals, shopping, eating, bathing, toileting, dressing and other grooming procedures, mobility (e.g., walking, standing, bending, climbing stairs, moving objects from place to place, using a pen or pencil, or other fine motor skills), and housekeeping chores (e.g., making a bed and washing dishes or clothes). Although geriatric patients should be encouraged to move toward greater independence in self-care, it is unrealistic to expect that all patients can function totally independently. The very process of hospitalization and conformity to the routine and procedures of the hospital environment fosters dependence on the part of the patient. Encouraging patients to become involved in their own care is important, since the more the patient can be reinforced for interdependence, the more his self-esteem will be enhanced. Realistic goals should be established and reevaluated periodically.

Positive support systems constitute one of the more critical factors in maintaining a sense of well-being throughout life. Nowhere is this more important than with the gerontological psychiatric patient. Two fifths of all elderly persons are not spending their final years with a spouse.[24] Therefore, as the number of significant contacts diminish, it is important that the remaining support systems are consistent and meaningful. The ethnic background of the patient may be an important factor in the determination of support systems and identification of significant others. Strong family/ethnic ties promote feelings of security. The elderly who live in isolation and are also without family ties generally encounter more serious problems in later life. These problems are not limited to financial instability, but may impact on the patient's desire to get well, by happy and content with his life, and maintain self-care activities whenever possible. Assessment of the support systems, to sustain the patient while in the hospital and on return home or to another institution, should be made on admission. Family and/or friends can assist in reducing the shock and stress of hospitalization and offer reassurance and comfort to the distressed elder. Studies have shown that relocation of the elderly is often a traumatic event. High mortality has been recorded for patients moved from one facility to another or from their familiar home environment to a nursing home or other long-term care facility.[9] The stress of relocation should be identified and anticipated for all geriatric patients and intervention planned to reduce the impact. Allowing the patient to have his own belongings, liberal visiting hours for family or friends, and careful explanations regarding the purpose and procedures of the hospital are but a few of the ways in which the stress of hospitalization can be minimized. Establishing an effective support system within the hospital environment may prevent the negative behavioral response often observed in isolated elders: apathy, depression, aggression, or hostility.

Mental status

Systematic and comprehensive assessment of cognitive function and psychiatric symptoms provides data for drawing diagnostic conclusions and planning intervention strategies. The appropriate use of standardized assessment instruments is an adjunct to the nursing history and interview.

THE MENTAL STATUS QUESTIONNAIRE.[26] The Mental Status Questionnaire (MSQ) has been extensively used in geriatric research and practice. The questionnaire contains 10 questions of orientation items regarding place, date, day of the week and month, age, and birthdate. The last two items cover current events and more distant events by questioning the patient's knowledge of the current and past presidents of the United States. Critics of this instrument suggest that the questions regarding the presidents are irrelevant and inappropriate for some elderly, particularly those in institutional settings and those isolated from the news of everyday happenings. The number of errors made by the patient in responding to the questions indicates the severity of the brain syndrome, which ranges from none or minimal to severe impairment. The MSQ was not designed to be used alone or as the only indicator of impairment. The instrument provides a gross measure of mental status and change in cognitive function. High reliability has been recorded with other measures of cognitive impairment.

THE SHORT PORTABLE MENTAL STATUS QUESTIONNAIRE.[15] The Short Portable Mental Status Questionnaire (SPMSQ) is also a 10-item questionnaire that tests orientation, remote and recent memory, practical skills (recalling a telephone number or street address), and mathematical ability (serial substraction from 20 by 3s). Developed as part of the Older Americans Resources and Services (OARS) at the Duke University Center for the Study of Aging and Human Development, the SPMSQ has high test-retest reliability. The instrument has been administered on both institutionalized and community-based elders. Scores range from 0 to 10 with four levels of disability (intact, mild, moderate, severe impairment) defined. Score adjustments are made for race and for education.

THE FACE-HAND TEST.[20] The Face-Hand Test is a test of organicity that has been widely used in gerontological research and practice for the last 20 years. The instrument was developed to distinguish patients with brain damage from those who are psychotic without an organic cause. The test requires that the individual recognize tactile stimulation on the cheek and palm of the hand. A rehearsal is allowed so that the individual can become familiar with the procedure. The last 4 of 10 paired stimuli count for the score. The individual sits facing the examiner, with the hands resting on the knees and the feet flat on the floor. The individual is touched simultaneously on one cheek and the dorsum of one hand in a specified order. The test is administered twice, once with the individual's eyes closed, then repeated with the individual's eyes open. Some degree of concentration and attention to the procedure must be tolerated by the patient. Anxiety and distraction from peripheral activities may prevent the patient from following the instructions.

THE MINI-MENTAL STATE EXAMINATION.[21] The Mini-Mental State Examination is a portable test of orientation (year, season, date, day, month, state, country, hospital, floor), registration (individually and collectively naming three objects), attention and calculation (counting backward by 7s from 100 or spelling "world" backward), recall (repeating three objects named earlier), and language (naming objects, repeating phrases, obeying three-step commands, writing a sentence, and copying a design). Measurement of cognitive function is the primary focus of the examination, and it is thorough in that area. Requiring only 5 to 10 minutes to administer, it is not tiring to the patient. Difficulty in writing or reading may necessitate adjustments by the nurse administering the tool (e.g., use large bold print when writing out sentences or instructions). Extensive use of this test has been made in distinguishing between patients with diagnoses of dementia, psychosis, and affective disorders (e.g., depression).

THE ZUNG SELF-RATING DEPRESSION SCALE.[44] This scale has the advantage of being a self-report test and the disadvantage of provoking wide interpretation and sensitivity on the part of the patient. The 20-item instrument consists of 10 negatively stated items (e.g., "I feel downhearted and blue") and 10 positively stated items (e.g., "My mind is as clear as it used to be"). The Likert-type scale ranges from "a little of the time" to "most of the time" and requires the individual to distinguish a choice on each item. Visual or language problems result in the test having to be administered orally. Although criticized by some researchers and clinicians as a potentially threatening test because of the sensitivity of the items, the scale takes minimal time to complete and provides an opportunity for the individual to participate in the assessment process by self-report.

THE SANDOZ CLINICAL ASSESSMENT—GERIATRIC.[35] The Sandoz Clinical Assessment—Geriatric (SCAG) specifies a rating of the patient on 18 dimensions and an overall impression score. Developed as part of psychopharmaceutical research, the SCAG necessitates interpretation and rating of the patient's presenting behavior and response to stimuli. Based on observations of the patient's behavior, the scale covers a broader area of assessment of mental status than the SPMSQ or the MSQ. Advanced clinical skill and experience are necessary for effective use of this instrument. As a supplement to other measurements of mental status, it provides data about mood, motivation, social ability, fatigue, and anxiety.

THE NURSES' OBSERVATION SCALE FOR INPATIENT EVALUATION.[25] This evaluation was developed for use with a chronic institutionalized schizophrenic population and is based on nursing observation of patient behavior over a 3-day interval. Observable responses of the patient, such as "talks freely with visitors," "hoards things," and "has temper outbursts," are objectively scored using Likert-type choices ("never" to "always"). Factors of social competence, social interest, cooperation, and psychotic depression represent some of the dimensions on the scale. Although only recently used to any extent with a nonpsychiatric geriatric population, the instrument has potential for providing systematical objective ratings of patient behavior. Interrater reliability is high, based on selected studies, compared to the SCAG and other more subjective rating scales.

Activities of daily living

Measures of physical functioning in the elderly vary in scope and emphasis. The use of measures of ADL along with measures of cognitive function and psychiatric symptoms, enables the nurse to develop a comprehensive data base on the patient. One or more of these instruments may constitute one component of the initial assessment interview in addition to being used throughout the intervention-evaluation phases of the nurse-patient relationship.

THE KATZ INDEX OF ACTIVITIES OF DAILY LIVING.[27] This index consists of dichotomous rating of six ADL functions: bathing, dressing, toileting, transfer, continence, and feeding. One point is assigned for each item of dependency observed. The dichotomous dependent-independent categories for each function are defined in observable terms ("gets clothes from closets and drawers"). This widely known and used instrument has the advantage of measuring change in ADL functions over time and as a result of rehabilitation.

PACE II.[40] PACE II focuses on evaluation of physical health of nursing home patients. Checklists are used to identify the presence of defined conditions (diagnosed), abnormal laboratory or other findings, risk factors, and other impairments and disabilities. Under each medically defined condition, the duration, type, or location of the problem is specified. Thoroughness of observations is necessary in this patient-planning tool, in addition to review and inclusion of the medical history and examination. PACE II has the advantage of providing for interdisciplinary assessment and planning for care.

Family-patient interaction

The manner in which family members relate to and support (or fail to support) each other has a profound influence on individuals within the family structure and the group as a whole. Nowhere is this influence more evident than when an older adult becomes the central focus of conflict or dysfunction for the family unit. Behavioral problems in the elderly may result from lack of the family's ability to deal with the losses and increasing dependence of an older member.

The inclusion of family members or significant others in the patient's life in the overall assessment process cannot be underestimated. In addition to verifying information supplied by the patient during the initial assessment process, the family's perceptions of their relationship with the patient adds yet another dimension to the understanding of the response of the patient to his own aging and disability.

The format for assessment of patient-family dynamics varies, depending on the setting (e.g., community clinic, home, or institution) and the behavior and needs of the patient. Two instruments for consideration in collection of data relevant to this area of assessment are described here.

THE FAMILY APGAR.[37] The family APGAR is designed to assist clinicians in systematically assessing an impression of family function from the perception of individual family members. Categories for rating include adaptation, partnership, growth, affection, and resolve. Sample questions for the categories include the following: "I am satisfied with the help that I receive from my family when something is troubling me" (adaptation), "I find that my family accepts my wishes to take on new activities and make changes in my life-style" (growth), and "I am satisfied with the way my family and I share time together" (resolve). Each family member indicates his degree of satisfaction or dissatisfaction with each item on a Likert-type 0 to 2 scale ("almost always, hardly ever"), or the clinician can verbally administer each question and score the response. A score of 3 or less (out of 10) indicates high dysfunction for the individual; a score of 4 to 6 would indicate moderate dysfunction. Discrepancies or low scores obtained by individual family members are indicators of problem areas and require further exploration and assessment. This usable practical tool was not developed specifically for assessing families dealing with an older member. As an indication of the patient's and his family's perception of each other, this instrument has potential for understanding the dynamics of the family's structure and function.

THE SOCIAL BEHAVIOR ASSESSMENT SCHEDULE.[34] This schedule utilizes the patient's more significant relative or friend to elicit information regarding the patient's social functioning ability. The instrument consists of a semistructured interview schedule focusing on the patient's behavior and psychosocial status. Adverse or dysfunctional effects on family function are explored. Patient behavior, such as withdrawal, forgetfulness, and indecisiveness are included in the inventory. Rating of the behavior consists of evaluation of the response as moderate to severe, frequency of occurrence, and time of onset. Twelve areas of social performance, such as household tasks, household management, and decision making, make up the social functioning rating. The onset of diminished performance and dysfunction observed are rated in a fashion similar to the rating of patient behavior. Additional categories in the instrument query adverse effects of others on the patient's behavior, concurrent events (e.g., physical illness, medications), and support to the informant received from neighbors, friends, and other family members. Nurses working with families in the home or community setting may find this instrument an important measure of baseline function of the patient as perceived by those involved in his care.

To date, nursing's use of standardized instruments in the data collection phase of the nursing process has been minimal. The selection of a tool depends on the setting, patient population, and purpose of the nursing assessment. The degree to which these tools are used alone or in conjunction with other forms of assessment (e.g., physical assessment and evaluation) varies with the presenting problems of the patient. Although skills required in the use of the instruments described here are easily learned, practice and verification with others providing care for the patient are necessary to develop confidence in the findings yielded by these measurement tools.

Nursing diagnosis

The nursing diagnosis is the culmination of the process of data collection and analysis regarding the patient's functional ability and resources. Behavioral interpretation of the patient's presenting needs and problems facilitates the nurse's role as intervenor in dysfunctional or disruptive processes. Both objective and subjective data are required to determine the extent of the patient's functional ability. Selective use of the data depends on the resources available to the patient and the nurse in collaboratively working toward resolution of the problem or problems.

The medical diagnosis is based on identification of the disease contributing to the patient's dysfunctional behavior. The medical diagnosis is complementary to the nursing diagnosis, since psychopathological conditions prevent the patient from functioning at his maximum potential and utilizing optimal capabilities. The relationship between the disease process and the behavioral response of the patient is not always clear since some of the same behaviors may be a result of different pathological processes. For example, mood swings and alterations in mood may be present in patients who are depressed and patients who are experiencing disruptions in cognitive function because of organic changes, as seen in Alzheimer's disease and related diseases.

Although the older adult may experience a wide range of psychiatric problems, consideration is given to those problems of greatest significance to the nurse and patient in the development of a helping therapeutic relationship.

Changes in cognitive function

MEMORY LOSS. One of the most distressing and often frustrating aspects of aging is the potential for progressive memory loss. Although memory loss may be the result of organic brain disease or depression, the onset does not necessarily imply an inherent disease process. With age, loss of short-term memory, recall for recent events, is more likely to occur than loss of remote memory, recall for events that occurred in the distant past. The conceptual network of past thoughts, images, ideas, and experiences that make up memory and remembering develops and matures over one's lifetime. Primary memory comprises the conscious control system for memory and appears stable over the life span. It is believed that few differences exist between ages in relation to primary memory. The speed of access appears to slow with increasing age.[36] Long-term memory (secondary memory) is the storage system for what is commonly understood as memory. Failure in retrieval, original acquisition, or learning may account for some of the loss experienced in secondary memory.[36]

Many factors contribute to alterations in memory in older adults. Stress or confrontation with crisis, depression, and a sense of worthlessness, loss of interest in present events, cerebrovascular changes that affect cerebral function, loss of neural cells because of disease or trauma, and sensory deprivation or isolation from verbal interactions are all situations or events one experiences with advancing age.[31] Sensory loss, including changes in vision and hearing, makes the older person vulnerable to the environment and to those around him, often resulting in avoidance of the situation at hand and withdrawal into a less threatening world. Comfort may be sought in old memories and experiences, replacing the need and desire to remain in touch with the present.

Institutionalized elders appear to have more difficulty in memory than older adults living at home or in other community settings. The institutional geriatric patient is portrayed as dull, listless, and uncommunicative. The environment often promotes this response and reinforces the "compliant" "cooperative" patient. A stimulating environment and therapeutic regimen can counteract and, in many situations, reverse withdrawal behavior in the gerontological psychiatric patient and revive interest in recall and participation in the present.

WITHDRAWAL. Withdrawal "is an adaptive or coping mechanism . . . involving physically pulling away from or psychologically losing interest in an anxiety-producing situation, person or stressful environment."[31] Multiple losses or fear of loss may precipitate withdrawal. Prolonged grief and hesitation about returning to an active life after the loss of a spouse, sibling, or child predisposes the elder to dysfunctional and nonresponsive behavior. The introverted adult may find adjusting to change and flexibility in response to new situations more difficult with advancing age, therefore it is important to understand the personality of the patient and his previous adaptive styles.

Sudden withdrawal and refusal to invest in relationships with others should alert the nurse to the possibility of physiological factors as potential causes; low-grade infection, pain, and toxicity or side effects of medications are but a few of the many precipitating events that could initiate changes in behavior. Careful assessment and evaluation are necessary.

The geriatric patient experiencing organic intellectual impairment (e.g., Alzheimer's disease and related disorders) frequently withdraws from social contacts, daily routines, and ADLs. He may deny the possibility of a problem, or because of difficulties with memory, fear the consequences of these changes. Withdrawal can become a defense mechanism, reinforcing the denial of perceived disability and further loss of functional ability.

CONFUSION. Confusion is a phenomenon only recently studied systematically by nurses. The term is used by nurses "to describe a constellation of client behaviors, including inattention and memory deficits, inappropriate verbalizations, disruptive behavior, noncompliance, and failure to perform activities of daily living."[42] Frequently, confusion is a nonspecific label imposed by staff on apathetic, withdrawn, or uncooperative patients. Wolanin and Phillips[41] suggest several categories of patients as particularly vulnerable to being perceived and labeled as confused: the problem patient, the patient with communication problems (slurred speech, expressive dysphasia), the patient who challenges personal values of the staff, the physically unattractive patient, the depressed patient, and the "troublemaker" (e.g., does not improve despite nursing interventions and ministrations).

Institutionalized elders are at particular risk for confusion. From 30% to 80% suffer from organic brain disease to some degree with concomitant disorientation regarding time, place and person, gross remote and recent memory loss, and inability to execute simple calculations. In many nursing homes and other long-term care facilities, over 30% of the patients experience severe confusion.[22] The precipitating factors in confusion vary and depend on both the physiological and psychological status of the patient.

Early morning confusion, appearing as a type of *sunrise syndrome,* may be due to the hangover effects of sedatives-hypnotics or other nighttime medications that interact with drugs for sleep. Sleep disruptions and insomnia are particularly bothersome to the elderly. Adverse reactions to drugs prescribed for sleep are not uncommon and should be considered. Increasing disorientation or confusion at night, resulting from loss of visual accommodation, is known as *sundown syndrome*.[9] Anticipation of the potential threats to the patient's safety during these times should alert the nurse to take special precautions to prevent falls and other mobility hazards.

The nurse should never assume that confusion and disorientation are natural consequences of changes in cognitive or physiological status. On the contrary, confusion is reversible in over half of the patients experiencing it. It is usually transient or of short duration and is one area in which the nurse has primary responsibility. The carefully planned, therapeutic nurse-patient relationship can be a significant factor in preventing and intervening in this distressing condition.

Although disorientation is often used analogously with confusion, care should be taken to differentiate between them. A disoriented patient is not necessarily confused, and a confused patient does not necessarily experience disorientation in all spheres. The mental status tests discussed earlier in the chapter differentiate disorientation in place, person, and time from components of confusion, such as alterations in memory, judgment, decision-making, and problem solving.

PARANOIA. Paranoia and fear are reactions by some older persons to loss, isolation, and loneliness. Classic psychopathological paranoia, demonstrated by a well-organized and elaborate system of superiority, is rare in older persons. Delusions and disturbances in mood, behavior, and thinking may be a transient condition experienced by the geriatric patient in reaction to sensory deprivation or sensory loss, imposed or voluntary isolation from social contacts, or as an adverse reaction to psychotropic or other drugs.[29]

Paranoid symptoms appear as diffuse or specific. The geriatric patient may perceive threat from certain persons (e.g., family, friends, neighbors) or at stressful times (e.g., night). Relocation to a new home, new room in the hospital or nursing home, or strange environment devoid of familiar belongings precipitates fears, anxiety, and for some, paranoid ideation.

The personality of the aging paranoid patient is characterized by withdrawal, aloofness, fearfulness, oversensitivity, and often secretiveness. As long as the patient does not call attention to himself or pose a threat to himself or others, he may go undetected for a long time. Once he is recognized as a potential threat to himself or others, institutionalization becomes a consideration. Older persons suffering from transient or chronic paranoia are at high risk for victimization by others, self-neglect, and abuse (e.g., refusal to eat, take prescribed medications, or attend to hygiene needs). Anticipation and assessment of the influence of paranoia on the patient's welfare constitutes an important aspect of the care of the patient.

Changes in affect

Disturbances in mood, mood swings, or oversensitive emotional reactions represent behaviors of older adults that are common to all age groups at one time or another. The reaction of an older person to physical limitations or disabilities, psychological loss (particularly a spouse or other significant other), or the possibility of institutionalization depends on previous coping styles, support systems, especially family, and present psychological and physiological strength.

Radical or abrupt alterations in mood indicate reaction to internal or external stress or inadequate coping mechanisms required to deal with progressive loss or dependency. When this behavior is evident in otherwise content, happy, and adjusted elderly people, physiological factors, including side effects of cardiovascular or psychotropic drugs, should be considered. Reassurance and support during evaluation are essential to reducing the anxiety and diminishing the threat perceived by the patient.

Depression and sadness are viewed by some as a natural phenomenon of aging, and depression is essentially a disorder of later life. Comfort[11] suggests scores on the Zung Self-Rating Depression Scale may reflect mild depression in many older people because of the bias of the instrument. The questionnaire emphasizes social usefulness and activity, which may be limited in some older adults. Although not limited to social impositions, depression, grief, and loss are common in later life.

Prolonged grief and mourning over a real or imagined loss should be recognized as depression and responded to as such. Symptoms common to the depressed geriatric patient include, but are not limited to, weight loss; anorexia;

undue fatigue; apathy; loss of interest in friends, family, and usual activities; and psychomotor retardation. None of the symptoms are precipitated by increasing age and should be considered problematical.

The older person's attitude toward his own aging and toward death and dying may greatly influence the degree to which the depression can be successfully treated. The "loss of hope" expressed by some older persons, particularly in the face of increasing disabilities, may precipitate or stem from a depressive reaction.

Undiagnosed depression may have serious consequences for the elderly, since the problem is always manifested in physical behavior. Many of the medications routinely prescribed for the older person may potentiate or enhance a depression. Examples include tranquilizers (major and minor), barbiturates, cardiotonics (digoxin), and steroids. A medication history is part of the evaluation and assessment.

When considering mood changes, grief, and depression in the geriatric patient, it is important to recognize and understand the significance of the patient's and family's attitude toward death and dying. The old differ from the young in facing death in several ways; older persons tend to integrate attitudes of death with their formal religious training, have more experience with death (e.g., peers, spouse), tend to be more accepting of death, and tend to approach problems primarily from an internal focus of activity. The state of the older person's health, in addition to the cues from observing peers or spouse who have died or are dying, signal that his life may be coming to an end. Awareness of the older person's "stage of dying" is important to understanding his needs and concerns.

Intentional deaths among the elderly are not uncommon. Of all suicides committed in this country annually 25% are persons over the age of 65 years. White males over the age of 85 are at particular risk. Other high-risk persons include the isolated elderly, experiencing loss of family or friends through death; elderly with changes in body function and decreased independence because of pain, weakness, immobility, and shortness of breath; elderly with changes in body structure because of surgery or stroke; or the prospect of a terminal illness. Examples of intentional deaths include excessive risk taking, imprudence in the management of ordinary affairs, refusal to eat, overuse or misuse of alcohol or drugs, and noncompliance with life-sustaining medical regimens, such as refusal to take insulin or digoxin, when these activities take place with the expectation that death will occur.

Elizabeth Kübler-Ross[28] has described five stages of the dying process that represent the coping mechanisms of dying. Her model is described in detail in Chapter 32. The family and significant others in the patient's life play an important role in the dying process. Nurses can encourage and support increased involvement of these support groups in the care of the patient. Assessment should be indirect and based on the cues from the patient that there is readiness to talk. Attentive listening alerts the nurse to the patient's need to express feelings or ventilate fears. Covert or overt references to death or thoughts concerning dying are early cues the patient may be making preparations for his own death.

Over 60,000 "living wills" have been distributed by America's Euthanasia Educational Council.[9] This reflects an increasing interest by consumers in how one's death will occur. It represents a person's choice in participating in the final decision to refuse heroic measures after there is no reasonable expectation for recovery. On admission, the existence of a "living will" should be ascertained, from either the patient, family, or guardian. The nurse should be well acquainted with the hospital's policy regarding the acknowledgment of this document and the procedures for sharing with all staff and for ensuring the patients' wishes are recognized.

Somatic responses

There is much overlap and interaction between hypochondriasis and depression. Overconcern and preoccupation with one's physical and emotional health and expression through body complaints are common with depressive feelings and introspection but may be present in the absence of a depressed mood.

The rationale underlying hypochondriasis characterizes the needs being expressed by the patient. As a symbol of the geriatric patient's sense of defectiveness and deterioration, somaticism communicates the distress surrounding and displacement of a diminished sense of worth. Escape into the "sick" role is a legitimate and socially acceptable way to deal with stress and anxiety. Support, concern, and interest are conveyed to the patient and he experiences a sense of control.

One of the real problems encountered by the

elder with a history of hypochondriasis is the tendency by health professionals to label the patient as a "crock" and dismiss complaints, even if based on organic pathological conditions. All complaints of the patient should be taken seriously and investigated thoroughly. One must never assume the problem is "just a response to some emotional distress" and can be dismissed. Whatever the reasons, the problem is real and the patient's discomfort is real.

Insomnia and anorexia may be symptoms or problems for the gerontological psychiatric patient. Many older adults experience chronic or semichronic sleep problems. Complaints of interrupted sleep, loss of sleep, or "poor sleep" with frequent awakenings and morning exhaustion are common. Daytime napping and drowsiness add to the problem.

Opinions regarding what is normal sleep with aging and the nature of normal sleep patterns in older adults vary and are often controversial. Some researchers suggest that older people need less sleep with increasing age. Chronic fatigue, physical illness, pain, and decreased mobility may result in a requirement for more sleep. Often, the geriatric patient expresses distress over the inability to sleep or stay asleep. Perceived lack of sleep becomes a cyclical reaction. Worry over the lack of sleep prevents the elder from falling asleep. Fatigue, the most common physical complaint of adults over the age of 75, contributes to much of the insomnia of this age group. Lack of exercise, limited mobility, and side effects of drugs are the potential factors contributing to insomnia.

The emotional effects of insomnia vary with the individual, but reinforcement of fatigue and depression are common. Recognition of insomnia as a reaction to emotional and physical disruptions and as a potential precipitator of other problems is the first step to an assessment of the nature of the problem.

Anorexia is common in depression but may be seen in confused or disoriented patients. Forgetting to eat or the inability to prepare one's meals may reinforce loss of appetite. Side effects of some drugs (e.g., dry mouth, change in taste) contribute to disinterest in food. The edentulous patient or the patient with gum disease avoids chewing when possible. The interaction of anorexia and emotional dysfunction should always be considered and included in the nutritional evaluation. Poor nutrition contributes to fatigue, listlessness, and immobility.

Planning and implementing nursing interventions

Nursing care strategies have been introduced throughout the chapter as part of the assessment and data collection process. Specific interventions will be considered as part of the total milieu for the patient. The elderly respond well to both individual and group psychotherapy. They need the opportunity to talk, have support in their efforts to deal with day by day problems, and plan for a meaningful future.

LIFE REVIEW THERAPY. Life review therapy was first described by Butler.[7] It has a positive psychotherapeutic function, providing an opportunity for the individual to reflect on his life to resolve, reorganize, and reintegrate troubling or disturbing concerns. The life review works well in both group and individual settings. Chubon[10] describes an innovative approach to life review with a 65-year-old woman who had experienced multiple disabilities. Using a novel describing people with lives similar to that of the patient's, the therapist assisted the patient in identifying with the characters, thereby reducing the emotional impact of reliving old conflicts and experiences. In a group setting, members may positively reinforce each other and stimulate the mutual learning process. Developing individual autobiographies to share within the group is one way to introduce commonalities among the members and to put the individuals at ease with sharing personal histories. The group cohesiveness and sharing can build self-esteem and a feeling of belonging, in addition to the cathartic atmosphere of the review itself.

REMINISCING GROUPS. Reminiscing groups resemble life review groups in that the focus is on recounting earlier life experiences and events. In reminiscence, sharing perceptions, historical life events, and generational attributes provides a common theme for the interaction. Individual reminiscing should be encouraged as much as possible and supported as an effort to assist the patient in discharging emotional and cognitive energy. Rambling does not constitute a therapeutic reminiscing experience, since the preoccupation with the dissociated thoughts may actually increase anxiety. Reminiscing is both a way of holding on to the past and letting go.[16]

REALITY ORIENTATION. Reality orientation was developed as a specific therapeutic program for institutionalized geriatric patients by James C. Folsom and colleagues in 1958.[39] Both 24-hour and classroom (structured) reality orientation have potential for preventing confusion, keeping patients oriented to time, place, person, and situation. The structure of the environment reinforces contact with reality, the here and now, when it is kept simple and focused. Physical props can assist by the inclusion of clocks, directional signs, calendars, and orientation boards (season of the year, weather, etc). The classroom reality orientation consists of an intensive small group experience, especially effective for the moderate to severely impaired elderly. It provides an opportunity to reinforce time, place, and person orientation with patients who have a short attention span and need extra verbal and visual stimulation. Reality orientation, along with a discussion of current events, stimulates the patient to maintain contact with reality and the outside world and his place in it. Current events discussions, used alone, may be more flexibly structured with sharing of newspaper headlines, special articles, or group viewing of television news programs. The scope and depth of the groups depend on the abilities of the patients and the other therapeutic modalities at hand.

COGNITIVE TRAINING. Much research is underway using cognitive training and stimulation.[43] Problem-solving situations, formal or didactic memory training, and memory exercises have proven effective in increasing attention span, efficiency of recall, and the ability to learn new skills (e.g., mathematical calculations, vocabulary). Intelligence does not decline with progressive age but may be dulled by depression, drugs, or lack of use. Cognitive training has promise for providing methods for keeping older adults active mentally, which in turn will enhance emotional well-being. The "use-it or lose-it" adage holds true for maintenance of intelligence as it does for physical functioning. Stimulating cognitive skills can challenge the nurse's creativity in relating to gerontological psychiatric patients. Capitalizing on the patient's interests and skills necessitates familiarity with the patient's past occupation, hobbies, and leisure activities. The nursing interview should focus on gathering as much of that information as possible on admission and adding to the data base as the nurse has the opportunity to build a trusting relationship with the patient.

RELAXATION THERAPY. Relaxation therapy is another therapeutic modality receiving increasing interest and research. In addition to promoting a sense of physical well-being, relaxation

has the potential for releasing tension and reducing stress, which are often viewed as barriers to relating with others. The steps in simple relaxation exercises are described in detail by Wolanin and Phillips and are presented in Chapter 7 of this text.[42] Relaxation, combined with mild isometric exercises, increases cardiovascular output, energy, and mobility and reduces stress. Relaxation and exercise strategies, used in group or individual contexts, do not require advanced skills of the nurse or the patient. They may begin with simple, basic tension-releasing muscle exercises, coupled with verbal instructions regarding breathing and concentration.

SUPPORT AND COUNSELING GROUPS. These groups offer therapeutic outlets for patients and families. Using a nondirective or unstructured format, the members can ventilate feelings, try out problem-solving approaches, and resolve conflicts in a rational systematical manner. Older adults respond well to a supportive group structure, increasing self-esteem, self-confidence, risk taking, and empathy for others. Caregiver groups are becoming very popular, since 80% of the older adults living at home are cared for by a spouse, sibling, or child. Many community agencies, clinics, and senior citizen centers are responding to the need of this group with special activities, training classes, and supportive groups.

Evaluation and future trends

Specific nursing interventions designed to promote optimum cognitive function and emotional well-being have been considered as part of the role of the gerontological psychiatric nurse. Increasingly, research is being initiated to determine the most appropriate strategy for the needs of the patient and the most effective modality for implementing that strategy.

Gerontological psychiatric nursing offers an exciting and challenging future for nurses interested in working with patients responsive to knowledgeable and creative care. In one sense, most nurses today practice gerontological/geriatric nursing without recognizing it as such, since a growing proportion of patients in all health care settings are elderly. The significance of this growing population will become even more evident as we move toward the twenty-first century. The establishment of chronic disease and other long-term care facilities will supercede the growth of acute care hospitals. The reliance on home care and the use of community resources to meet the health needs of all ages, but particularly the elderly, will grow in the next two decades. Advanced technology will permit shorter stays in acute care hospitals, quicker recovery periods, and less complicated disease courses.

Research in gerontological nursing has grown in the last 10 years. Without research, the direction and impact of practice remains unclear. Burnside[6] suggests several areas for research that stem from problems of concern to nurses working with the aged person: continence, sensory stimulation and deprivation, drug abuse, the use of touch and other communicative strategies with the elderly, effectiveness of treatment modalities in senile dementia, and promotion of wellness, to mention a few. The influence of nursing research on nursing practice will depend on the ability of clinicians and researchers to work together in identifying clinical problems of importance and designing projects collaboratively to investigate those problems. Only through collaboration will a body of nursing knowledge develop and grow.

Interprofessional activities in gerontology and geriatrics offer yet another avenue for nurses to impact on the care of the elderly. The funding by private and federal sources of teaching nursing home demonstration projects with a combined academic, clinical, and research focus promises greater cooperation between nursing, medicine, dentistry, pharmacy, and social work. The extent to which the academic nursing home is successful depends, to a great degree, on the strength of the individual groups participating in the effort.

The concept of nursing home without walls has grown in popularity over recent years.[32] The idea is to use the nursing home as a base for services for the elderly rather than a final resort, as it is now conceived. Maintenance of the patient in his home or other community setting as long as possible will become a reality by offering supportive and comprehensive services to the elder and his family. Patients will move into and out of the nursing home for intensive and episodical nursing care or as a respite for family members from their caregiver responsibilities.

The growing interest in and focus on gerontological/geriatric nursing in nursing education is promising and will assure the nurse of the future an opportunity to offer quality care to this age group.

Suggested cross-references

The phases of the nursing process are discussed in Chapter 4. Primary prevention and identification of the elderly as a high-risk group are discussed in Chapter 5. Disturbances of mood are discussed in Chapter 9. Nursing care of the patient with impaired cognition is discussed in Chapter 13. The mental status examination is discussed in Chapter 17.

SUMMARY

1. Sociodemographic factors of aging were presented with projections for the increase in this minority group over the next 20 years. Psychiatric and related disorders were defined and the statistical significance emphasized.

2. The evolution of the role of the gerontological psychiatric nurse was traced, beginning with changes in age distribution after World War II and the needs of an aging society. The gerontological nurse may function in a variety of roles, including patient-care manager in nursing homes or other long-term care settings, health assessor, primary care provider, independent practitioner, and researcher.

3. Several theories of aging and the consequences of aging were presented. Biological theories attempt to explain the reasons the body ages over time. De-liberate biological programming theory suggests that humans have a biological time clock in which the memory and capacity for terminating the life of a cell is stored in the cell itself. The wear-and-tear theory posits the notion that structure and function changes over time, which is accelerated by abuse and decelerated by care. The stress-adaptation theory presumes stress accelerates the aging process. Psychosocial and personality theories of aging focus on emotional response to the aging process. Disengagement theory postulates that mutual withdrawal by older adults and society is a normal and positive benefit of aging. Critics reacting to disengagement developed the activity theory, maintaining that active involved elders are healthier and happier. The life review, postulated by Butler, involves reminiscence and recall of past life

events with resulting release of anxiety, reduction of fear of the future, and successful reintegration of one's meaningful life experiences. Erikson's concept of ego integrity delineates the last developmental stage of life, in which one reflects on accomplishments and failures. Stability of personality (Costa and McCrae) persists over the life span regardless of external or internal stressors.

4. Nursing assessment of the gerontological psychiatric patient is a multifaceted process, consisting of the interview, functional assessment, and evaluation of mental status.

5. Standardized measurement tools for assessing the older adult were presented, including the Mental Status Questionnaire, the Short Portable Mental Status Questionnaire, the Face-Hand Test, the Mini-Mental Status Examination, the Zung Self-Rating Depression Scale, the Sandoz Clinical Assessment—Geriatric, the Nurses Observational Schedule for Inpatient Evaluation, the Katz Index of Activities of Daily Living, PACE II, the Family APGAR, and the Social Behavior Assessment Schedule. Discussion centered on the advantages and disadvantages of each of the tools as adjuncts to other assessment techniques.

6. Nursing diagnosis was differentiated from medical diagnosis. Behavioral approaches to nursing diagnosis with assessment and intervention strategies for each included consideration of memory loss, withdrawal, confusion, paranoia, mood swings, grief, loss, depression, perceptions of death and dying, hypochondriasis, insomnia, and anorexia. Emphasized throughout the discussion was the interrelationship between physiological and psychological factors impacting on optimum functioning.

7. The life review, as a therapeutic intervention, stressed the notion of context (group vs. individual) and innovative approaches to the technique. The similarity of reminiscence groups and the purpose of reminiscence as a therapeutic strategy were discussed.

8. Examples of therapeutic interventions with the elderly include reality orientation, cognitive training, and relaxation therapy.

9. Families and caregivers of the home-bound and home-care elderly respond well to supportive and counseling groups and are receiving increasing attention from nurses and other health care professionals.

10. New and innovative approaches to care of the elderly characterizes the future of gerontological nursing. The need for clinical research to build a body of nursing knowledge in gerontology is recognized by researchers and practitioners alike. Emphasis is being placed on interprofessional practice approaches to the care of the geriatric patient.

References

1. Abdellah, F.G.: Nursing care of the aged in the United States of America, J. Gerontol. Nurs. **7:**657, 1981.
2. American Nurses' Association: The American nurse, Kansas City, Mo., April 20, 1979, The Association.
3. Atchley, R.: Aging and suicide: reflection of the quality of life? In Haynes, S.G., and Feinleib, M., editors: Epidemiology of aging, second conference, U.S. Department of Health and Human Services, Washington, D.C., July 1980.
4. Brehm, H.P.: Organization and financing of health care for the aged: future implications. In Haynes, S.G., and Feinleib, M., editors: Epidemiology of aging, second conference, U.S. Department of Health and Human Services, Washington, D.C., July 1980.
5. Brown, E.L.: The professional role in community nursing. II. Nursing reconsidered: a study of change, Philadelphia, 1971, J.B. Lippincott Co.
6. Burnside, I., editor: Nursing and the aged, New York, 1981, McGraw-Hill, Inc.
7. Butler, R.N.: Re-awakening interest, Nurs. Homes **10:**8, Jan. 1961.
8. Butler, R.N.: Why survive? being old in America, New York, 1975, Harper & Row, Publishers, Inc.
9. Butler, R.N., and Lewis, M.R.: Aging and mental health: psychosocial and biomedical approaches, ed. 3, St. Louis, 1981, The C.V. Mosby Co.
10. Chubon, S.: A novel approach to the process of life review, J. Gerontol. Nurs. **6:**543, 1980.
11. Comfort, A.: Practice of geriatric psychiatry, New York, 1980, American Elsevier Publishing, Inc.
12. Cumming, E., and Henry, W.E.: Growing old: the process of disengagement, New York, 1961, Basic Books, Inc.
13. Davis, B.: A coming of age: a challenge for geriatric nursing, J. Am. Geriatr. Soc. **16:**1100, 1966.
14. Davis, B.: ANA and the geriatric nurse, Nurs. Clin. North Am. **3:**741, 1968.
15. Duke University Center for the Study of Aging and Human Development: Multidimensional functional assessment: the OARS methodology, Durham, N.C., 1978, Duke University.
16. Ebersole, P.P.: A theoretical approach to the use of reminiscence. In Burnside, I.M., editor: Working with the elderly: group processes and techniques, North Scituate, Mass., 1978, Duxbury Press.
17. Ehrman, J.: Elderly personalities remain stable over time, NIH Record **33:**3, Aug. 4, 1981.
18. Eisdorfer, C., and Feidel, R.O.: Cognitive and emotional disturbance in the elderly: clinical issues, Chicago, 1977, Year Book Medical Publishers, Inc.
19. Erikson, E.H.: Identity and the life cycle: psychological issues, New York, 1959, International Universities Press, Inc.
20. Fink, M., et al.: Face-hand test as a diagnostic sign of organic mental syndrome, Neurology **2:**46, Jan.-Feb. 1952.
21. Folstein, M.F. et al.: Mini-mental state: a practical method for grading the cognitive states of patients for the clinician, J. Psychol. Res. **12:**189, 1975.
22. Goldfarb, A.I.: Institutional care of the aged. In Busse,

E.W., and Pfeiffer, E., editors: Behavior and adaptation in late life, Boston, 1977, Little, Brown & Co.

23. Hayflick, L. et al.: The serial cultivation of human diploid cells, Exp. Cell Res. **25**:585, 1961.

24. Hendricks, J., and Hendricks, C.D.: Aging in mass society, ed. 2, Cambridge, Mass., 1981, Winthrop Publishers, Inc.

25. Honigfeld, G., and Klett, C.J.: The nurses' observation scale for inpatient evaluation: a new scale for measuring improvement in chronic schizophrenia, J. Clin. Psychol. **21**:65, Jan. 1965.

26. Kahn, R.L.: Brief objective measure for the determination of mental status in the aged, Am. J. Psychiatry **117**:326, 1960.

27. Katz, S. et al.: Sudies of illness in the aged. The index of ADL: a standardized measure of biological and psychosocial function, J.A.M.A. **185**:914, 1963.

28. Kübler-Ross, E.: On death and dying, London, 1970, Tavistock Publications, Ltd.

29. Lamy, P.P.: Prescribing for the elderly, Littleton, Mass., 1980, PSG Publishing Co., Inc.

30. Lowenthal, M.F. et al.: Four stages of life: a comparative study of women and men facing transitions, San Francisco, 1975, Jossey-Bass, Inc., Publishers.

31. Murry, R. et al.: The nursing process in later maturity, Englewood Cliffs, N.J., 1980, Prentice-Hall, Inc.

32. National Institute on Aging: National Advisory Council Meeting Minutes, Bethesda, Md., Oct. 1981, U.S. Department of Health and Human Services.

33. Ochsner, A.: Aging, J. Am. Geriatr. Soc. **24**:385, 1976.

34. Platt, S. et al.: Social behavior assessment schedule (SBAS): rationale, contents, scoring and reliability of a new interview schedule, Soc. Psychiatry **15**:43, 1980.

35. Shader, R.I. et al.: A new scale for clinical assessment in geriatric populations: Sandoz Clinical Assessment—Geriatric (SCAG), J. Am. Geriatr. Soc. **12**:107, March 1974.

36. Siegler, I.C.: The psychology of adult development and aging. In Busse, E.W., and Blazer, D.G., editors: Handbook of geriatric psychiatry, New York, 1980, Van Nostrand Reinhold Co.

37. Smilkstein, G.: The family APGAR: a proposal for a family function test and its use by physicians, J. Fam. Pract. **6**:1231, 1978.

38. Stone, V.: The nurse and the aged, R.N. **39**:21, Feb. 1976.

39. Taulbee, L., and Folsom, J.: Reality orientation for geriatric patients, Hosp. Community Psychiatry **17**:133, May 1966.

40. U.S. Department of Health, Education and Welfare: Working document on patient care management, Washington, D.C., 1978, U.S. Government Printing Office.

41. Wolanin, M.O., and Phillips, L.R.F.: Who's confused here? Geriatr. Nurs. **1**:122, July-Aug. 1980.

42. Wolanin, M.O., and Phillips, L.R.F.: Confusion: prevention and care, St. Louis, 1981, The C.V. Mosby Co.

43. Yesavage, J.A. et al.: Senile dementia: combined pharmacologic and psychologic treatment, J. Am. Geriatr. Soc. **29**:164, April 1981.

44. Zung, W.W.K.: A self-rating depression scale, Arch. Gen. Psychiatry **12**:63, Jan. 1965.

Annotated suggested readings

Brink, T.L.: Geriatric psychotherapy, New York, 1979, Human Sciences Press, Inc.

This introductory text in psychological gerontology is useful for all health professionals in applying psychotherapy skills with the elderly. Strategies and techniques of intervention include dream, group, family, milieu, behavioral, and psychopharmacological therapies.

Britnell, J., and Mitchell, K.: Inpatient group psychotherapy for the elderly, J. Psychiatr. Nurs. **19**:19, May 1981.

This is one of the few articles in the nursing literature on group psychotherapy for the elderly. It describes a theoretical framework and applies it to case examples.

Burnside, I.M., editor: Working with the elderly: group processes and techniques, North Scituate, Mass., 1978, Duxbury Press.

This volume of papers provides an overview of group work with the elderly, including reminiscence, reality orientation, remotivation, music, and art therapy. A practical "how to" approach is utilized.

Busse, E.W., and Blazer, D.G., editors: Handbook of geriatric psychiatry, New York, 1980, Van Nostrand Reinhold Co.

A multiauthored volume that provides an eclectic perspective to the field of geriatric psychiatry. The authors integrate basic biological and psychosocial knowledge into the diagnosis and clinical treatment of psychiatric disorders of late life.

Comfort, A.: Practice of geriatric psychiatry, New York, 1980, American Elsevier Publishing Inc.

A practical approach to geropsychiatry includes an overview and systematical discussion of every major category of geriatric mental disease. Both diagnostic and therapeutic data are included throughout the text.

Eisdorfer, C., and Friedel, R.O., editors: Cognitive and emotional disturbance in the elderly: clinical issues, Chicago, 1977, Year Book Medical Publishers, Inc.

A multiauthored book focused on the emerging developments in the field of cognitive and related emotional disturbances in the elderly. Particular attention is given to reversible dementia, differentiation of disease from normal aging, and the importance of combined medical and social management of the aging patient.

Ernst, P., and Shaw, J.: Touching is not taboo, Geriatr. Nurs. **1**:193, Sept.-Oct. 1980.

The physician/nurse co-authors suggest that touch provides a therapeutic intervention in treating disturbed and/or regressed elderly patients. Findings from clinical research studies provide the premise for examining the therapeutic elements of touch.

Hewes, C.J.: Role of the nursing coordinator on a geropsychiatric unit, J. Gerontol. Nurs. **7**:607, 1981.

The author is a nurse coordinator of a large neuropsychiatric institute in Southern California. Experimental role modeling for staff and patient advocacy are two of the many components of the role that are examined in this article.

Kane, R.A., and Kane, R.L.: Assessing the elderly: a practical guide to measurement, Lexington, Mass., 1981, Lexington Books.

The authors focus on specific areas of measurements addressing the particular needs of the aging individual. Criteria are included for instrument selection and for evaluating the reliability and validity of measurements presented.

Katzman, R., Terry, R.D., and Bick, K.L., editors: Alzheimer's disease: senile dementia and related disorders, Aging Series, vol. 7, New York, 1978, Raven Press.

This book provides detailed information on the current state of knowledge of Alzheimer's disease, senile dementia and other related cognitive/emotional disorders of the elderly. The contributors present conflicting views and criticisms and suggest a variety of specific research approaches to clinical problems in this area.

Pavkov, J.R., and Walsh, J.: For nursing homes: a mental health charting instrument, J. Gerontol. Nurs. **7:**13, Jan. 1981.

This article describes a standardized charting tool developed in a geriatric outpatient service unit of a community mental health center. The purpose of the tool is to define the role of the mental health consultant in the nursing home and to assist medical and nursing staff in the development of treatment plans.

Shraberg, D.: An overview of neuropsychiatric disturbances in the elderly, J. Am. Geriatr. Soc. **28:**422, 1980.

A brief overview of the relationship between neurology and psychiatry in geriatric medicine. Included are some of the myths regarding aging, normal changes in the aging nervous system, and criteria for differential diagnosis of dementia and pseudodementia.

Wahl, P.R.: Therapeutic relationships with the elderly, J. Gerontol. Nurs. **6:**260, 1980.

Components of a helping therapeutic relationship are posed. Special consideration of the needs of the elderly constitute the discussion of the phases of the relationship, goals, and outcome.

White, P.H.: Psychoactive medication noncompliance in a geropsychiatric outpatient agency, J. Gerontol. Nurs. **6:** 729, 1980.

A report of a descriptive study designed to examine the relationship between psychoactive medication noncompliance and intellectual impairment in a group of non-institutionalized geropsychiatric outpatients. Although no statistical significance was found between degree of impairment and rate of medication noncompliance, important questions are raised regarding the needs of outpatient geropsychiatric patients and the responsibility of the nurse in planning and evaluating patient care.

Wolanin, M.O., and Phillips, L.R.F.: Confusion: prevention and care, St. Louis, 1980, The C.V. Mosby Co.

This 1982 American Journal of Nursing Book of the Year for gerontological nursing focuses on confusion in the elderly. Using a multidimensional approach to assessment and intervention, the authors emphasize the impact of the diagnosis or misdiagnosis of confusion on the treatment selection and outcome for the elderly client.

Wolanin, M.O., and Phillips, L.R.F.: Who's confused here? Geriatr. Nurs. **1:**122, July-Aug. 1980.

The authors use case examples to illustrate how premature and biased labeling of patient behavior may lead to misinterpretation of the patient's problem and misdiagnosis. The consequence of misdiagnosis of confusion in the elderly is addressed, along with suggestions for more accurate assessment and nursing management.

Yesavage, J.A., Westphal, J., and Rush, L.: Senile dementia: combined pharmacologic and psychologic treatment, J. Am. Geriatr. Soc. **29:**164, April 1981.

The authors introduced either supportive counseling or cognitive training as adjuncts to pharmacological treatment of geriatric patients with moderate dementia. Multidimensional outcome measures were used to assess changes in cognitive function (memory and learning), behavioral responses, and depression. Despite the improved effect on memory in the group receiving cognitive training, there was no difference between the two experimental groups on measures of overall behavioral change or on depression. The implications of these findings are discussed in relationship to previous studies on cognitive function and behavior and affective disorders of the elderly.

Give sorrow words; the grief that does not speak whispers the o'er-fraught heart and bids it break.

William Shakespeare, Macbeth, Act IV

CHAPTER 32

INDIVIDUALS AND FAMILIES: CARING FOR THE DYING

Elizabeth Anne DeSalvo Rankin

Learning objectives

After studying this chapter, the student should be able to:

- *describe the influence of an individual's values, beliefs, and experiences on his attitudes toward death.*

- *analyze her own reactions to death based on her own values, beliefs, and past experiences.*

- *identify and describe the five psychological stages of dying as defined by Kübler-Ross.*

- *discuss the potential impact illness and death can have on the family.*

- *describe the importance of self-help groups and other community resources to the terminally ill and the bereaved.*

- *relate the child's understanding of death at various stages of development.*

- *assess the patient's understanding of his condition.*

- *plan nursing interventions based on the patient's understanding of his condition, psychological reactions, and preferred mode of communication.*

- *discuss the stages and characteristics of family adaptation to an impending death.*

- *identify ways in which nurses who are caring for the dying can be supported.*

- compare and contrast the care of the dying person in a traditional hospital and in an alternative care setting, such as a hospice or at home.

- identify suggested readings for future study.

Some of the most challenging situations faced by those in the caregiving professions involve dealing with grieving and dying individuals. These people must come to terms with various losses, the ultimate one being loss of life. To most effectively care for these individuals, each professional should have an understanding of the phenomena of dying and death and how to effectively interact within such situations. Yet the ultimate facilitator in dealing with grieving and dying persons is the actual experience. No one may fully understand the experiences of the dying without becoming involved in their care. To reach out and become involved is extremely difficult for most people, no matter what their position. To become aware of one's own perceptions, anxieties, and abilities to deal with grief and death is a necessary task of those professionals who dare to care for dying persons. To come to terms with the finality of life, for self and others, is a goal that requires the expenditure of much inner psychological energy. The person who can accomplish such a task is an asset to the health care team.

This chapter was developed to assist nurses in becoming aware of the processes involved in coming to terms with death, dying, and grieving. The first part provides background information of a more theoretical nature. The second part provides information relevant to actual interactions within situations in which persons are grieving or dying. Since there is a trend toward an increased incidence of terminal diseases, a major emphasis has been placed on dealing with individuals diagnosed as having a terminal disease and on working with their families. It should be noted that no matter what the specific situation, working through the processes of dying or grieving is similar from case to case. Also, recognition of the individuals' physical, psychological, cultural, and spiritual needs and preferences is especially important in dealing with the dying and the grieving. These factors greatly influence the death-work process and in so doing influence the interactions among nurses, patients, and families.

Thanatology, the study of dying and death, has undergone dramatic changes in the past few decades. These changes follow the increase in the length of the life span, the increase in the incidence of chronic debilitating diseases, the advent of organ transplant operations, and the secularization of dying. Death is no longer confined to or hidden in the hospital. There has been an increased appreciation of the complex nature of what constitutes death and the process of dying, sparking a concern for the refinement of the technical definitions of death. As an aspect of the general secularization of death, changes in hospital confinement of the terminally ill have occurred.

There is an increased awareness among professionals of the need for the specialization of careers in caring for the dying individual. There has also been a new concern with reconceptualizing the psychological dimensions of death based on a growing knowledge and understanding of the processes through which the dying individual and the family move. The current attitude toward death of the majority of Western cultures is ambivalent, with members viewing death as a taboo subject, yet insisting that it be discussed, and living a life constantly risking death (e.g., from automobiles, pollution, starvation) yet simultaneously loving and holding on to life.[14]

Philosophical perspectives

Attitudes toward death

Death is the most certain aspect of life. Human existence is finite and each individual must come to terms with this at some point in his life. Yet for most people any confrontation with death is dreaded and often circumvented. Fear of death is almost universal. It is not merely a cultural phenomenon but very much a part of being human. The unknown aspects of death, the termination of the experiences of living, and the conclusion of the relatively controllable activities of life all create a pervading dread of death. The "democracy of death" extends to all beings. Even before death occurs, it is an "absent presence."[2] To deny it or attempt to ignore it will distort life and holistic growth. It is essential to learn to deal with and become aware of the multiple facets of death to intensify one's awareness of life and to provide meaningful care for the dying.

There are no simple answers to the questions death poses. Perhaps this is one of the reasons that people are so frightened by the thought of their finality. It seems too difficult to contemplate or discuss. Few people can tolerate discussion of even natural physical deterioration or natural death. One reason for the rejection of the elderly is that they bring to mind death and the termination of life. Similarly, severely ill and dying persons arouse feelings, fears, and anxieties about one's own dying. It is as if being faced with dying and death casts a shadow on full ego functioning.

Death is treated as taboo in Western culture. Attitudes toward dying and death are evident in the euphemistic tendency to label the end of life as anything but death. It is "passing on" or "going to one's reward" and "to meet one's maker." In contrast to these soothing clichés, few individuals see death as a peaceful natural occurrence. Instead, death is generally conceptualized as a fearful catastrophic force overpowering the individual who has become powerless and cannot avoid destruction. Perhaps this anxiety-laden view can be associated with the advent of nuclear power making mass destruction so easily possible. This fear has been labeled the apprehension of megadeath or total annihilation.[14]

No matter how hard one tries to hide from the knowledge of his finite existence, he never quite succeeds. One's relationship to the world, to time, and to others is bound in a sense by inevitable termination. To learn not to be so fearful of death is an important step in learning to live. A willingness to die appears to be a necessary condition for life.[1] Only through integration of all aspects of one's existence, including its terminal stages, can the individual grow toward a high level of self-awareness. In essence, a recognition of one's limit is an aspect of maturity.

If one could learn to accept death as essential and a necessity, rather than to camouflage and demote it to a level of lesser importance, less time would be spent projecting fears. Energies bound up in attempts to repress the concept of death would be available for more constructive use—for living. However, to become comfortable with death takes time, deep introspection, and, often, pain. It is not an easy process.

Meaning of death

Attitudes toward death provide some understanding of the adaptational strategies used in coping with pain, stress, and crises. The types of reactions to dying or impending death are a function of multiple interrelated factors. Of par-

ticular importance are the psychological maturity and personality characteristics of the individual; one's coping repertoire, that is, the kinds of coping techniques and strategies available to the person; sociocultural variables such as ethnic origin, age, socioeconomic status, and religious orientation; the severity of any associated pathological organic process; and the attitudes of significant persons.[2]

Development of the concept of death is age related. There is little relevant meaning in the word death for the toddler who is ego centered and has limited understanding of cause and effect. The preschool child does not sense death as irreversible or inevitable and most often associates it with animals. The child may also misinterpret the deaths of family members and view them as wish fulfillment. A small child who is angry may fantasize that the object of his anger will go away or die. If the person then does go away or dies, the child feels responsible. The concept of death as a common terminal point for all living things is generally developed by the age of 8.[11] Then the child's focus is on physical aspects of death, such as body disintegration, and that adults they know may die. Eventually the finality of death and the abstract adult view become more evident. Yet, experiences with death provide the most meaningful learning situations.

The meaning of death is closely related to the experiences one has with death situations. The middle years of adult life become a time of heightened awareness of one's own mortality.[5] The individual becomes more aware of the decline in physical status and vulnerability. By this time most individuals have experienced the death of relatives, perhaps parents, and acquaintances. Death is a multifaceted concept that may vary in importance depending on the individual's development, the cultural context, and one's essential nature.

Death may represent a teaching of transcendental truths that are incomprehensible during life. For others, it is a friend or liberator who brings an end to pain. Some visualize death as an adventure, a new experience, whereas others perceive it as the great destroyer that should be opposed at all cost. In some cases, especially related to suicide, death may be a means of revenge, an escape from an unbearable situation, a narcissistic act granting unchallenged importance to the individual, or a form of self-punishment.[2]

Because of the societal tendency to avoid and repress any contact with death, the severely ill individual often faces progressive isolation and the development of a sense of aloneness. The dying person is not seen as an individual but as a symbol of what every human fears, and this prevents open communication. This tendency occurs not only among lay persons but also among persons in the helping professions, those to whom the care of the dying person is frequently given. Of these professionals, the nurse is likely to have the most contact with the dying person and his significant others. For this reason, it is essential for the nurse to deepen her understanding of death and the care of the dying person. Since dying is an experience that evokes intense emotions, the nurse must learn to recognize, respect, and deal with its behavioral manifestations. This means that each nurse must become aware of her own reactions toward the dying and their significant others.

The necessary insights and skills basic to compassionate care of the dying can be developed. If the nurse becomes competent in these skills, it is possible to provide the dying person with the necessary support and opportunity to express himself and to discuss feelings. The nurse who can overcome feelings of vulnerability and insecurity to listen to, and perhaps even to cry with, the dying person can learn what no one else can teach. Perhaps at this time, more than ever before, professional distance may be pathological in itself, further isolating and rejecting the dying person instead of giving freedom to the individual to grow in the experience.

Societal perspectives

Definitions of death

In view of the philosophical nature and complexity of the concept of death, it is important to examine how death is defined. The determination of death is a question with great societal implications in this age of organ transplants and fantastic "life-sustaining" machines. *When* is an organ donor dead? The sooner the organs are removed after death, the better the chance of the grafted organ surviving. *When* are the machines no longer of any use? *Who* shall decide when a person may leave the hospital or refuse further care? Is this the decision of the physician, the dying person, or the family members? Each of these questions raises ethical issues concerning the dignity and rights of the individual, the division between professional duty and personal requests, and the topic of euthanasia.

A medical definition of death is a requirement to certify that someone has ceased to live. Yet there is no unanimity as to what the criteria of death are. Following are several definitions:

- **Somatic death** Cessation of all vital functions such as heartbeat and respiration
- **Cardiac death** Cessation of heartbeat verified by electrocardiogram
- **Brain death** Unreceptivity and unresponsivity, no movements or breathing, no reflexes, and a flat electroencephalogram
- **Clinical death** Appearance of death signs on physical examination before technical pronouncement of death
- **Biological death** Cessation of cellular activity

Even when a combination of definitions is used, the pronouncement of death is imbued with multiple moral-ethical questions. Death is not an instantaneous process, and its initial phases are sometimes reversible. Vital processes may cease before cellular or biological death occurs. For instance, a person may collapse from a myocardial infarction and be apparently dead, lacking both respiratory movements and pulse. If modern methods of resuscitation are employed, it is possible to restore the heartbeat and respirations, bringing the person "back to life." If these processes are not restored, after a period of time tissue cells deteriorate and die. The United Nations Vital Statistics define death as the permanent disappearance of every sign of life, that is, somatic death.[9] There is some question whether this definition is sufficiently comprehensive, since it is possible to maintain respiration and pulse mechanically when they might otherwise spontaneously cease. If the definition of death goes beyond cardiac death to encompass brain death, then there is less of a question. Four criteria of brain death are unreceptivity and unresponsivity, lack of movements or breathing, lack of reflexes, and a flat electroencephalogram.[16] Still there is the moral and ethical question of whether a person in an irreversible coma or one who has lost the abilities to express himself or function at all within society is considered to be alive. If the brain ceases to function but other organs are functioning, is the individual dead? These issues combine technical and moral questions that confound medical and social responsibilities. These ethical issues must be brought into the awareness of all who care for the dying.

Temporal aspects

Associated with the actual occurrence of death, the time at which the individual ceased to live is often important, especially on the emotional level. The term "constructive death" is often used to refer to the death of an ill or injured person who could not have been kept alive without technological means. For example, a terminally ill, 90-year-old woman who goes into renal failure might be allowed to die without attempting dialysis. If a death occurs before the person's time of productivity has ended or before he has either achieved his goals or abandoned them with dignity, the term "premature death" is used. This is especially true for young people, as evidenced in the heroic efforts of physicians to prolong the life of youthful persons; a child's death is considered unjust and perhaps more emotionally draining than that of an adult.

Demographic aspects

Although statistical mortality varies somewhat from decade to decade, there have been some general trends. There has been a decline in mortality and an increase in life expectancy since 1900. The extent of the decline is somewhat understated, since there has been an increase in the high-mortality–risk age segments of the population.[8] Mortality is its lowest during the school-age period. It is higher during infancy and steadily increases from the adolescent age on, reaching the highest ratio for those over 85 years of age. There has also been a change in male-female mortality. Although the mortality for both males and females has declined, death rates for females have been decreasing more rapidly. It should also be noted that the male death rate has been and still is considerably higher than that of females of the same age.

The causes of death have also changed since the turn of the century, when communicable diseases ranked first and degenerative diseases ranked fourth. Now degenerative diseases, especially those of the heart, and malignant neoplasms rank first and second as leading causes of death. These are followed by vascular lesions affecting the central nervous system, accidents, communicable diseases, arteriosclerosis, diabetes mellitus, liver cirrhosis, and suicide.[8]

There appear to be conflicting data available concerning the precise relationship between socioeconomic status and mortality. However, some generalizations can be considered.[8] People in the lowest economic stratum have the highest death rates of all, especially from communicable diseases. This has been attributed to crowded living conditions, lack of economic resources to obtain personal health services, and a generally poorer nutritive and health status. The advent of financial assistance, Medicaid, and public health centers has been somewhat helpful, but these are still far from effective in many cases. In contrast, the upper stratum populace enjoys relatively adequate access to health care and has substantially lower mortality during infancy, childhood, and young adulthood.

During midlife and later years the mortality appears substantially higher than in the rest of the population, primarily as a result of degenerative diseases of the heart, cancer, and cerebrovascular accident. This may be caused by increased stresses and a lowered general resistance, which occur at midlife, as well as the tendency toward a sedentary existence. The middle stratum, the blue- and white-collar working class, appears to have the best overall mortality. During infancy and youth they have access to adequate medical care and therefore enjoy lower morbidity and mortality than does the lower socioeconomic class. Moreover, at midlife they seem to suffer fewer of the disabilities associated with affluence.

Over the past few decades there has also been a change in where people die. For the most part there has been a steady increase in the percent of deaths occurring in institutional settings as opposed to home settings. With the advances in medical technology there is a tendency to hospitalize people and attempt to prolong life. This may account for the increase in deaths occurring in institutions. Also, since the rate of degenerative diseases is increasing, the time between the onset of morbidity and demise may be sufficiently long to allow for hospitalization. With the growing awareness of the depersonalizing effects of hospitalization, many individuals are now choosing to leave the institutional settings to die within the familiar surroundings of home with their loved ones close by. This may become a trend.

Personal and interpersonal perspectives

Stages of dying

No matter how clinical or objective one tries to be when discussing dying, the subject will always have personal and interpersonal aspects. The intense emotions that are manifested by the dying person range from disbelief to hope, vacillating between calm and despair. Similar emotions are expressed by those close to the dying person. The individual may work through his thinking to the point where he states he is "ready" to die or accepts the death of a loved one. Then again, one may never reach that point. Some people demonstrate behaviors of anxiety, depression, or psychosomatic symptoms when faced with separations from loved ones.

Death work imposes a double burden: the intrapsychic tasks of preparing oneself for death and the interpersonal tasks of preparing oneself in relation to loved ones. These tasks are made all the more difficult by the pervasive emotional states of grief about the loss and separation from loved ones; anger at being impotent to change the outcome; and anxiety related to fear of pain, loss of competence, aloneness, and fear of the unknown. Yet there is always the intermittent upsurge of denial that death will occur. Denial is the unconscious defense employed to negate any portion of reality that is too threatening to accept. The purpose of denial is to avoid danger and also to prevent the loss of significant others.[18] The way one denies involves a complex of intrapsychic processes whereby an acknowledged threat is repudiated and replaced by a more innocuous thought or situation. This facilitates one's reorientation to reality.

There are varying degrees of denial. First-order denial is based on how the person perceives the primary facts of illness. This level of denial is usually easily identified because the discrepancy between the person's report and perceptions and those of the observer are apparent. For example, one elderly gentleman refused to accept his wife's death from cancer, insisting she was merely visiting her sister and that the body in the coffin was not hers. Although this is an extreme example, it is not unusual for individuals to deny primary facts of illness. One woman who had suffered several myocardial infarctions resisted efforts of her family to seek medical care when she suffered a series of fairly distressing chest pains. She insisted it was merely indigestion caused by overeating the previous evening.

Second-order denial follows first-order denial. When the facts have been denied, then the implications of the threat may be ignored. For example, a 57-year-old woman noticed a lump in her breast. Instead of having it checked, she avoided contact with the breast even to the point of using a thick sponge when showering so she would not feel the mass. In so doing, she also denied the implications for treatment and it was not until some time later that she sought medical help, which resulted in a mastectomy. Even after the operation, she attributed some soreness in the opposite axilla to minor problems, "just slight swollen glands." Thus each complaint was looked at independently, and a total composite of the illness was never seriously considered. However, there was some indication that she in fact had some knowledge of the dire consequences of her condition. She would refuse to comment about her future.

Third-order denial is the denial of extinction, of death itself. Patients may resist the conclusion that an incurable illness results in death. This degree of denial occurs among those who have already acknowledged the facts of illness and their extensions and face imminent confrontation with death. These individuals tend to discuss their future as if their present state would go on indefinitely. Often this later denial is assumed to be a sign of courage, hope, or some other more positive attribute. Third-order denial appears in selective situations and is communicated only to certain people with whom a person wants to maintain a relationship. Anyone faced with threats to survival is likely to use the strategy of denial. Denial is so closely affiliated with one's values and self-image that whenever illness threatens to be a humiliating, extended, and incapacitating experience, denial is likely.

Although denial is a major mechanism, Kübler-Ross[7] has gone further and delineated five psychological stages of dying. These are described in Table 32-1. These sets of reactions to

TABLE 32-1. Kübler-Ross's stages of dying

Stage	Characteristics
1. **Denial and isolation**	Disbelief, "No, not me," temporary state of shock
2. **Anger**	Rage, envy, resentment, anger displaced and projected, "Why me?"
3. **Bargaining**	Attempting to enter into an arrangement in the hope of postponing the inevitable, "If only I can . . . before I die"
4. **Depression**	Sense of loss, loss of status and esteem, "What's the use," preparatory grief for loss of life, increased silences
5. **Acceptance**	"It's okay now," quiet recognition of the inevitable, selective disengagement from social interactions

awareness of imminent death are categorized in terms of the coping mechanisms used at the time of a terminal illness. The first stage is that of *denial and isolation*. The typical reaction of most people to the awareness of a terminal illness or to the sudden death of a significant other is that it cannot be a reality. This stage is often called the "no, not me, it can't be true" stage. This denial, used to some degree by all those concerned, functions as a buffer, providing the shocked individual with time to collect thoughts and mobilize other less radical defenses. The degree of anxiety associated with the denial is variable and often a function of the abrupt presentation of the information. This is a difficult time because the reality of human finality is pressing.

Denial is usually a temporary defense that is replaced by partial acceptance in most cases. Most people vacillate between the ability and inability to discuss the reality of the situation. The person may talk about the relevant issues as far as his life is concerned, only to change the topic later or perhaps even to contradict his earlier statements. Frequently staff and family also use denial to cope with caring for dying persons. In response the dying person is almost forced to comply through behaviors manifesting denial. In such a case, the person may choose some individuals with whom he will discuss his impending death while maintaining the facade of recuperating with others who cannot tolerate the reality of the situation.

The second stage is that of *anger*, which is in evidence when denial is no longer maintained but is replaced by feelings of rage, resentment, and envy. The dying person questions "Why me?" In contrast to the stage of denial, this stage is a very difficult time. The patient, family, and staff all are uncomfortable because anger becomes displaced, projected, and misdirected onto the environment and those within it in a random and sometimes irrational manner. The nursing staff are most often the targets of this wrath if for no other reason than their proximity to the situation. The impending death has signaled an end to plans and activities; often all enjoyment of life seems to be robbed from the person. Then anger is showered on those who symbolize life and activity. The nurses symbolize busy, active, goal-directed people.

Wherever the patient looks, he finds grievances, since he truly is "grieved." At this stage the individual is an active complainer, often using complaints to receive attention and the assurance that he does matter and that he is yet alive and of importance. Unfortunately, such behavior serves to distance those to whom the patient most actively retaliates, the family and caregiving staff. The reactions of these significant others is to move away from the person when he is symbolically asking for their reassurances that he matters to them. Also, the dying person senses loss of control of his life or what is left of it, especially if hospitalized and during the later stages of terminal illness. Angry demands may be expressing the message of a need to regain some control over the situation. Still, it is difficult for the caregiver not to respond personally to the anger.

The third stage, although often brief, is characterized by *bargaining*. It is during this time that the individual seeks to enter into an arrangement of some sort, most frequently with God, in hopes of postponing the inevitable. The typical reaction is "If only I can do this or that before I die." The person uses such maneuvers in the hope that there is some chance that his wishes may prevail. Invariably the wish is for an extension of life or to be free of pain and discomfort. Bargaining is an attempt to postpone the inevitable. It usually involves asking for a reward for "good behavior" and a self-imposed deadline after which death will be viewed as timely. The implication is that such a request will occur only once. This is seldom the case, since almost every individual seeks to hold onto life as long as possible. The promises of "good behavior" may also be of a deeper significance, indicative of some feelings of guilt. If the individual is assisted to deal with the guilt, the emotional processes of coming to terms with one's finality may be facilitated.

The fourth stage occurs when the previous feelings give way to the gross sense of loss. This stage is the stage of *depression*. The individual is all too often faced with loss of esteem because of fatigue, loss of a job, extensive medical treatments, and hospitalization. The sense of loss of control is overwhelming. There are many things that seem to imply failure, such as being unable to finish a remodeling project or to send a child through college, perhaps because of the cost of the care that the individual requires. All these losses assist the individual in his grief as he prepares himself for his final separation from family, friends, and life. Thus the person responds in a depressed manner because of what he has lost and what he will lose.

The individual deserves to be allowed to express his grief at this time to reach an accepting stage. At the same time, when the individual begins to focus on the impending future losses, he may communicate less in a verbal manner, choosing instead to communicate through his silence. The person will mourn the impending loss of meaningful people and places and contemplate his end. The silence is difficult to understand for family members who often interpret it as rejection.

When the person has had sufficient time to work through the emotional processes to the point that he quietly expects the inevitable, then the fifth stage has been entered, the stage of *acceptance*. This is not a time of hopeless resignation but rather an acknowledgment of termination. The individual has found some sense of peace and rest. At this point the person disengages from most social interactions. This is a very difficult time for family members. The individual may seek to be assured of the presence of a few select individuals yet want few verbal interactions. At this time touching is frequently the most effective and desired form of interaction. Now, more than ever, silence is a meaningful communication. This stage is almost void of feelings. The individual who has expressed his rage and cried for his losses can usually come to the task of acceptance. There are those who fight the inevitable by continuing to deny, and for such persons, finding the peace of acceptance is very difficult. The one thing that persists throughout the ordeal is hope. If the individual loses hope, his despair can be so great that he is consumed in his own grief.

A simply resolved death, with all of one's death work completed, is rare even among the aged. Preparedness, acceptance and separation without anger are not easy. Invariably dying evokes regressive actions with whining, crying, clinging, and demanding behaviors. The individual is frightened and often can sense an abandonment even in the presence of family.[13] In the child, the stages are somewhat varied but involve similar behaviors. A child may first *protest,* exhibiting anger and searching for hope. Protest is followed by *despair* and depression and finally a sense of *detachment*. The sense of aloneness is, however, a characteristic of the process for all.

Family and others

The important role of family, friends, and staff in the maintenance of hope without engendering false aspirations cannot be ignored. The process of dying and of grieving encompasses the entire family. There are times when the family can hinder the grief work of the dying person. At other times they provide some of the necessary supports. Often the family and dying person are involved in mutual pretense, acting as if the person were going to live. To carry out this false situation, cooperative responses are required. An analysis of the pretense indicates that either party may initiate the situation and the others must comply with appropriate behaviors or else the illusion is destroyed.[4] The dying individual may be extremely perceptive of the behaviors and needs of others to deny or avoid the terminal nature of his illness and he may assist them in maintaining their pretense. The same person may flash cues to those with whom he interacts about his knowledge of his status, waiting for someone to react within the context of the real facts so that the facade of pretense can be broken. Each party shares the responsibility for maintaining or breaking the pretense. The transition to open awareness may be sudden or gradual. The pretense generally collapses when dangerous topics of discussion can no longer be avoided or when it is impossible to pretend any longer that nothing is awry, such as when one party can no longer hold up under the strain of the pretense.

Family members undergo different but similar stages of adjustment. They may deny the fact that their loved one is dying and frantically shop around from physician to physician, clinging to hope for a wrong diagnosis. Similarly to the dying person, the immediate family experiences the emotional reaction of anger. They, too, are angry with the physician for the diagnosis and with the personnel who never appear to care enough or do anything correctly. The family members often suffer from much guilt and wish to make up for past happenings. They, too, need to express their feelings and to work through their anger and guilt to begin their preparatory grief. If family members can share their feelings during their time of grieving, the impending separation can be dealt with more realistically and the family, too, can come to a state of acceptance.

No matter how long the anticipatory period, feelings of emptiness and loneliness are likely to present themselves after the death of the loved one. The loss of a loved one reactivates painful fears, the anguish of abandonment, and separation anxiety. No one wants to have these feelings recalled, and thus the mourner is often isolated and rejected by others under the pretense of their not wanting to impinge on privacy. Although it is true that those who are in the process of bereavement need separate time, they also must repeople their world. In some cases they must reconstruct relationships and need new skills to do so. Without an ongoing interaction there is no one to challenge the idealization of the deceased or to help resolve guilt. There is also the task of acknowledging those aspects of the deceased which the significant others have externalized while accepting the loss of the deceased. The inevitably slow mourning process can help the grieving family members find a new life. It is frequently the survivors who suffer the greatest pain of death.

Terminal illness invariably causes drastic changes in roles and demands within the family. Additional tasks must be assumed. A spouse or child may now be required to get involved in household management or child care activities. Along with concerns for the dying person, added work, responsibility, and loss of security create an uncomfortable emotional burden. These problems may be compounded by feelings of isolation, helplessness, anger, and resentment. The expected assistance from kin might be lacking. The way of life that was so comfortable has been snatched away. No matter what the particular circumstances, the family members can be assisted to explore and express their feelings. They must also be encouraged to continue with preillness activities; that is, illness should not be allowed to totally consume the household nor should it deprive family members of pleasurable activities. Some changes will occur, but the lives of the family members continue after the death of their loved one. Just as the fatally ill cannot face death 24 hours a day, neither can their family members.

Caring for dying children is even more emotionally challenging. Both nursing staff and family members react more strongly when the dying person is a child. It is hard to see a young exuberant life slowly ebb away. The parents are often overwhelmed by the prospect that someone so young, in whom they have entrusted so many hours of love and caring, might die. They have witnessed the unfolding of the youngster's life step by step through each stage of development. The feelings are present whether the death is caused by a terminal illness or a miscarriage of a yet unborn baby. Many parents, especially mothers, who have had the most intimate experience with their children, find the death work exhausting. They often have a greater knowledge of the personality, behaviors, likes, and dislikes of their children than they do of themselves. The death of their child is felt as if a part of themselves had died.

Often the parents, because of their personal anxiety and feelings of guilt, will attempt to satisfy every request of the child. In so doing, they become inconsistent in limit setting, which causes the child to begin to feel insecure. The pattern is then set for the child to express more anxiety and to become more demanding. The parents try to meet the excessive demands but often become frustrated, irritable, and hostile. The parents' recognition of their own hostility further compounds feelings of guilt, which leads to further decreased limit setting, increased insecurity and demands from the child, and still greater efforts by the parents to comply. To discourage this vicious cycle from developing, it is essential to explain to the parents the importance of making demands that are consistent with reality and setting reasonable limits which are consistently reinforced. If the nurses and the family treat the dying child as much like a well child as possible, the child feels more secure and more valued. Parents must also be urged to schedule time within the day for themselves to renew their strength and for their other family members. Too often parents become so tied to the ward that they neglect their own needs. This can be detrimental to all the family members, including the dying child.

Siblings may become resentful, since they have to assume additional tasks for their parents and at the same time receive little attention. The entire life-style of the family may be distorted as adaptations are made to secure a new family equilibrium. After the child has died, the surviving siblings often become the focus of maneuvers designed to alleviate guilt. There is an unspoken rule of silence about the deceased child or the circumstances related to death. There may be substitutions for the lost child or attribution of a surviving child with qualities of the deceased. Parents may become overprotective. The surviving siblings may find it difficult to compete with an incomparably precious memory.[6]

The traumatic nature of the death of a child is compounded when it occurs unexpectedly or when the cause is unknown. When a child suc-

cumbs to *sudden infant death syndrome (SIDS)*
the grief responses include shock, disbelief, and
anger. Parents, and sometimes siblings, are
overwrought with self-reproach and guilt. Extensive research on SIDS has pointed to a lack
of stability in state behaviors, such as breathing,
crying or reactions to environmental stimuli,
and developmental tasks, as characteristics of
SIDS infants. Yet the causes of this phenomenon are still unknown although several hypotheses have been formulated.[15] Since the child usually dies in its sleep, parents feel the brunt of
the responsibility, questioning their own integrity. Their behaviors are filled with self-reproach. They experience severe crisis, and it
takes months to regain a level of family organization and interpersonal relationships, especially
for the mothers who have been the major caregivers.

Nursing perspectives

Death: a necessary concern

By virtue of her proximity to the situation,
death is a necessary concern for the nurse.
Whether she functions as a staff nurse in a hospital setting, as a liaison nurse coordinating inpatient and outpatient services, or as a specialist
for the dying, the nurse can act as a facilitator
for the individual and his family. The complex
nature of the processes of dying and grieving is
invariably obscured by the emotional trauma experienced. Yet as caregivers, it is extremely important for nurses to assist all those affected
by the many factors involved. This also means
that dealing with death is a personal task, requiring self-knowledge and competence in managing one's own reactions effectively. This does
not mean to deny one's feelings but to acknowledge and express them as honestly as possible.
The impact of dying is powerful. Shock and a
sense of sorrow pervade the situation. The psychological manifestations of anxiety, anger, and
depression are often accompanied by psychophysiological reactions, including changes in
sleep or eating patterns, lethargy, restlessness,
and headaches.

Grieving occurs within the context of relatives, friends, co-workers, and associated professionals who are and have been involved with the
dying (or dead) individual and his family. Each
of these associated persons can be influential in
facilitating or hindering an individual's grief
work. They can provide supports and resources
for the family and the individual. Often the
family provides early supports to the individual.

Family members tend to use each other, other
kin, and professionals during the period in
which the person is dying. There are supportive
self-help groups in many communities, such as
widow-to-widow and bereaved spouse groups,
whose aims are to assist individuals and family
members with the anticipatory grieving process
and with the bereavement (postdeath) grief
work. The nurse may function in organizing
and directing such groups. After the actual
death of the individual, the survivors usually
find a sudden emergence of help from friends
and co-workers. The depth of desolation and
sorrow frequently is evident in the inability to
make realistic plans or adapt to new roles. At
this time self-help groups such as "widow's
groups" can be helpful, since few survivors
plan ahead; to do so signals the separation from
their loved one, which is too painful to acknowledge. To inform family members of the available
community resources is often a primary step in
aiding in the reorganization of their lives. After
a period of time the environmental-interpersonal
supports fade, leaving the survivors to resume
functioning within the community. Most survivors do adapt if they have been allowed and
are able to work through their grief. In cases
of unresolved grief, which is frequently evident
through various dysfunctions such as prolonged
withdrawal, prolonged insomnia, or decreased
intimate contact with spouses, psychotherapeutic interventions may be required. These are discussed in Chapter 9. Whatever the situation,
working with the dying and grieving is a challenge.

Importance of communicating

To say that communicating is difficult in such
situations is an understatement, since lack of
communication can be one of the most difficult
barriers to overcome. Communicating is especially a problem for the nurse who may be placed
in a position between the physician and patient.
The manner in which things are communicated
and the content of what is communicated must
be examined. Generally, the person and/or his
family may be informed of a terminal diagnosis.
The nurse, usually not present at the time that
the information is conveyed, lacks the detailed
knowledge of exactly what was said and the reactions. It is also difficult to know how much or
what exactly has been absorbed by those in-

formed. To effectively deal with the total situation, the nurse must have an understanding of the extent of the person's knowledge. Sometimes the individual will behave as if he knows nothing, yet the physician will report that he has informed the person of the situation. Often the converse may be experienced, with the individual conveying that he knows full well the terminal nature of his illness. This is often true because of the widespread knowledge about signs and symptoms of disease. Yet, if the nurse has been instructed not to discuss the terminal nature of his diagnosis, the anxiety associated with working with the fatally ill is compounded by the frustration of uncertainty, rendering the nurse uncomfortable, angry, or even helpless to deliver quality care.

As early as possible, the nurse should use her communication skills to ascertain the extent of the individual's knowledge of his condition, his understanding of the needed medical care or hospitalization, his past experiences with physicians and nurses, and his individual and family history. This can provide a vast amount of information to the nurse as to the individual's perceptions and fears about his present situation as well as any possible distortions of the facts. At the same time, she should be open to the subtle cues from the person that indicate how willing or unwilling he may be at the time to discuss his status. Such sensitivity to the metacommunication, the hidden messages, can become an asset for interactions with the dying and grieving. For example, if the person asks a question such as "I don't have cancer, do I?" using a negative questioning tone, he is probably asking that his fears be negated. The readiness to discuss his fate is probably lacking. If, on the other hand, he says, "I have cancer, don't I?" he is probably closer to accepting the reality of his fate. In either case gentle exploration of the person's concerns and meanings attached to the situation will usually lead to more definite signals as to whether or not the individual is ready and willing to learn of his actual fate. Hesitancy on the part of the individual to discuss his condition may simply mean he has not yet reached the point of recognition or that he is trying to deny the facts. In either case the individual usually eventually acknowledges the problem when he is able to sense that both he and the person to whom he is speaking are ready. In some cases the person never explicitly shares that he knows

his illness is terminal. This may be because he is better able to cope with the facade or because his family needs the charade so that the anxieties associated with dying are diminished. In any case, if the person is offered the opportunity to discuss his fate when he has indicated his readiness to do so, a primary nursing function has been carried out. The skills that the adept professional has to facilitate such communication are often developed only through interpersonal experiences in caring for the dying and grieving. A sensitive, skilled ability to listen is of great importance in facilitating such emotion-laden communication.

There are those, especially children, who cannot directly verbalize their concerns but can use symbolical communication. The universal language of touching and holding is the simplest of all symbolical communication. When a child senses the warmth, love, and security of a gentle touch, he can often begin to open up to that individual whom he feels can return his warmth. Children are quick to sense true sincerity and they will ventilate their feelings only to those who really can listen. They convey their messages in their own way.

Frequently, for younger children, drawings may serve as another form of symbolical nonverbal communication. It is not unusual for a dying child to draw a representation of death. For example, one child shared with her favorite nurse a drawing showing a large black catlike figure on one side of the page and across from it a small girl standing with her hand outstretched as if to signal "stop." The picture clearly depicted the feelings of helplessness the child sensed in the face of the "destructive" death. The child had selected this particular nurse to be the one with whom she would share her feelings and her awareness of her impending death. The best way to assist the child is to use the same mode of communication chosen. In this case to attempt to use the adult mode of verbal communication, asking the child to talk about the picture or forcing verbalization, would hinder the communication, since it is evident that the mode of nonverbal, symbolical communication was the child's choice. Instead, using drawings would be best. The nurse chose to draw a picture of the catlike figure facing the child, who was being accompanied by a woman holding the child's hand. Thus the nurse conveyed that although death was imminent, she would not leave the child to face it alone. On seeing the picture, the child clutched it tightly, said "thank you" and reached out to hold the nurse's hand.

There may come a time when the child can attempt to verbally express feelings, and if the nurse has been sincere and allowed the child to convey feelings and thoughts earlier, it will probably be easier for the child to talk about death in a personal way.

There are others, older children and some adults, who may indirectly verbalize their concerns; that is, they can use only a symbolical verbal communication. They, too, will carefully choose the person with whom they will convey their fears. Then they may discuss, or question that person about, things that can symbolically represent their predicament. Often the cue is in the topic. For example, one youngster asked the nurse what she would do when there was an earthquake. The nurse almost responded that never before were there earthquakes in the area, but she caught herself. The manifest content of the message included destruction that could not be stopped and the importance of the interpersonal relationship. The symbolical message was a question of whether the nurse would be there even when the child died. The nurse then reached for the child's hand, moved closer, and pressed her cheek against the child's face. Touching the child's chin, the nurse said, "Do you think this might help?" The youngster's reaction was to begin to cry and talk about the problem. She said she knew she was going to die but that her parents could not talk about it. They were grief ridden, but played a game to hide it. The importance of listening for the symbolical messages cannot be stressed enough. People are always afraid that they may say the wrong thing and have been socialized to maintain distance. However, when working with the dying and grieving, learning to trust one's inner feelings or "gut" reactions and to follow what seems intuitively right at any given moment will prove most facilitative. Being human, warm, and not afraid to touch are qualities that promote the process and progress of death work. The most important thing is not what the nurse says but how she feels within herself about it.

The role of the nurse in assisting the family of a dying child is similar to that with other dying individuals. However, the intense emotional strain on the parents makes them more demanding and insecure. They frequently use the nursing staff as the targets for their anger. The nurse can become an ally to the family if she allows them to express their emotions and assists them in understanding what is happening.

An additional aspect of dealing with parents of dying children is teaching parents about children's' real concepts of death.[11] If the nurse works with children, she, too, must have this knowledge. During the first 2 years of development the child has little understanding of death. He cannot conceptualize it. Still there are experiences within early childhood that imply a relationship to the state of nonbeing. As early as age 3 months the child may engage in the self-risking game of "peek-a-boo," during which he alternately experiences joy and the fear of loss. The young child's games of disappearance and return are also little experiments in nonbeing. The toddler experiences separation, loss, and nonbeing more than most people realize. Simple things such as throwing an object into the garbage can or losing a toy out of the car window serve to teach about finality and loss.

The preschool child begins to develop some ideas about death and to think more about death and related topics. The child is extremely curious about life and begins to ask questions. Yet he does not have a grasp of the concept of finality. The child regards death as a temporary state. For example, the 5-year-old might say that "Grandpa is dead and is asleep" or ask, "What will Grandpa eat when he's not asleep?" During these early years the child seems to regard death chiefly in terms of separation. The child also believes that death is accidental rather than inevitable and "just happens." At about age 4 to 6 the child begins to expand his ideas. He begins to understand death is final, inevitable, and universal. Personal experiences may become anxiety arousing because the child is likely to misinterpret information or to be given misinformation when he begins to question what death means or what causes death. At this time death is real but in an external and distant sense. The child often personifies death, referring to it as a "death man" who carries away the person.

It is not until age 9 or 10 that the child begins to conceptualize death. The child has developed the mental and emotional security to express an understanding of death as a final and inevitable outcome of life. At this age, differentiation between animate and inanimate objects occurs; most children have a concept of living and not living that approximates that of adults. As the child approaches adolescence, he is equipped with the intellectual tools to logically approach the topic of death. Death is explained as a natural phenomenon within a time, space, and causality framework. During adolescence the youngster develops his attitude or viewpoint about death. However, although he may explain death intellectually, emotionally and experientially the adolescent is just beginning to deal with death. The open discussion of the realities of death and dying with an adult who can offer his own constructive encounters with death can help the adolescent grow.

The most frequent question is how to tell the child that a parent has died or that the child himself is dying. There is no direct answer. It must be remembered that the child can understand only within the limits of his development. However, to give the child misinformation or to deny there is a problem only serves to confuse him. Often, by referring to the symptoms that the child is experiencing, it is possible to help him understand the nature of his illness. If a child asks "Will I die?" a great deal of concern is aroused. Strangely, children usually have a fairly accurate evaluation of the situation. The type of answer that allows the child to express his concerns is best. The nurse who responds in an open manner such as "Tell me what you are thinking" or "Why do you think you might die?" will allow the child a chance to express his concerns. Assisting parents to learn to help their dying children express fears is difficult.

Too frequently the parents cannot tolerate hearing the dying child speak of his own death. This only distorts the grief work and the child must carry the burden. Few parents can mask their anguish and the child readily perceives this. If the child and parents are helped to exchange feelings, a good deal of the emotional strain may be reduced. This can occur only when both the dying child and parents are at a point of readiness. The role of the nurse becomes one of facilitator in the grief work. This may be accomplished simply by providing the warmth of a receptive listener or the soothing touch of a caring person. More in-depth exploration of feelings can be accomplished through the use of other supportive services, such as of members of the clergy.

The needs of the family change throughout the duration of the illness and continue to do so after the person's death. Table 32-2 presents characteristics of family adaptation described by Giacquinta.[3] In the early stages the family reacts in a manner similar to the responses of the dying individual. They react to the feelings of despair, disbelief, and helplessness. They, too,

TABLE 32-2. Giacquinta's stages of family adaptation to impending death

Stage	Characteristics
1. Impact	Family reacts with despair and often retreats from their normal life-style; there are feelings of isolation, helplessness, and despair as they search for a meaning to the experience
2. Acknowledgment	Family acknowledges inevitable death of loved one; they begin to actively experience emotional facets of grieving experience, including fear of losing control
3. Reorganization	Family reorganizes role expectations and task distribution; they begin to reconstruct memories of dying member, putting their relationships with dying person into a continuum of person's living and dying
4. Separation	Family coalesces as dying person moves toward imminent death and loses awareness of environment; bereavement actively begins with the concomitant grief-guilt experiences; previous experiences of loss may resurface during this time of mourning
5. Resocialization	Family members begin to reenter their social environment after working through their grief; members experience changes in their relationships and become reinvolved in community

are vulnerable as they search for some meaning in the experience while trying to function. During these times the nurse can foster the expression of feelings and help the family members find security and strength, even a sense of cohesion, as they begin their problem-solving tasks. If this occurs, they can restructure and reorganize their life situation. At this time fostering cooperation and helping members to diminish competition best serves the interest of the family. It is during this period of reorganization that the family members begin to reflect on their lives with the dying person. This can be difficult because of their intense emotional involvement. It is also important for them to crystallize a picture of the dying person as he was prior to the illness to promote the identity of the person throughout his life span. As the family's image of the loved one is strengthened, they can come to depend less on his actual presence. This, then, facilitates their eventual separation and their mourning when the person dies.

As survivors, they need to continue their grief

work and bereavement. The nurse may be able to be a facilitator or to help the family members to find other supports at this time. The family members will need to begin to reestablish social interactions and relationships. Fostering relatedness may be difficult, but when grieving has been successful, the family members continue their lives with the memory of their loved one.

Nurses' own reactions

Nurses, in caring for the dying, know they are expected to provide not only physical care but also understanding, comfort, and emotional support for the individual and his family. However, our culture emphasizes youth, life, and avoidance of the taboo subject of death. Nurses have the same attitudes toward talking about dying as do lay people. Their educational experiences may have done little to change these attitudes. Thus nurses are faced with the contradiction of what they have experienced about avoiding dealing with death and what they have learned is important for quality nursing care. Many provide care but remain distant. Avoidance of involvement with the dying contributes to one of the patient's major problems, that is, loneliness and isolation. How, then, can this be resolved?

The first step is for the nurse to consciously become aware of her feelings and her behaviors in dealing with the dying. Few nurses have come to terms with their finality and are at peace with the concept of death. As a result they may project or transfer their fears and sorrows onto their patients. If one can face death and not be afraid, this peace can be conveyed to others. Yet the only way to reach this point is through actually experiencing the anguish of death-related situations, to learn from the dying how to grow. This is the ideal, the goal. The reality of the situation is that little is done to help the nurse (or any individual) learn about her reactions. Instead, many defense strategies for coping with the experiences are formulated. Nurses prepare themselves for conversations that might become threatening and manage their interactions with dying individuals and their families to minimize personal involvement. The behaviors used include limited contacts with the persons involved, talking on a superficial level, avoiding conversations altogether, and offering few details about physical signs and symptoms. Often these behaviors come under the guise of being extremely busy. The nurse begins to make use of selective listening, blocking out details of conversations that would draw her into closer contact with the person. The nurse may not speak until spoken to, say as little as possible, and diminish feedback to the person by refusing to pick up on invitations to talk about dying.

These are but a few of the coping maneuvers frequently used. Other maneuvers can be more facilitative. On a general level, continuing education seminars on death and dealing with the dying can begin to increase the cognitive awareness of those providing the care. Another suggestion is that a nursing specialist who has a good deal of knowledge, experience, and expertise about death and grieving be incorporated into the staff to help the personnel, the families, and the dying individuals. For example, by functioning as a co-caregiver, the specialist can help the nurse become aware of those behaviors which are not helpful to the individual. At the same time, the nurse has a colleague with whom she can discuss her feelings about working in the situation. While learning more positive methods of working within the situation, the nurse may still find it necessary to rely on some of those strategies described earlier. Yet it is important that the nurse be allowed to advance at a self-regulated pace in attaining awareness and the ability to work with the dying effectively and in an expressive manner. A specialist might also help all the staff by leading seminars related to giving care to the dying and by providing an outlet for the expression of feelings evoked by this kind of work. Another method of managing within the situation is to promote a degree of teamwork between the nursing staff and the family members. This helps relieve nursing personnel of some of their guilt about the limitations on time spent with individuals and also allows family members to feel less segregated from their loved one. Such a joint effort is dependent on the willingness of all concerned and must not be forced if any of the participants feel uncomfortable. Insistence would only cause feelings of resentment, compounding the existing emotional strain.

When nurses do invest time and emotional commitment in the care of the dying, the social skills that they use in other situations are of little help. They often identify with the dying person or his family members, making it difficult to forget the person. But this is not necessarily negative. In having dared to become close to the situation, they have shared the emotional ordeal, which can help them to grow to be much more effective caregivers. In such cases, in the postdeath time of acknowledging the death and of reorganization and integration, the nurse can be assisted to grow from the experience by being encouraged to express feelings related to the situation. If the work environment is one that will allow such expressions, then all those involved can share feelings together. Creating such an atmosphere is not an easy task and poses some practical problems.

Practical considerations

When considering care of the dying individual, the tendency is to focus first on the physical needs and second on interpersonal needs. Often other aspects of the person's being such as the psychological and spiritual needs are left unattended by the staff. Practical considerations of providing nursing care tend to center around physical aspects and then interpersonal or familial aspects. Too frequently the dying person is placed in a private room, often at some distance from the nursing station. This is rationalized as providing for quiet and privacy for the person. However rational this may be, it also tends to dramatically increase the nurse's distance from the dying person and thus increases the sense of loneliness and abandonment so common among the dying. Although they do not want to be in the thick of the ward activity, they do want to be acknowledged. After all, they are still living. One creative approach is to place two dying individuals in one semiprivate room so that they might strengthen each other and their families might support each other. When an individual has reached the point of acceptance in his death work, another human in a similar situation is not an imposition but a comrade. Using such an approach must, of course, be carefully evaluated with respect to the individuals, their diagnoses and prognoses, and the familial considerations. Regardless of the setting, a place that provides comfort and some privacy for the person and his grieving family is indispensable.

Another practical consideration that is often helpful to the dying person is the use of nursing measures which provide for rest. Persons who are aware they will die soon are frequently hesitant to sleep at night. Arranging for a subdued night-light and checking on them every 15 minutes can be helpful. The person comes to antici-

pate that someone is available who will be there and realizes that they are not alone. This can promote relaxation. Also, these brief encounters help the time pass more quickly, in a sense providing the person with a degree of time orientation. This can further reduce restlessness that accompanies the sleepless nights. The night, with its quietness, may become the time when the person can communicate his concerns to the nurse who has become his dependable contact with the world of the hospital.

The sense of abandonment can also occur when a nurse whom the person has come to know is no longer assigned to his care. Thus staffing practices present another practical problem. Good care for the dying requires the continued presence of the same helping persons. This enables the individual and his family to establish the necessary trust and a comfortable working relationship. Frequent changes in patient assignments or the use of part-time nursing staff to care for the dying is only useful to diminish the contact that the nurses have with death. For some nurses, especially those who cannot tolerate the dying and grieving process, such staffing patterns are a relief. However, these practices do little to serve the dying and grieving persons. Those nurses who cite their experiences with dying persons as traumatic memories should not be forced to care for the dying; without extensive supports the situation could become a cruel encounter for all involved.

Usually for one to be so traumatized by a death experience, several other conditions had to be present.[12] There was often a personal sense of inadequacy, immobilization, and negligence, causing extensive self-concern. There might have been overidentification with the person or his family or just a great deal of emotional involvement with them. There might have been personal associations with those for whom the nurse provided care. To the contrary, there may have been a genuine dislike of the individual so that there might be guilt associated with his death. Last, an unexpected or unforgettable sight at death might create a traumatic memory. Until the nurse works through her own feelings, she should not be expected to care for the dying. Such nurses would do better when assigned to areas of the hospital where death was not a frequent occurrence. They should also be provided with assistance to learn to work with the dying.

It must similarly be recognized that there is an immense emotional strain in constantly working with the dying and grieving. Nurses will need periodical relief from those wards where death often occurs. For example, rotating the staff about every 3 months between, for example, pediatric intensive care and postpartum and pediatric medicine would provide quite a change in the emotional investment accompanying the nursing care. Thus, to improve the care given to the dying and grieving, the nurse must have a commitment to engage in some degree of introspection to understand her own basic views of death and attitudes toward the dying. To accomplish this, one must have the support from colleagues, nursing educators, and nursing service administrators.

Alternative settings

There are some alternatives to typical hospital care of the dying. These include centers for the care of those with debilitating or terminal illnesses and at-home care. The former is a special type of institutional setting that often provides the care for the individual after a confirmed diagnosis has been established. Such centers are often called hospices and their approach is dedicated to removing the stigma of death.

A hospice is a coordinated program providing continuity of home and inpatient care for the dying and their family. The goals of the hospice are to maximize the person's functioning, maintain the individual as free from physical and emotional pain as possible, to reduce the sense of isolation, and to provide emotional support for the family, including bereavement follow-up. The aim is to care for the individual at home as long as possible and assist the person to retain his or her life-style, as far as possible, when staying in the hospice inpatient facility.[10] Outpatient services may be provided in the earlier phases in an effort to allow the person to maintain social contact with the everyday world and to remain close to family. Specialty centers tend to employ many of the most current ideas and are able to keep abreast of the changes in treatments for the specific disorders. Also, the staff can promote continuity in care, especially when a team approach is used. If that staff member with whom the family and individual have early contact either becomes part of the inpatient care team or actually performs the role of mediator in the transition to the ward setting, the feelings of anxiety and isolation caused by change and hospitalization may be lessened.

Specialty centers might also employ methods or implement policies that are not ordinarily used in the general hospital situation. For example, an unusual approach includes the an-

ticipatory prescription of sufficiently high doses of analgesics and anxiety-reducing drugs for the relief of pain. Staffing policies must be established that take into account the emotional drain of such work. Still, the atmosphere of these centers is generally different, more calm, as if death is acceptable. The peace associated with these centers gives the dying and grieving persons solace. The staff are less caught up in avoiding the issues. It takes a strong self-aware individual to choose to work within such a center. A drawback of such centers is that individuals and family members who are at different points in their grief work often find it extremely depressing to visit their loved ones, who may be surrounded by other dying persons.

The hospice setting offers the nurse an opportunity to practice individualized primary nursing to facilitate and promote self-care. Characteristics of hospice nurses include self-awareness, flexibility, awareness of self-limits, recognition that others' needs are separate from one's own needs, and a need for a balanced personal life.[17] The nurse is involved in individualized administration of care, initiating contact with individuals and families, as well as making home visits.

When the care is provided within the home situation, the person is within familiar and comfortable surroundings. A bedroom with familiar furniture looks and smells like home. An important aspect of home care is that loved ones, especially children, have access to the individual. Too often hospitals limit visiting hours and exclude younger children. For those who are dying, this can be distressing. They have a limited amount of time and energy and would like to spend it with those they love. As they progress toward death and they wish to see fewer persons, their loved ones are those chosen by the person to sit quietly with them. In our culture children are shielded from contacts with death. This may be a mixed blessing. Each experience with the dying promotes one's fuller understanding of his own demise. This can occur only if the atmosphere in the home is one of acceptance. When children are around their dying parent, they are given the opportunity to try to express their feelings. Also, because they are not excluded, they do not have to rely on verbal reports of what is happening to their parent. They can see for themselves the changes and the progression of the illness, thus holding in check their vivid imaginations. If the home setting is chosen because the dying individual requests it but the spouse or other family members cannot tolerate the demands of care or cannot bring themselves to use nursing personnel, then the atmosphere can become filled with discontent, anxiety, and anger.

The home is an alternative setting for care of the dying where creative nursing care may still be implemented. Managing care in a setting that is foreign to the nurse can be a challenge. Although the physical care may be more difficult, it is possible to provide good care and to incorporate family, when appropriate. Private duty nurses may be used. In some cases neighbors who are nurses may volunteer their time and services. Renting a hospital bed and other equipment is often the first thing that must be done. If these are worked into the familiar furniture of the bedroom, they can become unobtrusive. Then comes coordinating a schedule of care so that family can be included. Allowing family members time to visit, or, if possible, free access to come and go, maintains the pattern of family interaction. It may be easier to facilitate the psychological grief work of all those involved without the demands of the hospital setting. Death at home helps maintain some of the dignity of the dying and the family. The home therefore may be the setting of choice in some situations.

Suggested cross-references

Therapeutic relationship skills are discussed in Chapter 3. The phases of the nursing process and self-awareness of the nurse are discussed in Chapter 4. Primary prevention is discussed in Chapter 5. Nursing interventions with patients experiencing normal grief and disturbances of mood are discussed in Chapter 9.

SUMMARY

1. Although death is the most certain aspect of life, fear of it is universal. Because of this and because of their proximity to the situation of dying, death is a necessary concern for nurses.

2. Attitudes toward death are culturally learned. Personal reactions have their basis in the psychological maturity and personality characteristics of the individual. The individual's own values, beliefs, and experiences influence the cognitive aspects of dying.

3. Kübler-Ross described five psychological stages of dying: denial and isolation, anger, bargaining, depression, and acceptance.

4. Adaptation to changes within the existing family structure and interactions are invariably necessary. Change is difficult, and the family may require support from community resources. The dying of a child can be a shattering experience for the parents.

5. Although nurses are expected to provide physical care, comfort, understanding, and emotional support to the individual and the family, it must be recognized that there are limitations and immense emotional strains that pervade the caregiving situation.

6. Lack of communication is the most difficult barrier to overcome when dealing with dying individuals and their families. It is necessary to assess the person's understanding of the prognosis, reaction to the situation, and degree of readiness to discuss the prospect of death. Not all patients can verbally communicate and the nurse who uses the same mode of communication as the person can become an ally.

7. Understanding of the dying process is closely linked to the level of emotional maturity and cognitive abilities of the child and adult. Assisting children and parents to learn to express their fears about dying can help to diminish some of the emotional strain of grief work.

8. The needs of the family change throughout the duration of the illness and continue to do so after the death of the family member. The family progresses through stages of adaptation: impact, acknowledgment, reorganization, separation, and resocialization.

9. The nurse needs to have a cognitive grasp of the developmental aspects of the concept of death, the stages and processes associated with dying, and resources available to the individual and family. It is important to assess one's own viewpoints and attitudes toward death, since these often transfer over into the caregiving situation. Also, nurses caring for the dying need a professional support system of their own.

10. The nurse within the alternative care settings, such as a hospice or home, is a member of an interdisciplinary team with autonomous functions related to the care of dying individuals and family members.

References

1. Feifel, H., editor: The meaning of death, New York, 1967, McGraw-Hill Book Co.
2. Feifel, H.: Attitudes toward death: a psychological perspective. In Shneidman, E.S., editor: Death: Current perspectives, Palo Alto, Calif., 1976, Mayfield Publishing Co.
3. Giacquinta, B.: Helping families face the crisis of cancer, Am. J. Nurs. **77**:1585, 1977.
4. Glaser, B.G., and Strauss, A.L.: The ritual drama of mutual pretense. In Shneidman, E.S., editor: Death: current perspectives, Palo Alto, Calif., 1976, Mayfield Publishing Co.
5. Gould, P.I.: Transformation: growth and change in adult life, New York, 1978, Simon & Schuster, Inc.
6. Krell, R., and Rabkin, L.: The effects of sibling death on the surviving child: a family perspective, Fam. Process **18**:471, 1979.
7. Kübler-Ross, E.: On death and dying, New York, 1969, The MacMillan Co., Publishers.
8. Lerner, M.: When, why, and where people die. In Shneidman, E.S., editor: Death: current perspectives, Palo Alto, Calif., 1976, Mayfield Publishing Co.
9. Mant, A.K.: The medical definition of death. In Shneidman, E.S., editor: Death: current perspectives, Palo Alto, Calif., 1976, Mayfield Publishing Co.
10. Perrollaz, L.E., and Mollica, M.: Public knowledge of hospice care, Nurs. Outlook **29**:46, Jan. 1981.
11. Pugh, L.C.: The child and death, Issues Ment. Health Nurs. **2**:53, Dec. 1979.
12. Quint, J., and Strauss, A.L.: Nursing students, assignments and dying patients. In Browning, M., and Lewis, E., editors: The dying patient: a nursing perspective, New York, 1972, The American Journal of Nursing Co.
13. Renshaw, D.C.: The dying child, Proc. Inst. Med. Chic. **33**:59, April-June 1980.
14. Shneidman, E.S.: The deaths of man, Baltimore, 1974, Penguin Books, Inc.
15. Valdes-Dapena, M.A.: Sudden infant death syndrome: a review of the medical literature, 1974-1979, Pediatrics **66**:597, 1980.
16. Veatch, R.M.: Brain death. In Shneidman, E.S., editor: Death: current perspectives, Palo Alto, Calif., 1976, Mayfield Publishing Co.
17. Walborn, K.A.: A nursing model for the hospice: primary and self-care nursing, Nurs. Clin. North Am. **15**:205 March 1980.
18. Weisman, A.D.: On dying and denying: a psychiatric study of terminality, New York, 1972, Behavioral Publications, Inc.

Annotated suggested readings

Baird, S.B.: Nursing roles in continuing care: home care and hospice, Semin. Oncol. **7**:28, March 1980.

This thorough article delineates the parameters of continuing care and hospice programs for the terminally ill. It also includes conceptualization of multiple roles of the nurse in the delivery of care to patients and families in these alternative settings.

Browning, M., and Lewis, E., editors: The dying patient: a nursing perspective, New York, 1972, The American Journal of Nursing Co.

This is a compilation of articles that have appeared in nursing literature and has become a classic. Included are some reports of studies, as well as human interest pieces. Of particular note are the articles by Quint and Strauss, "Nursing Students, Assignments, and Dying Patients," and by Bright and France, "The Nurse and the Terminally Ill Child."

Caine, L.: Widow, New York, 1974, William Morrow & Co., Inc.

This book is a useful resource in assisting survivors in their grief work. It provides a look at the processes that the widow must work through. It is easily read and understood and is written for the population at large.

Deal, A.W., Bordeaux, B.R.: The phenomenon of SIDS, Pediatr. Nurs. **6**:48, Jan.-Feb. 1980.

Many salient questions about the SIDS phenomena are posed and briefly answered in the article. Information about the characteristics of SIDS infants, hypothesized causes from research, and resources available for the SIDS families are provided.

Feifel, H., editor: The meaning of death, New York, 1967, McGraw-Hill Book Co.

This classic work is a multifaceted approach to the theoretical and philosophical issues of death and dying. It is divided into four major areas: theoretical viewpoints, the developmental orientation toward death, cultural aspects, and clinical-experimental studies. Although of a sophisticated nature, it is highly recommended for those actively developing their understanding of the concepts of death and dying.

Giacquinta, B.: Helping families face the crisis of cancer, Am. J. Nurs. **77**:1585, 1977.

This article presents the author's systematized approach to dealing with the families of the terminally ill. It is recommended as a reading to lend perspective to working with the dying and their families.

Gill, D.: Quest: the life of Elizabeth Kübler-Ross, New York, 1980, Ballantine Books, Inc.

This biography is a fascinating account of the life thus far of Elizabeth Kübler-Ross. Nurses will identify easily with the problems she encountered as a woman physician confronting deficiencies in the care of the dying and their families. One is left with deep admiration for the accomplishments of this remarkable woman.

Glick, I.O., Weiss, R.S., and Parkes, C.M.: The first year of bereavement, New York, 1974, John Wiley & Sons, Inc.

As a reference directed toward the lay population, this book can be useful in helping survivors through their grief work. It focuses on the feelings, tasks, and obstacles often encountered during the first year of bereavement.

Kastenbaum, R.: Death, society, and human experience, ed. 2, St. Louis, 1981, The C.V. Mosby Co.

The author presents a responsible, informed, helpful, and humanistic exploration of death in its many related aspects. Its focus is on the individual in society, the quality of life, and the interplay of life and death in all levels of the social hierarchy.

Kübler-Ross, E.: On death and dying, New York, 1969, The Macmillan Co., Publishers.

This is a classic work representing some of the finest endeavors to describe the successive processes through which individuals move in their grief work. This reference is highly recommended for all nurses.

Kübler-Ross, E.: Death: the final stage of growth, Englewood Cliffs, N.J., 1975, Prentice-Hall, Inc.

This composite of readings on the subject of dying includes first-person psychosocial accounts of individuals involved in the dying and grieving processes. It represents an interesting overview of experiences and can be included as an additional reference to aid in one's own introspective processes.

Mills, G.C.: Books to help children understand death, Am. J. Nurs. **79**:291, 1979.

This excellent article reviews a broad spectrum of children's literature on the topic of death. Also included are suggestions on how to use books to facilitate discussion with the child. A complete bibliography includes prices.

Pincus, L.: Death and the family: the importance of mourning, New York, 1976, Vintage Books.

The author examines the experiences of coping with life after the death of a spouse. Included are case histories in which connections are made between how ways of grieving are related to ways of loving. The nature of the relationship provides the key to the mourning process. A valuable reading for those working with the grieving.

Pugh, L.C.: The child and death, Issues Ment. Health Nurs. **2**:53, Dec. 1979.

The author provides an overview of the developmental processes related to conceptualization of death, a synopsis of the coping stages of the dying and the grief responses of the survivors. These are taken into account in discussing nursing perspectives for the dying child.

Schiff, H.: Bereaved parents, New York, 1977, Crown Publishing Co.

This is a useful guide for professionals and parents to help them gain understanding of the trauma of the experience of death of a child. It provides a compilation of information about the process of mourning of parents and the effects on the other family members.

Shneidman, E.S.: The deaths of man, Baltimore, 1974, Penguin Books.

This is an extremely useful resource providing a sociophilosophical approach to the concept of death. Of particular interest are the sections on medical-legal aspects of death and the National Survey of the Attitudes Toward Death (1971).

Shneidman, E.S., editor: Death: current perspectives, Palo Alto, Calif., 1976, Mayfield Publishing Co.

This book is an extensive composite of literature on death and dying. Included are articles on such topics as cultural perspectives of death, social perspectives, personal perspectives, and interpersonal perspectives. The chapters on death with dignity present some creative approaches to caring for the dying. This fairly sophisticated text is recommended for the advanced student.

Tousley, M.M.: The use of family therapy in terminal illness and death, J. Psychosoc. Nurs. **20**:17, Jan. 1982.

The author applies the concepts of the family systems model of family therapy to a case study of a dying woman and her family. This is an excellent example of application of theory to nursing practice.

Walborn, K.A.: A nursing model for the hospice: primary and self-care nursing, Nurs. Clin. North Am. **15**:205, March 1980.

The philosophy and goals of hopsice care are described in light of the ideals of primary and self-care nursing. The characteristics of the nurse, as well as attitudes, knowledge, and skills necessary to design and carry out a nursing system for a hospice program are specified. Included is a partial design for hospice nursing with objectives, nursing actions, and rationale.

Winder, A., and Elam, J.: Therapist for the cancer patient's family: a new role for the nurse, J. Psychiatr. Nurs. **16**:22, Oct. 1978.

The authors suggest that the nurse therapist is in an ideal position to work with the terminally ill patient and his family. To support their view, they present a clinical illustration of their work with one family.

Wise, D.: Learning about dying, Nurs. Outlook **22**:42, Jan. 1974.

The author describes a learning experience she developed to help students give better nursing care to the dying. It includes cultural responses, self-awareness, and specific nursing interventions. This is a helpful article for nurse educators.

CHAPTER 33

THE
PRAGMATICS
OF PRIVATE
PRACTICE

SUZANNE SAYLE JIMERSON

There is a tide in the affairs of men,
Which, taken at the flood, leads on to fortune;
Omitted, all the voyage of their life
Is bound in shallows and in miseries:
And we must take the current when it serves,
Or lose our ventures.

William Shakespeare, *Julius Caesar*

Learning objectives

After studying this chapter, the student
should be able to:

- *determine the legality of independent practice by examining the relevant state nurse practice act.*

- *analyze various malpractice insurance policies and determine which provides the best coverage for psychiatric nursing practice.*

- *prepare a personal financial analysis and assess the resources necessary to initiate a practice.*

- *describe the factors to be considered when selecting a private office.*

- *identify the reasons for establishing a consultation contract with physicians who are specialists in psychiatry and internal medicine.*

- *discuss the importance of participating in clinical supervision by a more experienced psychotherapist and/or peers.*

- *determine the availability of third-party reimbursement for nurses in independent practice.*

- *discuss the considerations involved in establishing a system of record keeping.*

Private practice offers qualified nurses an opportunity to practice their skills in a setting of their own choice, thus maximizing their autonomy, independence, and decision-making skills. As such, it is viewed as a highly desirable manner of practice by an increasing number of nurses. To be qualified to function as a private practitioner, three requirements are usually necessary:

1. One must be a registered nurse with an active license to practice in that particular state.
2. One should be prepared at the graduate level as a clinical specialist in psychiatric nursing. The nurse's master's degree program should have provided her with a strong theoretical base in psychiatric nursing and supervised clinical experiences in various therapeutic modalities.
3. One must be able to document clinical competence through continuous clinical work, access to supervision or peer consultation, ongoing education, and preferably the attainment of certification as a psychiatric–mental health clinical specialist from the American Nurses' Association.

With these qualifications the nurse can open the door to the challenging, satisfying, and often uncertain world of private practice.

Engaging in private practice not only brings independence to nurses, but also direct accountability and a need to understand business arrangements. Accountability means that the quality of service provided by the nurse in private practice must be as good as or better than the same service delivered by a physician or other health care provider. Understanding business means that nurses must know how to make a living and provide for the future through self-employed pension plans as a sole proprietor in a complicated financial world. The nurse must not only provide a mechanism for collecting monies and budgeting for office operating costs, but she must also understand how to protect herself from malpractice, accidents at the office, and personal illness/disability—all those areas which are automatically taken care of with a job in a traditional setting such as a hospital. To get an idea of what running a business means, the interested nurse should write to the Small Business Administration for pamphlets on how to set up a business. It is also advisable to contract the professional help of a lawyer to ad-vise on insurance policies and an accountant to advise on tax credits. Gathering all the information before actually committing oneself to private practice will pave the way to making a successful decision.

Private practice as a career really means being totally responsible for patient care and self-care. Nurses in private practice need to feel secure and know that their functioning does not depend on praise or criticism from others. They need to be inner directed and feel sure enough of their own knowledge and judgment without closing doors to the learning process. Finally, it is necessary to answer the following questions: Who am I? What do I believe? What do I stand for? and What will I do or not do that differentiates me from my peers?[1]

Nurse practice act

Almost every state in America has a board of nursing that has adopted a legally binding position, or nurse practice act (NPA) on what a nursing license in that state allows a nurse to do. Once decided that private practice is a personally workable career choice, the first necessity is to read the relevant state's NPA to assure that practicing independently is legal. There are three different types of nurse practice acts; traditional, authorization, and administrative. The traditional NPA is based on the model definition of nursing formulated by the American Nurses' Association (ANA) in 1955 and does not include diagnosis, treatment, and prescription as functions of nurses. The authorization NPA defines exactly what the nurse can do beyond the traditional definition and is usually limited in scope, although this will vary from state to state. Finally, the administrative NPA recognizes the expanded role of the nurse, usually naming the provider, such as nurse practitioner or nurse anesthetist. Furthermore, the administrative NPA is accompanied by rules and regulations, usually jointly promulgated by the state boards of nursing and medicine and implemented by the board of nursing. These rules and regulations define the additional acts allowed by the extended role.[5] Thus an administrative NPA legalizes private practice, an authorization NPA probably does not, and a traditional NPA clearly makes private practice an illegal function of a nursing license.

Malpractice insurance

Malpractice insurance is a most important area in which to be informed. Most malpractice insurance will deny coverage for acts deemed outside the scope of the state's NPA. In addition, malpractice insurance will not cover for criminal acts. It is a law of public policy that coverage is not provided for acts that violate criminal law. If the relevant state law is such that the practice of medicine without a license is a criminal offense, the nurse will not be financially protected from the charge of this crime.[5] Thus it is extremely important that the nurse know what the insurance company defines as within her scope of practice or, in other words, their legal definition of the relevant state's NPA. An example of how nurses can be in legal jeopardy in this area is with the nursing function of diagnosis. Both the NPA and the insurance company must agree that diagnosis is also a nursing function, or the nurse is in danger of being accused of practicing medicine.

It is advisable to "shop around" for malpractice insurance and become totally familiar with coverage options. What needs to be particularly examined in a malpractice policy is the definitions of words used in the scope of coverage provision and the exclusion provisions. Will coverage be not only for malpractice/negligence, but also if a patient slips and falls on the sidewalk of the office premises? Does the insurance company define private practice as a small business enterprise and therefore not provide coverage? Does the insurance carrier guarantee in writing that the company will insure a nurse functioning independently without physician supervision? It may be necessary and comforting to go through the policy with a lawyer or someone familiar with the policy language to clarify policy advantages and limitations. The amount of coverage decided on depends, in part, on the site of the private practice and the clients to be served, however, it is advisable to purchase maximum dollar coverage.

Financial planning

Armed with a good lawyer, an accountant, and information from the Small Business Administration, the next step is to clearly delineate a proposed financial pattern.[2] To begin with, a personal financial statement subtracting debts from assets needs to be written (below). After this statement, a proposed monthly living expenses statement needs to be prepared (p. 932). Since the practice will probably not realize profit to cover the monthly expenses for 6 months to 1 year, money will have to be kept in reserve to pay basic living costs for that period of time. Simply multiply the total monthly expenses times 8 months to arrive at a necessary reserve and add $1000.00 for emergencies. Next, a projected initial start-up cost statement is necessary (p. 932), and these costs must also be set aside.

Starting a private practice does mean an initial reserve of quite a bit of money. If such a reserve of money seems formidable, there are two possibilities. One is to begin the practice at a home office and later move to rented space. The other

---

PERSONAL FINANCIAL STATEMENT*

Assets

Cash in bank and on hand
Securities (market value)
Home (market value)
Car (blue book value)
Cash value of life insurance
Savings bonds
Miscellaneous assets

TOTAL _____

Debts

Current household bills
Installment contracts: car, appliances, personal loans, charge accounts
Real estate mortgages
Other loans
Miscellaneous

TOTAL _____

Summary

Total assets minus total debts = net worth _____

---

*From Edmunds, M.: Nurse Pract. **5:**35, Sept.-Oct. 1980.

MONTHLY LIVING EXPENSES*

Regular monthly payments

Rent or mortgage payment, car payment (including insurance), appliance payments, home improvement loan payment, personal loan payment, health insurance plan, insurance premiums, miscellaneous payments   TOTAL _____

Household monthly operating expenses

Telephone, gas and electric, water, garbage, maintenance and repair   TOTAL _____

Tax expenses (monthly average)

Federal/state income tax, real estate taxes, miscellaneous taxes   TOTAL _____

Monthly family expenses (average)

Clothing, cleaning, laundry, drugs, physician, dentist, education, dues, gifts, contributions, travel, newspapers, publications, auto maintenance, gas, entertainment, miscellaneous expenses   TOTAL _____

Food expenses (monthly average)   TOTAL _____

Total monthly expenses _____

Times number of months until practice begins to return a profit _____

---

*From Edmunds, M.: Nurse Pract. **5:**35, Sept.-Oct. 1980.

ONE-TIME START-UP COSTS*

Decorating and remodeling
Furniture, fixtures, and equipment
Installation costs for fixtures and equipment
Answering machine
Supplies on hand
Deposits with utility companies
Initial stationery, announcements, office materials
Advance rent and cleaning deposit
Reserve for petty cash
Initial licenses and fees
Legal fees (cost of incorporation, partner, etc.)
Miscellaneous initial expenses

---

*From Edmunds, M.: Nurse Pract. **5:**35, 1980.

is to go into private practice on a part-time basis until a large enough clientele is possible to support total living expenses.

The final step in financial planning involves projecting the operating capital of the business (p. 933) on a monthly basis. Doing so allows the projection to consider vacation time, holidays, and other fluctuations in income and tax payment time; license and insurance renewal times; and other fluctuations in expenses. Hopefully, operating costs will remain relatively stable. In planning for operating costs, steps can be taken to keep them down. For instance, a phone-answering machine can be utilized rather than an answering service/receptionist; supplies can be purchased at discount stores rather than delivered to the office; and cleaning can be done by the practitioner or a friendly neighborhood young adult rather than a professional cleaning service.

If a home office is utilized, the one-time start-up costs will not include deposits with utility companies and advance rent and cleaning deposit. Operating capital will not include rent and utilities under fixed expenses. In addition, if

OPERATING CAPITAL*

		Month	Total Year
(A)	Expected income		
	Controllable expenses		
	Gross wages		_____
	Supplies		_____
	Repair and maintenance		_____
	Miscellaneous		_____
	Fixed expenses		
	Rent		_____
	Utilities		_____
	Insurance		_____
	Taxes and licenses		_____
	Depreciation		_____
	Interest		_____
(B)	TOTAL		
(C)	Net profit or loss (A − B = C)		_____

Determining when total expenses equals income will identify the break-even point in practice.

Total expenses for the time period before the projected break-even point will give you the amount of operating capital you will need for your practice.

*From Edmunds, M.: Nurse Pract. **5:**35, Sept.-Oct., 1980.

you are planning to run the practice alone, the gross wages can be eliminated. Calculating the start-up costs and operating capital both for a rented office and a home office will provide an accurate estimate of savings with a home office.

Office space

Choosing the office space to fit personal and practice needs requires much thought and knowledge of personal needs. The first choice to make is that between a home office or rented office space. A home office has certain advantages over rented office space in the following areas: (1) the cost of managing that space may be tax deductible, (2) there is no commuting, (3) if a patient does not keep the appointment, the nurse's time can easily be utilized elsewhere in the home, and (4) operating costs will be lower. A home office also means that the nurse will be responsible for upkeep, which means hiring someone to do it or taking the time to do it herself, such as shoveling snow and assuring adequate lighting, and this upkeep may not be tax deductible.

One major consideration with a home office is that of safety, not only of the nurse's home, but of the neighborhood in general. Seeing patients in a home office requires careful screening to assure that the patient is reality oriented and that there is no danger of pyromania, kleptomania, or other conditions that may cause the patient to act out in a destructive manner. Along with this concern is the view of one's home as a private, personal, or family space. The practitioner and her family must be comfortable with the decision to use the home for business. If the nurse has a family, she must also consider how much noise she can tolerate during patient hours and the effect on the family of trying to be more quiet. Children, especially, have difficulty with this. In addition, zoning laws in the community must also be checked to assure that operating a business is legal. Finally, availability of parking space may be a hindrance to a home office.

A rented office, on the other hand, relieves the nurse of concerns related to upkeep, safety, zoning, parking, and privacy and holds one other major advantage in that the location can be chosen according to where the practice might benefit the most people. For instance, the location might be situated on major bus routes and in an area that does not offer psychiatric services, but does offer family planning or general practitioner services. Both of these services might function as good sources of referral. However, a rented office will increase the operating cost of the practice, although some of these costs may be tax deductible, another reason for seeking the advice of an accountant.

Whichever office site is chosen, there are certain aspects to be looked for in setting up an office. Soundproofing is very important and often insulated ceilings and walls are necessary, as well as a double door to the office from the hallway to insulate sound from the hallway. Insulating the office space will not only decrease noise, but also serves to save energy through heat and cooling loss. It may also be tax deductible as an energy-saving improvement. In addition, an office where the furnace fan can be switched to automatic, creating "white noise," is an advantage. Sitting through a patient session listening to the family dog barking or the patient in the next office crying loudly is distracting to the therapeutic process, decreasing the amount of work both the patient and the practitioner can accomplish, and it should be avoided.

Unless patients can be scheduled 15 minutes or more apart, a waiting room with current magazines to browse through is necessary. If the practice includes children, a box of inexpensive children's toys and books is a thoughtful measure. Provision for bathroom facilities is comforting and, at times, also necessary. Finally, the care with which office space is utilized and decorated is a reflection of the practitioner's personality, and assuring patient privacy and comfort are important variables in the success of a practice.

Physician consultants

Although it is certainly possible to manage a private practice without a physician, it is necessary to have a contract, either formally or informally, with a psychiatrist and an internist. Nurses in private practice have a major advantage over other nonmedical mental health practitioners in their knowledge of medical matters and medication effects. It may, at some point, be necessary to refer a patient for medication, or the medication the patient is taking may need to be altered and the nurse should be able to readily provide this service. In addition, and particularly with somatic complaints, it may be necessary for a patient to have certain tests to rule out organic reasons for the complaint. Nurses should feel comfortable in seeking consultative advice from a psychiatrist or an internist whom they trust and with whom they have a good working relationship.

The other situation in which physician backup is essential is that of an emergency in which hospitalization is a necessity. Being able to respond to the patient's distress promptly not only is a legal responsibility of practice, but also potentially life saving. If the services of the backup psychiatrist are not available at the time needed, the nurse should know which hospital has a psychiatrist on call 24 hours a day so that the patient can be seen on an emergency basis. It is particularly important that the nurse be calm

and know what her alternatives are in dealing with a crisis situation.

Public relations

Obtaining those first patients in private practice is often the most difficult step. Ideally, a few patients (from the previous work setting) may continue treatment. Getting the practice off the ground requires good relations with churches, local colleges and universities, social and civic groups, and peers. Everywhere the nurse goes, she needs to discuss her role and services and hand out business cards with her name, qualifications, specialty, address (optional if starting a practice in the home), and phone number. It is advantageous for the nurse to be involved in the state nurses' association, health fairs, mental health conferences, local political activities, and community centers. In addition, sending out notices of the opening of the practice to all colleagues and the previously mentioned organizations is a good initial step. Going to the local newspaper for a small write-up on the services to be provided and the role served in the community can be quite helpful.

Furthermore, the American Nurses' Association has a Council of Specialists in Psychiatric and Mental Health Nursing that publishes a newsletter called *Pacesetter*, which can serve as a communiqué to other nurses. Belonging to the American Nurses' Association and to the council means that the nurse's name and practice specialty are published, and this is a good source for referrals for patients who are moving. In addition, the council has established a regional network of nurses in private practice concerned with third party reimbursement issues (Committee on Reimbursement) who also serve as good referral sources, as well as a source of help for third-party reimbursement problems. Another resource for out-of-town referrals is the National Directory of Psychiatric and Mental Health Nurses, which is published by Horizons in Health, Inc., of Cambridge, Massachusetts. Finally, in addition to becoming involved in these activities, ". . . the surest way to attract private practice is to become known for the quality of your practice, to be known to be consistently available and take on small and unremunerative cases as well as more lucrative ones."[3:32]

Supervision

One of the more difficult aspects about private practice is the tendency to become isolated, to stop learning. Supervision becomes important not only because it is a necessity for knowledgeable practice and at times a condition for reimbursement, but also to decrease the sense of isolation. Supervision can be acquired by contracting with a psychiatrist or other nurse specialist for individual or group supervision or by joining a peer group either comprised of other nurses or members of several of the core mental health disciplines. Individual supervision or involvement in a group with an identified leader usually involves payment of a fee; peer group supervision usually does not. Group supervision has advantages over individual supervision in that the practitioner is exposed to more cases than just her own. In addition, she is in contact with more peers, which facilitates gathering fresh ideas and alternatives to further her practice.

One other aspect of supervision which is taking on increasing importance is that to apply for certification as a psychiatric–mental health clinical specialist from the American Nurses' Association, the nurse must document 100 hours of supervision which cannot be accumulated in less than a year. Getting certified as a specialist from the American Nurses' Association is becoming an increasingly more important credential to have to qualify for third-party reimbursement.

Third-party reimbursement

Although the American Nurses' Association has been seeking third-party reimbursement for nurses since the 1950s, progress in that direction is slow. Mental health entered the third-party reimbursement field relatively late and, with emphasis on budget cutting, mental health coverage will see "a period of solidification of past gains rather than a continuation of expansion trends."[4] Nursing has traditionally had difficulty receiving third-party reimbursement, falling well behind psychologists and social workers.

Third-party reimbursement will probably not be possible for nurses in private practice unless the state has a freedom of choice law. A freedom of choice law basically guarantees that if the insurance policy covers the service, then the service is reimbursable when rendered by any legally licensed health care provider. However, insurance companies often find many ways around this law, for instance, claiming that the treatment is not medically necessary or claiming that their policy is part of an employee's benefit plan and as such is not regulated by state insurance laws. Also, an insurance company may agree that the service of psychotherapy is covered in the policy and therefore the freedom of choice law is legally binding, but when the provider is a nurse, they define the service as nursing, not as psychotherapy, and so avoid payment.

After assuring that the state has a freedom of choice law and that the client's policy covers the treatment, there are a few ways to increase the chances of reimbursement. First, the most common cause for rejection is paperwork problems. "The best way to avoid rejection is to follow directions exactly, be extra careful on diagnostic language and give a complete and accurate account of the treatment given."[4:3] Second, if rejected, calling or writing the claims manager with a protest, a copy of the state's freedom of choice laws, and a detailed description of why the claim is reimbursable can be effective. In addition, having the employer apply pressure on the claims manager often brings results, since the insurance company will not want to lose the contract with the employer. Finally, and if the patient is willing, the insurance commissioner of the state can be informed of the rejection and asked to judge the legitimacy of the rejection.

In all, getting reimbursed is a variable process, one company may reimburse for the services and another may not. Nurses in private practice will have a better chance of getting reimbursed if they are certified and can show ongoing evidence of supervision and continuing education.

Managing business arrangements

Perhaps the hardest area for the beginning nurse in private practice is that of setting a fee. The nurse needs to know what her maximum charge is as well as her minimum charge. To arrive at this figure, she can check with peers, as well as sample insurance companies, to ascertain what they consider to be acceptable fees. With the patient in the office, the urge not to talk about money is great. Nurses resist appearing mercenary and are reluctant to ask patients to consider what their services are worth. Money, however, is a powerful emotional force and failing to discuss it openly and without hesitation can often reinforce individual or family pathological conditions. Nurses have the responsibility to examine the factors that further the patient's need to remain sick, and discussing money issues often sheds light on these factors.

Setting the fee involves collecting a financial history from the patient, considering a similar format as that described on p. 931 in this chapter. With such a financial statement, the nurse and the patient can then agree on a mutually satisfactory fee. In addition, how the fee is to be paid should also be discussed. For example, payments monthly or after each visit should be decided, and the rules about uncancelled, but missed, appointments should be clearly delineated. The nurse may also want to discuss with the patient the use of telephone time. For example, if a phone call is longer than a few minutes, the nurse may charge for each 15 minutes utilized by taking one fourth of the original fee set. This then, would be added to the bill.

The nurse also needs to discuss with the patient how her phone answering service works, coverage should she be not available for an extended period of time, where the client can be reached should the nurse need to reach him, and rules about being late for appointments.

Record keeping

Although the information gathered at the initial evaluation will depend in part on the nurse's approach to therapy, it is useful to prepare a sheet of paper with certain essential information on it and use it as a guide for each patient seen (below). Writing notes at the end of each session is a necessity. However, how much is included in those notes is a hotly debated issue. Some nurses only note that the patient kept the appointment to protect the patient's confidentiality. On the other end of the continuum, some nurses describe the session in detail so as not to forget the therapeutic process. Checking with peers on their policies and coming up with what is personally comfortable is important. However, it must be kept in mind that patients' charts are legal records and can be subpoenaed

---

INITIAL INTAKE INTERVIEW

Date _____

Patient name _____

Age _____ Date of birth _____

Patient address _____

Occupation _____

Phone number: Home _____ Office _____

Significant medical history (operations, illnesses, medications, treatments) _____

Significant family history of medical problems (hypertension, cancer, heart disease) _____

Psychiatric history (past treatment, present client problem) _____

Significant psychiatric problems in family (include siblings, parents, grandparents) _____

Family position (sibling position, role in family) _____

Strengths _____

Limitations _____

Patient's goal for treatment _____

Diagnosis:

Projected treatment time:

Fee:

as evidence in court in malpractice suits. Therefore if a patient appears depressed, it is probably safest to include information on the depression, the assessment done to ascertain the patient's suicide potential, and the action taken to help the patient.

In a sense, the nurse's records are the most tangible evidence of a psychiatric nurse's practice. Properly done, they define the basis of her interventions, assure the proper treatment and referral of her patients, and protect her from claims of malpractice or negligence. They also reflect one outcome of the progressive documentation needed by the nurse who is attempting to establish a private practice and who must wrestle with nurse practice acts, financial planning, third-party reimbursement and public relations. But, unlike these tasks, record keeping

arises directly from caring for patients in a work context under the direct control of the nurse, and therein lies the compensation, reward, and satisfaction derived from establishing and maintaining a private practice in psychiatric nursing.

Suggested cross-references

The roles and functions of psychiatric nurses are discussed in Chapter 1. Legal aspects of psychiatric care are discussed in Chapter 16.

SUMMARY

1. Private practice by clinical specialists in psychiatric nursing offers independence and requires accountability and an understanding of business arrangements.

2. The legality of independent practice is determined by the nurse practice act of each state, which may be one of three types: traditional, authorization, and administrative. Only an administrative nurse practice act legalizes private practice.

3. The nurse in private practice must have a thorough understanding of malpractice insurance options, which may vary widely in their coverage.

4. Personal financial planning is necessary before initiating an independent practice. Several tools were presented to assist the nurse in this process.

5. There are numerous decisions to be made concerning the selection of an office, including location, safety, accessibility, cost, and physical characteristics.

6. Contractual consultative relationships with a psychiatrist and an internist are recommended to facilitate prescription of medication, work-ups for organic illnesses, and emergency hospital admissions.

7. Effective public relations are necessary to establish a referral network, and suggested contacts were described.

8. The nurse in independent practice is responsible for arranging to receive clinical supervision from a more experienced psychotherapist and/or peers. American Nurses' Association certification is recommended as a necessary credential to qualify for third-party reimbursement.

9. The nurse should investigate the availability of third-party reimbursement for nurse psychotherapists which varies from state to state. Ways to increase the nurse's chances for reimbursement were explored.

10. Business arrangements should be discussed with the patient, including fees, cancelled appointments, and communication arrangements, such as answering services.

11. Both therapeutic and legal aspects must be considered in making decisions about record keeping. The nurse's records are the most tangible evidence of her practice, and they can reflect on both her competence and effectiveness.

References

1. Alkon, N.: Preparing to individuate from team member to independent practitioner, J. Psychiatr. Nurs. **15**:31, June 1977.
2. Edmunds, M.: Financial planning for independent practice, Nurse Pract. **5**:35, Sept.-Oct. 1980.
3. Lewis, E.B.: Setting up in private practice: a guide for the newly appointed consultant, Anaesthesia **32**:158, Feb. 1977.
4. Managing your practice is your money, Psychother. Finances, p. 1, Aug. 1981.
5. Trandel-Korenchuk, D.K., and Trandel-Korenchuk, K.M.: Current legal issues facing nursing practice, Nurs. Admin. Q. **5**:37, Fall 1980.

Annotated suggested readings

Aiken, L.H., editor: Nursing in the 1980's: crises, opportunities, challenges, Philadelphia, 1982, J.B. Lippincott Co.

This book provides a wide variety of challenging viewpoints on nursing presented by a number of contemporary nurse leaders. The health care trends described will have great influence on future nursing practice and merit attention and consideration by nurses who seek to establish private practice.

Fagin, C.M.: Nursing as an alternative to high-cost care, Am. J. Nurs. **82**:56, 1982.

Current issues related to competition in the health care industry and the implications for nursing practice are presented by this author. It is critical that nurses who seek to practice independently be cognizant of the need to document the cost-effectiveness of mental health nursing care and to publicize these data to the public and to health care policy makers.

Ginzberg, C.: The economics of health care and the future of nursing, J. Nurs. Admin. **11**:28, March 1981.

This prominent economist analyzes nursing in terms of recent economic trends. He discusses issues related to nursing education, expanded practice, and collegial relationships with physicians. He poses a challenge to nurses to continue to progress in a time of decreased resources and increased competition.

Goldwater, M.: From a legislator: views on third-party reimbursement for nurses, Am. J. Nurs. **82**:411, 1982.

A state legislator who is also a nurse discusses her perception of the role of nurses in obtaining access to third-party reimbursement. She provides a very good review of the history of various reimbursement programs. She stresses the need for nurses to be politically active on their own behalf.

Griffith, H.M.: Strategies for direct third-party reimbursement for nurses, Am. J. Nurs. **82**:408, 1982.

This author describes the major issues that are involved as nurses struggle to become eligible for third-party reimbursement. She provides advice on the strategies that must be pursued to accomplish this goal. This article should be of interest to any nurse who is in private practice.

Hendrickson, D.E., Janney, S.P., and Fraze, J.E., editors, *Psychotherapy in Private Practice*, **1**:1, Fall 1982.

This is a new journal to be published quarterly that promises to provide practical information on the operation of a private practice. It merits review by nurses who are interested in issues related to the business aspect of their work.

Koltz, C.: Private practice in nursing: development and management, Rockville, Md., 1979, Aspen Systems Corp.

This is a basic book directed to the private nurse practitioner, but it does cover many areas pertinent to the psychiatric nurse, including state nursing laws, provision of services, promoting a practice, professional relations and financial management.

CHAPTER 34

ISSUES AND TRENDS IN PSYCHIATRIC–MENTAL HEALTH NURSING

Often do the spirits
Of great events stride on
before the events,
And in to-day already
walks tomorrow.

Samuel Taylor Coleridge, Wallenstein, Part II, Act V

MARY E. RERES

Learning objectives

After studying this chapter, the student should be able to:

- *state four issues that will be of concern to psychiatric nurses in the future.*

- *discuss the need for clear definition of the role and functions of the psychiatric–mental health nurse.*

- *analyze the role of the nurse in health planning and political action.*

- *identify the benefits of certification in psychiatric–mental health nursing.*

Nursing is the largest health care profession; its members totaling over 1,400,000 far exceed the disciplines of medicine, dentistry, or any allied health profession. From a political standpoint, if nurses were to act together, the impact of their force could be a major determinant in the direction of health care legislation. At this time, however, nursing is largely in a reactive stance to such measures. The majority of the members of the nursing profession choose not to participate in an organized collective way with one another and do not join the national association that speaks in their behalf. There is nonetheless a beginning momentum among nurses to speak as authorities on health and demand their being heard on major issues that affect health care delivery. It is a time when nurses are growing aware of their potential power as a group and also of the strength of the subgroups of nursing specialties.

Although psychiatric nurses make up only a small percentage of the total nursing population, they do form the group with the highest educational preparation. It is reasonable to assume that they will become the articulate spokeswomen for the profession and have a great impact on major health decisions. The focal issue, however, is whether psychiatric nursing will remain distinct in the field of mental health delivery. No social service–related activity can exist if it is not distinctly filling a great social service need. When any service is not specifically tailored to community need, it will soon be faced with extinction or have its role assumed by another group. It is not sufficient justification to cite the fact that one out of ten persons is in need of psychiatric care; rather, it is necessary that the mental health professions be able to demonstrate the impact their services are having on defined populations. Without such articulation a professional group soon loses a sense of its health target goals, and its treatment modalities are directed to the current fads or to outdated therapies more appropriate to other times and populations.

At the twenty-fifth anniversary of the National Mental Health Act, leaders of all behavioral fields related to the treatment of psychiatric or emotional disorders met in Washington, D.C., to discuss predictable outcomes for their disciplines in coming years. Although no major profession wished to relinquish its autonomy, it became obvious that much the same content was taught in preparing therapists in nursing, medicine, social work, and psychology. Functionally, in terms of graduate level preparations, all disciplines working in community mental health centers performed much the same tasks: family and group counseling, marital therapy, and supervision of other health professionals. Similarities and differences became a focus of concern, since each discipline was confronted with its own potential dissolution. A person's identity is intimately related to professional role, and the potential loss of the identity of one's distinct discipline is threatening not only to a group as a whole but also to the individual's sense of self. As a result, competition among disciplines has increased for visibility, power, and federal dollars. Nursing as a profession has not fared as well in such competition as have psychiatry, social work, and psychology. These three disciplines have been politically more adept at having roles in community mental health centers specifically earmarked for their group, at obtaining greater shares of the research and training monies, and at being officially recognized for receipt of third-party payments. Survival of psychiatric–mental health nursing is closely related to gearing itself to acquiring the roles and the image of a stable, independent discipline in twenty-first century mental health care.

As with any issue, there are two sides of the matter with equally sound factors. It is easy to intellectually grasp the fact that the keeping of distinct disciplines has produced recognizable overlaps in education. Psychiatry, psychiatric nursing, and all mental health disciplines each teach their own courses in such areas as growth and development, assessment skills, and therapeutic modalities. The cost factor to universities, which is passed on to the students and taxpayers, is enormous; each overlap has its own hidden duplication of faculty, administrative personnel, space, library facilities, and all other related resources. The disciplines in such situations come to maintain a distance of disdain, and new graduates of the professions have little or no real awareness of the learning experiences and skills of the related disciplines. However, by such separation the professions do maintain autonomy in educating their own members. Too frequently, however, the education follows the traditional mode of the past, rather than preparing the new careerists to meet the contemporary community problems. The time is steadily approaching when psychiatric nursing must prepare itself to assimilate the modes of operation and visibility of a distinct professional group if it is to remain one.

Psychiatric–mental health nursing must begin to actively proclaim and define its unique role in milieu management in inpatient settings, psychiatric liaison in health-related settings where disciplines other than medicine and nursing are incapable of health and medication assessment, and in CMHCs because of its developed skills in assessment of the home environment. By proclaiming and demonstrating how psychiatric–mental health nursing provides unique services in mental health compared to other behavioral disciplines and by learning and applying skills appropriate to short-term therapies in CMHCs this field of nursing may in all probability continue as a separate discipline.

The independent practice of psychiatric–mental health nurses is closely linked to the survival of the discipline because at the present time insurance companies' third-party payments for therapy are designated according to the professional roles and credentials of the therapist, rather than the therapeutic functions that are performed. The independent practitioner is identified by clients and paying institutions according to her professional group. The stronger and more visible the parent profession, the greater the practice potential of the independent practitioner. This is the reason that other disciplines with greater numbers of independent practitioners, such as medicine and psychology, have aligned so closely with the organization that nationally represents the parent profession—the American Medical Association, the American Psychiatric Association, or the American Psychologic Association. Such organizations have vigilantly protected the practice arena of their respective groups. They have demanded their involvement in all national health issues. Nursing, and its specialty of psychiatric–mental health nursing, cannot do less if the profession is to remain viable. There is a need for a clear understanding of the major national health and legislative issues and movements, since they too frequently determine the boundaries of independent, as well as group, practice. It is by studying such matters that one can begin preparation for the profession's tomorrows.

For example in 1981, the federal government undertook a study of the supply and distribution of physicians, which was published as the Report of the Graduate Medical Education National Advisory Committee (GMENAC) to the Secretary, Department of Health and Human Ser-

vices. As recorded, an oversupply of physicians exists in many specialties, which suggests a potential threat to the future economic income of that professional discipline. Recommendations have been made to limit the enrollment of students to medical schools, encourage physicians' specialization in programs of great demand, and maintain practice sites geographically distal to areas that are densely populated with physicians. A high level of anxiety arose among many physicians who read the portion of the report that suggested a potential economic threat to their careers. Such anxiety does not foster closer ties between the disciplines, but only further suggests that great effort will be exerted to ensure that physician prominence and domain prevail. As a result, third-party payment for nurse practitioners and nurse therapists now takes on even greater political undertones and meaning to the other disciplines.

Certainly the federal legislation that has had the most resounding impact on health care delivery in the decade was the National Health Planning and Resource Development Act of 1974. The professional organizations and the public as a whole were largely caught unaware by its quiet passage, which proceeded much like a dark cat on a foggy night. Since its enactment, however, no segment of our health care system has remained untouched. For the first time in our nation's history the consumer had the dominant voting voice on local and state health care decisions. The Health Manpower Law established the framework for a review process in the form, at the local level, of health service agencies (HSAs) to oversee local health planning, avoid costly duplication, and direct funding efforts to well-documented needs. Consumers nonaffiliated with the health professions were to make up at least 60% of both the local HSAs and the state's advisory health councils. All such regional and state agencies required approval by the federal Health Resources Administration.

The implications of the enactment of this law are still being experienced. Many health professionals realized that the average consumer was not prepared to define community or state major health planning needs; as a result, there was a massive scramble at every level by health professionals to be appointed to the HSAs and state councils. Nursing has not been well represented in the formulation of such groups. The reason is that nursing as a whole has not built its local base of political support to ensure its inclusion on governing boards. On the whole, the individual nurse was not aware of the power of this legislation, yet it is the individual who is appointed to such boards and councils. Nursing's image over time has become one of passive response and acceptance of major national health legislative decisions. Nursing is viewed mainly as a professional group that stands ready to implement at the patient care level decisions made. It is not seen as a creative and powerful political force at local, state, and national levels. It is not seen as a group that most state governors feel they must be accountable to in the assignment of political appointments.

However, it is essential that nursing be represented. Block grant mechanisms require that distribution of federal funds be determined at the local level. Such review processes will oversee and curtail duplication of use of both material and human resources. The impact on manpower development and assignment of health target facilities is slowly being experienced. In many areas no health facility (e.g., a hospital) can be built without local and state approval. Specialized health-related equipment can be authorized for purchase only according to specified need on a per capita basis. Such definitions ultimately direct where an individual has to go for a treatment and will also influence where training and employment of health professionals will occur. As the states develop their methods for allocating diminishing health care resources, health professionals will compete to have a voice in these difficult decisions. Such health professionals will have a distinct advantage in overseeing and protecting the viability of their own discipline as well as contributing to major decisions that will have an ongoing effect on health care delivery. The politics involved will make for a rough ride. At this time few nurses have even approached the track. Of those who have, there are few who are aware of nursing's role in community mental health.

Obviously now as never before there is a critical need to educate the consumer as to major health issues and definition of community health needs, with particular emphasis on community mental health needs. Health education has always been a stated function of nursing's professional role. Now, rather than the target being the individual learning about his health, it will be entire communities learning about need assessment and health delivery models to meet those needs. Of course, with public awareness of defined needs and the application of human and material resources to meet those needs, health professionals will be accountable as never before in terms of health care delivery and the effectiveness of designated manpower. In mental health particularly, the effectiveness of treatment modalities in reducing the incidence of various mental health problems will be under close evaluation. Such evaluation has the potential for being the best thing to occur for nursing. The opportunity will exist to demonstrate in terms of cost-effectiveness the role of the nurse as therapist. It is absolutely essential that nursing be specifically included in such manpower evaluation, rather than being categorized as "other allied professionals" in the data collection. Such data will have a major impact not only in terms of establishing the particular role of psychiatric nurses in CMHCs but also in demonstrating the cost-effectiveness of the nurse in private practice. Armed with these evaluation outcomes, the consumer will then probably join with nursing to exert pressure on insurance groups to recognize psychiatric–mental health nurses as primary therapists who should be designated for third-party payment of services. When psychiatric nursing has been so designated, then there will be greater economic stability for nurses in private practice and the community will be provided with greater selection of preferred therapists. Currently, however, it is the individual consumer who does battle with his insurance agency to obtain the fee for service of the nurse therapist. Thus it is essential that nursing fully involve itself in the manpower evaluation process.

The last decade has been marked by nursing steadily progressing in working with clients or patients to achieve a more autonomous role in the definition of their individual health care. Such linkage provides an important framework in the interaction between nursing and the community at large in approaching the Health Manpower Law. As a profession nursing has already complied with the intent of the law to ensure the rights and responsibility of the consumer with regard to health care. The task now is for the psychiatric–mental health nurse to become more political in her own behalf. This means having visibility at health planning meetings, only addressing major health issues from a nursing perspective, volunteering for community service activities and obtaining publicity for such activities, getting to know personally the state commissioner for mental health and seeking the assistance of that office in political appointments to support other qualified nurse leaders in their political aspirations. Enormous effort and expenditure of energy is needed to create a political base for nursing.

Federal block grants to individual states will require even greater concentrated political assertiveness by psychiatric nursing. Every discipline and health-related agency and community group will scramble for funding awards as distributed by the state. Unless psychiatric nursing can increase its visibility and power within the resident state, then potential federal funding to this discipline may not be a reality. Although direct federal grants from the NIMH are still obtainable, the monies have been greatly reduced, the projects highly specific to national priorities, and the competition keen. With block grants awarded to the states, there will be a return to the in-state political maneuvers of previous eras. The role of HSAs in the award of such federal funding has yet to be defined.

The women's movement is an assistance as this largely female profession begins to fully assert its role in the delivery of health care. Women have to a large extent held one another back in terms of achieving leadership roles. For too long one of the greatest risks in self-achievement was the potential alienation of one's own professional associates. When professionals are held back, no one looks inferior in comparison to the superior accomplishments of another. Such negative control by women of one another is diminishing, and it is important that this occur, since it is only through mutual respect and unity that nursing can effect its full political impact as a distinct profession. There is national expectation that women will assert themselves and will achieve positions of power and prestige. The time is ideal for nurses to not only acquire individual power but also to realize the collective power of the nursing profession. There is a focus in the women's movement on women's health care. As women proceed to take more political and power-related professional risks, they will experience stress to extremely heightened degrees. There will be an increase in stress-related diseases among women that used to occur primarily among men who were high achievers. Within the field of mental health, nursing can expand itself to identify these stressors and their expression among women. It is believed that nurse therapists would have a greater ad-

vantage in that area of therapy, since the majority of them are women who have undergone similar stress. Also nurse therapists have the knowledge related to physical, as well as mental, health assessment, which would allow them to assess the health in stress-associated physical health defects. If psychiatric–mental health nurses were to claim a major role in stress reduction in women's health care, they could become forerunners in this area. Certainly graduate education in nursing should address itself to meaningful clinical experience for its students in women's health care.

The routes taken by nurses in acquiring educational preparation to function within the mental health field are so diverse that those who choose to work in this area can no longer be termed psychiatric nurses merely by virtue of their area of employment. For some time the title psychiatric–mental health nurse has been relegated to those individuals with graduate preparation in clinical specialization of psychiatric–mental health nursing. Within our population, of course, persons assume the title who do not have advanced educational preparation in the area; someone who has been employed in a psychiatric setting merely labels herself a psychiatric nurse. Nurses prepared as clinical specialists have not asserted themselves in terms of the selective use of their title. As a result, we have persons thought to be psychiatric–mental health nurses who have no formal preparation beyond their basic educational experience. It is appalling to recognize that many of these individuals have not read a book, attended a workshop, or sought any additional formal learning during years of employment within a psychiatric setting. Funding provided at the national level sought to quickly increase the numbers of persons directly working in psychiatric settings. That funding was directed to the development of psychiatric technicians, who in their formalized learning program were presented with more information than many of the nurses with whom they worked. As a result, the identity and the stature of the psychiatric nurse has undergone a period of grave distortion. It has only been recently that clinical specialists are declaring that nurses who work in a psychiatric setting are not to be labeled psychiatric nurses unless they have the educational preparation that goes with the role. To ensure the comparability of the title on a national level, a source of national certification for the mental health nurse has been established by the parent professional organization, the American Nurses' Association. It is believed that certification will serve as an equalizer in terms of review of the graduates of the numerous graduate programs spread throughout the United States.

It is recognized that it is the responsibility of professional organizations to oversee members' abilities and to define major advances within the field. Certainly psychiatry is more advanced than the behavioral sciences in its articulated board certification examinations. Needless to remark, the whole certification issue had the potential to split the field of nursing in mental health apart. The professional organization was alert to the cries that came from those nurses who have learned experientially rather than by formalized educational programs in this field of care. The solomonic decision was to establish two certification examinations: one for the generalists in psychiatric–mental health nursing who did not possess graduate level credentials in the field and the other to be labeled the specialists examination for persons who did attain such levels of both educational and experiential preparation. The debate still rages as to whether the specialized examination should be directed to adult, child, family, or community mental health specializations.

Many argue that there should be only one examination that all may take regardless of preparation. Others believe that, being in disagreement with the American Nurses' Association's approach to certification, each individual state should develop its own certification examination. The latter approach certainly does not allow for national equalization of the title. With the mobility of the nursing population, individual certification by each state could mean nurses retaking the examination numerous times. Also, each state does not have at its disposal the hundreds of thousands of dollars that go into test construction.

One of the most pragmatic reasons for certification is certainly that it provides a hallmark for those nurses who can be designated as therapists. In terms of setting up a private practice in the field, such certification paves the way for designation of third-party payments. Without such credentials, third-party payments will be a long time in coming nationally to the field of psychiatric–mental health nursing. There is

absolutely no requirement that nurses take the certification examination, but reason suggests that careerists in the field want to have formal certification. The examination is not just a paper and pencil test but also provides for clinical evaluation of the nurse therapist's work. It recognizes the many roles of nurses within the field serving as supervisors for their own profession by providing ongoing approval of their work.

The days are quickly passing when the field of psychiatric–mental health nursing will have only psychiatrists or psychologists reviewing its work. The formal examinations were established and written by recognized national experts in the field of psychiatric–mental health nursing. The tests themselves involve all major areas related to this field of endeavor. Test items are compiled from nurses working in mental health from all over the United States. A test specification committee of recognized experts in psychiatric nursing has worked for several years with the Educational Testing Service of Princeton, New Jersey, in establishing a reliable tool. To receive certification in the field is no small achievement, and persons who have done so are understandably proud of their accomplishment. Within the next decade we will probably witness nurses assuming leadership roles in the field who are fully certified. Nationally, certification in nursing could not have come to a better time. The nation is rampant with therapist labels designated in all areas of dysfunction (e.g., marital therapists, sex therapists). Certification will serve to protect the formal title and role of the psychiatric–mental health nurse. It has been a long time in coming, and the heat of the battle has not yet cooled, but certification is established.

With certification comes the means of recognizing the basic equal competencies of graduates of often quite different clinical specialist programs in psychiatric–mental health nursing. Persons graduating from such programs in the next decade will be at the center of the career changes in the field. It is this group of graduates who will form the block of professionals electing private practice in psychiatric–mental health nursing. It is this group that politically will be greatly involved with the issue of national health insurance. It is these graduates who will not only be confronted with the tasks of working with persons with emotional dysfunction but will also be largely responsible for defining major methods of primary prevention in the field of mental health. It is essential that the graduate programs that are producing these professionals for tomorrow be politically current with the times and begin to teach the students how to meaningfully enter into the political social system. In order that federal monies be available and designated to graduate programs in nursing, there is a grave need for these programs to establish visibility on local and state levels. Furthermore, it is a necessity that there be national recognition of the faculty serving as directors or major professors in these programs. The faculty should be clinically competent and skilled in meeting today's mental health problems. Too frequently educators teach in the mode of their own previous learning experiences; too frequently the content taught is outdated; too frequently there is lack of recognition that many of the basic psychiatric and mental health preparations have already touched previous levels of the students' learning. Within nursing graduate programs there should be recognition that the major illnesses for the next generation will be largely stress related. As a result, every effort should be made to increase the student's ability to perform physical as well as mental health assessment. The student's behavioral knowledge should advance in tandem with her learnings in human physiology and its dysfunction. With the increase in patients' autonomy in their self-care, the nurse by means of biofeedback will be able to work independently of medical professionals because there will be reduced need for the prescription of medication.

This next plateau of psychiatric–mental health nursing will allow the profession to more formally distinguish itself from the behavioral disciplines of social service and psychology. When the profession can achieve fully independent practice, real collegiality with other disciplines will be truly possible. It is only when individuals fully experience autonomy that they can achieve interdependency with others. Without such autonomy professional individuals will find themselves still controlled in dependency patterns with other professions. There is every indication that this pattern of interaction among the professions will promote new growth as every discipline expands in terms of competency. Throughout the history of psychiatric–mental health nursing, in fact of all the behavioral disciplines, the focus has largely been on working with individuals or small groups to alleviate emotional pain, as well as to create new patterns of behavior. In the coming years the focus will shift to approaching and reducing large social emotional problems of the commu-

nity. The profession will find itself working in a consultant role to labor unions experiencing strife and frustration of workers; working with communities shocked by major national catastrophes; and working with communities experiencing alienation and apathy. The major learning supportive to such undertakings will have to include social system change. To date, most graduate programs have mainly focused on change in the self-system; they are now approaching the next plateau beyond working with the individual self or the small subsystem of the greater community. Graduate programs will also have to begin to prepare students in pragmatic ways for private practice. Courses in budgeting, cost-effectiveness, contract negotiation, and legal liabilities become necessary elements of learning for the products of the clinical specialist programs. No other time in the field of psychiatric–mental health nursing has been as exciting. It is hoped that the programs will so well prepare the graduates who will be faced with these major changes that they will experience the enthusiasm and the excitement of their new career, rather than being threatened with feelings of inadequacy.

National health insurance is without question a major issue within the United States today. The exorbitant costs to the consumer for health care, particularly related to catastrophic illness, was the genesis of this national movement. At this point, there is growing belief that some form of national health insurance will be passed by Congress. There is, however, grave concern about how it will be established. Debate currently rages concerning the potential astronomical cost to the consumer, the loss of the personal relationship between the physician and patient, the possible standardization of professional fees, the potential federal control of the professions, and the loss of private enterprise of insurance agencies. Nonetheless, the point has been reached at which the great costs of individual health care can no longer be absorbed by the average taxpayer. Since the professions and the organized institutions of health care delivery have not been able to control the rapid inflation that is consuming the health care system, it is believed that there will be national federal control. The independent practitioner in psychiatric–mental health nursing should be actively involved in the questioning process that will decide whether national health insurance fees will be based on the function performed for the client or patient or assessed by the label of the professional person performing them. It is imperative, if professional labeling is the means of fee payment, that psychiatric nursing be designated as one of the official groups for payment. Other major questions revolve about how the established insurance agencies will fit into a national framework of enrollment and payment. For example, will national health insurance deal only with costs related to catastrophic illness? The individual consumer is greatly concerned that he not lose the right of selecting the desired health care provider; that is, the taxpayer wants to continue selecting both the agency and the individual responsible for delivering his care. It is at times like these, when issues are still under debate and no one answer is the right answer, that professionals should be involved and visible in contributing to the data on which the ultimate decision will be based. It does not require great imagination to realize what will happen to the private practice of individual nurse therapists if they are not recognized as a distinct group for fee reimbursement with national health insurance. It is hoped that as a professional discipline psychiatric–mental health nursing will assume an active posture rather than a reactive stance as such issues and trends affect and determine the boundaries of the professional role in the twenty-first century.

Suggested cross-references

Issues of interest to the future of psychiatric nursing are discussed in Chapter 1.

Introduction

The purpose of *Standards of Psychiatric and Mental Health Nursing Practice** is to fulfill the profession's obligation to provide a means of improving the quality of care. The standards reflect the current state of knowledge in the field and are therefore provisional, dynamic, and subject to testing and subsequent change. Since standards represent agreed upon levels of practice, they have been developed to characterize, to measure, and to provide guidance in achieving excellence in care.

The present *Standards of Psychiatric and Mental Health Nursing Practice* are a revision of standards enunciated by the Division on Psychiatric and Mental Health Nursing Practice in 1973. They apply to any setting in which psychiatric and mental health nursing is practiced and to both generalists and specialists in psychiatric and mental health nursing. Standards V-F—Psychotherapy, of the nursing practice standards, and X—Community Health Systems, of the professional performance standards, specifically apply to the specialist. The standards are written within the framework of the nursing process, which includes data collection, diagnosis, planning, treatment, and evaluation. The treatment or intervention phase of the nursing process is elaborated upon in order to highlight the specific interventions or nursing care activities commonly carried out by psychiatric and mental health nurses: therapeutic interventions, health teaching, self-care, somatic therapies, therapeutic environment, and psychotherapy. In addition to the standards concerned with the nursing process, other standards address professional performance, such as use of theory, peer review, continuing education, interdisciplinary team collaboration, community health systems, and research. Accountability of the provider to the client, client rights, and client advocacy are implicit throughout the standards.

A rationale is provided for each standard, and criteria are developed to measure each standard. Criteria are divided into *structure, process,* and *outcome criteria.* Criteria are intended to provide a means by which attainment of the standard may be specifically measured. The criteria for each standard are not exhaustive.

The *Standards of Psychiatric and Mental Health Nursing Practice* should be used in conjunction with the following ANA publications:
1. *Standards of Nursing Practice*
2. *Statement on Psychiatric and Mental Health Nursing Practice*
3. *Nursing: A Social Policy Statement*
4. *Code for Nurses with Interpretive Statements*

*Reprinted with permission of the American Nurses' Association, Kansas City, Mo., 1982.

STANDARDS OF PSYCHIATRIC AND MENTAL HEALTH NURSING PRACTICE

Professional practice standards

STANDARD I—THEORY

The nurse applies appropriate theory that is scientifically sound as a basis for decisions regarding nursing practice.

Rationale

Psychiatric and mental health nursing is characterized by the application of relevant theories to explain phenomena of concern to nurses and to provide a basis for intervention and subsequent evaluation of that intervention. A primary source of knowledge for practice rests on the scholarly conceptualizations of psychiatric and mental health nursing practice and on research findings generated from intradisciplinary and cross-disciplinary studies of human behavior. The nurse's use of selected theories provides comprehensive, balanced perceptions of the clients' characteristics, diagnoses, or presenting conditions.

Structure criteria

1. Access to resource materials on theories is provided in the practice setting.
2. Continuing education programs on theories of human behavior are available and accessible.
3. Theory-based nursing actions are recognized within the practice setting and are congruent with overall agency philosophy.

Process criteria

The nurse:
1. Examines basic assumptions on the nature of persons
2. Corrects erroneous beliefs
3. Utilizes theory and critical thinking to:
   a. Formulate generalizations, e.g., opinion, speculation, and assumption
   b. Generate and test hypotheses
4. Utilizes inferences, principles, and operational concepts
5. Applies relevant theories

Outcome criterion

Measurable objectives and relevant interventions for clients are based on psychiatric and mental health nursing theory.

STANDARD II—DATA COLLECTION

The nurse continuously collects data that are comprehensive, accurate, and systematic.

Rationale

Effective interviewing, behavioral observation, and physical and mental health assessment enable the nurse to reach sound conclusions and plan appropriate interventions with the *client*.

Structure criterion

A means by which data are gathered, recorded, and retrieved is available in the practice setting.

Process criteria

The nurse:
1. Informs the client of their mutual roles and responsibilities in the data-gathering process
2. Uses clinical judgments to determine what information is needed. Health data undergirding the nursing process for psychiatric and mental health clients are obtained through assessing the following:
   a. Biophysical, developmental, mental, and emotional status
   b. Spiritual or philosophical beliefs
   c. Family, social, cultural, and community systems
   d. Daily activities, interactions, and coping patterns
   e. Economic, environmental, and political factors affecting the client's health
   f. Personally significant support systems, as well as unutilized but available support systems
   g. Knowledge, satisfaction, and change motivation regarding current health status
   h. Strengths that can be used in reaching health goals
   i. Knowledge of pertinent legal rights
   j. Contributory data from the family, significant others, the health care team, and pertinent individuals in the community

Outcome criteria

1. The client affirms the value of the data-gathering process. If illness precludes this capacity in the client, affirmation of the quality and ethical handling of the data is sought from the client's significant others and/or the nurse's peers.
2. The data base is synthesized and recorded in a standardized format.

STANDARD III—DIAGNOSIS

The nurse utilizes nursing diagnoses *and standard classification of mental disorders to express conclusions supported by recorded assessment data and current scientific premises.*

Rationale

Nursing's logical basis for providing care rests on the recognition and identification of those actual or potential health problems which are within the scope of nursing practice.

Structure criterion

In the practice setting opportunities are provided for validation of diagnosis by peers and exchange of information and research findings regarding the scientific premises underlying nursing diagnosis among peers.

Process criteria

The nurse:
1. Identifies actual or potential health problems in regard to:
   a. Self-care limitations or impaired functioning whose general etiology is mental and emotional distress, deficits in the ways significant systems are functioning, and internal psychic and/or developmental issues
   b. Emotional stress or crisis components of illness, pain, self-concept changes, and life process changes
   c. Emotional problems related to daily experiences such as anxiety, aggression, loss, loneliness, and grief
   d. Physical symptoms that occur simultaneously with altered psychic functioning, such as altered intestinal functioning or anorexia
   e. Alterations in thinking, perceiving, symbolizing, communicating, and decision-making abilities
   f. Impaired abilities to relate to others
   g. Behaviors and mental states that indicate the client is a danger to self or others or is gravely disabled
2. Analyzes available information according to accepted theoretical frameworks
3. Makes inferences regarding data from phenomena

Professional practice standards

STANDARD I—THEORY

The nurse applies appropriate theory that is scientifically sound as a basis for decisions regarding nursing practice.

STANDARD II—DATA COLLECTION

The nurse continuously collects data that are comprehensive, accurate, and systematic.

STANDARD III—DIAGNOSIS

The nurse utilizes nursing diagnoses and standard classification of mental disorders to express conclusions supported by recorded assessment data and current scientific premises.

STANDARD IV—PLANNING

The nurse develops a nursing care plan with specific goals and interventions delineating nursing actions unique to each client's needs.

STANDARD V—INTERVENTION

The nurse intervenes as guided by the nursing care plan to implement nursing actions that promote, maintain, or restore physical and mental health, prevent illness, and effect rehabilitation.

STANDARD V-A—PSYCHOTHERAPEUTIC INTERVENTIONS

The nurse (generalist) uses psychotherapeutic interventions to assist clients to regain or improve their previous coping abilities and to prevent further disability.

STANDARD V-B—HEALTH TEACHING

The nurse assists clients, families, and groups to achieve satisfying and productive patterns of living through health teaching.

STANDARD V-C—SELF-CARE ACTIVITIES

The nurse uses the activities of daily living in a goal-directed way to foster adequate self-care and physical and mental well-being of clients.

STANDARD V-D—SOMATIC THERAPIES

The nurse uses knowledge of somatic therapies and applies related clinical skills in working with clients.

STANDARD V-E—THERAPEUTIC ENVIRONMENT

The nurse provides, structures, and maintains a therapeutic environment in collaboration with the client and other health care providers.

STANDARD V-F—PSYCHOTHERAPY

The nurse (specialist) utilizes advanced clinical expertise in individual, group, and family psychotherapy, child psychotherapy, and other treatment modalities to function as a psychotherapist and recognizes professional accountability for nursing practice.

STANDARD VI—EVALUATION

The nurse evaluates client responses to nursing actions in order to revise the data base, nursing diagnoses, and nursing care plan.

Professional performance standards

STANDARD VII—PEER REVIEW

The nurse participates in peer review and other mean of evaluation to assure quality of nursing care provided for clients.

STANDARD VIII—CONTINUING EDUCATION

The nurse assumes responsibility for continuing education and professional development and contributes to the professional growth of others.

STANDARD IX—INTERDISCIPLINARY COLLABORATION

The nurse collaborates with interdisciplinary teams in assessing, planning, implementing, and evaluating programs and other mental health activities.

STANDARD X—UTILIZATION OF COMMUNITY HEALTH SYSTEMS

The nurse (specialist) participates with other members of the community in assessing, planning, implementing, and evaluating mental health services and community systems that include the promotion of the broad continuum of primary, secondary, and tertiary prevention of mental illness.

STANDARD XI—RESEARCH

The nurse contributes to nursing and the mental health field through innovations in theory and practice and participation in research.

PSYCHOSOCIAL
ASSESSMENT
TOOL

Facility _____

Assessor _____

Date _____

SOCIALPSYCHOLOGIC ASSESSMENT FORM*

1. Assessor's immediate thoughts, feelings, impressions of client on first meeting

Demographic and vital data

2. Name:
3. Present address:
4. When did you move to that address?
5. From where did you move?
6. Why did you move?
7. When were you born?
8. Where were you born?
9. Marital status: (circle) S M D W Sep.
10. Sex: (circle) F   M
11. Facial group: (circle)

    Caucasian   Mongoloid   Negro

Presenting data

12. Why are you here? (Voluntary or involuntary, referred, accompanied by whom, at whose urging, presenting difficulty whose perception?)
13. When did it all start?

Sociologic data

Now about your family . . .

14. Name the members and give their ages. Start with the oldest member. (Family is defined as whomever client perceives it to be.)

Name	Age	Relationship to client

15. Do you see them often? Where do they live?
16. Who talks to whom, about what, most of the time?
17. How open is your family to new ideas and new people?
18. Describe, in a few words, each family member.

Member	Description

19. How is your family reacting to your present difficulty?
20. In your family, who is more dependent and who is more independent in terms of money and emotionally (or psychologically)?

Now about your family's communication . . .

21. What problems or issues are discussed most in your family?
22. Are there members of the family who feel they are misunderstood? Explain.
23. Does your family seem to understand each other's hidden messages, i.e., can they read between the lines?
24. What patterns of nonverbal behavior have you noticed in the family, i.e., touch, facial grimaces, etc.?
25. Are there persons in your family who typically say one thing, but mean another?
26. Is there anyone in your family who tells you to do opposite things at the same time?

*From Francis, G., and Munjas, B.: Manual of socialpsychologic assessment, New York, 1976, Appleton-Century-Crofts.

27. What topics are hardest to talk about in your family?

Now about your family's togetherness . . .

28. Is your family close?
29. Do you like it that way?
30. Is this present difficulty bringing the family closer together or causing problems?
31. How does your family view you, e.g., wild, bookworm type, or what? Do *you* think you act your age?
32. How do *you* view your family?
33. What is the *central concern* in your family, e.g., success, education, or what?
34. Does your present difficulty interfere with that central concern in any way?
35. Are your family experiences broad or narrow, e.g., have they traveled much?
36. What illness or hospitalization has there been in other members of your family?
37. When there are problems in the family do the members seem to get focused on you?

Now about you and your family's resources for crises . . .

38. Do you feel that you cannot cope with your present situation or difficulty? (If "no" skip to item 46.)
39. Have you been in a crucial or decisive situation like this before?
40. How did you handle it?
41. How do you feel about this situation?
42. How will you handle those feelings?
43. Are you hopeful about solving the present situation? Why or why not?
44. What will you do about it?
45. Are there family or friends who will help you? How will they help?
46. What roles do different members of your family play generally? For example, is there a boss, a peacemaker, etc.?

    Member   *Role*

47. Do they like those roles? Do they play them well?
48. Do your family members seem to work against one another?
49. Are your physical needs met by your family?
50. Are your emotional needs met by your family?

51. Are there family goals which all members work toward?
52. Do you feel free to pursue an individual goal with which the family is in disagreement?

Now about you and your family's response to illness . . .

53. Is this the first time you have had these symptoms? If "no" discuss previous times.
54. How long have you had this difficulty before seeking help?
55. Are you the only family member with some difficulty at the present time?
56. Have you had other major illnesses or hospitalizations?
57. What jobs do you do in your family?
58. What jobs do the other family members do in the family?
59. Who does your family jobs when you cannot do them?
60. What occupations do your family members work at presently outside the home?

    Member   *Occupation*

61. Does your family see itself as a healthy family or a sick family?

Now about your occupation . . .

62. Describe the work you do. (If unemployed skip to item 70.)
63. How long have you been on the job?
64. Do you like it? Can you advance? Do you feel secure in it?
65. Do you get along with the people you work for and with?
66. Is the job what you pictured yourself doing when you were younger?
67. What does your family think of the job?
68. What effect will this present difficulty have on your job?
69. Do you think the job is in any way related to your present symptoms (go to item 73)?
70. Why are you *not* working?
71. Are you satisfied not to be working?
72. What does your family say about not working?
73. What have your jobs been since you left school?
74. Why did you leave them?

Now about your education . . .

75. How far did you go in school or college?
76. Are you satisfied with your education?
77. Are you in any educational program now, and how are you doing?
78. Are you studying on your own or teaching yourself anything now? Describe it.
79. How does your education compare with members of your family? If it is different, does it cause problems?
80. What made you decide to seek professional assistance?
81. Do you have suggestions for how your present difficulty can be managed?

Now about your leisure time . . .

82. How much leisure time do you have?
83. What are your favorite recreational pastimes? Can you afford them?
84. Are you satisfied with the way you spend your leisure time?
85. Do you and your family engage in recreational activities together, or is there disagreement on what you will do?

Now about where you live . . .

86. In what section of the city (county) is your home?
87. Do you like your neighborhood? Describe it.
88. Do you like your home? Is it big enough? Does it require a lot of work? Describe it.
89. How long have you lived there?
90. Have you moved much in your life and why?
91. How far do you live from here, and is getting here a problem?
92. Are there certain illnesses or health problems that seem to occur a lot in your neighborhood?

Now about your family's income . . .

93. What was your total family income last year? (Use a card and have client identify category if there is hesitancy.)
   _____ Under $5,000   _____ $15,000 to $19,999
   _____ $5,000 to $9,999   _____ Over $20,000
   _____ $10,000 to $14,999
94. Who contributes most of this?
95. Is the income enough to live on? Are you satisfied with it?
96. Are other family members satisfied with it?
97. Who pays the bills and makes the decisions about big expenditures?
98. Where do you usually go for professional health care?

99. Will this difficulty affect your family income in any way?
100. Did concern about the cost keep you from getting assistance sooner?

Now about your ethnic background . . .

101. Where did your parents or ancestors come from and when?
102. Was a language other than English spoken at home? What?
103. Do you hold to the values and customs of your ethnic group?
104. Do you have specific practices for treating sickness that you learned from your ethnic group? What are they?

Now about your religious background . . .

105. Are you a member of a church? What denomination?
106. Would you say you are a religious person? Why or why not?
107. Do your parents belong to your church? If not why the difference?
108. (If married and/or children) Do you all go to the same church? If not, why not? Does it create problems?
109. Are you satisfied with your church and religious life? If not, why not?
110. How do you view illness generally? Do you feel you have any control over it?
111. Do you have any religious beliefs or practices about the treatment of illness?

Now your beliefs about illness . . .

112. What do you think caused your present difficulty? Did you have anything to do with it? Could someone else have caused it?
113. Did you try to treat yourself before coming here?
114. Did you seek treatment (relief) from others before coming here? If "yes" describe it.
115. What are some of the home remedies you routinely use for illness?
116. Have you ever engaged in faith healing?
117. What do you think is the major cause of illness generally?

Now about your attitudes toward life . . .

118. What do you think about life in general?
119. Are you glad to be alive now? If not when would you liked to have lived?
120. Has life become better or worse as you have grown older? Why?
121. Are you generally a pessimist or an optimist?

122. Do you believe you could have prevented some of your difficulty if you had behaved differently? Why?

Now about your standard of living . . .

123. Describe your life-style, or how you live.
124. Do you think any of your possessions or behavior are extravagant? Why or why not?
125. Can you rank order the amount of your income spent on:

Housing _____ Religion and charity _____
Recreation and socializing _____ Health and illness _____
Shopping _____
Education _____

Now about your habits . . .

126. What and how much do you eat in a typical day?
127. Do you consider yourself a big, an average, or a small eater?
128. Where and with whom do you generally eat your meals?
129. What foods do you like and dislike most?
130. Do you have medical or religious food or drink restrictions?
131. Do you have any food or beverage allergies?
132. Do you get enough to eat?
133. Do you have any difficulty eating?
134. What beverages and how much of them do you drink each day?
135. How much alcohol do you drink in a day and when do you drink it? (If client does not drink alcohol skip to item 143.)
136. What is your favorite alcoholic beverage?
137. Do you usually drink alone or with others?
138. Do you find yourself drinking more when you are under stress?
139. Do you get intoxicated? How often? Do you black out?
140. Have you injured yourself or others while drinking?
141. Has your drinking ever interfered with your job?
142. Do you or your family worry about your drinking?
143. Do your family members drink alcohol? How much? Any problem drinkers?
144. What patent medicines do you take routinely? Why?
145. Do you have prescriptions from physicians? What are they for?
146. Do any of the medicines cause discomfort or do things they are not meant to do?
147. Have you been taking any medicine routinely for over a year? Why?
148. Do you smoke? How much? (If client does not smoke skip to item 151.)

149. When do you smoke?
150. Have you tried to stop smoking?
151. Do you feel as though you are dependent on coffee, tea, soft drinks, or alcohol?
152. Have you ever taken a narcotic drug for pain? How long?
153. Have you ever taken drugs to help you fall asleep or perk you up?
154. Have you taken drugs for depression?
155. Have you taken drugs for "kicks," or for the heck of it?
156. Have you taken medicine to control your appetite?
157. Have you been treated for taking too much of a drug, an overdose?
158. Have you ever gotten into trouble with the law from selling or using illegal drugs? What happened?
159. Do you believe that any of the medicines or drugs you have taken, or are taking now, are bad for your health?
160. Tell me about your bathing habits. How often do you bathe?
161. How often do you shampoo your hair?
162. Tell me about your sleeping habits. When do you go to bed? When do you get up?
163. Do you have difficulty falling asleep or waking up?
164. Do you sleep soundly or awaken a lot during the night? What awakens you?
165. Do you take naps during the day?
166. Do you feel you get enough sleep?
167. Have your sleeping patterns changed recently?
168. Do you wear glasses, contact lenses, or a hearing aid, and how do you feel about it?
169. Does your job present a danger to your sight or hearing? How do you protect yourself?
170. Do you have any problems with taste, smell, or touch?

Now some questions about your sexual behavior . . .

171. How do you see yourself as a man (woman)?
172. Do you ever wish you were a (the opposite sex)? What would the advantages be?
173. Have you ever felt discriminated against because you are a man (woman)?
174. Have you ever had to do things you did not want to do because you are a man (woman)?
175. Who was most influential in teaching you how to be a man (woman)?
176. Where and when did you learn about sexual behavior?
177. Do you know any of your parents' beliefs about sexual behavior?

178. In what ways are your beliefs and attitudes about sex different from your parents?
179. Tell me about your earliest sexual experiences. When did they occur? How did you feel about them?
180. (If above experiences were heterosexual) Have you had any homosexual experiences? Tell me about them.
181. Do you have any worries or difficulties about sex?
182. Do you and your (primary) sexual partner agree on the frequency and nature of your sexual activities? (Ask about masturbation.)
183. How frequently do you engage in sexual activity? Who initiates it?
184. (If male) Do you have difficulty maintaining an erection or with premature ejaculation?
185. Do you have difficulty reaching a climax or orgasm?
186. (If married) Do you engage in sexual activities with persons other than your spouse? Does it cause problems?
187. (If single) Do you engage in sexual activities? With more than one person?
188. Are you satisfied with your sexual behavior?
189. Have the difficulties that brought you here interfered with your sexual life?

Psychologic data

Now some questions about you as an individual, specifically your thinking . . .

Consciousness

190. Tell me again about your situation. What is the difficulty? How did you get here and what can I do for you?
191. Do you know or have you been told that you have dreamlike periods when you do things that you do not remember afterwards?
192. Do you believe or feel that you are another person doing things sometimes?
193. Do you walk in your sleep or write things automatically as though another person was doing it?

Orientation

194. What is today's date?
195. Tell me about your activities since you got up this morning.
196. Where are you now . . . exactly?
197. Who are you, and who are some of the persons close to you?

Attention

198. Do you ever find yourself concentrating on something so much that you cannot get on with other things?

199. Do you find yourself so excited sometimes that you cannot concentrate or pay attention to anything for very long?
200. Do you ever find you are in the middle of a sentence and forgot what you wanted to say?

Perception

201. Do you experience things differently from the way others say they are? Is there something there, but it appears different from what it is?
202. Do you see or hear things that others say are not there?
203. Do you ever smell or taste things that others say are imaginary?
204. Do you ever feel you are being touched when no one is there?
205. Do you believe you have ESP powers?

Apperception

206. I will ask you a question now. Tell me what I am asking, then answer it. (Ask, "Have you learned anything from the interview session so far?")

Thought content

207. Tell me, what sorts of things do you think about a lot?
208. Do you think about or dwell too much on one idea sometimes?
209. Do you have trouble falling asleep because you go over and over some thought?
210. Do you ever think about something so much and so long that you lose track of where you are and what you are doing?

Thought form

211. Do you spend a lot of time daydreaming so that you do not get the things done you should get done?
212. Do you ever have crazy thoughts that others laugh at, such as something you believe that no one else believes?
213. Do you have thoughts that run through your mind all the time that you cannot get out? Do they interfere with your life?
214. Do you have fears of certain things that bother you?

Thought progress

215. Do your thoughts ever come out so fast or so slow that you have difficulty making people understand you?
216. Does your thinking ever wander so much that you have trouble getting to the point?

Memory

217. Have you ever lost, or been told you lost, your memory for a while?
218. Is there a specific event in your life for which you have no memory?
219. (If older ask) Do you remember things from way back better than you remember things from yesterday?
220. Is there an event in your life that you remember extremely well and in great detail that you will never forget?
221. Do you ever get mixed up between what is real and what is not real, like thinking a dream is real?
222. Describe the person who spoke with you when you first came in here today.
223. Do you often believe or get the feeling that something you are experiencing has happened before?

Self-concept

224. What kind of a person would you say you are? Describe yourself.
225. Are your views of yourself mostly positive, mostly negative, or are you mixed up about how you see yourself?
226. Do you like yourself?
227. Do you seem to influence others, or do they usually influence you?
228. Are you more of a leader or a follower?
229. What was your life like generally during high school (13 to 18 years of age)?
230. Would you say you have reached or are reaching your life dreams and goals?
231. Has life been good to you?

Body image

232. What do you think of your body? Do you like it?
233. What part of your body displeases you the most?
234. Have you lost any part of your body (even teeth) that bother you?
235. (If not deformed from arthritis) Would deforming arthritis threaten you?
236. Have you ever thought that some part of your body was in the wrong place or somehow different from what it should be?
237. If you could change your body how would you change it?

Now some questions about how you feel and your moods . . .

238. Have you ever felt strangely unreal and separated from the real world so that you could sort of watch yourself as you would watch someone else?
239. Have you ever been so depressed that you gave up and wanted to die?

240. Have you ever been unusually depressed following some sort of loss?
241. Have you ever lost something or someone dear to you, but could not grieve over it?
242. Do you tend to get mild blue spells?
243. Have you experienced a lot of guilt throughout your life?
244. Do you have "ups" and "downs" a lot?
245. Are you a "moody" person?
246. Do you often feel two ways about something and cannot decide which way to go?
247. Do you often feel apathetic, detached, and indifferent to things?
248. Have you ever felt different from everyone else in a situation, such as thinking something was funny when everyone else was sad?
249. Do you experience a lot of anxiety, nervousness, or restlessness? When is it worse and what do you do about it?
250. Do you have any physical complaints that could be related to your anxiety or nervousness?
251. Would you say you are a nervous person?
252. Are your feelings easily hurt?

Aspects of conation (appearance, facies, voluntary and automatic motor activity, and communication) are to be observed and recorded in the space provided at the end of the interview session.

Antecedent data

Now some questions about what you remember of your early years . . .

253. Do you know anything about your family siutation when you were born? Were they able to take care of you? Who was there?
254. Are your parents still living and married to one another?
255. What do you know of your grandparents when you were born?
256. Do you believe you got any special attention or perhaps neglect?
257. Do you wish you had been born at a different time or into a different family?
258. Do you have any idea about what your parents thought or felt about you when you were born? Did they want you?
259. Do you remember your thoughts and feelings toward your parents? Are there positive memories of whomever raised you as far back as you can go?
260. (If brothers and sisters) How did you feel about your brothers and sisters when you were a child; how did they feel about you? Did you get along with them?

SOCIALPSYCHOLOGIC ASSESSMENT FORM—cont'd

261. (If older siblings) Did you have to wear and play with a lot of hand-me-downs?
262. Do you remember any other stories about yourself before you started school?
263. Has trusting people ever been a problem for you?
264. Do you know anything of when you learned to walk or were toilet trained?
265. Have you tended to doubt yourself a lot, or feel ashamed or embarrassed about yourself?
266. Do you know with whom you identified as a child?
267. Who was your favorite older person as you were growing up?
268. What do you remember of grade school? Did you do well? Did you make friends?
269. What was it like at home during your grade school years?
270. Did people tease you?
271. What are your most vivid memories of childhood?
272. Do you remember junior high school (middle school)? What was it like?
273. What was important during those years (hobbies, scouts, church)?
274. Were you satisfied with your grades and accomplishments?
275. Did you miss a lot of school? Why?
276. Did you get in trouble because of your behavior?
277. Did you learn anything about health or sex? Has it influenced you?
278. (If female) Tell me about your first menstrual period. Were you prepared? (If male) Do you remember your first ejaculations and painful testicles?
279. (If female) Do you remember when your breasts started to develop? Were you embarrassed?
280. Do you remember getting interested in boys (girls)? What were your earliest experiences with them? How did you feel about it?
281. What were your senior high school years like (dating, work)?
282. If you could sum up your whole school experience in a few words, what would they be?
283. How did you feel about your parents during high school years?
284. What about the years right after school, were you mixed up and undecided?

285. Was sex a problem area for you during that time? (Ask about pregnancies.)
286. Did you leave home, when and why?
287. Describe your first living arrangements away from home.
288. Describe your major relationship during that time.
289. Did you find it difficult to give and share? (If client never married skip to item 299.)
290. When and how did you meet your husband (wife)?
291. What attracted you to him (her)? Is that attraction still there?
292. What made you decide to marry? Who suggested it? How did he (she) respond?
293. Have either of you been married before? Are there children from previous marriages?
294. What did each set of in-laws think about the marriage? Do you all get along with each other?
295. Were there obstacles or problems surrounding the marriage?
296. Were your early expectations of one another met?
297. Have your plans for the future been working out?
298. Do you have any problems with your marriage now? (If client has no children skip to item 303.)
299. Tell me about your children. (If female ask about father of children.)
300. What do you believe about raising children? Have you been able to carry it out?
301. Were the children easy or hard to raise?
302. Are you satisfied with the way the children are turning out?
303. Describe a typical day in your life.
304. How much time do you spend with family members and relatives?
305. What has your biggest accomplishment been in life?
306. What major events have occurred in your life in the last 5 years; for example, has there been a(n):

Death _____ Marriage _____
Divorce _____ Job loss _____
Marital separation _____ Marital reconciliation _____
Someone in jail _____ Retirement _____
Injury or illness _____ Other _____

307. What was most stressful in life? How did you cope with it?
308. How do you feel about your life? Are you satisfied as you look back?

Observed conation data

309. Describe the appearance *and* expression of the client's face, noting traces of past action:

310. Describe the client's dress, noting jewelry:

311. Describe the client's posture:

312. Describe the client's motor activity noting whether underactive, overactive, and/or stereotypic:

313. Comment on the client's verbal communication generally:

314. Describe any nonverbal behavior (physical appearance, dress, facial expression, gestures, posture, and gait) and state your impression of messages you believe were being communicated:

315. Discussion and clinical judgment:

PHYSICAL
ASSESSMENT
TOOL

Facility _____
Assessor _____
Date _____

PHYSICAL HISTORY*

Biographical data

1. Name
2. Age
3. Race
4. Culture
5. Address
6. Marital status
7. Children and family in home
8. Occupation
9. Means of transportation to health care facility, if pertinent
10. Description of home; size and type of community

Reason for visit

One statement that describes the reason for the client's visit, or the chief complaint. State in the client's own words.

Present health status

1. General health status of the client in the past 1 year, 5 years, now
2. Client's current major health concerns
3. If illness is present, include (symptom analysis) history
   a. When was client last well
   b. Date of problem onset
   c. Character of complaint
   d. Nature of problem onset
   e. Course of problem
   f. Client's hunch of precipitating factors
   g. Location of problem
   h. Relation to other body symptoms, body positions, and activity

   i. Patterns of problem
   j. Efforts of client to treat
   k. Coping ability
4. Current medications
   a. Type (prescription, over-the-counter drugs, vitamins, etc.)
   b. Prescribed by whom
   c. Amount per day
   d. Problems

Current health statistics

1. Immunization status (note dates or year of last immunization)
   a. Tetanus, diphtheria
   b. Mumps
   c. Rubella
   d. Polio
   e. Tuberculosis tine test
   f. Influenza
2. Allergies (describe agent and reactions)
   a. Drugs
   b. Foods
   c. Contact substances
   d. Environmental factors
3. Last examinations (note physician/clinic, findings, advice, and/or instructions)
   a. Physical
   b. Dental
   c. Vision
   d. Hearing
   e. ECG
   f. Chest radiograph
   g. Pap smear (females)

*From Thompson, J., and Bowers, A.: Clinical manual of health assessment, St. Louis, 1980, The C.V. Mosby Co.

Past health status

Although each of the following is asked separately, the examiner must summarize and record the data *chronologically*.

1. Childhood illnesses: rubeola, rubella, mumps, pertussis, scarlet fever, chickenpox, strep throat
2. Serious or chronic illnesses: scarlet fever, diabetes, kidney problems, hypertension, sickle cell anemia, seizure disorders, blood infections
3. Serious accidents or injuries: head injuries, fractures, burns, other trauma
4. Hospitalizations: elaborate, reason for, location, primary care providers, duration
5. Operations: what, where, when, why, by whom
6. Emotional health: past problems, help sought, support persons
7. Obstetrical history
   a. Complete pregnancies: number, pregnancy course, postpartum course, and condition, weight, and sex of each child
   b. Incomplete pregnancies: duration, termination, circumstances (including abortions and stillbirths)
   c. Summary of complications

Family history

Family members include the client's blood relatives, spouse, and children. Specifically the interviewer should inquire about the client's maternal and paternal grandparents, parents, aunts, uncles, spouse, and children, as well as about the general health, stress factors, and illnesses of other family members. Questions should include a survey of the following:

Cancer	Retardation
Diabetes	Alcoholism
Heart disease	Endocrine diseases
Hypertension	Sickle cell anemia
Epilepsy (or seizure disorder)	Kidney disease
Emotional stresses	Unusual limitations
Mental illness	Other chronic problems

The most concise method to record these data is by a family tree.

Review of physiological systems

The purpose of this component of the data base is to collect information about the body regions or systems and their function.

1. General—reflect from client's previous description of current health status
   a. Fatigue patterns
   b. Exercise and exercise tolerance
   c. Weakness episodes
   d. Fever, sweats
   e. Frequent colds, infections, or illnesses
   f. Ability to carry out activities of daily living
2. Nutritional
   a. Client's average, maximum, and minimum weights during past month, 1 year, 5 years
   b. History of weight gains or losses (time element; specific efforts to change weight)
   c. Twenty-four–hour diet recall (helpful to mail client chart to fill in prior to visit)
   d. Current appetite
   e. Who buys, prepares food?
   f. Who does client normally eat with?
   g. Is client able to afford preferred food?
   h. Does client wear dentures? Is chewing a problem?
   i. Client's self-evaluation of nutritional status
3. Integumentary
   a. Skin
      (1) Skin disease or skin problems or lesions (wounds, sores, ulcers)
      (2) Skin growths, tumors, masses
      (3) Excessive dryness, sweating, odors
      (4) Pigmentation changes or discolorations
      (5) Pruritus (itching)
      (6) Texture changes
      (7) Temperature changes
   b. Hair
      (1) Changes in amount, texture, character
      (2) Alopecia (loss of hair)
      (3) Use of dyes
   c. Nails
      (1) Changes in appearance, texture
4. Head
   a. Headache (characteristics, including frequency, type, location, duration, care for)
   b. Past significant trauma
   c. Dizziness
   d. Syncope
5. Eyes
   a. Discharge (characteristics)
   b. History of infections, frequency, treatment
   c. Pruritus (itching)
   d. Lacrimation, excessive tearing
   e. Pain in eyeball
   f. Spots (floaters)
   g. Swelling around eyes
   h. Cataracts, glaucoma

i. Unusual sensations or twitching
j. Vision changes (generalized or vision field)
k. Use of corrective or prosthetic devices
l. Diplopia (double vision)
m. Blurring
n. Photophobia
o. Difficulty reading
p. Interference with activities of daily living

6. Ears
   a. Pain (characteristics)
   b. Cerumen (wax)
   c. Infection
   d. Hearing changes (describe)
   e. Use of prosthetic devices
   f. Increased sensitivity to environmental noise
   g. Vertigo
   h. Ringing and cracking
   i. Care habits
   j. Interference with activities of daily living

7. Nose, nasopharynx, and paranasal sinuses
   a. Discharge (characteristics)
   b. Epistaxis
   c. Allergies
   d. Pain over sinuses
   e. Postnasal drip
   f. Sneezing
   g. General olfactory ability

8. Mouth and throat
   a. Sore throats (characteristics)
   b. Lesions of tongue or mouth (abscesses, sores, ulcers)
   c. Bleeding gums
   d. Hoarseness
   e. Voice changes
   f. Use of prosthetic devices (dentures, bridges)
   g. Altered taste
   h. Chewing difficulty
   i. Swallowing difficulty
   j. Pattern of dental hygiene

9. Neck
   a. Node enlargement
   b. Swellings, masses
   c. Tenderness
   d. Limitation of movement
   e. Stiffness

10. Breast
    a. Pain or tenderness
    b. Swelling
    c. Nipple discharge
    d. Changes in nipples
    e. Lumps, dimples
    f. Unusual characteristics
    g. Breast examination: pattern, frequency

11. Cardiovascular
    a. Cardiovascular
       (1) Palpitations
       (2) Heart murmur
       (3) Varicose veins
       (4) History of heart disease
       (5) Hypertension
       (6) Chest pain (character and frequency)
       (7) Shortness of breath
       (8) Orthopnea
       (9) Paroxysmal nocturnal dyspnea
    b. Peripheral vascular
       (1) Coldness, numbness
       (2) Discoloration
       (3) Peripheral edema
       (4) Intermittent claudication

12. Respiratory
    a. History of asthma
    b. Other breathing problems (when, precipitating factors)
    c. Sputum production
    d. Hemoptysis
    e. Chronic cough (characteristics)
    f. Shortness of breath (precipitating factors)
    g. Night sweats
    h. Wheezing or noise with breathing

13. Hematolymphatic
    a. Lymph node swelling
    b. Excessive bleeding or easy bruising
    c. Petechiae, ecchymoses
    d. Anemia
    e. Blood transfusions
    f. Excessive fatigue
    g. Radiation exposure

14. Gastrointestinal
    a. Food idiosyncrasies
    b. Change in taste
    c. Dysphagia (inability or difficulty in swallowing)
    d. Indigestion or pain (associated with eating?)
    e. Pyrosis (burning sensation in esophagus and stomach with sour eructation)
    f. Ulcer history
    g. Nausea/vomiting (time, degree, precipitating and/or associated factors)
    h. Hematemesis
    i. Jaundice
    j. Ascites
    k. Bowel habits (diarrhea/constipation)
    l. Stool characteristics
    m. Change in bowel habits
    n. Hemorrhoids (pain, bleeding, amount)
    o. Dyschezia (constipation due to habitual neglect to respond to stimulus to defecate)

p. Use of digestive or evacuation aids (what, how often)
15. Urinary
    a. Characteristics of urine
    b. History of renal stones
    c. Hesitancy
    d. Urinary frequency (in 24-hour period)
    e. Change in stream of urination
    f. Nocturia (excessive urination at night)
    g. History of urinary tract infection, dysuria (painful urination, urgency, flank pain)
    h. Suprapubic pain
    i. Dribbling or incontinence
    j. Stress incontinence
    k. Polyuria (excessive excretion or urine)
    l. Oliguria (decrease in urinary output)
    m. Pyuria
16. Genital
    a. General
      (1) Lesions
      (2) Discharges
      (3) Odors
      (4) Pain, burning, pruritus (itching)
      (5) Venereal disease history
      (6) Satisfaction with sexual activity
      (7) Birth control methods practiced
      (8) Sterility
    b. Males
      (1) Prostate problems
      (2) Penis and scrotum self-examination practices
    c. Females
      (1) Menstrual history (age of onset, last menstrual period [LMP], duration, amount of flow, problems)
      (2) Amenorrhea (absence of menses)
      (3) Menorrhagia (excessive menstruation)
      (4) Dysmenorrhea (painful menses); treatment method
      (5) Metrorrhagia (uterine bleeding at times other than during menses)
      (6) Dyspareunia (pain with intercourse)
17. Musculoskeletal
    a. Muscles
      (1) Twitching
      (2) Cramping
      (3) Pain
      (4) Weakness
    b. Extremities
      (1) Deformity
      (2) Gait or coordination difficulties
      (3) Interference with activities of daily living
      (4) Walking (amount per day)
    c. Bones and joints
      (1) Joint swelling
      (2) Joint pain

      (3) Redness
      (4) Stiffness (time of day related)
      (5) Joint deformity
      (6) Noise with joint movement
      (7) Limitations of movement
      (8) Interference with activities of daily living
    d. Back
      (1) History of back injury (characteristics of problems, corrective measures)
      (2) Interference with activities of daily living
18. Central nervous system
    a. History of central nervous system disease
    b. Fainting episodes
    c. Seizure
      (1) Characteristics
      (2) Medications
    d. Cognitive changes
      (1) Inability to remember (recent vs. distant)
      (2) Disorientation
      (3) Phobias
      (4) Hallucinations
      (5) Interference with activities of daily living
    e. Motor-gait
      (1) Coordinated movement
      (2) Ataxia, balance problems
      (3) Paralysis (partial vs. complete)
      (4) Tic, tremor, spasm
      (5) Interference with activities of daily living
    f. Sensory
      (1) Paresthesia (patterns)
      (2) Tingling sensations
      (3) Other changes
19. Endocrine
    a. Diagnosis of disease states (thyroid, diabetes)
    b. Changes in skin pigmentation or texture
    c. Changes in or abnormal hair distribution
    d. Sudden or unexplained changes in height and weight
    e. Intolerance to heat or cold
    f. Exophthalmos
    g. Goiter
    h. Hormone therapy
    i. Polydipsia ($\uparrow$ thirst)
    j. Polyphagia ($\uparrow$ food intake)
    k. Polyuria ($\uparrow$ urination)
    l. Anorexia ($\downarrow$ appetite)
    m. Weakness
20. Allergic and immunological (Optional; use if client indicates allergic history. Note precipitating factors in each case.)
    a. Dermatitis (inflammation or irritation of skin)
    b. Eczema

PHYSICAL HISTORY—cont'd

c. Pruritus (itching)
d. Urticaria (hives)
e. Sneezing
f. Vasomotor rhinitis (inflammation and swelling of mucous membrane of nose; nasal discharge)
g. Conjunctivitis (inflammation of conjunctiva)
h. Interference with activities of daily living
i. Environmental and seasonal correlation
j. Treatment techniques
21. Does client have any other physiological problems or disease states not specifically discussed? If so, explore in detail (e.g., fatigue, insomnia, nervousness).

Health maintenance efforts

1. General statement of client's own physical fitness
2. Exercise (amount, type, frequency)
3. Dietary regulations; special efforts (describe in detail)
4. Mental health; special efforts such as group therapy, meditation, yoga (describe in detail)
5. Cultural or religious practices
6. Frequency of physical, dental, and vision health assessment

Environmental health

1. General statement of client's assessment of environmental safety and comfort
2. Hazards of employment (inhalants, noise, heavy lifting, psychological stress, machinery)
3. Hazards in the home (concern about fire, stairs to climb, inadequate heat, open gas heaters, inadequate toilet facilities, concern about pest control, inadequate space)
4. Hazards in neighborhood (noise, water, and air pollution, inadequate police protection, heavy traffic on surrounding streets, isolation from neighbors, overcrowding)
5. Community hazards (unavailability of stores, market, laundry facilities, drugstore; no access to bus line)

FAMILY
ASSESSMENT
TOOL

Facility _____

Assessor _____

Date _____

GUIDE TO FAMILY ANALYSIS*

Family genogram

1. Names, ages, ethnic and religious affiliation of all family members
2. Exact dates of birth, marriage, separation, divorce, death, and other significant life events
3. Notations with dates about occupation, grade in school, places of residence, illness, and changes in life course on the genogram itself
4. Information on three or more generations
5. Notation about frequency and type of contact (mail, telephone, visit, marriage, and funerals only)
6. Notation about closest and most distant relationships

Description of home environment

1. Characteristics of neighborhood, type of housing, ownership of housing, car
2. Adequacy of housing (safe, healthy, privacy, food preparation, temperature, space for children to play, yard)
3. Family satisfaction with housing, community
4. How does the family perceive the community's "attitude" toward it?
5. What are the private and public transportation facilities for the family? Are they a help or hindrance to their way of living?
6. What beauty exists in their environment? What efforts have they made to add beauty to the home?

Health and related factors

1. Physical level of growth and development, including developmental lags in the past
2. Past physical problems, including genetic and accidents
3. Current physical problems
4. Status of immunizations
5. Special physical abilities or hobbies, i.e., mechanical, gardening, sewing
6. What treatment does he rely upon before calling a physician?
7. How does he utilize medical resources (episodic or preventive)?
8. What is the family's usual source of health care, single or multiple?
9. What does the family's nutritional assessment reveal?
10. How susceptible to illness does the identified patient think he is? Does the family agree?
11. What is the identified patient's theory about his illness, i.e., to what does he attribute it? What is the family's theory?
12. How has the identified patient's illness changed the family's functioning? Who has been most involved in the care? Who has been most affected?
13. Mental abilities (social and/or academic performance, particular philosophical outlook, thought or language disorder)

*From Helm, P.E.: Guide to family analysis, New Haven, Conn., 1982, Yale University School of Nursing.

14. Sense of self-esteem of family members
15. Sense of humor of family members
16. Personal appearance and hygiene of family members

Financial status

1. What is the family's annual income? Who earns it? Where?
2. What work and homemaking skills are available to each person?
3. How is money managed in this family?
4. If the family doesn't have an adult who is working, why isn't the adult able to work and earn a living? (There is usually more than one reason.)
5. What consumer skills are available in the family? (Do they know how to comparison shop?) (Do they know how to determine what they need?) (Can they do home repair, sew, can food?)
6. Are there financial constraints on seeking health care?

Developmental stage in family life cycle

1. Is the family in a normative crisis of transition?
2. Are there outstanding emotional tasks from previous stages unsuccessfully completed and impeding current family functioning?
3. What are the major emotional tasks confronting the family at this stage in the family life cycle?
4. How is the identified patient's illness influencing the emotional process of the family life cycle?

Family structure

1. Are the boundaries in the family clearly delineated or diffuse between the following:
   a. The marital subsystem
   b. The parental subsystem
   c. The sibling subsystem
   d. Individual subsystems
   e. The grandparent subsystem
   f. The sexes
2. Are there identifiable coalitions or alliances? What are the key family triangles?
3. Are authority and responsibility clearly defined and/or delegated? Does the responsibility to the delegated member exceed his physical or maturational capacities?
4. Are subsystem functions being performed and subsystem interpersonal skills being developed?

Intrafamily relationships

1. How do family members converse with each other? Is communication direct, clear, tangential, amorphous, covert? What kind of information is communicated? Is there a "central switchboard"?
2. How are decisions made (about vacations, discipline, large purchases, personal problems)?
3. How do they have fun together? How do they share time, space, money?
4. How do family members encourage separateness, recognize privacy, among members?
5. How is nurturance, recognition, support given to each other?
6. How is the marital relationship (emotionally and sexually satisfying or distant and conflictual)?
7. How does each parent relate to the children? What child-rearing skills do the parents have or lack?
8. How are children being taught to problem solve, to develop independence and self-reliance?
9. How do family members interact with the outside world (neighbors, schools, work, agencies, church)?
10. What is the nature of extended family relationships? (Is one side or both distant or cut off? Is contact formal and obligatory? Is contact open, regular, and emotionally meaningful even if infrequent?)
11. Who are the most significant members in the extended families? How are they significant?

Sociocultural family context

1. What is the ethnic or cultural background of the family? In what ways is this apparent in their way of living? In household furnishing?
2. Is there a religious belief? Affiliation? How does this influence each one or the family?
3. Have members in any way altered the cultural, ethnic, or religious practices or beliefs? What has been the result of these changes?
4. What are the dominant attitudes toward health, the community, achievement in school and career, toward life?
5. What dominant stereotyped sex-role expectations are expressed or demonstrated between husband and wife, between parents and children?

Strengths and weaknesses of the family

1. As seen by the family
2. As seen by the nurse

Problems identified

1. By the family
2. By the nurse
3. Solutions tried by the family to resolve the problems

DRUG ABUSE
TERMS

This glossary* contains street language regarding the drugs of abuse. The same term may have different meanings in different areas.

a-boot Under the influence of drugs

Acapulco gold Mexican marijuana that contains about 1% or less of tetrahydrocannabinol (THC)

ace A marijuana cigarette

acid LSD (lysergic acid diethylamide)

acid head A user of LSD

ad Refers to an addict

all lit up Under the influence of a drug

amys Amyl nitrite ampules

angel dust Parsley leaves covered with phencyclidine; finely powdered hashish

Are you anywhere? Do you use marijuana?

around the turn Having gone through withdrawal period

artillery Equipment used for injecting and dissolving a powdered drug, or a solution of drugs

baby Marijuana

bad trip/bad acid An unpleasant reaction caused by a hallucinogenic drug, usually LSD; may be caused by taking a mixture of chemicals, resulting from an attempt at synthesis; emotions are dreadful and horrible; the images can be terrifying

bag (1) A package of drugs, usually marijuana or heroin; (2) a person's favorite "thing" or drug

bagman A person who supplies narcotics or other drugs; a pusher

ball Absorption of stimulants and cocaine through the genitalia

balloon A penny balloon that contains narcotics

bambita Desoxyn or amphetamine derivative

bammies A poor quality of marijuana

bang The injection of narcotics, usually heroin

banging Under the influence of drugs

barb(s) Barbiturates

barrels LSD tablets

batted out Apprehended by law

bean A capsule containing drugs

beat the gong Smoke opium

bedbugs Fellow addicts

behind the iron house Staying in jail

belongs On the habit

belted Under the influence of a drug

bending and bowing Under the influence of drugs

bennies Benzedrine tablets (amphetamines)

Bernice Cocaine

Bernie's flake Cocaine

bhang Marijuana

big bloke Cocaine

big C Cocaine

big D LSD

big John Police; law

big man A person who supplies drugs

big O Opium

bindle A package of narcotics (usually contains an ounce)

bingle A supplier of drugs

bingler A person selling narcotics

bingo The injection of drugs

biz Utensils used in dissolving and injecting narcotics and other drugs

black beauties Biphetamine capsules (amphetamines)

black magic LSD

black stuff Opium

blank Container of nonnarcotic powder that is sold as heroin

blast (1) Party, (2) a strong effect resulting from drug usage

blasted Under the influence of a drug

blow (1) To miss a vein when injecting, (2) to move from a place

blow Charlie or snow Sniff cocaine

blow horse Sniffing heroin

blow (pot) Smoke a cigarette that contains marijuana

blow your mind (1) To be high from a hallucinogenic drug, (2) to achieve a particular ecstatic mental level or high

blue acid LSD

blue angels, blue clouds, blue devils, blue heaven Amytal (amobarbital sodium) capsules

blue cheer LSD, methamphetamine, and strychnine tablets

blue heaven LSD

blue morphine Numorphan tablets (no longer made)

blue velvet (1) A mixture of Terpin Hydrate and

---

*From the Office of Training and Education for Addiction Services of the Maryland Department of Health and Mental Hygiene.

Codeine Elixir and Pyribenzamine (tripelenna-mine) (antihistamine), (2) a mixture of Paregoric and antihistamine

bluebirds Amytal (amobarbital sodium) capsules

blues Amytal (amobarbital sodium)

bo bo bush Marijuana

bomb Heroin that is highly potent and relatively un-diluted

bombida Methamphetamine

bombita An amphetamine injection, occasionally with heroin

boost Robbery

boxed Confined in jail

boy Heroin

brain pills Amphetamines

bread Money

brick Compressed block made of marijuana

broker A person who peddles dope to addicts

brown dots LSD

browns Multicolored capsules that are long-acting amphetamine sulfate

bull (1) A federal narcotics agent, (2) a police officer

bum trip A bad experience with psychedelics

bummer Another word for a "bad trip"

burn transaction Selling a substance as a certain drug when actually it is something else, e.g., goldenrod for marijuana

burned Getting cheated during a drug transaction

bush Marijuana

business Equipment used when injecting drugs

businessman's trip Dimethyltryptamine (DMT)

busted Arrested for possession of drugs

buttons Peyote buttons

buy A purchase of drugs

buzz Mild euphoric reaction to a drug

C Cocaine

C-joint A place where cocaine can be bought

cabbage head An individual who will use or experi-ment with any kind of drug

caca (1) Heroin; (2) an inferior quality of hashish, heroin, or LSD; (3) imitation or counterfeit heroin

cadet A new addict

California sunshine LSD

can A container that holds marijuana

candy Barbiturates

candy man A pusher

cannabis Marijuana

cap A gelatinous capsule that contains heroin or other drugs (usually one ounce or less)

Carrie Cocaine

cartwheels Amphetamine tablets

cashing a script Obtaining drugs by getting an illegal prescription filled

catch up A process of withdrawal

caught in a snow storm Being drugged by cocaine

CB Doriden (glutethimide) tablet

Cecil Cocaine

charge A quick drug effect

charged up Under the influence of drugs

chicken powder Some amphetamine powder

chief LSD

chip Use small injections occasionally

chipping Irregular use of small amounts of drugs

Christmas trees Tuinal (secobarbital sodium and amobarbital sodium) or Eskatrol (dextroampheta-mine sulfate and prochlorperazine)

chocolate chips LSD

Cholley Cocaine

Cibas Doriden (glutethimide)

Cibees Doriden (glutethimide)

clean Not using drugs any longer

cleared up A withdrawal method

clipped Getting arrested

coasting Under the influence of drugs

coast-to-coast Long-acting amphetamines

coffee habit A beginner in the use of narcotics

coke Cocaine

cokie Cocaine addict

cold turkey Sudden withdrawal from narcotics

coming down Recovering from a drug experi-ence or trip

connect To make a purchase of drugs

connection A drug supplier

contact lens LSD found on round gelatin flakes

cooker Bottle cap or spoon needed for heating and dissolving heroin in preparation for injection

cop To obtain drugs

cop a deuceway To buy a $2 pack of narcotics

cop man A supplier

cop out (1) Running away, (2) to leave, (3) to inform, (4) not participating, (5) to defect

cop-a-sneak To leave a place

co-pilots Amphetamine tablets

Corrine Cocaine

cotton shot When water is added to cotton to attempt to get remaining heroin out

crank Methamphetamine crystals

crashing Withdrawing from a drug experience

crashing pad Place where a user recovers from am-phetamine use

crinic, cris, Cristina Methamphetamine

croaker A physician

croaker joint A hospital

crossroads Amphetamine tablets

crusher A police officer

crutch A device for holding a marijuana cigarette butt

crystal Methamphetamine (Methedrine); cocaine

crystal palace A room, location, or house where meth-amphetamine is injected

cube juice Morphine

cubehead A person who uses LSD frequently

cupcakes LSD

cut (1) To dilute a powder drug, usually a narcotic; (2) to dilute the potency of marijuana

cut out To leave a certain place

D Doriden (glutethimide) tablets

dabble To use small amounts of drugs infrequently

dead on arrival Phencyclidine base

dealer (1) A person who supplies drugs, (2) a pusher

deck A package of narcotics (usually an ounce)

dexies Dexedrine (dextroamphetamine sulfate) tablets or capsules (amphetamines)

diet pills Include amphetamine tablets or capsules

dime bag $10 purchase, usually marijuana

dirty Have drugs on you; can be arrested if searched

do a bit To spend time in jail

do righters Nonaddicts

DOA Phencyclidine base

doin' Using some kind of drug, such as "He is doin' cocaine"

dollies Dolophine (methadone) tablets

DOM STP (2,5-dimethoxy-4-methylamphetamine)

domes LSD tablets

domino To complete a purchase of drugs

doojee Heroin

dope Includes any narcotics, sometimes extended to other drugs

dope fiend A heroin addict

doper Someone who uses drugs regularly

double trouble Tuinal (secobarbital sodium and amobarbital sodium) capsule

down, downer, downie (1) Barbiturates, (2) tranquilizers

down it To swallow a pill or capsule

dream Cocaine

dried up Off drugs, especially heroin

dripper Eyedropper

drop To take a capsule or tablet orally

drop acid To take LSD

drop out To leave a place

dujie Heroin

dummy (1) A purchase in which there are no narcotics, (2) a poor quality of merchandise

dust Heroin, cocaine

dust of angels Phencyclidine base

dynamite (1) A high quality of heroin and cocaine taken together, (2) a strong drug

eighth Heroin (⅛ ounce) that is diluted with some inert powder

emsel Morphine

eye openers Amphetamines

factory The equipment used when injecting drugs

fall To be arrested

fall out When an addict nods or falls asleep on and off after injecting

far out (1) Out of touch with reality, (2) under the influence of drugs

Feds Federal agents

fine stuff Marijuana that is finely cut or manicured

fix An injection of a narcotic

fixed Under the influence of a drug

flake Cocaine

flash A euphoric feeling following an injection

flashback When a previous drug user hallucinates without taking the drug again

flats LSD tablets

flea powder Poor-quality heroin or heroin that is greatly diluted

flip Become psychotic

floating Under the influence of drugs

flying high Under the influence of marijuana

fold up A withdrawal procedure

folding stuff Money

foolish powder Heroin

footballs Amphetamine tablets or capsules that are oval shaped

freak A regular user of a particular drug, e.g., acid freak

freak out An experience that is unpleasant and frightful, resulting from the use of a drug

freeze When a sale is turned down

fresh and sweet A person coming out of jail

front of the bread The money is put up first for a drug purchase

fu Marijuana

Fuzz (1) A policeman, (2) a detective

Fuzzy tail Police

gage Marijuana

garbage A poor-quality drug

gazer A federal agent

GBs Seconal (secobarbital), Tuinal (secobarbital and amobarbital), or Doriden (glutethimide)

gear Refers to drugs in general

gee head A person who uses paregoric

geetis Money

geezer A needle shot of any type of narcotic

get beat To buy a package that does not contain any heroin

get a gift To obtain some narcotics

get high To smoke a cigarette containing marijuana

get off To inject or use drugs

get the wind To leave a place or area

gimmicks Equipment with which a person injects drugs

girl Cocaine

give wings Give the first heroin injection to a friend

glad rag A handkerchief or cloth saturated with substances to be inhaled

glass eyes A narcotic addict

glued Arrested

gluey An individual who sniffs glue vapors

G-man A federal agent

go in sewer Inject a drug into a vein

gold A Mexican marijuana that has 1% or less of tetrahydrocannabinol (THC)

gold dust Cocaine

good go Purchase a fair amount of narcotics for the money

good trip Psychedelic drugs that cause good emotional feelings and pleasant imagery

goods (1) Narcotics, (2) includes any drugs

goofball Barbiturate

gorilla pills Doriden (glutethimide)

gow head Addict

gram The cube form of hashish

grape parfait LSD

grass Marijuana

green domes LSD tablets

greenies The mixture of barbiturates and amphetamines found in a green heart-shaped tablet

griefo Marijuana

gun (1) Eyedropper, (2) syringe, (3) hypodermic needle

H Heroin

hack Physician

hairy Heroin

half spoon Half a teaspoonful of heroin

hand-to-hand Paying for drugs when they are delivered

hang-up (1) A personal problem or personality problem, (2) a withdrawal

happy dust Cocaine

hard narcotics Includes all addicting narcotics

hard stuff Includes any addicting narcotic, e.g., heroin, morphine

harness bull Police

Harry Heroin

hash Hashish

hassle The procedure of buying drugs, preparing them, and taking the injection

Hawaiian sunshine LSD

hay Marijuana

head A person who depends on drugs

hearts Amphetamine tablets that are heart shaped

heat The police

heaven dust Cocaine

heavenly blue Morning glory seeds

heavy man Someone who possesses narcotics

hemp Marijuana

high Under the influence of drugs

hit To make a purchase of drugs

hitting the pipe, hitting the steam Smoking opium

hitting the stuff Under the influence of drugs

hitting up The act of injecting drugs

hocus Morphine

hog Vegetable material that has phencyclidine in it

holding To have drugs in one's possession

hooked Dependent on drugs

hop Opium

hop head A narcotic addict, mainly an opium addict

hoppie A narcotic addict

horner One who sniffs narcotics

horse Heroin

hot (1) Sought by police, (2) stolen articles, merchandise

hotshot A fatal injection of heroin, that may have been intentional

hot sticks Marijuana cigarettes

hustle (1) Prostitution, (2) any activity used to obtain money for heroin

hustler Prostitute

hype Addict

ice-cream habit Nonregular drug use

iced In jail

I'm beat I need a marijuana cigarette

I'm holding I am carrying drugs

I'm way down I need a marijuana lift

in high Under the influence of drugs

in a jam Wanted by the police

Indian bay, Indian hay Marijuana

into Involved with a drug, e.g., "She is into acid"

jab (1) To inject a drug, (2) a hypodermic shot

jag (1) Under the influence of drugs, (2) under the influence of amphetamines

jay Marijuana cigarette

jelly beans Tuinal (secobarbital sodium and amobarbital sodium)

jive Marijuana

jive sticks, joints Marijuana cigarettes

jolly beans Pep pills

Jones A habit

joy popping (1) Subcutaneously injecting a drug, (2) irregular drug habit

joy powder Cocaine

jump skid To leave a place

junk (1) Heroin, (2) can denote any drug

junker, junkie Addict (heroin)

kee A kilogram of a drug, usually heroin

keif Hashish

kick To get rid of a habit

kick the habit To stop using narcotics or drugs in general

kick sticks Marijuana cigarettes

kicking A withdrawal process

kicking the gong To be around an area where narcotics are sold

kilo A kilogram of drugs equivalent to 2.2 pounds

kit Equipment used when injecting drugs

knocking on the door When an addict is trying to stay away from other addicts while attempting to quit a habit

LA turnabouts Various colored capsules that are long-acting amphetamine sulfate

lay out (1) Equipment for injecting drugs, (2) opium smoker's outfit

laying on the hip Smoking opium

laying the hypo Receiving or taking a shot of narcotics

LBJ-336-JB-336 Methyl piperidyl benzilate (hallucinogen)

leader User of cocaine

leaping Under the influence of drugs

lemonade Poor-quality heroin or any merchandise

lettuce Money

lid A measure of marijuana in a sale

lid poppers Amphetamines

lid proppers Amphetamines

lie down To smoke opium

light artillery A hypodermic addict

Lipton tea Poor-quality merchandise

lit up Under the influence of drugs

load A quantity of 25 bags of heroin

loco weed Marijuana

log Marijuana cigarette

long green Money

love drug (1) MDA (methylene dioxyamphetamine), (2) methaqualone (soapers)

love weed Marijuana

LSD Lysergic acid diethylamide

m Morphine

machinery Utensils used when injecting drugs

magic mushroom A mushroom containing psilocybin

magic pumpkin seed An STP (2,5-dimethoxy-4-methylamphetamine) tablet shaped like a pumpkin seed

mainlining Shooting or injecting a drug directly into a vein

maintaining Keeping a particular level of a drug effect

make a croaker To trick a physician into giving narcotics

make a meet To make a buy

make a reader To get a physician to fill out a prescription

make the turn A withdrawal process

man (1) Policeman, (2) detective

manicure Removal of seeds, dirt, and stems from dried marijuana

Mary Jane, Mary Warner Marijuana

merchandise Narcotics or any drug in general

mesc Mescaline (hallucinogenic drug from the peyote cactus)

meth (1) Methamphetamine, (2) methadone, (3) methedrine, (4) methaqualone

meth head A regular use of methamphetamine

meth run Constant intravenous injection of methamphetamine

Mexican horse Mexican (brown) heroin

Mexican reds Secobarbital capsules

mezz Marijuana

Mickey Chloral hydrate

Mickey Finn The mixture of chloral hydrate plus alcohol

micro dots LSD

mikes Micrograms (millionths of a gram)

mind benders, mind blowers Hallucinogens

Miss Emma Morphine

MJ Marijuana

monkey A drug habit in which there is a physical dependence

monster Methamphetamine

mootos Marijuana cigarettes

mor-a-grifa Marijuana

morph, morphie, morpho Morphine

mouth worker A narcotic addict who swallows his drugs

Mr. Whiskers Federal agents

mud Asthmador mixed with a carbonated cola beverage

muggles Marijuana cigarettes

mule A supplier of drugs

mutah Marijuana

nail Needle

nailed Arrested

narc, narco Federal, state, or local narcotic officer

needle The syringe for injecting drugs

needle freak A person who enjoys using a needle

nibies Nembutal (pentobarbital sodium)

nickel bag (1) A $5 purchase of marijuana, (2) A measure of heroin

nimby (pentobarbital sodium)

noise Heroin

nose candy Cocaine

OD An overdose of drugs or narcotics, resulting in death or a coma

OJ Opium joint, a marijuana cigarette that has been dipped or smeared in opium

on ice In jail

on the beam Feeling good

on the blues Using Numorphan (oxymorphone hydrochloride)

on the bricks, on the ground Out of jail

on the nod The cycle of dozing and awakening when using heroin

on the street Out of jail

on a trip Under the influence of LSD

orange wedges LSD

oranges Heart-shaped amphetamine tablets containing Dexedrine (dextroamphetamine sulfate)

out of it Nonaddict

outfit Equipment used when injecting drugs

over the hump The completion of withdrawal

Owsley's acid LSD

pad A person's habitat or room

Pam freak Person who inhales aerosolized products

Panatella A large strong marijuana cigarette

panic man Addict who has lost his source of drugs

paper (1) A package of drugs (usually a quantity of 1 ounce), (2) prescription

PCP Phencyclidine

PCPA *p*-Chlorophenylalanine

pee Heroin powder

PG, PO Paregoric

peace (1) LSD tablets, (2) STP (2,5-dimethoxy-4-methylamphetamine)

peace pill Phencyclidine

peace tablet LSD tablets

peaches Benzedrine (amphetamine sulfate) tablets

peanuts Barbiturates

pearly gates Morning glory seeds

peddler Dealer in drugs

pep pills Amphetamine capsules or tablets

Pepsi Cola habit A small habit

Peter Chloral hydrate

pickup To buy drugs

piece (1) A measure of narcotics, (2) a holder of drugs

pig Policeman

piki A person who smokes opium

pillhead A person who often uses drugs, usually amphetamines and barbiturates

pillows Sealed polyethylene bags that contain drugs

pin yen Opium

pinks Seconal (secobarbital sodium) capsules

pipe (1) To look, (2) an opium utensil

plant A place to hide drugs

play around Irregular use of drugs

pod Marijuana

pop To inject drugs, usually below the skin

poppers Amyl nitrite ampules

pot Marijuana or hashish

pothead Marijuana user

product IV Combination capsules of PCP and LSD

purple barrels, purple haze, purple ozone LSD

purple rock A mixture of caffeine, barbiturates, heroin, and strychnine

push shorts To cheat a buyer of drugs; to sell short amounts of drugs

pusher A person who peddles drugs, narcotics, marijuana

R and R, ripple and reds Taking secobarbital capsules when drinking Ripple wine

rainbows Tuinal (secobarbital sodium and amobarbital sodium) capsules

red birds, red devils, red lilies, reds Secobarbital capsules

red rock Mixture of heroin and strychnine, barbiturates, and caffeine

reefer Marijuana cigarette

riding the wave Under the influence of narcotics

roach A marijuana cigarette butt

roach clip A device that holds a marijuana cigarette butt

robe Robitussin A-C cough syrup (guaifenesin and codeine phosphate)

robo, romo Codeine

rope Marijuana

roses Benzedrine (amphetamine sulfate) tablets

run Continuing the injection of methamphetamine

Sam Federal agent

satch cotton Cotton used to strain drugs before injection

sativa Marijuana

scag Heroin

scene Place where a person can buy drugs

schmack (1) Heroin, (2) cocaine

schoolboy Codeine

score To purchase drugs

scrap iron A bootleg drink made with a hypochlorite solution, alcohol, and mothballs

scratch Prescription

script Physician's prescription

script writer A person who forges prescriptions

seccy, seggy Seconal (secobarbital sodium) capsules

seeds Morning glory seeds

serenity, tranquility, and peace STP (2,5-dimethoxy-4-methylamphetamine)

sewer Vein

sex drug Methaqualone (soapers) or STP (2,5-dimethoxy-4-methylamphetamine)

sex juice An aphrodisiac

sharps Needles

shit (1) Heroin, (2) poor-quality heroin, hashish, or LSD, (3) drugs

shoot up To inject drugs

shooting gallery Location, room, or house where drugs are injected

shooting The injection of drugs

short go To take a small portion of narcotics

shot down Under the influence of drugs

shrink Psychiatrist

sizzling Sought by police

skee Opium

skid (1) Heroin, (2) to leave a place

skin popping The injecting of a narcotic underneath the skin

slammed In jail

sleepers, sleeping pills Barbiturates

sleigh ride Under the influence of drugs

smack (1) Heroin, (2) cocaine

smash Marijuana that has been cooked with acetone, the oil residue of which is added to hashish

smears LSD

smoke (1) Wood alcohol, (2) marijuana

snappers Amyl nitrite ampules

sniffer A narcotic addict who takes drugs through his nose

sniffing Inhaling solvents, cleaning fluid, etc.

snort The inhalation of cocaine or heroin through the nose

snorter A person who sniffs drugs through his nose

snow Cocaine crystals

snowbird Cocaine addict

soapers Methaqualone (sleeping pill)

sound Benactyzine

spaghetti sauce Robitussin A-C cough syrup (guaifenesin and codeine phosphate)

speed Amphetamines, usually methedrine

speed demon Methamphetamine user

speed freak Frequent methamphetamine user

speedball A mixture of heroin and cocaine that is taken intravenously

spike Hypodermic needle

splash Amphetamine powder

splim Marijuana

split To leave a place

splivins Amphetamine powder

spoon (1) A measure of heroin, (2) the spoon used for dissolving heroin over heat

spots Dextroamphetamine

squirrels LSD

square An individual who does not use drugs

star dust Cocaine

stash A safe place to keep drugs

station worker A user of narcotics who injects into his arms or legs

stick Marijuana cigarette

stinking Under the influence of drugs

stoned (1) Under the influence of drugs, (2) a relaxed, pleasant state of mind

stoolie Informer

stoppers Barbiturates

straight (1) Not using any drugs, (2) not having any drugs in one's possession

strawberry field LSD

street market Black market

strung out An amphetamine overdose

stuff Narcotics

stumblers (1) Barbiturates, (2) tranquilizers

sunshine LSD

superman pills Amphetamines

sweet Lucy Marijuana

swing man A supplier of drugs

syrup Codeine

TMA A combination of mescaline, LSD, and tetrahydrocannabinol

T-man A federal agent

take a powder, take the wind To leave a certain area

taking a main Injecting directly into the vein

tar Opium

taste A small amount of narcotics

tea Marijuana

tea pad The place where a group of people smoke marijuana

tea party A party where mostly everyone is smoking marijuana

teed up Intoxicated by a large quantity of drugs

Texas tea Marijuana

the bag The bag used to sniff airplane glue or cleaning fluid

the confidence drug Amphetamine

the one A material like hashish, supposedly natural tetrahydrocannabinol

thing A person's particular interest, often refers to a specific drug

three-day-habit The irregular use of drugs

TNT Heroin

toak (toke) A drag off a marijuana cigarette

to be off A process of withdrawal

toke pipe A short-stem pipe used for smoking marijuana

tooies Tuinal (secobarbital sodium and amobarbital sodium) capsules

tools Equipment used when injecting drugs

toy A small container of drugs

tracks Needle scars that result from frequent injecting of drugs

tranquility STP (2,5-dimethoxy-4-methylamphetamine)

travel agent LSD pusher

trey A purchase worth $3

trip A hallucinogenic drug experience

tripping out Under the influence of any hallucinogen

truck drivers Amphetamine tablets

tuies Tuinal (secobarbital sodium and amobarbital sodium)

turkey The absence of drugs or narcotics

turkey trots Scars and marks left from the use of a hypodermic needle

turn off To quit using drugs

turn on (1) To introduce a person to the use of drugs, (2) any stimulating experience caused by the use of drugs

turn up To feel the influence of a drug

turned on Under the influence of drugs

turps Terpin Hydrate and Codeine Elixir (a cough syrup)

twenty-five LSD

twist A marijuana cigarette

twisted Intense sedation caused by the use of drugs

uncle, Uncle Sam Federal narcotics agent

unkie Morphine

upper, ups Amphetamine tablets

viper's weed Marijuana

wake ups, washed ups Amphetamines

washed up A withdrawal process

wasted Under the influence of drugs

wedges (1) Dexedrine (dextroamphetamine sulfate) tablets, (2) LSD tablets

weed Marijuana

weekend habit The irregular use of drugs

wen shee Gum opium

whickers Federal agents

white junk Heroin

white lightening LSD

white merchandise, white stuff Morphine

whites Amphetamines

whiz bang A combination of morphine and cocaine, or heroin and cocaine, used by the old addicts

window glass A square gelatin flake that contains LSD

work the leather To leave an area

works Equipment used when injecting drugs

yellow birds Nembutal (pentobarbital sodium)

yellow dimples LSD

yellow jackets, yellow submarines, yellows Nembutal (pentobarbital sodium) capsules

yen hook The utensil used when smoking opium

yen shee The ashes from opium

yen sleep A period of restlessness and drowsiness during a withdrawal process

GLOSSARY

abreaction Ventilation of feelings that takes place when the patient verbally recounts emotionally charged areas. Awareness of affect is experienced, and tension reduction results.

absolute discharge A final and complete termination of the patient's relationship with the hospital.

abuse An act that deceives or puts to wrong or improper use so as to injure, damage, maltreat, or corrupt.

accountability Self-regulation and responsibility for the quality of one's nursing care.

acrophobia Fear of high places.

acting out Indirect expression of feelings through behavior, usually nonverbal, that attracts the attention of others.

action cues A category of nonverbal communication that consists of body movements and is sometimes referred to as kinetics.

activities of daily living When applied to the chronically mentally ill, refers to the skills necessary to live independently as an adult.

adolescence A stage of development occurring between the ages of 11 and 20 during which shifts in past developmental and learning processes occur.

adventitious crisis Accidental, uncommon, and unexpected crisis that results in multiple losses and gross environmental changes.

advocacy One method by which patients, mental health professionals, attorneys, and concerned citizens can work together to improve and protect the rights of all citizens to high-quality mental health care that is clinically and constitutionally appropriate.

affect Feeling; mood.

aggression Mental drive to action that encompasses both constructive and destructive activities.

agoraphobia Fear of open spaces.

akathisia A side effect of antipsychotic medication that is manifested by a feeling of restlessness, frequently accompanied by complaint of a twitching or crawling sensation in the muscles.

alcohol withdrawal delirium A medical diagnosis for a serious alcohol withdrawal syndrome that is characterized by agitation, disorientation, anorexia, paranoia, tremor, insomnia, and visual hallucinations. Associated physiological behaviors, including elevated temperature, tachycardia, tachypnea, hyperpnea, vomiting, diarrhea, and diaphoresis, may result in death if supportive intervention is not implemented.

alcoholic hallucinosis A medical diagnosis that refers to an alcohol withdrawal syndrome characterized by auditory hallucinations in the absence of any other psychotic symptoms.

alcoholism Any degree of dependency, physical or psychological, on alcohol to the extent that it interferes with normal life activities.

altruism A sense of concern for the welfare of others that can be expressed at the level of the individual or the larger social system.

ambivalence An inability to make decisions based on double approach-avoidance conflict feelings.

amnesia Loss of memory for a specific period of time or a loss of all past memories.

anaclitic depression A deprivational reaction in infants separated from their mothers in the second half of the first year of life. The reaction is characterized by apprehension, crying, withdrawal, psychomotor slowing, dejection, stupor, insomnia, anorexia, and gross retardation in growth and development.

analogical communication Relationship component of a message.

anger A feeling that is an expression of the anxiety that is aroused by a real or perceived threat to one's rights, possessions, values, or significant others.

anilingus Oral stimulation of the anal area.

anorexia nervosa An eating disorder in which the person experiences hunger, but refuses to eat based on a distorted body image leading to a self-perception of fatness. Starvation ensues.

anxiety A diffuse vague apprehension associated with feelings of uncertainty and helplessness. It is an emotion without a specific object, is subjectively experienced by the individual, and is communicated interpersonally. It occurs as a result of a threat to the person's being, self-esteem, or identity.

ascribed role An assigned role, such as age and sex, about which the individual has no choice.

assertiveness Behavior that is directed toward claiming one's rights without denying the rights of others.

assertiveness training An application of the behavioral model of psychiatric care. The patient is taught to stand up for his rights, while not infringing on the rights of others.

associationist model of learning A theory which defines learning as behavioral change that is a result of reinforced practice.

assumed role A role the individual selects or achieves by choice, such as occupation or marital roles.

attention The element of cognitive functioning that

refers to the maintenance of mental focus on a specific issue, activity, or object.

autism A preoccupation with the self and with inner experiences.

autistic thought Ideation that has a private meaning to individual.

autonomy The socially sanctioned condition that allows for the definition and control over one's work domain achieved through a negotiated process.

aversion therapy An application of the behavioral model of psychiatric care. A painful stimulus is given to create an aversion to another stimulus, which leads to a behavior that the individual wishes to change.

baseline behavior (or operant level) Specified rate (frequency and form) of a particular behavior during preintervention or preexperimental conditions.

baseline condition Environmental condition during which a particular behavior reflects a stable rate of responding, prior to the introduction of intervention or experimental conditions.

battered wife Any woman who is beaten by her mate, regardless of the legality of the marital relationship.

behavior Any observable, recordable, and measurable act, movement, or response of an individual.

behavior hierarchy A graded list of behavioral segments, beginning with the baseline behavior and gradually moving up to the terminal behavior.

behavior modification Changing and controlling behavior through the application of techniques derived from learning theory.

benzodiazepines A group of chemically related antianxiety drugs.

biofeedback A method of tension reduction in which electrodes are attached to the person's forehead, and he is then instructed to concentrate on relaxing, which will reduce the pitch of the biofeedback tone created by his tension. The lower the tone, the greater the muscle relaxation.

bipolar affective disorder A subgroup of the affective disorders that is characterized by the occurrence of at least one episode of manic behavior, with or without a history of episodes of depression.

blocking An interruption in the flow of speech due to the intrusion of distracting thoughts.

body image Sum of the conscious and unconscious attitudes the individual has toward his body. It includes present and past perceptions, as well as feelings about size, function, appearance, and potential.

body language The transmission of a message by body position or movement.

buccolinguomasticatory triad A complex of lips, tongue, jaw, and head movements that are associated with tardive dyskinesia.

bulimia An eating disorder that is characterized by uncontrollable binge eating, alternating with vomiting or dieting.

butyrophenones A group of chemically related antipsychotic drugs.

camisole restraint A straitjacket. A shirtlike garment that restrains the arms.

case management The identification, acquisition, and coordination of all social and health care resources needed by a patient.

catatonic A state of psychologically induced immobilization at times interrupted by episodes of extreme agitation.

catatonic excitement A state of extreme agitation that occurs when a person is unable to maintain catatonic immobility.

catatonic stupor An apparently unresponsive state that is related to a fear of loss of impulse control.

catharsis Release that occurs when the patient is encouraged to talk about things that bother him most. Fears, feelings, and experiences are brought out into the open and discussed.

cathexis Freud's term for the attachment of psychic energy to an object or mental construct.

certification The successful outcome of a formal review process of the clinical practice of a nurse specialist who is required to show a high degree of proficiency in interpersonal skills, use of the nursing process, and psychiatric, psychological, and milieu therapies.

child abuse Physical injury or sexual or emotional abuse that occurs when children are ignored, isolated, or continually shamed and demeaned.

circumstantial speech Inclusion of many nonessential details in a response.

clang associations A speech pattern characterized by rhyming.

claustrophobia Fear of closed places.

client-centered mental health consultation A format through which the consultant focuses on helping the consultee find the most effective treatment for a client.

cognition Process of logical thought.

cognitive model of learning A theory that defines learning as behavioral change based on the acquisition of information about the environment.

cohesiveness Force that attracts members to a group and causes them to remain in the group.

coitus Sexual intercourse with a partner of the opposite sex.

cold, wet sheet pack A form of somatic therapy in which the patient is swathed in cold, wet sheets, which then are warmed by body heat. The warmth and immobilization are soothing to very agitated people.

collective bargaining The use of collective action in negotiating patient care and economic issues with one's employer, including wages, hours, and conditions of work.

commitment Involuntary admission in which the request for hospitalization did not originate with the patient. When he is committed, he loses the right to leave the hospital when he wishes. It is usually justified on the grounds that the patient is dangerous to self or others and needs treatment.

communication Process of influencing the behavior of others by sending, receiving, and interpreting messages; feedback and consideration of the context complete the cycle.

community mental health centers (CMHCs) Institutions that provide comprehensive mental health services to meet the needs of all residents in a specific geographical area. Five basic services must be offered: (1) inpatient care, (2) partial hospitalization, (3) outpatient treatment, (4) emergency care, and (5) consultation and education.

compensation Process by which a person makes up for a deficiency in his image of himself by strongly emphasizing some other feature that he regards as an asset.

competent community A population that is aware of resources and alternatives, can make reasoned decisions about issues facing them, and can cope adaptively with problems. It parallels the concept of positive mental health.

compromise A task-oriented coping reaction that involves changing one's usual way of operating, substituting goals, or sacrificing aspects of one's personal needs. Compromise reactions are usually constructive and are frequently employed in approach-approach and avoidance-avoidance situations.

compulsion A recurring irresistible impulse to perform some act.

concreteness Use of specific terminology, rather than abstractions, in the discussion of the patient's feelings, experiences, and behavior.

conditional discharge A specified leave of absence or liberty from a psychiatric hospital in which certain things are expected from the patient and during which the commitment order is still in effect.

confabulation The manufacture of a response that is inaccurate but sounds appropriate. This is done to avoid embarrassment about memory loss.

confidentiality Term referring to disclosure of certain information to another specifically authorized person.

conflict Clashing of two opposing interests. The person experiences two competing drives and must choose between them.

confrontation An expression by the nurse of perceived discrepancies in the patient's behavior. It is an attempt by the nurse to bring to the patient's awareness the incongruence in his feelings, attitudes, beliefs, and behaviors.

confusion A nonspecific term used by nurses to describe a constellation of behaviors related to cognitive impairment, usually including disorientation, memory loss, loss of social skills, disruptive behavior, and difficulties with self-care.

congruent communication A communication pattern in which the sender is communicating the same message on both the verbal and nonverbal levels.

consensual validation Assuring understanding of the communication of another person by reaching agreement on the meaning of the message.

consequences Stimulus events following a behavior that strengthen or weaken the behavior. These are either reinforcers or punishers.

context Setting in which an event takes place.

continuous reinforcement A schedule of reinforcement in which each emission of a response is followed by the reinforcer.

conversion reaction See hysteria.

coping mechanisms Any effort directed at stress management. They can be task oriented and involve direct problem-solving efforts to cope with the threat itself or be intrapsychic or ego defense-oriented with the goal of regulating one's emotional distress.

coping resources Characteristics of the person, group, or environment that are helpful in assisting individuals in adapting to stress.

coprolalic A person who obtains sexual pleasure from using filthy language.

countertransference An emotional response of the nurse that is generated by the qualities of the patient and is inappropriate to the content and context of the therapeutic relationship or inappropriate in the degree of intensity of emotion.

crisis An internal disturbance that results from a stressful event or a perceived threat to self. Crises are self-limiting, and an adaptive or maladaptive resolution usually occurs in 6 weeks. Crises are a time of increased vulnerability and can produce increased personal growth.

crisis intervention A short-term active mode of psychotherapy that focuses on solving the patient's immediate problem and reestablishing psychological equilibrium.

cultural relativism The idea that health and normality emerge within a social context and that the content and form of mental health and mental illness will vary greatly from one culture to another. Differences are due to variations in stressors, symbolical interpretation, acceptance of expression and repression, and cohesion of social groups and their tolerance of deviation.

cunnilingus Oral stimulation of the female genitalia.

data base Sum total of information from which the patient's problems can be identified.

data collection A phase of the nursing process in which information about the health status of a patient is systematically obtained, communicated, and recorded.

defense mechanisms Coping mechanisms of the ego that attempt to protect the person from feelings of inadequacy and worthlessness and prevent awareness of anxiety. They are primarily unconscious in nature and involve a degree of self-deception and reality distortion.

deinstitutionalization At the individual patient level, the transfer to a community setting of a patient who has been hospitalized for an extended period of time, generally many years; at the mental health care system level, a shift in the focus of mental health care from the large long-term institution to the community, accomplished by discharging long-term patients and avoiding unnecessary admissions.

deliberate biological programming A theory of aging which proposes that the memory and capacity for terminating the life of a cell are stored within the cell itself.

delirium The medical diagnostic term that describes an organic mental disorder characterized by a cluster of cognitive impairments with an acute onset and the identification of a specific precipitating stressor.

delirium tremens A medical diagnostical term that has been replaced with the diagnosis "alcohol withdrawal delirium."

delusion A fixed false belief that may be persecutory, grandiose, or somatic in nature.

delusion of grandeur The false belief that one has great money, power, and prestige. It is frequently manifested in the belief that the individual is a famous person.

delusion of poverty The false belief that one is impoverished.

dementia The medical diagnostical term that describes an organic mental disorder characterized by a cluster of cognitive impairments which are generally of gradual onset and irreversible. The predisposing and precipitating stressors may or may not be identifiable.

denial Avoidance of disagreeable realities by ignoring or refusing to recognize them.

depersonalization A feeling of unreality and alienation from oneself. It is associated with a panic level of anxiety that produces a blocking off of awareness and a collapse in reality testing. The individual has difficulty distinguishing self from others, and his body has an unreal or strange quality about it. It is the subjective experience of the partial or total disruption of one's ego and the disintegration and disorganization of one's self-concept.

depot injection Intramuscular injection of medication in an oil suspension that results in sustained release over a period of several days.

depression An abnormal extension or overelaboration of sadness and grief. The term "depression" can be used to denote a variety of phenomena—a sign, symptom, syndrome, emotional state, reaction, disease, or clinical entity.

detoxification The removal of a toxic substance from the body, either naturally through physiological processes (e.g., hepatic or renal functions) or medically by the introduction of alternative substances and gradual withdrawal.

deviancy Failure to comply with a social norm.

direct nursing care functions Nursing actions that are focused on a particular patient, family, or group to whom the nurse is directly responsible and accountable.

direct self-destructive behavior Suicidal behavior.

discharge plan A formal written document that describes in detail the transition of the patient from one level of the mental health care system to another.

disengagement theory A theory of aging which postulates that older adults and society mutually withdraw from active exchange with each other.

disorientation Inability to correctly identify the self in relation to time, place, or person.

displacement Shift of an emotion from the person or object toward which it was originally directed to another, usually neutral or less dangerous, person or object.

dissociation The exclusion of anxiety-laden experiences or thoughts from awareness.

dissociative reaction Process by which a person blocks off part of his life from conscious recognition because of the threat of overwhelming anxiety.

diurnal mood variation Changes in mood that are related to the time of day.

divorce therapy A type of counseling that attempts to help couples disengage from their former relationship and malicious behavior toward each other or their children.

double bind Simultaneous communication of conflicting messages in the context of a situation that does not allow escape. See incongruent communication.

dream analysis A psychoanalytical therapeutic technique that requires the patient to report his dreams to the analyst who then interprets the meaning of the dream symbolism to assist the patient in understanding his unconscious mental functioning.

drug abuse Use of any chemical substance for reasons other than medical treatment.

dyspareunia Pain with sexual intercourse.

dystonia A side effect of antipsychotic medication that is characterized by muscle spasms, particularly of the head, neck, and tongue.

echolalia Repeating exactly whatever is heard.

echopraxia Imitation of the body position of another.

ego Element of the personality described by Freud that assesses reality and serves as a mediator between the opposing elements of the id and the superego.

ego boundaries An individual's perception of the boundary between himself and the external environment.

ego defense mechanisms See defense mechanisms.

ego state A transactional analysis term that refers to the role behaviors that an individual assumes in a particular unit of communication. It may be Adult, Parent, or Child.

ejaculatory incompetence Inability of a man to ejaculate intravaginally. It is also known as retarded ejaculation.

electroconvulsive therapy (ECT) Artificial induction

of a grand mal seizure by passing a controlled electrical current through electrodes applied to one or both temples. The patient is anesthetized and the seizure attenuated by administration of a muscle relaxant medication.

empathic understanding Ability to view the patient's world from his internal frame of reference. It involves the nurse's sensitivity to the patient's current feelings and the verbal ability to communicate this understanding in a language attuned to the patient.

enabler The role that is frequently assumed by the significant others of substance abusers, characterized by covert support of the substance abusing behavior.

encounter group therapy An application of the existential model of psychiatric care in a group setting. The focus is on here-and-now experience and the expression of real feelings verbally and nonverbally as members react to events in the group.

endorphins Naturally occurring peptides that have been found in the central nervous system and have a physiological effect similar to that of opiates.

enkephalins Naturally occurring peptides that have been found in the central nervous system and have a physiological effect similar to that of opiates.

enuresis Incontinence or involuntary urination. Bed wetting at night is particularly problematical for children.

environmental change Activities that have a social setting focus and require the modification of an individual's or group's immediate environment or the larger social system.

ethic A standard of valued behavior or beliefs adhered to by an individual or group. A goal to which one aspires.

ethical dilemma An issue for which moral claims conflict with one another. It can be defined as (1) a difficult problem that seems to have no satisfactory solution or (2) a choice between equally unsatisfactory alternatives.

evaluation A phase of the nursing process in which the patient's progress or lack of progress toward goal achievement is determined by the patient and nurse. This determination directs reassessment, reordering of priorities, new goal setting, and revision of the plan of nursing care.

exhibitionism Achievement of sexual pleasure by exposing one's sexual organs to another, usually a stranger.

existential A school of philosophical thought that focuses on the importance of experience in the present and the belief that man finds meaning in life through his experiences.

extinction A procedure in which reinforcement of a previously reinforced behavior is discontinued. This results in a decrease in the rate of responding.

extrapyramidal effects Side effects of an antipsychotic medication that resemble the symptoms of Parkin-

son's disease, including tremor, drooling, and altered gait.

face-hand test A psychomotor test used to assess the presence of organic mental disorders.

family APGAR An evaluation tool that focuses on family function as viewed by each member.

family therapy A therapy modality which focuses treatment on the process between family members that supports and perpetuates symptoms. It is a way of conceptualizing human relationship problems that focuses on the context in which an emotional problem is generated.

family violence The physical, psychological, sexual, material, or social violation of a person by a family member or their delegate. It is often described in terms of abuse or violence and both acts can exist in the same family.

fellatio Oral stimulation of the male genitalia.

female orgasmic dysfunction Inability of a female to achieve orgasm that may be primary or situational in origin.

fetishist A person who obtains sexual pleasure from an inanimate object, such as a shoe or leather garment.

fixation A psychoanalytical term referring to failure to resolve conflicts inherent in a stage of psychosocial development. Psychological energy (libido) is invested in these conflictual areas, inhibiting the person's ability to grow beyond that point.

flashback A phenomenon experienced by individuals who have taken hallucinogenic drugs in which they unexpectedly reexperience the effects of the drug.

flight of ideas A pattern of speech characterized by a rapid transition from one topic to another, frequently without completing the original thought. This behavior is characteristic of manic states.

free association A psychoanalytical therapeutic technique that requires the patient to repeat all of his thoughts without censorship, drifting naturally from one thought to the next.

freebasing A chemical process that is applied to cocaine to amplify the effect of the drug. It is then smoked.

frustration A feeling that results when something interferes with one's ability to attain a desired goal, satisfaction, or security.

functional disorder A mental or emotional impairment that is believed to be psychosocial in origin.

game In the context of transactional analysis, repetitive sets of ulterior transactions that are psychologically gratifying.

genuineness A quality of the nurse characterized by openness, honesty, and sincerity. The nurse is self-congruent and authentic and relates to the patient without a defensive facade.

geriatrics The study and treatment of diseases of old age.

gerontology The study of the phenomenon of aging.

gestalt therapy A therapeutic approach based on the existential model of psychiatric care. It was developed by Frederick Perls and focuses on the development of enhanced self-awareness.

grief An individual's subjective response to the loss of a person, object, or concept that is highly valued. Uncomplicated grief is a healthy, adaptive, reparative response.

group A collection of three or more individuals who have a relationship with one another, are interdependent, and who may share some common norms.

group maintenance Group functions directed toward satisfaction of members' psychosocial or emotional needs.

group-centered mental health consultation A format through which the consultant meets with a group to provide guidance regarding the consultees' work encounters.

habeas corpus A right retained by all psychiatric patients that provides for the release of an individual who claims he is being deprived of his liberty and detained illegally. The hearing for this determination takes place in a court of law in which the patient's sanity is at issue.

hallucination A sensory experience that is not the result of an external stimulus; may be visual, auditory, tactile, olfactory, or gustatory.

hallucinogens A class of abused drugs that cause a psychotic-like experience.

health education A teaching strategy related to health issues that involves the strengthening of individuals and groups through competence building.

helplessness A person's belief that no one will do anything to aid him.

homosexual A person whose sexual preference is for someone of the same sex.

homosexual panic A state of extreme agitation resulting from fear related to awareness of previously repressed homosexual impulses.

hopelessness An individual's belief that neither he nor anyone else can do anything to aid him.

hostility A feeling of anger and resentment characterized by destructive behavior.

hyperactive Unusually or excessively active.

hypochondriasis A reaction characterized by an exaggerated concern with one's physical health that is not based on real organic pathological conditions.

hypomania A clinical syndrome that is similar to, but less severe than, that described by the term manic or manic episode.

hysteria In this disorder, also known as conversion reaction, symptoms of physical illness appear without any underlying organic pathological condition.

id Element of the personality described by Freud that represents one's instinctual drives and primitive impulses and is largely unconscious in nature.

identification Process by which a person tries to make himself like someone else whom he admires by taking on the thoughts, mannerisms, or tastes of that individual.

identity Organizing principle of the personality system that accounts for the unity, continuity, uniqueness, and consistency of the personality. It is the awareness of the process of "being oneself" that is derived from self-observation and judgment and is the synthesis of all self-representations into an organized whole.

identity confusion Lack of clarity and consistency in one's perception of the self, resulting in a high degree of anxiety.

identity foreclosure Premature adoption of an identity that is desired by significant others without coming to terms with one's own desires, aspirations or potential.

illusion Misinterpretation of a sensory input.

immediacy State that occurs when the current interaction of the nurse and the patient is focused on.

implementation A phase of the nursing process in which nursing actions are carried out that assist the patient to maximize his health capabilities and provide for patient participation in health promotion, maintenance, and restoration.

impotence Failure to achieve an erection.

incest Act of having sexual relations with a close relative, such as one's mother, daughter, or son.

incompetency A legal status that must be proved in a special court hearing. As a result of the hearing the person can be deprived of many of his civil rights. Incompetency can be reversed only in another court hearing that declares the person competent.

incongruent communication A communication pattern in which the sender is communicating a different message on the verbal and nonverbal levels and the listener does not know to which level he should respond. See double bind.

indirect nursing care function Nursing activities in which some other person actually carries out the patient's care and that require the qualifications of a psychiatric and mental health nursing specialist.

indirect self-destructive behavior Any activity that is detrimental to the physical well-being of the person and potentially has the outcome of death, accompanied by lack of conscious awareness of the self-destructive nature of the behavior.

informal admission A type of admission to a psychiatric hospital in which there is no formal or written application and the individual is free to leave at any time.

informed consent Disclosure of a certain amount of information to the patient about the proposed treatment and the attainment of the patient's consent, which must be competent, understanding, and voluntary.

insanity defense Legal defense which proposes that a person who has committed an act that in a usual situation would be criminal should be held not guilty by reason of "insanity."

insulin shock therapy Induction of a coma by administration of insulin. The comatose state is allowed to last up to an hour and is then reversed by the administration of glucose or glucagon.

interdisciplinary health care team A group of health care workers who are members of different disciplines and who are involved in a formal arrangement to provide patient services while maximizing educational interchange.

intermittent reinforcement Noncontinuous reinforcement in which not every response is reinforced. Some emissions of a particular behavior are reinforced; others are not.

introjection An intense type of identification in which the person incorporates qualities or values of another person or group into his own ego structure.

involuntary admission See commitment.

irreversible brain syndrome Syndrome also known as dementia or chronic brain syndrome. A disorder related to a variety of biological stressors, characterized by deterioration of cognition. Recovery is not possible.

isolation Splitting off of the emotional component of a thought. It may be temporary or long term.

judgment Ability to make logical rational decisions.

judicial discharge A discharge granted by the courts.

Katz Index of Daily Living An instrument that is used to measure the individual's ability to bathe, dress, toilet, transfer, and feed himself and remain continent.

la belle indifference Term used to describe the patient's lack of concern or anxiety regarding his physical illness. It is used to describe the bland attitude characteristic of hysteria or conversion reactions.

labile Subject to frequent or unpredictable changes.

latency A stage of development occurring between the ages of 6 and 12 in which the major task is the achievement of a sense of competency.

learned helplessness A behavioral state and personality trait of a person who believes that he is ineffectual, his responses are futile, and he has lost control over the reinforcers in his environment.

learning A relatively stable, observable change in the frequency or form of behavior resulting from interaction with environmental antecedent and consequences.

lesbian A woman whose sexual preference is for another woman.

lethality An estimation of the probability that a person who is threatening suicide will succeed based on the method described, the specificity of the plan, and the availability of the means.

liaison nursing An interpersonal, coordinated problem-solving process between professionals who influence or participate in providing human services. The liaison nurse has a high degree of expertise in psychiatric nursing and an ability to integrate these skills with knowledge in medical-surgical nursing to provide expanded services.

libido Freud's term for psychic energy.

life review Reminiscence occurring in old age as a consequence of the realization of the inevitability of death.

life space interview An interaction between a child and adult that takes place outside the context of individual therapy. The focus is on improving the child's sense of self-identity and ego functioning with the developmental process.

limit setting Act of making a person aware of his rights and responsibilities, while communicating the expectation that he will respect the rules. Also, the application of appropriate sanctions if the person does not obey the rules.

logotherapy An approach to psychotherapy based on the existential model and developed by Viktor Frankl. The focus is on the search for meaning in present experiences.

loose associations A communication pattern characterized by lack of clarity of connection between one thought and the next.

malingering Deliberate and fraudulent imitation or exaggeration of an illness.

malpractice Failure of a professional person to give the kind of proper and competent care that is given by members of his profession in the community, which causes harm to the patient.

mania A condition which is characterized by a mood that is elevated, expansive, or irritable.

manipulation Controlling the behavior of others to achieve one's own goals.

masochism Achievement of pleasure, frequently sexual, from being physically or mentally hurt.

masturbation Act of achieving sexual arousal and orgasm through manual or mechanical stimulation of the sex organs.

maturational crisis Transitional or developmental periods within a person's life when his psychological equilibrium is upset.

mechanical restraints Any of several means of restricting a patient's freedom of movement. Includes camisoles, wrist and ankle restraints, sheet restraints, and sheet packs.

medical diagnosis The independent judgment of a physician of the health problems or disease states of the patient.

meditation A technique of tension reduction in which the person closes his eyes, relaxes the major muscle groups, and repeats a cue word silently to himself each time he exhales.

memory The ability to recall past events.

menarche First menstruation of a woman, which indicates that she may be capable of conceiving.

mental status examination A formal exploration of data relative to a patient's mental functioning in which information is collected about the patient's sensorium and intelligence, thought processes, mood and affect, and insight.

message A unit of communication.

metacommunication Messages about a communication pertaining to both the relationship and informational aspects.

Mini-Mental State Examination A brief psychological test designed to differentiate between dementia, psychosis, and affective disorders.

model A means of organizing a complex body of knowledge.

monoamine oxidase (MAO) inhibitors A group of chemically related antidepressant medications.

mood A prolonged emotional state that influences one's whole personality and life functioning.

mourning Includes all the psychological processes set in motion within the individual by a loss. The process of mourning is resolved only when the lost object is internalized, bonds of attachment are loosened, and new object relationships are established.

multidisciplinary health care team A group of health care workers who are members of different disciplines with each one providing specific services to the patient.

multiple personalities A type of dissociative reaction in which the person displays two or more complete personality systems that are usually dramatically different.

mutual support groups A type of group in which members organize themselves to solve their own problems. They are led by the group members who share a common experience, work together toward a common goal, and use their own strengths to gain control over their lives.

narcissism An exaggerated sense of self-importance manifested as extreme self-absorption.

narcotics A class of drugs that have powerful analgesic and euphoria-inducing properties.

necrophile A person who is sexually aroused by thoughts of death or sexual activity with a dead person.

need-fear dilemma An approach-violence conflict related to the need to experience closeness coupled with fear of the experience.

negative identity Assumption of an identity that is at odds with the accepted values and expectations of society.

negative punishment A punishment procedure in which the removal of a positive reinforcer immediately following the occurrence of a particular behavior results in a decrease in the rate of responding of that behavior.

negative reinforcement Refers to the procedure whereby the removal or termination of an aversive stimulus contingently follows the emission of a response and results in an increase in the rate of responding.

negative reinforcer A stimulus which, when presented immediately following the occurrence of a particular behavior, will decrease the rate of responding of that behavior. If antecedent to the emission of a particular behavior and terminated by that response, it will increase the rate of responding of that behavior.

neglect Condition that occurs when a parent is unable to or fails to provide minimal emotional and physical care to a child.

neologisms Words that are invented by the person and understood only by him.

networking A process of linking individuals or agencies with mutual interests to form a coalition and thereby more effectively effect social change.

neurasthenia A type of disorder characterized by chronic mental and physical fatigue and a variety of vague aches and pains, including weakness, headaches, and back pain. This reaction is not caused by overwork but is an attempt to reduce or mask areas of conflict.

neurotic behavior A behavioral dysfunction that is characterized by anxiety, but in which there is no distortion of reality.

neurotic disorders A category of health problems that is distinguished by the following characteristics: symptoms that are distressing and unacceptable to the individual, grossly intact reality testing; behavior that does not violate gross social norms, a disturbance that is relatively enduring or recurrent without treatment, and no demonstrable organic cause.

nihilistic delusion The false belief that the self, part of the self, or another object has ceased to exist.

noncompliance The failure of the individual to carry out the self-care activities prescribed in a health care plan.

nonverbal communication Transmission of a message without the use of words. It involves all of the five senses.

norm A culturally defined standard of behavior.

nurse practice act A state law that defines the legal limits of nursing practice and that must be adhered to by all licensed nurses.

nurses' observation scale for inpatient evaluation (NOSIE) A systematical, objective behavioral rating scale applied by nurses to patients' behavior.

nursing The diagnosis and treatment of human responses to actual or potential health problems.

nursing audit A type of clinical evaluation of nursing care that may focus on a nursing activity (process audit) or on the behavior of a patient in response to the nursing care that has been provided (outcome audit).

nursing diagnosis The independent judgment of a nurse of the patient's behavioral response to stress. It is a statement of the patient's nursing problems, which may be overt, covert, existing, or potential, and includes both the behavioral disruption or threatened disruption and contributing stressors.

nursing problems Aspects of the patient's health that may need to be promoted or with which the patient needs help in his biopsychosocial adaptation to stress.

nursing process An interactive, problem-solving process used by the nurse as a systematical and individualized way to fulfill the goal of nursing care. It includes the components of data collection, formulation of the nursing diagnosis, planning, implementation, and evaluation.

nursing therapeutic process The process by which the nurse strives to promote and maintain the adaptive coping responses of the patient, which involves the establishment of a therapeutic nurse-patient relationship and the use of the nursing process.

obesity A condition in which the individual weighs at least 20% more than his ideal weight.

object cues A category of nonverbal communication that includes the speaker's intentional and non-intentional use of all objects such as dress, furnishings, and possessions.

obsession A recurring thought that is unwanted but cannot be voluntarily excluded from consciousness.

oculogyric crisis A side effect of antipsychotic medication that is characterized by the uncontrollable rolling upward of the eyes.

operant behavior Behavior whose strength is controlled by the stimulus events that precede and follow it.

operant conditioning Modification of operant behavior by systematical manipulation of antecedents and consequences.

operant level Frequency or form of a performance under baseline conditions before any systematical conditioning procedures are introduced.

organic disorder A mental or emotional impairment that is believed to be physiological in origin.

orientation The ability to correctly relate the self to time, place, and person.

orthostatic hypotension A drop in blood pressure related to change in position. A common side effect of psychotropic medications.

PACE II An evaluation tool that focuses on the physical health of nursing home patients.

panic An attack of extreme anxiety that involves the disorganization of the personality. Distorted perceptions, loss of rational thought, and an inability to communicate and function are evident.

paranoia A behavioral manifestation representative of the unconscious operation of the mechanism of projection whereby the person attributes his ego-alien thoughts and impulses to others; a feeling of extreme suspicion.

paranoid delusion The false belief that one is being persecuted.

parapsychology The study of experiential phenomena that occur outside of the usual limits of sensory awareness, including extrasensory perception and precognition.

parkinsonian equivalents Side effects of antipsychotic medications that are behaviors characteristic of Parkinson's disease, including fine tremors, pill-rolling tremor of the fingers, drooling, and petit pas gait.

passive Behavior that subordinates the individual's own rights to the demands of others.

passive-aggressive Term describing indirect expression, verbal or nonverbal, of angry feelings.

pedophile A person whose sexual preference is for a child.

perception Sensory reception of a stimulus.

perseveration Repetition of a single word or phrase over and over.

phenothiazines A group of chemically related antipsychotic medications.

phobic reaction A persistent fear of some object or situation that presents no actual danger to the person or in which the danger is magnified out of proportion to its actual seriousness.

physical dependence A characteristic of drug addiction that is present when withdrawal of the drug results in physiological disruptions.

physical restraint Limitation of the individual's freedom of movement by immobilizing all or part of the body or by restricting the person to a confined space.

physiological conversions Physiological changes that accompany anxiety and serve no constructive purpose. They can, however, form the basis for pathological changes in function that may progress to structural changes and irreversible organic changes.

planning A phase of the nursing process in which goals are derived from the nursing diagnosis, priorities are set, and nursing approaches or measures to achieve the goals are prescribed.

positive punishment A punishment procedure in which the presentation of an aversive stimulus immediately following the occurrence of a particular behavior results in a decrease in the rate of responding of that behavior.

postvention Therapeutic intervention with the significant others of an individual who has committed suicide.

predisposing factors Conditioning factors that influence both the type and amount of resources which the individual can elicit to cope with stress. They may be biological, psychological, and sociocultural in nature.

premature ejaculation Inability of a man to delay ejaculation long enough for the female to achieve orgasm in at least 50% of his attempts at coitus.

primary appraisal of stressor The processing and comprehension of the stressful situation that takes place on many levels for the individual. It involves cognitive, affective, physiological, behavioral, and social responses.

primary gain A decrease in anxiety resulting from the individual's efforts to cope with stress.

primary prevention Biological, social, or psychological intervention that promotes health and well-being or reduces the incidence of illness in a community by altering the causative factors before they have an opportunity to do harm.

primary process thought Primitive thought processes that are normally kept unconscious by use of the coping mechanisms of repression; impulsive infantile ideation.

privileged communication A legal term that applies only in court-related proceedings and means that the right to reveal information belongs to the person who spoke and the listener cannot disclose the information unless the speaker gives permission. It exists between a patient and health professional only if a law specifically establishes it.

professionalization Evidence of a continuous attempt of a group in any community or society to gain more and more control over certain resources related to an occupational area.

program-centered consultation A format through which the consultant focuses on broader organizational and program areas in an attempt to help the consultee solve institution-wide issues.

projection Attributing one's own thoughts or impulses to another person. Through this process the individual can attribute his own intolerable wishes, emotional feelings, or motivations to another person.

pseudodementia A depressive condition of the elderly that is characterized by impaired cognitive functioning.

psychiatric nursing An interpersonal process that strives to promote and maintain behavior which contributes to integrated functioning. It employs the theories of human behavior as its science and purposeful use of self as its art. It is directed toward both preventive and corrective impacts on mental disorders and their sequelae and is concerned with the promotion of optimal mental health for society, the community, and those individuals who live within it.

psychiatric rehabilitation The process of enabling a mentally ill individual to return to his highest possible level of functioning.

psychoanalysis A therapeutic approach based on the belief that behavioral disorders are related to unresolved, anxiety-provoking, childhood experiences which are repressed into the unconscious. The goal of psychoanalysis is to bring repressed experiences into conscious awareness and to learn healthier means of coping with the related anxiety.

psychobiological resilience A concept which proposes that there is a recurrent human need to weather periods of stress and change throughout life. The ability to successfully weather each period of disruption and reintegration leaves the person better able to deal with the next change.

psychodrama Therapeutic use of dramatic techniques as developed by Moreno, enabling group members to act out and receive feedback about stressful life experiences.

psychological autopsy A retrospective review of the individual's behavior for the time preceding his death by suicide.

psychological dependence A characteristic of drug addiction that is manifested in a craving for the abused substance and a fear that it will not be available in the future.

psychological testing A diagnostical tool used by the psychologist to aid in assessment of the patient. It includes administration of a battery of cognitive and projective tests.

psychomotor retardation A slowing of motor activity related to a state of severe depression.

psychopharmacotherapy Treatment of psychiatric disorders with medication.

psychosomatic reactions Disorders in which the emotional tension is not discharged outwardly but is instead unconsciously channeled through the visceral organs.

psychosurgery Surgical interruption of selected neural pathways that involve the transmission of emotional impulses in the brain.

psychotherapy group A group developed for the purpose of treating emotional distress and disorder through means of a group method and group process.

psychotic behavior Severely dysfunctional behavior characterized by a panic level of anxiety, personality disintegration, and regressive behavior. The person experiences a reduced level of awareness and has great difficulty functioning adequately.

psychotic disorders A category of health problems distinguished by the following characteristics: severe mood disorder, regressive behavior, personality disintegration, reduced level of awareness, great difficulty in functioning adequately, and gross impairment in reality testing.

psychotomimetic Imitating a psychosis; refers to the effects of hallucinogenic drugs.

quality assessment measures Formal, systematical, organizational evaluation of overall patterns or programs of care, including clinical, consumer, and systems evaluation.

quality assurance activities Clinical evaluation of ongoing programs that include both evaluation and corrective action.

rape Legally defined as the forcible perpetration of the act of sexual intercourse on the body of a woman not one's wife. A more contemporary definition would include acts of oral and anal sodomy and allow for its occurrence within marriage as well.

rational-emotive therapy A therapeutic approach based on the existential model of psychiatric care developed by Albert Ellis. The emphasis is on risk taking and the assumption of responsibility for one's behavior.

rationalization Offering a socially acceptable or apparently logical explanation to justify or make acceptable otherwise unacceptable impulses, feelings, behaviors, and motives.

reaction formation Development of conscious attitudes and behavior patterns that are opposite to what one really feels or would like to do.

reality testing The ego function of determining the objective reality of experience, or a nursing action that validates objective reality for a patient who is unable to do so.

reality therapy A therapeutic approach based on the existential model of psychiatric care developed by William Glasser. The focus is on recognition and accomplishment of life goals with emphasis on development of the capacity for caring.

reasoning The ability to consider facts and arrive at a logical conclusion.

reciprocal inhibition A behavior modification technique that attempts to substitute a more adaptive behavior for a symptom by learning an alternative means of reducing anxiety.

regression A retreat in the face of stress to behavior characteristic of an earlier level of development.

reinforcement The response-contingent presentation of a positive reinforcer or to the termination of a negative reinforcer that results in the strengthening (or maintenance) of the behavior.

relatedness Process of establishing intimate relationships with others, including a meaningful balance among dependence, independence, and interdependence.

relaxation response A protective mechanism against stress that brings about decreased heart rate, lower metabolism, and decreased respiratory rate. It is the physiological opposite of the fight or flight, or anxiety, response.

relaxation therapy A behavior modification approach based on the principle of reciprocal inhibition. Consciously induced relaxation is experienced in conjunction with actual or fantasied anxiety-provoking experiences.

repression Involuntary exclusion of a painful or conflictual thought, impulse, or memory from awareness. It is the primary ego defense, and other mechanisms tend to reinforce it.

resistance Attempt of the patient to remain unaware of anxiety-producing aspects within himself. Ambivalent attitudes toward self-exploration in which the patient both appreciates and avoids anxiety-producing experiences are a normal part of the therapeutic process.

respect An attitude of the nurse that conveys caring for, liking, and valuing the patient. He is regarded as a person of worth and is accepted without qualification.

respite care The provision of temporary supervision in a community setting for a psychiatric patient who lives with his family to provide the family with relief from the demands for his care.

reversible brain syndrome Also known as delirium, or acute brain syndrome, this disorder is related to a variety of biological stressors and is characterized by a disruption of cognition. Recovery is possible.

role ambiguity A type of role strain that occurs when shared specifications set for an expected role are incomplete or insufficient to tell the involved individual what is desired or how to do it.

role clarification Gaining the knowledge, information, and cues needed to perform a role.

role conflict Frustration experienced by the individual because of role demands that are incompatible or incongruent or confusing regarding appropriate role behavior.

role overload A type of role strain which occurs when a person is faced with a role set that is too complex or overwhelms available resources.

role playing Acting out of a particular situation. It functions to increase the person's insight into human relations and can deepen one's ability to see a situation from another point of view.

role strain Stress, experienced as frustration, associated with expected roles or positions.

roles Set of socially expected behavior patterns associated with an individual's function in various social groups. Roles provide a means for social participation and a way to test out identities for consensual validation by significant others.

sadism Achievement of sexual pleasure by inflicting physical or mental pain on one's sexual partner.

Sandoz Clinical Assessment—Geriatric An examination of psychological functioning that is administered to the elderly to assist in the diagnostical process.

schizophrenia A manifestation of anxiety of psychotic proportions, primarily characterized by inability to trust other people and disordered thought processes, resulting in disrupted interpersonal relationships.

school phobia A child's state of anxiety related to separating him from his parents by his attending school. It is a form of separation anxiety; the child is not afraid of school per se.

script A transactional analysis term which refers to a life plan that originates in childhood perceptions and experiences.

seclusion A form of physical restraint in which the individual is placed in a single room, which may be locked, to decrease stimuli and allow the agitated patient to gain control of his behavior.

secondary gain Advantages other than a decrease in anxiety that are associated with the sick role, e.g., dependency need gratification, relief from responsibilities.

secondary prevention Type of prevention which seeks to reduce the prevalence of illness by interventions that provide for early detection and treatment of problems.

secondary process thought Conscious thought processes that are under the control of the ego and are characterized by logic.

security operations A term related to the interpersonal model of psychiatric care that refers to mental mechanisms which are developed to deal with anxiety-provoking experiences.

self-actualization Process of fulfilling one's potential.

self-concept All the notions, beliefs, and convictions that constitute an individual's knowledge of himself and influence his relationships with others.

self-destructive behavior Any behavior, direct or indirect, that if uninterrupted, will ultimately lead to the death of the individual.

self-disclosure Revelation that occurs when a person reveals information about his self, ideas, values, feelings, and attitudes.

self-esteem The individual's personal judgment of his own worth obtained by analyzing how well his behavior conforms to his self-ideal.

self-help groups See mutual support groups.

self-ideal The individual's perception of how he should behave based on certain personal standards. The standard may be either a carefully constructed image of the kind of person one would like to be or merely a number of aspirations, goals, or values that one would like to achieve.

self-system A term related to the interpersonal model of psychiatric care that refers to the self as perceived by the individual.

senility A nonspecific term that refers to impaired cognitive functioning in the elderly and is usually used in a derogatory sense.

sensitivity training group A group developed for the purpose of increasing self-awareness, increasing understanding of group process, or increasing awareness of the effects of one's behavior in groups.

separation anxiety A reaction in children caused by the temporary loss of a parent, especially under stressful circumstances.

set A predisposition to behave in a certain way.

sexuality A desire for contact, warmth, tenderness, and love, which includes all aspects of one's sense of self.

Short Portable Mental Status Questionnaire A short tool used to screen for cognitive impairment.

situational crisis Crisis that occurs when a specific external event upsets an individual's psychological equilibrium.

Social Behavior Assessment Scale A semistructured interview guide that elicits information from significant others regarding the patient's functioning.

social breakdown syndrome The progressive deterioration of the social and interpersonal skills of long-term psychiatric patients.

social learning theory A theory that explains the development of aggressive behavior as part of the socialization process.

social margin The total of resources available to the individual to cope with stress.

social networks See social support systems.

social support systems Those members of one's social environment who are perceived by the individual as "significant others" and who provide some degree of emotional support, task-oriented help, feedback and evaluation, social relatedness and integration, and access to new information.

somatic delusion The false belief that all or a part of the body is impaired in some way.

somatic therapies Treatment affecting one's physiological functioning.

somnambulism Dissociative manifestation of sleep-walking.

specialist in psychiatric and mental health nursing A psychiatric nurse who is characterized by graduate education, supervised clinical experience, and depth of knowledge, competence, and skill in practice.

stigma An irrational attribution of negative worth based on a person's behavior or experiences.

stimulus Any physical or environmental object, event, or condition, including one's own behavior and the behavior of others, that does or can influence.

stressors Stimuli that the individual perceives as challenging, threatening, or harmful. They require the use of excess energy and produce a state of tension and stress within the individual.

sublimation Acceptance of a socially approved substitute goal for a drive whose normal channel of expression is blocked.

substance abuse The use of any mind-altering agent to such an extent that it interferes with the individual's biological, psychological, or sociocultural integrity.

suicide Self-inflicted death.

suicide attempt Any action deliberately undertaken by the individual that, if carried to completion, will result in his death.

suicide gesture A suicide attempt that is planned to be discovered in an attempt to influence the behavior of others.

suicide threat A warning, direct or indirect, verbal or nonverbal, that the individual plans to attempt suicide.

sundown syndrome Increasing nighttime disorientation or confusion in the elderly related to loss of visual accommodation.

superego Element of the personality described by Freud that represents one's conscience and culturally acquired restrictions.

supervision A process whereby a therapist is helped to become a more effective clinician. The nurse supervisor serves as a provider of theoretical knowledge and therapeutic techniques, validates the use of the nursing process, and supports the working through of transference and countertransference reactions.

suppression A process that is the conscious analogy of repression. It is the intentional exclusion of material from consciousness.

synergistic A reaction between two or more substances in which after introduction into the body they enhance the physiological effects of each other.

systematical desensitization A technique of behavior therapy that involves the pairing of deep muscle relaxation with imagined scenes depicting situations that cause the patient to feel anxious. The assumption is that if the person is taught relaxation rather than anxiety while imagining such scenes, the real-life situation that the scene depicted will cause much less anxiety.

systems evaluation An evaluation of the organization of the health care delivery system that includes the components of systems analysis, economic analysis, and operations research. It is a supplement to clinical evaluation.

tangential speech Loss of goal direction in communication. Failure to address the original point.

tardive dyskinesia A serious side effect of antipsychotic medication characterized by the buccolinguomasticatory triad of head, jaw, and facial movements, athetoid and choreiform movement of the extremities, and tonic contractions of the back and neck muscles.

tertiary prevention Measures designed to reduce the severity, disability, or residual impairment resulting from illness through rehabilitation.

testamentary capacity A person's competency to make a will, which requires that he know that he is making a will, the nature and extent of his property, and who his friends and relatives are.

thanatology The study of dying and death.

themes Underlying issues or problems experienced by the patient that emerge repeatedly during the course of the nurse-patient relationship.

therapeutic community A concept proposed by Maxwell Jones in which the patient's social environment would be used to provide a therapeutic experience for him by involving him as an active participant in his own care and the daily problems of his community.

therapeutic group Group developed for the purpose of preventing emotional turmoil or disturbances through prevention, education, and providing support.

therapeutic impasses Roadblocks in the progress of the nurse-patient relationship. They arise for a variety of reasons and may take different forms, but they all create stalls in the therapeutic relationship.

therapeutic nurse-patient relationship A mutual learning experience and a corrective emotional experience for the patient in which the nurse uses herself and specified clinical techniques in working with the patient to bring about behavioral change.

therapeutic touch The nurse's laying-on of hands on or close to the body of an ill person for the purpose of helping or healing him.

third-party reimbursement Payment for health services by a government or private health insurance program.

token economy A behavior modification approach that uses positive reinforcement in the form of a tangible object to promote positive behavioral change.

tolerance A characteristic of drug addiction that refers to the progressive need for more of the abused substance to achieve the desired effect.

tort A civil wrong for which the injured party is entitled to compensation.

transactional analysis A therapeutic modality based on the communications model of psychiatric care and developed by Eric Berne. Therapy takes place through the identification and interpretation of communication units (transactions) leading to understanding of interpersonal games that underlie behavioral disturbances. The goal is to develop the ability to communicate directly without using games.

transference An unconscious response of the patient in which he experiences feelings and attitudes toward the nurse that were originally associated with significant figures in his early life.

transsexual A person who is genetically an anatomical male or female but expresses, with strong conviction, that he or she has the mind of the opposite sex, lives as a member of the opposite sex either part or full time, and seeks to change his or her original sex legally, through hormonal and surgical sex assignment.

transvestite A person who chooses to cross-dress or put on the garments of the opposite sex.

tricyclics A group of chemically related antidepressant medications.

undoing An act or communication that partially negates a previous one.

unidisciplinary health care team A group of health care workers who are all members of the same discipline.

urolognic A person who receives sexual stimulation from acts involving urine, such as watching people urinate or wishing to urinate on another.

vaginismus Involuntary contractions of the outer third of the vagina that prevent insertion of the penis.

value clarification A method whereby a person can discover his own values by assessing, exploring, and determining what his personal values are and what they hold in personal decision making.

values The concepts that a person holds worthy in his own personal life. They are formed as a result of one's life's experiences with family, friends, culture, education, work, and relaxation.

verbal communication Written or spoken transmission of a message.

violence Acting out of destructive aggression by assaulting people or objects in the environment.

vocal cues A category of nonverbal communication that includes all the noises and sounds which are extraspeech sounds. They are sometimes referred to as paralinguistic cues.

voluntary admission A type of admission to a psychiatric hospital in which the individual applies in writing and agrees to receive treatment and abide by the hospital rules. If the patient wishes to be discharged, he must give written notice to the hospital.

voyeurism Achievement of sexual pleasure by observing the nudity or sexual activity of others.

withdrawal The attempt to avoid interaction with others and thus avoid relatedness.

withdrawal syndrome Constellation of behaviors that occur when use of an abused substance is terminated. Behaviors are specific to the abused substance.

word salad A communication pattern characterized by a jumble of disconnected words.

working through Process by which repressed feelings are released and reintegrated into the personality.

zoophile A person whose sexual perference is for an animal.

Zung Self-Rating Depression Scale An instrument administered to determine the presence of depression.

INDEX